BOARD REVIEW

CLINICAL
PATHOLOGY
BOARD REVIEW

Steven L. Spitalnik, MD

Professor and Vice-Chairman, Pathology and Cell Biology
Columbia University Medical Center
Medical Director, Clinical Laboratories
New York-Presbyterian Hospital
New York, New York

Suzanne A. Arinsburg, DO

Instructor, Pathology and Cell Biology
Columbia University Medical Center
New York, New York

Jeffrey S. Jhang, MD

Director, Blood Bank and Transfusion Service
Associate Professor of Pathology
Mount Sinai Medical Center
New York, New York

ELSEVIER
SAUNDERS

SAUNDERS

1600 John F. Kennedy Blvd.
Ste 1800
Philadelphia, PA 19103-2899

CLINICAL PATHOLOGY BOARD REVIEW   ISBN: 978-1-4557-1139-0

Notices

Knowledge and best practice in this field are constantly changing. As new research and experience broaden our understanding, changes in research methods, professional practices, or medical treatment may become necessary.

Practitioners and researchers must always rely on their own experience and knowledge in evaluating and using any information, methods, compounds, or experiments described herein. In using such information or methods they should be mindful of their own safety and the safety of others, including parties for whom they have a professional responsibility.

With respect to any drug or pharmaceutical products identified, readers are advised to check the most current information provided (i) on procedures featured or (ii) by the manufacturer of each product to be administered, to verify the recommended dose or formula, the method and duration of administration, and contraindications. It is the responsibility of practitioners, relying on their own experience and knowledge of their patients, to make diagnoses, to determine dosages and the best treatment for each individual patient, and to take all appropriate safety precautions.

To the fullest extent of the law, neither the Publisher nor the authors, contributors, or editors, assume any liability for any injury and/or damage to persons or property as a matter of products liability, negligence or otherwise, or from any use or operation of any methods, products, instructions, or ideas contained in the material herein.

Library of Congress Cataloging-in-Publication Data
Clinical pathology : board review / editors, Steven L. Spitalnik, Suzanne A. Arinsburg, Jeffrey S. Jhang.
    p. ; cm.
Includes bibliographical references and index.
ISBN 978-1-4557-1139-0 (pbk. : alk. paper)
I. Spitalnik, Steven L., editor. II. Arinsburg, Suzanne A., editor. III. Jhang, Jeffrey S., editor.
[DNLM: 1. Pathology, Clinical–Examination Questions. QZ 18.2]
RB119
616.07076–dc23
                                            2014029527

Executive Content Strategist: William Schmitt
Content Development Specialist: Katy Meert
Publishing Services Manager: Patricia Tannian
Project Manager: Carrie Stetz
Design Direction: Louis Forgione

Printed in China

Last digit is the print number: 9 8 7 6 5 4 3 2 1

To Dr. Joseph G. Fink and Dr. Daniel J. Fink, our teachers, colleagues, and friends, who were both enthusiastically committed to medical education.

CONTRIBUTORS

Vimla Aggarwal, MBBS, FACMG
Assistant Professor of Pathology and Cell Biology
Columbia University Medical Center
New York-Presbyterian Hospital
New York, New York

Raphael Clynes, MD, PhD
Associate Professor of Pathology and Cell Biology
Columbia University Medical Center
New York, New York

Adriana I. Colovai, PhD, D(ABHI)
Associate Professor of Clinical Surgery
Albert Einstein College of Medicine
Director, Transplant Immunology Laboratory
Department of Surgery
Montefiore Medical Center
Bronx, New York

Serge Cremers, PharmD, PhD
Assistant Professor of Pathology and Cell Biology
Director, Biomarker Core Laboratory
Irving Institute for Clinical and Translational Research
Columbia University Medical Center
New York, New York

Phyllis Della-Latta, (D)ABMM, FAAM
Professor of Pathology
Director, Clinical Microbiology Service
Columbia University Medical Center
New York-Presbyterian Hospital
New York, New York

Kalpana Devaraj, MD, MHS
Assistant Professor of Pathology
University of Colorado, Anschutz Medical Campus
Denver, Colorado

Mark D. Ewalt, MD
Hematopathology Fellow
Stanford University Hospitals and Clinics
Stanford, California

Richard O. Francis, MD, PhD
Assistant Professor of Pathology and Cell Biology
Director, Special Hematology and Coagulation Laboratory
Columbia University Medical Center
New York-Presbyterian Hospital
New York, New York

Eldad A. Hod, MD
Assistant Professor of Pathology and Cell Biology
Columbia University Medical Center
New York-Presbyterian Hospital
New York, New York

Paul R. Hosking, MD
Assistant Professor of Pathology
Medical College of Wisconsin
Froedtert Hospital
Milwaukee, Wisconsin

Richard C. Huard, PhD, D(ABMM)
Assistant Professor of Pathology and Cell Biology
Columbia University Medical Center
New York-Presbyterian Hospital
New York, New York

Vaidehi Jobanputra, MS, PhD
Assistant Professor of Pathology and Cell Biology
Columbia University Medical Center
New York-Presbyterian Hospital
New York, New York

Alexander Kratz, MD, PhD, MPH
Associate Professor of Pathology and Cell Biology
Director, Core Laboratory and Point of Care Testing Service
Columbia University Medical Center
New York-Presbyterian Hospital
New York, New York

Brynn Levy, MSc(Med), PhD, FACMG
Professor of Pathology and Cell Biology
Co-Director, Personalized Genomic Medicine
Columbia University Medical Center
Director, Genetics Laboratory
New York-Presbyterian Hospital
New York, New York

Mahesh M. Mansukhani, MD
Associate Professor of Pathology and Cell Biology
Medical Director, Division of Personalized Genomic Medicine
Columbia University Medical Center
New York, New York

Vundavalli V. Murty, PhD
Associate Professor of Pathology and Cell Biology
Columbia University Medical Center
Director, Cancer Cytogenetics
New York-Presbyterian Hospital
New York, New York

Peter L. Nagy, MD, PhD
Assistant Professor of Pathology and Cell Biology
Director of Clinical Next-Generation Sequencing
Columbia University Medical Center
New York, New York

Ali Naini, PhD
Associate Professor of Pathology and Cell Biology
Columbia University Medical Center
New York, New York

Michael A. Pesce, PhD
Professor Emeritus of Pathology and Cell Biology
Columbia University Medical Center
New York-Presbyterian Hospital
New York, New York

Alex J. Rai, PhD, DABCC, FACB
Associate Professor of Pathology and Cell Biology
Columbia University Medical Center
New York-Presbyterian Hospital
New York, New York

Anjali Saqi, MD, MBA
Associate Professor of Pathology and Cell Biology
Columbia University Medical Center
New York-Presbyterian Hospital
New York, New York

Joseph (Yossi) Schwartz, MD, PhD
Associate Professor of Pathology and Cell Biology
Columbia University Medical Center
Director, Transfusion Medicine and Cellular Therapy
New York-Presbyterian Hospital
New York, New York

Jorge L. Sepulveda, MD, PhD
Associate Professor of Pathology and Cell Biology
Associate Medical Director of Clinical Laboratories
Columbia University Medical Center
New York-Presbyterian Hospital
New York, New York

Anthony N. Sireci, MD, MSc
Assistant Professor of Pathology and Cell Biology
Columbia University Medical Center
New York, New York

Patrice F. Spitalnik, MD
Associate Professor of Pathology and Cell Biology
Columbia University Medical Center
New York, New York

Brie Stotler, MD, MPH
Assistant Professor of Pathology and Cell Biology
Columbia University Medical Center
New York-Presbyterian Hospital
New York, New York

Yvette C. Tanhehco, MS, PhD, MD
Assistant Professor of Pathology and Cell Biology
Columbia University Medical Center
Assistant Director, Transfusion Medicine
New York-Presbyterian Hospital
New York, New York

Andrew Turk, MD
Assistant Professor of Pathology and Cell Biology
Columbia University Medical Center
New York, New York

Elena-Rodica Vasilescu, MD
Assistant Professor of Pathology and Cell Biology
Columbia University Medical Center
New York, New York

George Vlad, PhD
Assistant Professor of Pathology and Cell Biology
Columbia University Medical Center
New York, New York

Susan Whittier, PhD, D(ABMM)
Associate Professor of Pathology and Cell Biology
Associate Director, Clinical Microbiology Service
Columbia University Medical Center
New York-Presbyterian Hospital
New York, New York

Tilla S. Worgall, MD, PhD
Assistant Professor of Pathology and Cell Biology
Department of Pediatrics
Institute of Human Nutrition
Columbia University Medical Center
New York-Presbyterian Hospital
New York, New York

Fann Wu, MD, PhD
Assistant Professor of Pathology and Cell Biology
Columbia University Medical Center
Chief, Molecular Diagnostics and Epidemiology
Clinical Microbiology Services
New York-Presbyterian Hospital
New York, New York

PREFACE

We are pleased to have overseen the development of *Clinical Pathology Board Review* question book and edited its contents, which represent the efforts of more than 30 individuals who have been faculty members, residents, or fellows in the Division of Laboratory Medicine in the Department of Pathology and Cell Biology at Columbia University Medical Center/ New York-Presbyterian Hospital. As such, any strengths in our approach are due to the efforts of these individuals, and any weaknesses in organization or errors in the text are the responsibility of the editors. Although this book was developed based on the academic culture of the faculty members and residency/fellowship trainees at Columbia, given the magnitude of the project and the time interval required, several of these authors have since moved on to other opportunities.

Our goal is to help the reader prepare for the American Board of Pathology certification examination in Clinical Pathology. As such, the content of this book reflects practices currently in effect in the United States. It is also meant as a study guide, which, by the nature of the question or topic discussed, will encourage the board exam candidate to read more extensively. It is not meant as a substitute for broad and deep reading, training, and experience. As an initial guide to additional reading, relevant references are provided in the text for many of the questions. In addition, we recommend that the exam candidate read extensively in major textbooks relevant to Clinical Pathology. Examples of those we recommend for our residents include the following:

McPherson RA, Pincus MR: *Henry's Clinical Diagnosis and Management by Laboratory Methods,* ed 22, Philadelphia, 2011, Elsevier.

Klein HG, Anstee DJ: *Mollison's Blood Transfusion in Clinical Medicine,* ed 12, Blackwell, 2014.

Tille PM: *Bailey & Scott's Diagnostic Microbiology,* ed 13, Philadelphia, 2014, Elsevier.

Burtis CA, Ashwood ER, Bruns DE: *Tietz Textbook of Clinical Chemistry and Molecular Diagnostics,* ed 7, Philadelphia, 2014, Elsevier.

Nussbaum R, McInnes RR, Willard HF: *Thompson & Thompson Genetics in Medicine,* ed 7, Philadelphia, 2007, Elsevier.

In addition, although reference ranges are provided for specific analytes mentioned in each question, the reader may profit from referring to a resource listing reference ranges for virtually every analyte tested in clinical laboratories, such as:

Kratz A, Pesce MA, Basner RC, Einstein AJ: Laboratory values of clinical importance. In Longo DL, Fauci AS, Kasper DL, et al: *Harrison's Principles of Internal Medicine,* ed 18, New York, 2011, McGraw-Hill.

Each question in the text is original and was prepared "from scratch" by the authors. We prepared questions addressing a wide and comprehensive range of topics in modern Laboratory Medicine. However, given the "Columbia-centric" nature of the book, it is inevitable that consciously, or subconsciously, some topics were (over)emphasized due to the local interest and expertise of our faculty members. In addition, in some disciplines (e.g., clinical microbiology and genomics), the concepts, methods, and details are changing very quickly. Nonetheless, we endeavored to provide the most up-to-date information at the time the questions were prepared. Finally, we did not use recollections or reminiscences from prior board exams, either our own or those of our trainees, because this is unethical and illegal. A particularly good discussion of this issue can be found in the following editorial:

Davey DD: Recalled items and the American Board of Pathology Certification Examinations: what constitutes cheating? *Arch Pathol Lab Med* 2013;137:1540-1542.

Any similarities of our questions to those existing in the American Board of Pathology question bank, or the question bank maintained for the Resident in Service Exam (RISE) by the American Society of Clinical Pathology, are purely by chance.

Each question was designed to have only one correct answer, with five possible answers to choose from in almost every case. Whenever possible, the relevant clinical and scientific issues are illustrated by figures. A rationale is also provided for every possible answer explaining why it is correct or incorrect. We believe that this will help readers broaden their knowledge of each topic. In addition, one to five key points relating to the specific topic are identified as Major Topics of Discussion at the end of each question. We believe that these highlights will help readers focus their additional studying after they have answered all the questions. Finally, references are provided for many questions that help explain the concepts in more detail and serve as a jumping-off point for further reading. Thus, these are not necessarily meant to be the most recent relevant reference, nor the original description of the given topic.

To improve the book and address any inaccuracies, we created an email address to allow the reader to alert us to typographical errors, identify different points of view regarding medical and scientific issues, raise concerns, or ask us questions. Please contact us at CPQuestionBook@columbia.edu.

In conclusion, we would like to acknowledge the efforts and enthusiasm of the residents at Columbia who have received training in Clinical Pathology over the last 11 years.

Their curiosity and interest were major stimuli motivating the Laboratory Medicine faculty members to write this book. In addition, the inspiring efforts of our colleague, Dr. Jay Lefkowitch, including his enthusiasm for teaching and his leadership in preparing a prior question book for Anatomic Pathology, were important in encouraging us to embark on this task. Moreover, the clerical support of Ms. Ozaira Santana was invaluable. We also appreciate the patience and confidence of the staff at Elsevier (i.e., William Schmitt, Katy Meert, Carrie Stetz) in giving us this opportunity and shepherding us through the process. Moreover, we appreciate the support and patience of our families during this process. Finally, the continuous encouragement of Dr. Michael Shelanski has been critically important for all of our academic endeavors.

Steven L. Spitalnik
Suzanne A. Arinsburg
Jeffrey S. Jhang

CONTENTS

CHAPTER 1

LABORATORY MANAGEMENT:
General Principles, Statistics, and Test Interpretation

Alexander Kratz, Anthony N. Sireci, Brie Stotler, Jeffrey S. Jhang

QUESTIONS

1. In your annual performance evaluation meeting, your supervisor strongly suggests that you increase the productivity of your laboratory staff. Which one of the following represents the best path for you to take to address your supervisor's concern?
   A. Eliminate lunch breaks for your laboratory staff.
   B. Hire more technical full-time equivalents (FTEs).
   C. Reach out to the clinical staff of your hospital and ask them to limit the number of laboratory tests ordered.
   D. Try to bring in more business by expanding your outreach program, while exploring opportunities for decreasing staffing levels.
   E. Introduce strict controls on the use of copy paper and other office supplies.

2. Which one of the following is the best definition of a reagent rental (i.e., a "reagent lease")?
   A. The laboratory is billed for the reagents used. The price of the reagents includes the lease of the instruments. At the end of the lease period, the instruments belong to the laboratory.
   B. The laboratory is billed for reagents used. The price of the reagents includes the depreciation of the instruments.
   C. The laboratory pays the price of the reagents used; instruments are rented separately.
   D. The laboratory pays a rental fee for the instruments to the manufacturer; the rental fee includes free reagents for the duration of the rental period.
   E. The laboratory rents space for storing regents.

3. Your laboratory sends samples to a reference laboratory for analyses that are not performed in-house. Hospital administration notices that the charges associated with these tests have a significant impact on the laboratory budget and asks you to find ways to cut costs. You determine that, due to space and personnel constraints, you will not be able to bring most of these assays in-house. Which one of the following represents your best option in this situation?
   A. For every send-out test, find the cheapest send-out laboratory possible and send the samples there.
   B. Determine which other reference laboratories perform all (or most of) the testing you need. After determining which laboratories meet your quality standards, put out a request for proposals asking these laboratories to compete on price for your business.
   C. Find a reference laboratory that is close to your hospital; this will allow you to cut costs associated with sample transport.
   D. Ask all the ordering physicians at your institution which reference laboratory to use and then award the contract to the laboratory that received the most votes.
   E. Determine which reference laboratory can be electronically interfaced to your laboratory information system and then pick this laboratory. This will save on manual transcription costs.

4. Which one of the following is the best example of a semi-variable cost?
   A. The purchase of new laboratory equipment.
   B. A rental contract that has higher payments in the beginning (due to the higher value of new equipment) and lower payments at the end of the rental period (due to the lower remaining value of the equipment).
   C. Reagent rentals.
   D. Supervisory staffing in the laboratory.
   E. Hospital overhead allocated to the laboratory.

5. Which one of the following is true regarding high staff turnover in a clinical laboratory?
   A. It is desirable and a sign of a good laboratory.
   B. It allows a laboratory to keep costs down.
   C. It is almost impossible to quantify.
   D. It has a negative effect on the quality of work produced at a laboratory and on the cost of reporting laboratory results.
   E. It is entirely beyond the control of laboratory management.

6. As the laboratory director, you are planning to introduce a new laboratory test and want to determine the cost to your institution. Which one of the following sets of costs do you include in your calculation?
   A. Labor costs and material costs.
   B. Material costs, labor costs, and indirect costs.
   C. Labor costs and indirect costs.
   D. Material costs and indirect costs.
   E. Variable costs only.

7. Which one of the following intervals is the "true" or "total" turnaround time for a laboratory test?
   A. Accession-to-result time.
   B. Collection-to-result time.
   C. Collection-to-physician notification time.
   D. Order-to-physician notification time.
   E. Receipt-to-physician notification time.

8. Careful analysis of the turnaround times in your laboratory shows that there are significant delays between the arrival of samples in the laboratory and accessioning of samples in the laboratory information system. You decide that a redesign of your workflow is the best way to address the issue. Which one of the following represents a potential limitation of this approach?
   A. It will likely require a significant financial investment.
   B. It may only redistribute the delay to another step in the laboratory's preanalytical process.
   C. It will require hospital-wide cooperation from all ordering health care providers.
   D. It will require all samples received in the laboratory to arrive with a barcode label compatible with the laboratory information system.
   E. This approach has no limitations and will certainly work.

9. Which one of the following represents the largest expense in a typical clinical laboratory?
   A. Reagent costs.
   B. Utilities, such as electricity and water.
   C. Instrument purchasing and leasing costs.
   D. Salaries.
   E. Medical malpractice insurance.

10. Which one of the following statements best describes what a laboratory can do when billing for a basic metabolic panel (BMP)?
    A. Bill for each analyte separately or bill a lump sum for the entire panel using the appropriate Current Procedural Technology (CPT) code.
    B. Bill for each analyte separately; there is no CPT code for the entire panel.
    C. Bill for the entire panel with the CPT code for the panel; it is illegal to bill for each analyte separately.
    D. Bill for the entire panel for inpatients and bill for each analyte for outpatients, using the appropriate CPT code.
    E. Compare the reimbursement rates for individual tests versus the entire panel and bill the higher price using the appropriate CPT code.

11. For a clinical laboratory to be paid for performing a test, a CPT code and an International Classification of Diseases, Ninth Revision (ICD-9) code must be provided with every test. Which one of the following statements best describes the purpose of these codes?
    A. To provide accurate patient identification.
    B. To provide accurate identification of the patient's insurance carrier.
    C. To identify only the patient's medical condition.
    D. To identify only the test performed.
    E. To identify the test performed and the patient's medical condition.

12. Which one of the following statements best describes what is required for a physician to qualify as a laboratory director?
    A. Board certification in clinical pathology.
    B. Board eligibility in clinical pathology.
    C. Board certification in any medical specialty and a PhD in chemistry or a related field.
    D. A laboratory director certificate.
    E. One year of experience directing/supervising a nonwaived laboratory along with 20 continuing medical education (CME) credits in laboratory practice.

13. The expenses that a laboratory incurs for proficiency testing material are best described by which one of the following groups of costs?
    A. Indirect costs, fixed costs, and operating expenses.
    B. Direct costs, variable costs, and operating expenses.
    C. Indirect costs, variable costs, and operating expenses.
    D. Indirect costs, variable costs, and capital expenses.
    E. Direct costs, fixed costs, and operating expenses.

14. Using a laboratory information system's accession-to-result time as a proxy for the true turnaround time (TAT) may lead to which one of the following errors?
    A. An underestimation of the true TAT.
    B. An overestimation of the true TAT.
    C. A failure to capture tests not ordered electronically by the provider.
    D. A failure to capture critical result times.
    E. Using accession-to-result time as a proxy for the TAT will never lead to an error.

15. The obstetrical service of your hospital has asked you to offer a STAT test for fetal fibronectin. You currently do not have an instrument platform that could perform this test. The monthly lease for the new instrument would be $3000. Reagent costs would be $20 per reportable assay. Reimbursement for each fetal fibronectin test is $30. Assuming that there are no additional costs, which one of the following best describes the break-even monthly volume for this test?
    A. 100 tests per month.
    B. 150 tests per month.
    C. 300 tests per month.
    D. 600 tests per month.
    E. It is not possible to calculate the break-even volume with the information provided.

16. Which one of the following statements best describes a break-even analysis?
    A. It is the only factor laboratories use to decide if an assay should be brought in-house.
    B. It is based on the assumption that the selling price is variable.
    C. It can be used to help determine the price of a new assay.
    D. It has no connection to determining the profit or loss of a laboratory.
    E. It is only of importance in for-profit laboratories. Not-for-profit laboratories do not have to perform a break-even analysis, because they are not making a profit anyway.

17. Which one of the following statements best describes diagnosis-related groups (DRGs)?
    A. They are used to reimburse physicians for their services.
    B. They are used to reimburse hospitals for inpatient and outpatient services.
    C. They are used to reimburse hospitals for services provided for Medicare inpatients.
    D. They are used to reimburse hospitals and physicians for services provided to inpatients who have no insurance.
    E. DRG reimbursement rates are the same at every hospital in the United States.

18. You would like to determine the cost of performing a complete blood count in the laboratory. Which one of the following is an example of a direct cost?
    A. Custodial services.
    B. Lysing reagent.
    C. Security.
    D. Telephone service.
    E. Transporters.

19. You would like to determine the cost of performing a complete blood count in the laboratory. Which one of the following is an example of an indirect cost?
    A. Consumables.
    B. Hematology analyzer maintenance.
    C. Hematology technologist salary.
    D. Lysing reagent.
    E. Telephone service.

20. A 74-year-old man is admitted to an acute care hospital for community-acquired pneumonia. Which one of the following classification systems is used to determine the Medicare payment under the prospective payment system?
    A. Case-mix groups (CMGs).
    B. Diagnosis-related groups (DRGs).
    C. Home health resource groups (HHRGs).
    D. Resource utilization groups (RUG-III).
    E. Routine home care groups (RHCGs).

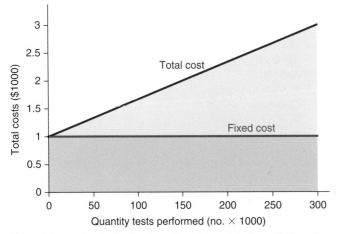

Figure 1-1 Total costs, fixed costs, and variable costs. This graph shows the total testing cost (*y*-axis) versus the number of tests performed (*x*-axis).

21. Your laboratory is planning to implement a new laboratory test. A graph of the total testing cost (*y*-axis) versus the number of tests performed (*x*-axis) is shown in Figure 1-1. The red line represents the total cost of the test and the blue line represents the fixed costs for performing the test. Which one of the following expenditures represents at least part of the cost shown in the beige area?
    A. Annual instrument maintenance contract.
    B. The medical director's malpractice insurance.
    C. Laboratory facility maintenance.
    D. Laboratory facility rental cost.
    E. Reagents.

22. Which one of the following statements best describes serum separator tubes (SSTs)?
    A. SSTs separate serum from plasma.
    B. SSTs are best suited for collecting samples for therapeutic drug monitoring.
    C. SSTs are best suited for collecting samples for endocrine testing.
    D. SSTs are often used to collect samples for serology testing.
    E. SSTs separate serum from blood cells upon centrifugation.

23. Compared with healthy ambulatory outpatients, which one of the following best describes the peripheral blood levels in healthy supine hospitalized patients?
    A. Lower glucose levels.
    B. Higher glucose levels.
    C. Lower albumin levels.
    D. Higher levels of protein-bound drugs.
    E. Higher cholesterol levels.

24. Prolonged application of a tourniquet (e.g., longer than 1 minute) before venipuncture can cause which one of the following?
    A. Hemodilution.
    B. An increase in blood pH.
    C. A decrease in serum protein levels.
    D. An increase in serum protein levels.
    E. A decrease in plasma lactate.

25. Optical interferences are major concerns in assays involving spectrophotometric analysis. The three most common interfering conditions are hemolysis, icterus, and lipemia. Which one of the following is the mechanism that explains these interferences?
    A. Hemoglobin and lipids scatter light; bilirubin absorbs particular wavelengths of light.
    B. Hemoglobin absorbs particular wavelengths of light; bilirubin and lipids scatter light.
    C. Lipids absorb particular wavelengths of light; bilirubin and hemoglobin scatter light.
    D. Hemoglobin, lipids, and bilirubin all scatter light.
    E. Hemoglobin and bilirubin absorb particular wavelengths of light; lipids scatter light.

26. Errors affecting laboratory results can be classified as preanalytical, analytical, or postanalytical. Which one of the following statements best describes the most frequent source of errors?
    A. Preanalytical errors.
    B. Analytical errors.
    C. Postanalytical errors.
    D. Errors occur with equal frequency in the preanalytical, analytical, and postanalytical phases.

E. It is very difficult to obtain accurate data on errors affecting the laboratory; therefore, it is not known in which phase errors occur most frequently.

27. Which one of the following best describes the effect(s) of high-protein, low-carbohydrate diets, such as the Atkins diet, on laboratory results?
    A. They have no effect on laboratory results.
    B. They increase urine ketones and increase blood urea nitrogen (BUN) levels in serum.
    C. They decrease urine ketones and decrease serum BUN levels.
    D. They decrease urine ketones and increase serum BUN levels.
    E. They increase urine ketones in the urine and decrease serum BUN levels.

28. Which one of the following statements best describes the use of gray-top tubes?
    A. They are used to collect samples for fluoride measurements.
    B. They are used to collect samples for sodium measurements.
    C. They contain no additives.
    D. They are used to collect samples for glucose measurements, especially when there is reason to expect a delay between sample collection and analysis.
    E. They can prevent glycolysis caused by bacterial septicemia.

Table 1-1

		True Disease Status	
		Present	Absent
Test Results	Positive	57	30
	Negative	3	130

A new assay has just been approved by the U.S. Food and Drug Administration. Table 1-1 details how the test performed in distinguishing between diseased and nondiseased individuals. Using this table, answer the following five questions.

29a. Which one of the following represents the sensitivity of this test?
    A. 0.95
    B. 0.81
    C. 0.66
    D. 0.24
    E. 0.98

29b. Which one of the following represents the specificity of this test?
    A. 0.98
    B. 0.81
    C. 0.95
    D. 0.66
    E. 0.24

29c. Which one of the following describes whether this test would be a good diagnostic screening test?
    A. Yes, the specificity is high.

B. No, the specificity is too low.
C. Yes, the sensitivity is high.
D. No, the specificity and the sensitivity are too low.
E. No, the sensitivity is too low.

29d. Which one of the following represents the positive predictive value of this test?
    A. 0.98
    B. 0.24
    C. 0.81
    D. 0.95
    E. 0.66

29e. Which one of the following represents the negative predictive value of this test?
    A. 0.98
    B. 0.24
    C. 0.81
    D. 0.95
    E. 0.66

Table 1-2

Result	Disease	No Disease	Total
Positive	160	40	200
Negative	10	190	200
Total	170	230	400

An assay was developed to detect anti-DNA antibodies in patients with lupus. The results of a pilot study correlating test results to disease status are shown below. Use this Table 1-2 to answer the following four questions.

30a. Which one of the following represents the sensitivity of this test?
    A. 83%.
    B. 94%.
    C. 80%.
    D. 90%.
    E. 99%.

30b. Which one of the following represents the specificity of this test?
    A. 94%.
    B. 96%.
    C. 80%.
    D. 90%.
    E. 83%.

30c. Which one of the following is the likelihood ratio of a positive result for this test?
    A. 88
    B. 1.1
    C. 5.5
    D. 0.88
    E. 7

30d. Which one of the following is the correct interpretation of the likelihood ratio for a positive result for this test?
    A. Lupus is 5.5 times more likely to occur in a patient with a positive result than it is in a patient with a negative result.

B. The prevalence of lupus in this patient population has increased 5.5 times above the national average.

C. A false-positive test result is 5.5 times more likely to occur using this assay compared with the gold standard.

D. A positive test result is 5.5 times more likely to occur in a patient with lupus compared with a patient without lupus.

E. The true-positive rate is 5.5 times the prevalence of the disease.

31. Which one of the following statements best describes test sensitivity for a given disease?
    A. The proportion of people without the disease who have a negative test result.
    B. The proportion of people with the disease who have a positive test result.
    C. The probability that someone with a negative test result does not have the disease.
    D. The probability that someone with a positive test result has the disease.
    E. The odds of having the disease when the test result is negative.

32. Which one of the following best describes test specificity?
    A. The proportion of people without the disease who have a negative test result.
    B. The proportion of people with the disease who have a positive test result.
    C. The probability that someone with a negative test result does not have the disease.
    D. The probability that someone with a positive test result has the disease.
    E. The odds of having the disease when the test result is negative.

33. You are evaluating precision at the high end of linearity for a thyroxin assay. The mean result value is 3.14 and the standard deviation (SD) is 0.09. What is the coefficient of variation (CV) of this test?
    A. 35%.
    B. 18%.
    C. 5.7%.
    D. 10%.
    E. 2.9%.

34. The prevalence of a disease has increased dramatically in the general population. Which one of the following statements best describes what this would do to the positive predictive value of a diagnostic test for this disease?
    A. The positive predictive value would remain the same.
    B. The increase in disease prevalence would decrease the positive predictive value of the test.
    C. The increase in disease prevalence would increase the positive predictive value of the test.
    D. Changing the disease prevalence does not affect the predictive value of the test.
    E. The positive predictive value would remain the same, but the test specificity would decrease.

35. Which one of the following statements best describes what the area under the receiver operating characteristic (ROC) curve represents?
    A. The overall sensitivity of the test as it varies with population prevalence range.
    B. The overall specificity of the test as it varies with population prevalence.
    C. The variation in the precision of the test over the entire technical linear range.
    D. The overall accuracy of the test over the entire range of sensitivity and specificity.
    E. The range of the coefficient of variation over all medical decision threshold values.

36. Proficiency testing for glucose yielded a mean value of 150 mg/dL with a standard deviation of 20 mg/dL. Your lab reported a result of 130 mg/dL. Which one of the following values is the standard deviation index (SDI) for your lab for this proficiency test?
    A. 0.13
    B. 0.15
    C. 1.0
    D. −1.0
    E. −0.15

A new point-of-care assay was developed for detecting HIV antibodies. The test sensitivity is 98% and the specificity is 95%. The test will be used by a mobile health care service that has clinics in two different developing countries. Country A has an HIV prevalence of 25%, and Country B has an HIV prevalence of 5%. Using this information, answer the following three questions.

37a. Which one of the following is the likelihood ratio of a positive test result for this test?
    A. 1.3
    B. 19.6
    C. 42.5
    D. 1.0
    E. 9

37b. Which one of the following is the post-test probability of true HIV infection if a patient from Country A tests positive?
    A. 51%.
    B. 25%.
    C. 5%.
    D. 87%.
    E. 98%.

37c. Which one of the following is the post-test probability of true HIV infection if a patient from Country B tests positive?
    A. 51%.
    B. 25%.
    C. 5%.
    D. 87%.
    E. 98%.

38. A new assay is developed for measuring anti–smooth muscle antibodies. The likelihood ratio of a positive test for this assay in

patients with primary sclerosing cholangitis is 7. Which one of the following statements is the correct interpretation of this likelihood ratio?

A. A likelihood ratio of 7 indicates no relationship between anti–smooth muscle antibodies and primary sclerosing cholangitis.

B. A likelihood ratio of 7 indicates no predictive ability of this assay in distinguishing disease from nondisease.

C. Anti–smooth muscle antibodies occur in 7% of patients with primary sclerosing cholangitis.

D. Primary sclerosing cholangitis is 7 times more likely to occur in a patient with a positive result compared with a patient with a negative result.

E. A positive test result is 7 times more likely to occur in a patient with primary sclerosing cholangitis than in a healthy patient.

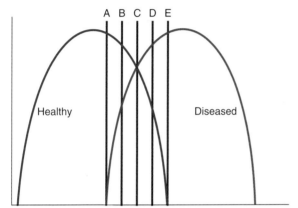

Figure 1-2 Healthy and diseased populations and test cutoffs. The image represents a test's result performance in populations of healthy and diseased individuals. Letters A through E represent possible test result cutoff levels for determining if the test is positive or negative.

Use Figure 1-2 answer the following four questions.

39a. Which letter best represents the test result cutoff value that would yield the highest sensitivity?

A. A
B. B
C. C
D. D
E. E

39b. Which letter represents the test result cutoff value that would yield the highest specificity?

A. A
B. B
C. C
D. D
E. E

39c. A disease is 100% curable if detected in the early stages. Which letter represents the best cutoff value to use for

this test, so that no affected patients would be missed during screening?

A. A
B. B
C. C
D. D
E. E

39d. A treatment for a disease has a 50% success rate at achieving disease remission, but this treatment also has a 25% mortality rate. Which letter represents the best cutoff value to use for a test to determine whether the patient undergoes this treatment?

A. A
B. B
C. C
D. D
E. E

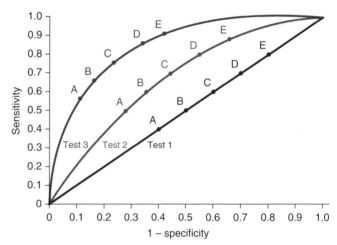

Figure 1-3 Receiver operating characteristic curve. Three receiver operating characteristic (ROC) curves for test 1 (red), 2 (blue), and 3 (green) are shown. Points A, B, C, D, and E are labeled on each curve. Sensitivity is plotted on the y-axis, and 1 – specificity is plotted on the x-axis.

40. Three tests were developed to detect the presence of hepatitis B antibodies in plasma. Using the receiver operating characteristics (ROC) curves in Figure 1-3, answer the following two questions regarding the performance of these three different tests.

40a. Which one of these tests is the most accurate?

A. Test 1.
B. Test 2.
C. Test 3.

40b. For Test 3, which point represents the cutoff with the most diagnostic accuracy?

A. A
B. B
C. C
D. D
E. E

41. You are determining the reference range for an analyte and have gathered test result data from 120 normal individuals. Which one of the data distributions in Figure 1-4 would be amenable to using the mean ± SD approach to determining a reference range that would encompass 95% of the healthy individuals' results?

A. Graph A.
B. Graph B.
C. Graph C.

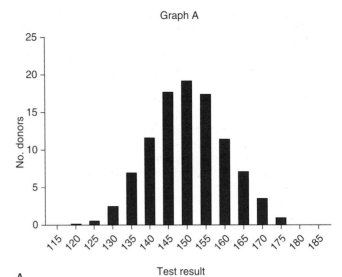

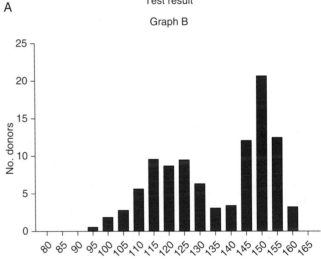

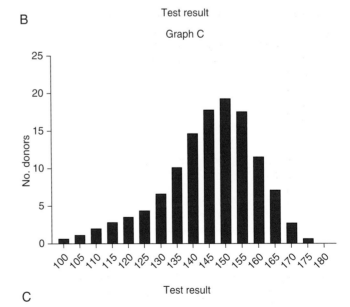

Figure 1-4　Three histograms (**A**, **B**, and **C**) show the number of subjects (i.e., the frequency) on the *y*-axis and the analytical result on the *x*-axis.

ANSWERS

1. A. Eliminate lunch breaks for your laboratory staff.
Rationale: Eliminating lunch breaks is unlikely to increase the number of results reported because of staff fatigue and dissatisfaction and will not decrease the number of FTEs.
B. Hire more technical full-time equivalents (FTEs).
Rationale: Hiring more FTEs will decrease the productivity of the laboratory staff.
C. Reach out to the clinical staff of your hospital and ask them to limit the number of laboratory tests ordered.
Rationale: Decreasing the number of laboratory tests performed may decrease expenditures for reagents but will not increase productivity.
D. Try to bring in more business by expanding your outreach program, while exploring opportunities for decreasing staffing levels.
Rationale: Expanding your outreach business will increase the number of tests performed, if this can be accomplished with the current size of your staff. Alternatively, decreasing staffing levels will allow you to do the testing with fewer FTEs, assuming that they can complete all of the testing requested.
E. Introduce strict controls on the use of copy paper and other office supplies.
Rationale: Decreasing the use of office supplies will decrease the overall expenditures of the laboratory but will not improve staff productivity.

Major points of discussion
- Productivity is defined as the number of products produced divided by the resources used to produce the product.
- In the case of the productivity of laboratory staff, the product is the billable laboratory result, and the resource is the technical FTEs needed to produce the result.
- Therefore, one can increase staff productivity by increasing the number of tests performed, reducing the number of FTEs, or both.
- Only BILLABLE tests count toward productivity; nonbillable tests, such as those performed for quality control and proficiency testing, do not count for this purpose.

2. A. The laboratory is billed for the reagents used. The price of the reagents includes the lease of the instruments. At the end of the lease period, the instruments belong to the laboratory.
Rationale: At the end of a reagent rental ("reagent lease"), the instruments belong to the manufacturer, not the laboratory.
B. The laboratory is billed for reagents used. The price of the reagents includes the depreciation of the instruments.
Rationale: This is the definition of a reagent rental ("reagent lease"). At the end of the rental period, the instruments still belong to the manufacturer.
C. The laboratory pays the price of the reagents used; instruments are rented separately.
D. The laboratory pays a rental fee for the instruments to the manufacturer; the rental fee includes free reagents for the duration of the rental period.
E. The laboratory rents space for storing regents.

Rationale: In a reagent rental ("reagent lease"), the laboratory is billed only for the reagents used. The price of the reagents includes the lease costs of the instruments. At the end of the lease period, the instruments still belong to the manufacturer.

Major points of discussion
- Clinical laboratories often have difficulty raising the capital required for purchasing laboratory instruments.
- Therefore, to enable the use of large, expensive instruments, laboratories often use reagent rentals (i.e., "reagent leases").
- The major advantage of a reagent rental is that the laboratory can use operational funds (as opposed to capital funds) to pay for the use of the instruments required to provide clinical laboratory testing.

3. A. For every send-out test, find the cheapest send-out laboratory possible and send the samples there.
Rationale: Choosing send-out laboratories based on price alone may lead to multiple issues, including assay quality, turnaround time, and the need to deal with multiple reference laboratories.
B. Determine which other reference laboratories perform all (or most of) the testing you need. After determining which laboratories meet your quality standards, put out a request for proposals, asking these laboratories to compete on price for your business.
Rationale: This method will allow you to choose a high-quality laboratory that meets your needs at the best possible price.
C. Find a reference laboratory that is close to your hospital; this will allow you to cut costs associated with sample transport.
Rationale: Although the physical proximity of a reference laboratory can be an advantage, it should not be the only determinant in choosing a reference laboratory.
D. Ask all the ordering physicians at your institution which reference laboratory to use and then award the contract to the laboratory that received the most votes.
Rationale: Although ordering physician input is very important in choosing a reference laboratory, it is unlikely that all ordering physicians at your institution will be sufficiently knowledgeable in this matter.
E. Determine which reference laboratory can be electronically interfaced to your laboratory information system and then pick this laboratory. This will save on manual transcription costs.
Rationale: The ability to electronically interface to a reference laboratory is very important. However, it should not be the only determinant in choosing a reference laboratory.

Major points of discussion
- Many factors influence the decision regarding which reference laboratory tests will not be performed in-house and will be sent to reference laboratories.
- These factors include the quality/reliability of the assays, turnaround times, the ability to electronically interface your laboratory information system with the reference laboratory, and price.

- No single issue should be the sole determining factor.
- It is important to obtain input from the ordering physician stakeholders at your institution when choosing a reference laboratory. For example, when choosing a reference laboratory for pediatric endocrinology assays, buy-in from the pediatric endocrinology physicians and staff is crucial.
- Electronically interfacing your laboratory information system with the reference laboratory will avoid manual transcription errors, decrease turnaround times, and save the salary of employees who would otherwise be needed for manually transcribing the results.

4. A. The purchase of new laboratory equipment.
Rationale: Purchasing new laboratory equipment is a fixed cost, not a semi-variable cost.
B. A rental contract that has higher payments in the beginning (due to the higher value of new equipment) and lower payments at the end of the rental period (due to the lower remaining value of the equipment).
Rationale: The rental contract described here does not meet the definition of semi-variable costs (see Major Points of Discussion).
C. Reagent rentals.
Rationale: Reagent rentals are variable costs, not semi-variable costs.
D. Supervisory staffing in the laboratory.
Rationale: Supervisory staffing of the laboratory is a good example of semi-variable costs; thus, when laboratory volumes increase, a given number of supervisors will be able to handle the increased volume up to a certain threshold. After this threshold is reached, additional supervisors will need to be hired.
E. Hospital overhead allocated to the laboratory.
Rationale: Hospital overhead allocated to the laboratory is a fixed cost, not a semi-variable cost.

Major points of discussion

- Semi-variable costs (also known as "step variable costs") are expenses that vary with test volume but not in direct proportion to the volume.
- Fixed costs do not vary over time and do not change with sample volume.
- Variable costs vary directly and proportionally with the volume of samples analyzed.
- Costs associated with performing a particular test can be fixed (e.g., the purchase of the equipment needed to perform the test), variable (e.g., the reagents used per test), or semi-variable (e.g., the salaries of the staff required to perform the test).

5. A. It is desirable and a sign of a good laboratory.
B. It allows a laboratory to keep costs down.
Rationale: High employee turnover in a clinical laboratory increases the costs of running the laboratory because there are significant costs associated with recruiting and training new staff.
C. It is almost impossible to quantify.
Rationale: The employee turnover rate can be calculated by dividing the number of separations and terminations by the total number of employees on staff at the end of a given time period.

D. It has a negative effect on the quality of work produced at a laboratory and on the cost of reporting laboratory results.
Rationale: New staff is more likely to be unfamiliar with all of the standard operating procedures (SOPs), which can lead to mistakes due to a lack of local experience. High staff turnover in a clinical laboratory leads to significant costs associated with recruiting and training new employees.
E. It is entirely beyond the control of laboratory management.
Rationale: The employee turnover rate of a laboratory can be decreased by increasing salaries and benefits, by addressing employee complaints in a timely manner, and by improving other workplace factors that determine employee satisfaction.

Major points of discussion

- Employee satisfaction is influenced by various factors, including compensation, benefits, working hours, and working conditions.
- High employee turnover can be evaluated by exit interviews to determine the causes of employee resignations and the success, or lack thereof, of targeted interventions.
- The employee turnover rate can be calculated by dividing the number of separations and terminations by the total number of employees on staff at the end of a given time period.
- New staff members are more likely to make mistakes due to lack of familiarity and experience with the laboratory's SOPs.

6. A. Labor costs and material costs.
B. Material costs, labor costs, and indirect costs.
C. Labor costs and indirect costs.
D. Material costs and indirect costs.
E. Variable costs only.
Rationale: The total cost of performing a laboratory test includes labor costs, material costs (e.g., reagents and other supplies), and indirect costs (i.e., overhead). Some of these costs are not variable but fixed; these fixed costs also need to be included in the calculation.

Major points of discussion

- It is important to include all costs in the cost accounting of laboratory tests.
- Accurate cost accounting allows accurate pricing of laboratory services.
- Accurate cost accounting also allows the laboratory to make informed decisions regarding whether to perform nonurgent testing in-house or to send these samples to a reference laboratory.

7. A. Accession-to-result time.
Rationale: The accession-to-result time does not measure the time from order to accessioning and from results to physician notification and, therefore, is not a "true" representation of the total turnaround time for laboratory tests.
B. Collection-to-result time.
Rationale: The collection-to-result time does not measure the time from ordering to collection and from results to physician notification and, therefore, is not a "true"

representation of the total turnaround time for laboratory tests.

C. Collection-to-physician notification time.
Rationale: The collection-to-physician notification time does not measure the time from ordering to collection and, therefore, is not a "true" representation of the total turnaround time for laboratory tests.

D. Order-to-physician notification time.
Rationale: The order-to-physician notification time measures all preanalytical, analytical, and postanalytical portions of the turnaround time and, therefore, is the best representation of the total turnaround time for laboratory specimens.

E. Receipt-to-physician notification time.
Rationale: The receipt-to-physician notification time does not measure the time from ordering to receipt in the laboratory and, therefore, is not the best representation of the "true" turnaround time for laboratory testing.

Major points of discussion

- Total turnaround times for laboratory samples consist of the sum of the preanalytical, analytical, and postanalytical intervals.
- The preanalytical interval consists of the time from ordering of the test to the beginning of sample analysis.
- The analytical interval consists of the time needed for analysis.
- The postanalytical interval consists of the time from completion of analysis to notification of the ordering clinician.
- It is important that laboratory turnaround reports include all relevant components of the total turnaround time.

8. A. It will likely require a significant financial investment.
Rationale: Redesigning workflow in the laboratory generally does not require a significant financial investment.

B. It may only redistribute the delay to another step in the laboratory's preanalytical process.
Rationale: If the laboratory staff in the preanalytical area is already working at full capacity, redesign of the workflow may lead to delays in other preanalytical steps.

C. It will require hospital-wide cooperation from all ordering health care providers.
Rationale: Cooperation from ordering providers is not required for redesign of the laboratory workflow.

D. It will require all samples received in the laboratory to arrive with a barcode label compatible with the laboratory information system.
Rationale: A redesign of the laboratory workflow does not necessarily require that all samples are received with a barcode label.

E. This approach has no limitations and will certainly work.
Rationale: If the laboratory staff in the preanalytical area is already working at full capacity, redesign of the workflow may lead to delays in other preanalytical steps.

Major points of discussion

- The preanalytical turnaround time interval consists of the time from ordering the test to the beginning of analysis.

- The preanalytical turnaround time interval includes the time intervals from ordering to collection, from collection to receipt in the laboratory, from receipt to accessioning, and from accessioning to completion of all necessary preanalytical steps (e.g., centrifugation, aliquotting), as well as the transport times within and between laboratory sections.
- Possible interventions for decreasing the preanalytical turnaround interval include introduction of electronic order entry, laboratory automation, addition of additional laboratory staff, and redesign of laboratory workflow.
- Introduction of electronic order entry requires a significant financial investment as well as cooperation from health care providers.
- Introduction of laboratory automation requires significant investment, the availability of suitable space, and appropriate infrastructure.

9. A. Reagent costs.
Rationale: Reagent costs are not the largest expense in laboratories. This status belongs to salary costs, which constitute 60% to 80% of most laboratories' budgets.

B. Utilities, such as electricity and water.
Rationale: Utility costs are not the largest expense in laboratories. This status belongs to salary costs, which constitute 60% to 80% of most laboratories' budgets.

C. Instrument purchasing and leasing costs.
Rationale: Instrument purchasing and leasing costs are not the largest expense in laboratories. This status belongs to salary costs, which constitute 60% to 80% of most laboratories' budgets.

D. Salaries.
Rationale: Salary expenses account for 60% to 80% of the budget of a typical clinical laboratory.

E. Medical malpractice insurance.
Rationale: Malpractice insurance costs are not the largest expense in laboratories. This status belongs to salary costs, which constitute 60% to 80% of most laboratories' budgets.

Major points of discussion

- Fringe benefits (Social Security, health insurance, pension plans, etc.) can represent an additional 16% to 28% expense above the salary base.
- Because salary expenses are generally fixed, it is important to strive for efficiency, productivity, and economies of scale.
- Costs are also associated with the recruitment, interview, and selection process for new staff.
- Once an employee is hired, orientation and training costs are also incurred.[6]

10. A. Bill for each analyte separately or bill a lump sum for the entire panel using the appropriate Current Procedural Technology (CPT) code.
Rationale: When billing for panels, the appropriate CPT code specific for the entire panel MUST be used. Coding for each individual test is considered "unbundling" and fraudulent.

B. Bill for each analyte separately; there is no CPT code for the entire panel.
Rationale: There are special codes for 10 identified panels, including the BMP. When billing for panels, the CPT code

specific for the entire panel MUST be used. Coding for each individual test is considered "unbundling" and fraudulent.
C. Bill for the entire panel with the CPT code for the panel; it is illegal to bill for each analyte separately.
Rationale: When billing for panels, the appropriate CPT code specific for the entire panel MUST be used. Coding for each individual test is considered "unbundling" and fraudulent.
D. Bill for the entire panel for inpatients and bill for each analyte for outpatients, using the appropriate CPT code.
Rationale: There is no difference between inpatients and outpatients with regard to billing for panels. When billing for panels, the appropriate CPT code specific for the entire panel MUST be used. Coding for each individual test is considered "unbundling" and fraudulent.
E. Compare the reimbursement rates for individual tests versus the entire panel and bill the higher price using the appropriate CPT code.
Rationale: When billing for panels, the appropriate CPT code specific for the entire panel MUST be used. Coding for each individual test is considered "unbundling" and fraudulent.

Major points of discussion
- CPT codes serve to identify the laboratory test performed.
- There are specific CPT codes for each of 10 frequently used panels.
- Coding for each individual assay in a panel (i.e., "unbundling"), as opposed to coding for the entire panel, is considered to be fraud.
- Reimbursement for panels is lower than for the sum total of the reimbursement for its components.
- These rules apply equally to inpatients and outpatients.

11. A. To provide accurate patient identification.
    B. To provide accurate identification of the patient's insurance carrier.
    C. To identify only the patient's medical condition.
    D. To identify only the test performed.
    E. To identify the test performed and the patient's medical condition.
    Rationale: The CPT code identifies the laboratory test performed; the ICD-9 code identifies the patient's medical condition or diagnosis, thereby establishing the medical necessity for the test. Both pieces of information are needed for billing. Neither code identifies the patient or the patient's insurance carrier.

Major points of discussion
- CPT codes identify the laboratory test performed.
- ICD-9 codes identify the patient's medical condition or diagnosis.
- The ICD-9 code establishes the medical necessity for a test; tests are reimbursed only if the medical condition justified the performance of that particular test.
- Both a CPT code and an ICD-9 code must be submitted for billing.
- A provider can order a test that is not medically necessary, but it will not be reimbursed.

12. A. Board certification in clinical pathology.
    Rationale: Board certification in clinical pathology is not necessary to become a laboratory director.
    B. Board eligibility in clinical pathology.

Rationale: Board eligibility in clinical pathology is not necessary to become a laboratory director.
C. Board certification in any medical specialty and a PhD in chemistry or a related field.
Rationale: Neither board certification nor a PhD is necessary to become a laboratory director.
D. A laboratory director certificate.
Rationale: CLIA does not require an individual to hold a laboratory director certificate to direct a clinical laboratory.
E. One year of experience directing/supervising a nonwaived laboratory along with 20 continuing medical education (CME) credits in laboratory practice.
Rationale: A physician with 1 year of experience directing/supervising a nonwaived laboratory along with 20 CME credits in laboratory practice qualifies to be a laboratory director.

Major points of discussion
- Laboratories that perform under a certificate of waiver are not required to have a laboratory director.
- Laboratories that perform moderately complex testing are required to have a laboratory director.
- The laboratory director is responsible for the overall management and direction of the laboratory.
- The director is responsible for the analytical performance of all assays and for determining the qualifications of individuals performing and reporting test results.

13. **A. Indirect costs, fixed costs, and operating expenses.**
    B. Direct costs, variable costs, and operating expenses.
    C. Indirect costs, variable costs, and operating expenses.
    Rationale: Operating expenses are costs incurred to produce a product or service, such as proficiency testing material. Therefore, proficiency testing expenses include indirect costs, fixed costs, operating expenses.
    D. Indirect costs, variable costs, and capital expenses.
    Rationale: To qualify as a capital expense, an item must last longer than 1 year, cost a certain minimum amount, and either replace existing equipment or be bought to support new products or services. Therefore, proficiency testing material is NOT a capital expense.
    E. Direct costs, fixed costs, and operating expenses.
    Rationale: Operating expenses are costs incurred to produce a product or service, such as proficiency testing material. Therefore, proficiency testing expenses include indirect costs, fixed costs, operating expenses.

Major points of discussion
- Indirect costs are not directly related to a billable test but are necessary for its production. This is the case for expenses for proficiency testing material. Variable costs change proportionately with the volume of tests; this does NOT apply to proficiency testing expenses.
- Direct costs are expenses that can be directly traced to an end product. This does NOT apply to proficiency testing expenses.
- Fixed costs do not change with the volume of tests performed.

14. **A. An underestimation of the true TAT.**
    B. An overestimation of the true TAT.

Rationale: Using accession-to-result time as a proxy for the true TAT will not measure the time from ordering to accessioning and from results to physician notification. Therefore, this will lead to an underestimation, not to an overestimation, of the "true" or "total" TAT.
C. A failure to capture tests not ordered electronically by the provider.
Rationale: Tests not ordered electronically by the provider will be ordered in the laboratory information system at the time of accessioning. Therefore, they will be captured on this type of TAT report.
D. A failure to capture critical result times.
Rationale: Critical result times are captured and evaluated independently of this type of TAT report.
E. Using accession-to-result time as a proxy for the TAT will never lead to an error.
Rationale: Using accession-to-result time as a proxy for the true TAT will not measure the time from ordering to accessioning and from results to physician notification. Therefore, this will lead to an underestimation, not to an overestimation, of the "true" or "total" TAT.

Major points of discussion
- Total turnaround times for laboratory samples consist of the sum of the preanalytical, analytical, and postanalytical intervals.
- The preanalytical interval consists of the time from ordering the test to the beginning of analysis.
- The analytical interval consists of the time needed for analysis.
- The postanalytical interval consists of the time from completion of analysis to notification of the ordering clinician.
- It is important that laboratory turnaround reports include all relevant components of the total turnaround time.

15. A. 100 tests per month.
B. 150 tests per month.
C. 300 tests per month.
D. 600 tests per month.
E. It is not possible to calculate the break-even volume with the information provided.
Rationale: The break-even volume for a laboratory assay is the "fixed cost" divided by the ("reimbursement rate" minus the "variable cost"). In this example, the monthly fixed cost is $3000. The reimbursement rate per test is $30, and the variable cost (reagents) is $20. Therefore, the break-even volume is 3000/(30 − 20) = 300. You will have to be successfully reimbursed for 300 tests per month to break even.

Major points of discussion
- Break-even analysis is the process of calculating the sales needed to cover costs so that there is zero profit or loss.
- In the laboratory, break-even analysis can be used as a screening tool to determine whether bringing a new assay in-house makes financial sense.
- A break-even analysis is not the only determining factor in the decision if a laboratory test should be performed in-house.
- Clinical needs and physician and patient satisfaction can override a break-even analysis.

- The break-even volume for a laboratory assay is calculated as the "fixed cost" divided by the ("reimbursement rate" minus the "variable cost").

16. A. It is the only factor laboratories use to decide if an assay should be brought in-house.
Rationale: A break-even analysis is only a screening tool to determine whether it makes sense financially to bring an assay in-house. Many other factors, including clinical needs and patient and physician satisfaction, influence the decision to bring a new assay in-house.
B. It is based on the assumption that the selling price is variable.
Rationale: Break-even analysis is generally based on the assumption that the selling price is constant, not varying.
C. It can be used to help determine the price of a new assay.
Rationale: Break-even analysis can be used to help determine the price of a new assay. However, because most insurance reimbursement rates are fixed, the prices charged by the laboratory will be less important than the reimbursement rates.
D. It has no connection to determining the profit or loss of a laboratory.
Rationale: Break-even analysis is important in the process of predicting possible profits or losses resulting from implementing a new laboratory test.
E. It is only of importance in for-profit laboratories. Not-for-profit laboratories do not have to perform a break-even analysis because they are not making a profit anyway.
Rationale: Break-even analysis is important for both for-profit and not-for-profit laboratories. Not-for-profit laboratories also have to balance their books!

Major points of discussion
- Break-even analysis is the process of calculating the sales needed to cover costs so that there is zero profit or loss.
- In the laboratory, break-even analysis can be used as a screening tool to determine whether bringing a new assay in-house makes financial sense.
- A break-even analysis is not the only determining factor in the decision regarding whether a laboratory test should be performed in-house.
- Clinical needs and physician and patient satisfaction can override a break-even analysis.
- Break-even analysis is usually based on the assumption that the selling price of a product (e.g., a laboratory test) is constant.

17. A. They are used to reimburse physicians for their services.
B. They are used to reimburse hospitals for inpatient and outpatient services.
C. They are used to reimburse hospitals for services provided for Medicare inpatients.
D. They are used to reimburse hospitals and physicians for services provided to inpatients who have no insurance.
Rationale: DRGs are only used to reimburse hospital costs for Medicare inpatients (Part A services). DRGs are not used to reimburse hospitals for outpatient services or to reimburse physicians for their services.
E. DRG reimbursement rates are the same at every hospital in the United States.

Rationale: The reimbursement rate for each DRG depends on the type of hospital, the hospital setting, and the hospital's location.

Major points of discussion

■ Each DRG is assigned a weight based on the severity of the diagnosis, the types of procedures performed, and the presence of comorbid conditions or complications.

■ Hospitals are reimbursed for each DRG by a rate determined with reference to the type of hospital, the hospital setting, and the hospital's location.

■ In DRG-based systems, hospitals receive a lump sum for treating each patient. There is no additional revenue provided for performing more laboratory tests for that patient.

18. A. Custodial services.
   B. Lysing reagent.
   Rationale: This is a direct cost.
   C. Security.
   D. Telephone service.
   E. Transporters.
   Rationale for A, C, D, and E: These are indirect costs, which are those costs that benefit more than one product or project. In most cases, the indirect costs are difficult to trace and it is not economically feasible to perform this tracing.

Major points of discussion

■ A direct cost is a cost associated with directly producing a product, in this case a complete blood count.

■ The attributes of a direct cost include being:
   1. An integral part of producing the product (not benefiting more than one product)
   2. Easily traceable
   3. Economically traceable (tracing the cost does not cost an unreasonable amount)

■ Examples of direct costs include technologist salaries, instrument supplies and reagents, and equipment maintenance.

■ Individual laboratories determine how the total cost of the test is calculated. Some include direct costs only; some include indirect and direct costs.

19. A. Consumables.
   B. Hematology analyzer maintenance.
   C. Hematology technologist salary.
   D. Lysing reagent.
   Rationale: This is a direct cost; these typically are an integral part of producing the product (and do not benefit more than one product), easily traceable, and economically traceable.
   E. Telephone service.
   Rationale: This is an indirect cost.

Major points of discussion

■ Indirect costs are those costs that benefit more than one product or project (i.e., overhead).

■ In most cases, the indirect costs are difficult to trace and assign to a specific product; therefore, it is often not economically feasible to perform this tracing.

■ The attributes of a direct cost include being:

1. An integral part of producing the product (not benefitting more than one product)
2. Easily traceable
3. Economically traceable (tracing these costs does not cost an unreasonable amount)

■ If any of these criteria is not met, then the cost is considered to be an indirect cost.

■ Examples of indirect costs include custodial services, building maintenance, telephone service, security, building rent, transport, and general administration.

■ Individual laboratories determine how the total cost of the test is calculated. Some include direct costs only; some include indirect and direct costs.

20. A. Case-mix groups (CMGs).
   Rationale: This classification is used for an inpatient rehabilitation hospital.
   B. Diagnosis-related groups (DRGs).
   Rationale: This classification is used for acute inpatient admissions.
   C. Home health resource groups (HHRGs).
   Rationale: This classification is used for care by a home health aide.
   D. Resource utilization groups (RUG-III).
   Rationale: This classification is used for skilled nursing facilities.
   E. Routine home care groups (RHCGs).
   Rationale: There is no classification for Medicare with this name.

Major points of discussion

■ The Centers for Medicare & Medicaid Services adopted the prospective payment system to control the amount of inpatient care expenditures for Medicare beneficiaries.

■ Under this system, a payment is made to the hospital to cover the expenses for the hospital admission over a defined period, regardless of the resources actually used to treat the patient.

■ Payment is based on the admission diagnosis, which is classified according to one of 535 DRGs.

■ There are some adjustments to the DRG-based payment based on the patient's age, gender, secondary medical problems, and other factors that add to treatment complexity.

■ Classification systems and prospective payments are now used for Medicare payments to skilled nursing facilities and rehabilitation hospitals and for home health care and hospice care.

21. A. Annual instrument maintenance contract.
   B. The medical director's malpractice insurance.
   C. Laboratory facility maintenance.
   D. Laboratory facility rental cost.
   Rationale: This is a fixed cost; these are expenses to the laboratory that do not change based on the volume of tests performed.[6]
   E. Reagents.
   Rationale: This is a variable cost; these are expenses to the laboratory that change with the volume of tests performed.

Major points of discussion

■ The total cost of performing a test includes both the fixed costs and the variable costs. In the figure, the total cost varies with the number of tests performed; it is represented by the red line.

■ Fixed costs are expenses to the laboratory that do not change based on the volume of tests performed. For example, rent, taxes, insurance, and maintenance all need to be paid regardless of how many tests are performed. The fixed cost does not vary with the number of tests performed; it is represented by the blue line.

■ Variable costs are expenses to the laboratory that change with the volume of tests performed. For example, the volumes of reagents, cuvettes, and other consumables increase when additional tests are performed, so they are considered variable costs.

■ The green shaded area represents the fixed costs. The yellow shaded area represents the variable costs (total cost minus fixed cost).

■ Wages can be fixed or variable depending on how staff members are paid. If the technologist is paid for a 40-hour work week regardless of how many tests are run, then the salary is considered a fixed expense. However, if the technologist is paid per manual differential performed, then it would be considered a variable cost.

22. A. SSTs separate serum from plasma.
Rationale: SSTs contain a gel that, during centrifugation, localizes between packed cells and the top serum layer. They separate cells from serum, not serum from plasma.
B. SSTs are best suited for collecting samples for therapeutic drug monitoring.
Rationale: The gel separator in SSTs can absorb certain drugs, such as phenytoin, phenobarbital, lidocaine, quinidine, and carbamazepine. Therefore, they should not be used to collect samples for therapeutic drug monitoring.
C. SSTs are best suited for collecting samples for endocrine testing.
Rationale: There are some reports that SSTs can interfere with endocrine testing. Therefore, SSTs are not the first choice for collecting samples to measure endocrine markers.
D. SSTs are often used to collect samples for serology testing.
Rationale: The gels in SSTs can interfere with immunologic reactions. Therefore, these tubes should not be used for blood bank serology or testing using immunologic methods.
E. SSTs separate serum from blood cells upon centrifugation.
Rationale: SSTs contain a gel that, during centrifugation, localizes between packed cells and the top serum layer. They separate cells from serum, not serum from plasma.

Major points of discussion
■ SSTs contain a gel that, during centrifugation, localizes between packed cells and the top serum layer. Therefore, they are used to separate cells from serum.
■ SSTs are mainly used in clinical chemistry for routine assays.

23. A. Lower glucose levels.
B. Higher glucose levels.
Rationale: Glucose moves freely between the interstitial space and the circulation. Therefore, glucose levels are little affected by posture.
C. Lower albumin levels.
D. Higher levels of protein-bound drugs.
E. Higher cholesterol levels.

Rationale: Standing leads to increased venous pressure in the lower parts of the body, increased capillary pressure, and, therefore, filtration of plasma into the interstitial space. This causes an increase in the intravascular concentration of protein molecules, which do not easily pass the capillary endothelium (which includes cholesterol circulating attached to lipoproteins). Therefore, cholesterol levels and blood levels of protein-bound drugs are lower in bed-bound patients.

Major points of discussion
■ Ambulatory patients have higher serum albumin levels than bed-bound patients.
■ For the same reason, substances that are partly or entirely protein bound, such as drugs, cholesterol, hormones, and some metal ions, are also higher in the blood, serum, and plasma of ambulatory patients.
■ In this setting (i.e., standing vs. supine), serum levels of ionized calcium are less affected than total calcium.[3]

24. A. Hemodilution.
Rationale: Prolonged application of a tourniquet results in hemoconcentration, not hemodilution.
B. An increase in blood pH.
Rationale: Prolonged application of a tourniquet leads to anaerobic glycolysis and a decrease in pH, not an increase.
C. A decrease in serum protein levels.
Rationale: Prolonged application of a tourniquet results in hemoconcentration. Therefore, protein levels are increased, not decreased.
D. An increase in serum protein levels.
Rationale: Prolonged application of a tourniquet results in hemoconcentration. This causes an increase in total protein levels.
E. A decrease in plasma lactate.
Rationale: Prolonged application of a tourniquet leads to anaerobic glycolysis and an increase in plasma lactate, not a decrease.

Major points of discussion
■ Prolonged application of a tourniquet before venipuncture causes hemoconcentration.
■ This hemoconcentration causes an increase in serum and plasma levels of total protein, iron, lipid, and cholesterol.
■ Anaerobic glycolysis leads to an increase in plasma lactate and a decrease in pH.
■ Repeated fist clenching during phlebotomy can also cause a 1- to 2-mEq/L increase in serum potassium levels.

25. A. Hemoglobin and lipids scatter light; bilirubin absorbs particular wavelengths of light.
Rationale: Hemoglobin interferes in spectrophotometric assays by absorbing light, not scattering it.
B. Hemoglobin absorbs particular wavelengths of light; bilirubin and lipids scatter light.
Rationale: Bilirubin interferes in spectrophotometric assays by absorbing light, not scattering it.
C. Lipids absorb particular wavelengths of light; bilirubin and hemoglobin scatter light.
Rationale: Bilirubin and hemoglobin interfere in spectrophotometric assays by absorbing light; they do not scatter it.

D. Hemoglobin, lipids, and bilirubin all scatter light.
Rationale: Hemoglobin and bilirubin absorb light at specific wavelengths; they do not scatter light.
E. Hemoglobin and bilirubin absorb particular wavelengths of light; lipids scatter light.
Rationale: Hemoglobin and bilirubin absorb light at specific wavelengths. In addition, increased levels of lipids scatter light and thereby block light transmission.

Major points of discussion
- The most common substances causing optical interferences in spectrophotometric assays are bilirubin, hemoglobin, and lipids.
- Bilirubin interferes in spectrophotometric assays due to high light absorbance (between 340 and 500 nm).
- Hemoglobin interferes in spectrophotometric assays due to high light absorbance, particularly surrounding the Soret band at 412 nm.
- Lipids interfere by scattering light and thereby blocking light transmission.
- Interference due to lipemia can be reduced by ultracentrifugation of the sample.

26. **A. Preanalytical errors.**
B. Analytical errors.
C. Postanalytical errors.
D. Errors occur with equal frequency in the preanalytical, analytical, and postanalytical phases.
E. It is very difficult to obtain accurate data on errors affecting the laboratory; therefore, it is not known in which phase errors occur most frequently.
Rationale: Most studies indicate that the majority of errors (~60%) occur in the preanalytical phase. The second most common (~20%) are errors in the postanalytical phase. Analytical errors are the least frequent (~15%).

Major points of discussion
- Based on strong evidence that medical errors are significant causes of morbidity and mortality, The Joint Commission and other regulatory agencies emphasize the avoidance of errors in all aspects of patient care, including laboratory testing.
- Errors affecting laboratory results can occur in the preanalytical, analytical, and postanalytical phases.
- Approximately 20% of errors occur in the postanalytical phase.
- Approximately 15% of errors occur in the analytical phase.

27. A. They have no effect on laboratory results.

B. They increase urine ketones and increase blood urea nitrogen (BUN) levels in serum.
C. They decrease urine ketones and decrease serum BUN levels.
D. They decrease urine ketones and increase serum BUN levels.
E. They increase urine ketones in the urine and decrease serum BUN levels.
Rationale: High-protein, low-carbohydrate diets increase urine ketones in the urine and increase BUN levels in serum.

Major points of discussion
- Physiologic factors that may affect laboratory results should be minimized before phlebotomy.
- Some types of physiologic factors include diurnal variation, exercise, fasting, diet, ethanol consumption, smoking, drug ingestion, and posture.
- An individual's diet can greatly affect laboratory results.
- These dietary effects are transient and easily controlled.
- High-protein, low-carbohydrate diets, such as the Atkins diet, increase urine ketones and increase serum levels of blood urea nitrogen.

28. A. They are used to collect samples for fluoride measurements.
B. They are used to collect samples for sodium measurements.
Rationale: Gray-top tubes contain a preservative, such as sodium fluoride, that prevents glycolysis. Because the tube contains sodium or fluoride, it is not suited for the collection of samples for sodium or fluoride measurements.
C. They contain no additives.
Rationale: Gray-top tubes contain a preservative. In contrast, red-top tubes contain no additives.
D. They are used to collect samples for glucose measurements, especially when there is reason to expect a delay between sample collection and analysis.
Rationale: They are used for collecting samples for glucose measurements, especially in outpatient settings, where many hours may pass between sample collection in the physician's office and analysis in the laboratory.
E. They can prevent glycolysis caused by bacterial septicemia.
Rationale: Gray-top tubes cannot prevent the glycolysis caused by bacterial septicemia.

Major points of discussion
- Gray-top tubes are used for collecting samples for glucose measurements, especially in outpatient settings, where many hours may pass between sample collection in the physician's office and analysis in the laboratory.
- When collecting a sample in a gray-top tube for glucose analysis, an additional sample in another tube (e.g., a gold-top tube or a red-top tube) must be obtained for running a basic metabolic panel.

29a. **A. 0.95**
Rationale: The sensitivity of the test = [true-positive results/ (true-positive results + false-negative results)]. In this example, sensitivity = 57/(57 + 3) = 0.95.
B. 0.81
Rationale: This is the test specificity.
C. 0.66
Rationale: This is the positive predictive value.
D. 0.24
Rationale: This is not the correct answer.
E. 0.98
Rationale: This is the negative predictive value.

29b. A. 0.98
Rationale: This is the negative predictive value.

B. 0.81
Rationale: The specificity of the test = [true-negative results/(true-negative results + false-positive results)]. In this example, specificity = 130/(130 + 30) = 0.81.
C. 0.95
Rationale: This is the test sensitivity.
D. 0.66
Rationale: This is the positive predictive value.
E. 0.24
Rationale: This is not the correct answer.

29c. A. Yes, the specificity is high.
Rationale: A test with high specificity correctly identifies people without the disease.
B. No, the specificity is too low.
Rationale: A test with low specificity will misclassify disease-free individuals as diseased.
C. Yes, the sensitivity is high.
Rationale: Generally speaking, a highly sensitive test is preferred for screening purposes because it is usually positive in the presence of disease; hence, few cases would be missed.
D. No, the specificity and the sensitivity are too low.
Rationale: The sensitivity is 95% and the specificity is 81%. For a screening test, high sensitivity is important so that the test will correctly classify diseased individuals as such (true positives).
E. No, the sensitivity is too low.
Rationale: The sensitivity is 95%, which generally speaking is not considered low.

29d. A. 0.98
Rationale: This is the test sensitivity.
B. 0.24
Rationale: This is not the correct answer.
C. 0.81
Rationale: This is the test specificity.
D. 0.95
Rationale: This is the test sensitivity.
E. 0.66
Rationale: The positive predictive value is the true-positive results divided by all positive test results. In this example, the positive predictive value = 57/(57 + 30) = 0.66.
The positive predictive value is the probability that someone with a positive test result actually has the disease. In this example, someone with a positive test result has a 0.66 probability of having the disease.

29e. A. 0.98
Rationale: The negative predictive value is the true-negative results divided by all negative test results. In this example, the negative predictive value = 130/(130 + 3) = 0.98. The negative predictive value is the probability that someone with a negative test result does not have the disease. In this example, someone with a negative test result has a 0.98 probability of not having the disease.
B. 0.24
Rationale: This is not the correct answer.
C. 0.81
Rationale: This is the test specificity.
D. 0.95
Rationale: This is the test sensitivity.
E. 0.66
Rationale: This is the positive predictive value.

Major points of discussion

		True Disease Status	
		Present	Absent
Test Results	Positive	TP	FP
	Negative	FN	TN

- Sensitivity (%) = $100 \times TP/(TP + FN)$.
- Specificity (%) = $100 \times TN/(TN + FP)$.
- Positive predictive value (%) = $100 \times TP/(TP + FP)$.
- Negative predictive value (%) = $100 \times TN/(TN + FN)$.
- A test with high sensitivity has a high negative predictive value, meaning that a negative test result most likely rules out the disease.[4]

30a. A. 83%.
Rationale: This is the specificity of the test.
B. 94%.
Rationale: The sensitivity of the test is 94%. Sensitivity = $100 \times 160/(160 + 10)$.
C. 80%.
Rationale: This is the positive predictive value.
D. 90%.
E. 99%.
Rationale: See Major Points of Discussion.

30b. A. 94%.
Rationale: This is the sensitivity of the test.
B. 96%.
Rationale: See Major Points of Discussion.
C. 80%.
Rationale: This is the positive predictive value.
D. 90%.
Rationale: See Major Points of Discussion.
E. 83%.
Rationale: The specificity of the test is 83%. Specificity = $100 \times 190/(190 + 40)$.

30c. A. 88
B. 1.1
C. 5.5
Rationale: The likelihood ratio of a positive result for this test is 5.5 = 0.94/(1 − 0.83).
D. 0.88
E. 7
Rationale for A, B, D, and E: See Major Points of Discussion.

30d. A. Lupus is 5.5 times more likely to occur in a patient with a positive result than it is in a patient with a negative result.
Rationale: The likelihood ratio is a measure of test performance, not disease status.
B. The prevalence of lupus in this patient population has increased 5.5 times above the national average.
Rationale: The likelihood ratio is not used to determine disease prevalence.
C. A false-positive test result is 5.5 times more likely to occur using this assay compared with the gold standard.
Rationale: The likelihood ratio gives odds of getting a test result, not a rate.

D. A positive test result is 5.5 times more likely to occur in a patient with lupus compared with a patient without lupus.
Rationale: The likelihood ratio is a measure of test performance and gives the odds of getting a test result in a patient.
E. The true-positive rate is 5.5 times the prevalence of the disease.
Rationale: The likelihood ratio gives odds of getting a test result, not a rate.

Major points of discussion
- Sensitivity (%) = $100 \times$ TP/(TP + FN).
- Specificity (%) = $100 \times$ TN/(TN + FP).
- Likelihood ratio of a positive test = sensitivity/ (1 − specificity).
- The likelihood ratio of a positive test result is the odds of getting a positive result in a diseased patient, and the likelihood ratio of a negative test result is the odds of getting a negative result in an unaffected patient.
- The likelihood ratio can be used to determine the post-test probability of a test result.
- Pretest odds (disease prevalence) × likelihood ratio = post-test odds.
- Post-test probability = post-test odds/(1 + post-test odds).[8]

31. A. The proportion of people without the disease who have a negative test result.
Rationale: This is test specificity.
B. The proportion of people with the disease who have a positive test result.
Rationale: This is test sensitivity.
C. The probability that someone with a negative test result does not have the disease.[8]
Rationale: This is the negative predictive value.
D. The probability that someone with a positive test result has the disease.
Rationale: This is the positive predictive value.
E. The odds of having the disease when the test result is negative.
Rationale: This is the odds of getting a false-negative result.

Major points of discussion
- Test sensitivity and specificity are measures of diagnostic accuracy.
- Sensitivity and specificity provide information regarding a test's ability to distinguish between a disease and nondisease state at a given result cutoff. Test sensitivity refers to a test's ability to detect disease and is expressed as the proportion of diseased individuals who will test positive.
- A test with a high sensitivity will identify a greater number of patients with the disease.
- Sensitivity (%) = $100 \times$ TP/(TP + FN).
- Test specificity refers to the ability of a test to detect truly disease-negative individuals. A test that is 90% specific will give negative results in 90% of patients without the disease.

32. **A. The proportion of people without the disease who have a negative test result.**
Rationale: Test specificity refers to the ability of a test to detect truly disease-negative individuals. A test that is 90%

specific will give negative results in 90% of patients without the disease.
B. The proportion of people with the disease who have a positive test result.
Rationale: This is test sensitivity.
C. The probability that someone with a negative test result does not have the disease.
Rationale: This is the negative predictive value.
D. The probability that someone with a positive test result has the disease.
Rationale: This is the positive predictive value.
E. The odds of having the disease when the test result is negative.
Rationale: This is the odds of getting a false-negative result.

Major points of discussion
- Specificity (%) = $100 \times$ TN/(TN + FP).
- Highly specific tests are used to rule-in a diagnosis, as these tests are unlikely to yield false-positive results.
- Sensitivity is the proportion of diseased individuals with a positive test result.
- The positive predictive value is the probability that someone with a positive test result actually has the disease.
- The negative predictive value is the probability that someone with a negative test result does not have the disease.

33. A. 35%.
B. 18%.
C. 5.7%.
D. 10%.
Rationale: See Major Points of Discussion.
E. 2.9%.
Rationale: The coefficient of variation (CV) (%) = $100 \times 0.09/3.14$. CV (%) = $100 \times$ standard deviation (SD)/mean.

Major points of discussion
- Precision, otherwise known as the reproducibility of a test, is expressed by using the CV.
- Determining the precision is accomplished by repeating the test approximately 20 times using the same sample and determining the range of variation.
- CV (%) = $100 \times$ SD/mean.
- SD is a measure of dispersion from the mean in a Gaussian normal distribution.
- The CV of a test can vary over the assay's analytical range and therefore should be determined at low, mid, and high range values.
- The "within-run" or "intra-assay" CV is determined by repeating the test using the same sample on 1 day, typically during one run. The "between-run" or "interassay" CV is determined by comparing the results obtained with the same assay on different days using the same sample. Typically, the within-run CV is smaller than the between-run CV.

34. A. The positive predictive value would remain the same.
Rationale: The positive predictive value varies with disease prevalence.
B. The increase in disease prevalence would decrease the positive predictive value of the test.

Rationale: An increase in disease prevalence increases the positive predictive value.

C. The increase in disease prevalence would increase the positive predictive value of the test.

Rationale: The predictive value of a test is influenced by the prevalence of the disease in the population. The positive predictive value of a test increases as the prevalence of the disease increases. Recall that:

Positive predictive value (%) = 100 × TP/(TP + FP).

Therefore, as the disease prevalence increases in the population being tested, the number of true-positives will increase more than the number of false-positives, as long as the sensitivity and specificity of the test remain unchanged.

D. Changing the disease prevalence does not affect predictive value of the test.

Rationale: Disease prevalence and predictive value of a test are associated.

E. The positive predictive value would remain the same, but the test specificity would decrease.

Rationale: Test specificity is not affected by disease prevalence.

Major points of discussion
■ Positive predictive value (%) = 100 × TP/(TP + FP).
■ The positive predictive value is the probability that someone with a positive test result actually has the disease.
■ Negative predictive value (%) = 100 × TN/(TN + FN).
■ The negative predictive value is the probability that someone with a negative test result does not have the disease.

35. A. The overall sensitivity of the test as it varies with population prevalence range.
B. The overall specificity of the test as it varies with population prevalence.
Rationale: The ROC curve does not graphically represent the population prevalence of a disease.
C. The variation in the precision of the test over the entire technical linear range.
Rationale: The ROC curve does not graphically display precision.
D. The overall accuracy of the test over the entire range of sensitivity and specificity.
Rationale: The ROC curve is a graphic representation of the sensitivities and specificities that are possible when varying the test result cutoff value.
E. The range of the coefficient of variation over all medical decision threshold values.
Rationale: The coefficient of variation is not graphically represented by the ROC curve.

Major points of discussion
■ The area under the ROC curve is a measure of the test's overall ability to discriminate between disease and nondisease.
■ An area under the ROC curve of 1 represents a perfect test, whereas an area of 0.5 represents a test with no ability to discriminate.
■ Generally speaking, an area under the ROC curve greater than 0.8 indicates good discriminatory power.

■ The ROC curve can also be used to compare two different test methods by comparing the area under the ROC curves. The test method with the larger area under the curve has better diagnostic ability.[2]

36. A. 0.13
B. 0.15
C. 1.0
D. −1.0
Rationale: The standard deviation index (SDI) = (130 − 150)/20 = −1.0.
The SDI = (lab result − peer group mean)/peer group standard deviation.
E. −0.15
Rationale for A, B, C, and E: See Major Points of Discussion.

Major points of discussion
■ The SDI is the distance an individual data point is away from the mean value divided by the standard deviation.
■ One common use of the SDI is to standardize the performance of a laboratory with regard to the proficiency testing performance of all laboratories.
■ An SDI of ±2.0 is sometimes used as a cutoff to identify labs with unacceptable performance on a proficiency testing sample.
■ The SDI = (lab result − peer group mean)/peer group standard deviation.
■ The standard deviation is a measure of dispersion from the mean in a Gaussian normal distribution.

37a. A. 1.3
B. 19.6
Rationale: The likelihood ratio of a positive result is 0.98/(1 − 0.95) = 19.6. Therefore, a positive result is 19.6 times more likely in a patient with HIV than in a patient without HIV.
C. 42.5
D. 1.0
E. 9
Rationale for A, C, D, and E: See Major Points of Discussion.

37b. A. 51%.
B. 25%.
C. 5%.
D. 87%.
Rationale: The post-test probability can be calculated using the disease prevalence and likelihood ratio of a positive result for this test. Post-test probability is 6.5/(1 + 6.5) = 87%.
E. 98%
Rationale for A, B, C, and E: See Major Points of Discussion.

37c. **A. 51%**
Rationale: The post-test probability can be calculated using the disease prevalence and likelihood ratio of a positive result for this test. The post-test probability is 51%.
B. 25%.
C. 5%.
D. 87%.
E. 98%.
Rationale: See Major Points of Discussion.

Major points of discussion

- The likelihood ratio of a positive result is the likelihood of a positive test result in a patient with disease compared with the likelihood of a positive result in a patient without the disease.
- The likelihood ratio can be used to determine the post-test probability of a test result.
- Country A:
  - The post-test probability can be calculated using the disease prevalence and likelihood ratio of a positive result for this test.
  - First, convert the disease prevalence to the pretest odds; for Country A, the HIV disease prevalence is 25%: pretest odds = [pretest probability/(1 − pretest probability)] = 0.25/(1 − 0.25) = 0.33.
  - Then, calculate the post-test odds and convert to a probability: post-test odds = pretest odds × likelihood ratio = 0.33 × 19.6 = 6.5.
  - Post-test probability is 6.5/(1 + 6.5) = 87%.
  - This is the predictive value of the test in this patient setting and is the probability of disease in the post-test situation using the population prevalence as the pretest probability.
- Country B:
  - The post-test probability can be calculated using the disease prevalence and likelihood ratio of a positive result for this test.
  - First, convert the disease prevalence to the pretest odds; for Country B, the HIV disease prevalence is 5%: pretest odds = [pretest probability/(1 − pretest probability)] = 0.05/(1 − 0.05) = 0.05.
  - Then, calculate the post-test odds and convert to a probability: post-test odds = pretest odds × likelihood ratio = 0.05 × 19.6 = 1.03.
  - Post-test probability is 1.03/(1 + 1.03) = 51%.
  - This is the predictive value of the test in this patient setting and is the probability of disease in the post-test situation using the population prevalence as the pretest probability.
- Likelihood ratio[1] of a positive test = sensitivity/(1 − specificity).

38. A. A likelihood ratio of 7 indicates no relationship between anti–smooth muscle antibodies and primary sclerosing cholangitis.
Rationale: The likelihood ratio is not used to assess the strength of association between analyte and disease.
B. A likelihood ratio of 7 indicates no predictive ability of this assay in distinguishing disease from nondisease.
Rationale: This is not the correct interpretation of the likelihood ratio.
C. Anti–smooth muscle antibodies occur in 7% of patients with primary sclerosing cholangitis.
Rationale: The likelihood ratio is a measure of test performance, not of symptom prevalence.
D. Primary sclerosing cholangitis is 7 times more likely to occur in a patient with a positive result compared with a patient with a negative result.
Rationale: The likelihood ratio is a measure of test performance, not of disease status.

E. **A positive test result is 7 times more likely to occur in a patient with primary sclerosing cholangitis than in a healthy patient.**
Rationale: The likelihood ratio gives the odds of the test result occurring in a diseased patient compared with a healthy patient.

Major points of discussion

- The likelihood ratio is used to assess test performance. It is the ratio between the probabilities of the test result when disease is present and the probability of the test result when the disease is absent.
- The likelihood ratio is not affected by disease prevalence.
- Likelihood ratio of a positive test = sensitivity/(1 − specificity).
- Likelihood ratio of a negative test = (1 − sensitivity)/specificity.
- The likelihood ratio can be used to determine the post-test probability of a test result.
- Pretest odds (disease prevalence) × likelihood ratio = post-test odds.
- Post-test probability = post-test odds/(1 + post-test odds).

39a. **A. A**
Rationale: Using the result cutoff value at Letter A, all patients with the disease would be categorized as positive; that is, 100% of the diseased individuals would test positive.
B. B
C. C
D. D
Rationale: A cutoff value at these points would result in both false-positive test results and false-negative test results.
E. E
Rationale: A cutoff value at this point would yield 100% specificity.

39b. **A. A**
Rationale: This point represents the cutoff value with the highest sensitivity.
B. B
C. C
D. D
Rationale: A cutoff value at these points would result in both false-positive test results and false-negative test results.
E. E
Rationale: Using a cutoff value at this point would yield a negative result in all patients who lack the disease; that is, 100% of nondiseased individuals would test negative. Therefore, the specificity would be 100%.

39c. **A. A**
Rationale: Letter A represents the cutoff value with the highest sensitivity (all diseased individuals would test positive). A highly sensitive test is preferred for screening purposes because it is positive in the majority of diseased individuals; hence, few cases would be missed. For a disease that is 100% curable if detected early, false-negative test results are unacceptable, as these results would lead to affected individuals not being treated.
B. B
C. C
D. D

Rationale: A cutoff value at these points would result in both false-positive test results and false-negative test results.

E. E

Rationale: A cutoff value at this point would yield 100% specificity.

39d. A. A

Rationale: A cutoff value at this point would yield 100% sensitivity.

B. B

C. C

D. D

Rationale: A cutoff value at these points would result in both false-positive test results and false-negative test results.

E. E

Rationale: Letter E represents the cutoff value with the greatest specificity. In this example, the disease state needs to be ruled-in with certainty because the treatment is potentially lethal. A highly specific test is likely to give a negative result in the absence of disease; therefore, an unaffected individual is unlikely to have a false-positive test result.

Major points of discussion
- Sensitivity is the proportion of diseased individuals with a positive test result.
- Specificity refers to the proportion of nondiseased individuals who have a negative test result.
- Specificity $(\%) = 100 \times TN/(TN+FP)$.
- Generally speaking, a test with high specificity has a high positive predictive value; that is, a positive test result rules in the diagnosis.
- Sensitivity $(\%)^7 = 100 \times TP/(TP+FN)$.

40a. A. Test 1.

Rationale: Test 1 has no diagnostic utility.

B. Test 2.

Rationale: Test 2 has a lower area under the curve, hence a lower sensitivity and specificity at all cutoffs.

C. Test 3.

Rationale: Test 3 has the greatest area under the curve and is the most accurate. It has the highest sensitivity for any given specificity.

40b. A. A

B. B

C. C

Rationale: Point C represents the optimal cutoff because the test has the greatest sensitivity at this value (i.e., ability to detect true-positive patients) while still maintaining a relatively low false-positive rate (1 – specificity).

D. D

E. E

Rationale for A, B, D, and E: This point does not represent the optimal cutoff, because this value does

not provide the greatest sensitivity (i.e., ability to detect true-positive patients) while still maintaining a relatively low false-positive rate (1 – specificity).

Major points of discussion
- The ROC curve is a graphic representation of all the sensitivities and specificities that are possible when varying the test result cutoff value.
- The area under the ROC curve is a measure of the test's overall ability to discriminate between disease and nondisease.
- Generally speaking, an area under the ROC curve of greater than 0.8 indicates good discriminatory power.
- The optimal cutoff point is determined by the cutoff with the maximum discriminatory power; that is, the point with the highest sensitivity and the lowest false-positive rate.
- An area under the ROC curve of 1.0 represents a perfect test, whereas an area under the ROC curve of 0.5 represents a test with no ability to discriminate between disease and nondisease. A 45-degree line represents a test with an area under the ROC curve of 0.5.[2,4]

41. **A. Graph A.**

Rationale: This test result distribution is normal shaped (Gaussian); therefore, calculating mean ± 2 SDs will capture 95% of the central data points.

B. Graph B.

Rationale: This test result distribution is bimodal; thus, calculating mean ± 2 SDs will not capture 95% of the data points.

C. Graph C.

Rationale: This test result distribution is skewed; thus, calculating mean ± 2 SDs will not capture 95% of the data points.

Major points of discussion
- When establishing a reference range, using a range where the majority of healthy individuals' results fall is the most acceptable method; ideally, no more than 5% of results from disease-free individuals should fall outside this range.
- If the test result distribution is normal shaped (Gaussian), then calculating mean ± 2 SDs will capture 95% of the central data points (Graph A).
- If the test result distribution is skewed, the central data points can be determined by taking results from the 2.5th percentile to the 97.5th percentile, which would exclude 2.5% of the results at both the upper and lower ends of the spectrum (Graphs B and C).
- If the test result distribution is skewed, another approach is to perform a logarithmic transformation of the skewed data, which may produce a more normal distribution.
- The Clinical Laboratories Standards Institute recommends using 120 individuals when developing new reference intervals.[5,7]

References

1. Bianchi MT, Alexander BM, Cash SS. Incorporating uncertainty into medical decision making: an approach to unexpected test results. Med Decis Making 2009;29:116–124.
2. Bossuyt X. Clinical performance characteristics of a laboratory test. A practical approach in the autoimmune laboratory. Autoimmun Rev 2009;8:543–548.
3. Dixon M, Patterson CR. Posture and the composition of plasma. Clin Chem 1978;24:824–826.
4. Fischer JE, Bachmann LM, Jaeschke R. A readers' guide to the interpretation of diagnostic test properties: clinical example of sepsis. Intensive Care Med 2003;29:1043–1051.
5. Nichols JH. Verification of method performance for clinical laboratories. Adv Clin Chem 2009;47:121–137.
6. Orsulak PJ. Stand-alone automated solutions can enhance laboratory operations. Clin Chem 2000;46:778–783.
7. Scott A, Greenberg PB, Poole PJ. Cautionary tales in the clinical interpretation of studies of diagnostic tests. Intern Med J 2008;38:120–129.
8. van Stralen KJ, Stel VS, Reitsma JB, Dekker FW, Zoccali C, Jager KJ. Diagnostic methods. I: sensitivity, specificity, and other measures of accuracy. Kidney Int 2009;75:1257–1263.

CHAPTER 2

LABORATORY MANAGEMENT:
Quality Management, Regulations, and Quality Control

Brie Stotler, Anthony N. Sireci

QUESTIONS

1. Which one of the following statements is true about the Three-Day Stay Rule of 1990?
   A. A hospital must include in its charges for the inpatient hospital stay the charges for all laboratory services performed in the 3-day period prior to hospital admission.
   B. It helps laboratories develop programs that promote highly ethical and lawful conduct, especially in terms of billing.
   C. It prevents physicians from referring Medicare patients to self-owned laboratories.
   D. It establishes that all clinical laboratories must be certified by the federal government with programs to ensure quality, appropriate personnel training, and regular proficiency assessment.
   E. It directs how health care information is managed.

2. Which one of the following statements describes an Advance Beneficiary Notice of Noncoverage?
   A. A legal notice provided to all uninsured patients before they receive any medical care.
   B. A legal notice provided to all Medicaid participants.
   C. A legal notice provided to all uninsured patients receiving outpatient chemotherapy.
   D. A legal notice provided to Medicare fee-for-service participants delineating services expected to not be covered under their Medicare insurance plan.
   E. A legal notice to all insured patients delineating services routinely not covered by major insurance carriers.

3. Which one of the following is a mission of the Agency for Healthcare Research and Quality (AHRQ)?
   A. To compare the effectiveness of new treatments.
   B. To direct the Department of Health and Human Services (DHHS).
   C. To oversee the National Institutes of Health (NIH) research programs.
   D. To be the largest source of funding for biomedical research.
   E. To provide health care to the elderly and indigent.

4. In method validation studies, Clinical Laboratory Improvement Amendments (CLIA) regulations state that a laboratory must test for analytical specificity. Which one of the following sets of experiments would satisfy this requirement?
   A. Running samples of a known analyte concentration spiked with prescription drugs that could potentially interfere with the measurement of the analyte of interest.
   B. Running samples without the analyte of interest (i.e., Matrix blanks), ensuring that a zero sample actually reads zero.
   C. Running both positive and negative samples and determining the specificity by taking true negatives and dividing by true negatives plus false positives.
   D. Running samples spiked with increasing concentrations of an analyte and determining the concentration of the analyte that most specifically discriminates diseased from healthy patients.
   E. Running samples spiked with the highest measurable concentration of the analyte of interest followed by a Matrix blank.

5. Which one of the following provides the best definition for analytical sensitivity?
   A. The false-negative rate of the assay.
   B. The value obtained when the number of true positives is divided by the sum of the true positives and the false negatives.
   C. The lowest possible concentration of an analyte that is accurately and reproducibly measured by an assay.
   D. The performance of the assay when measuring an analyte in the presence of an interfering substance.
   E. The formula that relates instrument response to analyte concentration.

6. The Centers for Disease Control and Prevention (CDC) classifies laboratories by biosafety level. Which one of the following represents the best example of a level 3 laboratory?
   A. A training laboratory for students.
   B. A clinical chemistry laboratory.
   C. A clinical hematology laboratory.
   D. A laboratory working with highly infectious fungal pathogens.
   E. A satellite clinical laboratory in an emergency department.

7. Which one of the following is the best definition of "calibration verification"?
   A. The process of testing and adjusting an assay so that the instrument measurements best correlate with the known analyte concentrations.
   B. The process of testing known concentrations of an analyte throughout the reportable range and confirming that the assay returns the appropriate value, within an established allowable error.
   C. The process of comparing the slope and y-intercept of the current calibration curve with the previous curves.
   D. The process of running previously assayed patient samples with a new lot of calibration material and comparing them with results obtained when the same samples were run using a previous lot of calibration material.
   E. The process of running samples of known high and low analyte concentrations and plotting them on a Levey-Jennings chart.

8. You are the director of a large hospital laboratory that is accredited by the College of American Pathologists (CAP). Which one of the following indicates how often your laboratory will be subject to a routine inspection by CAP?
   A. Every 6 months.
   B. Once every year.
   C. Once every 2 years.
   D. Once every 3 years.
   E. Once every 5 years.

9. A new lot of reagent arrives in the laboratory and after several days of concurrent analysis with the old lot of reagent, a significant positive shift in the value of the high quality control (QC) material using the new reagent lot relative to the same QC material using the old reagent lot is noted. The section supervisor thinks this is a differential matrix interaction of the new lot with the high control and that it will not affect patient results. Which one of the following is the best piece of experimental evidence to support this hypothesis?
   A. Patient samples spanning the analytical range of the assay are run using the old reagent lot and compared with the same samples using the new reagent lot. The correlation coefficient should be close to 1.
   B. Random patient samples are run using the old and new reagent lots and then compared. The correlation coefficient should be close to 1.
   C. Calibration standards dissolved in methanol are run across the full analytical range of the instrument using the old and new reagent lots and are then compared. The correlation coefficient should be close to 1.
   D. The analyte should be extracted from each level of control material using a solid-phase extraction procedure and then run using the old and new reagent lots. The correlation coefficient should be close to 1.
   E. The assay should be recalibrated; the control material should then be run and compared between both reagent lots.

10. Your laboratory currently runs a full menu of moderate-complexity testing and is accredited by CLIA under a certificate of accreditation. A treating physician asks you to add a test that the Food and Drug Administration (FDA) has classified as a "waived" test. Which one of the following statements is the appropriate course of action with regard to regulatory compliance?
   A. You must apply for a CLIA certificate of waiver.
   B. You must apply for a CLIA certificate of registration.
   C. You must apply for a CLIA certificate of compliance.
   D. No additional certificates are necessary.
   E. You cannot run a waived test in a laboratory that performs predominantly moderate-complexity testing.

11. Laboratory testing in the United States is regulated through the CLIA program. The program is overseen by which one of the following regulatory entities?
   A. The FDA.
   B. The AABB.
   C. The CAP.
   D. The Joint Commission.
   E. The Centers for Medicare and Medicaid Services (CMS).

12. At a minimum, before introducing a new FDA-approved assay into the laboratory, which one of the following groups of performance characteristics must be assayed during a method validation and compared with manufacturer claims, to be compliant with CLIA '88 regulations?
   A. Accuracy, precision, reportable range, and confirmation of the manufacturer's reference range.
   B. Accuracy, analytical sensitivity and specificity, reportable range, and a full reference range study with a minimum of 120 patient samples.
   C. Accuracy, clinical sensitivity and specificity, analytical specificity and sensitivity, full reference range study, and reportable range.
   D. Extraction efficiency, reportable range, full reference range study, QC material stability, and analytical sensitivity and specificity.
   E. Only accuracy and precision must be confirmed.

13. According to CLIA regulations, which one of the following best indicates how often laboratories must perform QC evaluation (i.e., assay QC samples) for most assays that are performed 24 hours a day?
   A. Once every 12 hours.
   B. Once every 24 hours.
   C. Every time the assay is performed.
   D. Once every 48 hours.
   E. Once every week.

14. You are the director of a newly established laboratory that will perform a mix of waived and nonwaived, moderate-complexity testing. Which one of the following best describes when you can begin testing?
   A. After you have applied, paid for, and received a certificate of registration, assuming your state Department of Health has no additional requirements.
   B. After you are inspected by your state Department of Health and have received your certificate of compliance.
   C. After you have been inspected by an approved accreditation agency and have received your certificate of accreditation.
   D. After your state Department of Health, or an approved accreditation agency, and CMS have both inspected your laboratory.
   E. Once you have validated your assays to your satisfaction.

15. A laboratory medical director is overseeing the implementation of a new hematology analyzer and is in the process of setting up delta checks for several complete blood cell count parameters. Which one of the following best describes a delta check?
    A. It is a comparison of reference ranges across laboratories.
    B. It is a quality measure by which a patient's previous result is compared with the current one.
    C. It is a quality measure by which samples are visually checked for hemolysis.
    D. It is a level of an analyte thought to be life-threatening to the patient, requiring verbal notification to the ordering provider.
    E. It is a quality measure that occurs when results fall above the analytical limit of an assay.

16. Which one of the following statements best describes the benefit(s) that the Family and Medical Leave Act (FMLA) provides to eligible individuals?
    A. The FMLA provides employees with up to 12 weeks of paid, job-protected leave per year.
    B. The FMLA provides employees with up to 16 weeks of paid, job-protected leave for the birth or care of a newborn child.
    C. The FMLA provides employees with up to 16 weeks of unpaid, job-protected leave for females and 12 weeks for males for the birth or care of a newborn child.
    D. The FMLA provides employees with up to 12 weeks of unpaid, job-protected leave per year leave for qualifying reasons.
    E. The FMLA provides employees with continuous health insurance coverage for up to 16 weeks.

17. In the United States, blood banks are regulated by which of the following entities?
    A. The AABB.
    B. The CAP.
    C. The CMS.
    D. The CDC.
    E. The FDA.

18. Which one of the following statements best describes the role of the FDA in the regulation of laboratory-developed tests (LDTs)?
    A. LDTs are not medical devices and therefore do not fall under the FDA's jurisdiction.
    B. LDTs are considered medical devices, and each laboratory must receive FDA approval before implementing an LDT.
    C. LDTs are considered medical devices, but the FDA has exercised enforcement discretion on LDTs.
    D. LDTs are not considered medical devices, but the FDA regulates them.
    E. LDTs may or may not be considered medical devices, and the FDA considers each assay on a case-by-case basis and decides whether to regulate.

19. During an interview with a potential laboratory technologist, which one of the following questions is appropriate to ask?
    A. Do you have any disabilities?
    B. Were you born in the United States?
    C. What is your native language?
    D. How old are you?
    E. Are you capable of performing all of the duties required by this position?

20. The International Organization for Standards (ISO) standard 15189:2007 deals with which one of the following?
    A. Standards for quality and competence in medical laboratories.
    B. Standards for pricing and reimbursement in medical laboratories.
    C. Laboratory services that must be covered under universal health insurance plans.
    D. Standard requirements for laboratory technologist school curricula.
    E. Standard requirements for retirement benefit packages.

21. As the director of a laboratory performing high-complexity testing, you are required to ensure that your laboratory is appropriately staffed with all required levels of qualified personnel whose duties and qualifications are clearly defined by CLIA. The laboratory director can assume the responsibility of which one of the following required positions given appropriate training and background?
    A. Technical supervisor.
    B. Clinical consultant.
    C. General supervisor.
    D. Testing personnel.
    E. The laboratory director can assume any and all of these positions.

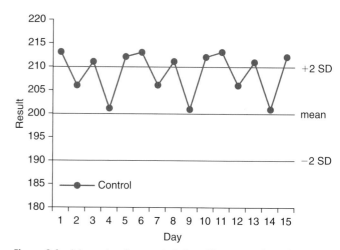

Figure 2-1 A Levey-Jennings control chart. The test result is plotted on the y-axis, and controls are performed on one shift per day (plotted on the x-axis).

22. The Levey-Jennings control chart for an assay performed in your laboratory is shown in Figure 2-1. The chart indicates which type of analytical problem for this assay?
    A. The assay is accurate but not precise.
    B. The assay is precise but not accurate.
    C. The assay is neither precise nor accurate.
    D. The assay is clinically useless.
    E. The assay is precise and accurate.

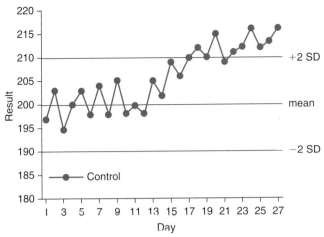

Figure 2-2 A Levey-Jennings control chart. The test result is plotted on the y-axis, and controls are performed on one shift per day (plotted on the x-axis).

23. Quality control (QC) material is run at the start of each shift (in this case, for one shift per day) for all assays before testing patient samples. The QC results for several days for one of the assays are plotted on a Levey-Jennings chart shown in Figure 2-2. Which one of the following best describes what this Levey-Jennings chart demonstrates?
    A. Positive trending of QC results.
    B. Negative trending of QC results.
    C. Result interference by an unknown substance.
    D. The use of an inappropriately narrow reference range.
    E. The need to change the technical range for the assay.

24. Which one of the following best describes how to plot a Levey-Jennings chart?
    A. The x-axis as "Average value" and the y-axis as "% Difference."
    B. The x-axis as the "Gold standard method" and the y-axis as "Test method."
    C. The x-axis as "Calibrator level" and the y-axis as "% CV."
    D. The x-axis as "Run #" and the y-axis as "Concentration."
    E. The x-axis as "Instrument response" and the y-axis as "Expected concentration."

25. In a method validation study, a sample at the proposed lower limit of quantification (LoQ) is run 20 times, 4 times daily for 5 days. Which one of the following answers best describes the performance parameters that can be determined from this experiment?
    A. Validation of LoQ.
    B. Validation of the LoQ, intraday and interday reproducibility, and accuracy at the LoQ.
    C. Validation of the LoQ and establishment of accuracy at the LoQ.
    D. Validation of the LoQ and establishment of the reportable range.
    E. Establishment of reproducibility at the LoQ.

26. A laboratory director is designing a validation experiment for quantifying a drug metabolite in urine by gas chromatography–mass spectrometry. She asks her laboratory technologist to run a blank urine sample spiked with the lowest clinically relevant value of the metabolite 20 times and to average the signal/noise ratio of the analyte peak at this concentration. The laboratory director is trying to establish which one of the following analytical performance parameters?
    A. Analytical specificity.
    B. Analytical sensitivity
    C. Clinical specificity.
    D. Clinical sensitivity.
    E. The lower limit of linearity.

27. Which one of the following entities administers the Medicaid insurance program?
    A. The CDC.
    B. The FDA.
    C. The American Medical Association.
    D. Individual states.
    E. Private insurance companies.

28. You are validating a high-complexity assay to measure analyte X. In a method comparison study, you choose 40 samples that span the analytical range of your method, analyze them by the new method, and compare your results with a reference, gold standard method at a reference laboratory. The resulting correlation analysis reveals a coefficient of determination (R^2) of 0.99, an intercept of +0.1, and a slope of 1.34 when the gold standard is plotted on the x-axis. Which one of the following statements best describes your assay?
    A. Your assay correlates poorly with the reference method.
    B. Your assay correlates well with the reference method but has a positive proportional bias.
    C. Your assay correlates well with the reference method but has a negative constant bias.
    D. Your assay correlates well with the reference method. No other statements can be accurately made.
    E. Your assay correlates poorly with the reference method and shows a positive proportional bias.

29. Which one of the following government agencies is responsible for developing standardized materials for calibration, weights, and measures?
    A. The FDA.
    B. The NIH.
    C. The CMS.
    D. The National Institute of Standards and Technology (NIST).
    E. The DHHS.

30. Which one of the following statements best describes a requirement(s) expected of employers by the Occupational Health and Safety Administration (OSHA)?
    A. Apply for state certification every 2 years and pay the annual membership fee.
    B. Provide subsidized health insurance for all employees and offer at least two separate insurance plans.
    C. Display an OSHA poster in the workplace informing employees about the Occupational Safety and Health Act.
    D. Require that all employees receive an annual physical health exam with urine drug screening.
    E. Receive state OSHA agency approval before increasing the number of employees.

31. Which one of the following is the best example of a postanalytical error?
    A. The patient results are manually entered into the wrong patient's medical record.
    B. The sample is drawn into an inappropriate tube.
    C. The sample is run using a reagent lot that has expired.
    D. The phlebotomist did not fill the tube completely on a sample sent for coagulation testing.
    E. The autosampling pipette was jostled and is now drawing only 1.3 µL of sample instead of 1.5 µL of sample.

32. Which one of the following statements best describes proficiency testing?
    A. A quality assessment tool that compares a patient's previous results with current results.
    B. A quality assessment tool that involves testing two levels of QC material before testing patient samples.
    C. A quality assessment tool by which laboratories test samples with unknown results and compare their results.
    D. A quality assessment tool that involves running calibrators every 6 months to ensure linear assay results.
    E. A quality assessment test given to all newly hired technologists to ensure appropriate training and competency.

33. Your laboratory receives a proficiency testing (PT) specimen from an approved provider of PT material for a particular analyte. Which one of the following choices best describes how the sample should be handled?
    A. The PT samples should be specifically marked and personally walked through the testing procedure by the laboratory director or his or her designee.
    B. The PT sample should be split; one aliquot should be run in your laboratory and the other aliquot should be sent to a reference laboratory to ensure concordant results.
    C. The PT sample should be entered into your laboratory's workflow and tested and resulted as with any other patient specimen.
    D. The PT sample should be treated as any other patient sample. If send-out is required as a reflex for this analyte, your laboratory should send it out as per protocol.
    E. The PT sample should be run multiple times during multiple days and the values averaged to minimize error.

34. Which one of the following is the best definition of "unsuccessful" participation or performance in PT?
    A. Failure to attain the minimum satisfactory score for an analyte, test, subspecialty, or specialty for a testing event.
    B. Failure to submit the results of a testing event in the requisite amount of time.
    C. A clerical error in reporting the results for a testing event.
    D. Repeated unsatisfactory test scores for an analyte or for the entire testing event in a particular specialty or subspecialty on two consecutive PT events or two of three testing events.
    E. This is not a term used in assessing performance in PT events.

35. The quality manager of your laboratory recommends that your laboratory register for a PT program for a test that the FDA has classified as "waived." Which one of the following best describes how you should you respond to this recommendation?
    A. You should agree. To maintain CLIA certification, *all* assays performed in your laboratory must be evaluated in a CLIA-approved PT program.
    B. You should agree. Although PT is not required for waived tests, if a valid PT program exists, participation will help ensure your laboratory's accuracy in result reporting.
    C. You should disagree. After looking through the CLIA regulations for PT, you notice the analyte you are measuring is not on the list of regulated analytes for which PT is required.
    D. You should disagree. The FDA does not require PT for tests it deems waived.
    E. You should disagree. PT will only highlight your laboratory's inaccuracy.

36. Which one of the following is most characteristic of root cause analysis (RCA), regardless of the method that is used?
    A. Identifies a single cause of the error.
    B. Favors the subjective opinion of experts.
    C. Results in an executable and quantifiable solution(s).
    D. Seeks to identify and blame the specific person or group responsible.
    E. Uses the Ishikawa fishbone diagram.

37. Which one of the following is a specific management infrastructure required for Six Sigma certification?
    A. Master "Black Belts" and "Green Belts."
    B. Merger and acquisitions attorneys.
    C. Only the chief executive officer commitment is required.
    D. Six Sigma consultants.
    E. Support of engineers.

38. Section 1877 of the Social Security Act (42 U.S.C. 1395) prohibits which one of the following?
    A. Billing Medicare and Medicaid for tests completed in a laboratory without a CLIA license.
    B. Professional billing for laboratory tests without a physician-documented order that includes the physician's signature.
    C. Physician patient referral to an entity for a designated health service from which the physician will financially benefit.
    D. Performing genetic tests without a signed consent form.
    E. Performing HIV tests without a signed consent form.

39. A supervisor informs you that the QC values for an assay performed in your laboratory have triggered the $8_{1.5s}$ Westgard rule. Which one of the following types of type of analytical error does this most likely indicate?
    A. Volume error.
    B. User error.
    C. Random error.
    D. Imprecision.
    E. A bias trend.

40. An area supervisor from your laboratory asks you to review your QC rules. She says that QC is failing too frequently using the 1_{2s} Westgard rule and troubleshooting reveals no errors in the method. This has been the case over multiple reagent lots. You would like to maintain the sensitivity of the rule with regard to error detection but would also like to

decrease the false-alert rate. Which one of the following is the most logical step?

A. Change to using the 1_{3s} rule.

B. Change to using the 8_{1s} rule.

C. Adopt a hybrid rule combining the 1_{3s} and 2_{2s} rules in a multirule scheme.

D. Rules are not necessary, and each QC value should be judged individually.

E. Ask the supervisor to change lots of QC material; the failure rate is likely due to a faulty batch.

41. Which one of the following is the most common type of CLIA certificate issued?

A. Certificate of waiver.

B. Certificate for provider-performed microscopy procedures.

C. Certificate of registration.

D. Certificate of compliance.

E. Certificate of accreditation.

Table 2-1

	Assay Result	Standard Deviation (SD)
Low control sample, mean concentration	5 mIU/mL	0.2 mIU/mL
High control sample concentration	50,000 mIU/mL	10 mIU/mL
Potentially contaminated sample (low control sample repeated), concentration	5.1 mIU/mL	

42a. A laboratory is validating a new β-human chorionic gonadotropin assay. Below are the results from a validation study assessing potential carryover. The acceptable limit for carryover was set at 2 times the SD for the low concentration mean. According to Table 2-1, the calculated percent carryover is:

A. 12%.

B. 2%.

C. 15%.

D. 10%.

E. 5%.

42b. Which one of the following statements best describes whether this amount of carryover acceptable?

A. This amount of carryover is acceptable because the result of the potentially contaminated sample falls in the range of 5.0 to 5.4 mIU/mL.

B. This amount of carryover is acceptable because it is less than 10 mIU/mL.

C. This amount of carryover is acceptable because it is less than 15% of the original sample.

D. This amount of carryover is not acceptable because it is more than 5% of the original sample.

E. This amount of carryover is not acceptable because it is more than 0.2 mIU/mL.

43. According to CLIA regulations, laboratories that hold a certificate of waiver must comply with which one of the following?

A. Follow Universal Precautions when testing patient samples.

B. Have a designated laboratory director who holds a medical degree.

C. Follow the test manufacturer's instructions.

D. Engage in CLIA-directed PT.

E. Record all patient test results in an electronic format.

44. Laboratory testing in the United States is regulated through CLIA. The CLIA program is overseen by which one of the following regulatory entities?

A. The FDA.

B. The AABB.

C. The CAP.

D. The Joint Commission.

E. The CMS.

45. CLIA quality system regulations require verification of a manufacturer's stated performance specifications for which one of the following categories of tests?

A. Waived tests approved by the FDA.

B. Provider-performed microscopy tests approved by the FDA.

C. Moderate-complexity tests approved by the FDA.

D. Waived, provider-performed microscopy, and moderate-complexity tests approved by the FDA.

E. All FDA-approved tests used for patient care.

46. Which one of the following is categorized as a waived test according to the CLIA classification?

A. Pinworm examination.

B. Fecal occult blood examination.

C. Urine sediment examination.

D. Fecal leukocyte examination.

E. The fern test.

47. According to CLIA regulations, cytology slide preparations must be retained for which one of the following periods of time?

A. 1 year.

B. 2 years.

C. 5 years.

D. 10 years.

E. Indefinitely.

48. According to CLIA regulations, clinical pathology test records must be retained for at least which one of the following periods of time?

A. 1 year.

B. 2 years.

C. 5 years.

D. 10 years.

E. Indefinitely.

49. Which one of the following methods best helps ensure the accuracy of a test?

A. Analyze samples from healthy subjects and determine the 95% prediction interval.

B. Analyze samples with no measurable analyte spiked with low concentrations of analyte.

C. Analyze samples with a high value followed by samples with a low value.

D. Analyze a sample 20 times and determine the mean and SD.

E. Compare samples between the test method and a reference method.

Answers

1. **A. A hospital must include in its charges for the inpatient hospital stay the charges for all laboratory services performed in the 3-day period prior to hospital admission.**
   Rationale: The Three-Day Stay Rule of 1990 states that a hospital must include in its charges for the inpatient hospital stay the charges for all laboratory services performed in the 3-day period prior to hospital admission.
   B. It helps laboratories develop programs that promote highly ethical and lawful conduct, especially in terms of billing.
   Rationale: This describes the Office of Inspector General (OIG) compliance guidelines.
   C. It prevents physicians from referring Medicare patients to self-owned laboratories.
   Rationale: This describes the physician self-referral ban (the Stark Act).
   D. It establishes that all clinical laboratories must be certified by the federal government with programs to ensure quality, appropriate personnel training, and regular proficiency assessment.
   Rationale: This describes Clinical Laboratory Improvement Amendments (CLIA) '88.
   E. It directs how health care information is managed.
   Rationale: This broadly describes the Health Insurance Portability and Accountability Act (HIPAA).

   Major points of discussion
   - CLIA '88 establishes that all clinical laboratories must be certified by the federal government with programs to ensure quality, appropriate personnel training, and regular proficiency assessment. Prior to this act, there was no federal regulation of diagnostic laboratory testing.
   - The physician self-referral ban, or Stark Act, prevents physicians from referring Medicare patients to self-owned laboratories.
   - HIPAA directs how health care information is managed.
   - The OIG compliance guidelines help laboratories develop programs that promote highly ethical and lawful conduct, especially in terms of billing. The OIG is responsible for identifying fraud and abuse in laboratory testing, as regulated by the CMS.

2. A. A legal notice provided to all uninsured patients before they receive any medical care.
   B. A legal notice provided to all Medicaid participants.
   C. A legal notice provided to all uninsured patients receiving outpatient chemotherapy.
   D. A legal notice provided to Medicare fee-for-service participants delineating services expected to not be covered under their Medicare insurance plan.
   Rationale: An Advance Beneficiary Notice of Noncoverage is a notice provided by independent laboratories, health care practitioners, and medical suppliers to Medicare participants for services when payment is expected to be denied if the patient receives the service/supply.

   E. A legal notice to all insured patients delineating services routinely not covered by major insurance carriers.
   Rationale for A, B, C, and E: An advance beneficiary notice is required for people who have Medicare insurance (not uninsured patients).

   Major points of discussion
   - An Advance Beneficiary Notice of Noncoverage must be provided by independent laboratories.
   - The Advance Beneficiary Notice of Noncoverage was formerly named the Advance Beneficiary Notice.
   - The law requires a provider to notify a beneficiary in advance if the service will likely be denied as "not reasonable and necessary." If an Advance Beneficiary Notice of Noncoverage is not given, providers may not bill Medicare or the individual patient for these services.
   - Medicare is a health insurance program for people 65 years or older, people younger than 65 years with certain disabilities, and people of all ages with end-stage renal disease.
   - Medicaid is a joint state-federal–administered health insurance program that provides health coverage for income-qualifying individuals. To participate in Medicaid, federal law requires states to cover certain population groups.[3,24]

3. **A. To compare the effectiveness of new treatments.**
   Rationale: The mission of the AHRQ is to improve the safety and quality of patient care. One way to meet this goal is to support research that compares the effectiveness of new treatments.
   B. To direct the Department of Health and Human Services (DHHS).
   Rationale: AHRQ is 1 of 12 agencies that are directed by the DHHS.
   C. To oversee the National Institutes of Health (NIH) research programs.
   Rationale: AHRQ provides research funding along with its sister agency, the NIH.
   D. To be the largest source of funding for biomedical research.
   Rationale: The NIH is the largest source of funding for biomedical research. AHRQ provides research funding for its initiatives, but not on the order of magnitude provided by the NIH.
   E. To provide health care to the elderly and indigent.
   Rationale: The DHHS is responsible for Medicare and Medicaid.

   Major points of discussion
   - The goals of AHRQ are to improve the quality, safety, effectiveness, and efficiency of patient care through its initiatives.
   - Its focus areas are the comparison of effectiveness of new treatments, quality improvement, patient safety, the use of health information technology in patient safety, and determining the cost effectiveness of health care.
   - AHRQ, like its sister agency the NIH, applies more than 80% of its budget for research. However, the NIH is the

largest source of funding for biomedical research in the United States.

- In addition, AHRQ publishes technology assessments to provide information to other agencies. For example, AHRQ provided a summary to the FDA on the scientific evidence on the quality of laboratory-developed tests (i.e., LDTs or "home brew" tests).[16]

4. **A. Running samples of a known analyte concentration spiked with prescription drugs that could potentially interfere with the measurement of the analyte of interest.**
Rationale: Analytical specificity refers to the assay's ability to (1) measure the analyte in question specifically and (2) not measure other interfering substances that may affect the result.
B. Running samples without the analyte of interest (i.e., Matrix blanks), ensuring that a zero sample actually reads zero.
Rationale: This is one method for establishing the analytical sensitivity or, equivalently, the lower limit of detection/quantification.
C. Running both positive and negative samples and determining the specificity by taking true negatives and dividing by true negatives plus false positives.
Rationale: This is the method used for determining clinical specificity, or the true-negative rate.
D. Running samples spiked with increasing concentrations of an analyte and determining the concentration of the analyte that most specifically discriminates diseased from healthy patients.
Rationale: This experiment could be used to establish the appropriate cutoff for a test.
E. Running samples spiked with the highest measurable concentration of the analyte of interest followed by a Matrix blank.
Rationale: This experiment could be used to establish carryover within the analytical system.

Major points of discussion
- Analytical specificity is a performance characteristic of an assay that quantifies a laboratory test's ability to measure a particular analyte in the presence of possible interfering substances.
- Possible interfering substances vary by analyte and analytical method but can include hemolysis, lipemia, icterus, hyperproteinemia, and prescription drug interferences.
- It is generally impossible to test for *all* possible interferences; thus, the most commonly encountered interfering substances should be determined and assayed.
- Analytical specificity is distinct from clinical specificity.
- Clinical specificity, which is sometimes part of method validation, is determined by taking the number of true negatives identified by the assay and dividing by the sum of the true negatives and false positives.

5. A. The false-negative rate of the assay.
Rationale: This would be determined by the subtracting the clinical sensitivity from 1.

B. The value obtained when the number of true positives is divided by the sum of the true positives and the false negatives.
Rationale: This is the clinical sensitivity.
C. The lowest possible concentration of an analyte that is accurately and reproducibly measured by an assay.
Rationale: See Major Points of Discussion.
D. The performance of the assay when measuring an analyte in the presence of an interfering substance.
Rationale: This is the analytical specificity.
E. The formula that relates instrument response to analyte concentration.
Rationale: This is the calibration curve.

Major points of discussion
- Analytical sensitivity is best defined as the lowest possible value of an analyte that is accurately and reproducibly measured by an assay.
- Analytical specificity is best defined as the performance of the assay when measuring an analyte in the presence of an interfering substance.
- The calibration curve is best defined as the formula that best correlates instrument response to analyte concentration.
- Clinical sensitivity is defined as the true-positive rate of an assay and is calculated as the ratio of true positives divided by the sum of true positives and false negatives.
- Clinical specificity is defined as the true-negative rate of an assay and is calculated as the ratio of true negatives dividied by the sum of true negatives and false positives.

6. A. A training laboratory for students.
Rationale: A training laboratory for student education typically deals only with samples that are not usually infectious and is classified as a level 1 laboratory.
B. A clinical chemistry laboratory.
Rationale: A clinical chemistry laboratory is classified as a level 2 laboratory.
C. A clinical hematology laboratory.
Rationale: A clinical hematology laboratory is classified as a level 2 laboratory.
D. A laboratory working with highly infectious fungal pathogens.
Rationale: A biosafety level 3 laboratory works with microbiological agents that may cause fatal disease through inhalation. A laboratory that works with highly infectious fungal pathogens meets this definition.
E. A satellite clinical laboratory in an emergency department.
Rationale: A satellite clinical laboratory in an emergency department usually performs only routine tests, including chemistry and hematology assays; therefore, it is classified as a level 2 laboratory.

Major points of discussion
- Biosafety level 1 laboratories are suitable for work involving well-characterized agents not known to consistently cause disease in healthy adult humans and are of minimal potential hazard to laboratory personnel and the environment.

- Biosafety level 2 laboratories are suitable for work involving agents of moderate potential hazard to personnel and the environment.
- Biosafety level 3 laboratories are suitable for work with indigenous or exotic agents that may cause serious or potentially lethal disease after inhalation.
- Biosafety level 4 laboratories are suitable for work with dangerous and exotic agents that pose a high individual risk of aerosol-transmitted laboratory infections. These include agents that cause severe to fatal disease in humans for which vaccines or other treatments are *not* available.

7. A. The process of testing and adjusting an assay so that the instrument measurements best correlate with the known analyte concentrations.
Rationale: This is the definition of "assay calibration." This should be done more frequently than every 6 months.
B. The process of testing known concentrations of an analyte throughout the reportable range and confirming that the assay returns the appropriate value, within an established allowable error.
Rationale: This is the correct definition of "calibration verification."
C. The process of comparing the slope and *y*-intercept of the current calibration curve with the previous curves.
Rationale: This is good practice. When recalibrating an assay, tracking the slope and intercept helps identify calibration shifts. However, this is not the definition of "calibration verification."
D. The process of running previously assayed patient samples with a new lot of calibration material and comparing them with results obtained when the same samples were run using a previous lot of calibration material.
Rationale: This is good laboratory practice when changing lots of calibration reagent. The patient samples should be chosen to span the analytical range of the assay. However, this is not the definition of "calibration verification."
E. The process of running samples of known high and low analyte concentrations and plotting them on a Levey-Jennings chart.
Rationale: This describes a quality control (QC) performance procedure and not calibration verification.

Major points of discussion
- Calibration verification should be performed on medium- and high-complexity assays every 6 months, unless the test system meets specific CLIA requirements.
- Calibration verification should also be performed after major servicing of the equipment, changing to a new lot of reagents, or when the performance of the assay is questionable.
- The goal of calibration verification is to ensure that your assay maintains accuracy across its analytical range.
- Calibration verification is a quality assurance measure.
- Calibration of an assay is best defined as the process of adjusting an instrument response to maximize the correlation with analyte concentration. This is distinct from calibration verification.
- A laboratory should establish, a priori, what tolerance limits it will allow for variation within calibration verification. These limits should be based on the clinical accuracy requirement of the assay.

- Comparing the slope and intercept of a current calibration line with previous lines is an additional piece of quality assurance that is distinct from calibration verification and will identify shifts in calibration in real time.[5]

8. A. Every 6 months.
B. Once every year.
Rationale: These are too frequent.
C. Once every 2 years.
Rationale: This is the normal frequency for inspections.
D. Once every 3 years.
Rationale: Regular CAP inspections occur more frequently than every 3 years.
E. Once every 5 years.
Rationale: Regular CAP inspections occur more frequently than every 5 years.

Major points of discussion
- The CAP offers a laboratory accreditation program that routinely inspects laboratories on a 2-year cycle.
- A CLIA-accredited laboratory is one that is inspected by accrediting organizations that have been approved by the CMS.
- An approved accrediting organization can inspect a laboratory in lieu of the CMS.
- CMS has granted the CAP Laboratory Accreditation Program deeming authority.
- CAP inspections are guided by detailed checklists created for different areas of the laboratory.[25]

9. A. **Patient samples spanning the analytical range of the assay are run using the old reagent lot and compared with the same samples using the new reagent lot. The correlation coefficient should be close to 1.**
Rationale: The key here is that the patient samples are preselected to span the analytical range of the assay.
B. Random patient samples are run using the old and new reagent lots and then compared. The correlation coefficient should be close to 1.
Rationale: Random patient samples would not be ideal because the majority of the analyte values will cluster within the normal range. To prove no effect on patient samples, one should select a panel of patient samples that span the analytical range of the assay.
C. Calibration standards dissolved in methanol are run across the full analytical range of the instrument using old and new reagent lots and are then compared. The correlation coefficient should be close to 1.
Rationale: Running standards out of their matrix would not prove that patient samples (in matrix) will quantify correctly using a new lot of reagent.
D. The analyte should be extracted from each level of control material using a solid-phase extraction procedure and then run using the old and new reagent lots. The correlation coefficient should be close to 1.
Rationale: This is a valid approach to prove that the matrix in the high-QC material is, in fact, causing the discrepancy. However, it does nothing to prove that patient samples, which are always in matrix, will react the same between different reagent lots.
E. The assay should be recalibrated; the control material should then be run and compared between both reagent lots.

Rationale: This could help, particularly if the QC run using the old reagent lot were quantified relative to a different calibration curve than the QC run using the new reagent lot. However, it does nothing to prove that patient samples, which are always in matrix, will react the same between different reagent lots.

Major points of discussion

- It is good laboratory practice to run a set of samples before and after reagent lot change to ensure that the reagent change does not cause a shift in analyte quantification.
- Samples should be both QC material and real patient samples (in matrix) that span the analytical range of the assay to prove that the new reagent lot reacts the same as the old lot in matrix and in the "pseudo-matrix" in which many QC materials are prepared.
- Differences in QC values using two different lots of reagent may be due to different reactions between the new lot and the pseudo-matrix of the QC material. This difference in reaction may extend to patient samples and should be excluded by running patient samples across the analytical range using both lots.
- New reagent lots should be "verified" in the above manner well before the old lot expires or runs out. This requires good inventory control.
- It is ultimately the responsibility of the laboratory director to ensure that good QC practices are followed in the laboratory.
- A priori, the laboratory should establish allowable differences in patient sample values between lots. These tolerance limits should be established based on the clinical accuracy needs of the assay.

10. A. You must apply for a CLIA certificate of waiver.
Rationale: This is issued to a laboratory that performs *only* waived testing. This certificate is not needed if the laboratory already operates under a certificate that allows for higher complexity testing.
B. You must apply for a CLIA certificate of registration.
Rationale: This certificate is issued to a laboratory to allow it to conduct nonwaived (i.e., moderate- and/or high-complexity) testing until the laboratory is surveyed (by the state Department of Health or an accreditation agency) to determine its compliance with CLIA regulations. Only laboratories that apply for a certificate of compliance or a certificate of accreditation will receive a certificate of registration. This is not needed for waived testing.
C. You must apply for a CLIA certificate of compliance.
Rationale: This certificate is issued to a laboratory once the state Department of Health conducts an inspection and determines that the laboratory is compliant with all applicable CLIA requirements. This type of certificate is issued to a laboratory that performs nonwaived testing and is not needed to add a waived test.
D. No additional certificates are necessary.
E. You cannot run a waived test in a laboratory that performs predominantly moderate-complexity testing.
Rationale: You can perform a waived test under either a certificate of compliance or a certificate of accreditation,

both of which allow the laboratory to conduct moderate- or high-complexity tests.

Major points of discussion

- A certificate of accreditation is issued to a laboratory on the basis of the laboratory's accreditation by an accreditation organization approved by CMS. This type of certificate is issued to a laboratory that performs nonwaived (i.e., moderate- and/or high-complexity) testing.
- There are six CMS-approved accreditation agencies:
  - AABB
  - American Osteopathic Association
  - American Society for Histocompatibility and Immunogenetics
  - COLA
  - CAP
  - The Joint Commission[7]

11. A. The FDA.
Rationale: The FDA does not directly oversee the CLIA program. However, the FDA is responsible for classifying laboratory test systems as waived, moderate-complexity, or high-complexity.
B. The AABB.
Rationale: The AABB publishes standard guidelines for blood banks, cell therapy, and transfusion services, not for general clinical laboratories.
C. The CAP.
Rationale: The CAP does not oversee the CLIA program. CAP does publish laboratory standards and offers a laboratory accreditation program, which is a voluntary program separate from CLIA.
D. The Joint Commission.
Rationale: The Joint Commission does not oversee CLIA. The Joint Commission does publish laboratory standards and offers an accreditation program for laboratories, which is a voluntary program separate from CLIA.
E. The Centers for Medicare and Medicaid Services (CMS).
Rationale: CMS oversees the enforcement of CLIA regulations.

Major points of discussion

- CLIA was passed by Congress in 1988.
- The CLIA program is designed to ensure quality laboratory testing.
- The CMS oversees the operation of the CLIA program.
- The CMS recognizes additional accrediting agencies and will issue a certificate of accreditation to laboratories that receive accreditation from the AABB, American Osteopathic Association, American Society for Histocompatibility and Immunogenetics, COLA, CAP, and The Joint Commission.
- There are five types of CLIA certificates: certificate of waiver, certificate for provider-performed microscopy procedures, certificate of registration, certificate of compliance, and certificate of accreditation.[4,7]

12. **A. Accuracy, precision, reportable range, and confirmation of the manufacturer's reference range.**
Rationale: These are the four performance characteristics that CLIA regulations require a laboratory to confirm prior to performing an FDA-approved moderate-complexity assay.

The reference range study does not have to be a full 120-patient study; rather, it is meant to confirm that manufacturer's ranges are appropriate for your patient population.
B. Accuracy, analytical sensitivity and specificity, reportable range, and a full reference range study with a minimum of 120 patient samples.
Rationale: A full reference range study requires 120 individuals in each demographic subset. This is not required to confirm the manufacturer's reference ranges. Generally, 20 to 40 healthy individuals will suffice for a reference range confirmation.
C. Accuracy, clinical sensitivity and specificity, analytical specificity and sensitivity, full reference range study, and reportable range.
Rationale: These are some of the more advanced performance parameters that laboratories introducing laboratory-developed tests would assess.
D. Extraction efficiency, reportable range, full reference range study, QC material stability, and analytical sensitivity and specificity.
Rationale: These are more detailed and assay-specific performance characteristics that some laboratories will establish when validating laboratory-developed tests.
E. Only accuracy and precision must be confirmed.
Rationale: There are four performance characteristics defined by CLIA. Accuracy and precision are two of them. The other two are reportable range and reference range.

Major points of discussion
- CLIA guidelines require laboratories to confirm the manufacturer's claims on assay performance prior to instituting the assay in the laboratory.
- Accuracy, reproducibility, reportable range, and reference range are the four performance characteristics of an FDA-approved, moderate-complexity assay that must, at a minimum, be confirmed.
- Laboratory-developed tests are considered high-complexity tests and are held to a different standard of validation by CLIA regulations. Additional performance parameters must be assessed.
- The purpose of a method validation is to assess the degree of uncertainty in the measurements made by the assay and to point out assay weaknesses and potential for error.
- Accuracy is usually validated by running standards of known concentrations and comparing the measured concentration as a percentage of the expected concentration.
- Precision or reproducibility (inter-run) is generally assessed by running at least two levels of an analyte in quadruplicate over 5 days. Precision is expressed as a % CV ([mean/SD] × 100%).
- The reportable range is established by running increasing concentrations of the analyte and choosing the range of concentrations in which instrument response increases *linearly* with analyte concentration. A linear regression procedure is usually used.

13. A. Once every 12 hours.
B. Once every 24 hours.
Rationale: QC samples must be assayed once every 24 hours, or more frequently if recommended by the manufacturer.
C. Every time the assay is performed.
Rationale for A and C: These are too frequent.
D. Once every 48 hours.
Rationale: QC must be run more often than every 48 hours if the test is offered continuously (i.e., 24 hours a day).
E. Once every week.
Rationale: QC samples must be assayed more often than once a week for tests that are offered 24 hours day.

Major points of discussion
- According to CLIA, QC samples must be assayed once every 24 hours, or more frequently if recommended by the manufacturer.
- Laboratories can assay QC samples more frequently if deemed necessary to ensure accurate results.
- QC samples should be assayed after calibration or maintenance of an analyzer to verify correct method performance.
- Blood gas measurements have separate, stricter QC requirements. CLIA requires at least one QC level to be assayed every 8 hours for blood gas measurements.
- In addition to running QC samples every 8 hours for blood gas measurements, CLIA also requires that a control sample be run with every patient sample, unless the analyzer calibrates itself every 30 minutes.[6]

14. **A. After you have applied, paid for, and received a certificate of registration, assuming your state Department of Health has no additional requirements.**
Rationale: The certificate of registration is an intermediate step that allows your laboratory to begin testing until the laboratory is inspected by either your state Department of Health or a deemed accreditation agency.
B. After you are inspected by your state Department of Health and have received your certificate of compliance.
C. After you have been inspected by an approved accreditation agency and have received your certificate of accreditation.
Rationale: Neither of these certificates is required to begin testing, unless otherwise specified by your state Department of Health.
D. After your state Department of Health, or an approved accreditation agency, and CMS have both inspected your laboratory.
Rationale: CMS inspects only a small number of laboratories on a random basis. This is not required to begin testing.
E. Once you have validated your assays to your satisfaction.
Rationale: You must apply for a CLIA license to provide patient testing results.

Major points of discussion
- CLIA requires all facilities that perform any tests (even waived) on "materials derived from the human body for the purpose of providing information for the diagnosis, prevention, or treatment of any disease or impairment of, or the assessment of the health of, human beings" to meet federal regulatory criteria. If a laboratory performs the aforementioned testing, it is considered a clinical laboratory and must apply for and obtain a certificate from the appropriate CLIA program, depending on the complexity of the testing offered.

- A certificate of registration is issued to a laboratory to allow it to conduct nonwaived (moderate- and/or high-complexity) testing until the laboratory is surveyed (inspected) to determine its compliance with CLIA regulations. Only laboratories that apply for a certificate of compliance or a certificate of accreditation will receive a certificate of registration.
- A certificate of provider-performed microscopy (PPM) is issued to a laboratory in which a physician, midlevel practitioner, or dentist performs specific microscopy procedures during the course of a patient's visit. A limited list of microscopy procedures is included under this certificate type; these are categorized as moderate-complexity.
- There are six CMS-approved accreditation organizations:
  - AABB
  - American Osteopathic Association
  - American Society for Histocompatibility and Immunogenetics
  - COLA
  - College of American Pathologists
  - The Joint Commission
- As defined by CLIA, waived tests are categorized as "simple laboratory examinations and procedures that have an insignificant risk of an erroneous result." The FDA determines the criteria for "simple" tests as those with a low risk of error and approves manufacturer's applications for test system waiver.[7]

15. A. It is a comparison of reference ranges across laboratories.
Rationale: Delta checks do not involve reference range comparisons.
B. It is a quality measure by which a patient's previous result is compared with the current one.
Rationale: Delta checks compare current result values with previous result values.
C. It is a quality measure by which samples are visually checked for hemolysis.
Rationale: A delta check is not a visual assessment for hemolysis.
D. It is a level of an analyte thought to be life-threatening to the patient, requiring verbal notification to the ordering provider.
Rationale: This is a critical value.
E. It is a quality measure that occurs when results fall above the analytical limit of an assay.
Rationale: A delta check does not assess the analytical limit of an assay.

Major points of discussion
- Delta checks compare current result values with previous result values and flag samples that have exceeded predefined acceptable limits for variation.
- Delta checks are intended to detect either preanalytic or analytic errors in testing, such as specimen mix-up errors, diluted samples, or analyzer malfunction.
- Laboratories individually determine (1) which assays will have delta checks and (2) the acceptable thresholds for intraindividual variation.
- An example of an assay that commonly has a delta check is the mean corpuscular red blood cell volume.
- Delta checks are an example of patient-derived QC procedures.[21,23]

16. A. The FMLA provides employees with up to 12 weeks of paid, job-protected leave per year.
B. The FMLA provides employees with up to 16 weeks of paid, job-protected leave for the birth or care of a newborn child.
Rationale: The FMLA does not enforce paid leave.
C. The FMLA provides employees with up to 16 weeks of unpaid, job-protected leave for females and 12 weeks for males for the birth or care of a newborn child.
Rationale: The FMLA does not have gender-specific standards.
D. The FMLA provides employees with up to 12 weeks of unpaid, job-protected leave per year leave for qualifying reasons.
Rationale: Employers must grant up to12 weeks of unpaid leave for qualifying reasons.
E. The FMLA provides employees with continuous health insurance coverage for up to 16 weeks.
Rationale: The FMLA provides health insurance coverage for only 12 weeks.

Major points of discussion
- The FMLA requires employers to offer 12 weeks of unpaid, job-protected leave per year for qualifying reasons.
- Qualifying reasons include the birth of a newborn child; placement of a child for adoption or foster care; care for an immediate family member with a serious health condition; or employee medical leave if unable to work because of a serious health condition.
- The FMLA applies to all public agencies, elementary and secondary schools, and companies with 50 or more employees.
- The FMLA is enforced by the U.S. Department of Labor's Employment Standards Administration, Wage and Hour Division.
- The FMLA requires health insurance to be maintained during the leave if insurance was provided before the leave was taken.
- Employees are eligible for leave if they have worked for their employer at least 12 months.[15]

17. A. The AABB.
B. The CAP.
Rationale: The AABB and CAP have accreditation standards for blood banks, but they do not set the federal regulations.
C. The CMS.
D. The CDC.
Rationale: The CMS and CDC do not regulate blood banks.
E. The FDA.
Rationale: The FDA oversees the regulations, and their compliance, for all blood banks.

Major points of discussion
- All blood-banking establishments must be licensed by the FDA. Blood products are regulated by the federal government as a pharmaceutical.
- The FDA conducts unannounced inspections of all blood banks on a periodic basis.

- The FDA promulgates criteria for blood donor eligibility.
- The CMS oversees the CLIA regulatory program.
- The AABB, CAP, and The Joint Commission have accreditation standards for blood banks and will conduct inspections.

18. A. LDTs are not medical devices and therefore do not fall under the FDA's jurisdiction.
Rationale: The FDA considers laboratory assays to be medical devices.
B. LDTs are considered medical devices, and each laboratory must receive FDA approval before implementing an LDT.
Rationale: Although LDTs are considered medical devices, the FDA exercises enforcement discretion on this issue to encourage rapid implementation of the newest, most-effective diagnostics into laboratories to improve public health.
C. LDTs are considered medical devices, but the FDA has exercised enforcement discretion on LDTs.
Rationale: Although LDTs are, indeed, laboratory devices, the FDA exercises enforcement discretion on this issue allowing laboratories to implement their assays after an in-house, CLIA-appropriate validation.
D. LDTs are not considered medical devices, but the FDA regulates them.
Rationale: The FDA does not regulate LDTs.
E. LDTs may or may not be considered medical devices, and the FDA considers each assay on a case-by-case basis and decides whether to regulate.
Rationale: The FDA is clear on its stance on the status of LDTs as medical devices over which it could exercise regulatory control, but chooses not to, in the interest of enhancing public health.

Major points of discussion
- The FDA considers LDTs medical devices and the laboratories producing them as manufacturers of medical devices.
- The definition of an LDT is a test designed in a laboratory for specific use *only* in that laboratory.
- The FDA exercises enforcement discretion with regard to LDTs to enable implementation of the newest diagnostics in clinical laboratories in a meaningful time period.
- The FDA's proposed jurisdiction over LDTs is the subject of debate, particularly from the CMS, which considers LDTs a service offered by the laboratory to ordering physicians without any reagents or devices crossing state borders. Therefore, they argue that the FDA has no authority in regulating LDTs.
- Although LDTs are not actively regulated by the FDA, CLIA has a strict set of performance criteria that must be established in method validation before releasing patient results. These include, but are not limited to, linearity, reproducibility, analytical sensitivity/specificity, reference range, and recovery/accuracy.
- LDT validation studies should be tailored to address issues specific to the technology being used. For example, ionization suppression experiments should always be included in methods using electrospray ionization–mass spectrometry, despite this not being specifically listed by CLIA regulations.[14,17]

19. A. Do you have any disabilities?
Rationale: Title 1 of the Americans with Disabilities Act makes it unlawful for an employer to discriminate against a qualified applicant based on disability.
B. Were you born in the United States?
C. What is your native language?
Rationale: Title VII of the Civil Rights Act of 1964 makes it illegal to discriminate against someone on the basis of race, color, religion, national origin, or gender.
D. How old are you?
Rationale: The Age Discrimination in Employment Act (ADEA) forbids age discrimination only against people who are age 40 years or older.
E. Are you capable of performing all of the duties required by this position?
Rationale: This is the best way to gather information about whether the potential employee is mentally and physically capable of performing the job. There is no need to ask about specific disabilities, age, or language fluency.

Major points of discussion
- Not everyone with a medical condition is disabled and, therefore, protected by the American with Disabilities Act. There are three ways to be considered disabled under the law:
  - A person may be disabled if he or she has a physical or mental condition that substantially limits a major life activity (such as walking, talking, seeing, hearing, or learning).
  - A person may be disabled if he or she has a history of a disability (such as cancer that is in remission).
  - A person may be disabled if he or she is believed to have a physical or mental impairment that is not transitory (lasting or expected to last 6 months or less) and minor (even if he or she does not have such an impairment).
- The Age Discrimination in Employment Act of 1967 protects people who are age 40 years or older from discrimination because of age. The law also makes it illegal to retaliate against a person because the person complained about discrimination, filed a charge of discrimination, or participated in an employment discrimination investigation or lawsuit.
- Title VII of the Civil Rights Law of 1964 makes it illegal to retaliate against a person because the person complained about discrimination, filed a charge of discrimination, or participated in an employment discrimination investigation or lawsuit. The law also requires that employers reasonably accommodate applicants' and employees' sincerely held religious practices, unless doing so would impose an undue hardship on the operation of the employer's business.
- Title I of the Americans with Disabilities Act of 1990 makes it illegal to discriminate against a qualified person with a disability, in the private sector or in state and local governments. The law also makes it illegal to retaliate against a person because the person complained about discrimination, filed a charge of discrimination, or participated in an employment discrimination investigation or lawsuit. The law also requires that employers reasonably accommodate the known physical or mental limitations of an otherwise qualified individual

with a disability who is an applicant or employee, unless doing so would impose an undue hardship on the operation of the employer's business.

■ The Genetic Information Nondiscrimination Act of 2009 makes it illegal to discriminate against employees or applicants because of genetic information. Genetic information includes information about an individual's genetic tests and the genetic tests of an individual's family members, as well as information about any disease, disorder, or condition of an individual's family members (i.e., an individual's family medical history). The law also makes it illegal to retaliate against a person because the person complained about discrimination, filed a charge of discrimination, or participated in an employment discrimination investigation or lawsuit.

20. A. Standards for quality and competence in medical laboratories.
Rationale: ISO 15189:2007 is the "Medical laboratories—Particular requirements for quality and competence" standards.
B. Standards for pricing and reimbursement in medical laboratories.
Rationale: ISO 15189:2007 does not regulate laboratory test pricing.
C. Laboratory services that must be covered under universal health insurance plans.
Rationale: ISO 15189:2007 does not regulate health insurance.
D. Standard requirements for laboratory technologist school curricula.
Rationale: ISO 15189:2007 does not regulate laboratory technologist training.
E. Standard requirements for retirement benefit packages.
Rationale: ISO 15189:2007 does not regulate employee work benefits.

Major points of discussion
■ The ISO is a nongovernment organization that develops standards for a variety of disciplines in business, government, and society.
■ ISO is a network of the national standards institutes of 163 countries.
■ International Standards for technical regulations on products, production methods, and services help ensure a certain level of performance and safety worldwide.
■ Adherence to ISO standards is voluntary. ISO has no legal authority to enforce its standards unless countries have incorporated them into their national laws.
■ ISO 15189:2007 ("Medical laboratories—Particular requirements for quality and competence") is designed specifically for clinical and medical laboratories and includes quality management standards, technical competence standards, and test reliability standards.[20]

21. A. Technical supervisor.
Rationale: A high-complexity laboratory requires a technical supervisor whose training requirements and responsibility are defined in CLIA Subpart M Section 493.1449 Standard; Technical supervisor qualifications.

B. Clinical consultant.
Rationale: A high-complexity laboratory requires a clinical consultant whose training requirements and responsibility are defined in CLIA Subpart M Section 493.1455 Standard; Clinical consultant qualifications.
C. General supervisor.
Rationale: A high-complexity laboratory requires a general supervisor whose training requirements and responsibility are defined in CLIA Subpart M Section 493.1461 Standard: General supervisor qualifications.
D. Testing personnel.
Rationale: A high-complexity laboratory requires a testing personnel whose training requirements and responsibility are defined in CLIA Subpart M Section 493.1489 Standard; Testing personnel qualifications.
E. The laboratory director can assume any and all of these positions.
Rationale: Although all of the positions described in answers A through D are required by CLIA to operate a high-complexity laboratory, the regulations do not require that separate individuals fill each role. Indeed, as long as the laboratory director meets the qualification standards in Subpart M for each position, he or she may fill any and all of the positions.

Major points of discussion
■ CLIA '88 requires that a laboratory performing high-complexity testing be staffed by personnel who can fulfill the qualifications and responsibilities of a technical and general supervisor, testing personnel, and a clinical consultant.
■ If the laboratory performs a mix of moderate- and high-complexity testing, only those employees working on high-complexity testing must meet the above requirements.
■ These four positions can be filled by one person (i.e., the laboratory director) as long and he or she meets the qualifications and is able to meet the established responsibilities defined in Subpart M of CLIA.
■ It is the laboratory director's responsibility to ensure that appropriate personnel work in the laboratory.
■ The personnel requirements for a laboratory are determined by the level of complexity of the assays run in the laboratory.

22. A. The assay is accurate but not precise.
Rationale: Accuracy refers to how closely an assay result value matches the true value of the analyte. This chart would show scatter around the expected value.
B. The assay is precise but not accurate.
Rationale: Precision refers to the reproducibility of the results.
C. The assay is neither precise nor accurate.
Rationale: The QC results are scattered, representing a large SD, and there is a bias trend away from the expected mean value. This suggests imprecision and inaccuracy.
D. The assay is clinically useless.
Rationale: Levey-Jennings control charts do not assess the clinical utility of laboratory tests but, rather, assess if the assay is performing as expected.
E. The assay is precise and accurate.

Rationale: A precise and accurate assay would have an observed mean value close to the expected mean value and a small SD.

Major points of discussion

- A Levey-Jennings control chart plots QC results around their expected mean value.
- Acceptable limits for the deviation of the QC results from the expected value are determined by the laboratory.
- This is often achieved through the use of the Westgard rules, which are QC interpretive rules for statistical monitoring of assay accuracy and precision.
- Accuracy can be assessed by measuring an analyte in reference material and comparing the result with the known certified concentration.
- Precision is the agreement between result values obtained by repeat measurements of a given quantity of the analyte.[18,30]

23. A. Positive trending of QC results.
Rationale: These QC results trend at approximately 2 SDs above the mean value.
B. Negative trending of QC results.
Rationale: These QC results trend in a positive direction, above the mean value, not in a negative direction.
C. Result interference by an unknown substance.
Rationale: Levey-Jennings charts are not used to analyze interference.
D. The use of an inappropriately narrow reference range.
Rationale: Levey-Jennings charts are not used to analyze reference ranges.
E. The need to change the technical range for the assay.
Rationale: Levey-Jennings charts are not used to determine the technical range of an assay.

Major points of discussion

- QC procedures are used to detect errors that occur because of test system failure. They are used to monitor the accuracy and precision of laboratory tests.
- For all tests classified as CLIA nonwaived tests, a minimum of two levels of controls must be run on each day that patient testing is performed.
- Levey-Jennings charts show QC results over time and plot how far each point lies from the mean expected value.
- Just by chance, QC values should fall outside 2 SDs from the mean 5% of the time.
- There are many Levey-Jennings rules that are used to flag a QC violation. For example, if a QC value falls 2 SDs beyond the mean, then it would be denoted a 1_{2s} violation. If it falls 3 SDs beyond the mean, it is denoted 1_{3s}.
- An action plan should be in place to evaluate QC violations.[6]

24. A. The x-axis as "Average value" and the y-axis as "% Difference."
Rationale: This is typical for a Bland-Altman or bias plot.
B. The x-axis as the "Gold standard method" and the y-axis as "Test method."
Rationale: This is an example of a method comparison plot.

C. The x-axis as "Calibrator level" and the y-axis as "% CV."
Rationale: This is a nice way of visualizing trends in reproducibility with increasing analyte concentration.
D. The x-axis as "Run #" and the y-axis as "Concentration."
Rationale: This is the classic Levey-Jennings chart. Often, the expected, average value for the control material and the ±2 SD limits are also noted as dashed or dotted lines on the plot.
E. The x-axis as "Instrument response" and the y-axis as "Expected concentration."
Rationale: This is a calibration curve.

Major points of discussion

- Levey-Jennings charts are a graphic way of plotting QC data to monitor test quality.
- The graphic representation allows for quick trend spotting and identification of rule violations.
- The typical Levey-Jennings chart has the QC Run # on the x-axis and the QC result on the y-axis.
- At least two levels of QC are typically run on an assay, and different levels should be graphed on separate Levey-Jennings chart.
- It is often useful to denote the expected/average value of the QC material and then ±2 SDs on the Levey-Jennings chart to help spot rule violations.

25. A. Validation of LoQ.
Rationale: If the reproducibility (CV <15%) and accuracy (>80%) meet a prespecified value, the LoQ is validated. However, there is additional information available from these experiments.
B. Validation of the LoQ, intraday and interday reproducibility, and accuracy at the LoQ.
Rationale: The within-day and between-day reproducibility are determined by running the same sample multiple times per day for multiple days. The values of these 20 runs can then be averaged to obtain a value for the sample that can be compared with the "known" value of the sample to establish accuracy at the LoQ. As long as these two measures fall within preestablished criteria, the proposed LoQ has been verified.
C. Validation of the LoQ and establishment of accuracy at the LoQ.
Rationale: The intraday and interday reproducibility is also determined by this experiment.
D. Validation of the LoQ and establishment of the reportable range.
Rationale: The reportable range is generally established by running samples across the hypothesized range and assessing linearity, usually by linear regression methods.
E. Establishment of reproducibility at the LoQ.
Rationale: Reproducibility is established at the LoQ, but additional information is also available.

Major points of discussion

- To validate a proposed LoQ, the accuracy and reproducibility at this concentration should fall within prespecified limits.
- By FDA method validation guidelines, the CV at the LoQ should be less than 15%.
- By FDA method validation guidelines, the accuracy at the LoQ should be greater than 80%.

- An appropriate LoQ is a value below the lowest, clinically relevant value of the analyte.
- If no proposed LoQ is provided in the literature or from experience, the LoQ of the assay can be determined by either:
  - Establishing the analyte value for which the signal/noise ratio is more than 10, or
  - Running a matrix blank 20 times and adding 5 SDs to the average value obtained in this experiment.[19]

26. A. Analytical specificity.
Rationale: Analytical specificity refers to an assay's ability to discriminate the analyte of interest from possible interferences.
B. Analytical sensitivity.
Rationale: Analytical sensitivity defines the lowest value of an analyte that can reproducibly and accurately be measured by an assay. The higher the sensitivity, the lower is the possible concentration of analyte that it can measure.
C. Clinical specificity.
Rationale: Clinical specificity is defined as the true-negative rate—that is, how often the assay categorizes samples from patients without disease as "healthy."
D. Clinical sensitivity.
Rationale: Clinical sensitivity is defined as the true-positive rate—that is, how often the assay categorizes samples from patients with disease as "diseased."
E. The lower limit of linearity.
Rationale: Although the lower limit of linearity may be the same as the lower limit of detection/quantification, more often, it is a lower value. Lower limits of linearity are usually determined by running serial dilutions of a standard and then analyzing the results using linear regression.

Major points of discussion
- Analytical sensitivity defines the lowest concentration of an analyte that can accurately and reproducibly be measured by an assay. This is also known as the lower limit of quantification or the lower limit of detection (for nonquantitative or semiquantitative assays).
- There are several ways to determine this value. One way is to average the ratio of analyte signal to background noise. For the limit of quantification, the signal/noise ratio is typically more than 10. For lower limits of detection, the signal/noise ratio is typically more than 3.
- Another approach to establish a lower limit of quantification is by running a matrix sample without analyte (i.e., matrix blank) 20 times. To the average concentration of the blank, 4 to 5 times the SD of the multiple runs is added. This sum is now the lower limit of quantification.
- Clinical sensitivity is the true-positive rate of an assay, which differs from analytical sensitivity.
- Clinical specificity is the true-negative rate of an assay and differs from the analytical specificity. For laboratory-developed assays, CLIA regulations require that analytical specificity be established during test validation. There is no specific regulation for clinical specificity.[19]

27. A. The CDC.
Rationale: The CDC primarily focuses on infectious disease epidemiology and research.

B. The FDA.
Rationale: The FDA primarily regulates food safety, dietary supplements, medications, vaccines, blood transfusions, medical devices, and veterinary products.
C. The American Medical Association.
Rationale: The American Medical Association is a physician trade association.
D. Individual states.
Rationale: Individual states establish and administer their own Medicaid programs.
E. Private insurance companies.
Rationale: Medicaid is not a form of private health insurance.

Major points of discussion
- Medicaid is jointly funded by the federal government and state governments.
- To participate in Medicaid, states are required to offer the health insurance coverage to certain population groups.
- States can expand the health insurance coverage to additional population groups if they deem this appropriate.
- States receive federal matching funds to provide the benefits.[25]

28. A. Your assay correlates poorly with the reference method.
Rationale: The R^2 value is 0.99, which indicates excellent correlation.
B. Your assay correlates well with the reference method but has a positive proportional bias.
Rationale: The slope greater than 1 implies that for every unit increase in concentration detected in the gold standard method, your method detects an increase of 1.34 concentration units. This is proportional and positive bias. The R^2 value of 0.99 implies excellent correlation.
C. Your assay correlates well with the reference method but has a negative constant bias.
Rationale: A negative constant bias would be reflected in a negative intercept term.
D. Your assay correlates well with the reference method. No other statements can be accurately made.
Rationale: Although your assay does correlate well with the reference method, the slope and *y*-intercept provide additional data that can and must be interpreted in this method correlation experiment.
E. Your assay correlates poorly with the reference method and shows a positive proportional bias.
Rationale: The two assays correlate very well with one another.

Major points of discussion
- A method correlation study between your laboratory's proposed method and a gold standard or reference method should always be part of a method validation for a high-complexity, laboratory-developed test (subject to the availability of a reference method).
- Classically, the reference method is plotted on the *x*-axis and your laboratory's method on the *y*-axis.
- If the plot is classically drawn, a slope greater than 1 implies a positive and proportional bias of your method relative to the reference method.
- If plotted classically, a *y*-intercept term greater than 0 implies a constant positive bias.

- Both constant and proportional biases may coexist in a method comparison study.
- An R^2 value approaching 1 indicates that the linear regression line drawn between the two methods is an excellent fit. However, high coefficient of determination does not rule out bias in your method.

29. A. The FDA.
Rationale: The FDA is a part of the DHHS and regulates the manufacture of biologics, medical devices, and test kits.
B. The NIH.
Rationale: The NIH is an agency of the DHHS, the main aim of which is the performance and funding of biomedical research.
C. The CMS.
Rationale: CMS sets quality standards and reimbursement rates that apply to laboratories. These rates are often then adopted by other third-party payers.
D. The National Institute of Standards and Technology (NIST).
Rationale: The NIST is a branch of the U.S. Department of Commerce. Among other things, the NIST develops and distributes standardized calibration materials for a finite list of analytes.
E. The DHHS.
Rationale: This federal agency oversees the CMS, FDA, and OIG. It is not involved in developing standards for calibration.

Major point of discussion
- The DHHS oversees the CMS, FDA, and OIG.

30. A. Apply for state certification every 2 years and pay the annual membership fee.
Rationale: There is no application process for OSHA.
B. Provide subsidized health insurance for all employees and offer at least two separate insurance plans.
Rationale: OSHA does not mandate that employees provide health insurance.
C. Display an OSHA poster in the workplace informing employees about the Occupational Safety and Health Act.
Rationale: Employers are required to display a poster prepared by the Department of Labor containing this information.
D. Require that all employees receive an annual physical health exam with urine drug screening.
Rationale: OSHA does not mandate health exams or drug testing.
E. Receive state OSHA agency approval before increasing the number of employees.
Rationale: OSHA does not regulate staffing numbers.

Major points of discussion
- The Occupational Safety and Health Act was passed by Congress in 1970 and requires employers to provide a safe workplace.
- The OSHA, which enforces the Occupational Safety and Health Act, is part of the U.S. Department of Labor.
- OSHA standards are rules that employers must follow to protect employees from hazards.
- These standards limit hazardous chemical exposure, require certain safety practices and equipment, require

monitoring hazards, and require keeping records of workplace injuries.
- All employers are required to display a poster prepared by the Department of Labor informing employees of their protections under the Occupational Safety and Health Act.
- OSHA regulates occupational exposure to hazardous chemicals in laboratories.[26]

31. A. **The patient results are manually entered into the wrong patient's medical record.**
Rationale: This is an example of postanalytical error.
B. The sample is drawn into an inappropriate tube.
C. The sample is run using a reagent lot that has expired.
D. The phlebotomist did not fill the tube completely on a sample sent for coagulation testing.
Rationale for B and D: These are examples of preanalytical errors.
E. The autosampling pipette was jostled and is now drawing only 1.3 µL of sample instead of 1.5 µL of sample.
Rationale for C and E: These are examples of analytical errors.

Major points of discussion
- Anything involving specimen acquisition, transport, and processing is part of the preanalytical phase of testing.
- The analytical phase of testing is defined by those procedures dealing with sample manipulation, reagent preparation, calibration, measurement, and instrument readout.
- The postanalytical phase involves recording test results, interpretation of results, and transmission of reports.
- Errors can occur in any and all phases of the total testing process.
- Manual result entering and reporting increase the risk of postanalytical errors, such as the one described in this question.[30]

32. A. A quality assessment tool that compares a patient's previous results with current results.
Rationale: This is a delta check.
B. A quality assessment tool that involves testing two levels of QC material before testing patient samples.
Rationale: This describes standard QC procedures that ensure real-time test accuracy.
C. A quality assessment tool by which laboratories test samples with unknown results and compare their results.
Rationale: PT is an external assessment tool used to grade laboratory testing quality.
D. A quality assessment tool that involves running calibrators every 6 months to ensure linear assay results.
Rationale: PT does not involve recalibration of analyzers.
E. A quality assessment test given to all newly hired technologists to ensure appropriate training and competency.
Rationale: PT occurs on a regular basis and is not restricted to newly hired individuals.

Major points of discussion
- PT involves testing samples with a quantity unknown to the laboratory and then comparing these results across laboratories that use similar methodology.

- Proficiency samples should be tested in the same manner as patient samples.
- Proficiency samples cannot be sent to reference laboratories for result correlation.
- Laboratories should not discuss test results with other laboratories prior to the deadline for submission.
- PT ensures accuracy and reliability of laboratory testing.
- Delta checks compare current result values with previous result values for a given patient and flag samples that have exceeded predefined acceptable limits for variation.
- Delta checks are intended to detect either preanalytical or analytical errors in testing, such as specimen mix-up errors, diluted samples, or analyzer malfunction.[10]

33. A. The PT samples should be specifically marked and personally walked through the testing procedure by the laboratory director or his or her designee.
Rationale: PT samples should be entered into your laboratory's normal workflow and run by regular testing personnel (i.e., treated like a patient sample).
B. The PT sample should be split: one aliquot should be run in your laboratory and the other aliquot should be sent to a reference laboratory to ensure concordant results.
Rationale: PT samples should never be sent out to a reference laboratory or to any other laboratory.
C. The PT sample should be entered into your laboratory's workflow and tested and resulted as with any other patient specimen.
Rationale: This is the correct answer.
D. The PT sample should be treated as any other patient sample. If send-out is required as a reflex for this analyte, your laboratory should send it out as per protocol.
Rationale: If your laboratory protocol requires a reflex test, which is offered only at a reference laboratory as a send-out, the PT sample *should never* be sent out for analysis. Instead, check the box on the proficiency test result form that indicates "would send out" or "confirmatory testing not performed in house."
E. The PT sample should be run multiple times over multiple days and the values averaged to minimize error.
Rationale: PT samples should be evaluated as if they were routine patient samples. Unless your laboratory averages multiple runs to obtain a patient value, this is an incorrect answer.

Major points of discussion
- PT samples should never be sent out to another laboratory even if your laboratory's protocol calls for reflex testing at an outside laboratory.
- The purpose of PT is to ensure the accuracy and reliability of your laboratory with regard to other laboratories performing the same or comparable assays.
- To maintain a CLIA certificate, a laboratory must participate in a CLIA-approved PT program for all regulated moderate- and high-complexity tests performed under the CLIA certificate.
- If a moderate- or high-complexity analyte does not fall under the "regulated" category established by CLIA, the laboratory must establish a semiannual program by which accuracy and reliability are checked.[10]

34. A. Failure to attain the minimum satisfactory score for an analyte, test, subspecialty, or specialty for a testing event.

Rationale: This is the definition of an unsatisfactory PT performance.
B. Failure to submit the results of a testing event in the requisite amount of time.
Rationale: Although this is counted as a score of 0 for the analyte for that testing event and is, therefore, an unsatisfactory performance and/or an unsuccessful performance, this is not the correct definition.
C. A clerical error in reporting the results for a testing event.
Rationale: Although this is counted as an incorrect result and is, therefore, an unsatisfactory PT performance for the analyte in question and, depending on previous performance, may also be an unsuccessful performance, this is not the correct answer.
D. Repeated unsatisfactory test scores for an analyte or for the entire testing event in a particular specialty or subspecialty on two consecutive PT events or two of three testing events.
Rationale: This is the definition of unsuccessful participation/performance in PT.
E. This is not a term used in assessing performance in PT events.
Rationale: This is indeed a term used to express multiple unsatisfactory performances for an analyte or within a specialty/subspecialty.

Major points of discussion
- An unsuccessful performance/participation in PT means repeated unsatisfactory test scores for an analyte, or for the entire testing event in a particular specialty or subspecialty, on two consecutive PT events or two of three testing events.
- An unsatisfactory performance in PT means failure to attain the minimum satisfactory score for an analyte, test, subspecialty, or specialty for a testing event.
- Clerical errors in entering PT results are counted as incorrect results and, therefore, as unsatisfactory performance for the analyte in question.
- Failure to report the results of PT within the allotted time frame will cause the laboratory to receive a score of 0 for that event.
- If a laboratory receives a nonpassing score for an analyte, the laboratory must investigate the cause of the error and consider, implement, and document corrective actions.[10]

35. A. You should agree. To maintain CLIA certification, *all* assays performed in your laboratory must be evaluated in a CLIA-approved PT program.
Rationale: PT program registration is required only for a defined number of moderate- and high-complexity tests specified in CLIA '88 Subpart I (Proficiency Testing of Nonwaived Testing).
B. You should agree. Although PT is not required for waived tests, if a valid PT program exists, participation will help ensure your laboratory's accuracy in result reporting.
Rationale: This answer reflects the best laboratory medicine practice. Although PT is not required for waived tests, the purpose of PT is to ensure quality and accuracy. If a PT program is available and your laboratory can feasibly participate, it should.
C. You should disagree. After looking through the CLIA regulations for PT, you notice the analyte you are measuring

is not on the list of regulated analytes for which PT is required.

Rationale: This test is not subject to PT requirements because it is a waived test, not because it does not appear on the list of CLIA regulated analytes. "Regulated" analytes (defined under subpart I of CLIA regulations) are, by definition, tested using moderate- or high-complexity methods.

D. You should disagree. The FDA does not require PT for tests it deems waived.

Rationale: The FDA does not regulate PT; this is handled by CMS through CLIA.

E. You should disagree. PT will only highlight your laboratory's inaccuracy.

Rationale: The purpose of PT is to help a laboratory identify areas in which it needs improvement in terms of analytical accuracy.

Major points of discussion

- To maintain valid CLIA certification, your laboratory must enroll in PT programs for those moderate- and high-complexity tests listed in Subpart I of the CLIA regulations.
- FDA-waived tests need not participate in PT programs.
- The purpose of PT programs is to ensure quality, accuracy, and reliability of your laboratory results.
- CMS provides a list of approved PT programs in which your laboratory can enroll to meet PT regulatory criteria.
- PT participation is required for each CLIA certificate, not for each test site. Therefore, if you have multiple testing locations under one CLIA certificate, you need to register only for one PT program for any one regulated analyte.
- Importantly, even if a moderate- or high-complexity test is not listed as a regulated analyte in Subpart I, CLIA requires that the accuracy of the test be confirmed at least twice annually.[10]

36. A. Identifies a single cause of the error.
Rationale: A single cause of error is rarely identified. It is usually a system of errors that contributes to an adverse event.
B. Favors the subjective opinion of experts.
Rationale: An RCA should be supported by evidence.
C. Results in an executable and quantifiable solution(s).
Rationale: The solution(s) from an RCA should be executable and should be monitored by a quantitative method.
D. Seeks to identify and blame the specific person or group responsible.
Rationale: An RCA should not seek to place blame on any individual or group. Rather, it usually identifies multiple systemic errors that contribute to an event.
E. Uses the Ishikawa fishbone diagram.
Rationale: A fishbone diagram is a specific tool that can be, but is not always, used to identify specific reasons an error occurred.

Major points of discussion

- An RCA is a managerial tool that improves the quality of patient care by identifying errors that lead to an adverse event. It then seeks to define solutions.
- An RCA assumes that errors are best reduced by identifying and preventing the root cause(s) of an error.
- There are many methods and tools used in performing an RCA:

- Methods: Event and causal factor mapping, tree diagrams, etc.
- Tools: Ishikawa fishbone diagram, change analysis, Pareto analysis, etc

- All methods for performing RCAs have limitations. For example, a Pareto analysis requires data to be collected to track the frequency of certain errors. If the database is inaccurate or incomplete, the RCA will not result in an appropriate solution.
- All RCAs share common characteristics regardless of the method or tools that are used:
  1. The adverse event or the problem is clearly identified.
  2. No blame is placed on a single individual or group because adverse events are usually due to a chain of errors.
  3. Specific causes and effects are identified; typically it identifies a system of errors rather than a single cause.
  4. These causes and effects are supported by evidence.
  5. Results in a clearly defined, executable, quantifiable solution(s) that can be monitored quantitatively.

37. A. Master "Black Belts" and "Green Belts."
Rationale: Master "Black Belts" and "Green Belts" champion Six Sigma initiatives.
B. Merger and acquisitions attorneys.
Rationale: Attorneys may be needed for certain projects but are not required for implementation of Six Sigma.
C. Only the chief executive officer commitment is required.
Rationale: A commitment from all employees in the organization is required for Six Sigma to be effective.
D. Six Sigma consultants.
Rationale: Six Sigma consultants may be useful in initiatives but are not required.
E. Support of engineers.
Rationale: All employees of an organization must commit to Six Sigma, but not all organizations have engineers.

Major points of discussion

- Six Sigma is a method of quality management that was developed in the manufacturing industry. Six sigma (i.e., 6 SDs or 3.4/1,000,000) refers to the goal of minimizing the number of defects.
- Six Sigma seeks to minimize the number of defects by eliminating the cause(s) of the defects.
- This management style requires the full commitment of upper management, as well as all employees involved in the manufacturing process.
- Six Sigma is characterized by champions called "Black Belts" and "Green Belts," who lead initiatives to identify errors and develop executable solutions.
- Six Sigma has been applied to health care for cost savings and quality improvement. However, some experts feel that the method may not be as effective as it has been in the manufacturing industry.[22]

38. A. Billing Medicare and Medicaid for tests completed in a laboratory without a CLIA license.
B. Professional billing for laboratory tests without a physician-documented order that includes the physician's signature.
Rationale: Section 1877 of the Social Security Act does not address laboratory CLIA licensing or physician laboratory test ordering.

C. Physician patient referral to an entity for a designated health service from which the physician will financially benefit.
Rationale: This is commonly known as the Stark Law. This law prohibits a physician from making referrals for designated health services payable by Medicare to an entity with which he or she or an immediate family member has a financial relationship, unless a specific exception applies.
D. Performing genetic tests without a signed consent form.
E. Performing HIV tests without a signed consent form.
Rationale: Section 1877 of the Social Security Act does not address legal issues surrounding patient consent.

Major points of discussion

- The Stark Law was enacted in 1989. This law also makes it illegal to bill Medicare (or anyone else) for designated health services that arise as the result of a prohibited referral. If payments are issued, the entity in question must refund all payments collected that were associated with the prohibited referral(s).
- The following are considered designated health services: clinical laboratory services, physical and occupational therapy services, outpatient speech-language pathology services, radiology services, radiation therapy services, durable medical equipment and supplies, parenteral/ enteral nutrients and supplies, orthotics and prosthetic devices and supplies, home health services, outpatient prescription drugs, and inpatient and outpatient hospital services.
- There are three CLIA test categories: waived, moderate-complexity, and high-complexity testing.
- The most commonly issued CLIA certificate is a waived certificate.
- All laboratories must have a CLIA license to test patient samples legally.[9]

39. A. Volume error.
Rationale: It is unlikely that a volume error would produce this pattern of QC results.
B. User error.
Rationale: It is unlikely that user error would produce this pattern of QC results.
C. Random error.
Rationale: Eight sequential QC results falling 1.5 SDs above or below the mean expected value does not suggest random error but rather a systemic problem.
D. Imprecision.
Rationale: Imprecision would be suggested by a wide range of QC results for the same level of QC material.
E. A bias trend.
Rationale: Eight sequential results that exceed 1.5 SDs of the expected mean value suggest a bias trend in the results.

Major points of discussion

- The $8_{1.5s}$ Westgard rule means that eight sequential QC results were at least 1.5 SDs from one side of the expected mean value. This suggests that there is a systematic bias trend (either negative or positive, depending on the direction of the trend) in the QC results.
- Common causes for a bias trend in QC results include a need for recalibration of the analyzer or an error in reconstituting the QC material.

- A wide scatter of QC values suggests imprecision or poor reproducibility of results.
- Westgard rules are QC interpretive rules used by laboratories for statistical monitoring of the accuracy and precision of their assays.
- The Levey-Jennings control chart is used to plot QC data results.[23,31]

40. A. Change to using the 1_{3s} rule.
Rationale: This would definitely decrease your false-alert rate, but it would also decrease your sensitivity for error detection.
B. Change to using the 8_{1s} rule.
Rationale: This would decrease false-alert rates but would lack the real-time sensitivity for error detection. This rule also is made to detect systematic errors that may develop subtly over time.
C. Adopt a hybrid rule combining the 1_{3s} and 2_{2s} rules in a multirule scheme.
Rationale: This combines the sensitivity of a 2_{2s} rule and the false-alert rate of the 1_{3s} rule. Combination rules (i.e., multirules) are often used to combine the sensitivity and specificity of individual rules.
D. Rules are not necessary, and each QC value should be judged individually.
Rationale: Every laboratory should have clearly stated QC interpretation rules that it follows daily.
E. Ask the supervisor to change lots of QC material; the failure rate is likely due to a faulty batch.
Rationale: The supervisor's complaint was not lot specific but more of a trend she noticed in QC over time.

Major points of discussion

- The most popular way of expressing QC interpretive rules is the use of a shortened nomenclature introduced to laboratories by Westgard in 1981.
- Westgard developed power functions in 1979 to express the probability that a particular QC interpretive rule would detect systemic error biases at a variety of magnitudes.
- A 1_{2s} rule (i.e., one value >2 SDs above or below the mean), although very sensitive for detecting systematic error biases, even small ones, also has a fairly high false-alert rate.
- To improve the efficiency of QC interpretative rules, a combination of rules applied simultaneously may be considered (i.e., multirules).
- A combination such as the $1_{3s}/2_{2s}$ rule would trigger investigation if either rule is broken. This combines the sensitivity and specificity of each individual rule.[29]

41. A. Certificate of waiver.
Rationale: The most commonly issued type of CLIA certificate is the certificate of waiver. This allows providers to perform only waived tests and is effective for 2 years after the date of issue.
B. Certificate for provider-performed microscopy procedures.
Rationale: This is the second most commonly issued certificate. It is issued to providers that want to perform only approved microscopy procedures but no other moderately complex tests.

C. Certificate of registration.
D. Certificate of compliance.
Rationale: These two certificates are issued to laboratories that perform moderate- or high-complexity testing after inspection that determines their compliance with CLIA requirements.
E. Certificate of accreditation.
Rationale: This certificate is issued to laboratories accredited by an organization other than CLIA, such as the CAP.

Major points of discussion

- The CLIA was passed by Congress in 1988 for the purpose of establishing quality standards for laboratory testing.
- The number of laboratories issued a certificate of waiver has grown to more than 50% of the approximate 225,000 laboratories enrolled as of 2011.
- CLIA is user-fee funded; the biennial certificate fee is based on the type of certificate and the test volume of the performing entity.
- Provider-performed microscopy procedures are considered moderately complex.
- The certificate of compliance and certificate of accreditation are issued to laboratories that perform nonwaived (i.e., moderate- and/or high-complexity) testing. These two certificates also confer the ability to perform waived and provider-performed microscopy tests.[4,5]

42a. A. 12%.
Rationale: 12% carryover of this sample would correspond to a concentration of 0.6 mIU/mL.
B. 2%.
Rationale: Percent carryover equals [(Results from potentially contaminated low sample – Original results from the uncontaminated low sample)/(Original results from the uncontaminated sample)] multiplied by 100. In this example, it is $(5.1 - 5.0)/5.0 \times 100 = 2\%$.
C. 15%.
Rationale: 15% carryover of this sample would correspond to a concentration of 0.75 mIU/mL.
D. 10%.
Rationale: 10% carryover of this sample would correspond to a concentration of 0.5 mIU/mL.
E. 5%.
Rationale: 5% carryover of this sample would correspond to a concentration of 0.25 mIU/mL.

42b. **A. This amount of carryover is acceptable because the result of the potentially contaminated sample falls in the range of 5.0 to 5.4 mIU/mL.**
Rationale: The acceptable limit for the carryover study was determined to be 2 times the SD of the original low control result. The SD is 0.2 mIU/mL; therefore, the acceptable range is 5.0 to 5.4 mIU/mL. This corresponds to no more than an 8% increase over the original result of 5.0 mIU/mL.
B. This amount of carryover is acceptable because it is less than 10 mIU/mL.
Rationale: 10 mIU/mL is above the acceptable amount of carryover. The acceptable amount of carryover in this example was determined to be no greater than 0.4 mIU/mL. This is twice the SD of the low control result mean. This corresponds to an acceptable result value up to 0.4 mIU/mL above the "true" result.

C. This amount of carryover is acceptable because it is less than 15% of the original sample.
Rationale: 15% of the original sample corresponds to 0.75 mIU/mL (15% of 5.0), which is more than the acceptable amount of carryover.
D. This amount of carryover is not acceptable because it is more than 5% of the original sample.
Rationale: The amount of carryover is not greater than 5% of the original sample (0.1 mIU/mL of carryover corresponds to 2% of 5.0 mIU/mL).
E. This amount of carryover is not acceptable because it is more than 0.2 mIU/mL.
Rationale: This limit is too low.

Major points of discussion

- *Carryover* refers to the transfer of a quantity of an analyte from one reaction into the next subsequent reaction.
- Carryover of an analyte could potentially cause a false elevation in patient results and, therefore, should be assessed when validating a new test system, if applicable to the methodology.
- Accuracy can be assessed by measuring an analyte in reference material with a known concentration and comparing the result with the certified value.
- Precision is the agreement between result values obtained by repeat measurements of a quantity.
- The limit of detection is the lowest concentration of an analyte in a sample that can be reliably detected.[1,13,28]

43. A. Follow Universal Precautions when testing patient samples.
Rationale: Universal Precautions are not addressed in the CLIA requirements for the certificate of waiver.
B. Have a designated laboratory director who holds a medical degree.
Rationale: There is no special training or education required to apply for a certificate of waiver.
C. Follow the test manufacturer's instructions.
Rationale: The CLIA requirements for waived testing include enrolling in the CLIA program; paying the certificate fee every 2 years; following the manufacturer's instructions on how to perform the test; notifying the appropriate state agency of any changes in ownership, name, address, or directorship; and permitting inspections by the CMS.
D. Engage in CLIA-directed PT.
Rationale: PT is not required for waived tests.
E. Record all patient test results in an electronic format.
Rationale: Electronic test reporting is not required by CLIA.

Major points of discussion

- There are three levels of testing recognized by CLIA: waived, moderate complexity, and high complexity.
- The available CLIA certificates are the certificate of waiver, certificate for provider-performed microscopy procedures, certificate of registration, certificate of compliance, and certificate of accreditation.
- The CMS-approved laboratory accreditation organizations include the AABB, COLA, American Society for Histocompatibility and Immunogenetics, CAP, and The Joint Commission.

- Waived tests are defined as "simple laboratory examinations and procedures that have an insignificant risk of an erroneous result."
- The FDA is responsible for determining the level of test complexity for approved testing platforms.[8]

44. A. The FDA.
Rationale: The FDA does not directly oversee the CLIA program; however, the FDA is responsible for classifying laboratory test systems as waived, moderate complexity, or high complexity.
B. The AABB.
Rationale: The AABB publishes standard guidelines for blood banks, not general clinical laboratories.
C. The CAP.
Rationale: The CAP does not oversee the CLIA program. CAP does publish laboratory standards and offers a laboratory accreditation program, which is a voluntary program and is separate from CLIA.
D. The Joint Commission.
Rationale: The Joint Commission does not oversee CLIA. The Joint Commission does publish laboratory standards and offers an accreditation program for laboratories, which is a voluntary program and separate from CLIA.
E. The CMS.
Rationale: The CMS oversees the enforcement of the CLIA regulations.

Major points of discussion
- CLIA was passed by Congress in 1988.
- The CLIA program is designed to ensure laboratory testing quality.
- The CMS oversees the operation of the CLIA program.
- The CMS recognizes additional accrediting agencies and will issue a certificate of accreditation to laboratories that receive accreditation from the AABB, American Osteopathic Association, American Society for Histocompatibility and Immunogenetics, COLA, CAP, and/or The Joint Commission.
- There are five types of CLIA certificates: certificate of waiver, certificate for provider-performed microscopy procedures, certificate of registration, certificate of compliance, and certificate of accreditation.[4,7]

45. A. Waived tests approved by the FDA.
Rationale: CLIA requires entities performing waived tests to follow the manufacturer's instructions. Performance verification is not required.
B. Provider-performed microscopy tests approved by the FDA.
Rationale: Performance verification is not required for provider-performed microscopy procedures.
C. Moderate-complexity tests approved by the FDA.
Rationale: The Quality System Regulations became effective in 2003. These regulations require laboratories to verify the manufacturer's stated performance for accuracy, precision, reportable range, and reference ranges for moderate-complexity tests (other than provider-performed microscopy) that the laboratory wishes to perform. This helps ensure that the test performs as the manufacturer intended.
D. Waived, provider-performed microscopy, and moderate-complexity tests approved by the FDA.

Rationale: Performance verification is not required for waived or provider-performed microscopy tests.
E. All FDA-approved tests used for patient care.
Rationale: Performance verification is not required for tests classified as waived.

Major points of discussion
- CLIA Quality System Regulations were implemented in 2003.
- Measuring accuracy determines whether the test results are correct. This can be tested by analyzing samples with known concentrations.
- Precision ensures that comparable results are obtained when the same sample is tested repeatedly.
- The reportable range of a test is the result range that is accurate. Values above or below this range should not be reported.
- Records of performance verification of the test system must be retained while the test is in use and for 2 years after discontinuing the test.[12,13]

46. A. Pinworm examination.
Rationale: This is a provider-performed microscopy test.
B. Fecal occult blood examination.
Rationale: Fecal occult blood examination is a waived test. Other common waived tests include urine pregnancy tests by visual color comparison, blood glucose tests that use glucose monitoring devices cleared by the FDA for home use, and dipstick or tablet reagent urinalysis. All of the other choices are categorized as provider-performed microscopy procedures. These include vaginal, cervical, or skin wet mounts; potassium hydroxide preparations; pinworm examinations; fern tests; postcoital qualitative examinations of vaginal or cervical mucus; microscopic urinalysis; fecal leukocyte examination; semen analysis for presence and/or motility of sperm; and nasal smears for eosinophils.
C. Urine sediment examination.
D. Fecal leukocyte examination.
E. The fern test.
Rationale: These are provider-performed microscopy tests.

Major points of discussion
- Waived tests are defined as "simple laboratory examinations and procedures that have an insignificant risk of an erroneous result."
- The FDA determines the classification category for all CLIA-regulated tests.
- CLIA-regulated tests fall into one of three categories: waived, moderate complexity, or high complexity.
- Provider-performed microscopy procedures are considered moderate-complexity tests and include vaginal, cervical, or skin wet mounts; potassium hydroxide preparations; pinworm examinations; fern tests; postcoital qualitative examinations of vaginal or cervical mucus; microscopic urinalysis; fecal leukocyte examination; semen analysis for presence and/or motility of sperm; and nasal smears for eosinophils.
- A certificate for provider-performed microscopy procedures is available from CLIA and confers the permission to perform any waived test, or any moderate-

complexity test, as long as it is a provider-performed microscopy procedure.[4,7,11]

47. A. 1 year.
B. 2 years.
C. 5 years.
D. 10 years.
E. Indefinitely.
Rationale: According to the Code of Federal Regulations, Title 42, section 493.1105 Standard: Retention requirements, laboratories must retain cytology slide preparations for at least 5 years from the date of examination.

Major points of discussion

- According to CLIA, laboratories must retain test requisitions, PT records, testing standard operating procedures after discontinuation, and quality system assessment records (i.e., QC records) for at least 2 years.
- Histopathology slide preparations must be retained for 10 years after the date of examination.
- The CAP requires blood bank QC records be kept for a minimum of 5 years.
- The CAP requires retention of QC records for the general laboratory for 2 years.
- Flow cytometry plots and histograms must be kept for 10 years.[2,27]

48. A. 1 year.
B. 2 years.
C. 5 years.
Rationale: Cytopathology slide preparations must be retained for 5 years from the date of examination.
D. 10 years.
Rationale: Histopathology slide preparations must be retained for 10 years after the date of examination.
E. Indefinitely.
Rationale for A, B, and E: According to the Code of Federal Regulations, Title 42, section 493.1105 Standard: Retention requirements, laboratories must retain or be able to retrieve a copy of the original test report (including final, preliminary, and corrected reports) for at least 2 years after the date of reporting.

Major points of discussion

- Additional retention regulations state that laboratories must retain test requisitions, PT records, test retired standard operating procedures, and quality system assessment records (i.e., QC records) for at least 2 years.
- The CAP requires all peripheral blood smears/body fluid smears to be retained for 7 days.
- The CAP requires all stained slides for microbiology (i.e., Gram stains) be kept for 7 days.[2,27]

49. A. Analyze samples from healthy subjects and determine the 95% prediction interval.
Rationale: This determines the reference range.
B. Analyze samples with no measurable analyte spiked with low concentrations of analyte.
Rationale: This determines the analytical sensitivity of the test—that is, the lower limit of detection.
C. Analyze samples with a high value followed by samples with a low value.
Rationale: This assesses for analyte carryover.
D. Analyze a sample 20 times and determine the mean and SD.
Rationale: This assesses the precision of the test.
E. Compare samples between the test method and a reference method.
Rationale: Accuracy refers to how close a measured value is to the actual concentration of the analyte in the sample.

Major points of discussion

- Accuracy can be assessed by measuring an analyte in reference material and comparing the result with the known certified concentration.
- Accuracy can also be assessed by comparing the test results from one method with the results from a reference method, using the same samples.
- The analytical range of an assay refers to the interval between the highest and lowest concentrations of the analyte in which precision, accuracy, and linearity have been demonstrated to be acceptable.
- The limit of detection is the lowest concentration of an analyte that can be reliably detected.[13,18]

References

1. Araujo P. Key aspects of analytical method validation and linearity evaluation. J Chromatogr B Analyt Technol Biomed Life Sci 2009;877:2224–2234.
2. College of American Pathologists. Available at www.cap.org/.
3. Centers for Medicare and Medicaid Services. Beneficiary Notices Initiative (BNI). Available at www.cms.gov/BNI/02_ABN.asp.
4. Centers for Medicare and Medicaid Services. CLIA Update, December 2013. Available at www.cms.gov/CLIA/downloads/statupda.pdf.
5. Centers for Medicare and Medicaid Services. Clinical Laboratory Improvement Amendments (CLIA). Available at www.cms.gov/CLIA/08_Certificate_of_%20Waiver_Laboratory_Project.asp.
6. Centers for Medicare and Medicaid Services. Equivalent Quality Control Procedures Brochure #4. Available at www.cms.gov/CLIA/downloads/6066bk.pdf.
7. Centers for Medicare and Medicaid Services. Equivalent Quality Control Procedures Brochure. How to Obtain a CLIA Certificate. Available at www.cms.gov/CLIA/downloads/HowObtainCLIACertificate.pdf.
8. Centers for Medicare and Medicaid Services. How to Obtain a CLIA Certificate of Waiver. Available at www.cms.gov/CLIA/downloads/HowObtainCertificateofWaiver.pdf.
9. Centers for Medicare and Medicaid Services. CMS.gov. 2011. Physician Self Referral. Available at www.cms.gov/Medicare/Fraud-and-Abuse/PhysicianSelfReferral/index.html?redirect=/physicianselfreferral/.
10. Centers for Medicare and Medicaid Services. Proficiency Testing: Dos and Don'ts. Available at www.cms.gov/CLIA/downloads/CLIAbrochure8.pdf.
11. Centers for Medicare and Medicaid Services. Tests Granted Waived Status Under CLIA. Available at www.cms.gov/CLIA/downloads/waivetbl.pdf.
12. Centers for Medicare and Medicaid Services. Updated Regulations Brochure #1. Available at www.cms.gov/CLIA/downloads/6063bk.pdf.
13. Centers for Medicare and Medicaid Services. Verification of Performance Specifications Brochure #2. Available at www.cms.gov/CLIA/downloads/6064bk.pdf.

14. Danzis SD, Flannery EJ. *In vitro diagnostic: a complete regulatory guide.* Washington, DC: Food and Drug Law Institute, 2010, pp. 115–123.

15. U.S.Department of Labor. Leave Benefits: Family & Medical Leave. Available at www.dol.gov/dol/topic/benefits-leave/fmla.htm.

16. ECRI Institute. Evidence-based Practice Center. Quality, regulation and clinical utility of laboratory-developed molecular tests. Available at www.cms.gov/Medicare/Coverage/DeterminationProcess/downloads/id72TA.pdf.

17. FDA Rule on Analyte Specific Reagents 62 FR 62243. Federal Register Nov. 21, 1997;62:62243–62249.

18. Feinberg M. Validation of analytical methods based on accuracy profiles. J Chromatogr A 2007;1158:174–183.

19. U.S. Department of Health and Human Services. Food and Drug Administration. Guidance for Industry: Bioanalytical Method Validation, May 2001. Available at www.fda.gov/downloads/Drugs/GuidanceComplianceRegulatoryInformation/Guidances/ucm070107.pdf.

20. International Organization for Standardization. Available at www.iso.org/iso/home.htm.

21. Kazmierczak SC. Laboratory quality control: using patient data to assess analytical performance. Clin Chem Lab Med 2005;41:617–627.

22. Llopis MA, Trujillo G, Llovet MI, et al. Quality indicators and specifications for key analytical-extranalytical processes in the clinical laboratory. Five years' experience using the Six Sigma concept. Clin Chem Lab Med 2011;49:463–470.

23. McPherson RA, Pincus MR. Henry's clinical diagnosis and management by laboratory methods. 22nd ed. Philadelphia: Elsevier; 2011.

24. Centers for Medicare and Medicaid Services. Eligibility. Available at www.medicaid.gov/Medicaid-CHIP-Program-Information/By-Topics/Eligibility/Eligibility.html.

25. Centers for Medicare & Medicaid Services. Medicaid information by topic. Available at www.medicaid.gov/Medicaid-CHIP-Program-Information/By-Topics/By-Topic.html.

26. U.S. Department of Labor. Occupational Safety and Health Administration. United States Department of Labor. Available at www.osha.gov/index.html.

27. Code of Federal Regulations, Public Health. Standard: Retention requirements. Title 42, Pt. 493.1105, 2003.

28. Rambla-Alegre M, Esteve-Romero J, Carda-Broch S. Is it really necessary to validate an analytical method or not? That is the question. J Chromatogr A 1232:101–109, 2012.

29. Westgard JO. Basic QC, practices. 3rd edition. Madison, WI: Westgard QC; 2010.

30. Westgard JO, Groth T. Power functions for statistical control rules. Clin Chem 1979;25:863–869.

CHAPTER 3

GENERAL LABORATORY:
Instrumentation, Analytic Techniques, Automation, Point of Care Testing, and Informatics

Alexander Kratz, Michael A. Pesce, Jeffrey S. Jhang

QUESTIONS

1. Which one of the following statements best describes the requirements of the College of American Pathologists (CAP) regarding competency assessment for all operators for waived and nonwaived point-of-care tests (POCTs)?
   A. Within the first 4 weeks after hire and annually thereafter.
   B. Every 6 months during the first 2 years and annually thereafter.
   C. Every 6 months.
   D. Before the operator performs patient testing, semiannually during the first year, and annually thereafter.
   E. Before the operator performs patient testing.

2. Chemiluminescence immunoassays can be used to measure a wide variety of biomarkers. Which one of the following best describes a chemiluminescence assay?
   A. Measurement of the amount of light absorbed at two different wavelengths.
   B. Measurement of the amount of emitted light after a molecule is chemically excited from the ground to the excited state.
   C. Measurement of the amount of emitted light after a molecule is biologically excited from the ground to the excited state.
   D. Measurement of the amount of emitted light when a molecule in a triplet state returns to the ground state.
   E. Measurement of the amount of emitted light after a molecule is excited from the ground to the excited state by a short pulse of light.

3. The cloned enzyme donor immunoassay (CEDIA) is a homogeneous assay that is used to quantify small molecules. The reagents consist of two different inactive fragments of the enzyme beta-galactosidase. One fragment is bound to the antigen and is known as the enzyme donor (ED), whereas the other fragment is the enzyme acceptor (EA). The ED fragment must combine with the EA fragment to produce an active enzyme. In the CEDIA assay, which one of the following best explains how the labeled antigen that is bound to the antibody is differentiated from the labeled antigen that is not bound to the antibody?

A. The enzyme-labeled antigen that is bound to the antibody is inhibited by changing the pH of the solution.
B. The enzyme-labeled antigen that is bound to the antibody reacts at a slower rate with the EA to form the active enzyme than the enzyme-labeled antigen that is not bound to the antibody.
C. The enzyme-labeled antigen that is bound to the antibody reacts with the EA to form the active enzyme.
D. The enzyme-labeled antigen that is bound to the antibody is physically separated from the enzyme-labeled antigen that is not bound to the antibody and reacts with the EA to form the active enzyme.
E. The enzyme-labeled antigen that is bound to the antibody is inhibited from reacting with the EA. The enzyme-labeled antigen that is not bound to the antibody reacts with the EA to form the active enzyme.

4. The majority of laboratory testing errors occur at which one of the following stages?
   A. During the ordering of tests.
   B. During the preanalytical phase of testing.
   C. During the analytical phase of testing.
   D. During the reporting of the test results.
   E. During physician interpretation of the test results.

5. Which one of the following is the best definition of the Stokes shift?
   A. Quenching of fluorescence in the excited state.
   B. Difference between the wavelengths of the excitation light and emitted light in a fluorescence assay.
   C. Rate of formation of an antibody-antigen complex.
   D. Difference between detection time of the internal standard and the compound of interest in a high-performance liquid chromatography (HPLC) assay.
   E. Distance between the solvent front and the compound of interest in a thin-layer chromatography (TLC) assay.

6. Time-resolved fluorescence immunoassays have been used to measure serum hormone levels. Which one of the following reasons best describes the advantage of time-resolved

fluorescence immunoassays over conventional fluorescence immunoassays?

A. The fluorescence lifetime of the molecule is decreased, resulting in an increase in analytical sensitivity and a decrease in background fluorescence.

B. The fluorescence lifetime of the molecule is increased, resulting in an increase in analytical sensitivity and a decrease in background fluorescence.

C. The small Stokes shift that is observed with time-resolved fluorescent immunoassays increases the sensitivity of the assay.

D. Fluorescence measurements are rapid, which reduces the background fluorescence.

E. Fluorescence is quenched, which reduces the background fluorescence.

7. A 57-year-old man arrived in the emergency department with acute chest pain. He has a history of heavy alcohol use, hypertension, and hyperlipidemia. His electrocardiogram was normal throughout his hospital stay. A chest radiograph showed clear lung fields and no evidence of acute cardiopulmonary pathology. Serum levels of troponin I were measured with a two-site immunometric assay to determine if there was cardiac damage. On admission, his troponin I level was 41 μg/L, and on day 2, his troponin I level was 40 μg/L (reference range: <0.04 μg/L). Total serum levels of creatine kinase (CK) activity and CK-MB were normal on both days. Which one of the following provides the best explanation of why this patient's troponin I level was elevated?

A. The hook effect caused a false-positive troponin I result.

B. Heterophile antibodies interfered with the troponin I assay, causing a false-positive result.

C. The patient was correctly diagnosed with an acute myocardial infarction.

D. The patient was correctly diagnosed with congestive heart failure.

E. There was cross-reactivity of troponin T with the troponin I method.

8. The enzyme-multiplied immunoassay technique (EMIT) is a homogeneous immunoassay that is used to measure low molecular weight molecules. In an EMIT assay, which one of the following best explains how the enzyme-labeled antigen that is bound to the antibody is distinguished from the non–antibody-bound, free enzyme-labeled antigen?

A. The enzyme-labeled antigen activity is inhibited by changing the pH of the reaction.

B. The antibody-bound enzyme-labeled antigen complex is not as stable as the free, non–antibody-bound enzyme-labeled antigen complex, and the enzyme activity is measured by a kinetic rate reaction.

C. Antibody binding to the enzyme-labeled antigen enhances the enzyme activity.

D. Antibody binding to the enzyme-labeled antigen sterically inhibits the enzyme activity.

E. The free, non–antibody-bound enzyme-labeled antigen is fluorescent.

9. The fluorescent polarization immunoassay (FPIA) is a homogeneous assay for measuring low molecular weight molecules, such as drugs. In the quantification of a drug level by FPIA, which one of the following best explains how the non–antibody-bound fluorescent-labeled drug is

differentiated from the antibody-bound fluorescent-labeled drug?

A. No fluorescence is observed when antibody binds to the fluorescent-labeled drug.

B. Rotation of the non–antibody-bound fluorescent-labeled drug is slower than the antibody-bound fluorescent-labeled drug and depolarizes the emitted light.

C. The antibody-bound fluorescent-labeled drug emits less polarized light than the non–antibody-bound fluorescent-labeled drug.

D. The antibody-bound fluorescent-labeled drug emits polarized light. The non–antibody-bound fluorescent labeled drug depolarizes the emitted light.

E. Rotation of the non–antibody-bound fluorescent-labeled drug is faster than the antibody-bound fluorescent-labeled drug and emits more polarized light.

10. The presence of heterophile antibodies, which usually are human anti-mouse antibodies (HAMA), may interfere with the measurement of an analyte using a competitive binding immunoassay. Which one of the following is the most likely cause of the erroneous analytical result?

A. Binding of the HAMA to the analyte that is being measured, thereby causing a falsely elevated result.

B. Binding of the HAMA to the analyte that is being measured, thereby causing a falsely lower result.

C. Binding of the HAMA to the capture antibody, thereby causing a falsely elevated result.

D. Binding of the HAMA to the capture antibody, thereby causing a falsely lower result.

E. Binding of HAMA to the labeled analyte, thereby causing a falsely lower result.

11a. An 18-year-old girl presents to the emergency department with a 2-week history of nausea, vomiting, and vaginal spotting. Serum human chorionic gonadotropin (hCG) was measured with a one-step, two-site immunometric assay and was 20 IU/L (reference range: <25 IU/L). In this case, the physician called the laboratory director and suggested that the hCG result was incorrect because the patient was diagnosed as having a hydatidiform mole and should have an extremely high circulating hCG level. Which one of the following best explains this false-negative serum hCG result?

A. Interference by heterophile antibodies (i.e., HAMAs).

B. The hook effect.

C. A matrix effect.

D. Inhibition of hCG by maternal antibodies.

E. Binding of hCG to human immunoglobulin (Ig) G.

11b. In this case, which one of the following is the best approach the laboratory can take to ensure that the correct hCG result is reported (which turned out to be an hCG level of 3,500,000 IU/L)?

A. Repeat the hCG assay using another serum sample.

B. Measure the hCG level using a different method.

C. Precipitate the interfering heterophile antibodies in the sample using polyethylene glycol and remeasure the hCG level.

D. Perform a serial dilution of the sample and remeasure the hCG levels using the diluted samples.

E. Add mouse immunoglobulins to the sample to remove the interference from heterophile antibodies and remeasure the hCG level.

12. Which one of the following best describes reflectance photometry?
    A. Reflectance photometry is used to detect serum electrolyte concentrations.
    B. Reflectance photometry is used in DNA testing.
    C. Reflectance photometry measures the light intensity emitted from the excited state of the molecule.
    D. In reflectance photometry, there is a linear relationship between the intensity of light reflected and concentration of the analyte.
    E. In reflectance photometry, the sample concentration is calculated by comparing the reflectance of a white standard to the light reflected by the sample.

13. A falsely increased result for a given analyte in samples containing a heterophile antibody, usually a HAMA, can be obtained with some two-site immunometric assays. This can best be explained by which one of the following mechanisms?
    A. Binding of HAMA to the capture antibody.
    B. Binding of HAMA to the analyte being measured.
    C. Binding of HAMA to both the capture antibody and the labeled antibody.
    D. Binding of the HAMA to the labeled antibody.
    E. Binding of the HAMA to both the capture antibody and the analyte that is being measured.

14. Which one of the following statements is true about the activated clotting time (ACT)?
    A. The test is sensitive to deficiencies in coagulation factors in the extrinsic and final common pathways.
    B. The test is sensitive to deficiencies in coagulation factors in the intrinsic and final common pathways.
    C. The test is performed on plasma.
    D. Clotting times are usually between 50 and 100 seconds.
    E. The test is often used for managing outpatients treated with Coumadin.

15. Heparin therapy during cardiac surgery can be monitored using either the ACT or heparin assays. Which one of the following statements best describes the principle(s) on which these two assays are based?
    A. Both assays are based on adding a strong contact activator of the clotting cascade to whole blood. The only difference is the amount of activator added.
    B. Both assays are based on adding large amounts of thromboplastin to the sample.
    C. The ACT assay is based on adding a strong contact activator of the clotting cascade to whole blood. The heparin assay is based on titrating the amount of protamine needed to neutralize the heparin present in the sample.
    D. The ACT assay is based on adding kaolin or Celite to the sample. The heparin assay is based on adding glass beads to the sample.
    E. The ACT assay is based on adding a strong contact activator of the clotting cascade to whole blood. The heparin assay use antibodies specific for heparin to determine heparin levels.

16. Which one of the following statements is true about the microscopic detection of amniotic fluid crystallization?
    A. It is classified as a waived test.
    B. It is positive in the presence of amniotic fluid at any gestational age.

C. It is more sensitive for the presence of amniotic fluid than the nitrazine paper test.
D. It is more specific for the presence of amniotic fluid than the nitrazine paper test.
E. It is rendered unreliable by the presence of even small amounts of blood.

17. Which one of the following is the best example of an advantage of point-of-care testing (POCT), as opposed to testing in a centralized laboratory?
    A. Improved turnaround time for the test.
    B. Enhanced competency of the operator performing the assay.
    C. Decreased test cost.
    D. Improved test accuracy.
    E. Improved test precision.

18. Many modern POCT devices have built-in barcode readers. Which one of the following best describes the purpose of these barcode readers?
    A. Patient identification only.
    B. Operator identification only.
    C. Reagent and/or cartridge identification only.
    D. Quality control material identification only.
    E. Identification of patients, operators, reagents, cartridges, and quality control material.

19. The appropriate definition, reporting, and documentation of critical values are important issues in the management of clinical laboratories. Which one of the following statements best describes critical values in the context of POCT?
    A. The concept of critical values is not applicable to POCT because a care provider usually either performs the test or is present at the testing site.
    B. Critical values from POCTs performed in hospitals are the responsibility of the performing clinical care provider, not of the clinical laboratory.
    C. Critical values in POCT, and the intervention taken in response to them, must be documented.
    D. Critical values in POCT are never repeated.
    E. The documentation of critical values from POCT instruments always requires a separate entry in the patient's medical record.

20. POCT programs in hospitals are routinely inspected by which one of the following?
    A. The Department of Health of the state in which the hospital is located.
    B. A "deemed" organization, such as The Joint Commission or the College of American Pathologists.
    C. The Centers for Medicare and Medicaid Services.
    D. A professional organization, such as the American Association for Clinical Chemistry.
    E. The Food and Drug Administration.

21. Which one of the following statements best describes the use of POC glucose meters?
    A. They should not be used to manage diabetes because they are not sufficiently accurate.
    B. They should not be used to screen for diabetes.
    C. They should not be used to diagnose diabetes.
    D. Their results are not affected by lipemia.
    E. They all use the same chemical reaction for measuring glucose.

22. According to the Clinical Laboratory Improvement Amendments of 1988 (CLIA'88), POCT programs must keep records of all quality control activities for which one of the following time intervals?
    A. At least 2 years.
    B. At least 1 year.
    C. As long as the program is active.
    D. At least 5 years.
    E. For the amount of time required by state law.

23. Many modern POCT instruments can be connected to a hospital's data network. The connection can be either through docking stations or through a wireless connection. Which one of the following currently represents the best advantage of a wireless connection versus a cable-based docking connection?
    A. Setting up wireless connections is always cheaper.
    B. A wireless network is safer.
    C. Wireless connections provide faster availability of results in the electronic medical record.
    D. The wireless connection can be bidirectional and allow both uploading of patient data and physician orders to the POCT device.
    E. A wireless connection can be turned off more easily if the security of the network has been compromised.

24. Provider-performed microscopy procedures are tests performed by a health care provider using a microscope. Which one of the following statements best describes how these procedures are usually performed?
    A. After the patient leaves the provider's office.
    B. By physicians and nurses.
    C. For the determination of white blood cell differentials in peripheral blood smears.
    D. On specimens that require only limited sample handling or processing.
    E. With bright-field, fluorescence, or phase-contrast microscopy.

25. The nitrazine paper test is used to detect the presence of amniotic fluid and to confirm the premature rupture of membranes. Which one of the following is a true statement about this test?
    A. The nitrazine paper test has a wide pH range.
    B. The nitrazine paper test has a sensitivity and specificity of greater than 95%.
    C. The nitrazine paper test has a sensitivity of 40% and a specificity of greater than 75%.
    D. The nitrazine paper test has a sensitivity of 95% and a specificity of greater than 40%.
    E. The reasons for false-positive nitrazine tests are unknown.

26. Many POCT analyzers use conductivity-based methods for determining hemoglobin and hematocrit. Which one of the following best describes the major limitation of this method compared with the optical method?
    A. Conductivity-based methods take longer to perform than optical methods.
    B. Conductivity-based methods are more difficult to calibrate than optical methods.
    C. Conductivity-based methods can be significantly influenced by plasma composition, including electrolyte and protein concentrations.
    D. Conductivity-based methods are less accurate at higher hematocrit levels.
    E. Conductivity-based methods are less accurate at lower hematocrit levels.

27. Which one of the following statements best describes the relationship between hematocrit and POCT blood glucose measurements?
    A. A high hematocrit leads to underestimation of blood glucose levels; a low hematocrit leads to overestimation of blood glucose levels.
    B. A high hematocrit leads to overestimation of blood glucose levels; a low hematocrit leads to underestimation of blood glucose levels.
    C. High and low hematocrit levels both lead to overestimation of blood glucose levels.
    D. High and low hematocrit levels both lead to underestimation of blood glucose levels.
    E. There is no effect of hematocrit on blood glucose determination using POCT devices.

28. Which one of the following statements best describes the limitation of both thromboelastography and thromboelastometry?
    A. They do not measure platelet function and platelet count.
    B. They do not measure fibrinogen levels.
    C. They do not measure the final common pathway of the coagulation cascade.
    D. They cannot be performed on citrated blood samples.
    E. Results obtained with these methods often do not correlate well with results obtained by standard coagulation tests, such as the prothrombin time and the partial thromboplastin time.

29. Hospital-wide electronic order entry systems with onsite label printing and specimen collection scanning facilitate electronic capture of various time element(s) of the preanalytical process. Which one of the following best describes what is possible using this approach?
    A. Capturing accession times.
    B. Capturing order and collection times.
    C. Capturing critical value result times.
    D. Identifying result corrections and capturing result update times.
    E. Capturing accession, order, and collection times.

30. The clinical staff members at your hospital complain that it takes too long to receive laboratory test results from the primary reference laboratory you use. You investigate and determine that the reference laboratory faxes results to your laboratory in a timely fashion; however, due to your own staffing issues, there are major delays in the transcription of these results into your laboratory information system (LIS). You determine that direct electronic interfacing of your LIS with the reference laboratory would eliminate these delays. However, hospital administration informs you that the money needed for this interface is not available in the current budget. Which one of the following contains the best arguments you should make to hospital administration?
    A. Electronic interfacing of the LIS with the reference laboratory will decrease the number of tests sent to the reference laboratory, thereby saving the hospital money.

B. Electronic interfacing of the LIS with the reference laboratory will eliminate the need for laboratory employees to manually transcribe results; this will reduce overtime and/or staffing costs and, thereby, save the hospital money. In addition, by decreasing the turnaround times for these results, patients may be discharged faster and the average length of stay may decrease, thereby allowing the hospital to improve revenue.

C. Electronic interfacing of the LIS with the reference laboratory will decrease courier costs.

D. Electronic interfacing of the LIS with the reference laboratory will decrease the time required to transport samples to the reference laboratory.

E. Electronic interfacing of the LIS with the reference laboratory will increase transcription errors in preanalytical functions in your laboratory.

31. A byte is a unit of measurement for information storage on computers. How many unique combinations of letters, numbers, or special characters can 1 byte produce?
    A. 2.
    B. 8.
    C. 64.
    D. 128.
    E. 256.

32. Which one of the following is an advantage of adding computerized physician order entry (CPOE) to an existing electronic health record (EHR) system versus implementing a new EHR with CPOE?
    A. Faster implementation.
    B. Greater cost of supporting an older system.
    C. Greater disruption of operations.
    D. Greater variety of options.
    E. Increased number of user devices required.

33. Which one of the following would be the final step in purchasing a new LIS?
    A. Determine functional requirements.
    B. Form a working group.
    C. Negotiate the contract.
    D. Send out a request for information (RFI).
    E. Send out a request for proposals (RFP).

34. If all power sources to a computer are turned off, which one of the following storage devices is most likely to lose its data?
    A. Compact disc.
    B. Hard disk drive.
    C. Solid-state drive.
    D. Random-access memory (RAM).
    E. Read-only memory (ROM).

35. Which one of the following is an example of an output device?
    A. Camera.
    B. Keyboard.
    C. Monitor.
    D. Mouse.
    E. Scanner.

36. Which one of the following is the best example of an input device?
    A. Hard drive.
    B. Label printer.

C. LCD projector.
D. Monitor.
E. Scanner.

37. In your laboratory, the Cockcroft-Gault equation for creatinine clearance is calculated in the laboratory information system and reported along with the serum creatinine. Which one of the following best describes how accuracy checks for calculations should be performed?
    A. Accuracy of the calculations and reports should be reviewed on a periodic basis.
    B. Accuracy of the calculations and reports need to be checked only when a system change is made.
    C. Calculations shared by multiple hospitals using the same laboratory information should be checked by every site.
    D. Checks of calculation accuracy do not have to be performed if calculations are made by middleware.
    E. Checks of calculation accuracy do not have to be performed if calculations are made by the analyzer.

38. Which one of the following best describes the purpose of Logical Observation Identifiers Names and Codes (LOINC)?
    A. Links human-readable terms to concepts.
    B. Standard used for the transfer of information associated with blood transfusion.
    C. Communications protocol used for sending and receiving data across the Internet.
    D. Seventh level of the seven-layer communications model for open systems interconnection.
    E. Universal identifiers for laboratory and other clinical observations.

39. Which one of the following best describes the main function of the Massachusetts General Hospital Utility Multi-Programming System (MUMPS)?
    A. It is a utility software to optimize a computer system.
    B. It allocates computer resources to more than one application (i.e., multitasking).
    C. It is an Internet protocol.
    D. It is a laboratory information system.
    E. It is a programming language.

40. Which one of the following applications is best solved by a neural network?
    A. Autoverification.
    B. Delta check.
    C. Calculations.
    D. Image-based white blood cell differential.
    E. Reflex test ordering.

41. Which one of the following is the preferred method for inputting data into an electronic health record (EHR)?
    A. Automated interface to other systems.
    B. Free text manual data entry.
    C. Scanning documents with subsequent optical character recognition translation.
    D. Structured form manual data entry.
    E. Transcription of physician dictation.

42. Which one of the following represents the best advantage of an EHR over a paper-based system?
    A. Smaller financial investment.

B. Fewer organizational challenges.

C. Catastrophic loss of all patient data.

D. Smaller time commitment for physician entry.

E. Increased availability of records.

43. Which one of the following best describes the Health Information Technology for Economic and Clinical Health (HITECH) Act?

A. Assigns the National Institute of Standards and Technology (NIST) to manage all federal, nonmilitary information systems.

B. Promotes the adoption and meaningful use of electronic health records.

C. Protects identifiable patient information from being used to identify patient safety events.

D. Requires all federal employees to take an information security awareness program.

E. Requires federal agencies to develop, document, and implement security of information systems.

44. Which one of the following best describes the seventh level of the seven-layer communications model for Open Systems Interconnection (OSI)?

A. Application layer.

B. Data layer.

C. Network layer.

D. Physical layer.

E. Session layer.

45. Packet-filtering routers and an application gateway are two types of firewalls. Which one of the following represents the best advantage of packet-filtering over application gateway firewalls?

A. Easier auditing of incoming traffic.

B. Less processing overhead.

C. Easier logging of incoming traffic.

D. Better security.

E. Ability to relay packets without examining them.

46. Which one of the following best describes the purpose of the Federal Information Security Management Act of 2002 (FISMA)?

A. Assigns the NIST to create a national standard for protecting health care information against cyber attacks.

B. Establishes national standards for the security and maintenance of confidentiality of protected health information.

C. Requires all EHRs to maintain a log of users who access a health record and what the user accessed.

D. Requires federal agencies to develop and implement plans to ensure information and information system security.

E. Requires all hospitals to be certified by a federal agency prior to implementing an EHR.

47. Middleware versions must have a short cycle time to adjust to rapid changes in which one of the following?

A. OSI.

B. LIS upgrades.

C. Instrument interface engine upgrades.

D. User-defined expert rules.

E. Server hardware upgrades.

48. Which one of the following issues must be resolved before implementation of total laboratory automation?

A. Multiple different types of specimen containers are used throughout the hospital.

B. Many samples arrive hand-labeled accompanied by a paper requisition.

C. The available capital budget does not contain enough funds to purchase the automation line.

D. The Laboratory Information System (LIS) assigns the same specimen number to all specimens collected from a single patient phlebotomy.

E. The laboratory desires to continue to use instrumentation from different vendors in different sections of the laboratory.

49. Which one of the following represents the best reason to implement total laboratory automation in a clinical laboratory?

A. It does not require a major financial investment.

B. Little planning is required for implementation.

C. It can increase production capacity severalfold without adding space or personnel.

D. Usually, no architectural work is required.

E. Organizational changes are usually not required.

ANSWERS

1. A. Within the first 4 weeks after hire and annually thereafter.
B. Every 6 months during the first 2 years and annually thereafter.
C. Every 6 months.
D. Before the operator performs patient testing, semiannually during the first year, and annually thereafter.
Rationale: The CAP checklist specifically states: "The competency of each person to perform the duties assigned must be assessed following training before the person performs patient testing. Thereafter, during the first year of an individual's duties, competency must be assessed at least semiannually. After an individual has performed his/her

duties for 1 year, competency must be assessed annually. Retraining and reassessment of employee competency must occur when problems are identified with employee performance."
E. Before the operator performs patient testing.
Rationale for A, B, C, and E: The CAP requires competency assessment before the operator performs patient testing, semiannually during the first year, and annually thereafter.

Major points of discussion
■ According to the CAP checklist, competency can be assessed by the following:

1. Direct observations of routine patient test performance, including, as applicable, patient identification and preparation; and specimen collection, handling, processing, and testing.
2. Monitoring the recording and reporting of test results, including, as applicable, reporting critical results.
3. Review of intermediate test results or worksheets, quality control records, proficiency testing results, and preventive maintenance records.
4. Direct observation of performance of instrument maintenance and function checks.
5. Assessment of test performance through testing previously analyzed specimens, internal blind testing samples, or external proficiency testing samples.
6. Evaluation of problem-solving skills.

- Other elements of competency may be assessed, as applicable. For nonwaived tests, all six elements described above must be assessed at each assessment event. For waived tests, it is not necessary to assess all elements at each assessment event; the laboratory may select which elements to assess.
- Ongoing supervisory review is an acceptable method of assessing competency for certain elements (as examples, direct observation of test performance, instrument maintenance, and problem-solving skills). Competency assessment may be documented in various ways, including a checklist completed by a supervisor.[21]

2. A. Measurement of the amount of light absorbed at two different wavelengths.
Rationale: This is the definition of a bichromatic measurement of an analyte.
B. Measurement of the amount of emitted light after a molecule is chemically excited from the ground to the excited state.
Rationale: This is the definition of chemiluminescence
C. Measurement of the amount of emitted light after a molecule is biologically excited from the ground to the excited state.
Rationale: This is the definition of bioluminescence
D. Measurement of the amount of emitted light when a molecule in a triplet state returns to the ground state.
Rationale: This is the definition of phosphorescence.
E. Measurement of the amount of emitted light after a molecule is excited from the ground to the excited state by a short pulse of light.
Rationale: This is the definition of fluorescence.

Major points of discussion
- The first step in a chemiluminescence assay occurs when the electrons in an organic molecule (e.g., luminol, isoluminol, adamantyl-1,2-dioxetane, acridinium esters) are transitioned to an excited state due to a chemical reaction.
- The chemical reactions must be exothermic to generate the energy required for this transition. The reactions usually involve an oxidation step using hydrogen peroxide or other strong oxidants to provide the high energy needed to excite the electrons.
- When the electrons return to the ground state, the amount of light generated is measured. In chemiluminescence assays, electrons are in an excited state without the absorption of radiation.

- A heterogeneous chemiluminescence immunoassay assay involves the addition of the sample containing the antigen, the capture antibody, and the antigen labeled with an organic molecule. After incubation and separation of the bound from the free labeled antigen, hydrogen peroxide is added, which reacts with the organic molecule and raises the electrons to the excited state. The amount of light emitted is related to the concentration of the analyte in the sample.
- One major advantage of a chemiluminescence assay is increased analytical sensitivity. Because there is no need for radiation of the sample, the problems associated with light scattering are eliminated, thereby resulting in a low background. Another advantage is that chemiluminescence assays usually have a wide linear range.[5,25]

3. A. The enzyme-labeled antigen that is bound to the antibody is inhibited by changing the pH of the solution.
Rationale: This homogeneous reaction occurs at a single pH.
B. The enzyme-labeled antigen that is bound to the antibody reacts at a slower rate with the EA to form the active enzyme than the enzyme-labeled antigen that is not bound to the antibody.
Rationale: The enzyme-labeled antigen that is bound to the antibody does not react with the EA at all.
C. The enzyme-labeled antigen that is bound to the antibody reacts with the EA to form the active enzyme.
Rationale: The enzyme-labeled antigen that is bound to the antibody is inhibited from binding to the EA.
D. The enzyme-labeled antigen that is bound to the antibody is physically separated from the enzyme-labeled antigen that is not bound to the antibody and reacts with the EA to form the active enzyme.
Rationale: There is no physical step separating the bound antigen from the free antigen because the CEDIA assay is a homogeneous immunoassay.
E. The enzyme-labeled antigen that is bound to the antibody is inhibited from reacting with the EA. The enzyme-labeled antigen that is not bound to the antibody reacts with the EA to form the active enzyme.
Rationale: See Major Points of Discussion.

Major points of discussion
- CEDIA is an automated competitive homogeneous immunoassay that is used to measure low molecular weight antigens.
- By using genetic engineering, two inactive fragments of the enzyme beta-galactosidase are produced by *Escherichia coli.* These fragments include an EA that lacks the complementary enzyme donor (ED) fragment required for enzyme activity. Combination of the EA and ED fragments is needed for enzyme activity.
- In the CEDIA assay, the antigen is bound to the ED fragment and competes with free antigen in the sample for binding sites on the antigen-specific antibody.
- When the antigen that is bound to the ED binds to the antibody, the combination of the ED with the EA fragment to produce the active enzyme is inhibited. However, if the antigen bound to the ED does not bind to the antibody, then the ED will combine with the EA to produce the active enzyme, which then reacts with the enzyme substrate to produce a chromagen.

■ With the CEDIA assay, there is a direct relationship between the concentration of the free antigen (i.e., the low molecular weight analyte to be quantified) and the amount of chromagen produced. Higher levels of the free antigen in the sample lead to higher levels of non–antibody-bound ED fragment, which combine with the EA to produce higher levels of active enzyme.[3,15]

4. A. During the ordering of tests.
Rationale: Approximately 1% to 2% of errors occur when laboratory tests are ordered.
B. During the preanalytical phase of testing.
Rationale: Most errors (68% to 75%) occur in the preanalytical phase of testing.
C. During the analytical phase of testing.
Rationale: Approximately 10% to 32% of errors occur during the analytical testing phase.
D. During the reporting of the test results.
Rationale: Approximately 2% to 5% of errors occur when test results are reported.
E. During physician interpretation of the test results.
Rationale: Approximately 3% to 5% of errors occur because of physician misinterpretation of test results.

Major points of discussion

■ Errors can occur in any of the three phases of laboratory testing: (1) preanalytical, which begins with the patient and ends with preparation of the sample for testing; (2) analytical, which includes all steps involved in performing a laboratory test; and (3) postanalytical, which begins with reporting the results to the health care provider and ends with actions taken by the health care provider based on the test results.

■ Most laboratory errors occur during phlebotomy and front-end processing of samples. The manual phlebotomy process—which involves collecting specimen labels, identifying the patient by examining the wristband, matching the labels with the patient, collecting blood using the correct order of draw, and correctly labeling the tubes—is highly susceptible to error. Standardizing the phlebotomy process can greatly reduce these errors.

■ The most common sample processing errors are mislabeling the sample, incorrectly preparing aliquot samples (e.g., pouring from the wrong sample), mislabeling aliquot tubes, and misplacing samples in the laboratory. Automation of sample processing eliminates most of these errors.

■ Errors in physician orders commonly happen because of the similarity of test names, lack of ordering physician knowledge about tests, duplicate orders, and transcription errors. The key to improving test ordering accuracy is to implement computerized order entry by the physician.

■ Delays in transporting the specimen to the laboratory can compromise test results. To minimize postcollection variation, specimens should be delivered, processed, and stored promptly after collection. For example, glucose levels decrease at a rate of 5% to 7% per hour in whole blood maintained at room temperature. Transportation of specimens to the laboratory often significantly delays processing. Mechanical transport systems, typically with pneumatic tubes, are used by some laboratories to expedite specimen delivery.

■ The concept of "critical values" refers to a pathophysiological state that can be life threatening for a patient unless appropriate therapy is initiated rapidly. Failure to report critical values expeditiously can compromise patient care and result in legal actions against the physician, the hospital, and the laboratory.

■ Misinterpretation of test results means that the health care provider received the correct result but did not take the correct action based on the result. Interpretive reports can prevent this type of error and should include a description of the abnormal result, possible reasons for an abnormal result, suggestions for further testing, and a statement of need for treatment.[4,7]

5. A. Quenching of fluorescence in the excited state.
Rationale: Quenching is the loss of fluorescence due to interactions between the fluorophore and its molecular environment.
B. Difference between the wavelengths of the excitation light and emitted light in a fluorescence assay.
Rationale: The Stokes shift should be large for the design of a useful clinical assay.
C. Rate of formation of an antibody-antigen complex.
Rationale: This kinetic rate is not the Stokes shift.
D. Difference between detection time of the internal standard and the compound of interest in a high-performance liquid chromatography (HPLC) assay.
Rationale: In HPLC, the internal standard should elute close to the compound of interest.
E. Distance between the solvent front and the compound of interest in a thin-layer chromatography (TLC) assay.
Rationale: In TLC, the retention factor value is the distance traveled by the compound, divided by the distance traveled by the solvent front. This is a useful characteristic of every compound that can be separated by TLC.

Major points of discussion

■ In fluorescence, when a molecule absorbs a photon of energy, electrons are transferred from the ground to the excited state. While in the excited state, the molecule will lose some energy due to interaction with other molecules and drop to a lower energy level.

■ When the electrons return to the ground state, the energy of the photon emitted is lower than the one that was initially absorbed and emits light at a longer wavelength.

■ The Stokes shift is the difference between the excitation and emission wavelengths.

■ If the Stokes shift is small, the excitation and emission spectra can overlap, causing an increase in background fluorescence due to the scattering effects of the excitation light.

■ A large Stokes shift will reduce the amount of incident light arriving at the detector and will improve the sensitivity of the assay. The difference between the excitation and emission wavelengths should be at least 50 nm but ideally should be more than 200 nm.[14]

6. A. The fluorescence lifetime of the molecule is decreased, resulting in an increase in analytical sensitivity and a decrease in background fluorescence.
Rationale: The fluorescence lifetime is significantly increased in time-resolved fluorescence assays.

B. The fluorescence lifetime of the molecule is increased, resulting in an increase in analytical sensitivity and a decrease in background fluorescence.
Rationale: This is the main advantage of time-resolved fluorescence assays.
C. The small Stokes shift that is observed with time-resolved fluorescent immunoassays increases the sensitivity of the assay.
Rationale: There is a large Stokes shift with time-resolved fluorescence assays.
D. Fluorescence measurements are rapid, which reduces the background fluorescence.
Rationale: Fluorescence measurements are prolonged in time-resolved fluorescent immunoassays.
E. Fluorescence is quenched, which reduces the background fluorescence.
Rationale: Quenching is not a significant issue in time-resolved fluorescence immunoassays.

Major points of discussion

- In time-resolved fluorescent immunoassays, a lanthanide ion (usually europium [Eu^{3+}]) is used. The fluorescence of the Eu^{3+} ion alone is weak and is, therefore, bound to an organic ligand, which significantly enhances its fluorescence.
- When the Eu^{3+} organic complex is excited by light irradiation, the organic ligand absorbs energy and electrons are raised from the ground to a singlet excited state. While in the excited state, these electrons can pass to a triplet state.
- If the ligand is chelated to Eu^{3+}, there can be an energy transfer from the triplet excited state of the ligand to the Eu^{3+} ion, which then can move to an excited singlet state and emit fluorescence that is characteristic of Eu^{3+}.
- The major advantage of time-resolved immunoassay is its long fluorescence lifetime. In conventional fluorescence assays, the fluorescence lasts about 1 μsec, whereas in time-resolved assays, the fluorescence can be measured at intervals of 400 to 800 μsec. This prolonged fluorescence eliminates the noise created by background fluorescence in biological samples, cuvettes, and solvents. As a result, the sensitivity of the assay is increased.
- Another advantage of time-resolved fluorescent assays is the long Stokes shift. The Stokes shift in some time-resolved assays can be greater than 200 nm. As a result, there is no overlap between the excitation and emission wavelengths. For example, the excitation and emission wavelengths for a Eu^{3+} organic complex are 295 and 612 nm, respectively.[28,29]

7. A. The hook effect caused a false-positive troponin I result.
Rationale: The hook effect would produce a lower-than-expected result
B. Heterophile antibodies interfered with the troponin I assay, causing a false-positive result.
Rationale: The heterophile antibodies are human anti-animal antibodies that bind to the reagent antibodies used in the assay, thereby interfering with their function.
C. The patient was correctly diagnosed with an acute myocardial infarction.
Rationale: The patient did not have an acute myocardial infarction because the troponin I value did not change with time and the CK, CK-MB, and electrocardiogram were all normal.

D. The patient was correctly diagnosed with congestive heart failure.
Rationale: Measurement of brain natriuretic peptide (BNP) or N-terminal prohormone-BNP (NT-proBNP) are used to assess patients for congestive heart failure.
E. There was cross-reactivity of troponin T with the troponin I method.
Rationale: Troponin I methods are very specific and measure only troponin I with little or no cross-reactivity for troponin T.

Major points of discussion

- Heterophile antibodies are defined as antibodies in serum that bind antibodies of other species. Human anti-mouse antibodies (HAMAs) are the most common type of heterophile antibody. Human anti-rabbit, -goat, -cow, -horse, and -sheep heterophile antibodies have also been identified. These HAMAs can cause either a positive or negative interference with immunochemical assays. A falsely elevated analytical result is the most common effect of a heterophile antibody.
- Heterophile antibodies can arise from
  - Administering mouse monoclonal antibodies for diagnostic imaging or therapeutics
  - Exposure to animals
  - Vaccination
  - Blood transfusions
  - Maternal transfer across the placenta to an unborn child
- The prevalence of heterophile antibodies in healthy blood donors can range from 0.7% to 3.1% and is approximately 3% to 4% in hospitalized populations.
- HAMAs interfere with some assays for analytes, such as cancer antigen 125 (CA-125), troponin I, troponin T, CK-MB, thyroid-stimulating hormone (TSH), T_4, T_3, luteinizing hormone (LH), follicle-stimulating hormone (FSH), human chorionic gonadotropin (hCG), carcinoembryonic antigen (CEA), prostate-specific antigen (PSA), prolactin, hepatitis B surface antigen, C-reactive protein (CRP), progesterone, and alpha-fetoprotein (AFP).
- The clinical laboratory can detect the presence of a heterophile antibody by measuring the analyte using another immunochemical method that does not use the same antibodies that were used in the original method. If a heterophile antibody is present, a much lower analytical result will typically be obtained with the second method.
- Heterophile antibodies can also be identified by serially diluting the sample. Heterophile antibody–positive samples frequently yield aberrant dilution results.
- The heterophile antibody can also be removed by using protein G or protein A immobilized on agarose (Sepharose) beads or by precipitation with polyethylene glycol.[6,9,19]

8. A. The enzyme-labeled antigen activity is inhibited by changing the pH of the reaction.
Rationale: This homogeneous assay is performed at a single pH.
B. The antibody-bound enzyme-labeled antigen complex is not as stable as the free, non–antibody-bound enzyme-

labeled antigen complex, and the enzyme activity is measured by a kinetic rate reaction.
Rationale: The enzyme-labeled antibody complex is stable and the enzyme activity is not measured by a kinetic assay.
C. Antibody binding to the enzyme-labeled antigen enhances the enzyme activity.
Rationale: Actually, antibody binding sterically inhibits the enzymatic activity of the antigen-labeled enzyme.
D. Antibody binding to the enzyme-labeled antigen sterically inhibits the enzyme activity.
Rationale: See Major Points of Discussion.
E. The free, non–antibody-bound enzyme-labeled antigen is fluorescent.
Rationale: No fluorescence measurements are involved in EMIT assays.

Major points of discussion

- The EMIT assay is an automated homogeneous enzyme immunoassay that is used primarily for measuring drugs.
- An enzyme (usually glucose-6-phosphate dehydrogenase) is labeled with a drug (i.e., enzyme-bound antigen) and competes with the free drug in the sample (i.e., the free antigen) for binding sites on a drug-specific antibody. After the reaction is complete, enzyme substrate is added and the amount of enzyme product produced is measured spectrophotometrically.
- The enzyme-labeled drug that is bound to the antibody is sterically inhibited from reacting with the enzyme substrate. Only the free, non–antibody-bound enzyme-labeled drug reacts with the enzyme substrate.
- The concentration of the drug in the patient sample is directly related to the amount of enzyme product produced.
- The EMIT assay can be used with any spectrophotometer and is the most common procedure used for quantifying serum drug levels.[22]

9. A. No fluorescence is observed when antibody binds to the fluorescent-labeled drug.
Rationale: Fluorescence is observed when the fluorescent-labeled drug is bound to the antibody.
B. Rotation of the non–antibody-bound fluorescent-labeled drug is slower than the antibody-bound fluorescent-labeled drug and depolarizes the emitted light.
Rationale: Rotation of the free, non–antibody-bound fluorescent-labeled drug depolarizes the emitted light because it rotates faster than the antibody-bound fluorescent-labeled drug.
C. The antibody-bound fluorescent-labeled drug emits less polarized light than the non–antibody-bound fluorescent-labeled drug.
Rationale: The antibody-bound fluorescent-labeled drug rotates slowly and emits polarized light. Rotation of the non–antibody-bound fluorescent-labeled drug depolarizes the emitted light.
D. The antibody-bound fluorescent-labeled drug emits polarized light. The non–antibody-bound fluorescent labeled drug depolarizes the emitted light.
Rationale: See Major Points of Discussion.

E. Rotation of the non–antibody-bound fluorescent-labeled drug is faster than the antibody-bound fluorescent-labeled drug and emits more polarized light.
Rationale: Rotation of the non–antibody-bound fluorescent-labeled drug depolarizes the emitted light.

Major points of discussion

- FPIA is a homogeneous automated assay based on the amount of polarized fluorescent light detected when the fluorescent label is excited with polarized light.
- If a fluorescent molecule absorbs polarized light to produce the excited state, the emitted light will also be polarized if the fluorophore does not rotate during its time in the excited state. If the fluorophore rotates in the excited state before fluorescence emission takes place, the emitted light will be depolarized.
- The principle of FPIA involves competition between a fluorescent-labeled antigen (i.e., the drug; fluorescein is the most common fluorophore) and the antigen (i.e., free drug) in the sample for binding sites on an antigen-specific (i.e., drug-specific) antibody.
- The antibody-bound fluorescent-labeled antigen is a large molecule and rotates slowly in the excited state. Therefore, the polarization of the emitted light is not significantly changed from the polarized light that was used to excite the molecule.
- The non–antibody-bound fluorescent-labeled antigen is a small molecule and rotates rapidly in the excited state before fluorescence light is emitted. In this case, the emitted light is depolarized.
- In an FPIA assay, the amount of polarized light emitted is inversely related to the sample concentration of the analyte to be measured. At low analyte concentrations, more of the fluorescent-labeled antigen will bind to the antibody, resulting in a large amount of emitted polarized light.[27]

10. A. Binding of the HAMA to the analyte that is being measured, thereby causing a falsely elevated result.
Rationale: Binding of HAMA to an analyte is not a common occurrence.
B. Binding of the HAMA to the analyte that is being measured, thereby causing a falsely lower result.
Rationale: HAMA usually will not bind to an analyte.
C. Binding of the HAMA to the capture antibody,[6,19] thereby causing a falsely elevated result.
Rationale: See Major Points of Discussion.
D. Binding of the HAMA to the capture antibody, thereby causing a falsely lower result.
Rationale: Binding of HAMA to the capture antibody will cause an elevated result.
E. Binding of HAMA to the labeled analyte, thereby causing a falsely lower result.
Rationale: HAMA usually will not bind to a nonimmunoglobulin analyte.

Major points of discussion

- Competitive binding immunoassays are based on reactions in which the number of antigen-binding sites is limited. The analyte that is being measured and a labeled derivative of the analyte compete for binding to the capture antibody.

■ There is an inverse relationship between the amount of labeled analyte that binds to the capture antibody and the concentration of analyte in the sample. At low analyte concentrations, more of the labeled analyte binds to the capture antibody and a high signal is observed.

■ If a HAMA is present and binds to the capture antibody, it prevents formation of the labeled analyte–capture antibody complex, thereby resulting in a lower than expected signal and a higher than expected analytical result.

■ The interference of HAMA with competitive binding assays is not as frequent as with two-site immunometric assays because of the greater affinity of the analyte for the antibody binding sites.

■ Falsely elevated results have been observed for competitive binding assays for free T_4, T_4, and inhibin A. Addition of blocking agents (e.g., mouse or animal immunoglobulins) is used to prevent binding of HAMA to the capture antibody.

11a. A. Interference by heterophile antibodies (i.e., HAMAs).
Rationale: If heterophile antibodies are present, a higher-than-expected result is usually obtained.
B. The hook effect.
Rationale: The hook effect describes the situation when a sample with an extremely high analyte concentration produces a result below that of the highest calibrator.
C. A matrix effect.
Rationale: This will usually not cause the very low levels of hCG observed with this sample.
D. Inhibition of hCG by maternal antibodies.
Rationale: hCG is usually not inhibited by maternal antibodies.
E. Binding of hCG to human immunoglobulin (Ig) G.
Rationale: hCG is usually not bound to IgG.

11b. A. Repeat the hCG assay using another serum sample.
Rationale: A similar hCG result would be obtained by simply repeating the process.
B. Measure the hCG level using a different method.
Rationale: Because the correct hCG result is very high, measuring hCG with another method would most likely also yield a lower-than-expected hCG result.
C. Precipitate the interfering heterophile antibodies in the sample using polyethylene glycol and remeasure the hCG level.
Rationale: Because heterophile antibodies are not present, this would not affect the hCG result.
D. Perform a serial dilution of the sample and remeasure the hCG levels using the diluted samples.
Rationale: When hydatiform moles are present, serum hCG levels are very high and a hook effect can be observed. Serial dilutions of the sample are used to determine the correct hCG level.
E. Add mouse immunoglobulins to the sample to remove the interference from heterophile antibodies and remeasure the hCG level.
Rationale: The same hCG result would be obtained because heterophile antibodies are not the cause of these low hCG values.

Major points of discussion

■ Definition of the hook effect: A sample with an extremely high analyte concentration that produces a result below that of the highest calibrator. It can occur with hCG, prolactin, luteinizing hormone (LH), follicle-stimulating hormone (FSH), prostate-specific antigen (PSA), alpha-fetoprotein (AFP), and CA-125 immunoassays.

■ The high-dose hook effect occurs in one-step immunometric assays when the sample and signal antibody are simultaneously added to the capture antibody and incubated. The presence of large amounts of the antigen in the sample limits the number of antigen-antibody complexes that can be formed because excess antigen saturates the capture and signal antibodies and blocks the formation of the antigen-antibody complex, which then results in a lower signal than expected. If the concentration level obtained falls in the linear range of the assay, the sample is not diluted and a falsely low concentration will be reported.

■ In this case, the sample was serially diluted with the zero concentration hCG calibrator. The hCG level obtained after dilution was 3,500,000 IU/L. Because of this very high hCG level, very little of the antibody-antigen complex was formed, resulting in a normal hCG level.

■ The use of a two-step immunometric assay could eliminate the high-dose hook effect. It involves adding the sample to the capture antibody, an incubation step, and a subsequent washing step that removes the excess antigen. Adding the signal antibody in the second step of the assay would result in a signal that is above the linear range of the assay.

■ In this case, the sample would be diluted and the correct result reported. However, manufacturers are reluctant to use this technique because they would have to change the reagent formulation, which would increase the reporting time for the analyte and would involve approval by the FDA.

■ If the hook effect is undetected, a significantly lower analyte value will be reported, which can result in patient mismanagement. The laboratory should have a dilution protocol to test for the hook effect when using these types of assays.[1,2]

12. A. Reflectance photometry is used to detect serum electrolyte concentrations.
Rationale: Serum electrolytes are measured using ion-specific electrodes.
B. Reflectance photometry is used in DNA testing.
Rationale: DNA testing typically uses other types of methods, such as those involving capillary electrophoresis, polymerase chain reaction, etc.
C. Reflectance photometry measures the light intensity emitted from the excited state of the molecule.
Rationale: This defines fluorescence.
D. In reflectance photometry, there is a linear relationship between the intensity of light reflected and concentration of the analyte.

Rationale: There is a nonlinear relationship between the intensity of the reflected light and sample concentration.

E. In reflectance photometry, the sample concentration is calculated by comparing the reflectance of a white standard to the light reflected by the sample.

Rationale: See Major Points of Discussion.

Major points of discussion

■ In reflectance photometry, the sample is added to a reagent strip or to a dry film slide, which contains all the reagents needed for the chemical reaction to occur. The instrumentation used in reflectance photometry is similar to that in spectrophotometry.

■ Light from a lamp passes through a filter wheel that selects the wavelength of interest. The light is directed to the test surface of the reagent strip or dry film slide. Some light is absorbed by the chromophore on the test surface and some light is reflected. The amount of light reflected is focused onto a photomultiplier.

■ In reflectance photometry, light can be directed onto the reagent strip at a 45-degree angle and the reflected light detected at a 90-degree angle. The amount of the reflected light depends on the amount of chromophore formed and is related to the concentration of the analyte in the sample.

■ The relationship between the amount of reflected light and the concentration of the analyte is not linear. To calculate the sample concentration, the signal from the reflected light of the sample is compared with the signal from a reference white standard. The signal from the white standard is set to 100% because all light is reflected. The reflection density, which is the ratio of the reflected light from the white standard and the light reflected by the sample, is obtained and an algorithm is used to linearize the relationship of this reflectance signal/concentration ratio.

■ Reflectance photometry is used in POC testing, in urinalysis testing using reagent strips, in automated analyzers (e.g., the Vitros system from Ortho Diagnostics, which uses dry-film slide technology for measuring routine chemistry analytes), and in therapeutic drug monitoring.[8]

13. A. Binding of HAMA to the capture antibody.
Rationale: HAMA must bind to both the capture and labeled antibody to produce a signal.
B. Binding of HAMA to the analyte being measured.
Rationale: HAMA does not typically bind to nonimmunoglobulin analytes.
C. Binding of HAMA to both the capture antibody and the labeled antibody.
Rationale: In this case, a signal will be generated and a falsely increased result will be reported.
D. Binding of the HAMA to the labeled antibody.
E. Binding of the HAMA to both the capture antibody and the analyte that is being measured.
Rationale D and E: To produce a signal, the HAMA needs to bind to both the capture and labeled antibodies.

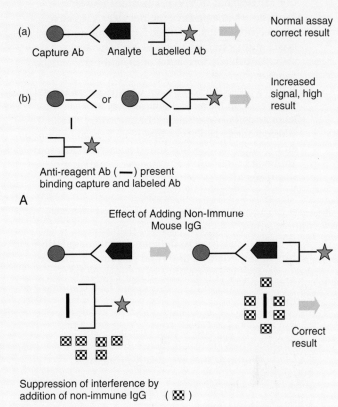

Figure 3-1 **A** and **B**, Schematic diagram of mechanisms of interference of reagent antibodies by heterophile antibodies. *Ab,* antibodies; *IgG,* immunoglobulin G.

Major points of discussion

■ The normal reaction of an analyte with both the capture and labeled antibodies in a two-site immunometric assay is shown in Figure 3-1, *A*, in reaction scheme a. Sample and labeled antibody are added to a capture antibody, thereby resulting in an antibody-antigen complex. The concentration of the analyte in the sample is directly related to the amount of antibody-antigen complex that is formed. The positive interference from heterophile antibodies (e.g., HAMA) is shown in Figure 3-1, *A*, in reaction scheme b. The heterophile antibody will bind to both the capture and labeled antibodies at either the Fc or Fab positions on the reagent IgG molecules and cause a falsely elevated result.

■ The interference from heterophile antibodies can be removed, in most cases, by adding blocking agents (usually animal immunoglobulins) to the reagent system. For example, adding mouse immunoglobulin binds the HAMA and usually prevents the binding of this type of heterophile antibody to the capture and labeled antibodies. The reaction scheme is shown in Figure 3-1, *B*.

■ Although reagent manufacturers use blocking reagents to reduce the interference from heterophile antibodies, interferences still can be seen, especially when the heterophile antibody titer is high or when the blocking reagents do not bind the heterophile antibody.

- Heterophile antibodies can also produce a negative interference, but this occurs at a much lower incidence than a positive interference. A negative interference occurs when the heterophile antibody binds to the capture or labeled antibody and sterically inhibits formation of the antibody-antigen complex
- When a physician receives an unexpected analytical result with an immunochemical assay and calls the laboratory for consultation, the laboratory should consider the possibility of interference from heterophile antibodies. Not detecting interference from heterophile antibodies can result in misdiagnosis and unnecessary treatment.[6,9,19]

14. A. The test is sensitive to deficiencies in coagulation factors in the extrinsic and final common pathways.
B. The test is sensitive to deficiencies in coagulation factors in the intrinsic and final common pathways.
Rationale: The ACT is sensitive to deficiencies in coagulation factors in the intrinsic and final common pathways.
C. The test is performed on plasma.
Rationale: The test is performed on whole blood.
D. Clotting times are usually between 50 and 100 seconds.
Rationale: Clotting times are usually greater than 100 seconds.
E. The test is often used for managing outpatients treated with Coumadin.
Rationale: The ACT is used for monitoring patients receiving heparin therapy.

Major points of discussion
- The activated clotting time (ACT) is a whole-blood coagulation test.
- It monitors both the intrinsic and common pathways of the coagulation cascade.
- Strong activators such as kaolin or Celite are used for monitoring high-dose heparin therapy.
- Activators such as glass beads are used for monitoring low-dose heparin therapy.
- Depending on the activators used, different reference ranges need to be applied.[26]

15. A. Both assays are based on adding a strong contact activator of the clotting cascade to whole blood. The only difference is the amount of activator added.
B. Both assays are based on adding large amounts of thromboplastin to the sample.
C. The ACT assay is based on adding a strong contact activator of the clotting cascade to whole blood. The heparin assay is based on titrating the amount of protamine needed to neutralize the heparin present in the sample.
D. The ACT assay is based on adding kaolin or Celite to the sample. The heparin assay is based on adding glass beads to the sample.
E. The ACT assay is based on adding a strong contact activator of the clotting cascade to whole blood. The heparin assay use antibodies specific for heparin to determine heparin levels.
Rationale: The ACT assay is based on adding a strong contact activator of the clotting cascade to whole blood. Heparin assays are based on titrating the amount of protamine needed to neutralize the heparin present in the sample, using a semiquantitative titration method.

Major points of discussion
- Strong contact activators include substances such as Celite, kaolin, and glass beads.
- The ACT assay does not correlate well with heparin levels in patients undergoing cardiopulmonary bypass.
- This allows the calculation of the heparin concentration in the sample, as well as the calculation of the amount of protamine needed to reverse heparinization.[26]

16. A. It is classified as a waived test.
Rationale: The fern test is classified as provider-performed microscopy; therefore, it is not a waived test.
B. It is positive in the presence of amniotic fluid at any gestational age.
Rationale: The fern test becomes positive only after 20 weeks of gestation.
C. It is more sensitive for the presence of amniotic fluid than the nitrazine paper test.
Rationale: The fern test is not more sensitive for the presence of amniotic fluid than the nitrazine paper test.
D. It is more specific for the presence of amniotic fluid than the nitrazine paper test.
Rationale: The fern test is more specific than the nitrazine paper test for the presence of amniotic fluid.
E. It is rendered unreliable by the presence of even small amounts of blood.
Rationale: Blood at a dilution of less than 1:1 does not interfere with the fern test.

Major point of discussion
- Amniotic fluid crystallization (i.e., "ferning") can be used to detect amniotic fluid after premature rupture of the fetal membranes.[17]

17. A. **Improved turnaround time for the test.**
Rationale: This is a distinct advantage of POCT versus testing in a centralized laboratory; POCT usually has a shorter turnaround time with the results rapidly available at the "point of care."
B. Enhanced competency of the operator performing the assay.
Rationale: Professional laboratory technologists are better trained at performing laboratory assays compared with non–laboratory-affiliated POCT operators.
C. Decreased test cost.
Rationale: For a given test, it is usually more efficient and cheaper to perform testing in a centralized laboratory.
D. Improved test accuracy.
Rationale: Most tests performed in a centralized laboratory are more accurate than their POCT equivalents.
E. Improved test precision.
Rationale: Most tests performed in a centralized laboratory are more precise than their POCT equivalents.

Major points of discussion
- POCT typically has a much shorter turnaround time than analysis of samples in a centralized laboratory.
- POCT is often significantly more expensive than testing in a centralized laboratory.

- It can be challenging to ensure appropriate training and continuous competency assessment of POCT operators.
- Enforcement of performance of quality control analysis in POCT can be challenging.
- In general, POCT methods tend to be less accurate and less precise than assays performed in a centralized laboratory.

18. A. Patient identification only.
Rationale: Barcode readers on POCT instruments can be used to scan barcodes on patients' wristbands, thereby ensuring correct identification of the patient to be tested. However, barcode readers can also be used for identification of operators, reagents, and quality control material.
B. Operator identification only.
Rationale: Barcode readers on POCT instruments can be used to scan barcodes on operators' identification tags. This can be used to ensure that only operators who have been properly trained and whose competency assessment is up-to-date will perform the testing. However, barcode readers can also be used for identification of patients, reagents, and quality control material.
C. Reagent and/or cartridge identification only.
Rationale: Barcode readers on POCT instruments can be used to scan barcodes on cartridge and/or reagent packages. This can be used to ensure that only reagents lots and/or cartridges that are not expired and have been validated by the POC service are used for testing. However, barcode readers can also be used to identify the patient, operator, and quality control material.
D. Quality control material identification only.
Rationale: Barcode readers on POCT instruments can be used to scan barcodes on quality control material packages. This can be used to ensure that only lots of quality control material that are not expired and have been validated by the POC service are used for testing. However, barcode readers can also be used to identify patients, operators, reagents, and cartridges.
E. Identification of patients, operators, reagents, cartridges, and quality control material.
Rationale: Barcode readers on POCT devices can be used to scan barcodes on patients' wristbands, on operator identification tags, on reagents and cartridges, and on quality control material. Therefore, they can ensure correct patient identification, the performance of assays by trained operators, and the exclusive use of reagents lots, cartridges, and quality control material that are not expired and have been validated by the POC service.

Major points of discussion

- Many modern POCT devices have built-in barcode readers.
- These barcode readers can be used for patient identification, operator lock-outs, and prevention of the use of nonvalidated or expired reagents lots, cartridges, or quality control material.
- By scanning barcodes on patients' wristbands, the correct identification of these patients can be ensured.
- By requiring the scanning of barcodes on operators' identification tags, operators without appropriate training or competency assessment can be prevented from using the POCT system.

- Barcode readers on POCT instruments can be used to scan barcodes on cartridges, reagent lots, and control material packages. This can ensure that only lots that are not expired and have been validated by the POC service are used for testing.

19. A. The concept of critical values is not applicable to POCT because a care provider usually either performs the test or is present at the testing site.
Rationale: Critical values are very much applicable in POCT. Critical values (e.g., for glucose and hematocrit) need to be defined, and the interventions taken in response to critical values must be documented.
B. Critical values from POCTs performed in hospitals are the responsibility of the performing clinical care provider, not of the clinical laboratory.
Rationale: Critical values from all laboratory tests, including POCTs, are the responsibility of the clinical laboratory.
C. Critical values in POCT, and the intervention taken in response to them, must be documented.
Rationale: Critical values in POCT, as in any other area of clinical laboratory testing, must be documented together with the ensuing intervention.
D. Critical values in POCT are never repeated.
Rationale: Many institutions have standard operating procedures that require critical values obtained by POCT methods to be repeated in the central laboratory.
E. The documentation of critical values from POCT instruments always requires a separate entry in the patient's medical record.
Rationale: Many modern POCT devices allow for documentation of critical values on the instrument, with direct transmission of an annotation of the result to the electronic medical record, along with the critical result.

Major points of discussion

- Critical values in POCT (e.g., for glucose and hematocrit) need to be defined, and the interventions taken in response to critical values must be documented.
- Many POCT devices also allow settings that block the user from proceeding to the next patient before acknowledging a critical value and documenting the response.

20. A. The Department of Health of the state in which the hospital is located.
Rationale: Some states do not routinely inspect POCT programs.
B. A "deemed" organization, such as The Joint Commission or the College of American Pathologists.
C. The Centers for Medicare and Medicaid Services.
Rationale: Usually, inspections of hospitals are performed by "deemed" organizations, such as The Joint Commission or the College of American Pathologists, and not directly by the Centers for Medicare and Medicaid Services.
D. A professional organization, such as the American Association for Clinical Chemistry.
E. The Food and Drug Administration.
Rationale for B, D, and E: "Deemed" organizations, such as The Joint Commission or the College of American Pathologists, usually inspect POCT programs in hospitals.

Major points of discussion
- All laboratory testing, including POCT, is regulated by the Clinical Laboratory Improvement Amendments of 1988 (CLIA'88).
- Laboratory inspections in hospitals are usually performed by the College of American Pathologists or by The Joint Commission.
- Although the College of American Pathologists uses a system of peer-review inspections, The Joint Commission uses full-time inspectors.
- The Food and Drug Administration regulates laboratory methods and reagents.
- In some, but not all, states, the Department of Health also inspects hospitals.[10]

21. A. They should not be used to manage diabetes because they are not sufficiently accurate.
Rationale: Point-of-care glucose meters are sufficiently accurate for managing diabetes.
B. They should not be used to screen for diabetes.
Rationale: Point-of-care glucose meters are sufficiently accurate for screening for diabetes.
C. They should not be used to diagnose diabetes.
Rationale: Point-of-care glucose meters are not recommended for diagnosing diabetes; they are approved only for screening and managing diabetes.
D. Their results are not affected by lipemia.
Rationale: Lipemia can interfere with the results obtained using point-of-care glucose meters.
E. They all use the same chemical reaction for measuring glucose.
Rationale: Different point-of-care glucose meters use different chemical reactions for measuring glucose.

Major points of discussion
- Point-of-care glucose meters (i.e., glucometers) are approved only for screening and managing diabetes.
- Point-of-care glucose meters may not perform well in neonates at the 40-mg/dL threshold.
- Elevated levels of hematocrit and lipids and the presence of glycolysis inhibitors may interfere with the results obtained using point-of-care glucose meters.
- Point-of-care glucose meter test strips can be damaged by heat or freezing.[23]

22. **A. At least 2 years.**
B. At least 1 year.
C. As long as the program is active.
D. At least 5 years.
E. For the amount of time required by state law.
Rationale: According to the Clinical Laboratory Improvement Amendments of 1988 (CLIA'88), POC testing programs must keep their records of all quality control activities for at least 2 years.

Major points of discussion
- In hospitals, inspections for compliance are usually performed by the College of American Pathologists or The Joint Commission.
- Inspections are usually unannounced and take place every 2 years.
- Failure to comply with requirements can lead to discontinuation of the POCT program.

- It is the responsibility of the laboratory director to ensure compliance.[10]

23. A. Setting up wireless connections is always cheaper.
Rationale: Setting up wireless connections is not necessarily cheaper. There can be significant costs associated with the implementation of a wireless network if the institution presently does not own one.
B. A wireless network is safer.
Rationale: A wireless network needs data encryption to maintain patient confidentiality.
C. Wireless connections provide faster availability of results in the electronic medical record.
Rationale: Downloading data from POC devices via a wireless network allows the results to be available in the patient's electronic medical record immediately and avoids delays caused by devices being docked only at the end of the shift or at the end of the day.
D. The wireless connection can be bidirectional and allow both uploading of patient data and physician orders to the POC device.
Rationale: Both a wireless connection and a cable-based docking connection can be bidirectional and allow the uploading of patient data and physician orders to the POC device.
E. A wireless connection can be turned off more easily if the security of the network has been compromised.
Rationale: A cable-based network and a wireless network can both be turned off if security has been compromised.

Major points of discussion
- Many modern POC devices can be connected to hospital networks.
- The connection can be by docking stations requiring data lines or by a wireless network.
- When docking stations are used, results are often downloaded only at the end of rounds, at the end of the shift, or at the end of the day. This leads to delays in the availability of results in the electronic medical record.
- Both wired and wireless connections can be used to download results to the hospital network and to upload patient data and physician orders for testing.

24. A. After the patient leaves the provider's office.
Rationale: For provider-performed microscopy procedures, the specimen must be examined during the patient visit.
B. By physicians and nurses.
Rationale: Nurses are not allowed to perform provider-performed microscopy procedures.
C. For the determination of white blood cell differentials in peripheral blood smears.
Rationale: Only labile samples qualify for provider-performed microscopy procedures.
D. On specimens that require only limited sample handling or processing.
Rationale: Provider-performed microscopy procedures are usually performed on specimens that require only limited sample handling or processing.
E. With bright-field, fluorescence, or phase-contrast microscopy.
Rationale: Provider-performed microscopy procedures can only be performed using bright-field or phase-contrast microscopy.

Major points of discussion

- Analyte lability can compromise test accuracy for certain specimens.
- Because of analyte lability, federal law created the special category of provider-performed microscopy procedures.
- A physician, dentist, midlevel practitioner, or physician assistant must personally perform these tests.
- A certificate for provider-performed microscopy procedures is required. Under this certificate, the laboratory may also perform waived tests.
- Provider-performed microscopy procedures include wet mounts, all potassium hydroxide preparations, pinworm examinations, fern tests, postcoital direct qualitative examinations, vaginal or cervical mucus evaluations, nasal smears for granulocytes, fecal leukocyte examinations, and qualitative semen analyses.[18]

25. A. The nitrazine paper test has a wide pH range.
Rationale: The nitrazine paper test has a narrow pH range, with a color change occurring at a pH of 6.4 to 6.8.
B. The nitrazine paper test has a sensitivity and specificity of greater than 95%.
Rationale: See Major Points of Discussion.
C. The nitrazine paper test has a sensitivity of 40% and a specificity of greater than 75%.
D. The nitrazine paper test has a sensitivity of 95% and a specificity of greater than 40%.
Rationale: The nitrazine paper test has a sensitivity and specificity of greater than 95%.
E. The reasons for false-positive nitrazine tests are unknown.
Rationale: False-positive nitrazine tests can occur in the presence of blood, soaps, or infection.

Major points of discussion

- The nitrazine paper test is used to detect the presence of amniotic fluid and confirm the premature rupture of membranes
- The test is based on the determination of the pH of the fluid to be tested: amniotic fluid is alkaline; urine is usually acidic.[17]

26. A. Conductivity-based methods take longer to perform than optical methods.
Rationale: There is no significant difference in the time it takes to obtain hematocrit results with conductivity-based methods compared with optical methods.
B. Conductivity-based methods are more difficult to calibrate than optical methods.
Rationale: There is no significant difference in calibration with conductivity-based methods compared with optical methods.
C. Conductivity-based methods can be significantly influenced by plasma composition, including electrolyte and protein concentrations.
Rationale: Conductivity-based methods for measuring hemoglobin/hematocrit levels can be significantly influenced by plasma composition, including electrolyte and protein concentrations.
D. Conductivity-based methods are less accurate at higher hematocrit levels.
Rationale: Conductivity-based methods are not less accurate at higher hematocrit levels.

E. Conductivity-based methods are less accurate at lower hematocrit levels.
Rationale: Conductivity-based methods are not less accurate at lower hematocrit levels.

Major points of discussion

- Manufacturers of POC testing instruments are aware of this problem and suggest that hematocrit measurements outside the normal plasma protein range be adjusted appropriately.
- This issue makes it difficult to use hematocrit/ hemoglobin measurements in critically ill patients when conductivity-based methods are used.
- Therefore, many hospitals have disabled the hematocrit/ hemoglobin function in intensive care units and operating rooms.
- Because most centralized clinical laboratories use the optical method for hemoglobin measurement, results obtained with POC instruments using conductivity-based methods will not always correlate with the results obtained in the central laboratory.[16]

27. **A. A high hematocrit leads to underestimation of blood glucose levels; a low hematocrit leads to overestimation of blood glucose levels.**
B. A high hematocrit leads to overestimation of blood glucose levels; a low hematocrit leads to underestimation of blood glucose levels.
C. High and low hematocrit levels both lead to overestimation of blood glucose levels.
D. High and low hematocrit levels both lead to underestimation of blood glucose levels.
E. There is no effect of hematocrit on blood glucose determination using POCT devices.
Rationale: A high hematocrit leads to underestimation of blood glucose levels; a low hematocrit leads to overestimation of blood glucose levels.

Major points of discussion

- Abnormally high and low hematocrit levels can influence POC blood glucose measurements.
- This phenomenon is especially important in neonates, who can have very high hematocrit levels (i.e., up to 63%).
- Older glucometers often gave unreliable results in hospitalized patients with high or low hematocrit levels.
- Newer glucometers measure hematocrit and glucose simultaneously and adjust the glucose measurement for the measured hematocrit.[12]

28. A. They do not measure platelet function and platelet count.
Rationale: Thromboelastography and thromboelastometry results do reflect platelet function and platelet count.
B. They do not measure fibrinogen levels.
Rationale: Thromboelastography and thromboelastometry results do reflect fibrinogen levels.
C. They do not measure the final common pathway of the coagulation cascade.
Rationale: Thromboelastography and thromboelastometry results do reflect the functioning of the final pathway of the coagulation cascade.
D. They cannot be performed on citrated blood samples.

Rationale: Citrated blood can be used for both thromboelastography and thromboelastometry.

E. Results obtained with these methods often do not correlate well with results obtained by standard coagulation tests, such as the prothrombin time and the partial thromboplastin time.

Rationale: Results obtained with thromboelastography and thromboelastometry often do not correlate well with results obtained by standard coagulation testing, such as the prothrombin time and the partial thromboplastin time.

Major points of discussion

- Thromboelastography and thromboelastometry are used to assess perioperative coagulation disorders by means of viscoelastic analysis of clotting in vitro.
- Results are typically available within 10 minutes, allowing for immediate guidance of coagulation therapy during surgery.
- These methods provide several parameters that have different levels of correlation with standard coagulation assays, such as the prothrombin time, the partial thromboplastin time, and platelet function assays.
- The prothrombin time and the partial thromboplastin time cannot be used interchangeably with thromboelastography and thromboelastometry parameters.
- The results of both thromboelastography and thromboelastometry are affected by various factors, including platelet count, platelet function, and fibrinogen level.

29. A. Capturing accession times.
Rationale: Hospital-wide electronic order entry systems do not enhance the electronic capture of the accession time. They do, however, enhance the electronic capture of the order and collection times.
B. Capturing order and collection times.
Rationale: An electronic order entry system that interfaces with the laboratory information system enables the capture of the test order time and the collection time.
C. Capturing critical value result times.
Rationale: Hospital-wide electronic order entry systems do not enhance the electronic capture of the critical value result time. They do, however, enhance the electronic capture of the order and collection times.
D. Identifying result corrections and capturing result update times.
Rationale: Hospital-wide electronic order entry systems do not enhance the electronic capture of the result correction and result update times. They do, however, enhance the electronic capture of the order and collection times.
E. Capturing accession, order, and collection times.
Rationale: Hospital-wide electronic order entry systems do not enhance the electronic capture of the accession time. They do, however, enhance the electronic capture of the order and collection times.

Major points of discussion

- Hospital-wide electronic order entry systems allow providers to place electronic orders and print sample labels containing barcodes, the latter of which can be read by scanners in clinical departments, in the laboratory, and on laboratory instruments.
- Such systems allow the electronic capture of the order and collection times.
- Electronic capture of order and collection times allows for the generation of more accurate turnaround time reports.
- Electronic capture of order and collection times facilitates troubleshooting of delays in various preanalytical steps.
- Electronic order entry enhances patient care by eliminating both transcription errors on order entry in the laboratory and the mislabeling of specimens by laboratory employees.
- By eliminating the need for data entry in the laboratory, electronic order entry decreases the turnaround time for laboratory testing.

30. A. Electronic interfacing of the LIS with the reference laboratory will decrease the number of tests sent to the reference laboratory, thereby saving the hospital money.
Rationale: Electronic interfacing of the LIS with the reference laboratory is unlikely to decrease the number of samples sent to the reference laboratory.
B. Electronic interfacing of the LIS with the reference laboratory will eliminate the need for laboratory employees to manually transcribe results; this will reduce overtime and/or staffing costs and, thereby, save the hospital money. In addition, by decreasing the turnaround times for these results, patients may be discharged faster and the average length of stay may decrease, thereby allowing the hospital to improve revenue.
Rationale: These are valid reasons to electronically interface a reference laboratory with the LIS.
C. Electronic interfacing with the LIS to the reference laboratory will decrease courier costs.
Rationale: Electronic interfacing the LIS with the reference laboratory will not decrease courier costs required to send the samples to the reference laboratory.
D. Electronic interfacing of the LIS with the reference laboratory will decrease the time required to transport samples to the reference laboratory.
Rationale: Electronic interfacing of the LIS with the reference laboratory will not decrease the time required to transport samples to the reference laboratory.
E. Electronic interfacing of the LIS with the reference laboratory will increase transcription errors in preanalytical functions in your laboratory.
Rationale: Electronic interfacing of the LIS with the reference laboratory will decrease transcription errors in preanalytical functions in your laboratory.

Major points of discussion

- Whenever possible, reference laboratories should be electronically interfaced with your LIS.
- Electronic interfacing of reference laboratories with your LIS eliminates the possibility of transcription errors associated with manual result entry.
- Electronic interfaces also allow easy transmission of long, complex interpretative comments, which would otherwise not be available to the ordering physician.
- Electronic interfacing of reference laboratories with your LIS eliminates delays in turnaround time

caused by waiting for manual transcription to be completed.
- Electronic interfacing of reference laboratories with your LIS eliminates the need to pay for transcriptionists or other similar personnel, thereby saving money for your hospital.
- Electronic interfacing of reference laboratories with your LIS decreases turnaround times and allows earlier discharge of patients, thereby allowing hospitals to increase revenue.

31. A. 2.
Rationale: A bit is the smallest unit of measurement. It can hold a 0 or 1, which would be two unique letters, numbers, or special characters (2^1).
B. 8.
Rationale: Eight unique letters, numbers, or special characters can be produced in 3 bits (2^3).
C. 64.
Rationale: Sixty-four unique letters, numbers, or special characters can be produced in 6 bits (2^6).
D. 128.
Rationale: One hundred twenty-eight unique letters, numbers, or special characters can be produced in 7 bits (2^7).
E. 256.
Rationale: Eight bits is equal to 1 byte. Two hundred fifty-six unique letters, numbers, or special characters can be produced by 1 byte (8 bits; 2^8).

Major points of discussion
- Information is stored on computers in digital form (i.e., 0 or 1). Binary digits (bits) are the smallest unit of measurement of computer storage; the bit can store either a 0 or 1.
- A byte consists of 8 bits and can therefore produce one of 256 (i.e., 2^8) combinations of 0s and 1s.
- Two hundred fifty-six characters, numbers, or special characters can be assigned a unique binary number, which is called "binary code." It takes 1 byte of storage to store one character in an 8-bit (1-byte) binary code
- Examples:
  - 1011 0000 may represent "A."
  - 1011 0010 may represent "B."
- Standardized binary codes consisting of a different number of bits (e.g., 7 or 8) can encode a different number of characters. For example, ASCII is a binary code using 7 bits to produce 128 unique number combinations. UTF-32 is a 32-bit (4-byte) binary code and requires 4 bytes to store one character.

32. **A. Faster implementation.**
Rationale: It is faster to add CPOE to an existing system than to implement both a new EHR and CPOE.
B. Greater cost of supporting an older system.
Rationale: Supporting an existing EHR may or may not be more expensive.
C. Greater disruption of operations.
Rationale: Implementing a new EHR and CPOE is a greater disruption to operations than adding CPOE to an existing, legacy system.
D. Greater variety of options.
Rationale: Implementing a new EHR and CPOE allows for a greater number of options in the EHR and CPOE. Adding a

CPOE system to an existing EHR may limit the functions available.
E. Increased number of user devices required.
Rationale: The number of user devices should not change or would not necessarily be predictable based on whether adding CPOE alone or implementing a new EHR along with CPOE.

Major points of discussion
- Computerized physician order entry (CPOE) is a highly desirable component of electronic health record (EHR) systems.
- CPOE allows for enhancements that can influence laboratory orders such as decision support, alerts, and reminders.
- Implementing CPOE requires support at the highest level of administration and the information technology partners, as well as the laboratory director and staff.
- CPOE can be added to an existing EHR system or the entire EHR can be replaced with a new EHR that has CPOE capability.
- Although adding CPOE to an existing system is faster with less disruption to the organization, it may limit the number of enhancements that are available and may not even meet the minimal requirements for the institution. Purchasing a new EHR system with CPOE will likely have greater cost of implementation, more disruption of operations, and take more time.

33. A. Determine functional requirements.
Rationale: This should be an early step in the process of procuring a new LIS.
B. Form a working group.
Rationale: This should be one of the first steps in the process of procuring a new LIS.
C. Negotiate the contract.
Rationale: Contracts should be negotiated after determining the requirements of the LIS, qualifying the vendor(s), reviewing the proposals, and then choosing the final vendor.
D. Send out a request for information (RFI).
Rationale: RFIs are simply a request to vendors to share information in order to determine the types of LIS and LIS enhancements that are available. This step precedes the request for proposals (RFP) and contract negotiation processes. A vendor that has submitted information in response to an RFI may or may not receive an RFP.
E. Send out a request for proposals (RFP).
Rationale: Once the RFI and requirements of the LIS have been reviewed, the appropriate vendors will be asked to submit proposals. Contracts can then be negotiated with the desired vendor.

Major points of discussion
- Purchasing a new LIS is a very large undertaking that requires the commitment and support from the highest level of administration and the entire laboratory.
- The process starts with high-level administrators and laboratory directors who develop a strategic and financial plan for the LIS. The plan for the LIS must fit into the overall strategic plan for the hospital system.

- An LIS working group is then formed to determine the current and future needs of the laboratory and to develop intermediate plans to meet the strategic goals.
- The LIS working group may request information from vendors (i.e., an RFI) to determine what current offerings are available. The working group then chooses which vendors are able to meet the needs of the laboratory.
- The RFP process is initiated after all the requirements for the LIS are listed. The vendors can then create a proposal to meet those requirements and may also include pricing at that time.
- After the proposals are reviewed, the laboratory will choose the "best fit" LIS. Contract negotiations are completed and then LIS implementation can begin.

34. A. Compact disc.
Rationale: Data are stored on compact discs by using a laser to burn "pits" or "bumps" to represent bits. If power is turned off, the data physically remain on the polycarbonate disc.
B. Hard disk drive.
Rationale: A motor spins a platter below an arm that holds an apparatus that writes and reads magnetic signals on the platter. When power is turned off, the magnetic domains remain on the platter.
C. Solid-state drive.
Rationale: Unlike random-access memory (RAM), solid-state drives are nonvolatile, rewritable storage devices that use transistors rather than magnetic domains to store data.
D. Random-access memory (RAM).
Rationale: RAM is a volatile storage device and will lose data if power is turned off. Some computers may have an alternate power source to maintain power to RAM, but if all power is turned off, RAM will lose the stored data.
E. Read-only memory (ROM).
Rationale: ROM is used in computers and other electronic devices and is preprogrammed with specific data by the manufacturer. In computers, these data are known as firmware.

Major points of discussion
- Data can be stored on many different storage devices such as ROM, RAM, hard disk drives, solid-state drives, compact discs, and many others.
- Hard-disk drives store data on platters using an arm with an apparatus that reads and writes data by changing the magnetic domains. These data remain on the disk until they are overwritten or reformatted. Disk drives can be removed and installed on another computer without losing data.
- Solid-state drives, unlike hard disk drives, use integrated circuits and store data on a foundation of transistors that form grids. The data are nonvolatile and rewritable. Solid-state drives can be removed and moved to another computer without losing data.
- Compact discs (CDs) and digital video discs (DVDs) use similar technology to store data on polycarbonate plastic discs. A laser burns "pits" and "bumps" into the plastic, which can then be later read by an optical system. The CD or DVD can be removed, stored, and then read again by a CD/DVD player.
- ROM is a nonvolatile storage device that is preprogrammed with data and programs by the manufacturer of a specific device. In computers, firmware

is stored on ROM. ROM is generally not modified within the functioning life of the device. Non-rewritable CDs can also be considered a form of a read-only storage device.
- RAM is a volatile memory device that is often referred to as "computer memory." It allows storage of data that can be quickly and easily accessed. The design on integrated circuits allows the data to be accessed in a random fashion rather than reading and writing in a predetermined order, such as with hard disks and CDs. Data are stored on capacitors. These capacitors will discharge when power is no longer supplied and the data will be lost.

35. A. Camera.
B. Keyboard.
C. Monitor.
Rationale: This is an output device.
D. Mouse.
E. Scanner.
Rationale for A, B, D, and E: These are input devices.

Major points of discussion
- Output devices take the results of computer processing and present them to humans (i.e., the end user) using different methods.
- Input devices provide data and control signals from the end user to the computer for processing.
- Examples of output devices used in the laboratory include computer monitors, printers, label printers, speakers, and other audible signals.
- Examples of output devices that may not be found in a clinical laboratory include headphones, LCD projector, Braille embossers, and three-dimensional printers.
- Examples of input devices include a mouse and keyboards, microphones, cameras, touch screens, and scanners.

36. A. Hard drive.
Rationale: This is a storage device.
B. Label printer.
C. LCD projector.
D. Monitor.
Rationale: These are output devices.
E. Scanner.
Rationale: This is an input device.

Major points of discussion
- Input devices provide data and control signals from the end user to the computer for processing.
- Output devices take the results of computer processing and present them to humans (i.e., the end user) to observe.
- Storage devices receive input and produce output. However, they do not interact directly with the end user. Storage devices interact with the central processing unit.
- Examples of input devices include a mouse and keyboards, microphones, cameras, touchscreens, and scanners.
- Examples of output devices used in the laboratory include computer monitors, printers, label printers, speakers, and other audible signals.

37. **A. Accuracy of the calculations and reports should be reviewed on a periodic basis.**
B. Accuracy of the calculations and reports need to be checked only when a system change is made.

Rationale: Accuracy of calculations should be checked at installation and then every 2 years thereafter, or after every system change that may affect the calculation.
C. Calculations shared by multiple hospitals using the same laboratory information should be checked by every site.
Rationale: If multiple hospitals use the same calculation using the same laboratory information system, then it only has to be checked at one site; the documentation should then be reviewed, approved, and filed at every other site.
D. Checks of calculation accuracy do not have to be performed if calculations are made by middleware.
E. Checks of calculation accuracy do not have to be performed if calculations are made by the analyzer.
Rationale: Accuracy checks should be performed if the calculation is made in the instrument, middleware, or the laboratory information system.

Major points of discussion
- Calculations using laboratory values can be performed in instruments, middleware, or laboratory information systems.
- These calculations can be simple, such as calculating the blood urea nitrogen/creatinine (BUN/Cr) ratio by simple division.
- These calculations can be more complicated, such as reporting creatinine clearance, which requires incorporation of age, weight, gender, and creatinine, as well as additional modifications depending on the patient's age and ideal body weight.
- Calculations that are reported in the patient's medical record should be validated for accuracy at the time of implementation and after major system changes are made.
- In addition, calculations should be reviewed periodically, usually once every 2 years.

38. A. Links human-readable terms to concepts.
Rationale: SNOMED (the Systematized Nomenclature of Medicine) links human-readable terms to concepts.
B. Standard used for the transfer of information associated with blood transfusion.
Rationale: ISBT128 is a standard used for the transfer of information associated with blood transfusion.
C. Communications protocol used for sending and receiving data across the Internet.
Rationale: The Internet protocol communications protocol is used to send and receive data across the Internet.
D. Seventh level of the seven-layer communications model for open systems interconnection.
Rationale: The Health Level Seven (HL7) communications protocol is used for health care communications. The "7" refers to the seventh level of the seven-layer communications model for open systems interconnection.
E. Universal identifiers for laboratory and other clinical observations.
Rationale: LOINC coding is a standard that assigns universal identifiers for laboratory and other clinical observations.

Major points of discussion
- The Logical Observation Identifiers Names and Codes (LOINC) system was developed by the Regenstrief Institute, which is associated with Indiana University.

- The purpose of LOINC is to assign universal codes for communicating clinical and laboratory observation across independent electronic medical record systems.
- Internally, an institution may share its observations across internal systems using a local coding system for laboratory results. These messages are sent by a coding protocol such as Health Level Seven (HL7). However, when sending to an external, independent system, this code must be "translated" by the receiving system.
- LOINC solves this translation problem by setting a universal code for these observations, so that sending and receiving systems can use the same encoding of these observations without the need to translate between local encoding systems.
- The record fields included for each test or observation are the name of the analyte (e.g., hemoglobin), standard units (e.g., g/dL), time (e.g., 24-hour urine), sample type (e.g., serum), type of data (e.g., quantitative, qualitative, nominal), and method.[20]

39. A. It is a utility software to optimize a computer system.
Rationale: Utility software analyzes, troubleshoots, protects, maintains, and optimizes a computer system. Antivirus, backup, disk fragmenter, disk space optimizer, and system monitors are examples of utility software.
B. It allocates computer resources to more than one application (i.e., multitasking).
Rationale: MUMPS has multitasking functions, but it has a broader application as a programming language.
C. It is an Internet protocol.
Rationale: MUMPS is a programming language, not a protocol for sending information over the Internet.
D. It is a laboratory information system.
Rationale: Many laboratory information systems are built on MUMPS programming language. However, financial systems are also programmed using MUMPS.
E. It is a programming language.
Rationale: MUMPS is a programming language originally developed at the Massachusetts General Hospital for the health care industry, but the language is also used in the financial industry.

Major points of discussion
- Many well-known laboratory information systems and electronic health records are built on MUMPS, including those of the Veterans Administration, MEDITECH, Sunquest, and many others.
- MUMPS was developed for writing database-driven applications, and much of the programming supports seamless integration of database management.
- MUMPS was one of the earliest adopters of multitasking, which allows multiple tasks to be worked on at the same time.
- MUMPS was designed for multiple users, so it has built-in controls to prevent multiple users from accessing the same files.

40. A. Autoverification.
Rationale: Autoverification can be built as an expert system following a simple set of rules. These rules are usually available as part of a laboratory information system.
B. Delta check.

Rationale: Delta checks are usually available as part of a laboratory information system and require the laboratory information system to follow a simple set of rules.
C. Calculations.
Rationale: Calculations can be simply implemented as rules and numerical calculations in a laboratory information system.
D. Image-based white blood cell differential.
Rationale: Analyzing images to perform a differential count requires more programming than a set of rules. Neural networks are better suited to "learn" from the experience of identifying cell types.
E. Reflex test ordering.
Rationale: Reflex test ordering is usually available as part of a laboratory information system; it requires the laboratory information system to follow a simple set of rules.

Major points of discussion
- Expert systems perform functions based on a simple or complex set of rules. These rules capture the approach a human would take to perform the task.
- For example, an expert system may have the following rule: If the prothrombin time and/or partial thromboplastin time is abnormal, then reflexively order a mixing study.
- Neural networks do not work by a set of rules; instead, these systems try to modify their output based on "experience" or "learning." After a neural network has been developed, it "learns" on a set of known examples.
- For example, the neural network would examine 100 normal neutrophils. Each time the system identifies or misidentifies a neutrophil, its programming is adjusted automatically. Then, the system is put to use on unknown cases.
- The advantage of a neural network versus an expert system is that the expert system must have its rules adjusted to better fit the approach taken by experts, whereas a neural network is constantly adjusting itself during its learning process.
- The disadvantage of a neural network is its high processing and storage requirements. In addition, computer analysts are not able to reproduce "how" or "why" the neural network came to a particular conclusion (e.g., identified a white blood cell as a particular type).

41. **A. Automated interface to other systems.**
   Rationale: Automated interfaces are fast and less prone to errors.
   B. Free text manual data entry.
   C. Scanning documents with subsequent optical character recognition translation.
   Rationale: Scanning documents is time consuming and labor intensive. Optical character recognition is not perfect at reading typed text and much less accurate when analyzing handwriting.
   D. Structured form manual data entry.
   E. Transcription of physician dictation.
   Rationale for B, D, and E: Manual data entry is time consuming and labor intensive, and it is prone to errors. Structured forms or coding may be preferable to free text entry.

Major points of discussion
- There are three methods for entering data into an electronic health record: manual, interfaced, and scanned.
- Manual data entry can be direct entry of free text, entry of coded or structured data, or transcription of dictated or written notes.
- Scanned data entry allows for the paper-based medical record to be entered into the EHR. However, to structure and search the data, optical character recognition is required, which is also prone to errors.
- Data entry into the EHR by an interface to another system is the ideal method for inputting information.
- Laboratory information systems are commonplace systems that interface with EHRs. The data are rapidly transferred after the results have been verified. The results can be updated, if necessary. In addition, if tested appropriately, the data should transfer without the risk of transcription errors.

42. A. Smaller financial investment.
   Rationale: EHRs have a higher initial financial investment due to the need to purchase hardware, software, and perform training.
   B. Fewer organizational challenges.
   Rationale: The EHR has greater organizational challenges to overcome. Physicians, nurses, and staff must be trained on how to use the EHR; information technology departments must technically support the system; and higher-level management must maintain the system and develop enhancements.
   C. Catastrophic loss of all patient data.
   Rationale: This is an advantage of a paper-based system versus an EHR. An EHR can catastrophically fail and all electronic data can be lost permanently.
   D. Smaller time commitment for physician entry.
   Rationale: Physicians spend a greater amount of time entering patient data when an EHR is used.
   E. Increased availability of records.
   Rationale: Records can be accessed by one or more users at the site of the system, or remotely, when an EHR is used.

Major points of discussion
- Electronic health records (EHRs) are increasingly used by hospitals to increase the overall quality of patient care.
- EHRs increase patient safety and quality of care by allowing access of a patient's medical records by one or more users at multiple sites. These records are comprehensive, legible, and structured.
- EHRs are useful for research and quality improvement because the structured data can be retrieved and analyzed for trends and for evaluating the effect of interventions.
- The advantage of EHRs include better access to records, legibility, structured data, comprehensiveness, long-term availability, and the ability to add enhancements such as decision support, computer-based physician order entry, and prescription writers.
- There are several disadvantages of EHRs, as follows:
  - There is a high initial financial investment and organizational investment. Hardware, software, and

training must be purchased, and the system must be maintained and regularly updated by an information technology department.
- The organizational workflow must be changed, and the culture of the medical staff, nursing, and ancillary staff must be changed to incorporate the EHR into this new workflow.

43. A. Assigns the National Institute of Standards and Technology (NIST) to manage all federal, nonmilitary information systems.
Rationale: This was not part of the HITECH Act. The Federal Information Security Act of 2002 assigned NIST to coordinate the security of all federal, nonmilitary information systems.
B. Promotes the adoption and meaningful use of electronic health records.
Rationale: Promotion of the meaningful use of electronic health records was one of the main goals of the HITECH Act.
C. Protects identifiable patient information from being used to identify patient safety events.
Rationale: This requirement is for patient privacy, which is not covered under the HITECH Act.
D. Requires all federal employees to take an information security awareness program.
Rationale: This not a requirement of the HITECH Act, although it is a good practice.
E. Requires federal agencies to develop, document, and implement security of information systems.
Rationale: This is a requirement of the Federal Information Security Act of 2002, not HITECH.

Major points of discussion
- The Health Information Technology for Economic and Clinical Health (HITECH) Act is part of the American Recovery and Reinvestment Act of 2009.
- The United States Department of Health and Human Services is spending billions of dollars to promote the use of information technology in health care, in particular, the use of electronic health records.
- The HITECH Act financially rewards physicians who implement electronic health records in a way such that the implementation has "meaningful use."
- "Meaningful use" includes information technology functions, such as computerized order entry to pharmacies (e.g., electronic prescription writer), medication reconciliation, active problem lists, lists of allergies, clinical rules (e.g., drug-drug interactions and reminders), clinical notes, and many others.
- Hospitals and physicians are encouraged to increase the compatibility of electronic health records so that information can be exchanged easily across different systems.

44. **A. Application layer.**
Rationale: The application layer is the seventh layer of OSI. It is the level closest to the user. The OSI and the user interact with the application
B. Data layer.
Rationale: The data layer is the second layer of OSI. This level outlines the way data are transferred within the same network.
C. Network layer.

Rationale: The network layer is the third layer of OSI. This level defines the way data are routed between networks.
D. Physical layer.
Rationale: The physical layer is the first layer of OSI. It outlines physical and electrical specifications.
E. Session layer.
Rationale: The session layer is the fifth layer of OSI. It defines the way systems start, maintain, and end a dialog across a network.

Major points of discussion
- The Open Systems Interconnection (OSI) model is an international standard under the International Organization for Standardization (ISO). The seven-layer OSI model of networking is an abstract model of networking.
- Each of the seven layers supports the layer above it and interacts with only one level below it.
- The seven layers are physical, data, network, transport, session, presentation, and application.
- This standard, although abstract, provides a guide to manufacturers so that their systems are more likely to be able to interact with systems designed by another manufacturer.
- Some examples are as follows:
  - Physical: The RS-232 standard defines the signal and pins for physical connections such as computer serial ports.
  - Application: Health Level 7 (HL7) defines the way health information is structured and then exchanged between computer applications (e.g., laboratory instrument to laboratory information system).[13]

45. A. Easier auditing of incoming traffic.
Rationale: Auditing incoming traffic is easier at the application level in the application gateway firewall.
B. Less processing overhead.
Rationale: There is more processing overhead in an application gateway firewall and a separate proxy must be set up for each service.
C. Easier logging of incoming traffic.
Rationale: Logging incoming traffic is easier at the application level in the application gateway firewall.
D. Better security.
Rationale: Application gateway firewalls are more secure.
E. Ability to relay packets without examining them.
Rationale: Both types of firewalls examine packets before relaying them.

Major points of discussion
- A firewall is a software- or hardware-based system that is implemented to protect a private network from a wide-area network (WAN) or the Internet. The goal is to prevent malware from entering the private network and cyber attacks.
- Firewalls work by implementing a set of rules to determine whether incoming or outgoing traffic is to be trusted.
- Packet-filtering routers were one of the earliest forms of a firewall. Incoming traffic is examined, and if the packet passes a predefined screening process, it is relayed into the private network. If the packet does not meet criteria, it is either dropped or rejected.

■ Application layer filtering is performed at the application layer (Open Systems Interconnection layer 7) and, therefore, can examine packets for specific applications. Logging and auditing of incoming traffic are easier with application layer filtering, but it comes at a cost of higher processing overhead.

■ Proxy servers are an intermediary between secure networks. A client will request a service from the proxy server; the proxy server then determines whether the request and connection should be trusted.

46. A. Assigns the NIST to create a national standard for protecting health care information against cyber attacks.
Rationale: NIST was assigned the task of coordinating the development of guidelines for nonnational security federal agencies to protect information systems against cyber attacks.
B. Establishes national standards for the security and maintenance of confidentiality of protected health information.
Rationale: Health information protection falls under the Health Insurance Portability and Accountability Act of 1996 (HIPAA).
C. Requires all EHRs to maintain a log of users who access a health record and what the user accessed.
Rationale: This is good security practice to protect the privacy of patients but is not part of FISMA.
D. Requires federal agencies to develop and implement plans to ensure information and information system security.
Rationale: FISMA requires all federal agencies not involved in national security to develop and implement procedures to protect information systems.
E. Requires all hospitals to be certified by a federal agency prior to implementing an EHR.
Rationale: This is not a requirement of FISMA.

Major points of discussion
■ The purpose of the Federal Information Security Management Act of 2002 (FISMA) was to require federal agencies not involved in national security to develop and implement procedures to protect information systems.
■ The National Institute of Standards and Technology (NIST) was assigned the task of overseeing the development of standards and guidelines for the protection of information systems against cyber attacks.
■ NIST was assigned the task of coordinating the federal agencies and ensuring that the standards are consistent with national security–related federal agencies as much as possible.
■ The Department of Defense and the Central Intelligence Agency were excluded from this act because they are the main federal national security agencies.
■ The director of a federal agency is responsible for developing and implementing standards that protect information systems.[11]

47. A. OSI.
Rationale: Although the OSI model is often referenced, the TCP/IP (Transmission Control Protocol/Internet Protocol) is the standardized network protocol. TCP/IP is a standard with a long cycle time and it does not drive rapid changes to middleware.

B. LIS upgrades.
Rationale: LIS versions have a long cycle time and are expensive to purchase and validate. Middleware's rapid versioning is able to fill the gaps between upgrades.
C. Instrument interface engine upgrades.
Rationale: New instruments require quick adoption of new interface engines; frequent patches to these interface engines are often required.
D. User-defined expert rules.
Rationale: Expert rules are if-then statements that are written for the middleware. Middleware versioning is not driven by the need for additional rule-based functions as it is for interface engines.
E. Server hardware upgrades.
Rationale: Hardware upgrades are performed to improve performance. Hardware is upgraded approximately every 3 years.

Major points of discussion
■ Middleware is a bundle of software that is layered between laboratory instruments and the LIS. Generally, middleware allows interfacing of multiple instruments and information systems using different communication protocols.
■ Middleware can meet the needs of the laboratory by applying rule-based algorithms (e.g., if-then statements) for quality control rules, autoverification, delta checks, critical value flags, reflex test ordering, and specimen archiving. These rule-based algorithms are also known as "expert-systems."
■ Total laboratory automation requires middleware to operate as the controller of specimen routing, load balance, and specimen archiving and retrieval.
■ Just as all LISs are different, middleware products are also different. Selection of the appropriate middleware products will depend on the functions of the laboratory information systems and the types of enhancements that are needed.

48. A. Multiple different types of specimen containers are used throughout the hospital.
Rationale: Although it is highly desirable to use as few different types of specimen containers as possible, different containers can often coexist, as long as the manufacturer of the system supports them.
B. Many samples arrive hand-labeled accompanied by a paper requisition.
Rationale: Although it is extremely desirable to receive all samples in the laboratory with barcodes, samples can be relabeled with barcode labels in the laboratory prior to placement on the automated line.
C. The available capital budget does not contain enough funds to purchase the automation line.
Rationale: Instrumentation can often be leased or obtained on reagent rental, instead of purchased outright.[21]
D. The Laboratory Information System (LIS) assigns the same specimen number to all specimens collected from a single patient phlebotomy.
Rationale: If the LIS assigns the same specimen number to all specimens from the same phlebotomy from an individual patient, the system will not be able to distinguish between different sample tube types. For example, it will not know whether to perform a complete blood cell count or a basic metabolic panel on a given sample.

E. The laboratory desires to continue to use instrumentation from different vendors in different sections of the laboratory.
Rationale: Many automation lines allow connection of analytical instruments from multiple vendors.

Major points of discussion

- For total laboratory automation, the LIS must be able to assign unique identifiers to each sample container.
- Instrumentation from different vendors can often be connected to the same automation line.
- For automation to be successful, (almost) all samples must have barcode labels.
- Early involvement of the LIS team in the selection and implementation planning of laboratory automation is an important key to success.
- It may be possible to lease automation equipment or obtain it by reagent rental. Therefore, it does not have to be purchased outright.

49. A. It does not require a major financial investment.
Rationale: Laboratory automation requires major financial investments for equipment and computerization.
B. Little planning is required for implementation.
Rationale: Total laboratory automation requires major space and personnel planning for implementation.
C. It can increase production capacity severalfold without adding space or personnel.

Rationale: Total laboratory automation can significantly improve laboratory efficiency and productivity.
D. Usually, no architectural work is required.
Rationale: The introduction of laboratory automation often requires major architectural work to allow placement of large, robotic instruments.
E. Organizational changes are usually not required.
Rationale: Introduction of laboratory automation often requires far-reaching organizational changes—for example, in the way samples are handled and employees pursue their tasks.

Major points of discussion

- Introduction of total laboratory automation almost always requires major financial investments, substantial planning, major architectural work, and far-reaching organizational changes.
- Total laboratory automation allows the consolidation of work and personnel.
- Total laboratory automation can allow laboratories to increase production capacity severalfold without adding space or personnel.
- Centralized accessioning of patient samples is a precondition for total laboratory automation to succeed.
- A modern laboratory information system with unique specimen identifiers is a precondition for the success of total laboratory automation.[24]

References

1. Akamstsu S, Tsukazaki H, Inoue K, et al. Advanced prostate cancer with extremely low prostate-specific antigen value at diagnosis: an example of high dose hook effect. Int J Urol 2006;13:1025–1027.
2. Al-Mahdili HA, Jones GRD. High-dose hook effect in six automated human chorionic gonadotropin assays. Ann Clin Biochem 2010;47:383–385.
3. Armbruster DA, Hubster EC, Kaufman MS, et al. Cloned enzyme donor immunoassay (CEDIA) for drugs-of-abuse screening. Clin Chem 1995;1:92–98.
4. Astion Ml, Kaveh G, Shojania MD, et al. Classifying laboratory incident reports to identify problems that jeopardize patient safety. Am J Clin Pathol 2003;120:18–26.
5. Baeyens WRG, Schulman SG, Calokerinos AC, et al. Chemiluminescence-based detection: principles and analytical applications in flowing streams and in immunoassays. J Pharm Biomed Anal 1998;6–7:941–953.
6. Bjerner J, Nustad K, Norum LF, et al. Immunometric assay interference: incidence and prevention. Clin Chem 2002;48:613–621.
7. Bonini P, Piebani M, Ceriotti F, et al. Errors in laboratory medicine. Clin Chem 2002;48:691–698.
8. Curme HG, Columbus RL, Dappen GM, et al. Multilayer film elements for clinical analysis: general concepts. Clin Chem 1978;24:1335–1342.
9. Despres N, Grant AM. Antibody interference in thyroid assays: a potential for clinical misinformation. Clin Chem 1998;44:440–454.
10. Ehrmeyer SE, Laessig RH. Regulation, accreditation, and education for point-of-care testing. In Kost GJ, ed. Principles and practice of point-of-care testing. Philadelphia: Lippincott, 2002, pp. 434–443.
11. National Institute of Standards and Technology. Federal Information Processing Standards Publication 200. Minimum security requirements for federal information and information systems. March 2006. Available at http://csrc.nist.gov/publications/fips200/FIPS-200-final-march.pdf.
12. Haas T, Spielmann N, Mauch J, et al. Comparison of thromboelastometry (ROTEM®) with standard plasmatic coagulation testing in paediatric surgery. Br J Anaesth 2012;108:36–41.
13. Health Level Seven International. Available at www.hl7.org.
14. Hemmila I. Fluoroimmunoassays and immunofluorometric assays. Clin Chem 1985;3:359–570.
15. Henderson DR, Friedman SB, Harris JD, et al. CEDIA, a new homogeneous immunoassay system. Clin Chem 1986;9:1637–1641.
16. Hopfer SM, Nadeau FL, Sundra M, et al. Effect of protein on hemoglobin and hematocrit assays with a conductivity-based point-of-care testing device: comparison with optical methods. Ann Clin Lab Sci 2004;34:75–82.
17. Kiechle FL, Gauss I. Provider performed microscopy. Clin Lab Med 2001;21:375–387.
18. Kiechle FL. Point-of-care testing for body fluids. In Kost GJ, ed. Principles and practice of point-of-care testing. Philadelphia: Lippincott; 2002, pp. 174–194.
19. Kricka LJ. Human anti-animal antibody interference in immunological assays. Clin Chem 1999;45:942–956.
20. Logical Observation Identifiers Names and Codes (LOINC). Available at www.loinc.org.
21. Melanson EF, Lindeman NI, Jarolim P. Selecting automation for the clinical chemistry laboratory. Arch Pathol Lab Med 2007;131:1063–1069.
22. Mendru DR, Chou PP, Soldin SJ. An improved application of the enzyme multiplied immunoassay technique for caffeine, amikacin, and methotrexate assays on the Dade-Behring dimension RxL Max Clinical Chemistry System. Ther Drug Monit 2007;5:632–637.

23. Nichols JH. Point-of-care testing. In Lewandrowski K, ed. Clinical chemistry. Philadelphia: Lippincott, 2002, pp. 174–194.
24. Orsulak PJ. Stand-alone automated solutions can enhance laboratory operations. Clin Chem 2000;46:778–783.
25. Rongen HAH, Hoetelmans RMW, Bult A, et al. Chemiluminescence and immunoassays. J Pharm Biomed Anal 1994;4:433–462.
26. Santrach PJ. Point-of-care hematology, hemostasis, and thrombolysis testing. In Kost GJ, ed. Principles and practice of point-of-care testing. Philadelphia: Lippincott Williams & Wilkins, 2002, pp. 157–180.

27. Smith DS, Eremin SA. Fluorescence polarization immunoassays and related methods for simple, high-throughput screening of small molecules. Anal Bioanal Chem 2008;5:1499–1507.
28. Sterinkamp T, Karst U. Detection strategies for bioassays based on luminescent lanthanide complexes and signal amplification. Anal Bioanal Chem 2004;1:24–30.
29. Yuan J, Wang G. Lanthanide complex-based fluorescence label for time-resolved fluorescence bioassay. J Fluoresc 2005;4:559–568.

CHAPTER 4

CLINICAL CHEMISTRY:
Endocrine (Thyroid, Pituitary, Adrenal, Bone, Pancreas, Reproductive) and Catecholamines

Serge Cremers, Jorge L. Sepulveda, Andrew Turk

QUESTIONS

During a diagnostic workup for hypertension and weight gain, a patient's midnight salivary cortisol is found to be elevated (40 µg/dL; reference range, <0.100 µg/dL) with a borderline decreased plasma adrenocorticotropic hormone (ACTH). The diagnosis of primary hyperadrenalism (Cushing's syndrome) is considered.

1a. Which one of the following is the most likely next diagnostic step to confirm primary hyperadrenalism?
  A. Measure urinary free cortisol.
  B. Measure a repeat salivary cortisol in the morning.
  C. Low-dose dexamethasone suppression test (DST).
  D. Measure plasma aldosterone.

1b. A diagnosis of Cushing's syndrome is confirmed, and abdominal computed tomography (CT) reveals a 5-cm mass over the right adrenal gland. A high-dose DST is performed. Which one of the following is the most likely result of this testing?
  A. Greater than 50% reduction in serum cortisol.
  B. No suppression of serum cortisol.
  C. An elevation in serum cortisol.
  D. Suppression of serum metanephrines.

A mother brings her 8-year-old son to the pediatrician for his annual checkup. She states that he seems to be struggling in school. Physical examination shows short stature and a palpable goiter. There is a family history of short stature and learning difficulties. The pediatrician performs thyroid function tests consisting of serum free thyroxine (FT_4), free triiodothyronine (FT_3), and thyroid-stimulating hormone (TSH). The results prompt additional workup. Ultimately, the boy is diagnosed with resistance to thyroid hormone (RTH). Use this scenario to answer the following four questions.

2a. Which one of the following choices most likely reflects this patient's thyroid function studies?
  A. Normal TSH, decreased FT_4, decreased FT_3.
  B. Normal TSH, elevated FT_4, elevated FT_3.
  C. Elevated TSH, decreased FT_4, decreased FT_3.
  D. Elevated TSH, normal FT_4, normal FT_3.
  E. Elevated TSH, elevated FT_4, elevated FT_3.

2b. Given the physical examination findings (i.e., goiter) and the ultimate diagnosis of resistance to thyroid hormone (RTH), which one of the following mutations was most likely identified by genetic analysis?
  A. Inactivating mutation of the thyrotropin-releasing hormone receptor (TRHR) gene.
  B. Inactivating mutation of the thyroid stimulating hormone receptor (TSHR) gene.
  C. Inactivating mutation of the TSH β-chain gene.
  D. Inactivating mutation of the thyroxine-binding globulin (TBG) gene.
  E. Inactivating mutation of the thyroid hormone receptor (TR) β gene.

2c. Which one of the following statements is correct regarding the relative metabolic activity of thyroxine (T_4), triiodothyronine (T_3), and reverse triiodothyronine (rT_3)?
  A. T_4 is more metabolically active than T_3, which is more metabolically active than rT_3.
  B. T_4 is more metabolically active than rT_3, which is more metabolically active than T_3.
  C. T_3 and rT_3 are approximately equally metabolically active. These hormones are more metabolically active than T_4.
  D. T_3 is more metabolically active than T_4, which is more metabolically active than rT_3.
  E. T_3 is more metabolically active than rT_3, which is more metabolically active than T_4.

2d. Certain organs show greater impairment than others in the setting of hypothyroidism. Which one of the following organs is likely to show the *least* functional impairment in a hypothyroid patient?
  A. Liver.
  B. Kidney.
  C. Spleen.
  D. Skeletal muscle.
  E. Heart.

During his annual checkup, a 34 year-old white man complains of a chronically low libido to his primary care physician. The patient's history includes acute leukemia during his early childhood, which was treated with chemotherapy. Physical examination reveals tall stature and gynecomastia. Laboratory workup reveals a serum total testosterone level of 150 ng/dL (reference range, 270 to 1070 ng/dL). Use this scenario to answer the following four questions.

3a. Careful physical examination of this patient is most likely to show which one of the following features?
  A. Decreased fat deposition in the hips, buttocks, and thighs.
  B. Increased fat deposition in the face, abdomen, and waist.
  C. Decreased facial and body hair.
  D. Decreased hair on the temporal aspect of the scalp.
  E. A diamond-shaped escutcheon (pubic hair pattern), rather than a triangular escutcheon.

3b. Serum total testosterone levels are most likely to be normal in patients with which one of the following genetic conditions?
  A. Klinefelter's syndrome.
  B. XYY syndrome.
  C. Kallmann's syndrome.
  D. Loss-of-function mutations in the gene encoding GPR54.
  E. CHARGE syndrome.

3c. Which one of the following statements best explains this patient's tall stature?
  A. Androgens stimulate increased secretion of insulin-like growth factor 1 (IGF-1), which in turn causes growth.
  B. Estrogens ultimately terminate growth by causing closure of the epiphyses of the long bones.
  C. Androgens have a net anabolic effect in terms of protein metabolism (i.e., androgens increase protein synthesis and decrease protein degradation).
  D. Androgens increase the deposition of calcium salts and the rate of bone growth.
  E. Boys who undergo precocious puberty (i.e., onset of puberty before age 9 years) typically have tall stature as adults.

3d. Regarding demographic and physiologic parameters that affect normal serum testosterone levels in adult men, which one of the following statements is true?
  A. Serum total testosterone levels decrease with age, whereas serum free testosterone levels remain relatively constant with age.
  B. The quantitative relationship between serum total testosterone and serum free testosterone depends primarily on the serum concentration of albumin.
  C. Serum testosterone levels are inversely proportional to body mass index (BMI).
  D. Serum testosterone levels have no quantitative relationship with central obesity (i.e., waist/hip ratio).
  E. Serum total testosterone levels are higher in young white men compared with young black men.

A 35-year-old woman was brought to the emergency department after developing psychosis. Laboratory studies performed in the emergency department revealed hyperglycemia and hypokalemia. Further studies performed during her subsequent hospital course revealed increased 24-hour urine free cortisol (5796 nmol; reference range, 55 to 193 nmol), consistent with Cushing's syndrome. Imaging studies revealed a left adrenal mass. Use this scenario to answer the following four questions.

4a. Which one of the following statements is true?
  A. The combination of hypokalemia, elevated urine free cortisol, and an adrenal mass indicates a neoplasm of adrenal cortical origin and rules out the possibility of a pheochromocytoma.
  B. The increased urine free cortisol indicates a functional adrenal cortical neoplasm and effectively rules out the possibility of a malignant neoplasm.
  C. Cushing's syndrome caused by ectopic production of ACTH occurs more frequently than ACTH-independent Cushing's syndrome.
  D. The patient's psychosis is probably related to her adrenal mass.
  E. The patient's hypokalemia is probably due to increased intracellular potassium uptake caused by high serum cortisol levels.

4b. Given the patient's elevated urine free cortisol, additional laboratory testing would likely show increased levels of other glucocorticoids and glucocorticoid precursors. Which one of the following molecules is a mineralocorticoid precursor, rather than a glucocorticoid, glucocorticoid precursor, or biosynthetic precursor of cortisol?
  A. Pregnenolone.
  B. Progesterone.
  C. 11-Deoxycortisol.
  D. Corticosterone.
  E. Cortisone.

4c. Which one of the following statements explains hyperglycemia within the context of Cushing's syndrome?
  A. Cortisol decreases hepatic gluconeogenesis by inhibiting protein synthesis, thereby increasing the amounts of amino acid substrates for gluconeogenesis.
  B. Cortisol decreases hepatic gluconeogenesis by accelerating protein degradation, thereby increasing the amounts of amino acid substrates for gluconeogenesis.
  C. Cortisol directly activates key hepatic gluconeogenic enzymes and increases the activity of hepatic glycogen synthetase.
  D. Cortisol increases the uptake and phosphorylation of glucose by peripheral tissues.

4d. Which one of the following statements regarding hormones produced by adrenal tumors is true?
  A. Primary hyperaldosteronism (Conn's syndrome) is characterized by hyperkalemia and hypotension (among other features) and is almost always due to an adenoma of the adrenal cortex.
  B. Virilizing tumors of the adrenal gland occur rarely, cause clinical changes in women but not in men, and are associated with low levels of dehydroepiandrosterone sulfate (DHEA-S) in serum and 17-ketosteroids in urine.
  C. Pheochromocytomas are associated with multiple endocrine neoplasia syndrome, types IIa (MEN IIa) and IIb (MEN IIb), von Hippel–Lindau syndrome, familial paraganglioma syndrome, and neurofibromatosis I.
  D. Neuroblastoma is a well-differentiated tumor of childhood that rarely produces catecholamines.

A 36-year-old man sought help from a reproductive endocrinologist for a workup of infertility. Physical examination showed normal male genitalia. Hormonal analysis revealed markedly increased levels of serum 17-hydroxyprogesterone and reduced levels of serum 11-deoxycortisol. Circulating levels of other hormones were with normal limits. Semen analysis showed a reduced percentage of viable sperm and a reduced percentage of morphologically normal sperm. Sperm concentration and percentage of motile sperm were within normal limits. Use this scenario to answer the following three questions.

5a. Which one of the following is the most likely diagnosis?
A. Addison's disease.
B. 21-Hydroxylase deficiency.
C. 11-β-Hydroxylase deficiency.
D. 3-β-Hydroxylase deficiency.
E. Androgen insensitivity syndrome (AIS).

5b. Thorough evaluation of this patient would most likely reveal increased levels of which one of the following hormones?
A. 17-Hydroxypregnenolone.
B. Aldosterone.
C. 18-Hydroxycorticosterone.
D. Corticosterone.
E. Cortisol.

5c. Which one of the following features would most likely characterize a female patient with this condition?
A. Decreased serum levels of pregnenolone.
B. Increased serum levels of 11-deoxycorticosterone.
C. Decreased serum levels of dehydroepiandrosterone.
D. Decreased serum levels of progesterone.
E. An abnormal physical examination.

A 38-year-old woman with polycystic ovarian syndrome (PCOS) consulted with a reproductive endocrinologist regarding in vitro fertilization (IVF). After a comprehensive review of the patient's history and a thorough physical examination, the physician ordered a battery of laboratory tests. Use this scenario to answer the next four questions.

6a. Which one of the following hormones is most likely to be within normal limits in this patient's serum?
A. Testosterone.
B. Androstenedione.
C. Luteinizing hormone (LH).
D. Follicle-stimulating hormone (FSH).
E. Insulin.

6b. Additional workup revealed abnormalities of anti-Müllerian hormone (AMH). Which one of the following options most accurately describes abnormalities associated with AMH in patients with PCOS?
A. AMH levels are elevated in serum but not in ovarian follicular fluid.
B. AMH levels are elevated in ovarian follicular fluid but not in serum.
C. AMH levels are elevated in serum and in ovarian follicular fluid.
D. AMH levels are not elevated in serum or ovarian follicular fluid.
E. In patients with PCOS, the abnormality of AMH is qualitative rather than quantitative.

6c. Which one of the following is likely to show abnormalities of AMH similar to those associated with PCOS?
A. Pelvic inflammatory disease (PID).
B. Salpingitis isthmica nodosa (SIN).
C. Endometriosis.

D. Pelvic adhesions from prior surgery.
E. Granulosa cell tumors.

6d. Which one of the following explanations has been proposed to account for the chronic anovulatory state of patients with PCOS?
A. FSH levels in these patients are too high to initiate the maturation process among primordial follicles.
B. Low serum LH levels prevent primordial follicles from initiating the process of maturation.
C. AMH activity prevents primordial follicles from initiating the process of maturation.
D. AMH stimulates aromatase activity within granulosa cells, thereby reducing production of estradiol.

A 45-year-old woman underwent surgical resection of a granulosa cell tumor, a representative image of which is shown in Figure 4-1. Use this scenario to answer the following three questions.

7a. Which one of the following statements is correct in terms of the hormones secreted by these tumors?
A. Granulosa cell tumors secrete steroid hormones; secretion of peptide hormones by these tumors has not been reported.

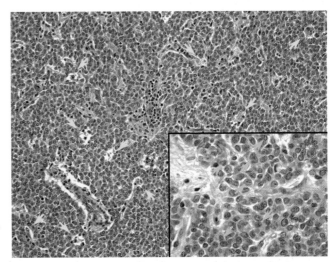

Figure 4-1 Micrograph showing the characteristic features of an adult-type granulosa cell tumor. The lesion consists of neoplastic granulosa cells that proliferate in a microcystic pattern, forming Call-Exner bodies (*yellow arrows*). The inset shows the tumor's cytomorphology. The tumoral granulosa cells have scant cytoplasm and ovoid nuclei with characteristic longitudinal grooves (*blue arrows*).

B. Granulosa cell tumors secrete peptide hormones; secretion of steroid hormones by these tumors has not been reported.
C. Granulosa cell tumors secrete steroid hormones (including estrogen, testosterone, progestins, and inhibin), as well as peptide hormones (including AMH).
D. Granulosa cell tumors secrete steroid hormones (including estrogen, testosterone, and progestins), as well as peptide hormones (including AMH and inhibin).
E. Granulosa cell tumors are generally poorly differentiated neoplasms, and production of functional hormones by these lesions is exceedingly rare.

7b. Granulosa cell tumors are most likely to cause elevation of which one of the following tumor markers?

A. α-Fetoprotein (AFP).
B. β-Human chorionic gonadotropin (β-hCG).
C. Carcinoembryonic antigen (CEA).
D. Lactate dehydrogenase (LDH).
E. CA-125.

7c. Which one of the following options most accurately conveys the clinical features of granulosa cell tumors?
A. Granulosa cell tumors frequently behave aggressively in middle-aged and postmenopausal patients but generally follow a benign course in children and young adults.
B. Granulosa cell tumors frequently behave aggressively in children and young adults but generally follow a benign course in middle-aged and postmenopausal patients.
C. Granulosa cell tumors frequently behave aggressively in younger and older patients alike.
D. Granulosa cell tumors generally follow a benign course in younger and older patients alike.
E. Granulosa cell tumors generally follow a benign course in middle-aged and postmenopausal patients; these tumors have not been described in children and young adults.

Table 4-1

	Patient	Reference Range	Units
Na	142	136-146	mmol/L
K	2.6	3.5-5.0	mmol/L
Cl	92	102-109	mmol/L
CO_2	32	22-30	mmol/L

A 35-year-old man is found on routine examination to have a blood pressure of 165/110 mm Hg without any other symptoms. Laboratory values are shown in Table 4-1. Urine electrolyte measurements resulted in sodium excretion of 216 mmol/24 hours (reference range, 40 to 220 mmol/24 hr) and potassium 135 mmol/24 hours (reference range, 25 to 125 mmol/24 hr). Use this scenario to answer the following three questions.

8a. Which one of the following disorders best explains these results?
A. Addison's disease.
B. Graves' disease.
C. Conn's syndrome.
D. Mild congenital adrenal hyperplasia.
E. Panhypopituitarism.

8b. Which one of the following laboratory test results is most consistent with the diagnosis?
A. Elevated plasma renin activity (PRA) and decreased aldosterone.
B. Suppressed PRA and elevated aldosterone.
C. Elevated 17-hydroxyprogesterone and low aldosterone.
D. Elevated FT_4 and suppressed TSH.
E. Low TSH and low FT_4.

8c. Which one of the following confirmatory test results is most consistent with the patient's diagnosis?
A. Continued suppression of aldosterone after stimulation with adrenocorticotropic hormone.
B. Failure to increase TSH after stimulation with thyroid-releasing hormone.
C. Maintained aldosterone elevation after infusion of 2000 mL of isotonic saline.

D. Elevated 17-hydroxyprogesterone after ACTH stimulation.
E. Failure to increase cortisol after insulin-induced hypoglycemia.

9. A 17-year-old woman was referred to the endocrinologist for primary amenorrhea. On physical examination, she had minimal axillary and pubic hair and Tanner stage II breast development. Which one of the following laboratory results would have the highest diagnostic value?
A. FSH.
B. DHEA-S.
C. Androstenedione.
D. Progesterone.
E. β-hCG.

10. A 45-year-old woman presents with lack of menstruation for 7 months, proptosis, headaches, and personality changes. A pregnancy test result was repeatedly negative. Laboratory evaluation was remarkable for a prolactin level of 65 ng/mL (reference range, 3.8 to 23.2 ng/mL). Magnetic resonance imaging (MRI) of the head revealed a 3-cm mass in the base of the skull. Which one of the following most likely explains the patient's symptoms and elevation in prolactin levels?
A. Large prolactinoma and hook effect.
B. Non–prolactin-secreting tumor and macroprolactin.
C. Stress-associated hyperprolactinemia.
D. Graves' disease.
E. Unreported opiate use.

11. A 20-year-old woman was diagnosed with primary amenorrhea. On physical examination, she had a normal female habitus and voice, normal breast development, and absent axillary and pubic hair. Family history was unremarkable. Pelvic ultrasound showed absence of a uterus and ovaries and the presence of undescended testes. Her karyotype was 46,XY. Which one of the following laboratory results is most consistent with the patient's diagnosis?
A. Decreased testosterone.
B. Decreased LH and FSH.
C. Low estradiol.
D. Elevated 17-hydroxyprogesterone.
E. Mutated androgen receptor.

12. As part of her bone health checkup, C-terminal telopeptide (CTX) and N-terminal propeptide of type I collagen (PINP) are measured by automated chemiluminescent (CLIA) and radioimmunoassay (RIA) in a morning serum sample of a 62-year-old woman with postmenopausal osteoporosis (bone mineral density T-score, −2.8). CTX was 0.738 ng/mL (reference range, 0.115 to 0.748 ng/mL) and PINP was 60 ng/mL (reference range, 19 to 83 ng/mL). One month later, these bone markers are remeasured, this time in a morning fasting sample tested by a reference laboratory rather than your hospital laboratory. CTX was 1.032 ng/mL and PINP was 62 ng/mL. The patient has been taking vitamin D supplements for more than 2 years. Which one of the following is the most likely explanation for why CTX is higher while PINP is relatively unchanged?
A. CTX reflects significant improvement in osteoporosis, whereas N-terminal PINP does not respond to vitamin D treatment.
B. CTX reflects significant improvement in osteoporosis, whereas PINP is falsely elevated because of the influence of food intake and circadian variability on PINP levels.

C. The difference between the two CTX levels is within the expected analytical variability.

D. Influence of food intake on CTX levels and circadian variability in CTX levels.

E. Intralaboratory variability in CTX and PINP results.

13. A 32-year-old woman is admitted to the hospital with paresthesia and seizures. A total calcium level, determined in plasma ethylenediaminetetraacetic acid (EDTA) by a colorimetric method using arsenazo III, is 8.5 mg/dL (reference range, 8.6 to 10.1 mg/dL). Albumin is 3.8 mg/dL (reference range, 3.5 to 5.2 g/dL). Which one of the following would be the most appropriate next step in the management of this patient?

A. The patient should be treated for hypocalcemia.

B. The sample should be sent to a reference laboratory to determine calcium by atomic absorption spectrometry (AAS).

C. The measurement should be repeated using serum.

D. The patient should not be treated for hypocalcemia

E. Ionized calcium should be measured in the EDTA sample.

A 35-year-old pregnant woman with a history of hyperthyroidism (Graves' disease) was assessed for the presence of TSH receptor (TSHR) antibodies (TRAb) during a third-trimester prenatal evaluation. Her thyroid-binding inhibitory immunoglobulin (TBII) levels measured by quantitative chemiluminescence immunoassay were 15.0 U/mL (reference range, <1.75 U/mL), and her thyroid peroxidase (TPO) antibody levels were 150 U/mL (reference range, <9 U/mL). Her FT_4 levels were 1.45 ng/dL (reference range, 0.70 to 1.24 ng/dL), and her TSH levels were less than 0.01 mIU/L (reference range, 0.32 to 4.04 mIU/L). Use this scenario to answer the following three questions.

14a. Which one of the following statements is most consistent with these findings?

A. The patient has active Graves' disease.

B. This patient has gestational thyrotoxicosis.

C. The presence of anti-TPO antibodies rules out Graves' disease.

D. This patient is undergoing effective anti-thyroid drug treatment.

E. This patient has Hashimoto's thyroiditis and not Graves' disease.

14b. Which one of the following statements regarding the risk for neonatal thyroid disease in this case is correct?

A. The risk for neonatal thyroid disease is the same as in the general population.

B. The fetus is at risk for neonatal hyperthyroidism due to transplacental transport of TRAb.

C. The fetus is at risk for neonatal hypothyroidism due to transplacental transport of thyroid-blocking antibodies.

D. The fetus is at risk for hypothyroidism due to overtreatment of the mother's hyperthyroidism with antithyroid medications.

E. The fetus is at risk for neonatal hypothyroidism due to Hashimoto's thyroiditis.

14c. The mother was treated with 100 mg of propylthiouracil (PTU) four times per day, resulting in normalization of FT_4 and TSH levels and delivery of a normal infant. PTU treatment was discontinued postpartum. Six months postpartum, the patient complained of facial puffiness, depression, lack of

energy, and insomnia. Evaluation of thyroid function showed FT_4 levels of 0.20 ng/dL (reference range, 0.70 to 1.24 ng/dL), TSH levels of 290 mIU/L (reference range, 0.4 to 5.0 mIU/L), thyroid-binding inhibitory immunoglobulin levels of 10.75 U/mL (reference range, <1.75 U/mL), and anti—thyroid peroxidase antibody levels of 15 U/mL (reference range, <9 U/mL). A cell culture assay for thyroid-stimulating antibodies (TSAb) in the patient's serum showed levels of 5% (reference range, <11%). Which one of the following statements is most consistent with these findings?

A. The patient has postpartum depression but is euthyroid.

B. The patient has atrophic hypothyroidism due to overtreatment with PTU.

C. The patient now has hypothyroidism due to autoimmune thyroiditis.

D. The patient developed anti-TSH antibodies.

E. This patient now has thyroid-blocking antibody-induced hypothyroidism.

A 67-year-old man with multiple health problems sought medical attention for difficulty sleeping. Physical examination revealed markedly reduced vibratory sensation in his legs. Laboratory workup showed low TSH (<0.03 mIU/L; reference range, 0.4 to 5.0 mIU/L), high free thyroxine (T_4) (2.42 ng/dL; reference range, 0.70 to 1.24 ng/dL), negative anti—thyroid peroxidase (anti-TPO) antibodies, normal white blood cell count (4.1 × 10^9/L; reference

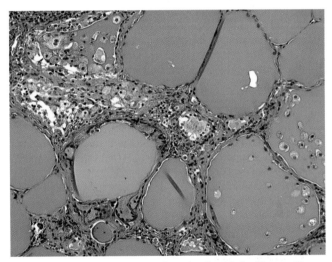

Figure 4-2 Representative section from the thyroid of a 67-year-old man after total thyroidectomy. This section of thyroid shows follicles (some of which are disrupted) associated with foamy macrophages.

range, 3.5 to 9.1 × 10^9/L), and normal erythrocyte sedimentation rate (13 mm/hr; reference range, 1 to 15 mm/hr). Nuclear medicine studies showed low radionuclide uptake. Collectively, these findings indicate thyrotoxicosis without underlying hyperthyroidism. He underwent total thyroidectomy, a representative image of which is shown in Figure 4-2. Use this scenario to answer the following three questions.

15a. Which one of the following drugs did this patient most likely receive before the development of his symptoms?

A. Interferon-α.

B. Interleukin-2.

C. Amiodarone.

D. Minocycline.

15b. Which one of the following forms of thyroiditis would most likely be associated with the clinical scenario and laboratory findings described above (i.e., thyrotoxicosis without underlying hyperthyroidism)?
   A. Acute thyroiditis.
   B. Subacute thyroiditis.
   C. Hashimoto's thyroiditis.
   D. Riedel's thyroiditis.

15c. Which one of the following hyperplastic or neoplastic conditions (or sequelae thereof) would most likely be associated with the clinical scenario and laboratory findings described above?
   A. Diffuse follicular epithelial hyperplasia.
   B. Follicular adenoma.
   C. Infarcted adenoma.
   D. Medullary thyroid carcinoma.

16. 25(OH)-Vitamin D is measured in the serum of a 6-month-old boy using three different techniques: DiaSorin Liaison TOTAL (CLIA), Immunodiagnostics-iSYS (CLIA), and liquid chromatography/tandem mass spectrometry (LC-MS/MS). Using the latter, the concentration of 25(OH)-vitamin D_2 was below the level of detection of 1 ng/mL and the concentration of 25(OH)-vitamin D_3 was 35 ng/mL. The 25(OH)-vitamin D serum concentrations measured with the DiaSorin Liaison TOTAL and the Immunodiagnostics-iSYS instruments were 25 and 26 ng/mL, respectively. Which one of the following reasons best explains the discrepancy between the results obtained by LC-MS/MS and those obtained by the automated immunochemistry analyzers?
   A. Because of cross-reactivity, immunoassays generally give higher results than mass spectrometry–based assays.
   B. The DiaSorin Liaison TOTAL and the Immunodiagnostics-iSYS CLIA methods both detect 25(OH)-vitamin D_2 and 25(OH)-vitamin D_3.
   C. The DiaSorin Liaison TOTAL and the Immunodiagnostics-iSYS CLIA methods do not detect 25(OH)-vitamin D_2.
   D. The DiaSorin Liaison TOTAL and the Immunodiagnostics-iSYS CLIA methods detect both the 25(OH)-vitamin D_3 C3-epimer and 25(OH)-vitamin D_3.
   E. Most mass spectrometry–based assays do measure the 25(OH)-vitamin D_3 C3-epimer but cannot distinguish it from 25(OH)-vitamin D_3.

17. Which one of the following best describes serum hCG levels in pregnancy?
   A. In an ectopic pregnancy, serum hCG levels double every 2 days during the first 5 to 6 weeks after implantation of the embryo.
   B. Molar pregnancies are associated with lower than expected serum hCG levels.
   C. In a normal pregnancy, maximum serum hCG levels are reached at or near the end of the first trimester.
   D. In a normal pregnancy, serum hCG levels return to nonpregnant levels within 2 to 3 days after a normal delivery.
   E. In a normal pregnancy, serum hCG levels are at their highest in the third trimester.

Table 4-2

Test	Result	Reference Range	Units
Calcium	11	9-10.5	mg/dL
Creatinine	1.0	0.6-1.2	mg/dL
Intact PTH	8	10-60	pg/mL
25(OH)-vitamin D	64	20-50	ng/mL
25(OH)-vitamin D	72	18-78	pg/mL

Table 4-3

Test	Result	Reference Range	Units
Calcium	90	100-250	mg/day
Phosphate	1220	400-1300	mg/day
Uric acid	400	<750	mg/day
Protein	210	<150	mg/day
β_2-Microglobulin	0.7	<0.3	µg/mL

18. An 18-year-old man presents with renal colic. A calcium oxalate kidney stone is passed several days later. His serum levels are shown in Table 4-2 and his 24-hour urine levels are shown in Table 4-3. Which one of the following answers contains the best explanation for this patient's hypercalciuric nephrolithiasis and the biochemical test that should be done to support this diagnosis?
   A. Decreased CYP24A1 activity. Measure serum 24,25(OH)-vitamin D.
   B. Hypoparathyroidism. Measure parathyroid hormone (PTH) with a third-generation assay.
   C. Cancer. Measure PTH-related peptide.
   D. Chronic kidney disease. Measure neutrophil gelatinase–associated lipocalin (NGAL).
   E. Familial hypocalciuric hypercalcemia. Measure serum phosphate.

19. An otherwise healthy 28-year-old woman has incompletely understood symptoms suggestive of hypomagnesemia. However, a total serum magnesium (Mg) level determined colorimetrically was normal. Now, an ionized serum Mg level is requested to acquire additional information. Which one of the following reasons would be the best explanation of a falsely low ionized Mg level in this patient?
   A. There is a weak relationship between ionized and total Mg levels in serum.
   B. Interference by cotinine in the serum from cigarette smoking by the patient.
   C. Interference by thiocyanate in the serum from cigarette smoking by the patient.
   D. Vitamin C intake by the patient.
   E. The presence of hypoalbuminemia.

20. At 3 to 5 weeks of gestation, which one of the following is the predominant form of hCG that is detected in serum?
   A. Hyperglycosylated hCG.
   B. Intact hCG.
   C. Free β-hCG.
   D. Nicked hCG.
   E. Pituitary hCG.

21. Several bone turnover markers are measured in the serum and urine of a cancer patient. Serum levels (nonfasting, collected at 2 PM) are as follows:
   - Carboxy-terminal collagen cross-links (serum CTX) = 0.730 ng/mL (reference range, 0.112 to 0.738 ng/mL)
   - Bone alkaline phosphatase = 18.7 U/L (reference range, 11.5 to 29.6 U/L)

   Levels in a 24-hour urine sample are as follows:
   - N-telopeptide cross-links/creatinine (urinary NTX/Cr) = 87 nmol bone collagen equivalents (BCE)/mmol (reference range, 5 to 65 nmol BCE/mmol)

   Given these findings, which one of the following types of cancer is most likely present in this patient?
   A. Prostate cancer with bone metastasis.
   B. Breast cancer with bone metastasis.
   C. Multiple myeloma with osteolytic lesions.
   D. Renal carcinoma with bone metastasis.
   E. Bone metastases from non–small cell lung carcinoma.

Table 4-4

Test	Result	Reference Range	Units
Na	141	136-145	mmol/L
K	4.3	3.5-5.0	mmol/L
Cl	107	98-106	mmol/L
HCO_3	25	20-29	mmol/L
BUN	13	10-20	mg/dL
Cr	0.7	0.6-1.2	mg/dL
Glucose	90	75-115	mg/dL
Albumin	4.3	3.5-5.5	g/dL
Phosphorus	3.2	3-4.5	mg/dL
Calcium	9.6	9-10.5	mg/dL
Aspartate aminotransferase (AST)	25	0-35	U/L
Alanine aminotransferase (ALT)	23	0-35	U/L
Alkaline phosphatase (ALP)	150	30-120	U/L
25(OH)-vitamin D	22	20-50	ng/mL

22. A 57-year-old white man has been complaining for 2 years about pain in his right humerus. The skin overlying the painful bone feels warm. The bone itself feels smooth. Otherwise, the patient is healthy and does not show any skeletal deformations. To his knowledge there is no family history of bone disease. Serum levels are shown in Table 4-4. X-rays show focal osteolysis with coarsening of the trabecular pattern, bone expansion, and cortical thickening. A technetium-99 m (^{99m}Tc) diphosphonate bone scan shows increased uptake in the upper part of the right humerus. Which one of the following is the most likely diagnosis?
   A. Melorheostosis.
   B. Multiple myeloma.
   C. Paget's disease of bone.
   D. Male osteoporosis.
   E. Van Buchem's disease.

23. A 46-year-old woman in good health was seeing her internist as part of a routine physical examination. Because she reported 6 months of amenorrhea, serum and urine hCG levels were measured to rule out pregnancy. The serum hCG level was 10 IU/L (reference range, 5 to 20 IU/L), and a positive urine hCG result was obtained. Serum hCG was measured in another sample 7 days later and was 12 IU/L. When hCG was measured with a different immunochemical method, the serum hCG result was 11 IU/L. The patient's serum FSH level was 130 IU/L (reference range, ≥45 IU/L). Which one of the following is the most probable cause of the detectable hCG level in this patient?
   A. Positive interference from human anti-animal antibodies.
   B. Normal intrauterine pregnancy.
   C. Ectopic pregnancy.
   D. Synthesis and release of hCG from the pituitary gland.
   E. Presence of a hydatidiform mole.

24. Intact PTH is measured in a plasma sample from a 42-year-old man using an RIA (Scantibodies, Santee, CA). The concentration is 75 pg/mL (reference range, 14 to 66 pg/mL). Whole PTH is also measured in the same plasma sample using an RIA (Scantibodies). The concentration is 37 pg/mL (reference range, 6 to 32 pg/mL). The patient's height, body weight, and serum creatinine are 186 cm, 85 kg, and 0.8 mg/dL (reference range, 0.6 to 1.2 mg/dL), respectively. Serum calcium and albumin are 10.3 mg/dL (reference range, 9 to 10.5 mg/dL) and 4.5 mg/dL (reference range, 3.5 to 5.5 g/dL), respectively. Which one of the following statements best explains these results?
   A. The patient has primary hyperparathyroidism.
   B. The patient has hyperparathyroidism secondary to kidney disease.
   C. The patient has a parathyroid carcinoma.
   D. Intact PTH assays always give a higher result than the whole PTH assays.
   E. RIA methods are unreliable for measuring PTH levels.

Table 4-5

Test	Result	Reference Range	Units
Calcium	10.8	9-10.5	mg/dL
Phosphorus	3.2	3-4.5	mg/dL
Magnesium	1.8	1.8-3	mg/dL
Creatinine	0.9	0.6-1.2	mg/dL
Intact PTH	21	10-60	pg/mL
25(OH)-vitamin D	20	20-50	ng/mL
1,25(OH)-vitamin D	35	18-78	pg/mL

25. A 59-year-old man with a history of type 2 diabetes and hyperlipidemia is referred to your hospital for evaluation of recently discovered hypercalcemia. His laboratory results from blood samples are shown in Table 4-5. In addition, his liver function tests, thyroid function tests, urine metanephrines, serum angiotensin-converting enzyme (ACE) activity, and serum and urine protein and electrophoresis analyses are all normal. The intact PTH level was measured by an immunochemiluminescent assay (ICMA). Ultrasonography of the neck did not reveal any abnormalities of the thyroid or parathyroid glands, but a ^{99m}Tc-sestamibi scan suggests the presence of a parathyroid adenoma. Bone mineral densities by dual x-ray absorptiometry (DXA) scanning of the lumbar spine, femoral neck, and radius are −1.7, −1.3, and −1.7, respectively, indicating osteopenia. Which one of the following is the best explanation for the unusual combination of results for calcium and intact PTH in this case?
   A. Serum samples were kept on ice during transport.
   B. Vitamin D deficiency.
   C. Circulating variant forms of PTH.

  D. Hypermagnesemia.
  E. The hook effect.

Table 4-6

Test	Result	Reference Range	Units
Na	141	136-145	mmol/L
K	4.3	3.5-5.0	mmol/L
Cl	106	98-106	mmol/L
BUN	5	10-20	mg/dL
Cr	0.9	0.6-1.2	mg/dL
Glucose	91	75-115	mg/dL
Albumin	4.3	3.5-5.5	g/dL
Phosphorus	5.1	3-4.5	mg/dL
Calcium	8.5	9-10.5	mg/dL
Magnesium	2.1	1.8-3	mg/dL
25(OH)-vitamin D	28	20-50	ng/mL
1,25(OH)-vitamin D	37	18-78	pg/mL
Parathyroid hormone	321	10-60	pg/mL
Free T_4	0.7	5-12	μg/dL
TSH	4.5	0.4-5.0	mIU/L
C-terminal collagen cross-links	0.821	0.115-0.748	ng/mL
N-terminal propeptide of human procollagen type I	92	22-87	pg/mL

Table 4-7

Test	Result	Reference Range	Units
Creatinine	1050	1000-2500	mg/day
Calcium	90	100-250	mg/day
Phosphorus	1400	400-1300	mg/day

26. An 18-year-old obese man with short stature, a round face, subcutaneous ossifications, and brachydactyly undergoes a biochemical workup by an endocrinologist. His laboratory results from blood samples under fasting conditions are shown in Table 4-6. His laboratory results from a 24-hour urine collection are shown in Table 4-7. Which one of the following is the most likely diagnosis in this patient?
   A. Primary hyperparathyroidism.
   B. Secondary hyperparathyroidism.
   C. Hypoparathyroidism.
   D. Pseudohypoparathyroidism.
   E. Pseudopseudohypoparathyroidism.

27. In which one of the following situations is 1,25(OH)-vitamin D expected to be elevated?
   A. Secondary hyperparathyroidism.
   B. Hypoparathyroidism.
   C. Postmenopausal osteoporosis.
   D. Sarcoidosis.
   E. Hypercalcemia of malignancy.

28. A 52-year-old morbidly obese man underwent bariatric surgery in 2005. Three years later, he was seen by an ophthalmologist for progressive loss of vision and night blindness. Blood work performed as part of a routine checkup showed mild hypercalcemia and mild hyperparathyroidism. Measuring which one of the following is the most appropriate and most specific test to account for his impaired night vision?
   A. Retinol.
   B. 25(OH)-vitamin D.
   C. 1,25(OH)-vitamin D.
   D. Total protein.
   E. Albumin.

29. You are asked to measure the zinc (Zn) level in a specimen from a 23-year-old woman to confirm suspected Zn deficiency. You measure Zn in your laboratory by flame atomic absorption spectroscopy (AAS). Which one of the following settings could lead to higher Zn levels?
   A. An acute-phase reaction.
   B. The use of prednisone by the patient.
   C. Obtaining a blood sample in the evening.
   D. Measuring Zn in serum rather than plasma.
   E. Recent food intake.

ANSWERS

1a. A. Measure urinary free cortisol.
B. Measure a repeat salivary cortisol in the morning.
Rationale: Choices A and B alone would simply confirm the diagnosis of hyperadrenalism.
C. Low-dose dexamethasone suppression test (DST).
Rationale: The low-dose DST is useful in testing which portion of the hypothalamic-pituitary-adrenal axis is impaired in hyperadrenalism. The normal response to 2 days of low-dose dexamethasone is suppression of serum cortisol levels. Lack of suppression suggests primary hyperadrenalism, or Cushing's syndrome.
D. Measure plasma aldosterone.
Rationale: Choice D has no role in this diagnostic workup of *glucocorticoid* excess.

1b. A. Greater than 50% reduction in serum cortisol.
Rationale: This is the definition of suppression in the high-dose DST and would be seen in patients with Cushing's disease (*secondary hyperadrenalism*).
B. No suppression of serum cortisol.
Rationale: The high-dose DST is used to differentiate the cause of Cushing's syndrome as ACTH dependent or independent. Given the patient's CT finding, the patient most likely has an adrenal adenoma or carcinoma and the Cushing's syndrome is ACTH independent. The patient's serum cortisol will therefore not be suppressed with high-dose dexamethasone.
C. An elevation in serum cortisol.
Rationale: An elevation in serum cortisol is possible but is not generally seen in the DST.
D. Suppression of serum metanephrines.
Rationale: Serum metanephrines would not be expected to change with the DST because they are not under the control of ACTH.

Major points of discussion
- Cushing's syndrome is characterized by truncal obesity, thin extremities hypertension, weakness, fatigue, hirsutism, amenorrhea, purple striae, glucosuria, and osteoporosis.
- There are multiple etiologies for Cushing's syndrome, but all result in excess production of cortisol by the adrenal glands or hyperadrenalism.
- Laboratory testing reveals increased levels of serum cortisol, urinary free cortisol, lack of suppression of cortisol production after administration of low-dose dexamethasone overnight, and hyperglycemia.
- Cushing's syndrome may result from multiple etiologies, including iatrogenic administration, ectopic production of corticotropin-releasing hormone (CRH) or ACTH, adrenal carcinoma or adenoma, and an ACTH-producing pituitary adenoma or Cushing's disease. The treatment and prognosis are dependent on the etiology.
- Screening tests for hyperadrenalism include 24-hour urinary free cortisol, overnight low-dose DST, and a midnight salivary cortisol.
- The low-dose DST is useful in testing to determine which portion of the hypothalamic-pituitary-adrenal axis is impaired in hyperadrenalism. The normal

response to 2 days of low-dose dexamethasone is suppression of serum cortisol levels. Lack of suppression suggests primary hyperadrenalism, or Cushing's syndrome.
- In cases of hyperadrenalism with borderline depressions in ACTH, the best diagnostic test is the low-dose DST.
- A high-dose overnight DST is used to help differentiate between the different causes of Cushing's syndrome. Suppression of cortisol production with increased ACTH suggests Cushing's disease or ectopic production of ACTH. Demonstration of a pituitary mass on MRI or CT is diagnostic of Cushing's disease. If a pituitary mass is not present, CT of the chest and abdomen may demonstrate an ACTH-producing neoplasm. Failure to suppress after high-dose dexamethasone and increased ACTH levels suggests ectopic ACTH production, and CT of the chest and abdomen is warranted. Failure to suppress after high-dose dexamethasone and low ACTH levels suggests the hyperadrenalism may be of adrenal origin. CT of the adrenals may demonstrate an adrenal tumor.

2a. A. Normal TSH, decreased FT_4, decreased FT_3.
B. Normal TSH, elevated FT_4, elevated FT_3.
C. Elevated TSH, decreased FT_4, decreased FT_3.
D. Elevated TSH, normal FT_4, normal FT_3.
E. Elevated TSH, elevated FT_4, elevated FT_3.
Rationale: Reduced end-organ responsiveness to thyroid hormone would result in a compensatory *increase* in TSH, FT_4, and FT_3.

2b. A. Inactivating mutation of the thyrotropin-releasing hormone receptor (TRHR) gene.
Rationale: This patient's goiter likely results from increased stimulation of the thyroid by TSH, which in turn results from reduced end-organ responsiveness to thyroid hormone. This mutation would not lead to increased TSH and would not affect end-organ responsiveness to thyroid hormone.
B. Inactivating mutation of the thyroid stimulating hormone receptor (TSHR) gene.
Rationale: This mutation would *decrease* the effectiveness of TSH (i.e., TSH would bind to a nonfunctional TSHR) and would not affect end-organ responsiveness to thyroid hormone.
C. Inactivating mutation of the TSH β-chain gene.
Rationale: This mutation would lead to a *decrease* in the functionality of TSH and would not affect end-organ responsiveness to thyroid hormone.
D. Inactivating mutation of the thyroxine-binding globulin (TBG) gene.
Rationale: This mutation would not lead to increased TSH and would not affect end-organ responsiveness to thyroid hormone.
E. Inactivating mutation of the thyroid hormone receptor (TR) β gene.
Rationale: In the context of this mutation, end-organ responsiveness to thyroid hormone would be reduced. Goiter would form as a result of a compensatory increase in TSH.

2c. A. T_4 is more metabolically active than T_3, which is more metabolically active than rT_3.
Rationale: T_3 is more metabolically active than T_4.
B. T_4 is more metabolically active than rT_3, which is more metabolically active than T_3.
C. T_3 and rT_3 are approximately equally metabolically active. These hormones are more metabolically active than T_4.
D. T_3 is more metabolically active than T_4, which is more metabolically active than rT_3.
E. T_3 is more metabolically active than rT_3, which is more metabolically active than T_4.
Rationale: T_3 is the most metabolically active of these hormones, followed by T_4 and then rT_3.

2d. A. Liver.
Rationale: Liver is among the most thyroid-responsive tissues.
B. Kidney.
Rationale: Kidney is among the most thyroid-responsive tissues.
C. Spleen.
Rationale: Spleen is considered relatively thyroid unresponsive.
D. Skeletal muscle.
Rationale: Skeletal muscle is among the most thyroid-responsive tissues.
E. Heart.
Rationale: Heart is among the most thyroid-responsive tissues.

Major points of discussion
- Congenital hypothyroidism results from various causes. These etiologies consist of five main categories: (1) defects in the hypothalamic-pituitary-thyroid axis; (2) defects in thyroid ontogeny; (3) defects in thyroid hormone formation; (4) abnormal thyroid hormone transport; and (5) reduced responsiveness of target tissues to thyroid hormone.
- Among the various etiologies of congenital hypothyroidism, errors that decrease the quantity or functionality of TSH (including errors that are "upstream" of TSH) and errors that affect thyroid hormone transport do not cause goiter. In general, this applies to categories (1), (2), and (4), as outlined above.
- Congenital hypothyroidism caused by errors in thyroid hormone synthesis and action (e.g., RTH) generally result in goiter formation, owing to a compensatory increase in TSH. This applies to categories (3) and (5) as outlined above.
- RTH is a rare syndrome of reduced end-organ responsiveness to thyroid hormone. Because of a compensatory feedback mechanism, patients with RTH have elevated T_4, T_3, and serum rT_3.
- T_4 is three to four times more metabolically active than T_3. T_4 is a precursor hormone that can be transformed into T_3 by type I or type II iodothyronine deiodinase. Type III iodothyronine deiodinase inactivates T_4 and T_3 by producing rT_3.
- Liver, kidney, and skeletal muscle are among the most thyroid-responsive tissues. Spleen, testes, and (adult) brain are relatively thyroid unresponsive.[28,37]

3a. A. Decreased fat deposition in the hips, buttocks, and thighs.
Rationale: This patient exhibits features of hypogonadism, likely secondary to chemotherapy during his childhood. Men with hypogonadism that began before puberty typically demonstrate a female fat distribution pattern, which includes *increased* fat deposition in the hips, buttocks, and thighs.
B. Increased fat deposition in the face, abdomen, and waist.
Rationale: Men with hypogonadism that began before puberty typically demonstrate a female fat distribution pattern, which includes *decreased* fat deposition in the face, abdomen, and waist.
C. Decreased facial and body hair.
Rationale: Decreased facial and body hair are typical findings in men with hypogonadism.
D. Decreased hair on the temporal aspect of the scalp.
Rationale: Men with hypogonadism typically do not undergo temporal hair recession.
E. A diamond-shaped escutcheon (pubic hair pattern), rather than a triangular escutcheon.
Rationale: Men with hypogonadism that began before puberty typically demonstrate a female (inverted triangular) escutcheon, rather than a male (diamond-shaped) escutcheon.

3b. A. Klinefelter's syndrome.
Rationale: Klinefelter's syndrome is the most common genetic cause of primary hypogonadism in men.
B. XYY syndrome.
Rationale: Testosterone levels are normal in 47, XYY males.
C. Kallmann's syndrome.
Rationale: Kallmann's syndrome (anosmic hypogonadotropic hypogonadism) is a cause of central hypogonadism.
D. Loss-of-function mutations in the gene encoding GPR54.
Rationale: These mutations are associated with idiopathic hypogonadotropic hypogonadism.
E. CHARGE syndrome.
Rationale: Mutations of the gene *CHD7*, which is associated with the CHARGE syndrome (*c*oloboma, *h*eart anomalies, choanal *a*tresia, *r*etardation of growth and development, and *g*enital and *e*ar anomalies), have been identified in patients with hypogonadism.

3c. A. Androgens stimulate increased secretion of insulin-like growth factor 1 (IGF-1), which in turn causes growth.
B. Estrogens ultimately terminate growth by causing closure of the epiphyses of the long bones.
Rationale: Estrogens are derived from androgens. Patients with prepubertal hypogonadism undergo delayed epiphyseal closure and consequently have tall stature.
C. Androgens have a net anabolic effect in terms of protein metabolism (i.e., androgens increase protein synthesis and decrease protein degradation).
D. Androgens increase the deposition of calcium salts and the rate of bone growth.
Rationale for A, C, and D: These statements are true but do not explain the tall stature of a patient with decreased androgen levels.

E. Boys who undergo precocious puberty (i.e., onset of puberty before age 9 years) typically have tall stature as adults.
Rationale: Boys who undergo precocious puberty typically have short stature as adults. Estrogens, which are derived from androgens, ultimately terminate growth by causing closure of the epiphyses of the long bones. Boys with precocious puberty, therefore, undergo premature epiphyseal closure.

3d. A. Serum total testosterone levels decrease with age, whereas serum free testosterone levels remain relatively constant with age.
Rationale: Serum total testosterone levels *and* serum free testosterone levels decrease with age.
B. The quantitative relationship between serum total testosterone and serum free testosterone depends primarily on the serum concentration of albumin.
Rationale: The quantitative relationship between serum total testosterone and serum free testosterone levels depends primarily on the serum concentration of sex hormone–binding globulin.
C. Serum testosterone levels are inversely proportional to body mass index (BMI).
Rationale: Cross-sectional epidemiologic studies have shown an *inverse* relationship between BMI and circulating testosterone levels.
D. Serum testosterone levels have no quantitative relationship with central obesity (i.e., waist/hip ratio).
Rationale: Cross-sectional epidemiologic studies have shown an *inverse* relationship between central obesity and circulating testosterone levels.
E. Serum total testosterone levels are higher in young white men compared with young black men.
Rationale: Results of studies comparing serum testosterone levels of white and black men have been mixed. Some studies demonstrate that serum testosterone levels are higher in black men compared with white men, especially among younger adult men, whereas other studies have not shown any difference between the two groups even at younger ages.

Major points of discussion
- The cause of hypogonadism may be primary or central. In primary hypogonadism, the testes themselves do not function properly. Some causes of primary hypogonadism include genetic and developmental disorders (e.g., Klinefelter's syndrome, androgen resistance, germinal cell aplasia), autoimmune disorders, infection, chemotherapy, and radiation.
- In central hypogonadism, the hypothalamus and/or pituitary does not function properly. Some causes of central hypogonadism include genetic and developmental disorders (e.g., Kallmann's syndrome), central nervous system tumors, nutritional deficiencies, infection, medications (e.g., steroids, opiates), radiation, and trauma.
- Men with hypogonadism with onset before puberty typically demonstrate tall stature, decreased facial and body hair, gynecomastia, a female or triangular escutcheon (rather than a male

or diamond-shaped escutcheon), a female fat distribution pattern (increased fat deposition in the hips/buttocks/thighs, decreased fat deposition in the face/abdomen/waist), and lack of temporal hair recession. These men are also at increased risk for osteoporosis later in life.
- Androgens affect bone growth during puberty by various mechanisms. Androgens increase the amplitude of the "spikes" in the pulsatile secretion of growth hormone. This effect increases secretion of IGF-1, which in turn causes growth. Androgens also facilitate bone growth by increasing protein synthesis, decreasing protein degradation, and increasing the deposition of calcium salts. These effects account for the growth changes seen in boys during puberty. Estrogens, which are derived from androgens, ultimately terminate growth by causing closure of the epiphyses of the long bones.
- In healthy adult men, serum total testosterone and serum free testosterone levels decrease with age. The quantitative relationship between serum total testosterone and serum free testosterone levels depends primarily on the serum concentration of sex hormone–binding globulin. Cross-sectional epidemiologic studies have shown an inverse relationship between BMI and serum testosterone levels, as well as an inverse relationship between waist/hip ratio and serum testosterone levels.[26,60]

4a. A. The combination of hypokalemia, elevated urine free cortisol, and an adrenal mass indicates a neoplasm of adrenal cortical origin and rules out the possibility of a pheochromocytoma.
Rationale: Pheochromocytomas associated with Cushing's syndrome are well-documented entities.
B. The increased urine free cortisol indicates a functional adrenal cortical neoplasm and effectively rules out the possibility of a malignant neoplasm.
Rationale: Functional tumors are not necessarily benign. Functional adrenal cortical carcinomas and catecholamine-producing malignant pheochromocytomas are well-documented entities.
C. Cushing's syndrome caused by ectopic production of ACTH occurs more frequently than ACTH-independent Cushing's syndrome.
Rationale: ACTH-independent Cushing's syndrome caused by adrenal tumors is approximately twice as common as ACTH-dependent Cushing's syndrome caused by ectopic production of ACTH.
D. The patient's psychosis is probably related to her adrenal mass.
Rationale: Clinical features of Cushing's syndrome include various psychiatric symptoms.
E. The patient's hypokalemia is probably due to increased intracellular potassium uptake caused by high serum cortisol levels.
Rationale: Cortisol possesses some mineralocorticoid activity. In the context of Cushing's syndrome, hypokalemia results from increased renal secretion of potassium mediated by cortisol.

4b. **A. Pregnenolone.**
Rationale: Pregnenolone is a biosynthetic precursor of cortisol.
B. Progesterone.
Rationale: Progesterone is a biosynthetic precursor of cortisol.
C. 11-Deoxycortisol.
Rationale: 11-Deoxycortisol is a glucocorticoid precursor.
D. Corticosterone.
Rationale: Corticosterone is a mineralocorticoid precursor, rather than a glucocorticoid precursor.
E. Cortisone.
Rationale: Cortisone is a glucocorticoid (like cortisol) and exists in equilibrium with cortisol.

4c. A. Cortisol decreases hepatic gluconeogenesis by inhibiting protein synthesis, thereby increasing the amounts of amino acid substrates for gluconeogenesis.
Rationale: Cortisol *increases* hepatic gluconeogenesis by inhibiting protein synthesis, thereby increasing the amounts of amino acid substrates for gluconeogenesis.
B. Cortisol decreases hepatic gluconeogenesis by accelerating protein degradation, thereby increasing the amounts of amino acid substrates for gluconeogenesis.
Rationale: Cortisol *increases* hepatic gluconeogenesis by accelerating protein degradation, thereby increasing the amounts of amino acid substrates for gluconeogenesis.
C. Cortisol directly activates key hepatic gluconeogenic enzymes and increases the activity of hepatic glycogen synthetase.
Rationale: Cortisol increases glycogen stores in the liver, or gluconeogenesis, and decreases uptake of glucose by peripheral tissues, leading to hyperglycemia.
D. Cortisol increases the uptake and phosphorylation of glucose by peripheral tissues.
Rationale: Cortisol *decreases* the uptake and phosphorylation of glucose by peripheral tissues.

4d. A. Primary hyperaldosteronism (Conn's syndrome) is characterized by hyperkalemia and hypotension (among other features) and is almost always due to an adenoma of the adrenal cortex.
Rationale: Primary hyperaldosteronism (Conn's syndrome) is characterized by hypokalemia and hypertension (among other features) and is almost always due to an adenoma of the adrenal cortex.
B. Virilizing tumors of the adrenal gland occur rarely, cause clinical changes in women but not in men, and are associated with low levels of dehydroepiandrosterone sulfate (DHEA-S) in serum and 17-ketosteroids in urine.
Rationale: Virilizing tumors of the adrenal gland occur rarely, cause clinical changes in women but not in men, and are associated with high levels of DHEA-S in serum and 17-ketosteroids in urine.
C. Pheochromocytomas are associated with multiple endocrine neoplasia syndrome, types IIa (MEN IIa) and IIb (MEN IIb), von Hippel–Lindau syndrome, familial paraganglioma syndrome, and neurofibromatosis I.
Rationale: All answer choices are correct.
D. Neuroblastoma is a well-differentiated tumor of childhood that rarely produces catecholamines.

Rationale: Neuroblastoma is a poorly differentiated tumor of childhood, and catecholamine production is seen in more than 90% of cases.

Major points of discussion

- Clinical features of Cushing's syndrome include abnormal fat distribution and dermatologic, hematologic, and musculoskeletal changes related to increased protein catabolism, diabetes mellitus, hypertension, and various psychiatric symptoms. Cortisol possesses some mineralocorticoid activity. In the context of Cushing's syndrome, hypokalemia results from increased renal secretion of potassium mediated by cortisol.
- Cortisol facilitates the net conversion of protein to glycogen. Cortisol simultaneously increases glycogen stores in the liver (by increasing the activity of glycogen synthetase), as well as production of glucose by the liver. Cortisol increases hepatic glucose production by facilitating gluconeogenesis (i.e., by inhibiting protein synthesis, accelerating protein degradation, and directly activating gluconeogenic enzymes). Cortisol also decreases the uptake and phosphorylation (i.e., catabolism) of glucose by peripheral tissues.
- Steroid hormones produced by the adrenal gland (e.g., cortisol) are ultimately derived from cholesterol. Cholesterol is converted into pregnenolone, which is in turn converted into progesterone. Progesterone, 17-hydroxyprogesterone, and 11-deoxycortisol are considered glucocorticoid precursors. 11-Deoxycortisol is converted into cortisol, which is in turn converted into cortisone; cortisol and cortisone are considered active glucocorticoids.
- Pheochromocytomas can mimic functional adrenal cortical tumors in terms of their clinical features (e.g., by causing the clinical scenario described in this case). Functional tumors are not always benign; hormone-producing adrenal cortical carcinomas and catecholamine-producing malignant pheochromocytomas are well-documented entities. ACTH-independent Cushing's syndrome caused by adrenal tumors is approximately twice as common as ACTH-dependent Cushing's syndrome caused by ectopic production of ACTH.
- Various other tumors arising in the adrenal gland produce hormones. Primary hyperaldosteronism (Conn's syndrome) is almost always due to an adenoma of the adrenal cortex. Virilizing tumors of the adrenal occur rarely, cause clinical changes in women but not in men, and are associated with high levels of DHEA-S in serum and 17-ketosteroids in urine. Neuroblastoma is a poorly differentiated neoplasm derived from neural crest cells, usually occurring in infants and small children. From 50% to 80% arise in the adrenal gland, and more than 90% produce catecholamines.[35,36,56]

5a. A. Addison's disease.
Rationale: 17-Hydroxyprogesterone levels would not be increased in a patient with Addison's disease.
B. 21-Hydroxylase deficiency.
Rationale: 21-Hydroxylase converts progesterone into 11-deoxycorticosterone (a precursor of aldosterone) and 17-hydroxyprogesterone into 11-deoxycortisol

(a precursor of cortisol). Patients with 21-hydroxylase deficiency have markedly increased levels of serum 17-hydroxyprogesterone and reduced levels of serum 11-deoxycortisol.
C. 11-β-Hydroxylase deficiency.
Rationale: Patients with 11-β-hydroxylase deficiency have increased levels of serum 11-deoxycortisol.
D. 3-β-Hydroxylase deficiency.
Rationale: 17-Hydroxyprogesterone levels would not be increased in a patient with 3-β-hydroxylase deficiency.
E. Androgen insensitivity syndrome (AIS).
Rationale: Normal male genitalia are inconsistent with AIS.

5b.　A. 17-Hydroxypregnenolone.
Rationale: 17-Hydroxypregnenolone is a precursor of 17-hydroxyprogesterone.
B. Aldosterone.
C. 18-Hydroxycorticosterone.
D. Corticosterone.
Rationale: Patients with 21-hydroxylase deficiency have relatively low levels of mineralocorticoids (which are downstream of progesterone).
E. Cortisol.
Rationale: Patients with 21-hydroxylase deficiency have relatively low levels of the glucocorticoids downstream of 17-hydroxyprogesterone (i.e., 11-deoxycortisol and cortisol).

5c.　A. Decreased serum levels of pregnenolone.
Rationale: Serum levels of pregnenolone would likely be increased in a patient with 21-hydroxylase deficiency.
B. Increased serum levels of 11-deoxycorticosterone.
Rationale: Serum levels of 11-deoxycorticosterone would likely be decreased in a patient with 21-hydroxylase deficiency.
C. Decreased serum levels of dehydroepiandrosterone.
Rationale: Serum levels of dehydroepiandrosterone would likely be increased in a patient with 21-hydroxylase deficiency.
D. Decreased serum levels of progesterone.
Rationale: Serum levels of progesterone would likely be increased in a patient with 21-hydroxylase deficiency.
E. An abnormal physical examination.
Rationale: In female patients with 21-hydroxylase deficiency, high levels of dehydroepiandrosterone and androstenedione may cause virilization and hirsutism.

Major points of discussion
- Each individual adrenal gland actually consists of two glands (the cortex and medulla) with different embryologic derivation, cellular composition, hormonal products, and regulatory mechanisms. In terms of their function, the adrenal cortex and medulla both mediate various aspects of normal homeostasis, as well as the stress response.
- The adrenal cortex derives from intermediate mesoderm and produces steroid hormones. The cortex consists of three layers (from outermost to innermost: the zona glomerulosa, zona fasciculata, and zona reticularis). The renin-angiotensin system modulates the function of the zona glomerulosa, whereas the hypothalamic-pituitary axis regulates the zona fasciculata and zona reticularis.

- The adrenal medulla derives from neural crest (ectoderm) and produces peptide hormones (i.e., catecholamines, enkephalins, chromogranins, and others). The splanchnic nerve regulates the function of the medulla.
- Adrenal cortical cells produce three types of steroid hormones: mineralocorticoids, glucocorticoids, and sex hormones. Mineralocorticoids, synthesized primarily in the zona glomerulosa, mediate renal tubular reabsorption of sodium and water. Glucocorticoids, produced primarily in the zona fasciculata, facilitate the net conversion of protein to glycogen (among myriad other functions). Sex hormones (androgens and estrogens) are the major products of the zona reticularis.
- Mineralocorticoids include aldosterone, 18-hydroxycorticosterone, corticosterone, and 11-deoxycorticosterone. Glucocorticoids (e.g., cortisol, 11-deoxycortisol, 17-hydroxyprogesterone, and 17-hydroxypregnenolone) consist of 21 carbons and are hydroxylated at position 17. Androgens (e.g., dehydroepiandrosterone, androstenedione, androstenediol, and testosterone) contain 18 carbons, whereas estrogens (e.g., estrone and estradiol) contain 17 carbons. Estrogens also possess aromatic A rings.
- Enzymatic deficiencies that affect the biosynthesis of cortisol are collectively known as congenital adrenal hyperplasia. These disorders include 21-hydroxylase deficiency, 11-β-hydroxylase deficiency, 3-β-hydroxylase deficiency, 17-β-hydroxylase deficiency, and lipoid hyperplasia. The manifestations of these disorders are heterogeneous and depend on the severity of the patient's enzymatic defect.
- 21-Hydroxylase converts progesterone into 11-deoxycorticosterone (a precursor of aldosterone) and 17-hydroxyprogesterone into 11-deoxycortisol (a precursor of cortisol). Patients with 21-hydroxylase deficiency consequently have relatively low levels of mineralocorticoids (which are downstream of progesterone) and relatively low levels of the glucocorticoids downstream of 17-hydroxyprogesterone (i.e., 11-deoxycortisol and cortisol). Laboratory findings associated with this condition include elevated serum and urinary 17-hydroxyprogesterone.
- In patients with 21-hydroxylase deficiency, shunting of precursor molecules along remaining functional pathways results in a relative increase in dehydroepiandrosterone and androstenedione. In female patients, this phenomenon results in virilization, hirsutism, amenorrhea, and infertility. Manifestations in male patients include precocious puberty and infertility.
- 11-β-Hydroxylase converts 11-deoxycorticosterone into corticosterone and 11-deoxycortisol into cortisol. Patients with 11-β-hydroxylase deficiency consequently have relatively low levels of corticosterone, aldosterone, and cortisol. Laboratory findings associated with this condition include elevated serum 11-deoxycorticosterone and 11-deoxycortisol.
- 3-β-Hydroxylase converts pregnenolone into progesterone, 17-hydroxypregnenolone into 17-hydroxyprogesterone, and dehydroepiandrosterone into androstenedione. Patients with 3-β-hydroxylase

deficiency consequently have relatively low levels of progesterone (and all mineralocorticoids), 17-hydroxyprogesterone (and all downstream glucocorticoids), and androstenedione. Laboratory findings associated with this condition include elevated serum pregnenolone, 17-hydroxypregnenolone, and dehydroepiandrosterone.

- Addison's disease refers to primary adrenal insufficiency. In the United States, this condition most frequently results from autoimmune adrenalitis.

- AIS, also known as testicular feminization syndrome, causes male pseudohermaphroditism. AIS results from end-organ resistance to androgens, usually caused by qualitative or quantitative abnormalities of the androgen receptor. Androgen biosynthesis and testicular development are normal in patients with this syndrome. The karyotype of these patients is 46,XY.[21,43]

6a. A. Testosterone.
Rationale: Testosterone levels are generally elevated in patients with PCOS.
B. Androstenedione.
Rationale: Androstenedione levels are generally elevated in patients with PCOS.
C. Luteinizing hormone (LH).
Rationale: LH levels are generally elevated in patients with PCOS.
D. Follicle-stimulating hormone (FSH).
Rationale: FSH levels are usually within normal limits in PCOS but may be low in some cases.
E. Insulin.
Rationale: Insulin levels are generally elevated in patients with PCOS because of the strong association between PCOS and insulin resistance.

6b. A. AMH levels are elevated in serum but not in ovarian follicular fluid.
B. AMH levels are elevated in ovarian follicular fluid but not in serum.
C. AMH levels are elevated in serum and in ovarian follicular fluid.
D. AMH levels are not elevated in serum or ovarian follicular fluid.
Rationale: In patients with PCOS, AMH levels are elevated in serum and in ovarian follicular fluid.
E. In patients with PCOS, the abnormality of AMH is qualitative rather than quantitative.
Rationale: In patients with PCOS, AMH is qualitatively normal.

6c. A. Pelvic inflammatory disease (PID).
B. Salpingitis isthmica nodosa (SIN).
C. Endometriosis.
Rationale: Endometriosis is not associated with increased levels of AMH in serum or ovarian follicular fluid.
D. Pelvic adhesions from prior surgery.
Rationale for A, B, and D: Infertility due to "tubal factors" (e.g., PID, SIN, or pelvic adhesions) is not associated with increased levels of AMH in serum or ovarian follicular fluid.
E. Granulosa cell tumors.
Rationale: AMH levels may be very high in patients with granulosa cell tumors.

6d. A. FSH levels in these patients are too high to initiate the maturation process among primordial follicles.
Rationale: FSH levels in these patients are too low to initiate the maturation process among primordial follicles.
B. Low serum LH levels prevent primordial follicles from initiating the process of maturation.
Rationale: High serum LH levels prevent primordial follicles from initiating the process of maturation.
C. AMH activity prevents primordial follicles from initiating the process of maturation.
Rationale: AMH levels may be markedly increased in PCOS.
D. AMH stimulates aromatase activity within granulosa cells, thereby reducing production of estradiol.
Rationale: AMH inhibits aromatase activity within granulosa cells, thereby reducing production of estradiol.

Major points of discussion

- Folliculogenesis begins in a female fetus at gestational age 14 to 20 weeks. At birth, the ovaries of female babies contain approximately 400,000 primordial follicles. Of these, only approximately 400 mature to ovulation. The remaining 99.9% undergo the degenerative process of atresia.

- Maturation of follicles, eventually resulting in ovulation, proceeds as follows: During the luteal phase of the menstrual cycle, a cohort of primary follicles begins the maturation process. Each primary follicle consists of a primary oocyte surrounded by a single layer of granulosa cells. Primary follicles mature into secondary/preantral follicles; each secondary follicle has a zona pellucida around its oocyte, surrounded by three to five layers of granulosa cells. Secondary follicles then mature into tertiary/antral/vesicular follicles, each of which contains a fluid-filled antrum and is surrounded by a theca interna and theca externa. Tertiary follicles proceed to become mature/Graafian mature follicles, each of which has an eccentrically located oocyte surrounded by a cumulus oophorus consisting of granulosa cells.

- By the mid to late luteal phase of each menstrual cycle, fewer than four follicles from that cycle's cohort persist as mature follicles. The other follicles from each cohort digress into atresia during the maturation process. Of these few mature follicles, only one will become that cycle's preovulatory follicle. Relative to the other mature follicles, the preovulatory follicle has higher intrafollicular levels of FSH and higher aromatase activity. These properties enable the preovulatory follicle to continue the maturation process, driven by estradiol (synthesized by aromatase) and FSH.

- Plasma LH levels rise during the late proliferative phase of the endometrial cycle. This change stimulates production of androstenedione by theca cells. Aromatase converts this androstenedione into estradiol, which further drives maturation of the preovulatory follicle.

- Granulosa cells of early developing follicles produce AMH, also known as Müllerian-inhibiting substance. Although this hormone's action is incompletely understood, proposed functions include inhibition of initial recruitment of primordial follicles and inhibition of aromatase activity. Accordingly, studies have shown an inverse relationship between serum levels of AMH and estradiol. Studies have also shown an inverse relationship between serum levels of AMH and FSH.

- In healthy women, serum levels of AMH undergo minor fluctuations during the menstrual cycle, presumably in concert with cyclic growth of small follicles, and loss of follicles via atresia.
- In patients with PCOS, recruitment and initial growth of follicles proceeds normally, but selection of a dominant preovulatory follicle does not occur. Consequently, the ovaries of these patients contain multiple small Graafian follicles. AMH levels are markedly increased in patients with PCOS.
- Patients with PCOS are at increased risk for development of endometrial hyperplasia and malignancy as the result of chronic anovulation.[14,18,38]

7a. A. Granulosa cell tumors secrete steroid hormones; secretion of peptide hormones by these tumors has not been reported.
B. Granulosa cell tumors secrete peptide hormones; secretion of steroid hormones by these tumors has not been reported.
C. Granulosa cell tumors secrete steroid hormones (including estrogen, testosterone, progestins, and inhibin), as well as peptide hormones (including AMH).
Rationale: Inhibin is a peptide hormone, not a steroid hormone.
D. Granulosa cell tumors secrete steroid hormones (including estrogen, testosterone, and progestins), as well as peptide hormones (including AMH and inhibin).
E. Granulosa cell tumors are generally poorly differentiated neoplasms, and production of functional hormones by these lesions is exceedingly rare.
Rationale: Secretion of steroid hormones (e.g., estrogens, progestins) and/or peptide hormones (e.g., inhibin, AMH) by granulosa cell tumors is a well-recognized phenomenon.

7b. **A. α-Fetoprotein (AFP).**
Rationale: Increased AFP has been reported in the context of juvenile granulosa cell tumor.
B. β-Human chorionic gonadotropin (β-hCG).
Rationale: β-hCG levels are generally normal in patients with granulosa cell tumors.
C. Carcinoembryonic antigen (CEA).
Rationale: CEA levels are generally normal in patients with granulosa cell tumors.
D. Lactate dehydrogenase (LDH).
Rationale: LDH levels are generally normal in patients with granulosa cell tumors.
E. CA-125.
Rationale: CA-125 levels are generally normal in patients with granulosa cell tumors.

7c. **A. Granulosa cell tumors frequently behave aggressively in middle-aged and postmenopausal patients but generally follow a benign course in children and young adults.**

B. Granulosa cell tumors frequently behave aggressively in children and young adults but generally follow a benign course in middle-aged and postmenopausal patients.
C. Granulosa cell tumors frequently behave aggressively in younger and older patients alike.
D. Granulosa cell tumors generally follow a benign course in younger and older patients alike.
E. Granulosa cell tumors generally follow a benign course in middle-aged and postmenopausal patients; these tumors have not been described in children and young adults.
Rationale: The granulosa cell tumor group includes the adult type and the juvenile type. The adult type occurs in middle-aged to postmenopausal women and behaves aggressively. Juvenile granulosa cell tumors are encountered predominantly during the first three decades of life and generally follow a benign clinical course.

Major points of discussion

- Ovarian tumors consist of three main categories: epithelial, stromal, and germ cell tumors. Epithelial tumors tend to predominate in adults, whereas germ cell tumors predominate in pediatric patients.
- Granulosa cell tumors belong to the category of ovarian sex cord–stromal tumors. This category accounts for approximately 8% of ovarian neoplasia. As outlined by the World Health Organization, this category encompasses tumors composed of granulosa cells, theca cells, Sertoli cells, Leydig cells, and fibroblasts of stromal origin.
- Granulosa cell tumors represent 1% to 2% of ovarian tumors overall and 6% to 10% of ovarian malignancies.
- The granulosa cell tumor group includes the adult type and the juvenile type. The adult type occurs in middle-aged to postmenopausal women. The granulosa cells have a round to ovoid nucleus with a longitudinal groove. Juvenile granulosa cell tumors are encountered predominantly during the first three decades of life. Almost all nuclei lack grooves. The adult type frequently recurs and behaves invasively, whereas the juvenile type generally follows a benign clinical course.
- Granulosa cell tumors may produce steroid hormones (e.g., estrogens, progestins) and/or peptide hormones (e.g., inhibin, AMH).
- Fibromas are the most common sex cord–stromal tumors; these lesions represent approximately 4% of ovarian tumors. They are most common in middle-aged women (patients' mean age is 48 years). They occur only occasionally in children.[30,47]

8a. A. Addison's disease.
Rationale: Hypoadrenalism leads to hypotension, hyperkalemia, and metabolic acidosis.
B. Graves' disease.
Rationale: Hyperthyroidism can be associated with hypertension but usually not hypokalemia because of renal loss.
C. Conn's syndrome.

Rationale: Hyperaldosteronism causes renal loss of potassium and protons. resulting in hypokalemia and hypochloremic metabolic alkalosis.

D. Mild congenital adrenal hyperplasia.

Rationale: Deficiency in adrenocorticoid synthesis pathways can lead to hypoaldosteronism, typically compensated in mild cases by increased ACTH and consequent adrenal hyperplasia.

E. Panhypopituitarism.

Rationale: Pituitary or hypothalamic lesions can lead to secondary or tertiary adrenal insufficiency, not hyperadrenalism.

8b. A. Elevated plasma renin activity (PRA) and decreased aldosterone.

Rationale: Primary hypoaldosteronism can result in hypotension and compensatory increased renin.

B. Suppressed PRA and elevated aldosterone.

Rationale: Primary hyperaldosteronism leads to salt retention, expanded blood volume, hypertension, and feedback suppression of renin production by the juxtaglomerular apparatus.

C. Elevated 17-hydroxyprogesterone and low aldosterone.

Rationale: These are findings consistent with congenital adrenal hyperplasia caused by defective 21-hydroxylase (CYP21A2) or 11-β-hydroxylase (CYP11B1/B2).

D. Elevated FT_4 and suppressed TSH.

Rationale: These are findings in Graves disease.

E. Low TSH and low FT_4.

Rationale: These are consistent with secondary hypothyroidism.

8c. A. Continued suppression of aldosterone after stimulation with adrenocorticotrotpic hormone.

Rationale: Inability to produce aldosterone after multiday ACTH stimulation is consistent with primary hypoaldosteronism (e.g., Addison's disease).

B. Failure to increase TSH after stimulation with thyroid-releasing hormone.

Rationale: This is a response consistent with pituitary insufficiency.

C. Maintained aldosterone elevation after infusion of 2000 mL of isotonic saline.

Rationale: A confirmatory test for Conn's syndrome is failure to suppress aldosterone production (plasma aldosterone >10 ng/dL) after expansion of intravascular volume with infusion of 300 to 2000 mL of isotonic saline over a period of 4 hours, indicating autonomous aldosterone production.

D. Elevated 17-hydroxyprogesterone after ACTH stimulation.

Rationale: This is consistent with congenital adrenal hyperplasia.

E. Failure to increase cortisol after insulin-induced hypoglycemia.

Rationale: This is consistent with secondary or tertiary hypoadrenalism.

Major points of discussion

- Conn's syndrome is defined as primary hyperaldosteronism caused by autonomous production of mineralocorticoids by the adrenal cortex. About 50% of the cases are due to an aldosterone-producing adrenal adenoma, whereas bilateral hyperplasia of the zona glomerulosa accounts for 45% and adrenal carcinoma for 5% of the cases.

- Hyperaldosteronism should be suspected in patients with refractory hypertension (e.g., receiving more than three anti-hypertensive agents) and in patients with spontaneous hypokalemia (<3.5 mmol/L), especially when associated with metabolic alkalosis. When patients are treated with diuretics, hyperadrenalism should be suspected when the potassium is less than 3.0 mmol/L and when it fails to normalize 2 to 4 weeks after stopping diuretics. Although potassium can be normal in up to 50% of patients with adrenal hyperplasia, the 24-hour urine potassium levels are almost always higher than 30 mmol/24 hr.

- Screening tests include simultaneous measurement of plasma aldosterone and renin levels. In the case of primary hyperaldosteronism, the plasma aldosterone will be high-normal or elevated (>8 to 15 ng/dL), whereas the plasma renin will be low, resulting in a aldosterone/renin ratio higher than 20 to 50 (depending on the laboratory).

- Plasma aldosterone and renin measurements should be made with careful attention to patient preparation because any condition interfering with plasma volume and the renin-angiotensin-aldosterone-potassium axis can complicate interpretation of the results. Examples include discontinuation of drugs such as spironolactone, ACE inhibitors, diuretics, nonsteroidal anti-inflammatory drugs, β-blockers, and similar agents for at least five half-lives. Other important considerations are correction of hypokalemia with potassium chloride before testing and collection of the blood sample from a seated patient the morning after ambulation for more than 30 minutes.

- Renin can be measured by its enzymatic activity (PRA) because it cleaves angiotensinogen to form angiotensin 1, which is then measured by an immunoassay. Issues with this approach include avoidance of refrigeration of the sample to prevent cold activation of renin and variability in plasma angiotensinogen levels. Recently, renin mass immunoassays have been developed and will provide a measure of renin levels independent of its activity.

- Aldosterone immunoassays are also subject to interferences by other sterols, such as in patients with adrenal hyperplasia and elevated levels of 21-deoxyaldosterone, as well as other uncharacterized substances. Measuring aldosterone with a liquid chromatography–mass spectrometry method can largely obviate these issues.[46,51,52]

9. A. FSH.

Rationale: FSH and LH levels establish whether primary amenorrhea is caused by failure of the gonads (levels are high) or hypothalamic-pituitary axis (levels are low).

B. DHEA-S.

Rationale: DHEA-S may be elevated in PCOS and other conditions associated with hyperandrogenism, which accounts for less than 5% of cases of primary amenorrhea.

C. Androstenedione.

Rationale: Androstenedione may be elevated in PCOS and other conditions associated with hyperandrogenism and hirsutism, which accounts for less than 5% of cases of primary amenorrhea.

D. Progesterone.

Rationale: Progesterone levels are not usually helpful in the diagnosis of primary amenorrhea.

E. β-hCG.

Rationale: Pregnancy is a major cause of secondary amenorrhea but not primary amenorrhea.

Major points of discussion

■ Primary amenorrhea is defined as the absence of menarche (first menstruation) by age 15 or 16 years in the presence of normal secondary sexual development or within 5 years of normal breast development if breast development occurs before 10 years of age, or lack of breast development by age 13 years.

■ The American Society for Reproductive Medicine classification of primary amenorrhea includes three main groups:
  1. Primary amenorrhea with normal Tanner stage
  2. Primary amenorrhea with low Tanner stage and high FSH level
  3. Primary amenorrhea with low Tanner stage and normal or low FSH level

■ In primary amenorrhea with normal Tanner stage, it is important to ascertain whether Müllerian structures (fallopian tubes, uterus, cervix) are present. If the uterus is present, particularly in patients with periodic abdominal pain, outlet abnormalities such as cervical stenosis, vaginal aplasia, vaginal septum, and imperforate hymen are likely. Rarely, primary amenorrhea in a patient with fully developed external female genitalia and normal Müllerian structures with 46,XY karyotype is due to pure gonadal dysgenesis, caused by mutations in genes involved in testis development, including *SRY*, steroidogenic factor 1 (*NR5A1*), *DAX1* (*NR0B1*), desert hedgehog (*DHH*), *WT1*, *WNT4*, and *SOX9*.

■ In primary amenorrhea with normal Tanner stage in the absence of Müllerian structures, a karyotype will distinguish the two most common causes: Müllerian agenesis and complete androgen insensitivity. A normal karyotype and LH and FSH levels within the reference range indicate Müllerian agenesis. Complete androgen insensitivity (testicular feminization), caused by mutations in the androgen receptor, will present with 46, XY karyotype with an external female phenotype with normal breast development, undescended testes, normal or elevated LH and FSH, and testosterone levels in the normal to high male range.

■ Low Tanner staging with elevated LH and FSH indicate delayed puberty caused by hypergonadotropic hypogonadism (gonadal dysgenesis). The most common cause is Turner's syndrome, defined by a 45,XO karyotype in a female. These patients lose their germ cells during gestation and are at high risk for cardiac, renal, thyroid, and ear abnormalities. Other congenital causes of hypergonadotropic hypogonadism include fragile X, Noonan's, and Swyer's syndromes. Causes of acquired primary hypogonadism include premature ovarian failure (idiopathic, trauma, surgery, radiation, chemotherapy, mumps, autoimmune disease); resistant ovary syndrome; and aromatase, 17-hydroxylase, and 17,20-lyase deficiencies.

■ Patients with hypogonadotropic hypogonadism present with low levels of FSH, LH, and estradiol. Elevated prolactin suppresses gonadotropin-releasing hormone and can occur with defects in the hypothalamic-pituitary axis, including pituitary adenomas, brain tumors, infections, hemochromatosis, sarcoidosis, aneurysms, trauma, hypothyroidism, and medications. Other causes include Kallmann's syndrome (congenital GnRH deficiency), thyroid disease, anorexia nervosa, malnutrition, stress, excessive exercise, and several chronic debilitating diseases. Occasionally, early onset of PCOS, Cushing's syndrome, ovarian or adrenal tumor, or late-onset congenital adrenal hyperplasia can cause primary amenorrhea with signs of hyperandrogenism such as acne and hirsutism. Hypogonadism with low FSH and LH, a family history of delayed puberty, and exclusion of other diseases can be due to constitutional delay of puberty, when puberty occurs later than 2.5 deviations from the population mean.

■ Physical examination, patient and family history, and laboratory measurements of FSH, LH, and prolactin can identify the most common causes of primary amenorrhea. Depending on the clinical situation, other useful tests include pelvic ultrasonography, head MRI, karyotype, TSH, testosterone, estradiol, DHEA-S, androstenedione, and 17-hydroxyproges-terone.[39,58]

10. A. Large prolactinoma and hook effect.

Rationale: Given the discrepancy between her prolactin levels and a biopsy-confirmed prolactin-secreting macroadenoma, the serum was repeatedly diluted and revealed a prolactin level of 8000 ng/mL.

B. Non–prolactin-secreting tumor and macroprolactin.

Rationale: Macroprolactin usually presents with elevations greater than 90 ng/mL. Tumors and lesions affecting the hypothalamus can cause mild hyperprolactinemia by interfering with the dopaminergic inhibition of prolactin secretion.

C. Stress-associated hyperprolactinemia.

Rationale: Stress can lead to mild hyperprolactinemia, rarely exceeding 40 ng/mL, but is insufficient to explain all the patient's findings.

D. Graves' disease.

Rationale: Hypothyroidism, but not hyperthyroidism, is frequently associated with hyperprolactinemia and amenorrhea.

E. Unreported opiate use.

Rationale: Opiates can interfere with dopaminergic pathways and lead to mild hyperprolactinemia, but this is insufficient to explain all the patient's findings.

Major points of discussion

■ Secondary amenorrhea is defined as the absence of menstruation for more than three cycles or six months in a woman who previously has had menses.

■ Excluding pregnancy, the causes of secondary amenorrhea can be classified into five main groups:
  1. Hypogonadotropic hypogonadism (low/normal FSH about 46% of the cases); for example, malnutrition, anorexia, depression, chronic anovulation, hypothyroidism, Cushing's syndrome, and hypothalamic and pituitary lesions.

2. Hypergonadotropic hypogonadism (high FSH; about 12%); for example, premature ovarian failure, autoimmune oophoritis, 46,XY karyotype, and fragile X syndrome.
3. Hyperprolactinemia (13%).
4. Anatomic (Asherman's syndrome, 7%).
5. Hyperandrogenic states (22%); for example, PCOS, ovarian tumors, and late-onset congenital adrenal hyperplasia.

■ The initial laboratory tests for evaluation of secondary amenorrhea should include FSH, LH, TSH, and prolactin levels.

■ Hyperprolactinemia can usually be explained by one of these mechanisms:
1. Physiologic stimulation of prolactin secretion; for example, pregnancy, high estrogen, stress, meals, sleep, sexual intercourse, nipple stimulation.
2. Decreased dopaminergic inhibition of prolactin secretion:
   a. Damage to hypothalamus or pituitary (e.g., tumors, neurosarcoidosis, trauma, surgery, non-lactotroph adenomas).
   b. Drugs interfering with dopaminergic pathways (e.g., antipsychotics, metoclopramide, methyldopa, reserpine, verapamil, selective serotonin uptake inhibitors).
3. Prolactin-secreting tumor: pituitary lactotroph adenomas.
4. Miscellaneous pathologic causes: hypothyroidism, chest wall injury, chronic renal failure.
5. Macroprolactinemia: prolactin complexed with immunoglobulins (or rarely polymers of prolactin ranging up to 500 kDa) causes decreased renal clearance and elevated concentrations of nonfunctional prolactin.

■ Because a large number of physiologic variables and medications can raise prolactin levels, it is recommended that prolactin testing be repeated to confirm the increased level. It is also recommended to treat the serum with a method that removes macroprolactin (either gel filtration or polyethylene glycol precipitation) in samples with prolactin levels higher than 90 to 100 ng/mL.

■ In women with persistent hyperprolactinemia, the prevalence of a pituitary tumor is approximately 50% to 60%, justifying follow-up with imaging. Microadenomas (<1 cm) usually have levels below 200 ng/mL, whereas macroadenomas (>2 cm) typically present with levels above 1000 ng/mL.

■ The hook effect occurs when very high levels of prolactin overwhelm the binding capacity of the reagent antibodies in the immunoassay, causing single antibody-antigen complexes instead of the required "sandwich" (capture antibody-antigen-detection antibody) and a falsely low result. Serial dilution of the antigen before adding the reagents is required to accurately determine the antigen concentration.[20,32,39]

11. A. Decreased testosterone.
Rationale: This patient has AIS, which is characterized by testosterone and other androgens in the normal to elevated male range with a female phenotype.
B. Decreased LH and FSH.

Rationale: These tend to be elevated in AIS because feedback inhibition by androgens is absent.
C. Low estradiol.
Rationale: There is no ovarian hormone production, but elevated testosterone is converted to estradiol by aromatase in extragonadal tissues. These patients can present with normal testosterone and elevated estradiol.
D. Elevated 17-hydroxyprogesterone.
Rationale: This is seen in a form of congenital adrenal hyperplasia with elevated adrenal androgens.
E. Mutated androgen receptor.
Rationale: This is the cause of AIS.

Major points of discussion
■ AIS is caused by mutations in the androgen receptor leading to reduced or absent virilization despite the presence of testes and normal testosterone production during puberty. Depending on the degree of impairment of the receptor function, various phenotypes can be observed.
■ Complete androgen insensitivity (CAIS, testicular feminization) will present with 46,XY karyotype with an external female phenotype, primary amenorrhea, no Müllerian structures (uterus, fallopian tubes, cervix), normal breast development, undescended testes, elevated LH levels, normal or elevated FSH levels, testosterone levels in the normal to high male range, and normal to high estradiol levels.
■ Less severe defects in the androgen receptor cause partial androgen insensitivity (PAIS) with incomplete virilization ranging from female phenotype with clitoromegaly or posterior labial fusion to male phenotype with minor virilization defects such as azoospermia, gynecomastia, and scant facial and pubic hair. In PAIS, abnormalities in sex hormones are less pronounced, and LH, testosterone, and estradiol levels may be normal.
■ Phenotypes similar to PAIS (but without normal breast development) can occur with defects in testosterone synthesis. In these cases, testosterone and estradiol levels are low, LH and FSH levels are elevated with a higher LH/FSH ratio, and precursors proximal to the synthetic defect will be elevated. The most common defect is in *HSD17B3*, which codes for 17β-hydroxysteroid dehydrogenase. 17β-Hydroxysteroid dehydrogenase converts androstenedione to testosterone in the testes, resulting in accumulation of androstenedione. Most of these patients present with some degree of virilization due to the action of extragonadal androgens.
■ Patients with gonadal dysgenesis and a 46,XY karyotype can also present with a female phenotype. These cases are also characterized by low testosterone and estradiol, high LH/FSH ratio, and low Müllerian inhibitory hormone levels, which result in the formation of normal Müllerian structures.
■ Complete failure of testosterone production can be distinguished from CAIS because postpubertal testosterone will be low in the former and normal to high in the latter. However, partial or incomplete defects are not always easy to distinguish. In prepubertal children with intact testosterone production, a stimulation test with hCG will typically result in an increase in testosterone levels of greater than 200 ng/dL.

■ Laboratory testing for testosterone in children and women should use methods that are sufficiently specific and sensitive at the low concentrations expected in normal individuals; for example, liquid chromatography—mass spectrometry.[22,34,39]

12. A. CTX reflects significant improvement in osteoporosis, whereas N-terminal PINP does not respond to vitamin D treatment.
Rationale: Vitamin D improves bone health and alters levels of bone turnover markers. However, the patient was taking vitamin D supplements for more than 2 years during both occasions, so the described change is unlikely to be related to vitamin D treatment.
B. CTX reflects significant improvement in osteoporosis, whereas PINP is falsely elevated because of the influence of food intake and circadian variability on PINP levels.
Rationale: The influence of food intake on N-terminal PINP levels is minimal. Circadian variability in PINP levels is low.
C. The difference between the two CTX levels is within the expected analytical variability.
Rationale: The minimum significant change for CTX measured by CLIA is 27%.
D. Influence of food intake on CTX levels and circadian variability in CTX levels.
Rationale: Fasting substantially increases CTX levels. During fasting, there is also substantial circadian variability in CTX levels with high levels in the morning, followed by decreasing levels during the day.
E. Intralaboratory variability in CTX and PINP results.
Rationale: Intralaboratory variability using automated CLIA is low. Interlaboratory variability can be high.

Major points of discussion
■ Relative to an 8 AM sample (fasting or nonfasting), CTX in a sample collected later in the day is lower by up to 50%. Relative to nonfasting, CTX in a sample collected during fasting, especially randomly collected throughout the day, is higher (Figure 4-3, *A*).

■ Food intake substantially decreases the level of the bone resorption marker serum CTX collected at 9 AM. The level of bone formation markers such as serum N-terminal PINP in such a sample is not significantly altered by food intake (Figure 4-3, *B*).
■ Bone formation markers such as PINP, osteocalcin, and bone alkaline phosphatase show relatively small circadian variability.
■ Bone resorption markers such as CTX and NTX show substantial circadian variability.
■ Considerable interlaboratory variability exists despite efforts to standardize bone turnover marker assays and the introduction of proficiency testing. To some extent, this variability is related to different methodologies for the same markers and lack of standardization.
■ Other sources of variability in bone turnover levels are renal function, age, gender, adolescence, menopause, exercise, and recent fracture.
■ Analytical variability is reduced by using automated assays rather than manual assays. The minimum significant change for serum CTX has been reported as 37% for enzyme-linked immunosorbent assay (ELISA)[9] and 27% for electrochemiluminescent immunoassay (ECLIA).[21]
■ Whether an increase or a decrease in the level of bone formation and/or resorption markers reflects an improvement in bone health is determined by bone disease and treatment.[9,10,21,40]

13. A. The patient should be treated for hypocalcemia.
Rationale: The patient's symptoms and the calcium level suggest hypocalcemia. However, the measured value of the total calcium might be lower because of a matrix effect.
B. The sample should be sent to a reference laboratory to determine calcium by atomic absorption spectrometry (AAS).
Rationale: AAS is less prone to the matrix effect from EDTA than the photometric methods. However, turnaround times for even the best reference laboratories are too long in this case.

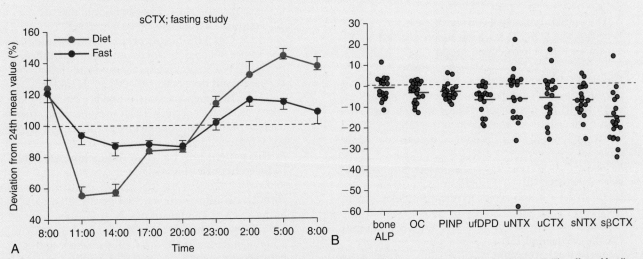

Figure 4-3 **A,** Serum carboxy-terminal collagen cross-links (sCTX) in premenopausal women on a normal diet and during fasting. **B,** The effect of feeding on bone turnover markers in individual subjects as a percentage difference (fed minus fasting). Each circle represents one subject. The *horizontal line* indicates the mean percentage difference for each marker. (**A,** From Qvist P, Christgau S, Pedersen BJ, et al. Circadian variation in the serum concentration of C-terminal telopeptide of type I collagen (serum CTx): effects of gender, age, menopausal status, posture, daylight, serum cortisol, and fasting. *Bone* 2002;31[1]:57–61. **B,** From Clowes JA, Hannon RA, Yap TS, et al. Effect of feeding on bone turnover markers and its impact on biological variability of measurements. *Bone* 2002;30[6]:886–890.)

C. The measurement should be repeated using serum.
Rationale: Serum is the preferred sample for measuring calcium by photometric methods.
D. The patient should not be treated for hypocalcemia.
Rationale: The corrected calcium is normal (8.7 mg/dL). The low calcium is due to a matrix effect and suggests that the patient does not have hypocalcemia. However, it is best to first repeat the measurement using serum.
E. Ionized calcium should be measured in the EDTA sample.
Rationale: In this case, it is best to first repeat the total calcium measurement using serum. In addition, EDTA interferes with ionized calcium measurements and calcium measurements should be performed on serum.

Major points of discussion
- Total calcium can be measured photometrically using the *o*-cresolphthalein complexone method or the arsezano III method. AAS can also be used to measure calcium.
- Serum and heparinized plasma are the preferred specimens for measuring total calcium. Citrate, oxalate, and EDTA anticoagulants should not be used for photometric methods because they interfere by forming complexes with calcium.
- Corrected total calcium (mg/dL) = total calcium (mg/dL) + $0.8 \times (4 - \text{albumin [g/dL]})$.
- Free (ionized) calcium can be measured using ion selective electrodes (ISEs). Citrate, oxalate, and EDTA anticoagulants should not be used for photometric methods because they interfere by forming complexes with calcium. Heparin may also interfere and, therefore, serum is the preferred specimen.
- pH influences the binding of calcium by proteins. Free calcium changes by approximately 5% for each 0.1 unit of change in pH.
- Hemolysis, lipemia, icterus, paraproteinemia, and magnesium can interfere with photometric methods for total calcium.

14a. **A. The patient has active Graves' disease.**
Rationale: The high FT_4 level and suppressed TSH are consistent with active Graves' disease.
B. This patient has gestational thyrotoxicosis.
Rationale: Gestational thyrotoxicosis presents typically in the first trimester with hyperemesis gravidarum, high FT_4, and low TSH, but it is not associated with TRAb. High levels of hCG contribute to stimulation of the TSHR.
C. The presence of anti-TPO antibodies rules out Graves' disease.
Rationale: Anti-TPO antibodies are present in more than 80% of patients with Graves' disease.
D. This patient is undergoing effective anti-thyroid drug treatment.
Rationale: Effective treatment should result in decreased FT_4 and normalized TSH.
E. This patient has Hashimoto's thyroiditis and not Graves' disease.
Rationale: Hashimoto's autoimmune thyroiditis is usually associated with hypothyroidism, although it can manifest with thyrotoxicosis, particularly early in the natural course of the disease. It is also characterized by the presence of

thyroid antibodies, particularly anti-TPO. In contrast to Graves' disease, Hashimoto's thyroiditis is only rarely associated with anti-TSHR antibodies.

14b. A. The risk for neonatal thyroid disease is the same as in the general population.
Rationale: The presence of hyperthyroidism in the mother that is associated with TSHR antibodies (TRAb) increases the risk for transplacental crossing of thyroid-stimulating antibodies (TSAb).
B. The fetus is at risk for neonatal hyperthyroidism due to transplacental transport of TRAb.
Rationale: The risk for neonatal hyperthyroidism is about 2% to 10% in pregnancies with high levels of TRAb (>3.25 U/L by this assay), even if the mother is euthyroid.
C. The fetus is at risk for neonatal hypothyroidism due to transplacental transport of thyroid-blocking antibodies.
Rationale: In rare cases, thyroid-blocking antibodies can cause neonatal hypothyroidism. However, in this patient, a preponderance of TSAb is more likely.
D. The fetus is at risk for hypothyroidism due to overtreatment of the mother's hyperthyroidism with antithyroid medications.
Rationale: Although this scenario is possible, in this case the mother is not being overtreated.
E. The fetus is at risk for neonatal hypothyroidism due to Hashimoto's thyroiditis.
Rationale: Although anti-thyroid peroxidase (TPO) antibodies can cross the placenta and appear transiently in the newborn's circulation, anti-TPO antibodies do not typically cause thyroiditis in the newborn.

14c. A. The patient has postpartum depression but is euthyroid.
Rationale: Low FT_4 and elevated TSH are not consistent with a euthyroid state.
B. The patient has atrophic hypothyroidism due to overtreatment with PTU.
Rationale: PTU treatment (in contrast with radioiodine therapy) is unlikely to cause thyroid atrophy and persistent hypothyroidism after discontinuation.
C. The patient now has hypothyroidism due to autoimmune thyroiditis.
Rationale: Given the history of Graves' disease and the persistence of high levels of thyroid-binding inhibiting immunoglobulins, autoimmune thyroiditis is unlikely.
D. The patient developed anti-TSH antibodies.
Rationale: Although anti-TSH antibodies can result in falsely elevated or decreased TSH measurements, the overall clinical laboratory picture in this patient is more consistent with hypothyroidism.
E. This patient now has thyroid-blocking antibody-induced hypothyroidism.
Rationale: Although rare, this is a possibility in patients with Graves' disease when the levels of TSAb decline and/ or the levels of TBAb markedly increase. The chemiluminescence assay for thyroid-binding inhibiting immunoglobulins (TBII) measures the ability of the patient's antibodies to compete with a labeled monoclonal antibody for binding to immobilized TSHR. It does not distinguish between TSAb and TBAb, which requires a biologic assay. In this case, the biologic assay for TSAb showed normalization in the presence of high TBII, suggesting the presence of TBAb.

Major points of discussion

- TRAb can be classified as stimulating (TSAb), blocking (TBAb), or neutral antibodies. Initially described by Adams and Purves in 1956 as "long-acting thyroid stimulator" antibodies linked to Graves' disease, TSAb bind to the TSHR in a conformation similar to the native TSH and are able to activate the receptor, resulting in stimulation of thyroid hormone production. In contrast, TBAb bind to the TSHR in a competitive manner with TSH, resulting in lower signaling activity and reduced thyroid hormone production. Neutral TRAbs are also present in Graves' disease but do not interfere with thyroid production. However, they may have some noncanonical signaling effects of the TSHR.

- Current automated immunoassays can detect TRAb in about 95% to 97% of patients with Graves' disease. These assays are based on a competition between a labeled anti-TSHR monoclonal antibody and the patient's immunoglobulins for binding to a solid-phase–bound TSHR. These assays are also called thyroid-binding inhibiting immunoglobulins (TBII) because of their ability to compete with TSH for binding to the TSHR. This assay does not differentiate between TSAb and TBAb.

- The effect of the TRAb on the TSHR activity can be measured by biologic assays using cultured cells expressing the TSHR and the ability to stimulate (TSAb) or inhibit (TBAb) cyclic adenosine monophosphate (cAMP) production (or luciferase expression under the control of a cAMP-responsive promoter) induced by TSH. The balance of activities of TSAb and TBAb, which depends on their relative concentration and binding affinity, correlates with thyroid function in patients with Graves' disease. Patients can alternate between periods of hyperthyroidism (high TSAb), euthyroidism, and rarely hypothyroidism (high TBAb with low TSAb). Total TBII levels do not correlate with symptoms or severity of Graves' disease.

- Transplacental transport of TSAb can cause neonatal hyperthyroidism even when the mother is euthyroid (2% to 10% risk). Very rarely, transplacental TBAb can cause transient hypothyroidism. Therefore, evaluation of TRAb in pregnant females during the third trimester (22 to 26 weeks of gestation) is indicated in females with a history of Graves' disease or a previous delivery of an infant with neonatal hyperthyroidism. In the first trimester, testing for TRAb is useful in patients with active Graves' disease undergoing treatment, as well as to distinguish between gestational thyrotoxicosis and Graves' disease.

- TRAb testing may also be useful to establish hyperthyroidism when other tests are unclear, to distinguish Graves' disease from other causes of thyrotoxicosis, and to evaluate patients with suspected thyrotoxic orbitopathies.

- In general, TRAb show poor predictive value for monitoring of recurrence of Graves' disease and are not currently recommended for that purpose.

- Isolated TBAb are an extremely rare cause of hypothyroidism associated with thyroid gland atrophy.

Anti–thyroid peroxidase antibodies (anti-TPO) are present in 90% to 100% of patients with Hashimoto thyroiditis, the most common cause of hypothyroidism. Anti-TPO antibodies are also present in 75% to 80% of patients with Graves' disease, but because of poor clinical predictivity, specificity, and sensitivity, they are not recommended for diagnosis or follow-up in Graves' disease.[27,33]

15a. A. Interferon-α.
Rationale: Patients receiving interferon-α may develop painless or "silent" thyroiditis, hypothyroidism, or Graves' disease. The clinical, laboratory, and/or pathologic findings in these conditions would likely differ from those described above.
B. Interleukin-2.
Rationale: Patients receiving interleukin-2 may develop painless or silent thyroiditis. The laboratory and pathologic findings in this condition would likely differ from those described above.
C. Amiodarone.
Rationale: This clinical scenario and these laboratory findings are consistent with amiodarone-induced destructive thyroiditis.
D. Minocycline.
Rationale: Minocycline appears to inhibit thyroid peroxidase activity and is associated with specific pathologic findings (see Major Points of Discussion). Use of this drug would not likely result in the scenario described above.

15b. A. Acute thyroiditis.
Rationale: In acute thyroiditis, the erythrocyte sedimentation rate and the white blood cell count are usually increased, and thyroid function is generally normal.
B. Subacute thyroiditis.
Rationale: Destruction of follicles during the initial thyrotoxic phase of subacute thyroiditis would cause release of thyroid hormones (thyrotoxicosis) without underlying hyperthyroidism.
C. Hashimoto's thyroiditis.
Rationale: Hashimoto's thyroiditis is rarely associated with thyroid-stimulating immunoglobulins. In these rare patients, however, thyrotoxicosis results from hyperthyroidism.
D. Riedel's thyroiditis.
Rationale: Thyroid dysfunction is uncommon in Riedel's thyroiditis.

15c. A. Diffuse follicular epithelial hyperplasia.
Rationale: Diffuse hyperplasia of the thyroid (Graves' disease) is hyperthyroidism due to thyroid-stimulating immunoglobulins. Radionuclide uptake would be increased.
B. Follicular adenoma.
Rationale: These lesions are usually asymptomatic. A minority of adenomas ("toxic" adenomas) are associated with hyperthyroidism.
C. Infarcted adenoma.
Rationale: Infarction of an adenoma would cause release of thyroid hormones (thyrotoxicosis) without underlying hyperthyroidism.

D. Medullary thyroid carcinoma.
Rationale: Medullary thyroid carcinoma is a neoplastic process of the parafollicular cells of the thyroid gland and is not typically associated with increased levels of thyroid hormones. Patients with follicular or papillary thyroid carcinoma usually present with asymptomatic thyroid nodules and elevated levels of thyroid hormones.

Major points of discussion

- Thyrotoxicosis refers to elevated levels of thyroid hormone. Hyperthyroidism refers to excessive thyroid function. Thyrotoxicosis can, but does not necessarily, result from hyperthyroidism.
- Thyrotoxicosis without hyperthyroidism (destructive thyroiditis) results from thyroid destruction; for example, due to amiodarone, subacute thyroiditis, and infarction of an adenoma.
- Amiodarone exerts various effects on thyroid function and causes thyrotoxicosis through multiple different mechanisms. In individuals without underlying thyroid abnormalities, amiodarone-induced thyrotoxicosis manifests as destructive thyroiditis resulting from lysosomal activation. The pathologic hallmark of this condition is accumulation of foamy macrophages within thyroid follicles.
- Subacute thyroiditis (also known as de Quervain's thyroiditis, granulomatous thyroiditis, or viral thyroiditis) characteristically involves a thyrotoxic phase, followed by a hypothyroid phase, followed by a recovery phase. Destruction of follicles during the initial thyrotoxic phase causes release of thyroid hormones (thyrotoxicosis) without underlying hyperthyroidism.
- Patients receiving interferon-α or interleukin-2 may develop painless or silent thyroiditis. This condition is associated with development of anti-TPO antibodies and follows a clinical course similar to that of subacute thyroiditis. Minocycline appears to inhibit thyroid peroxidase and is associated with deposition of granular black pigment in follicular epithelial cells, colloid, and macrophages.
- Acute thyroiditis is rare and results from suppurative infection of the thyroid; thyroid function is generally normal in this condition. Hashimoto's thyroiditis is the most common cause of chronic hypothyroidism. Patients with Riedel's thyroiditis (idiopathic fibrosis of the thyroid) typically present with symptoms related to compression of local structures; thyroid dysfunction is uncommon in this condition.
- Etiologies of primary hyperthyroidism include Graves' disease, toxic goiter, and toxic adenoma. Etiologies of secondary hyperthyroidism include pituitary adenoma and gestational thyrotoxicosis.[54,57]

16. A. Because of cross-reactivity, immunoassays generally give higher results than mass spectrometry–based assays.
Rationale: Generally, immunoassays give higher results than mass spectrometry–based assays, which is often related to cross-reactivity. However, this does not explain the discrepancy seen here.
B. The DiaSorin Liaison TOTAL and the Immunodiagnostics-iSYS CLIA methods both detect 25(OH)-vitamin D_2 and 25(OH)-vitamin D_3.

Rationale: Both assays indeed detect 25(OH)-vitamin D_2 and 25(OH)-vitamin D_3 and report the sum of these two, but this does not explain the discrepancy.
C. The DiaSorin Liaison TOTAL and the Immunodiagnostics-iSYS CLIA methods do not detect 25(OH)-vitamin D_2.
Rationale: Both assays TOTAL do detect 25(OH)-vitamin D_2 as well as 25(OH)-vitamin D_3.
D. The DiaSorin Liaison TOTAL and the Immunodiagnostics-iSYS CLIA methods detect both the 25(OH)-vitamin D_3 C3-epimer and 25(OH)-vitamin D_3.
Rationale: Both assays detect 25(OH)-vitamin D_3 but not the 25(OH)-vitamin D_3 C3-epimer.
E. Most mass spectrometry–based assays do measure the 25(OH)-vitamin D_3 C3-epimer but cannot distinguish it from 25(OH)-vitamin D_3.
Rationale: The 25(OH)-vitamin D_3 C3-epimer is not distinguished from 25(OH)-vitamin D_3 by most routine LC-MS/MS assays.

Major points of discussion

- Epimeric forms of 25(OH)-vitamin D_3, as well as of 1,25(OH)-vitamin D_3, have recently been identified in infant, pediatric, and adult populations and provide a challenge for clinical laboratories.
- The epimers of 25(OH)-vitamin D_3, 24,25(OH)-vitamin D_3, and 1,25(OH)-vitamin D_3 are formed through an epimerization pathway that parallels the standard metabolic pathway of vitamin D. In the epimerization pathway, the hydroxyl group at position C-3 of the A-ring is converted from the alpha to the beta conformation.
- The physiologic function of 3-epimer forms of vitamin D appears to be the suppression of parathyroid hormone (PTH) expression, without inducing other classic vitamin D effects.
- Although still subject to debate, it is the general consensus that 25(OH)-vitamin D_3 C3-epimer should be quantified in infant and pediatric populations because the levels can be substantial in those populations relative to levels of 25(OH)-vitamin D_3.
- Most routine LC-MS/MS assays do not separate these isomers and, therefore, do not distinguish between 25(OH)-vitamin D_3 C3-epimer and 25(OH)-vitamin D_3 because they have the same retention time and the same mass transitions.
- A 2011 vitamin D External Quality Assessment Scheme proficiency survey showed that, whereas most LC-MS/MS and high-performance liquid chromatography methods, as well as the Roche Total 25(OH)-vitamin D assay, detect the C3 epimer, most other immunoassays (e.g., Abbott Architect, IDS enzyme immunoassay, IDS iSYS, DiaSorin Liaison TOTAL, DiaSource, and DiaSorin radioimmunoassay) did not detect this epimer.[4]

17. A. In an ectopic pregnancy, serum hCG levels double every 2 days during the first 5 to 6 weeks after implantation of the embryo.
Rationale: In an ectopic pregnancy, serum hCG levels increase, but do not double every 2 days.
B. Molar pregnancies are associated with lower-than-expected serum hCG levels.
Rationale: In molar pregnancies, serum hCG concentrations are higher than expected.

C. In a normal pregnancy, maximum serum hCG levels are reached at or near the end of the first trimester.
Rationale: This is the correct answer.
D. In a normal pregnancy, serum hCG levels return to nonpregnant levels within 2 to 3 days after a normal delivery.
Rationale: Serum hCG levels return to baseline in 1 to 2 weeks after a normal delivery.
E. In a normal pregnancy, serum hCG levels are at their highest in the third trimester.
Rationale: In a normal pregnancy, serum hCG levels decrease after reaching a maximum level in the first trimester.

Major points of discussion
- hCG is a glycoprotein consisting of an α- and β-subunit. The α-subunit is identical to the α-subunits of LH, FSH, and TSH. hCG is produced by placental syncytiotrophoblastic cells and is used as a marker for pregnancy detection and monitoring of pregnancy. hCG is also produced by trophoblast cells in hydatidiform moles and choriocarcinoma and in patients with germ cell carcinomas. The pituitary gland is also a source of hCG.
- In a normal pregnancy, hCG levels rise exponentially, doubling about every 2 days for about 8 weeks after implantation of the embryo. Maximum levels are reached at 8 to 10 weeks after the last menstrual period, and hCG levels higher than 100,000 IU/L can be obtained.
- After the first trimester, hCG levels decrease and remain at a constant level during the third trimester. A wide range of hCG values can be obtained during pregnancy. Serum hCG levels can take up to 4 weeks to return to baseline after a normal delivery.
- In an ectopic pregnancy, lower-than-expected serum hCG values are obtained compared with a normal pregnancy. In addition, serum hCG levels increase at a slower rate than in a normal pregnancy and do not double every 2 days. Low serum hCG levels and a lack of doubling every 2 days are suggestive of an ectopic pregnancy.
- Hydatidiform moles occur in approximately 1 in 1500 to 2000 pregnancies in the United States. Patients with hydatidiform moles present with a uterus larger than expected for gestational age, absence of fetal heart tones, dark brown to bright red vaginal discharge in the fourth or fifth month of pregnancy, expulsion of cystic vesicles, markedly elevated serum hCG levels, severe nausea and vomiting during pregnancy, and pregnancy-induced hypertension before 24 weeks of gestation. Patients with a complete hydatidiform mole can have serum hCG levels higher than 1,000,000 IU/L.[5,11]

18. A. Decreased CYP24A1 activity. Measure serum 24,25 (OH)-vitamin D.
Rationale: Idiopathic infantile hypercalcemia is caused by loss of function mutations in *CYP24A1,* leading to low 24-hydroxylase activity and high levels of 25(OH)-vitamin D and 1,25(OH)-vitamin D. 24,25(OH)-vitamin D levels are low in these patients.
B. Hypoparathyroidism. Measure PTH with a third-generation assay.

Rationale: Hypoparathyroidism is usually characterized by hypocalcemia.
C. Cancer. Measure PTH-related peptide.
Rationale: Urinary calcium can be high in patients with malignancy-associated hypercalcemia. However, urinary phosphate levels tend to be lower.
D. Chronic kidney disease. Measure neutrophil gelatinase–associated lipocalin (NGAL).
Rationale: Chronic kidney disease usually leads to hyperparathyroidism and low 1,25(OH)-vitamin D levels. NGAL is a marker of acute kidney injury.
E. Familial hypocalciuric hypercalcemia. Measure serum phosphate.
Rationale: This patient is not hypocalciuric.

Major points of discussion
- The differential diagnosis of hypercalcemia includes primary hyperparathyroidism, tertiary hyperparathyroidism, malignancy-associated hypercalcemia, granulomatous diseases (e.g., sarcoidosis, tuberculosis, and berylliosis), vitamin D intoxication, lymphoma, chronic kidney disease treated with calcium and 1,25(OH)-vitamin D or its analogs, thyrotoxicosis, pheochromocytoma, thiazide diuretics, milk-alkali syndrome, hypervitaminosis A, immobilization, familial hypocalciuric hypercalcemia, and idiopathic infantile hypercalcemia.
- Idiopathic infantile hypercalcemia is caused by a loss-of-function mutation in the gene encoding for the CYP24A1 enzyme, which is also known as 24-hydroxylase. The enzyme inactivates 1,25(OH)-vitamin D to 1,24,25(OH)-vitamin D and also metabolizes 25 (OH)-vitamin D to 24,25(OH)-vitamin D. Loss of activity of the enzyme leads to relatively high levels of 25(OH)-vitamin D, and 1,25(OH)-vitamin D and, therefore, vitamin D toxicity, which includes hypercalcemia.
- Idiopathic infantile hypercalcemia is characterized by low levels of 1,24,25(OH)-vitamin D and 24,25(OH)-vitamin D. There is no good method available to measure 1,24,25(OH)-vitamin D, but 24,25(OH)-vitamin D can be measured by LC-MS/MS. The serum concentration of 24,25(OH)-vitamin D is low (i.e., <1.5 ng/mL) in idiopathic infantile hypercalcemia.
- The patient described had hypercalciuria. Monogenic forms of hypercalciuric nephrolithiasis include various syndromes, such as Bartter's syndrome, Dent's disease, Lowe's disease, and autosomal dominant hypocalcemia with hypercalciuria.
- Several loss-of-function mutations of *CYP24A1,* encoding a 24-hydroxylase, have been described.
- The possibility of a 24-hydroxylase loss of function mutation should be considered in the differential diagnosis of nephrolithiasis and idiopathic hypercalciuria, particularly when hypercalcemia or a positive family history is present.[16,17,49]

19. A. There is a weak relationship between ionized and total Mg levels in serum.
Rationale: A weak relationship per se does not explain falsely low ionized Mg levels.
B. Interference by cotinine in the serum from cigarette smoking by the patient.

Rationale: Although smoking can lead to falsely low Mg serum concentrations, this is not caused by cotinine.

C. Interference by thiocyanate in the serum from cigarette smoking by the patient.
Rationale: Thiocyanate in circulating in serum due to smoking can cause falsely low free Mg concentrations when some free Mg assays are used.

D. Vitamin C intake by the patient.
Rationale: Ascorbic acid is not known to interfere with any of the free Mg assays.

E. The presence of hypoalbuminemia.
Rationale: Hypoalbuminemia correlates with high ionized Mg levels.

Major points of discussion

- Measuring ionized (i.e., "free") Mg may be useful in certain conditions, such as inflammatory bowel disease, cardiac surgery, stroke, head injury, renal dysfunction, alcoholism, liver disease, and eclampsia. However, in contrast to total Mg (i.e., protein-bound, complexed, and free), ionized Mg is not often measured. The relationship between total Mg and ionized Mg is weak and is influenced by factors such as albumin.
- Ionized Mg can be measured in serum using ISEs. These are available from several manufacturers and interferences are model specific.
- Current ISEs for Mg have insufficient selectivity for Mg over calcium (Ca). Free Ca is simultaneously determined and used chemometrically with the signal from the Mg electrode to calculate free Mg concentrations.
- Many of the factors that affect the free Ca levels also affect the free Mg levels.
- Certain silicones, other tube additives, and zinc heparin interfere with free Mg determinations.
- Thiocyanate from smoking (and from foods in the diet, such as cabbage) leads to falsely low free Mg levels when measured using some ISE models.[7,25,42]

20. A. Hyperglycosylated hCG.
Rationale: Most of the hCG that is detected in serum at 3 to 5 weeks of pregnancy is hyperglycosylated.

B. Intact hCG.
Rationale: Intact hCG is detected in serum at 3 to 5 weeks of pregnancy but at lower levels than hyperglycosylated hCG.

C. Free β-hCG.
Rationale: Free β-hCG is present at low concentrations in serum at 3 to 5 weeks of pregnancy.

D. Nicked hCG.
Rationale: Nicked hCG is present at very low concentrations in serum at 3 to 5 weeks of pregnancy.

E. Pituitary hCG.
Rationale: Pituitary hCG is not detected in serum at 3 to 5 weeks of pregnancy.

Major points of discussion

- Intact hCG is a glycoprotein consisting of a 92–amino acid α-subunit and a 145–amino acid β-subunit with a molecular weight of about 37.9 kDa. The β-subunit determines the biologic activity of hCG. The α-subunit of hCG has the same amino acid sequence as in TSH, LH, and FSH. The β-subunit of hCG has a slightly different amino acid sequence compared with the β-subunits of

TSH, LH, and FSH; this differentiates hCG from these other glycoprotein hormones.
- Hyperglycosylated hCG is a glycosylated variant of hCG. Hyperglycosylated hCG consists of 42% carbohydrate by molecular weight compared with 30% in intact hCG. Hyperglycosylated hCG is the major hCG molecule that is produced between 3 and 5 weeks of pregnancy and accounts for about 87% of the total hCG in the third week of pregnancy.
- Intact hCG accounts for most of the remaining hCG at 3 weeks of pregnancy. The amount of hyperglycosylated hCG rapidly decreases after 3 weeks, and at 6 weeks intact hCG is the predominant form of circulating hCG. The amount of hyperglycosylated hCG in the second and third trimesters is less than 1% of total hCG.
- Intact hCG promotes progesterone production during the first 3 weeks of pregnancy. Hyperglycosylated hCG stimulates implantation and the growth of placenta. Intact hCG and hyperglycosylated hCG together are believed to be responsible for implantation of the embryo in early pregnancy.
- Hyperglycosylated hCG is also the major form of hCG in choriocarcinoma. Nicked hCG is formed from the β-subunit of hCG, usually by enzymatic cleavage of the peptide bonds at positions 47 to 48. Nicking inactivates hCG. Nicked hCG may be present in serum after removal of a hydatidiform mole or in postgestational choriocarcinoma. Free β-hCG levels are used in the first trimester as part of a screening protocol for Down syndrome. Free β-hCG levels in serum are a sensitive marker for testicular cancer.[11,29]

21. A. Prostate cancer with bone metastasis.
Rationale: Although metastases are predominantly osteoblastic in prostate cancer, evidence of both bone resorption and formation is usually seen.

B. Breast cancer with bone metastasis.
Rationale: Although metastases are predominantly osteolytic in breast cancer, evidence of both bone resorption and formation is usually seen.

C. Multiple myeloma with osteolytic lesions.
Rationale: In multiple myeloma, markers of bone resorption are elevated, but markers of bone formation may be normal or low. Serum carboxy-terminal collagen cross-link levels are subject to circadian variation and vary depending on food intake, which explains the normal level seen in the nonfasting sample collected at 2 PM.

D. Renal carcinoma with bone metastasis.
Rationale: In renal carcinoma with metastatic bone disease, evidence of both bone resorption and formation is usually seen.

E. Bone metastases from non–small cell lung carcinoma.
Rationale: In non–small cell lung carcinoma with metastatic bone disease, evidence of both bone resorption and formation is usually seen.

Major points of discussion

- Bone turnover markers are usually elevated in patients with solid tumors with metastatic bone disease.
- The levels of these markers are related to the risk for skeletal related events, which include spinal cord compression, pathologic fractures, a need for radiation therapy or surgery, and hypercalcemia of malignancy.

■ The levels of these markers are also related to the extent of skeletal disease, such as the number of metastases.

■ In multiple myeloma, there is increased activation of osteoclasts and suppression of osteoblast function. Bone resorption markers such as urinary N-telopeptide cross-links and serum carboxy-terminal collagen cross-links (CTX) are usually elevated. Results for bone formation markers are more variable, but multiple studies have shown normal-low bone alkaline phosphatase levels in a substantial proportion of these patients.

■ Serum CTX levels show circadian variation and are influenced by food intake. Circadian levels reach a nadir at approximately 1 to 2 PM. Relative to fasting levels, the nadir is even lower when nonfasting samples are obtained.[12,55,59]

22. A. Melorheostosis.
Rationale: Melorheostosis is a rare progressive developmental disease that presents with extremity deformity and stiffness, pain, and decreased range of motion due to thickening of cortical bone. This hyperostosis has a radiographic appearance resembling wax that has dripped off a candle and shows increased uptake on a bone scan. This hyperostosis can often be felt through the warm skin. Alkaline phosphatase is normal in this setting.
B. Multiple myeloma.
Rationale: Multiple myeloma typically does not show increased uptake on bone scan. Serum alkaline phosphatase is often normal or decreased in multiple myeloma.
C. Paget's disease of bone.
Rationale: The clinical presentation, imaging, and laboratory findings suggest that this patient has monostotic Paget's disease of bone.
D. Male osteoporosis.
Rationale: Male osteoporosis typically does not show increased uptake on bone scan, nor does it show increased serum levels of alkaline phosphatase.
E. Van Buchem's disease.
Rationale: Van Buchem's disease is a hereditary sclerosing dysplasia of bone. The autosomal dominant form is benign and presents with jaw bone enlargement. The recessive form is more severe with hyperostotic bone causing cranial nerve impingement. Facial palsy is common in these patients. Serum alkaline phosphatase levels are often increased in the recessive form.

Major points of discussion
■ Paget's disease of bone (osteitis deformans) is a common disorder characterized by focal areas of increased and disorganized bone remodeling affecting one or more bones throughout the skeleton. The disease is rare before the age of 55 years and predominantly affects individuals of European descent. The cause of the disease is unknown. Viral infection of osteoclasts and environmental factors have been linked to this disease, and several rare inherited forms are recognized.

■ The diagnosis of Paget's disease of bone can usually be made on the basis of a radiograph. The extent of the disease is best determined by radionuclide scans. Laboratory testing should include assessment of renal function, measurement of levels of calcium, albumin, alkaline phosphatase, and 25(OH)-vitamin D. Liver function should be assessed to rule out increases of

alkaline phosphatase resulting from liver disease. Typically, patients with Paget's disease present with an isolated elevated alkaline phosphatase activity with otherwise normal biochemical testing.

■ Normal alkaline phosphatase levels do not rule out the diagnosis of Paget's disease. Monostotic disease, in particular, can present with normal levels.

■ The use of more specific biochemical markers of bone turnover (i.e., bone alkaline phosphatase, type I PINP, osteocalcin, urinary N-telopeptide cross-links/creatinine ratio (uNTX/Cr) or serum carboxy-terminal collagen cross-links [sCTX]) can be useful in cases with concomitant liver disease but otherwise offer little advantage for diagnosis and monitoring of treatment.

■ Bisphosphonates, which inhibit osteoclast-mediated bone resorption, are first-line treatment for patients with Paget's disease. Markers of bone resorption and bone formation are expected to decrease after initiation of bisphosphonate therapy. After biochemical markers of bone turnover normalize, they can remain suppressed for long periods of time (i.e., years) depending on the extent of disease. Relapse is usually defined as an increase in biochemical markers of bone turnover or symptoms.[41]

23. A. Positive interference from human anti-animal antibodies.
Interference from human anti-animal antibodies can be eliminated because different immunochemical methods for measuring hCG use antibodies from different animal sources.
B. Normal intrauterine pregnancy.
Rationale: A normal intrauterine pregnancy can be eliminated because there was no change in serum hCG levels after a 7-day interval.
C. Ectopic pregnancy.
Rationale: Ectopic pregnancy can be eliminated because of the low level of serum hCG.
D. Synthesis and release of hCG from the pituitary gland.
Rationale: hCG levels increase with age. The decrease in ovarian production of estrogen and progesterone leads to an increase in GnRH synthesis. GnRH stimulates the release of pituitary hCG and could be the cause of the low levels of hCG seen in some perimenopausal and postmenopausal women.
E. Presence of a hydatidiform mole.
Rationale: A very high serum hCG level would be observed in a patient with a hydatidiform mole.

Major points of discussion
■ hCG was first identified in the pituitary gland in 1976. Pituitary hCG has the same amino acid structure as the intact hCG that is secreted during pregnancy. Pituitary hCG is produced at low levels during the menstrual cycle and is a sulfated variant of hCG.

■ hCG levels increase with increasing age. In perimenopausal and postmenopausal women, ovarian steroid synthesis decreases. As a result, the negative feedback control on GnRH decreases, and the GnRH pulse significantly increases. GnRH stimulates the release of pituitary hCG and could be the cause of the low levels of hCG seen in some perimenopausal and postmenopausal women.

- Pituitary hCG can be excluded in perimenopausal and postmenopausal women as the source of the low hCG level by treating the patient with estrogen-progesterone hormone replacement therapy. If the source of the hCG is the pituitary, then the hCG level will be suppressed.
- FSH levels can also be used to investigate the source of the hCG. FSH levels are suppressed during pregnancy and increased in perimenopausal and postmenopausal women. In perimenopausal women (41 to 55 years old), the FSH reference range is 45 IU/L or greater. In pregnancy, the FSH level is significantly lower. If a low hCG level is obtained in perimenopausal women, reflex FSH testing should be performed. The FSH of 130 IU/L in this patient suggests that the patient is not pregnant and that the pituitary gland is probably the source of the low hCG level.
- Human anti-animal antibodies (HAAAs) have a molecular mass of more than 120 kDa and are not excreted into the urine. Therefore, a positive urine hCG result, together with obtaining essentially the same serum hCG result using two different immunochemical methods with a different set of antibodies to measure hCG, suggests that HAAAs are not the cause of the low hCG level that was obtained in this patient.[11,48]

24. **A. The patient has primary hyperparathyroidism.**
Rationale: Intact PTH and whole PTH are both high. The ratio of the two is less than 0.8. Renal function is normal, and serum calcium is slightly elevated. Taken together, these results suggest that the patient has primary hyperparathyroidism.
B. The patient has hyperparathyroidism secondary to kidney disease.
Rationale: Renal function is normal in this patient.
C. The patient has a parathyroid carcinoma.
Rationale: A ratio of intact PTH to whole PTH of 0.8 would suggest a parathyroid carcinoma.
D. Intact PTH assays always give a higher result than the whole PTH assays.
Rationale: This is not always the case. Indeed, a ratio of intact PTH to whole PTH could be greater than 0.8 in cases of parathyroid carcinoma.
E. RIA methods are unreliable for measuring PTH levels.
Rationale: RIAs are approved by the U.S. Food and Drug Administration and are sufficiently reliable for patient care–related measurements.

Major points of discussion
- Intact PTH assays, also known as second-generation assays, measure both the 1-84 form of the PTH molecule as well as several truncated fragments. Whole PTH assays, also known as biointact PTH assays or third-generation assays, selectively measure the 1-84 form of the PTH molecule.
- It is assumed that the whole PTH assays would be more useful in chronic kidney disease because results are not influenced by cross-reacting truncated forms of PTH 1-84 that accumulate because of decreased renal excretion. This potential advantage remains the subject of debate.
- Some patients with a parathyroid carcinoma present with overproduction of nontruncated amino-terminal PTH, a post-transcriptionally modified form of PTH 1-84. This is usually detected by an elevated intact PTH/whole PTH

ratio. The exact ratio depends on the assays used, but for the Scantibodies assays, it is greater than 0.8.
- If left untreated, primary hyperparathyroidism might lead to hypercalcemia, which formerly was one of the first biochemical findings leading to a diagnosis of primary hyperparathyroidism. Presently, with PTH assays readily available, a first indication of this disorder can be the PTH level itself. In addition, whereas primary hyperparathyroidism was formerly seen in the presence of hypercalcemia, so-called normocalcemic primary hyperparathyroidism is now also observed.
- Typically, in the milder form of primary hyperparathyroidism, seen in most countries now, bone density by DXA and detailed analyses of iliac crest bone biopsies by histomorphometry and microcomputerized tomography show detrimental effects in cortical bone, whereas the trabecular site (lumbar spine by DXA) and the trabecular compartment (by bone biopsy) appear to be relatively well preserved. Despite these findings, the fracture risk at both vertebral and nonvertebral sites is increased in primary hyperparathyroidism.[6,8,50]

25. A. Serum samples were kept on ice during transport.
Rationale: Breaking the cold chain could lead to decreased levels of serum and plasma levels of intact PTH.
B. Vitamin D deficiency.
Rationale: High levels of vitamin D can suppress PTH levels. 25(OH)-vitamin D and 1,25(OH)-vitamin D levels were normal in this patient.
C. Circulating variant forms of PTH.
Rationale: Biologically active post-translationally modified forms of PTH and biologically active fragments of PTH that are not detected by intact PTH assays have been described.
D. Hypermagnesemia.
Rationale: Hypomagnesemia would be a possible explanation of the findings seen in this patient.
E. The hook effect.
Rationale: Although possible when an immunoradiometric assay is used to measure intact PTH, the hook effect is uncommonly seen when using ICMA.

Major points of discussion
- Assays for intact PTH do not detect all biologically active forms of PTH that may be present in the circulation. On occasion, biologically active variant forms of PTH circulate in patients with parathyroid adenomas. These patients can have clinical symptoms of hyperparathyroidism in the absence of elevated PTH levels as measured by intact PTH assays or second-generation PTH assays.
- Other potential reasons for normal-low intact PTH levels in the presence of hypercalcemia are listed below:
  1. Failure to keep the sample on ice during transport or breaking of the "cold chain"
  2. Coexistent sarcoidosis and/or vitamin D toxicity, hypomagnesemia
  3. The hook effect
  4. PTH–related protein (PTHrP) secretion by a parathyroid carcinoma
- Magnesium is necessary for the synthesis, secretion, and function of intact PTH.

- PTHrP can be secreted by various tumors, leading to the humoral hypercalcemia syndrome. PTHrP is also present in the circulation during lactation and fetal life.
- PTH is a heat-labile peptide. When PTH is measured in serum, the specimen should be kept on ice or frozen from the time of collection to measurement (cold chain), thereby preventing degradation of the peptide.
- The hook effect, or prozone effect, which can be seen with immunoassays, occurs when a false-negative or falsely low result is obtained in the presence of high levels of analyte. Excess analyte saturates antibody binding sites, preventing lattice or sandwich formation and loss of a measurable signal. The hook effect can be observed using various types of assays, and its occurrence is highly assay dependent.[3,31,44]

26. A. Primary hyperparathyroidism.
Rationale: The clinical findings, as well as the chemistry results (especially the hypocalcemia), indicate that this patient does not have primary hyperparathyroidism.
B. Secondary hyperparathyroidism.
Rationale: The clinical findings, as well as the chemistry results (such as the normal creatinine and the presence of hypocalcemia), suggest that this patient does not have secondary hyperparathyroidism.
C. Hypoparathyroidism.
Rationale: The clinical findings in this patient, as well as the chemistry results (e.g., elevated intact PTH, elevated markers of bone turnover), suggest that this patient does not have hypoparathyroidism.
D. Pseudohypoparathyroidism.
Rationale: The clinical findings in this patient (suggestive of Albright's hereditary osteodystrophy), combined with functional hypoparathyroidism (hypocalcemia and hyperphosphatemia) in the presence of high PTH levels and normal magnesium and vitamin D levels, are consistent with pseudohypoparathyroidism.
E. Pseudopseudohypoparathyroidism.
Rationale: The clinical findings in this patient (suggestive of Albright's hereditary osteodystrophy) could be consistent with pseudopseudohypoparathyroidism. However, because the clinical chemistry results are abnormal, this instead suggests that this patient has pseudohypoparathyroidism.

Major points of discussion
- Pseudohypoparathyroidism (PHP) is a rare endocrine disease characterized by resistance to the peripheral action of PTH, a key regulator of calcium homeostasis that mediates its action through a G-protein–coupled receptor. Several variants of the disease have been described and classified as PHP type 1a, PHP type 1b, PHP type 1c, and PHP type 2 based on associated phenotypes and pathogenesis. Alterations at the GNAS locus, the genomic localization of the *GNAS* gene (20q13.32), which encodes the α-subunit of the heterotrimeric G protein ($G_S\alpha$), are associated with PHP type 1.
- PHP should be considered in any patient with functional hypoparathyroidism (e.g., with hypocalcemia and hyperphosphatemia) and an elevated plasma concentration of PTH. Hypomagnesemia and vitamin D deficiency can also produce biochemical features of PTH resistance in some patients and should be investigated.

- PPHP (or pseudopseudohypoparathyroidism) may be suspected in patients who present with somatic features of Albright hereditary osteodystrophy. These include short stature, round facies, brachydactyly of hands and/or feet, mild mental retardation, subcutaneous ossification, and obesity.
- Modifications of the Ellsworth-Howard (PTH infusion) test facilitate the diagnosis of PHP. This test consists of measuring creatinine and phosphorus in serum samples and cAMP, phosphorus, and creatinine in urine samples collected during several hours after administration of PTH (or PTH 1-34). Patients with hypoparathyroidism show a robust increase in urinary excretion of both cAMP and phosphorus. Patients with PHP type 1 fail to show an appropriate increase of both cAMP and phosphorus, whereas subjects with the less-common PHP type 2 show a normal increase of cAMP, but not of phosphorus.
- $G_S\alpha$ mediates the stimulation of adenylate cyclase regulated by various peptide hormones (e.g., PTH, TSH, gonadotropins, ACTH, GnRH, antidiuretic hormone (ADH), glucagon, and calcitonin). Patients with PTH and TSH resistance, along with Albright hereditary osteodystrophy, are clinically diagnosed with PHP type 1a.
- Genotyping can be useful in the diagnosis of PHP.[15,19,44]

27. A. Secondary hyperparathyroidism.
Rationale: Secondary hyperparathyroidism is the excessive secretion of PTH in response to hypocalcemia caused by chronic renal failure. 1,25(OH)-vitamin D is low in this setting because of decreased 1-α-hydroxylase activity.
B. Hypoparathyroidism.
Rationale: 1,25(OH)-vitamin D is low in this setting because of decreased 1-α-hydroxylase activity.
C. Postmenopausal osteoporosis.
Rationale: 1,25(OH)-vitamin D is not specifically elevated in this setting.
D. Sarcoidosis.
Rationale: Sarcoidosis is accompanied by increased 1-α-hydroxylase activity and increased serum concentrations of 1,25(OH)-vitamin D.
E. Hypercalcemia of malignancy.
Rationale: In hypercalcemia of malignancy, 1,25(OH)-vitamin D levels are expected to be low.

Major points of discussion
- Decreased serum levels of 1,25(OH)-vitamin D are seen in renal failure, hyperphosphatemia, hypomagnesemia, hypoparathyroidism, PHP, vitamin D–dependent rickets (type I), and hypercalcemia of malignancy.
- Increased levels of 1,25(OH)-vitamin D are seen in granulomatous diseases (e.g., sarcoidosis), primary hyperparathyroidism, lymphoma, 1,25(OH)-vitamin D intoxication, and vitamin D–dependent rickets (type II).
- 25(OH)-vitamin D has a relatively long half-life (i.e., 2 weeks), is bound tightly to vitamin D–binding protein (VDBP), and is used to determine a patient's vitamin D status. Renal production of 1,25(OH)-vitamin D is normally tightly regulated by PTH, serum calcium and phosphate levels, and fibroblast growth factor 23 (FGF23). 1,25(OH)-vitamin D has a relatively short half-life (0.5 day) and is bound less tightly to VDBP than 25(OH)-vitamin D. 1,25(OH)-vitamin D measurements are

indicated only in certain cases, such as those mentioned above.

■ 1,25(OH)-vitamin D can be measured in serum and plasma by RIA, ELISA, and LC-MS/MS.

■ The mechanism producing elevated 1,25(OH)-vitamin D levels in sarcoidosis is increased conversion of 25(OH)-vitamin D to 1,25(OH)-vitamin D by extrarenal 1-α-hydroxylase, which is expressed in activated macrophages.[1,23,61]

28. A. Retinol.
Rationale: Vitamin A deficiency, which is commonly seen after bariatric surgery because of malabsorption, leads to impaired dark adaption.
B. 25(OH)-vitamin D.
Rationale: Low 25(OH)-vitamin D levels caused by malabsorption after bariatric surgery could explain the mild hyperparathyroidism and hypercalcemia but do not explain his impaired night vision.
C. 1,25(OH)-vitamin D.
Rationale: Low 1,25(OH)-vitamin D levels would lead to decreased calcium absorption and bone turnover and increased PTH levels, but they have not been related to impaired night vision.
D. Total protein.
Rationale: Low total protein may be observed after bariatric surgery, but this does not directly explain his impaired vision.
E. Albumin.
Rationale: Low albumin may be observed after bariatric surgery, but this does not directly explain his impaired vision.

Major points of discussion
■ Vitamin A is the nutritional term for the group of compounds with a 20-carbon structure containing a methyl-substituted cyclohexenyl ring and an isoprenoid side chain with a hydroxyl group (retinol), an aldehyde group (retinal), a carboxylic group (retinoic acid), or an ester group (retinyl ester) at the terminal C15.
■ Vitamin A plays a critical role in immune function, bone growth, maintenance of epithelial linings, reproduction, and vision, especially dark adaptation.
■ The earliest symptoms of vitamin A deficiency involve impaired dark adaptation, recognized simply as night blindness. Eye disorders caused by vitamin A deficiency fall under the category of xerophthalmia. Bitot spots are dry, scaly patches on the conjunctiva that are usually foamy in appearance. They are specific for vitamin A deficiency and are areas of keratinized epithelial cells with mucosal and submucosal edema. Keratin admixed with corynebacteria accounts for the foamy appearance.
■ Vitamin A status can be assessed by measuring retinol in plasma by high-performance liquid chromatography with ultraviolet detection (HPLC-UV) or LC-MS/MS. However, this is not an ideal indicator of low vitamin A stores because values do not decline until liver stores become critically depleted (i.e., at <20 μg/g liver). Retinol

in plasma circulates as a 1:1:1 complex with retinol-binding protein and transthyretin; the reference range is 20 to 100 μg/dL.
■ Retinopathy after bariatric surgery can be related to vitamin A deficiency caused by decreased absorption of lipid-soluble vitamins. Treatment could include oral supplementation of lipid-soluble vitamins.[13,53]

29. A. An acute-phase reaction.
Rationale: An acute phase reaction leads to decreased plasma Zn levels.
B. The use of prednisone by the patient.
Rationale: Corticosteroids lower plasma Zn levels.
C. Obtaining a blood sample in the evening.
Rationale: Plasma Zn concentrations are negatively related to the time of blood sampling.
D. Measuring Zn in serum rather than plasma.
Rationale: Zn levels in serum can be higher than in plasma.
E. Recent food intake.
Rationale: Nonfasting Zn levels are lower than fasting levels.

Major points of discussion
■ The plasma or serum Zn concentration is widely used to assess Zn status. It can be measured using several methods, including flame AAS, inductively coupled plasma mass spectrometry, inductively coupled plasma atomic emission spectroscopy, and colorimetry.
■ Zn has multiple biochemical functions (e.g., there are more than 300 Zn-containing metalloenzymes). Therefore, the clinical presentation of Zn deficiency is highly variable. Signs and symptoms include depressed growth, increased incidence of infection, skin lesions, and alopecia. An autosomal recessive inborn error affecting Zn absorption is called acrodermatitis enteropathica.
■ Although measured in both serum and plasma, Zn is usually measured in plasma because of possible Zn contamination from erythrocytes, platelets, and leukocytes induced by clotting and centrifugation. Zn can also be measured in urine and hair.
■ The reference range for Zn in plasma is 80 to 120 μg/dL. Fasting morning samples lower than 70 μg/dL on several occasions require further investigation, whereas results lower than 30 μg/dL suggest deficiency.
■ Zn serum concentrations are influenced by gender, age, use of steroid-based medications including oral contraceptives, time of blood collection, and fasting status. Zn levels decrease during acute-phase reactions because of the redistribution of albumin (and, therefore, of protein-bound Zn) into interstitial spaces and an induction of hepatic metallothionein synthesis with subsequent sequestration of Zn. Therefore, Zn levels should be interpreted in conjunction with markers of an acute-phase reaction. Zn concentrations can also be elevated because of artifactual contamination from the blood collection tubes.[2,24]

References

1. Adams J, Hewinson M. Extrarenal expression of the 25-hydroxyvitamin D-1-hydroxylase. Arch Biochem Biophys 2012;523:95–102.

2. Arsenault JE, Wuehler SE, de Romana DL, et al. The time of day and the interval since previous meal are associated with plasma zinc concentrations and affect estimated risk of zinc deficiency in young children. Eur J Clin Nutr 2011;65:184–190.

3. Badhada SK, Cardenas M, Bhansali A, et al. Very low or undetectable intact parathyroid hormone levels in patients with surgically verified parathyroid adenomas. Clin Endocrinol 2008;69:382–385.

4. Bailey D, Veljkovic K, Yazpanpanah M, Adeli K. Analytical measurement and clinical relevance of vitamin D3 C3-epimer. Clin Biochem 2013;46:190–196.

5. Barnhart KT. Clinical practice. Ectopic pregnancy. N Engl J Med 2009;361:379–387.

6. Boudou P, Ibrahim F, Cormier C, et al. Third- or second-generation parathyroid hormone assays: a remaining debate in the diagnosis of hyperparathyroidism. J Clin Endocrinol Metab 2005;90:6370–6372.

7. Burtis C, Ashwood ER, Burns DE, editors: Tietz Textbook of Clinical Chemistry and Molecular Diagnostics, 4th ed. St. Louis: Elsevier, 2006, pp 1909–1912.

8. Caron P, Simonds WF, Maiza J-C, et al. Nontruncated amino-terminal parathyroid hormone overproduction in two patients with parathyroid carcinoma: a possible link to *HRTP2* gene inactivation. Clin Endocrinol 2011;74:694–698.

9. Christgau S, Bitsch-Jensen O, Hanover Bjarnason N, et al. Serum CrossLaps for monitoring the response in individuals undergoing antiresorptive therapy. Bone 2000;26:505–511.

10. Clowes JA, Hannon RA, Yap TS, et al. Effect of feeding on bone turnover markers and its impact on biological variability of measurements. Bone 2002;30:886–890.

11. Cole LA. Biological functions of HCG and HCG-related molecules. Reprod Biol Endocrinol 2010;8:1–14.

12. Coleman RE, Major P, Lipton A, et al. Predictive value of bone resorption and formation markers in cancer patients with bone metastases receiving the bisphosphonate zoledronic acid. J Clin Oncol 2005;23:4925–4935.

13. De Salvo G, Maguire JI, Lotery AJ. Vitamin A deficiency-related retinopathy after bariatric surgery. Greafes Arch Clin Exp Ophthalmol 2012;250:941–943.

14. de Vet A, Laven JSE, de Jong FH, et al. Antimullerian hormone serum levels: a putative marker for ovarian aging. Fertil Steril 2002;77:357–362.

15. Dekelbab BH, Aughton DJ, Levine MA. Pseudohypoparathyroidism type 1a and morbid obesity in infancy. Endocrine Pract 2009;15:249–253.

16. Dinour D, Beckerman P, Ganon L, et al. Loss-of-function mutations of CYP24A1, the vitamin D 24-hydroxylase gene, cause long-standing hypercalciuric nephrolithiasis and nephrocalcinosis. J Urol 2013;190:552–557.

17. Endres D. Investigation of hypercalcemia. Clin Biochem 2012;954–963.

18. Fallat ME, Siow Y, Marra M, et al. Mullerian-inhibiting substance in follicular fluid and serum: a comparison of patients with tubal factor infertility, polycystic ovary syndrome, and endometriosis. Fertil Steril 1997;67:962–965.

19. Fernandez-Rebollo E, Lecumbri B, Gaztambide S, et al. Endocrine profile and phenotype-(epi)genotype correlation in Spanish patients with pseudohypoparathyroidism. J Clin Endocrinol Metab 2013;98:E996–1006.

20. Frieze TW, Mong DP, Koops MK. "Hook effect" in prolactinomas: case report and review of literature. Endocr Pract 2002;8:296–303.

21. Garnero P, Borel O, Delmas PD. Evaluation of a fully automated serum assay for C-terminal cross-linking telopeptide of type I collagen in osteoporosis. Clin Chem 2001;47:694–702.

22. Hiort O. Clinical and molecular aspects of androgen insensitivity. Endocr Dev 2013;24:33–40.

23. Holick M. Vitamin D, deficiency. N Engl J Med 2007;357:266–281.

24. Holtz C, Peerson JM, Brown KH. Suggested lower cutoffs of serum zinc concentrations for assessing zinc status: reanalysis of the second National Health and Nutrition Examination Survey data (1976–1980). Am J Clin Nutr 2003;78:756–764.

25. Johansson M, Whiss PA. Weak relationship between ionized and total magnesium in serum of patients requiring magnesium status. Biol Trace Elem Res 2007;117:13–21.

26. Kaiser UB, Kuohung W. KiSS-1 and GPR54 as new players in gonadotropin regulation and puberty. Endocrine 2005;26:277–284.

27. Kamath C, Adlan MA, Premawardhana LD. The role of thyrotrophin receptor antibody assays in Graves' disease. J Thyroid Res 2012;2012:525936.

28. Knobel M, Medeiros-Neto G. An outline of inherited disorders of the thyroid hormone generating system. Thyroid 2003;13:771–801.

29. Lempiainen A, Stenman UH, Blomqvist C, et al. Free β-subunit of human chorionic gonadotropin in serum in a diagnostically sensitive marker of seminomatous testicular cancer. Clin Chem 2008;54:1840–1843.

30. Long W-Q, Ranchin V, Pautier P, et al. Detection of minimal levels of serum anti-Mullerian hormone during follow-up of patients with ovarian granulosa cell tumor by means of a highly sensitive enzyme-linked immunosorbent assay. J Clin Endocrinol Metab 2000;85:540–544.

31. McCauley LK, Martin TJ. Twenty-five years of PTHrP progress: from cancer hormone to multifunctional cytokine. J Bone Mineral Res 2012;27:121–1239.

32. McCudden CR, Sharpless JL, Grenache DG. Comparison of multiple methods for identification of hyperprolactinemia in the presence of macroprolactin. Clin Chim Acta 2010;411:155–160.

33. McLachlan SM, Rapoport B. Thyrotropin-blocking autoantibodies and thyroid-stimulating autoantibodies: potential mechanisms involved in the pendulum swinging from hypothyroidism to hyperthyroidism or vice versa. Thyroid 2012;23:14–24.

34. Mendonca BB, Domenice S, Arnhold IJ, et al. 46, XY disorders of sex development (DSD). Clin Endocrinol 2009;70:173–187.

35. Newell-Price J, Bertagna X, Grossman AB, et al. Cushing syndrome. Lancet 2006;367:1605–1617.

36. Nijhoff MF, Dekkers OM, Vleming LJ, et al. ACTH-producing pheochromocytoma: clinical considerations and concise review of the literature. Eur J Intern Med 2009;20:682–685.

37. Olateju TO, Vanderpump MPJ. Thyroid hormone resistance. Ann Clin Biochem 2006;43:431–440.

38. Pigny P, Merlen E, Robert Y, et al. Elevated serum level of anti-Mullerian hormone in patients with polycystic ovary syndrome: relationship to the ovarian follicle excess and to the follicular arrest. J Clin Endocrinol Metab 2003;88:5957–5962.

39. Practice Committee of the American Society for Reproductive Medicine. Current evaluation of amenorrhea. Fertil Steril 2008;90:S219–225.

40. Qvist P, Christgau S, Pedersen BJ, et al. Circadian variation in the serum concentration of C-terminal telopeptide of type I collagen (serum CTx): effects of gender, age, menopausal status, posture, daylight, serum cortisol, and fasting. Bone 2002;31:57–61.

41. Ralston SH. Clinical practice. Paget's disease of bone. N Engl J Med 2013;368:644–650.

42. Rehak NN, Cecco SA, Niemela JE, et al. Thiocyanate in smokers interferes with the Nova magnesium ion-selective electrode. Clin Chem 1997;43:1595–1600.

43. Reisch N, Flade L, Scherr M, et al. High prevalence of reduced fecundity in men with congenital adrenal hyperplasia. J Clin Endocrinol Metab 2009;94:1665–1670.

44. Rubin MR, Levine MA. Hypoparathyroidism and pseudohypo-parathyroidism. In: Rosen CJ, Compston JE, Lian JB, editors: Primer on the Metabolic Bone Diseases and Disorders of Mineral Metabolism, 7th ed. Washington, DC: American Society for Bone and Mineral Research, 2008, pp 354–361.

45. Rubin MR, Silverberg SJ, D'Amour P, et al. An N-terminal molecular form of parathyroid hormone (PTH) distinct from hPTH(1-84) is overproduced in parathyroid carcinoma. Clin Chem 2007;53:1470–1476.

46. Schirpenbach C, Seiler L, Maser-Gluth C, et al. Automated chemiluminescence-immunoassay for aldosterone during dynamic testing: comparison to radioimmunoassays with and without extraction steps. Clin Chem 2006;52:1749–1755.

47. Schultz KAP, Sencer SF, Messinger Y, et al. Pediatric ovarian tumors: a review of 67 cases. Pediatr Blood Cancer 2005;44:167–173.

48. Snyder JA, Shannon H, Parvin CA, et al. Diagnostic considerations in the measurement of human chorionic gonadotropin in aging women. Clin Chem 2005;51:1830–1835.

49. Stechman MJ, Loh NY, Thakker RV. Genetic causes of hypercalciuric nephrolithiasis. Pediatr Nephrol 2009;24:2321–2332.

50. Stein EM, Silva BC, Boutroy S, et al. Primary hyperparathyroidism is associated with abnormal cortical and trabecular microstructure and reduced bone stiffness in postmenopausal women. J Bone Mineral Res 2013;28:1029–1040.

51. Stowasser M, Ahmed AH, Pimenta E, et al. Factors affecting the aldosterone/renin ratio. Horm Metab Res 2012;44:170–176.

52. Stowasser M, Taylor PJ, Pimenta E, et al. Laboratory investigation of primary aldosteronism. Clin Biochem Rev 2010;31:39–56.

53. Stroh C, Weiher C, Hohman U, et al. Vitamin A deficiency (VAD) after a duodenal switch procedure: a case report. Obes Surg 2010;20:397–400.

54. Taurog A, Dorris ML, Doerge DR. Minocycline and the thyroid: antithyroid effects of the drug, and the role of thyroid peroxidase in minocycline-induced black pigmentation of the gland. Thyroid 1996;6:211–219.

55. Terpos E, Dimopoulos MA, Sezer O, et al. The use of biochemical markers of bone remodeling in multiple myeloma: a report of the international myeloma working group. Leukemia 2010;24:1700–1712.

56. Terzolo M, Ali A, Pia A, et al. Cyclic Cushing's syndrome due to ectopic ACTH secretion by an adrenal pheochromocytoma. J Endocrinol Invest 1994;17:869–874.

57. Thompson LD. Diffuse hyperplasia of the thyroid gland (Graves' disease). Ear Nose Throat J 2007;86:666–667.

58. Winter WE, Sokoll LJ, Jialal I. Handbook of Diagnostic Endocrinology. Washington, DC: AACC Press, 2008, pp 211–220.

59. Wood SJ, Brown JE. Skeletal metastasis in renal cell carcinoma: current and future management options. Cancer Treatment Rev 2012;38:284–291.

60. Wu AH, Whittemore AS, Kolonel L, et al. Serum androgens and sex hormone–binding globulins in relation to lifestyle factors in older African-American, white, and Asian men in the United States and Canada. Cancer Epidemiol Biomark Prev 1995;4:735–741.

61. Zhang JTW, Chan C, Kwun SY, et al. A case of severe 1,25-dihydroxyvitamin D-mediated hypercalcemia due to a granulomatous disorder. J Clin Endocrinol Metab 2012;97:2579–2583.

CHAPTER 5

CLINICAL CHEMISTRY:
Liver, Gastrointestinal, Pancreas, Biliary Tract

Anthony N. Sireci, Kalpana Deveraj, Jorge L. Sepulveda

QUESTIONS

1. A 3-day-old, ex 32-week, male infant is noted to have tarry black stools in his diaper on the third day of life. The clinical team is concerned about gastrointestinal bleeding, and an Apt-Downey test is ordered on a sample of the infant's stool. After addition of 1% sodium hydroxide, the stool extract remains pink. Which one of the following is the best interpretation of these results?
   A. Fetal hemoglobin is more resistant to denaturation by alkali, and the persistent pink color of the sample implies a maternal source of blood.
   B. Fetal hemoglobin is more resistant to denaturation by alkali, and the persistent pink color of the sample implies a fetal source of blood.
   C. Fetal hemoglobin is less resistant to denaturation by alkali, and the persistent pink color of the sample implies a maternal source of the blood.
   D. Fetal hemoglobin is less resistant to denaturation by alkali, and the persistent pink color of the sample implies a fetal source of the blood.
   E. Adult hemoglobin and fetal hemoglobin react equivalently under basic conditions, and the persistent pink color of the sample is inconclusive.

2. A 34-year-old woman presents to her primary care physician with weight loss and complaints of intermittent diarrhea and constipation. The physician's differential diagnosis includes celiac disease. Which one of the following tests is the most sensitive and specific serum biomarker for celiac disease?
   A. Anti-smooth muscle antibody (SMA).
   B. Anti-endomysial antibody.
   C. HLA-DQ2.
   D. Total immunoglobulin A (IgA) levels.
   E. Anti-thyroglobulin antibody.

3. A 54-year-old man recently underwent resection of an insulinoma located in the tail of the pancreas. At initial presentation, serum chromogranin A levels were 10 times the upper limit of the reference range at 2000 ng/mL, and the patient suffered from severe hypoglycemic episodes. After resection, chromogranin A levels dropped to within the reference range and have been normal since the surgical resection. On his 1-year postoperative visit, the patient's chromogranin A level was found to have increased to 450 ng/mL, which is twice the upper limit of the reference range and much higher than the patient's recent baseline. The patient denied any symptoms of tumor recurrence (e.g., hypoglycemia, flushing, or diarrhea). He admits to frequent dyspepsia, which he has been treating with an over-the-counter medication. However, he cannot recall the name of the medication. Which one of the following is the best next step in the management of this patient?
   A. Repeat the chromogranin A measurement after 4 to 5 half-lives have passed since discontinuing the over-the-counter medication.
   B. Send the patient for a positron emission tomography (PET) scan and magnetic resonance imaging (MRI) of the abdomen.
   C. Send the patient immediately to the operating room for an additional pancreatic resection.
   D. Do nothing; this change is within the normal, intraindividual variation of chromogranin A.
   E. Order a serum CA 19-9 level.

4. Serum levels of pepsinogen type I below the reference range in healthy adults are used in screening at-risk populations for which one of the following diseases?
   A. Chronic atrophic gastritis.
   B. Gastric cancer.
   C. Celiac disease.
   D. Gastroesophageal reflux disease.
   E. Peptic ulcer disease.

5a. A 23-year-old man of Ashkenazi Jewish descent presents to his primary care physician with a 4- to 5-month history of abdominal pain, intermittent diarrhea, and constipation. He reports a 5-pound unintentional weight loss. He denies any travel history. His physician submits blood samples for a perinuclear antineutrophil cytoplasmic antibody screen (P-ANCA) and a test for anti–Saccharomyces cerevisiae antibody (ASCA). Only the ASCA test result was positive. Which one of the following disorders is most consistent with this serologic pattern?
   A. Irritable bowel syndrome.
   B. Ulcerative colitis.
   C. Crohn's disease.
   D. Celiac disease.
   E. Sarcoid.

5b. By routine testing, this patient is also found to be anemic (hemoglobin =11 g/dL; reference range, 13.3 to 16.2 g/dL) with a mean corpuscular volume (MCV) of 103 fL (reference range, 80 to 100 fL). Ileal involvement by the patient's underlying disease is thought to be the cause. To confirm this hypothesis, a two-step Schilling test is performed. After oral loading with radiolabeled vitamin B_{12}, the patient receives an intravenous bolus of unlabeled vitamin B_{12}. Urinary measurement of radiolabeled B_{12} is performed. The same test is then repeated with the addition of oral intrinsic factor (IF). If the patient's pathology involves impaired ileal absorption of vitamin B_{12}, the results of this two-part Schilling test would show which one of the following patterns?

  A. Less than 5% of the radiolabeled vitamin B_{12} in the urine after both steps 1 and 2.

  B. Less than 5% of the radiolabeled vitamin B_{12} in the urine after step 1 and an increase in urinary radiolabeled vitamin B_{12} after step 2.

  C. 15% urinary radiolabeled vitamin B_{12} after step 1 and 15% urinary radiolabeled vitamin B_{12} after step 2.

  D. 15% urinary radiolabeled vitamin B_{12} after step 1 and a decrease to less than 5% radiolabeled vitamin B_{12} after step 2.

  E. The Schilling test is not the appropriate test.

6. A patient with exocrine pancreas insufficiency is tested for enteric causes of malabsorption using the D-xylose test. After an overnight fast, the patient is given a dose of oral D-xylose, and his urinary levels of this analyte are monitored. Which one of the following comorbidities would affect your interpretation of the D-xylose test results?

  A. Type 1 diabetes.

  B. Crohn's disease.

  C. Cystic fibrosis.

  D. Chronic renal insufficiency.

  E. Hyperthyroidism.

7. An 8-year-old girl with cystic fibrosis (i.e., a positive sweat test and homozygous for the cystic fibrosis transmembrane regulator gene *(CFTR)* ΔF508 mutation) is transferring her care to a new pediatrician. The patient had a diagnosis of pancreatic insufficiency for which she has been treated with oral pancreatic enzyme replacement therapy. The physician wants to confirm the diagnosis of pancreatic insufficiency and collects a stool sample for fecal elastase testing. The stool is watery and poorly formed. Which one of the following reasons would cause the laboratory to reject this specimen?

  A. Fecal elastase measurements should be performed only on adult patient samples because pediatric reference ranges do not exist.

  B. Fecal elastase measurements should not be performed on patients who are receiving pancreatic replacement therapy.

  C. Fecal elastase measurements should be performed only on well-formed stools.

  D. Fecal elastase measurement is not indicated for the diagnosis of pancreatic insufficiency.

  E. Fecal trypsin, not fecal elastase, measurement should be performed.

8. A 58-year-old man from India presents to his primary care physician with a complaint of postprandial dyspepsia. His symptoms began 6 months ago after a trip to India. The patient has been self-medicating with bismuth subsalicylate, usually needed immediately after meals. The primary care physician is highly suspicious for *Helicobacter pylori* infection and orders serologic testing, which comes back positive. However, a follow-up urea breath test is negative. Endoscopy with biopsy demonstrates the presence of *H. pylori.* Which one of the following is the most likely cause of these discrepant results?

  A. Urease breath testing for *H. pylori* is notoriously inaccurate and should not be used in clinical testing protocols.

  B. The endoscopic biopsy was contaminated with *H. pylori.*

  C. The patient's use of bismuth subsalicylate caused a false-negative test result.

  D. The patient was infected with a non–urease-producing strain of *H. pylori.*

  E. Urease breath testing is not useful in patients of Indian descent.

9. A patient suspected of having lactose intolerance is given a lactose tolerance test. After an overnight fast, the patient is given a 50-g oral bolus of lactose in 400 mL of water. Serum glucose levels are monitored 30, 60, and 120 minutes after ingestion. In a patient with severe lactase deficiency, which one of the following changes in serum glucose would you expect to see?

  A. A large spike in glucose concentrations because the lactose is absorbed and broken down into its constituent monosaccharides in the serum by serum lactase.

  B. A small increase in serum glucose caused by residual lactase activity, but most lactose will not by hydrolyzed by lactase in the intestinal brush border.

  C. A small increase in serum glucose because of cross-reactivity between lactose and glucose.

  D. A large decrease in serum glucose concentrations because most assays are inhibited by lactose.

  E. A small decrease in serum glucose concentrations because most assays are inhibited by lactose.

10. A 65-year-old man presents to a gastroenterologist with 2 weeks of abdominal cramping and foul-smelling diarrhea that floats. He also reports a recent 10-pound unintentional weight loss after a trip in the local mountains. The doctor characterizes his diarrhea as steatorrhea based on history alone but would like to characterize the cause of the fat malabsorption as either pancreatic (pancreatic insufficiency perhaps secondary to malignancy) or enteric (e.g., ileal disease or infection). He performs a two-step C^{14}-glycerol trioleate breath test and measures the C^{14} content of expired CO_2 as a percentage of total CO_2, with and without oral pancreatic enzyme replacement. Which one of the following testing patterns would be seen if the patient's malabsorption is a result of pancreatic insufficiency?

  A. A low percentage of C^{14} on the first round of testing and a relative increase in C^{14} percentage when C^{14} is coadministered with pancreatic enzymes.

  B. A low percentage of C^{14} on the first round of testing without any change in C^{14} percentage after administration of pancreatic enzymes.

  C. A high percentage of C^{14} on the first round of testing without any change in C^{14} percentage after administration of pancreatic enzymes.

  D. A high percentage of C^{14} on the first round of testing with a decrease in C^{14} percentage after administration of pancreatic enzymes.

  E. A low percentage of C^{14} on the first round of testing with a decrease in C^{14} percentage after administration of pancreatic enzymes.

11a. A 31-year-old African American man presents to his primary care physician with a 3-month history of bloating and diarrhea. The symptoms occur only after certain meals, but he cannot pinpoint any additional specific triggers. A stool sample is collected and sent for multiple studies, including an examination for ova and parasites, stool osmolality, and stool pH.

    Which one of the following would be a classic finding on stool osmolality and pH studies in a patient with lactase deficiency?

A. A stool osmotic gap of less than 50 mOsm/kg (low) and pH less than 5.5.

B. A stool osmotic gap of more than 125 mOsm/kg (high) and pH greater than 5.5.

C. A stool osmotic gap of 80 mOsm/kg (normal) and pH less than 5.5.

D. A stool osmotic gap of more than 125 mOsm/kg (high) and pH of 7.

E. The stool osmotic gap is not a useful assay to discriminate between secretory and osmotic diarrhea.

11b. The patient later divulges that he had taken some antibiotics he had saved from a previous sinus infection. He thought it might help treat his diarrhea. Which one of the following stool studies ordered is most affected by coadministration of antibiotics?

A. Stool water sodium level.

B. Stool water potassium level.

C. Stool pH.

D. Stool osmotic gap.

E. Stool water chloride level.

12. A 64-year-old woman presents with the chief complaint of dyspepsia. She experiences burning discomfort after most meals. She denies the use of nonsteroidal antiinflammatory drugs or aspirin, and she has never used an antacid or a proton pump inhibitor (PPI). She has no personal or family history of pancreatic lesions, parathyroid adenoma, or pituitary adenoma. Her last meal, right before her appointment, precipitated the same symptoms. A serum gastrin level is ordered to rule out Zollinger-Ellison syndrome and is reported as 300 ng/L (reference range, <100 ng/L). Which one of the following is the best interpretation of this test result?

A. Gastrin-secreting tumor secondary to Zollinger-Ellison syndrome.

B. Falsely elevated result caused by prolonged storage at room temperature before testing.

C. Atrophic gastritis.

D. Normally elevated postprandial serum gastrin levels.

E. Serum gastrin is not the appropriate biomarker for Zollinger-Ellison syndrome.

13. A patient with stage 4 cirrhosis, decreased synthetic function (low total protein and albumin; coagulopathy), and hepatic encephalopathy is found to have a serum sodium level of 124 mEq/L (reference range, 135 to 145 mEq/L). Which one of the following is the most likely cause of the patient's hyponatremia?

A. Activation of the renin-aldosterone system.

B. Overhydration.

C. Assay interference by elevated bilirubin.

D. Nutritional imbalance.

E. Normal variation in serum sodium.

14a. A 56-year-old woman presents with severe abdominal pain that radiates to her back. She vomited once. The symptoms began approximately 48 hours ago; she has had minimal oral intake since then. Her physical examination shows dry mucous membranes, normal bowel sounds, mild abdominal guarding, but no rebound tenderness or tympany. Her past medical history includes hypertension; hypercholesterolemia, which is well controlled with a statin; and gallstones treated electively by cholecystectomy several years ago. The patient does not have a history of weight loss or alcohol abuse. She is sent by her primary care physician to the local emergency department for a computed tomography (CT) scan of the abdomen for suspected acute pancreatitis. The CT scan findings are consistent with acute pancreatitis, with possible necrosis, and no masses are observed. Laboratory testing shows a white blood cell count of 19.2×10^9/L (reference range, 4.5 to 11.0×10^9/L), bicarbonate 12 mmol/L (reference range, 21 to 28 mmol/L), blood urea nitrogen 41 mg/dL (reference range, 10 to 20 mg/dL), calcium 7.2 mg/dL (reference range, 9.0 to 10.5 mg/dL), glucose 276 mg/dL (reference range, 75 to 115 mg/dL), aspartate aminotransferase (AST) 310 U/L (reference range, 0 to 35 U/L), alanine aminotransferase (ALT) 280 U/L (reference range, 0 to 35 U/L), and lactate dehydrogenase (LDH) 400 U/L (reference range, 100 to 190 U/L). Pancreatic enzyme levels are as follows: amylase 172 U/L (reference range, 60 to 180 U/L) and lipase 165 U/L (reference range, 0 to 150 U/L). Cholesterol and triglyceride levels were within normal limits. The specimen was drawn into a lavender-top tube and stored at room temperature for 4 hours before analysis. Which one of the following reasons best explains the normal serum amylase despite a clear clinical diagnosis of acute pancreatitis?

A. Acute or chronic alcohol abuse.

B. Interference by statins.

C. Collection of the patient's blood sample in heparin anticoagulant.

D. Collection of the patient's blood sample in K_2-EDTA.

E. Storage of the sample at room temperature for 4 hours.

14b. If the physician wanted to be certain that the patient did not have alcohol-induced pancreatitis, which one of the following tests would be the best to use?

A. Serum amylase.

B. Lipase/amylase ratio greater than 3.

C. Carbohydrate-deficient transferrin.

D. Total and direct bilirubin.

E. Trypsinogen-1.

15. A 21-year-old man is diagnosed with celiac sprue based on a small intestinal biopsy and positive serologic testing for serum anti-endomysial immunoglobulin G (IgG) antibodies. His physician prescribes a gluten-free diet. At a follow-up appointment, the patient states that he tries to follow the diet but is uncertain whether he is always choosing gluten-free products. In addition to providing additional nutrition education, which one of the following is the best next diagnostic step to determine diet adherence and treatment efficacy?

A. Perform a repeat small intestinal biopsy.

B. Measure serum anti-endomysial IgA antibodies.

C. Measure serum anti-endomysial IgG antibodies.

D. Measure fecal fat and fecal leukocytes.

E. Measure serum anti-gliadin IgG antibodies.

16a. A 4-year-old white boy of Scandinavian descent is referred to a children's hospital for a history of multiple upper respiratory tract infections. He was delivered by spontaneous vaginal delivery, notable only for meconium. The patient has had difficulty feeding since birth, and his growth and weight have been below the 20th percentile for age. Currently, the patient has swelling of the face and lower extremities and frothy urine. The referring outside hospital performed a chloride sweat test, which was 20 mmol/L (reference range, 4 to 60 mmol/L). They also reported a creatinine of 1.8 mg/dL (reference range, <1.5 mg/dL) and an albumin of 3.0 mg/dL (reference range, 3.5 to 5.5 mg/dL). Despite the negative chloride sweat test, the pediatrician at the children's hospital wants to rule out cystic fibrosis by genetic testing. Which one of the following factors could best explain a false-negative sweat chloride test result in this patient?
  A. Focal segmental glomerulosclerosis.
  B. Malnutrition.
  C. Minimal change disease.
  D. Glucose-6-phosphate dehydrogenase (G6PD) deficiency.
  E. Previous fludrocortisone administration.

16b. The physician recommends molecular testing for cystic fibrosis for this child. The patient's mother is well educated about cystic fibrosis and questions the relevance of this test because of its high cost. She is already certain that her child has cystic fibrosis and believes that a great uncle probably had the disease based on his symptoms. She asks if the test is an effective screening tool for cystic fibrosis, especially because her child is not of Ashkenazi Jewish descent. Which one of the following is the correct information that the physician could provide to the patient's family about the sensitivity of molecular testing for cystic fibrosis?
  A. The sensitivity is 80% even in African Americans.
  B. The sensitivity is 75% to 90% in non-Ashkenazi white North Americans.
  C. The sensitivity is below 50% in non-Ashkenazi white North Americans.
  D. The chance that one of the mutations in a 25-allele–screening panel is a deletion of the codon for phenylalanine 508 (Phe-508) in *CFTR* is 70%.
  E. Molecular testing for cystic fibrosis is a better screening strategy than the sweat chloride test.

17. A 53-year-old man has a history of multiple admissions for abdominal pain, nausea, vomiting, and dehydration, and one episode of metabolic acidosis with severe hypoxia. Acute pancreatitis was diagnosed at each admission. The patient says that he drinks a maximum of two 12-ounce beers per day, but his family relates that it is much more, which the patient is afraid to admit. The medical team is concerned about chronic pancreatitis and requests endoscopic retrograde cholangiopancreatography (ERCP). They contact the laboratory director about available laboratory tests that would support ERCP findings of chronic pancreatitis. Which one of the following combinations of ERCP results and fecal elastase-1 test results would best support the diagnosis?
  A. Fecal elastase-1 of less than 100 μg pancreatic elastase/gram of stool and an abnormal ERCP.
  B. Fecal elastase-1 of more than 200 μg pancreatic elastase/gram of stool and a normal ERCP.
  C. Fecal elastase-1 between 100 and 200 μg pancreatic elastase/gram of stool and normal ERCP.

  D. Fecal elastase-1 of less than 100 μg pancreatic elastase/gram of stool and normal ERCP.
  E. Fecal elastase-1 of greater than 200 μg pancreatic elastase/gram of stool and an abnormal ERCP.

18a. A patient is suspected of having a gastrin-secreting tumor. The physician drew the blood sample 2 days ago and stored it at 4°C. Now the physician calls to ask the laboratory where to deliver the specimen and whether overnight storage will affect the result. Which one of the following answers is the best response?
  A. Gastrin levels will remain unchanged, but the sample should be analyzed immediately.
  B. Gastrin levels remain at 95% of their physiologic levels, and the sample is stable for another 5 days.
  C. Gastrin levels will be decreased by about 50%, and the test results will be inaccurate.
  D. Gastrin levels will be decreased by about 95%, and the test results will be inaccurate.
  E. Gastrin levels will be decreased, but the sample should be analyzed immediately for accurate results.

18b. In this case, the physician says that the specimen was collected within 5 hours of the patient's last meal. She asks the laboratory if this will affect the result. Which one of the following is the best response?
  A. No, all gastrin isoform levels are unaffected by meals.
  B. No, G17 and G34 gastrin isoform levels, but not the G14 isoform level, are unaffected by meals.
  C. Yes, the patient must fast for at least 24 hours before specimen collection.
  D. Yes, the patient must fast for 8 hours before specimen collection.
  E. No, high-molecular-weight gastrin isoform levels are the most stable and are unaffected by meals.

19. A 44-year-old man visits his primary care physician complaining of several weeks of diarrhea and upper abdominal discomfort. His stools are slightly loose, larger than normal, and sometimes bloody, typically with dark blood. The patient, who is overweight (body mass index [BMI] = 29 kg/m²), has been trying to lose weight and began running at least 5 miles most days of the week. He now watches his diet closely, eating lean protein only once per week, but has had difficulty decreasing his caffeine intake, ingesting 3 to 5 cups of coffee per day. His medications include a multivitamin, vitamin C, and ibuprofen (at least 800 mg) daily for running-related injuries. A family history includes an uncle with polyps and a grandfather who died from complications of colon cancer. The physician thinks that the diarrhea is stress related but is concerned about the family history. Guaiac-smear tests on three consecutive stools are performed. Fecal material is spotted onto guaiac-smear slides, which the physician asks the nurse to read while he sees more patients. The nurse accidentally forgets and reads the slides the next day. Each test was positive for fecal occult blood. A colonoscopy is performed and shows no abnormalities. Hemorrhoids are not seen. The pathology of random biopsies showed unremarkable mucosa. The patient's abdominal discomfort worsens, particularly with meals. His complete blood cell count shows no change in hemoglobin. The guaiac-smear test is repeated, the same as previously, and with the same result. Which one of the following reasons best explains the positive guaiac-smear test result?

A. Failure to rehydrate guaiac-smear slides.
B. Ingestion of chicken.
C. Ingestion of large amounts of vitamin C.
D. Ibuprofen-induced gastroesophageal reflux disease.
E. Lack of red meat ingestion.

20. A 55-year-old man with a past medical history of hypertension, hyperlipidemia, and a benign salivary gland tumor resected 10 years previously is seen by his primary care physician for his annual examination. His only complaint is minor abdominal discomfort unrelated to eating. There is no nausea, vomiting, loss of appetite, weight loss, or change in bowel habits. His family medical history is remarkable for his father having pancreatic cancer. He does not smoke and only drinks alcohol once a month. Medications include simvastatin and aspirin daily. His physician orders several laboratory tests. Results for the complete blood cell count, basic metabolic panel, lipid studies, and liver function tests (LFTs) are within normal limits. Amylase is elevated at 275 U/L (reference range, 60 to 180 U/L), and lipase is within normal limits (reference range, 0 to 150 U/L). Urine amylase is measured and is below the reference range. CT imaging of the abdomen is performed and shows no pancreatic lesions. Type 1 macroamylasemia is suspected. Which one of the following laboratory tests would confirm type 1 macroamylasia?
    A. Amylase clearance/creatinine clearance ratio (C_{am}/C_{Cr}).
    B. Trypsinogen 2.
    C. Lipase/amylase ratio.
    D. Urine trypsinogen activation peptide.
    E. Carbohydrate-deficient transferrin.

21. A gastroenterologist sees a 53-year-old woman with persistent diarrhea. The complete blood cell count, chem-20 (serum sodium, potassium, carbon dioxide, chloride, blood urea nitrogen, creatinine, glucose, AST, ALT, total protein, albumin, total and direct bilirubin, calcium, phosphorus, γ-glutamyl transpeptidase, alkaline phosphatase, total cholesterol, uric acid, LDH), and abdominal radiograph are unremarkable. Colonoscopy findings are consistent with laxative abuse. The patient reveals that she uses a magnesium laxative because of bouts of constipation. Which one of the following sets of laboratory test results best supports this diagnosis?
    A. Stool sodium of 60 mOsm/kg, potassium of 80 mOsm/kg, and osmolality of 290 mOsm/kg.
    B. Stool sodium of 10 mOsm/kg, potassium of 20 mOsm/kg, and osmolality of 290 mOsm/kg.
    C. Elevated serum gastrin levels.
    D. More than 5 g of stool lipids over 24 hours.
    E. Presence of fecal leukocytes and blood.

22. A 63-year-old woman returns to her physician because of continued gnawing epigastric pain. She previously was treated with a PPI and antibiotics for suspected peptic ulcer disease. She discontinued the antibiotics after half the course because the pain did not improve. She is now experiencing too much discomfort and returned for further workup. A nonradioactive hydrogen breath test is performed and is negative. Which one of the following is the best next step in confirming this patient's diagnosis?
    A. Continue the PPI treatment and repeat the breath test after completing antibiotic therapy.
    B. Repeat the hydrogen breath test.
    C. Perform endoscopy and biopsy of the esophagus and stomach.

D. Perform a urease test on a stomach and esophageal biopsy.
E. Culture the stomach or esophageal biopsy tissue at 25°C.

23. A physician wants to confirm a diagnosis of ulcerative colitis. Which one of the following sets of results would provide the best evidence for the diagnosis of ulcerative colitis and would effectively exclude Crohn's disease?
    A. Positive serum P-ANCA and negative serum ASCA.
    B. Negative serum P-ANCA and positive serum ASCA.
    C. Negative serum perinuclear P-ANCA and negative serum ASCA.
    D. Colon and small intestinal biopsy showing discontinuous presence of granulomas, crypt abscesses, and transmural inflammation.
    E. Low levels of serum vitamin B_{12}.

24. A 47-year-old white male farmworker presents to his physician with joint pain and a 10-pound weight loss over several years. Further questioning reveals that he has had diarrhea many days of the week for several years. The patient is also HIV positive, but his disease is well controlled with highly active antiretroviral therapy (HAART). A small intestinal biopsy reveals periodic acid-Schiff (PAS)-positive, diastase-resistant, lipid-laden macrophages in the lamina propria. Which one of the following is the best next step in this patient's management?
    A. Request microbial culture of the small intestinal tissue.
    B. Discontinue abacavir therapy for HIV.
    C. Order a polymerase chain reaction (PCR) test of small intestinal tissue.
    D. Initiate treatment with metronidazole.
    E. Measure serum anti-endomysial immunoglobulin A antibodies.

25. A 46-year-old woman with a past medical history of hypertension, Paget's disease, and alcoholism presents with abdominal and back pain. Diagnostic radiology shows features consistent with Paget's disease and possible gallstones. Results of routine laboratory evaluation include elevated alkaline phosphatase (ALP) and gamma-glutamyl transferase (GGT). Based on the above information, which one of the following statements is most correct?
    A. The patient most likely does not have alcoholic liver disease if the ALT and AST levels are normal.
    B. The patient's 5′-nucleotidase activity would add no additional diagnostic information.
    C. The patient's ALP would show at least partial heat lability on heat fractionation.
    D. The patient has an elevated Regan isoenzyme.
    E. The patient is expected to have an increased indirect bilirubin.

26. A patient with stage 4 cirrhosis, decreased synthetic function (low total protein, albumin, and coagulopathy) and hepatic encephalopathy is found to have a serum sodium level of 124 mEq/L (reference range, 135 to 145 mEq/L). Which one of the following is the most likely etiology for the patient's hyponatremia?
    A. Activation of the renin-aldosterone system.
    B. Overhydration.
    C. Assay interference by elevated bilirubin.
    D. Nutritional imbalance.
    E. Normal variation in serum sodium.

27. Which one of the following best describes the pathophysiology of Dubin-Johnson syndrome?
    A. Autoimmune hepatitis.
    B. Bile duct obstruction.
    C. Cirrhosis.
    D. Defective organic anion transporter.
    E. Acute viral hepatitis.

28a. A 59-year-old man with a history of pulmonary hypertension and alcohol abuse presents to the emergency department with progressively worsening shortness of breath, increasing abdominal girth, and jaundice. Examination is positive for elevated jugular venous distention, abdominal fluid wave, and 2+ pitting edema bilaterally. Scleral icterus is also noted. Neurologic examination is unremarkable. A hepatic function panel is ordered because of the scleral icterus and shows minimal elevations in AST, ALT, total bilirubin, and ALP. His total protein and albumin are normal. Which one of the following choices represents the most likely pathology explaining the abnormal LFT results?
    A. Cirrhosis.
    B. Hepatocellular carcinoma.
    C. Passive congestion.
    D. Fulminant hepatic failure.
    E. Normal variation in liver function.

28b. Which one of the following cardiac markers, if elevated in this patient, would support your conclusions about the patient's hepatic pathology diagnosed in the previous question?
    A. Myoglobin.
    B. Troponin T.
    C. Ischemia-modified albumin.
    D. Brain natriuretic peptide.
    E. LDH.

29. A 28-year-old man sought the care of his primary care physician when he developed tremors and became unsteady on his feet. On further questioning, his physician learned that the patient's friends had noted that his behavior had become increasingly erratic over the past year. Routine laboratory evaluation revealed mildly elevated AST and ALT, at which point the patient was referred to a hepatologist. The hepatologist's subsequent workup revealed serum and urine chemistry abnormalities as well as fibrosis and increased quantitative copper in liver biopsy material, resulting in the patient being treated with penicillamine. Which one of the following combinations of laboratory test results would be most consistent with diagnosis?
    A. Increased serum ceruloplasmin, increased serum total copper, decreased 24-hour urine copper.
    B. Decreased serum ceruloplasmin, increased serum total copper, increased 24-hour urine copper.
    C. Decreased serum ceruloplasmin, decreased serum total copper, decreased 24-hour urine copper.
    D. Decreased serum ceruloplasmin, decreased serum total copper, increased 24-hour urine copper.
    E. Increased serum ceruloplasmin, increased serum total copper, increased 24-hour urine copper.

30. A 35-year-old obese man presents to the emergency department with epigastric pain radiating to the back and lower abdomen, nausea, and vomiting. Physical examination shows abdominal tenderness, distention, guarding, unstable blood pressure averaging 135/80 mm Hg, tachycardia, and

temperature of 37.8°C. Which one of the following statements is true concerning the laboratory diagnosis of this patient with acute pancreatitis?
    A. A glucose level of 60 mg/dL indicates a poor prognosis.
    B. Amylase is released earlier than lipase and therefore is more sensitive for acute pancreatitis.
    C. Lipase is more specific than amylase for acute pancreatitis.
    D. Most commercially available amylase assays are immunoassays.
    E. Elastase assays are commonly used to rule out acute pancreatitis.

31. Which one of the following tests helps distinguish the origin of an elevated serum ALP level?
    A. AST.
    B. ALT.
    C. Anti–hepatitis B core antibody.
    D. GGT.
    E. Ammonia.

32. AST and ALT tests are often ordered together. Which one of the following statements is true?
    A. ALT is more abundant in the liver than AST.
    B. ALT is more specific than AST for liver disease.
    C. The AST/ALT ratio is usually lower than 2 in severe alcoholic liver disease.
    D. The AST/ALT ratio is usually lower than 2 during the acute phase of viral hepatitis.
    E. AST half-life in plasma is significantly longer than that of ALT.

33. A 54-year-old male heavy smoker presented to the oncology clinic for follow-up 4 months after surgical resection of a stage III, well-differentiated adenocarcinoma of the ascending colon. After surgery, the patient was treated with adjuvant chemotherapy, including 5-fluorouracil, leucovorin, and oxaliplatin for 3 months. Preoperative plasma levels of carcinoembryonic antigen (CEA) were 5.5 ng/mL (reference range, <5.0 ng/mL) and 3 months after initiation of chemotherapy, the levels of CEA were 9.6 ng/mL. Which one of the following statements best describes the interpretation of this test?
    A. Preoperative elevation of CEA indicates a poor prognosis.
    B. Increased CEA after the procedure is highly suggestive of treatment failure.
    C. An early increase of more than 15% in CEA levels during chemotherapy indicates a better prognosis.
    D. CEA has good accuracy for screening of early-stage (Dukes A) colon cancer.
    E. Significant CEA elevations (>10 ng/mL) are specific for colon cancer.

34a. Many laboratories use the diazo method for measuring bilirubin. Which one of the following is the end product that is measured when using this technique?
    A. Unconjugated bilirubin.
    B. Azobilirubin.
    C. Nicotinamide adenine dinucleotide phosphate (NADP).
    D. Nicotinamide adenine dinucleotide (NAD).
    E. Uridine diphosphate (UDP) glucuronyltransferase.

34b. The addition of accelerants such as caffeine to the diazo method for bilirubin testing facilitates the measurement of which one of the following compounds?
    A. UDP glucuronyltransferase.
    B. Albumin.

C. Unconjugated bilirubin only.
D. Conjugated bilirubin only.
E. Total bilirubin.

35. A 65-year-old man with colon cancer is hospitalized with a diagnosis of sepsis caused by *Clostridium perfringens*. The collection of a blood sample was difficult because of poor vascular access. On centrifugation, a sample of serum appeared hemolyzed. Which one of the following tests would be least likely to be affected by in vitro hemolysis and therefore more likely to help in the diagnosis of intravascular hemolysis?
A. Plasma hemoglobin levels.
B. Plasma potassium levels.
C. Plasma AST levels.
D. Plasma LDH levels.
E. Plasma haptoglobin levels.

36. A patient has a plasma total bilirubin of 2.3 mg/dL (reference range, 0.1 to 0.4), direct bilirubin of 0.2 mg/dL (reference range, ≤0.2), and a urinalysis showing negative bilirubin and strongly positive urobilinogen. Which one of the following disorders is the patient most likely to have?
A. Hemolytic anemia.
B. Gilbert syndrome.
C. Crigler-Najjar syndrome.
D. Liver cirrhosis.
E. Extrahepatic cholestasis.

37. A 55-year-old man with a long history (>10 years) of heavy drinking presents with weakness, ascites, splenomegaly, gynecomastia, and pitting edema (both feet). Which one of the following laboratory tests is most consistent with severe liver cirrhosis?
A. ALT of 10,500 U/L (reference range, <45) and AST of 8500 U/L (reference range, <35).
B. ALP of 650 U/L (reference range, 110 to 390) and GGT of 35 U/L (reference range, 7 to 49).
C. Albumin of 3.2 g/dL (reference range, 3.4 to 4.8) and total protein of 10.4 g/dL (reference range, 6.4 to 8.3).
D. Total bilirubin of 4.3 mg/dL (reference range, 0.2 to 1.1) and direct bilirubin of 3.2 mg/dL (reference range, <0.2).
E. Prothrombin time of 12.2 seconds (reference range, 12.0 to 14.3) and platelet count of 350×10^9/L (reference range, 150 to 400).

38. Which one of the following is the most sensitive and specific laboratory test for primary biliary cirrhosis?
A. Total bilirubin.
B. Anti-SMAs.
C. ALP.
D. Immunoglobulin M (IgM).
E. Antimitochondrial antibodies.

39. A patient was admitted with a 6-day history of jaundice, fever, malaise, anorexia, and lower back pain. Physical examination showed icterus, a temperature of 38.8°C, heart rate of 115 beats/min, and a blood pressure of 110/60 mm Hg. Laboratory values on admission showed albumin of 4.4 g/dL (reference range, 3.5 to 4.5), ALP of 2300 U/L (reference range, 33 to 96), GGT of 345 U/L (reference range, 6 to 37), AST of 120 U/L (reference range, 12 to 38), ALT of 110 U/L (reference range, 7 to 41), total bilirubin levels of 21.2 mg/dL (reference range, 0.1 to 0.4), "direct" bilirubin levels of 18.5 mg/dL (reference range, 0.2 to 0.9), and positive urinary

bilirubin. Abdominal ultrasound results were normal, but MRI findings were consistent with osteomyelitis at the left sacroiliac joint. The patient was treated with broad-spectrum antibiotics, which were switched to intravenous flucloxacillin after blood cultures grew *Staphylococcus aureus*. The patient recovered quickly and was discharged from the hospital 12 days after admission. Twenty days after admission, the patient was asymptomatic, physical examination was normal, and laboratory results included normal albumin, AST, ALT, ALP, and GGT. Total bilirubin was elevated at 5 mg/dL, and direct bilirubin was 4.2 mg/dL. Which one of the following is the most likely explanation for the persistent hyperbilirubinemia?
A. Gilbert syndrome.
B. Persistent intrahepatic cholestasis.
C. Persistent hemolysis.
D. Delayed clearing of albumin-bound bilirubin (delta fraction).
E. Heterophilic antibody interference with bilirubin assay.

40. A 62-year-old woman presents with fatigue and progressive abdominal distention. Her past medical history includes type 2 diabetes and hypertension. She denies smoking and drinks less than one standard alcoholic drink per day. Physical examination shows a grossly distended abdomen, without tenderness and with shifting dullness. CT reveals hepatomegaly and ascites. Echocardiography is unremarkable. Abnormal laboratory tests include hemoglobin of 9.4 g/dL (reference range, 12.5 to 16.2), MCV of 88 fL (reference range, 79 to 93), albumin of 2.9 g/dL (reference range, 3.5 to 4.5), (GGT) of 180 U/L (reference range, 7 to 64), ALP of 350 U/L (reference range, 25 to 100), and total bilirubin of 1.1 mg/dL (reference range, 0.2 to 1.1). Which one of the following autoantibodies would be most sensitive for the diagnosis of primary biliary cirrhosis?
A. Antinuclear antibodies (ANAs) with a diffuse pattern.
B. Anti-SMA.
C. ANCA.
D. Anti–pyruvate dehydrogenase (PDC-M2) antibodies.
E. Anti–glutamic acid decarboxylase antibodies (GADA).

41. An assay for total hepatitis A virus (HAV) antibodies is used as a first-line screen for the laboratory diagnosis of hepatitis A. Which one of the following is the most appropriate reflex test for a positive result?
A. No reflex test is needed.
B. Hepatitis A IgM testing.
C. Hepatitis A IgA testing.
D. Hepatitis D IgG testing.
E. Hepatitis A nucleic acid testing.

42. Which one of the following is the most appropriate test for the diagnosis of acute hepatitis B virus (HBV) infection?
A. Hepatitis B surface antigen.
B. Anti–hepatitis B core total antibodies (IgG+IgM).
C. Anti–hepatitis B surface antibodies.
D. Anti–hepatitis B envelope antibodies.
E. Hepatitis B genotyping.

43. Which one of the following is the first-line screening test for hepatitis C virus (HCV) infection?
A. Recombinant immunoblot assay (RIBA) test for HCV.
B. HCV genotyping.
C. Anti-HCV immunoglobulin M (IgM) antibodies.
D. Anti-HCV immunoglobulin G (IgG) antibodies.
E. Hepatitis C surface antigen.

Answers

1. A. Fetal hemoglobin is more resistant to denaturation by alkali, and the persistent pink color of the sample implies a maternal source of blood.
B. Fetal hemoglobin is more resistant to denaturation by alkali, and the persistent pink color of the sample implies a fetal source of blood.
C. Fetal hemoglobin is less resistant to denaturation by alkali, and the persistent pink color of the sample implies a maternal source of the blood.
D. Fetal hemoglobin is less resistant to denaturation by alkali, and the persistent pink color of the sample implies a fetal source of the blood.
Rationale for C and D: Adult hemoglobin is less resistant than fetal hemoglobin to denaturation by alkali. If the blood had been from fetal ingestion of maternal blood, the sample would turn yellow-brown because adult hemoglobin denatures under basic conditions.
E. Adult hemoglobin and fetal hemoglobin react equivalently under basic conditions, and the persistent pink color of the sample is inconclusive.
Rationale for A, B, and E: Fetal hemoglobin is more resistant than adult hemoglobin to denaturation by alkali; this forms the basis of the Apt test. The persistent pink color of the sample implies that the hemoglobin has maintained its native conformation and is likely of fetal origin. If the blood had been from fetal ingestion of maternal blood, the sample would turn yellow-brown because adult hemoglobin denatures under basic conditions.

Major points of discussion
■ The source of blood in the stool of a newborn must be differentiated between an ingestion of maternal red cells during labor, an ingestion of maternal red cells during breastfeeding, and an actual gastrointestinal bleed in the newborn.
■ The Apt test is performed by adding water to the stool sample, washing out the red cells, and lysing them. A 1% NaOH solution is then added to the supernatant.
■ The Apt test capitalizes on the intrinsic stability of fetal hemoglobin in the presence of a base (i.e., sodium hydroxide).
■ If the sample maintains its pink color, the source of the blood is most likely of fetal origin.
■ If the sample turns yellow-brown, that implies that the hemoglobin is denatured and that the blood is derived from a maternal source.[22]

2. A. Anti–smooth muscle antibody (SMA).
Rationale: Anti-SMAs are associated with autoimmune hepatitis.
B. Anti-endomysial antibody.
Rationale: Testing for anti-endomysial immunoglobulin A (EMA) antibodies is the most sensitive and specific serologic test for celiac disease. However, these antibodies are detected by labor-intensive immunofluorescence assays that are expensive and technically difficult to perform.
C. HLA-DQ2.
Rationale: A large percentage of patients with celiac disease have the HLA-DQ2 allele (90% to 95%). However, this allele is present in approximately 30% to 40% of the general population. Therefore, this tool is not specific enough for diagnosis of this disorder.
D. Total immunoglobulin A (IgA) levels.
Rationale: Celiac disease is associated with IgA deficiency. However, rather than having diagnostic utility, this test result should be used for appropriate interpretation of negative EMA serologies. Thus, a total IgA level should always be ordered along with this specific serologic test.
E. Anti-thyroglobulin antibody.
Rationale: Although there are associations between celiac disease and other autoimmune disorders, this is not a sensitive or specific biomarker for this disorder.

Major points of discussion
■ EMA autoantibody is the most sensitive and specific marker for active celiac disease.
■ The target antigen for EMA is tissue transglutaminase.
■ Testing for EMA is typically done by an immunofluorescence assay on tissue sections of human umbilical cord. It is technically challenging to perform and interpret.
■ Because EMA is an IgA antibody and IgA deficiency is also associated with celiac disease, it is important to interpret EMA results in the context of total serum IgA levels.
■ The gold standard for the diagnosis of celiac disease is endoscopic biopsy showing lymphoepithelial lesions and blunting of the small intestinal villi.
■ Patients with untreated celiac disease are at higher risk for developing lymphoma.[1]

3. **A. Repeat the chromogranin A measurement after 4 to 5 half-lives have passed since discontinuing the over-the-counter medication.**
Rationale: The patient's over-the-counter medication is likely to be a proton pump inhibitor (PPI). PPIs are known to stimulate secretion of chromogranin A and cause falsely elevated levels. The chromogranin A measurement should be repeated after most of this medication has been cleared from the circulation (~4 to 5 half-lives of the drug). Omeprazole is a common over-the-counter PPI.
B. Send the patient for a positron emission tomography (PET) scan and magnetic resonance imaging (MRI) of the abdomen.
Rationale: Although this is not an illogical approach, the likelihood of recurrence is low given the patient's lack of constitutional signs and symptoms. The biochemical abnormality more likely results from a biologic false-positive test result and not true pathology.
C. Send the patient immediately to the operating room for an additional pancreatic resection.
Rationale: The patient has no signs or symptoms of a recurrent insulinoma to justify an immediate resection.
D. Do nothing; this change is within the normal, intraindividual variation of chromogranin A.
Rationale: Although there are assay-to-assay, interindividual, and intraindividual variations in chromogranin A levels, the patient has been "within normal range" for an entire year. He now presents with a twofold elevation. This is not compatible with intraindividual biologic variation.
E. Order a serum CA 19-9 level.
Rationale: This is a marker of pancreatic adenocarcinoma.

Major points of discussion

- Chromogranin A is elevated in patients with various neuroendocrine tumors, including functional and nonfunctional islet cell tumors of the pancreas; foregut, midgut, and hindgut carcinoid tumors; pheochromocytoma; medullary thyroid cancers; and neuroblastoma.
- Chromogranin A levels, in conjunction with measuring plasma serotonin and urinary 5-hydroxyindoleacetic levels, are particularly useful in the diagnosis and follow-up of carcinoid tumors.
- Chromogranin A levels are increased by the use of proton pump inhibitors and by kidney failure.
- Chromogranin A is measured by immunoassay and is, therefore, subject to interfering substances such as heterophile antibodies.
- There is no standard reference material for chromogranin A.[35]

4. **A. Chronic atrophic gastritis.**
Rationale: Serum pepsinogen levels correlate with parietal cell mass. Decreased serum pepsinogen is associated with a decrease in parietal cells, as is seen in atrophic gastritis. Chronic atrophic gastritis is a known precursor to gastric carcinoma. Screening high-risk populations, such as is done in Japan, aims to identify a group of patients with chronic atrophic gastritis who will be followed aggressively by endoscopy for the early detection of cancer.
B. Gastric cancer.
Rationale: Although serum pepsinogen levels are lower in patients with gastric carcinoma, screening programs aim to detect an at-risk population in need of more aggressive follow-up. Screening programs using serum pepsinogen are not used to diagnose patients with gastric cancer.
C. Celiac disease.
Rationale: Celiac disease involves the small intestine and is not expected to affect parietal cell mass.
D. Gastroesophageal reflux disease.
Rationale: Gastroesophageal reflux disease may result from hypersecretory states associated with increased serum pepsinogen levels.
E. Peptic ulcer disease.
Rationale: Generally, serum gastrin and secretin levels are elevated in patients with peptic ulcer disease. Parietal cell mass may theoretically be affected, but serum pepsinogen is not used to screen for this disease.

Major points of discussion

- Pepsinogens are produced in two distinct isoforms, types I and II. They are activated by enzymatic cleavage at acidic pH and degraded at alkaline pH.
- Only about 1% of secreted pepsinogens enter the circulation and can be measured in serum.
- Serum levels correlate with parietal cell mass; therefore, in states of decreased parietal cell mass, such as atrophic gastritis, pepsinogen levels are below the reference interval. High levels of pepsinogen are seen in hypersecretory states such as Zollinger-Ellison syndrome, duodenal ulcer disease, and gastrinoma.
- Severe atrophic gastritis increases the risk for the subsequent development of gastric carcinoma.
- Pepsinogen I levels in serum are measured by immunoassay and range from 20 to 107 µg/L in healthy adults.[23]

5a. A. Irritable bowel syndrome.
Rationale: Serologic testing is generally negative in irritable bowel syndrome.
B. Ulcerative colitis.
Rationale: Although this serologic pattern can be seen in a small percentage of patients with ulcerative colitis, these patients will more commonly test P-ANCA positive and ASCA negative.
C. **Crohn's disease.**
Rationale: ASCA is positive in 65% of patients with Crohn's disease and in 15% of patients with ulcerative colitis. P-ANCA is positive in only 20% of patients with Crohn's disease and in 70% of patients with ulcerative colitis. Therefore, the serologic pattern of ASCA positive and P-ANCA negative is most consistent with Crohn's disease.
D. Celiac disease.
Rationale: Celiac disease is serologically characterized by the presence of EMA autoantibodies.
E. Sarcoid.
Rationale: This disorder is characterized by elevated serum angiotensin-converting enzyme (ACE) levels.

5b. **A. Less than 5% of the radiolabeled vitamin B_{12} in the urine after both steps 1 and 2.**
Rationale: This is the classic finding in patients with ileal dysfunction caused by Crohn's disease (as in this patient). Radiolabeled vitamin B_{12} is not absorbed in the ileum caused by the disease, and the addition of intrinsic factor does not correct the problem. A cutoff of less than 5% of the dosed radiolabeled vitamin B_{12} in the urine is generally used to define malabsorption.
B. Less than 5% of the radiolabeled vitamin B_{12} in the urine after step 1 and an increase in urinary radiolabeled vitamin B_{12} after step 2.
Rationale: This is the pattern seen in pernicious anemia. In this setting, parietal cells do not produce intrinsic factor caused by gastric pathology (e.g., atrophic gastritis, carcinoma). Intrinsic factor is required to absorb vitamin B_{12} in the ileum. Therefore, addition of exogenous intrinsic factor corrects the vitamin malabsorption.
C. 15% urinary radiolabeled vitamin B_{12} after step 1 and 15% urinary radiolabeled vitamin B_{12} after step 2.
Rationale: This pattern is seen in patients without vitamin B_{12} malabsorption.
D. 15% urinary radiolabeled vitamin B_{12} after step 1 and a decrease to less than 5% radiolabeled vitamin B_{12} after step 2.
Rationale: This is a difficult pattern to explain pathophysiologically; therefore, the test should probably be repeated.
E. The Schilling test is not the appropriate test.
Rationale: The Schilling test is helpful in differentiating ileal causes of vitamin B_{12} malabsorption from parietal cell causes (i.e., pernicious anemia).

Major points of discussion

- ASCA test results are positive in 65% of patients with Crohn's disease and in only 15% of patients with ulcerative colitis.

- P-ANCA screening results are positive in 70% of patients with ulcerative colitis and in only 20% of patients with Crohn's disease.
- Irritable bowel syndrome is serologically negative more than 95% of the time.
- Because of the diffuse nature of the lesions in Crohn's disease, the ileum may be affected and ileal absorptive function may be compromised.
- The Schilling test, in two parts (i.e., without and with the addition of oral IF), can help localize the mechanism of vitamin B_{12} malabsorption.
- Vitamin B_{12} deficiency results in a macrocytic anemia, often accompanied by hypersegmented neutrophils and neurologic symptoms (e.g., decreased proprioception).[2]

6. **A. Type 1 diabetes.**
Rationale: Disorders of the endocrine pancreas do not generally affect the exocrine function of the gland.
B. Crohn's disease.
Rationale: Crohn's disease may alter gastrointestinal absorption of D-xylose, thereby causing decreased urinary D-xylose. This is the reason the D-xylose test is performed: to check for defects in enteric absorption.
C. Cystic fibrosis.
Rationale: In cystic fibrosis, the classic finding is insufficiency of the exocrine pancreas. D-Xylose does not require any pancreatic enzymes for absorption. This is how the test differentiates between enteric and pancreatic causes of malabsorption.
D. Chronic renal insufficiency.
Rationale: The D-xylose test depends on the ability of absorbed D-xylose to pass, unaltered, from the blood into the urine. In patients with chronic renal insufficiency, urinary D-xylose is affected by the renal dysfunction, thereby making it difficult to interpret the test results appropriately.
E. Hyperthyroidism.
Rationale: This disorder has no known effect on D-xylose test results.

Major points of discussion
- In the D-xylose test, the patient is given an oral dose of D-xylose after an overnight fast, and then urinary excretion of this molecule is monitored.
- The purpose of this test is to differentiate enteric causes of malabsorption (e.g., ileal dysfunction) from pancreatic causes (e.g., tumor, fibrosis, surgery).
- In patients with malabsorption caused by pancreatic insufficiency (or in a healthy patient), the urinary level of D-xylose should be elevated after the bolus because this sugar does not require pancreatic enzymes for absorption.
- In patients with malabsorption caused by enteric pathology, very little to no D-xylose will be absorbed; therefore, it will not be excreted in the urine.
- Any renal impairment will affect clearance of D-xylose and, therefore, interferes with proper interpretation of the test results.[3]

7. A. Fecal elastase measurements should be performed only on adult patient samples because pediatric reference ranges do not exist.
Rationale: Reductions in fecal elastase indicate pancreatic insufficiency in children older than 2 weeks.

B. Fecal elastase measurements should not be performed on patients who are receiving pancreatic replacement therapy.
Rationale: Pancreatic enzyme replacement therapy does not interfere with the measurement of fecal elastase.
C. Fecal elastase measurements should be performed only on well-formed stools.
Rationale: Fecal elastase must be performed on well-formed stools or the results have little interpretive value.
D. Fecal elastase measurement is not indicated for the diagnosis of pancreatic insufficiency.
Rationale: Fecal elastase is an extremely good marker for the diagnosis of severe pancreatic insufficiency. It is less sensitive for the detection of milder forms of pancreatic insufficiency.
E. Fecal trypsin, not fecal elastase, measurement should be performed.
Rationale: Fecal elastase is the best marker of pancreatic insufficiency; it is better than measuring other pancreatic enzymes.

Major points of discussion
- Fecal elastase is stable during transit through the bowel.
- Fecal elastase is concentrated in well-formed stools by fourfold to fivefold.
- The test is adequate for the diagnosis of severe pancreatic insufficiency but loses sensitivity in the setting of milder deficiencies.
- Fecal elastase is a better biomarker for pancreatic insufficiency than other pancreatic enzymes in stool.
- This biomarker is not affected by exogenous oral enzyme replacement.[39]

8. A. Urease breath testing for *H. pylori* is notoriously inaccurate and should not be used in clinical testing protocols.
Rationale: When performed correctly, urease breath testing is a specific and noninvasive method to confirm positive serologic testing for *H. pylori*. This is its appropriate clinical use.
B. The endoscopic biopsy was contaminated with *H. pylori*.
Rationale: Although this thought is not unreasonable, it is highly unlikely. On biopsy, *H. pylori* organisms are seen deep within the gastric gland pits and are unlikely to be a contaminant.
C. The patient's use of bismuth subsalicylate caused a false-negative test result.
Rationale: Bismuth-containing compounds are notorious for lowering the burden of *H. pylori* in patients to below the technical limits of the urease breath test assay. However, these compounds do not eradicate *H, pylori* and the patient's bacterial load will rebound, which leads to persistent infection.
D. The patient was infected with a non–urease-producing strain of *H. pylori*.
Rationale: Although this is possible, these strains are quite rare.
E. Urease breath testing is not useful in patients of Indian descent.
Rationale: There is no evidence of a differential utility of urease breath testing by patient ethnicity.

Major points of discussion
- *H. pylori* infection is the major cause of peptic ulcer disease worldwide.
- Other causes of peptic ulcer disease include chronic nonsteroidal antiinflammatory drug (NSAID) use and hypersecretory states.

- Chronic persistent *H. pylori* infection predisposes patients to increased risk for gastric carcinoma and gastric mucosal associated lymphoid tissue (MALT) lymphomas.
- False-negative results of the urease breath test include use of bismuth-containing antacids, PPIs, and antibiotics and testing the patient too soon after the completion of a treatment course. All of these settings may decrease the infecting load of *H. pylori* below the limits of detection but do not eradicate the infection.
- Urease-negative strains of *H. pylori* exist but are quite rare.[29]

9. A. A large spike in glucose concentrations because the lactose is absorbed and broken down into its constituent monosaccharides in the serum by serum lactase.
Rationale: Lactose cannot be absorbed as a disaccharide and must be hydrolyzed by lactase in the intestinal brush border.
B. A small increase in serum glucose caused by residual lactase activity, but most lactose will not by hydrolyzed by lactase in the intestinal brush border.
Rationale: Most lactose-intolerant individuals have some residual enzymatic activity resulting in a small spike in serum glucose levels. This increase must be less than 20 mg/dL to be diagnostic for lactose intolerance.
C. A small increase in serum glucose because of cross-reactivity between lactose and glucose.
D. A large decrease in serum glucose concentrations because most assays are inhibited by lactose.
E. A small decrease in serum glucose concentrations because most assays are inhibited by lactose.
Rationale: No lactose is absorbed.

Major points of discussion
- Lactose intolerance is caused by a decrease in the amount or function of the enzyme lactase in the brush border on the apical surface of small intestinal epithelial cells.
- Lactase acts on the disaccharide lactose to cleave it into its constituent monosaccharides: glucose and galactose. These sugars are then absorbed.
- The gold standard for the diagnosis of lactase deficiency is enzymatic testing of an endoscopically obtained biopsy of the small intestinal mucosa.
- A large percentage of otherwise normal adults are lactose intolerant. They are typically diagnosed by symptoms alone and managed by avoiding dairy products.
- Lactose intolerance is more common in patients of African or Asian descent.[13]

10. **A. A low percentage of C^{14} on the first round of testing and a relative increase in C^{14} percentage when C^{14} is coadministered with pancreatic enzymes.**
Rationale: This is the typical pattern seen in pancreatic insufficiency. The first round of testing involves having the patient fast overnight and administering an oral bolus of lipids with a C^{14}-labeled glycerol backbone. In steatorrhea of any etiology, very little C^{14} will be absorbed and metabolized to C^{14}-CO_2. The percentage of total CO_2 will be low. However, in cases of pancreatic insufficiency with addition of pancreatic lipases, the glycerol is liberated and absorbed and metabolized to CO_2, thereby increasing the relative percentage of C^{14}-labeled CO_2 that is expired.
B. A low percentage of C^{14} on the first round of testing without any change in C^{14} percentage after administration of pancreatic enzymes.

Rationale: This is the pattern seen in enteric causes of fat malabsorption.
C. A high percentage of C^{14} on the first round of testing without any change in C^{14} percentage after administration of pancreatic enzymes.
Rationale: This is the pattern seen in a normal patient with no fat malabsorption.
D. A high percentage of C^{14} on the first round of testing with a decrease in C^{14} percentage after administration of pancreatic enzymes.
E. A low percentage of C^{14} on the first round of testing with a decrease in C^{14} percentage after administration of pancreatic enzymes.
Rationale: It is difficult to interpret these results. If these results are obtained, the tests should be repeated.

Major points of discussion
- Steatorrhea is the term given to malabsorption of fats.
- Typically, steatorrhea presents with flatulence, bloating, and foul-smelling diarrhea with high fat content that floats on water.
- Generally, 93% of dietary fats are absorbed in a healthy gastrointestinal tract. In steatorrhea, as much as 40% of dietary fat is not absorbed and is passed in the stool.
- The causes of fat malabsorption can be divided into those that are primarily pancreatic in nature (e.g., a lesion obstructing the pancreatic duct or ampulla of Vater) or enteric (e.g., primary small intestinal pathologies).
- A common cause of steatorrhea, particularly in a patient with a camping history, is infection with *Giardia lamblia*.[25]

11a. A. A stool osmotic gap of less than 50 mOsm/Kg (low) and pH less than 5.5.
Rationale: A stool osmotic gap of less than 50 is typically seen in secretory diarrheas.
B. A stool osmotic gap of more than 125 mOsm/kg (high) and pH greater than 5.5.
Rationale: In osmotic diarrheas, the nonabsorbable material alters the osmotic gradient, drawing water into the lumen. This decreases the stool water sodium and potassium concentrations and increases the stool osmotic gap (normally, 80 mOsm/kg). A stool pH less than 5.5 (acidic) is classically seen in carbohydrate malabsorptive diarrhea.
C. A stool osmotic gap of 80 mOsm/kg (normal) and pH less than 5.5.
Rationale: A normal osmotic gap with an acidic pH is not typical of an osmotic diarrhea.
D. A stool osmotic gap of more than 125 mOsm/kg (high) and pH of 7.
Rationale: Although this osmotic gap correlates with an osmotic diarrhea, the neutral pH is not classic for a carbohydrate malabsorptive processs, which is generally characterized by an acidic stool caused by increases in various organic acids in the gut owing to bacterial metabolism of the carbohydrates.
E. The stool osmotic gap is not a useful assay to discriminate between secretory and osmotic diarrhea.
Rationale: The large differences in classic osmotic gaps between these two types of diarrhea make osmotic gap testing ideal for this differential diagnosis.

11b. A. Stool water sodium level.

B. Stool water potassium level.

C. Stool pH.

Rationale: Stool pH values cannot be interpreted in the setting of coadministered antibiotic therapy because of changes in gut flora that might dampen the effect of bacterial carbohydrate metabolism on stool pH.

D. Stool osmotic gap.

E. Stool water chloride level.

Rationale for A, B, D, and E: Unless the antibiotic is known to affect electrolyte balance in the intestine, there should be no effect of the coadministered antibiotics on this analyte.

Major points of discussion

- Stool osmotic gap is calculated by taking a value of 290 (a value of stool osmolality that approximates that in the blood) and subtracting from it 2 times the value of the sodium and potassium measured in the stool water. The factor of two accounts for the paired anions for sodium and potassium. A normal stool osmotic gap is 80 mOsm/kg.
- An osmotic gap greater than 125 mOsm/kg suggests an osmotic diarrhea (e.g., malabsorptive processes).
- An osmotic gap less than 50 mOsm/kg is seen in secretory diarrheas.
- In carbohydrate malabsorption, the stool pH is generally less than 5.5. It is acidic because of organic acids (including lactic acid) produced by bacterial metabolism of the poorly absorbed carbohydrate (e.g., lactose).
- Stool osmolality increases if the specimen is stored at room temperature, causing a false decrease in the osmotic gap. Therefore, the sample must be assayed immediately after collection.[6]

12. A. Gastrin-secreting tumor secondary to Zollinger-Ellison syndrome.

Rationale: Serum gastrin levels in patients with Zollinger-Ellison syndrome are generally greater than 1000 ng/mL. The diagnosis of Zollinger-Ellison syndrome is made not on gastrin levels alone but also after measuring gastric pH and imaging the pancreas.

B. Falsely elevated result caused by prolonged storage at room temperature before testing.

Rationale: Gastrin levels in serum should be run immediately or be immediately frozen at $-70°C$ to prevent proteolytic degradation of the enzyme. In fact, after 48 hours at $4°C$, 50% of the gastrin immune reactivity is lost.

C. Atrophic gastritis.

Rationale: Although gastric atrophy does lead to higher gastric pH and an increase in circulating gastrin levels, this is not the most likely answer in this clinical setting.

D. Normally elevated postprandial serum gastrin levels.

Rationale: Peptide fragments produced by digestion of proteins in food induce gastrin secretion. These are two to four times higher after a meal. Representative gastrin levels should be drawn on a fasted sample.

E. Serum gastrin is not the appropriate biomarker for Zollinger-Ellison syndrome.

Rationale: The triad of peptic ulcer disease, elevated serum gastrin levels, and hyperchlorhydria are diagnostic for Zollinger-Ellison syndrome.

Major points of discussion

- One cause of elevated gastrin levels in patients is Zollinger-Ellison syndrome. This entity is defined as a triad of elevated serum gastrin levels (usually >1000 ng/mL), peptic ulcer disease, and hyperchlorhydria.
- Serum gastrin levels increase with age as a result of progressive gastric atrophy.
- Gastrin secretion is highest at a gastric pH of 5 to 7. Gastrin secretion decreases by a negative feedback mechanism at pH less than 2.
- Increases in serum gastrin levels are common in patients taking PPIs whose gastric pH is generally elevated. However, gastric pH testing would reveal the absence of a hypersecretory state.
- After a meal, gastrin levels increase to two to four times of the upper limit of the reference range.[16]

13. **A. Activation of the renin-aldosterone system.**

Rationale: Patients with end-stage cirrhosis can have severe ascites and third spacing caused by low plasma oncotic pressure. This depletes their intravascular volume and activates the renin-aldosterone system to preserve volume. As a result, electrolyte disturbances, including hyponatremia or hypernatremia, are common in this patient population.

B. Overhydration.

Rationale: Overhydration is possible but is not the most common mechanism for electrolyte disturbances in patients with liver failure.

C. Assay interference by elevated bilirubin.

Rationale: Assay interference is possible but is not the most common mechanism for electrolyte disturbances in patients with liver failure.

D. Nutritional imbalance.

Rationale: Nutritional imbalance very rarely causes hyponatremia.

E. Normal variation in serum sodium.

Rationale: Serum sodium is very tightly regulated and is not subject to wide intraindividual variation.

14a. A. Acute or chronic alcohol abuse.

Rationale: This patient has acute pancreatitis. There are no laboratory signs of alcohol abuse, including a normal AST/ALT ratio of about 1. In addition, the lipase level would be expected to be fivefold greater than the amylase level.

B. Interference by statins.

Rationale: This patient has acute pancreatitis. There is no association between statin use and interference with serum amylase activity. Hypertriglyceridemia could cause a false decrease in serum amylase activity, but this patient has normal lipid studies.

C. Collection of the patient's blood sample in heparin anticoagulant.

Rationale: Serum amylase measurement depends on its enzyme activity, which requires calcium. Heparin tubes are recommended to avoid calcium chelation because amylase enzyme activity requires calcium and its chelation would lower this activity.

D. Collection of the patient's blood sample in K_2EDTA.

Rationale: Serum amylase measurement depends on its enzyme activity, which requires calcium. EDTA and citrate

anticoagulants chelate calcium; collection in these tubes could give a false normal or low activity. Therefore, amylase should be checked again using blood collected in a heparinized tube.
E. Storage of the sample at room temperature for 4 hours.
Rationale: Specimens collected for amylase and lipase can be stored for up to 14 days at room temperature.

14b. A. Serum amylase.
Rationale: Amylase can be normal in alcohol-induced acute pancreatitis.
B. Lipase/amylase ratio greater than 3.
Rationale: A lipase/amylase ratio greater than 5 is diagnostic for alcohol-induced acute pancreatitis.
C. Carbohydrate-deficient transferrin.
Rationale: Excessive alcohol consumption leads to elevated carbohydrate-deficient transferrin levels for several days to weeks after binge drinking. It is a useful test for patients who deny alcohol use, but in whom the physician still suspects it.
D. Total and direct bilirubin.
Rationale: Bilirubin studies are nonspecifically elevated depending on the severity of acute pancreatitis. In fact, an elevated direct bilirubin, indicative of obstruction, would support a diagnosis of biliary pancreatitis, rather than alcohol-induced pancreatitis.
E. Trypsinogen-1.
Rationale: Trypsinogen-1 elevation, as well as serum amylase and lipase elevation, suggests biliary pancreatitis. However, some data support the concept that elevated trypsinogen-2 and α_1-antitrypsin levels support the diagnosis of alcohol-induced pancreatitis.

Major points of discussion

- Many conditions can cause elevated serum amylase; these most commonly include conditions such as diabetic ketoacidosis (~60% of cases), cholecystitis, and peptic ulcer, following episodes of viral hepatitis or ruptured ectopic pregnancy, or after procedures such as gastric resection or renal transplantation.
- Normal serum and urine amylase is present in 20% of cases of acute pancreatitis. These can be false-negative results, such as that noted in Question 14a, but there are common clinical causes. For example, hyperlipidemia is thought to suppress serum amylase activity.
- In acute pancreatitis, serum lipase levels rise slightly earlier (4 to 8 hours) and peak sooner (24 hours) than serum amylase (rises at 2 to 12 hours, peaks at 48 hours).
- Prolonged elevation of serum lipase longer than 14 days suggests a poor prognosis or a pseudocyst.
- Elevated serum amylase and lipase can occur following abdominal trauma. Thus, a diagnosis of acute pancreatitis should be made only if it is supported by the total clinical picture.
- Pancreatic amylase (i.e., P-type) has a molecular weight of 54,000, whereas that of salivary amylase (S-type) can be larger. The enzymatic assay for salivary amylase requires the presence of 10 mmol/L of chloride. Interestingly, both serum and urine P-type amylase are elevated in acute pancreatitis, whereas S-type amylase

activity is decreased in chronic relapsing pancreatitis and cancer of the head of the pancreas.
- The Ranson criteria are useful for predicting the severity of acute pancreatitis. Thus, on admission, severity is predicted by factors such as age older than 55 years, white blood cell count greater than 16,000 cells/mm^3, blood glucose higher than 200 mg/dL, serum AST higher than 250 IU/L, and serum LDH higher than 350 IU/L. As in this patient, severity at 48 hours is predicted by factors such as calcium lower than 8.0 mg/dL, hematocrit decreased by more than 10%, hypoxemia with Po$_2$ less than 60 mm Hg, blood urea nitrogen increased by *at least* 5 mg/dL after administration of intravenous fluids, base deficit more than 4 mEq/L, and sequestration/third spacing of fluids greater than 6 L.[28]

15. A. Perform a repeat small intestinal biopsy.
Rationale: Although a biopsy would show mucosal and submucosal changes that indicate effective treatment (i.e., decreased intraepithelial inflammation and reversal of villous flattening), this is an unnecessarily invasive test. Serologic studies of anti-endomysial immunoglobulin A (IgA) antibodies are less invasive, have a diagnostic sensitivity of 89% to 100% in adults, and disappear after diet modification.
B. Measure serum anti-endomysial IgA antibodies.
Rationale: Serum anti-endomysial IgA antibodies disappear after effective treatment of celiac sprue.
C. Measure serum anti-endomysial IgG antibodies.
D. Measure fecal fat and fecal leukocytes.
Rationale: Although celiac sprue can cause steatorrhea and fecal leukocytes may be present, they are not used to monitor dietary modification. Multiple factors can change fecal fat and leukocytes. Therefore, serologic studies for serum anti-endomysial IgA antibodies are more specific.
E. Measure serum anti-gliadin IgG antibodies.
Rationale for C and E: Serum anti-gliadin IgG antibodies are accurate for diagnosing celiac sprue but inaccurate for monitoring treatment response. In general, IgG serologies for celiac sprue are not useful for monitoring dietary modification.

Major points of discussion

- Four serum antibodies can be used to diagnose celiac sprue: anti-gliadin IgA and IgG, anti-endomysial IgA and IgG, serum anti-reticulin (ARA) IgA, and serum transglutaminase (tTG) IgA. Of those, anti-endomysial IgA has the highest sensitivity and specificity.
- Serum anti-gliadin IgG is currently the most accurate alternative serologic test in patients who have IgA deficiency. However, small intestinal biopsy is still the gold standard.
- Anti-endomysial antibody detection is performed by allowing the antibodies to bind connective tissue that surrounds smooth muscle. Current tests use human umbilical cord sections as a substrate.
- Biopsy of small intestine is the gold stand for diagnosing celiac sprue.
- Nonspecific hematologic and biochemical abnormalities secondary to enteropathy and malabsorption can be present in patients with celiac sprue.

16a. A. Focal segmental glomerulosclerosis.
Rationale: This child has signs of renal failure and nephrotic syndrome with edema secondary to protein loss and low albumin. However, focal segmental glomerulosclerosis causes nephrotic syndrome primarily in adults.
B. Malnutrition.
Rationale: Malnutrition is one manifestation of cystic fibrosis, secondary to pancreatic insufficiency. However, it causes an elevated chloride sweat test (i.e., >60 mmol/L). Thus, if this patient does not have cystic fibrosis but is poorly nourished, a false-positive sweat chloride test result is possible.
C. Minimal change disease.
Rationale: False-negative chloride sweat test results have been reported in cases of hypoproteinemic edema which, in this case, is caused by nephrotic syndrome. Minimal change disease is the most common cause of nephrotic syndrome in the pediatric setting.
D. Glucose-6-phosphate dehydrogenase (G6PD) deficiency.
Rationale: G6PD deficiency causes elevated sweat chloride to levels above 60 mmol/L. The patient does not have signs and symptoms of G6PD deficiency. Whites of Northern European descent rarely have G6PD deficiency; it is most common among those of African, Southeast Asian, and Mediterranean descent.
E. Previous fludrocortisone administration.
Rationale: Fludrocortisone is sometimes used during chloride sweat testing for cystic fibrosis. It decreases sweat chloride in patients without cystic fibrosis but does not affect sweat chloride in patients with cystic fibrosis. The patient does not have signs of adrenal insufficiency (e.g., hypokalemia) that would indicate the use of fludrocortisone. In addition, the patient clinically shows signs of cystic fibrosis, including a history of upper respiratory infections. Therefore, it is unlikely that the child would have been given steroids, which could cause immunosuppression.

16b. A. The sensitivity is 80% even in African Americans.
Rationale: The sensitivity of molecular testing for cystic fibrosis in this population is approximately 50%.
B. The sensitivity is 75% to 90% in non-Ashkenazi white North Americans.
Rationale: The sensitivity of molecular testing for cystic fibrosis in this population is actually 75% to 90%. Although it is not absolutely necessary in this patient, it could be useful because this child has nephrotic syndrome and the sweat chloride test result is falsely low. Furthermore, there seems to be a family history of cystic fibrosis. The mother can refuse the test, and an elevated sweat chloride test result should be followed after the nephrotic syndrome resolves. Thus, the main role of the physician in this case is to accurately educate the patient's family.
C. The sensitivity is below 50% in non-Ashkenazi white North Americans.
Rationale: With the most current 25-allele–screening panel, the sensitivity of molecular testing for cystic fibrosis is 75% to 90% in non-Ashkenazi white North Americans, 97% in Ashkenazi Jews, 60% in Hispanic Americans, 50% in African Americans, and less than 10% in Asians.
D. The chance that one of the mutations in a 25-allele–screening panel is a deletion of the codon for phenylalanine 508 (Phe-508) in *CFTR* is 70%.
Rationale: Deletion of the three-nucleotide codon for Phe-508 (ΔF508) accounts for 70% of *CFTR* mutations in cystic fibrosis. However, currently, there are more than 1300 known additional mutations. Most are rare, and screening for all of them would be very expensive. In the current 25-allele screen, only 7 mutations in addition to the ΔF508 mutation account for at least 1% of cystic fibrosis mutations.
E. Molecular testing for cystic fibrosis is a better screening strategy than the sweat chloride test.
Rationale: Although molecular testing for cystic fibrosis confirms the diagnosis, many mutations are rare, still unknown, or not available for testing. Thus, a negative molecular test does not exclude the diagnosis, particularly if the sweat chloride test result is positive and the patient has signs and symptoms of cystic fibrosis.

Major points of discussion

- A sweat chloride test result of greater than 60 mmol/L on two separate occasions is diagnostic of cystic fibrosis.
- The actual test uses pilocarpine injected into the skin by iontophoresis, stimulating local sweat gland secretion. Sweat is collected by filter paper or gauze (≤100 μL), and 20 μL is analyzed using a chloride ion–selective electrode analyzer.
- Preanalytical variables are the most common causes of sweat chloride test errors.
- Sweat chloride tests in adults should be evaluated with caution. Random levels in men can vary up to as high as 70 mmol/L. Cyclic fluctuations occur in premenopausal women, peaking 5 to 10 days before menses.
- Chronic lung disease and malabsorption are the primary clinical problems seen in patients with cystic fibrosis.

17. **A. Fecal elastase-1 of less than 100 μg pancreatic elastase/gram of stool and an abnormal ERCP.**
B. Fecal elastase-1 of more than 200 μg pancreatic elastase/gram of stool and a normal ERCP.
Rationale: A fecal elastase-1 of greater than 200 μg pancreatic elastase/gram of stool is normal. In conjunction with a normal ERCP, this would argue against a diagnosis of chronic pancreatitis. Fecal elastase-1 is most useful in severe chronic pancreatitis, the most likely diagnosis in this case. ERCP is the radiologic test of choice for chronic pancreatitis.
C. Fecal elastase-1 between 100 and 200 μg pancreatic elastase/gram of stool and normal ERCP.
Rationale: A fecal elastase-1 between 100 and 200 μg pancreatic elastase/gram of stool is consistent with mild to moderate pancreatitis. However, a normal ERCP and nonspecific CT scan would not be diagnostic of chronic pancreatitis. Fecal elastase-1 is most useful in severe chronic pancreatitis, the most likely diagnosis in this case. ERCP is the radiologic test of choice for chronic pancreatitis.
D. Fecal elastase-1 of less than 100 μg pancreatic elastase/gram of stool and normal ERCP.
Rationale for A and D: A fecal elastase-1 of less than 100 μg pancreatic elastase/gram of stool is abnormally low.

However, an abnormal radiologic result is required before diagnosing chronic pancreatitis. ERCP is the best radiologic test for chronic pancreatitis. Fecal elastase 1 is most useful in severe chronic pancreatitis, the most likely diagnosis in this case.

E. Fecal elastase-1 of greater than 200 µg pancreatic elastase/gram of stool and an abnormal ERCP.
Rationale: A fecal elastase-1 of greater than 200 µg pancreatic elastase/gram of stool is normal. A low fecal elastase and abnormal ERCP would better support a diagnosis of chronic pancreatitis when combined with ERCP. Chronic pancreatitis is the most likely diagnosis in this case.

Major points of discussion

- A fecal elastase-1 cutoff of less than 200 µg pancreatic elastase/gram of stool has a positive predictive value of only 50%. Thus, radiology and clinical signs and symptoms are also necessary for the diagnosis of chronic pancreatitis.
- The sensitivity of fecal elastase-1 testing in chronic pancreatitis depends on disease severity: It is 100% in severe cases, 77% to 100% in moderate cases, and 0% to 63% in mild cases.
- Compared with chymotrypsin, another assay for pancreatic exocrine function, exogenous enzymes do not interfere with fecal elastase-1 assays. Exogenous enzymes are enzymes in the intestinal tract that come from ingestion of food and enzyme replacement therapy.
- Nonpancreatic gastrointestinal diseases—short gut syndrome, Crohn's disease, and gluten-sensitive enteropathy—cause false-positive results.
- Current literature indicates that fecal elastase-1 assay is unreliable in patients who have type 1 diabetes mellitus.[5,11]

18a. A. Gastrin levels will remain unchanged, but the sample should be analyzed immediately.
B. Gastrin levels remain at 95% of their physiologic levels, and the sample is stable for another 5 days.
Rationale: Gastrin levels decrease by about 50% after storage at 4°C for 48 hours. Serum specimens for quantifying gastrin levels (which is performed using an immunoassay) should be frozen immediately at −70°C because activity and stability are lost after storage at 4°C.
C. Gastrin levels will be decreased by about 50%, and the test results will be inaccurate.
D. Gastrin levels will be decreased by about 95%, and the test results will be inaccurate.
Rationale: This is a serum test, and specimens should be collected in a nonadditive glass tube or a serum separator tube. Specimens for quantifying gastrin levels, which is performed using an immunoassay, should be frozen immediately at −70°C and analyzed immediately after thawing. Stability is lost after storage at 4°C, and gastrin levels decrease by about 50% after 48 hours.
E. Gastrin levels will be decreased, but the sample should be analyzed immediately for accurate results.
Rationale for A and E: Serum specimens for quantifying gastrin levels (which is performed using an

immunoassay) should be frozen immediately at −70°C because activity and stability are lost after storage at 4°C. Gastrin levels decrease by about 50% after storage at 4°C for 48 hours.

18b. A. No, all gastrin isoform levels are unaffected by meals.
B. No, G17 and G34 gastrin isoform levels, but not the G14 isoform level, are unaffected by meals.
C. Yes, the patient must fast for at least 24 hours before specimen collection.
D. Yes, the patient must fast for 8 hours before specimen collection.
Rationale: The G17 and G34 gastrin isoform levels increase after meals (G17 quadruples and G34 doubles). Therefore, a patient must fast for at least 8 hours before specimen collection.
E. No, high-molecular-weight gastrin isoform levels are the most stable and are unaffected by meals.
Rationale: The opposite is true: High-molecular-weight and incompletely processed isoforms of gastrin, when pathologically increased, cannot be detected by conventional assays. In addition, big gastrin, known as G34, doubles after a meal.

Major points of discussion

- Gastrin has three isoforms in blood and tissues: G34 (big gastrin), G17 (little gastrin), and G14 (mini gastrin).
- All gastrin isoforms are derived from preprogastrin, which is cleaved by trypsin.
- The sensitivity of intraoperative gastrin assays is as high as 88%.
- The optimal pH range for gastrin activity is 5 to 7.
- Gastrin levels higher than 1000 ng/L are diagnostic for a gastrinoma. Zollinger-Ellison syndrome usually causes elevations up to 2000 ng/L.
- False-positive gastrin level results can occur secondary to H_2-antagonists and PPIs.
- Gastrin is measured by an enzyme-linked immunosorbent assay (ELISA).

19. A. Failure to rehydrate guaiac-smear slides.
Rationale: Rehydration increases the sensitivity (and lowers the specificity), leading to more false-positive guaiac-smear test results. The slides can be analyzed within 7 days of collection without rehydration and provide accurate results. Furthermore, in this patient, NSAID use and caffeine intake have probably caused gastroesophageal reflux disease, possibly leading to a low-grade bleeding ulcer. Some reports show an association between NSAID use and positive guaiac-smear test when no colon malignancy is present (i.e., false-positive results).
B. Ingestion of chicken.
Rationale: There is no association with white meats and false-positive results on guaiac-smear tests; this is seen only with red meats and some fruits and vegetables.
C. Ingestion of large amounts of vitamin C.
Rationale: Ingestion of large amounts of vitamin C is associated with false-negative guaiac-smear test results. Furthermore, in this patient, NSAID use and caffeine intake have probably caused gastroesophageal reflux disease, possibly leading to a low-grade bleeding ulcer. Some reports show an association between NSAID use and positive guaiac-

smear test when no colon malignancy is present (i.e., false-positive result).

D. Ibuprofen-induced gastroesophageal reflux disease.
Rationale: Several drugs can cause a positive guaiac-smear test result. Common ones include NSAIDs, anticoagulants, aspirin, and colchicines. Medications should always be considered if a false-positive test result is suspected.
E. Lack of red meat ingestion.
Rationale: Ingestion of red meat should be avoided because the guaiac-smear test detects the pseudo-peroxidase activity of heme and is, therefore, nonspecific with regard to hemoglobin from humans and animals.

Major points of discussion
- The sensitivity of fecal occult blood testing is 30% to 50%, but an accurate number is uncertain because patients with false-negative results typically do not undergo colonoscopy for confirmation. Thus, we do not know how many test results are truly falsely negative.
- The lower limit of detection for guaiac-smear tests is a 20-mL/day blood loss. A drop in hematocrit or hemoglobin is unnecessary in the setting of a true positive test result. For example, a 1 g/dL hemoglobin decrease over 1 day is more than enough blood loss (i.e., ~250 to 300 mL) to yield a positive guaiac-smear test result if the source of bleeding is the gastrointestinal system.
- Fecal occult blood testing should be performed on three consecutive stools, by using two slides each time. Positivity requires a positive result on only one of the two slides.
- Bleeding gums (i.e., ingestion of blood) can lead to false-positive fecal occult blood test results.
- The U.S. Preventive Services Task Force "recommends screening for colorectal cancer (CRC) by using fecal occult blood testing, sigmoidoscopy, or colonoscopy, in adults, beginning at age 50 years and continuing until age 75 years. The risks and benefits of these screening methods vary."[36]

20. **A. Amylase clearance/creatinine clearance ratio (C_{am}/C_{Cr}).**
Rationale: This ratio is very low in type 1 macroamylasemia (<1%) because it is caused by formation of amylase–macromolecule complexes, which are too large for excretion into the urine.
B. Trypsinogen 2.
Rationale: Trypsinogen 2 is elevated in, but has limited use for, the diagnosis of acute pancreatitis. It is not useful for the diagnosis of macroamylasemia.
C. Lipase/amylase ratio.
Rationale: This ratio has limited utility for the diagnosis of acute alcoholic pancreatitis when the ratio is 5 or greater because of low sensitivity. A minimally elevated ratio is not diagnostic of macroamylasemia.
D. Urine trypsinogen activation peptide.
Rationale: This peptide is elevated in the urine in the early stage of acute pancreatitis and has a 100% negative predictive value in this setting.
E. Carbohydrate-deficient transferrin.
Rationale: Excessive alcohol consumption leads to elevated levels of carbohydrate-deficient transferrin for several days to weeks after binge drinking. It is a useful test for patients

who deny alcohol use if the physician remains suspicious. It does not confirm or exclude macroamylasemia.

Major points of discussion
- Macroamylasemia is a disorder of elevated levels of serum amylase without clinical symptoms.
- There are three types of macroamylasemia, differentiated by high (type 1), moderately high (type 2), and trace (type 3) levels of serum macroamylase. The C_{am}/C_{Cr} ratio is low in all three, but very low in type 1.
- The key differential diagnosis for macroamylasemia includes disorders of elevated serum amylase, including pancreatic hyperamylasemia and salivary hyperamylasemia. In the latter two settings, serum macroamylase would be absent.
- The C_{am}/C_{Cr} ratio is not a reliable marker for macroamylasemia when acute or chronic renal failure is present along with an elevated serum amylase. The identification of serum macroamylase itself would be a more accurate diagnostic test in this setting.
- The assay for serum macroamylase uses ultracentrifugation or chromatography.

21. A. Stool sodium of 60 mOsm/kg, potassium of 80 mOsm/kg, and osmolality of 290 mOsm/kg.
Rationale: The patient has factitious diarrhea, best diagnosed by a good clinical history and the presence of an osmotic gap. Osmotic gap = $290 - \{2 \times ([Na] + [K])\}$, where less than 50 mOsm/kg indicates a secretory diarrhea, whereas more than 125 mOsm/kg indicates an osmotic diarrhea. Magnesium laxatives cause an osmotic diarrhea. For these laboratory results, the osmotic gap is 10 mOsm/kg, which would support a secretory diarrhea. Sodium phosphate laxatives cause a secretory diarrhea.
B. Stool sodium of 10 mOsm/kg, potassium of 20 mOsm/kg, and osmolality of 290 mOsm/kg.
Rationale: The patient has factitious diarrhea. For these laboratory results, the osmotic gap is 230 mOsm/kg, which is more than 125 mOsm/kg and supports an osmotic diarrhea as caused by magnesium laxatives.
C. Elevated serum gastrin levels.
Rationale: The patient has factitious diarrhea. Elevated gastrin levels are found in Zollinger-Ellison syndrome, which causes a secretory diarrhea.
D. More than 5 g of stool lipids over 24 hours.
Rationale: The patient has factitious diarrhea. The gold standard for steatorrhea is the 24-hour fecal lipid test. Normal is less than 5 g over 24 hours. Steatorrhea is defined as more than 5 g of lipids over 24 hours. Steatorrhea can result from malabsorption syndrome and does not differentiate between osmotic and secretory diarrhea, especially in this case.
E. Presence of fecal leukocytes and blood.
Rationale: The patient has factitious diarrhea. These laboratory results would be consistent with an inflammatory diarrhea caused, for example, by *Shigella* species.

Major points of discussion
- Secretory, osmotic, malabsorption, maldigestion, and inflammatory are the main types of diarrhea.
- Not only do active ingredients of certain drugs cause diarrhea, but carrier components do so as well. For example, sorbitol, which acts as a carrier, is one such ingredient.

- Chronic diarrhea is defined as more than three loose stools per day for more than 4 weeks. Acute diarrhea lasts less than 2 weeks and rarely requires diagnostic testing.
- Bloody or exudative diarrhea suggests an inflammatory cause (e.g., infectious, inflammatory bowel disease, ischemic colitis, radiation-induced colitis).
- Stool osmotic gap can be calculated, if given the stool sodium and potassium, using the following equation: Osmotic gap $290 - \{2 \times ([Na] + [K])\}$, where less than 50 mOsm/kg indicates a secretory diarrhea and more than 125 mOsm/kg indicates an osmotic diarrhea.

22. A. Continue the PPI treatment and repeat the breath test after completing antibiotic therapy.
B. Repeat the hydrogen breath test.
C. Perform endoscopy and biopsy of the esophagus and stomach.
D. Perform a urease test on a stomach and esophageal biopsy.
E. Culture the stomach or esophageal biopsy tissue at 25°C.
Rationale: The patient appears to have peptic ulcer disease, which is most commonly caused by *H. pylori*. Histology is the gold standard for diagnosis. In addition, *H. pylori* grows at 37°C. PPIs and antibiotics can lower the bacterial load and yield a false-negative hydrogen breath test result. However, the patient did not complete the full course of antibiotics, and therefore, she is not completely treated. Histology and serologic testing would be better approaches because this patient has already started therapy for *H. pylori* before confirmatory diagnosis. Accurate diagnosis is necessary for proper treatment. Persistent epigastric pain, even with therapy, could indicate a neoplasm, which requires biopsy.

Major points of discussion
- *H. pylori* grows at 37°C. In addition, it is oxidase, catalase, and urease positive. On susceptibility testing, it is resistant to nalidixic acid and sensitive to cephalothin.
- Warthin-Starry and Giemsa stains of tissue biopsies are alternatives to immunohistochemistry for the identification of *H. pylori*.
- Always consider NSAID use as a cause of peptic ulcer disease.
- *H. pylori* should be excluded before initiating PPI and antibiotic therapy because treatment can obscure the diagnosis, causing false-negative results if subsequent diagnostic tests are conducted. In practice, PPI therapy is often initiated before confirmation.
- A low bacterial load in general, even without treatment, can yield false-negative test results.

23. **A. Positive serum P-ANCA and negative serum ASCA.**
Rationale: This would help confirm ulcerative colitis because 70% of patients who have ulcerative colitis have a positive serum P-ANCA compared with 15% of those who have Crohn's disease.
B. Negative serum P-ANCA and positive serum ASCA.
Rationale: This would actually exclude ulcerative colitis because only 20% of patients who have ulcerative colitis have a positive serum ASCA compared with 65% of those who have Crohn's disease.
C. Negative serum P-ANCA and negative serum ASCA.

Rationale: Less than 5% of patients who have irritable bowelsyndrome have negative P-ANCA and ASCA serologies.
D. Colon and small intestinal biopsy showing discontinuous presence of granulomas, crypt abscesses, and transmural inflammation.
Rationale: Both ulcerative colitis and Crohn's disease can have granulomas and crypt abscesses. Transmural inflammation and discontinuous lesions (i.e., skip lesions) are consistent with Crohn's disease.
E. Low levels of serum vitamin B_{12}.
Rationale: Low levels of serum vitamin B_{12} would suggest damage to the ileum. Crohn's disease affects the mucosa anywhere from the mouth to the anus, whereas ulcerative colitis affects colon and rectal mucosa. Thus, low levels of vitamin B_{12} would be more consistent with Crohn's disease.

Major points of discussion
- The sensitivity of serum P-ANCA and ASCA for ulcerative colitis and Crohn's disease are low.
- Histologic diagnosis is the gold standard for diagnosing inflammatory bowel disease.
- The presence of fecal leukocytes is consistent with an inflammatory etiology of diarrhea.
- Always note a patient's clinical signs and symptoms when the diagnostic tests are inconclusive. These will usually support one diagnosis rather than the other.
- Anemia and elevated inflammatory markers (e.g., C-reactive protein and erythrocyte sedimentation rate) are nonspecific inflammatory markers that can be present in both ulcerative colitis and Crohn's disease.

24. A. Request microbial culture of the small intestinal tissue.
B. Discontinue abacavir therapy for HIV.
C. Order a polymerase chain reaction (PCR) test of small intestinal tissue.
D. Initiate treatment with metronidazole.
E. Measure serum anti-endomysial immunoglobulin A antibodies.
Rationale: This patient has Whipple disease caused by *Tropheryma whipplei*, an organism that is not readily cultured. Serum anti-endomysial antibody serologic tests are used to confirm celiac sprue, which also causes a malabsorption diarrhea. PCR of the infected tissue, which is the small intestine in this case, confirms the diagnosis of Whipple disease. Treatment includes penicillin, ampicillin, tetracycline (uncommon now), cotrimoxazole, and more recently, doxycycline and hydroxychloroquine. Sulfonamides can be added if neurologic symptoms are present, indicating infection of the central nervous system. Metronidazole, among other uses, is used to treat diarrhea secondary to *Clostridium difficile*.

Major points of discussion
- Whipple disease is most common among whites, particularly those from rural areas.
- A duodenal biopsy showing foamy macrophages in the lamina propria that are PAS positive, diastase resistant is pathognomonic for Whipple disease.
- PAS-positive macrophages may also be seen in patients with AIDS who are infected with *Mycobacterium avium*

complex. Therefore, PCR testing of the infected tissue is a better confirmatory test.

■ *T. whipplei* can infect the central nervous system, causing neurologic symptoms. Central nervous system infection requires longer-term antibiotic therapy.

■ Fifty percent of patients with Whipple disease have lymphadenopathy and hyperpigmentation. Arthropathy, malabsorption, and diarrhea are also common symptoms.

25. A. The patient most likely does not have alcoholic liver disease if the ALT and AST levels are normal.
Rationale: Serum GGT is often elevated in both alcoholic liver disease and alcoholism without liver disease. GGT levels decline with the cessation of alcohol use. ALT and AST levels may be normal in end-stage liver disease with or without alcohol use as the cause.
B. The patient's 5′-nucleotidase activity would add no additional diagnostic information.
Rationale: 5′-Nucleotidase is very rarely elevated in bone disease and not associated with alcohol use and therefore may help determine whether the elevated ALP is caused in part by biliary obstruction or bone disease alone.
C. The patient's ALP would show at least partial heat lability on heat fractionation.
Rationale: The patient would be expected to have an elevated ALP isoenzyme derived from bone, which is the most heat-labile ALP, compared with those from placenta, intestine, and liver.
D. The patient has an elevated Regan isoenzyme.
Rationale: Regan isoenzyme is placental ALP, which is sometimes elevated in malignancy.
E. The patient is expected to have an increased indirect bilirubin.
Rationale: The presence of gallstones puts the patient at risk for extrahepatic biliary obstruction, which would result in increased conjugated (direct) bilirubin rather than unconjugated (indirect) bilirubin. Alcoholic liver disease and cirrhosis can also result in increased conjugated bilirubin.

Major points of discussion
■ ALP is a hydrolase enzyme produced in liver, bone, kidney, intestine, and placenta. It is most commonly elevated in liver or bone disease. In the liver, the enzyme is found on the canalicular surface of hepatocytes, and therefore elevated ALP indicates biliary obstruction, cholestasis, or space-occupying lesions. Bone ALP is produced by osteoblasts and is elevated in Paget's disease, metastatic tumors, and metabolic bone disease, among others.

■ ALP isoenzymes can be separated by electrophoresis to distinguish the tissue of origin. In addition, heat fractionation can be used to distinguish the tissue source, with placental ALP being the most heat resistant and bone ALP being the most heat labile. Liver-derived ALP is moderately stable. Remember, "bone burns."

■ Placental ALP is known as Regan isoenzyme and is known to be produced by a number of malignancies, including germ cell and urinary tract tumors. Regan isoenzyme is heat stable.

■ Both GGT and 5′-nucleotidase help distinguish between an elevated ALP caused by liver versus bone disease and generally may be used interchangeably. However, GGT is

also associated with chronic alcohol use and alcoholic liver disease. Therefore, in this case, given that both the elevated ALP and GGT can be explained by other underlying conditions (Paget's disease and alcoholism, respectively), further laboratory evaluation for hepatobiliary disease is warranted, including AST, ALT, bilirubin, albumin, and prothrombin time.

■ The presence of gallstones puts the patient at risk for extrahepatic biliary obstruction, which would result in increased conjugated (direct) bilirubin rather than unconjugated (indirect) bilirubin. Alcoholic liver disease and cirrhosis can also result in increased conjugated bilirubin. Obstruction caused by gallstones would result in elevated ALP, 5′-nucleotidase, and GGT with or without mild elevation in ALT and AST.

■ Patients with cirrhosis of any cause often have normal or decreased levels of AST and ALT because ongoing hepatocyte injury is absent. However, the abnormal liver architecture of cirrhosis can result in regional intrahepatic obstruction of bile flow, resulting in elevated ALP, GGT, and 5′-nucleotidase.

26. **A. Activation of the renin-aldosterone system.**
Rationale: Patients with end-stage cirrhosis, as described in this patient, generally have severe ascites and third spacing caused by low plasma oncotic pressure. This depletes their intravascular volume and activates the renin-aldosterone system to preserve volume. As a result, electrolyte disturbances, including hyponatremia or hypernatremia, are common in this patient population.
B. Overhydration.
Rationale: Overhydration is possible, but it is not the most common mechanism for electrolyte disturbances in patients with liver failure.
C. Assay interference by elevated bilirubin.
Rationale: Assay interferences are possible, but they are not the most common mechanism for electrolyte disturbances in liver failure patients.
D. Nutritional imbalance.
Rationale: Nutritional imbalance very rarely causes hyponatremia.
E. Normal variation in serum sodium.
Rationale: Serum sodium is very tightly regulated and is not subject to wide intraindividual variation.

Major points of discussion
■ Patients with end-stage cirrhosis have severe ascites and third spacing caused by low plasma oncotic pressure. This depletes their intravascular volume, activating the renin-aldosterone system to preserve volume. As a result, electrolyte disturbances, including hyponatremia or hypernatremia, are common in this patient population.

■ Overhydration is possible, but it is not the most common mechanism for electrolyte disturbances in patients with liver failure.

■ Interference in the sodium assay by hyperbilirubinemia is possible, but it is not the most common mechanism for electrolyte disturbances in patients with liver failure.

■ Nutritional imbalance very rarely causes hyponatremia.

■ Serum sodium is very tightly regulated and is not subject to wide intraindividual variation.

27. A. Autoimmune hepatitis.
Rationale: Autoimmune hepatitis is inflammation of the liver of unknown cause.
B. Bile duct obstruction.
Rationale: Bile duct obstruction can be caused by primary sclerosing cholangitis, mass, or gallstone.
C. Cirrhosis.
Rationale: Cirrhosis is a common endpoint for many liver diseases. It does not cause Dubin-Johnson syndrome.
D. Defective organic anion transporter.
Rationale: A mutation in the canalicular multidrug resistance protein 2 (MRP2) leads to defective anion transport and defective biliary excretion.
E. Acute viral hepatitis.
Rationale: Hepatitis A, B, and C infections lead to hepatocyte injury.

Major points of discussion
- Dubin-Johnson syndrome is a rare autosomal recessive disorder, most commonly seen in the Sephardic Jewish population, associated with persistently elevated conjugated (direct) bilirubin. Patients with Dubin-Johnson syndrome typically have subtle clinical signs and symptoms, most commonly icterus, but also intermittent jaundice and/or constitutional complaints. These clinical features may be apparent only with other concurrent illnesses.
- Dubin-Johnson syndrome is caused by mutations of the gene encoding a multispecific organic anion transporter protein (*MRP2*). This protein transports organic anions such as conjugated bilirubin into the bile canaliculus from the hepatocytes.
- Although patients with Dubin-Johnson syndrome have elevated conjugated bilirubin, they do not have elevated transaminases, ALP, or GGT. Elevations in those enzymes would suggest intrahepatic cholestatic disease (e.g., medication-related toxicity, infiltrative disease, cholangitis) or extrahepatic obstruction.
- Unconjugated hyperbilirubinemia (elevated indirect bilirubin) may be prehepatic or hepatic. Prehepatic etiologies include increased bilirubin production such as hemolysis or dyserythropoiesis. Hepatic causes include neonatal jaundice, as well as heritable disorders such as Gilbert and Crigler-Najjar syndromes. Of all the heritable bilirubin metabolic disorders, Crigler-Najjar syndrome type I is the most serious and is often fatal, presenting as severe jaundice and kernicterus in neonates.
- Rotor syndrome is similar to Dubin-Johnson syndrome in that it is also a rare genetic disease with a benign course and presents as elevated conjugated bilirubin and normal LFTs. However, the underlying mechanism is defective storage rather than defective transport of organic anions (conjugated bilirubin). In addition, the liver appears unremarkable compared with the dense pigmentation seen in Dubin-Johnson syndrome. Different patterns of urine coproporphyrin excretion can also help discriminate between these two entities.

28a. A. Cirrhosis.
Rationale: Although patients with this clinical scenario in a chronic setting may develop cirrhosis, you would expect normal to low AST/ALT ratio and abnormal markers of synthetic function resulting from replacement of liver parenchyma with fibrosis.
B. Hepatocellular carcinoma.
Rationale: Hepatocellular carcinoma and other space-occupying lesions would likely show a marked increase in ALP and biliary obstruction.
C. Passive congestion.
Rationale: Passive congestion produces mild elevations in hepatocellular markers (AST/ALT ratio) and biliary markers (total bilirubin/ALP). However, synthetic function remains unaltered.
D. Fulminant hepatic failure.
Rationale: Finally, in fulminant hepatic failure, AST and ALT would be markedly elevated (100 times the upper limit of normal). Synthetic function would also be compromised.
E. Normal variation in liver function.
Rationale: Mild elevations in LFTs generally indicate pathology.

28b. A. Myoglobin.
B. Troponin T.
C. Ischemia-modified albumin.
Rationale: Although there may be a small degree of cardiac injury leading to increases of the other three biomarkers, the main elevation will be in brain natriuretic peptide.
D. Brain natriuretic peptide.
Rationale: The patient is clearly suffering from right heart failure, and elevations in brain natriuretic peptide as a result of right ventricular overloading would be expected.
E. LDH.
Rationale: LDH may be elevated in both myocardial and hepatic pathologies. However, this laboratory value would not help elucidate the mechanism of the liver dysfunction in this case.

Major points of discussion
- The pattern of hepatocellular and biliary biomarkers in a patient sample helps determine which hepatic compartment is abnormal.
- Elevated brain natriuretic peptide secondary to ventricular overload suggests congestive heart failure, particularly in this clinical vignette.
- In hepatic cirrhosis, the AST/ALT ratio will be low to normal, and synthetic function will be abnormal because of replacement of liver parenchyma with fibrosis.
- In fulminant hepatic failure, AST and ALT are markedly elevated, sometimes 100 times the upper limit of normal. Synthetic function is compromised.
- Passive congestion, as occurs in right heart failure, produces mild elevations in hepatocellular markers (AST/ALT ratio) and biliary markers (total bilirubin/ALP). Synthetic function remains unaltered.

29. A. Increased serum ceruloplasmin, increased serum total copper, decreased 24-hour urine copper.
Rationale: Serum ceruloplasmin would be decreased and 24-hour urine copper increased in Wilson's disease.
B. Decreased serum ceruloplasmin, increased serum total copper, increased 24-hour urine copper
Rationale: Serum copper is decreased in Wilson's disease.

C. Decreased serum ceruloplasmin, decreased serum total copper, decreased 24-hour urine copper.
Rationale: The 24-hour urine copper is increased in Wilson's disease.
D. Decreased serum ceruloplasmin, decreased serum total copper, increased 24-hour urine copper.
E. Increased serum ceruloplasmin, increased serum total copper, increased 24-hour urine copper.
Rationale: In Wilson's disease, there is a decrease in both serum ceruloplasmin and serum total copper (a measurement that includes bound and unbound copper) and an increase in urinary copper excretion.

Major points of discussion
- Wilson's disease can present clinically as a progressive neurologic disease, liver disease (typically chronic but occasionally acute), or a psychological disorder. Typically, patients present in childhood or young adulthood.
- Wilson's disease is an autosomal recessive disease caused by mutation of the *ATP7B* gene, located on chromosome 13, which encodes transmembrane copper-exporting adenosine triphosphatases localized to the canalicular membrane of hepatocytes. Defective copper exportation results in accumulation of copper within hepatocytes as well as ineffective formation of ceruloplasmin, the major carrier of copper in the blood. Approximately 90% of total serum copper consists of ceruloplasmin. Therefore, both serum ceruloplasmin and total serum copper are decreased in Wilson's disease. Conversely, the serum non–ceruloplasmin-bound copper concentration is elevated, as reflected in increased 24-hour urine copper, which measures free copper excretion.
- Ceruloplasmin is an acute-phase reactant and therefore may be normal or elevated in patients with Wilson's disease. Furthermore, ceruloplasmin may be low owing to other causes such as renal disease or non–Wilson's disease-related end-stage liver disease. Therefore decreased serum ceruloplasmin and serum total copper are not sensitive or specific laboratory tests to confirm the diagnosis of Wilson's disease. Increased urinary excretion of copper, although a useful screening modality in diagnosing Wilson's disease, may be increased in other liver diseases such as autoimmune hepatitis.
- Serum ceruloplasmin less than 20 mg/dL with increased hepatic copper of more than 250 µg/g dry weight is diagnostic of Wilson's disease. Genetic testing for *ATP7B* mutations has limited diagnostic utility because more than 30 mutations have been identified.
- Administration of D-penicillamine during the 24-hour urine copper excretion test results in increased copper excretion and can be helpful in distinguishing Wilson's disease from other causes of increased copper excretion.
- Untreated Wilson's disease results in development of advanced liver fibrosis and cirrhosis, as well as neuropsychiatric complications, and is ultimately fatal. The mainstay of treatment involves copper chelation therapy, such as with penicillamine, and liver transplantation when necessary.[30]

30. A. A glucose level of 60 mg/dL indicates a poor prognosis.
Rationale: Acute pancreatitis is often associated with defective insulin release and hyperglycemia. A glucose level higher than 200 mg/dL is an adverse prognostic factor in acute pancreatitis.

B. Amylase is released earlier than lipase and therefore is more sensitive for acute pancreatitis.
Rationale: Both amylase and lipase are released 3 to 8 hours after the initiation of the symptoms and persist for several days after recovery, with amylase tending to normalize in 3 to 6 days and lipase often persisting for 1 to 2 weeks. Lipase in most studies was found to be more sensitive than amylase for the diagnosis of acute pancreatitis.
C. Lipase is more specific than amylase for acute pancreatitis.
Rationale: Lipase is more specific for acute pancreatitis, although elevations can occasionally be seen in other pancreatic and gastrointestinal disorders and in renal failure. Amylase can be elevated in a wide variety of conditions, including salivary disease, gastrointestinal disorders, hepatitis, cirrhosis, gynecologic diseases, chronic alcoholism, pregnancy, trauma, burns, head injury, and renal failure. Because of its poor specificity and slightly lower sensitivity, amylase is no longer recommended for the diagnosis of pancreatitis, except in situations of high suspicion with normal lipase.
D. Most commercially available amylase assays are immunoassays.
Rationale: Most amylase assays rely on enzymatic hydrolysis of starch or starchlike substrates such as hepta-maltose. Immune inhibition with antibodies against salivary amylase, followed by an amylase enzymatic assay, has been used occasionally to measure pancreatic amylase more specifically, but these assays are not widely available.
E. Elastase assays are commonly used to rule out acute pancreatitis.
Rationale: Pancreatic elastase is elevated in acute pancreatitis, but its diagnostic efficiency is not better than lipase, and therefore it is not commonly used. However, decreased levels of fecal elastase can be of value in diagnosing chronic pancreatic insufficiency because it remains un-degraded in stool.

Major points of discussion
- Acute pancreatitis is a common cause of abdominal pain in patients presenting to the emergency department and represents a diagnostic challenge because of variable clinical presentation and lack of specificity of laboratory tests.
- The most common causes are cholelithiasis and alcohol use, with genetic factors playing an important predisposing role. Variants in the following genes have been strongly implicated in susceptibility to pancreatitis: cationic trypsinogen (*PRSS1*), anionic trypsinogen (*PRSS2*), serine protease inhibitor Kazal 1 (*SPINK1*), *CFTR*, chymotrypsinogen C (*CTRC*), and calcium-sensing receptor (*CASR*). Rare causes (<1%) include hypertriglyceridemia, hypercalcemia, malignancy, autoimmune disorders, vascular abnormalities, and hereditary enzymatic defects.
- Age greater than 55 years is associated with an adverse prognosis. Laboratory values indicating an adverse prognosis include age greater than 55 years, blood glucose higher than 200 mg/dL, white blood cell count (WBC) more than 16×10^9/L, AST higher than 250 U/L, LDH more than 700 U/L, creatinine more than 2 mg/dL, C-reactive protein more than 150 mg/dL, procalcitonin greater than 1.8 ng/mL, albumin less than 2.5 mg/dL, and calcium less than 8.5 mg/dL.

- Various professional organizations, including the American Gastroenterological Association and American Academy of Family Physicians, have published guidelines for the diagnosis of acute pancreatitis and unanimously recommend the use of lipase instead of amylase for initial diagnosis of pancreatitis. Most guidelines recommend a threshold of greater than two to four times the upper limit of normal (ULN), while stressing that early elevation (less than three times normal) should be interpreted in the context of the clinical evolution.
- A recent study[7] examined the diagnostic accuracy of lipase and amylase for acute pancreatitis in 3451 patients presenting to the emergency department with acute abdominal pain. Elevations of lipase greater than threefold ULN showed sensitivity, specificity, and area under the curve of 95%, 99%, and 0.996, respectively, whereas the corresponding values for amylase were 64%, 99%, and 0.992, respectively.
- Amylase assays rely on enzymatic hydrolysis of starch or starchlike substrates such as hepta-maltose. A dry-chemistry method uses the natural substrate starch coupled to a dye, which is released by amylase and diffuses to the reagent layer, where it is measured by reflectance spectrophotometry. Some liquid chemistry methods use a series of enzymes to convert the product of the amylase reaction (usually one or more maltose residues) to a measurable compound (usually reduced nicotinamide adenine dinucleotide [NADH] from a G6PD reaction). Other methods use chromogenic maltose oligomers that release a measurable dye, such as 4-nitrophenyl, on reaction with amylase.
- Lipases hydrolyze triglycerides and diglycerides to monoglycerides or glycerol and free fatty acids and typically are assayed by measuring hydrolysis of diglyceride substrates. In some methods, production is measured through a series of reactions leading to production of H_2O_2. Other methods use special diglyceride substrates that, on lipase reaction, release a chromogen. In addition to pancreatic lipase, other lipases released in the blood include lipoprotein lipase, intestinal lipase, and hepatic lipase. The latter two prefer short-chain fatty acid substrates, whereas pancreatic lipase and lipoprotein lipase can hydrolyze long-chain fatty acids. Lipoprotein lipase interference is eliminated by incorporation of bile acids and a pancreatic lipase cofactor, colipase.[7,19,27]

31. A. AST.
Rationale: AST is a marker for hepatocyte injury and can be normal in conditions causing canalicular injury.
B. ALT.
Rationale: ALT is a marker for hepatocyte injury and can be normal in conditions causing canalicular injury.
C. Anti–hepatitis B core antibody.
Rationale: This test assesses exposure to HBV.
D. GGT.
Rationale: Concurrent elevations in GGT suggest the elevated ALP is of biliary tract origin.
E. Ammonia.
Rationale: Ammonia levels will be elevated in patients with liver failure, but this test is not used to discriminate origins of ALP.

Major points of discussion
- ALP is present in many tissues, including bone and liver.
- In the liver, ALP is located on the canalicular surface of the hepatocyte, and elevations are seen in patients with cholestatic disease.
- GGT is an enzyme involved in amino acid transport across cell membranes. Elevations occur in cholestatic disease.
- If GGT and ALP are both elevated, the source of the ALP is likely to be the biliary tract.
- Posthepatic biliary obstruction will lead to elevations in ALP, GGT, and 5′-nucleotidase. Causes of posthepatic biliary obstruction include cholelithiasis, primary biliary cirrhosis, and primary sclerosing cholangitis.

32. A. ALT is more abundant in the liver than AST.
Rationale: In general, AST is more sensitive than ALT for liver injury because it is about two to three times more abundant in liver than ALT.
B. ALT is more specific than AST for liver disease.
Rationale: ALT is expressed predominantly in liver, although it is present in smaller amounts in other tissues such as kidney, skeletal muscles, heart, adrenal gland, adipose tissue, neurons, endocrine pancreas, and prostate. AST is widely expressed and therefore less specific for liver disease. Despite its presence in other tissues, isolated ALT elevations are rarely seen in the absence of liver disease.
C. The AST/ALT ratio is usually lower than 2 in severe alcoholic liver disease.
Rationale: Typically, patients with alcoholic hepatitis or severe alcohol-induced liver disease such as cirrhosis have an AST/ALT ratio (De Ritis ratio) greater than 2. Possible mechanisms for the elevation of this ratio include decreased hepatic production of ALT, mitochondrial oxidative damage leading to release of mitochondrial AST, and extrahepatic damage with AST release.
D. The AST/ALT ratio is usually lower than 2 during the acute phase of viral hepatitis.
Rationale: In acute viral or toxic hepatitis, aminotransferase levels are typically quite elevated (>300 U/L), and the AST/ALT ratio tends to be less than 1.
E. AST half-life in plasma is significantly longer than that of ALT.
Rationale: In general, the half-life of ALT is much higher (about 2 days) than that of AST (<24 hours), and therefore ALT may predominate after recovery of liver injury.

Major points of discussion
- Two different genes code the AST enzyme. *GOT1*, which codes for cytosolic AST, is most abundant in red cells and in cardiac and skeletal muscles. *GOT2* codes for a mitochondrial form of AST, which is most abundant in hepatocytes. The cytosolic form predominates in the plasma of normal individuals and patients with mild liver disease, whereas the mitochondrial form is released with advanced or severe liver disease.
- Two different genes code the ALT enzyme. *GPT* codes for the cytosolic form (ALT1), predominantly expressed in the liver, whereas *GPT2* codes for a mitochondrial form expressed in skeletal muscle and heart. The *GPT* gene can be induced in the liver by peroxisome proliferator–activated receptor (*PPAR*) α agonists, such as

fenofibrate, and by conditions associated with increased neoglucogenesis, such as fasting, insulin resistance, type 2 diabetes, the metabolic syndrome, and obesity.

- Both AST and ALT are sensitive markers of liver disease. ALT is more specific and AST is more sensitive for mild liver damage.
- Factors affecting the AST/ALT ratio (De Ritis ratio) include (1) extent of extrahepatic disease, affecting AST more than ALT; (2) severity of damage, with more severe disease leading to release of mitochondrial AST; (3) half-life of AST (<24 hours) versus ALT (about 2 days); (4) liver synthetic dysfunction, affecting ALT more than AST; (5) extent of ALT induction (e.g., drugs, insulin resistance); (5) levels of circulating pyridoxal-5′-phosphate (P5P) in circulation. Because P5P is an essential cofactor for the aminotransferase reaction with assays that do not supplement the reaction with exogenous P5P, this becomes a rate-limiting factor; the ALT enzyme is more susceptible to low levels of P5P seen, for example, with chronic alcoholism, malnutrition, and renal failure.
- The AST/ALT ratio can be helpful to differentiate causes of liver damage. In normal individuals, the De Ritis ratio is about 0.7 to 1.4. In general, the ratio is increased in acute ischemic, toxic, or alcoholic hepatitis, cirrhosis, liver metastasis, primary biliary cirrhosis, Reye syndrome, and Wilson disease. The De Ritis ratio is usually less than 2 in viral hepatitis (often <1), autoimmune hepatitis, cholangitis, hemochromatosis, infectious mononucleosis, non-alcoholic steatosis, and in the recovery phase of acute hepatitis.[8,26,32]

33. A. Preoperative elevation of CEA indicates a poor prognosis.
Rationale: Although elevations of CEA greater than 5 ng/mL are associated with the possibility of distant metastasis, particularly in patients with stage III colon cancer, this patient is a heavy smoker, and therefore mild elevations of CEA may be associated with smoking. About 5% of smokers have CEA elevations greater than 5 ng/mL. In these patients, a cutoff of 10 ng/mL may be more indicative of poor prognosis.
B. Increased CEA after the procedure is highly suggestive of treatment failure.
Rationale: Chemotherapy is often associated with a temporary increase in CEA, possibly released from dying cancer cells. CEA elevations should not be interpreted as failure to respond during the first 4 to 6 months of chemotherapy.
C. An early increase of more than 15% in CEA levels during chemotherapy indicates a better prognosis.
Rationale: CEA elevation during chemotherapy may be associated with a better prognosis because it indicates susceptibility to the chemotherapy. For example, a "CEA flare," defined as at least a 15% increase of 4 ng/mL or greater followed by a decrease of 15% or greater, had an objective response rate of 73% compared with 11% for patients with CEA increasing at least 15% in two consecutive measurements (Strimpakos, 2010).
D. CEA has good accuracy for screening of early-stage (Dukes A) colon cancer.
Rationale: CEA is more often normal in early-stage (Dukes A) colon cancer, with sensitivity ranging from 8% to 52% and specificity ranging from 55% to 100%. Use of CEA for screening and detection of early colon cancer in healthy individuals is not recommended because of poor sensitivity and specificity.
E. Significant CEA elevations (>10 ng/mL) are specific for colon cancer.
Rationale: CEA elevations are seen in a variety of benign and malignant gastrointestinal diseases, including esophageal and gastric cancer, diverticulitis, gastric ulcer, atrophic gastritis, pancreatitis, inflammatory bowel diseases, hepatobiliary diseases, chronic renal failure, chronic lung disease, cystic fibrosis, pneumonia, sarcoidosis, and other tumors (e.g., lung, breast, ovary, uterus, salivary).

Major points of discussion
- CEA is a glycoprotein abundantly expressed in the fetal gastrointestinal tract, but its expression is shut down in most adult cells. However, it can be re-expressed at high levels in epithelial carcinomas. The CEA protein is anchored to the cell membrane by a glycosyl phosphatidyl inositol tail and is easily cleaved from the membrane by phospholipases expressed in cancer cell, resulting in solubilization of CEA and consequent release into circulation.
- CEA is the only tumor marker recommended by several expert organizations for clinical use in gastrointestinal tumors. Moreover, these guidelines recommend that CEA measurements should be used for staging, therapy monitoring, and recurrence prediction in patients with colorectal cancer.
- CEA should not be used for screening of early-stage colon cancer in healthy individuals because of poor sensitivity and specificity. However, it may be of some value in individuals at high risk for epithelial cancer, with the caveat that more than 90% of the positive CEA results in asymptomatic individuals are a result of benign conditions.
- Pretreatment elevations of CEA are increasingly common with advancing colon cancer stage, ranging from 8% to 52% for Dukes A, 22% to 59% for Dukes B, 38% to 72% for Dukes C, and 69% to 96% for Dukes D. Significant elevations (>5 ng/mL in nonsmokers or >10 ng/mL in smokers) should prompt evaluation for the presence of metastatic cancer.
- The major role of CEA testing is evaluation of patients with colon cancer after treatment, with the goals of (1) documenting the effectiveness of treatment and (2) monitoring for recurrence or metastatic disease. It is important to note that CEA should not be the sole test used for these purposes because sensitivity is about 64% to 84%, whereas specificity varies between 73% and 91%. Most important, the vast majority of CEA elevations are false positive in the absence of positive imaging studies and should not be used in isolation to determine aggressive therapy. Conversely, a combination of CEA and imaging should provide more than 90% sensitivity for detection of postsurgical colon cancer recurrences.
- Successful surgical treatment of colon cancer should result in a decrease of CEA 3 to 4 weeks after surgery. In contrast, if chemotherapy with certain agents such as 5-fluorouracil, levamisole, irinotecan, and oxaliplatin is used, temporary "CEA flares" may be observed and should not be equated with treatment failure. Success of

chemotherapy should result in decreases in CEA levels after 6 months of therapy.

- Most guidelines recommend CEA measurement every 2 to 3 months in patients with stage II to IV disease for 2 to 3 years, if they are candidates for surgery or systemic treatment in the event of cancer recurrence or metastatic disease. After 2 to 3 years, monitoring every 6 months for another 2 to 5 years is appropriate.[31,33,34]

34a. A. Unconjugated bilirubin.
Rationale: Unconjugated bilirubin is usually not directly measured but rather is calculated by subtracting the direct from the total bilirubin values.
B. Azobilirubin.
Rationale: Azobilirubin is produced when bilirubin present in the patient's sample reacts with a diazotized sulfanilic acid. Azobilirubin absorbs light at 540 nm.
C. Nicotinamide adenine dinucleotide phosphate (NADP).
Rationale: NADP will absorb ultraviolet light at a specific wavelength; however, the production of NADP is not used in this reaction methodology.
D. Nicotinamide adenine dinucleotide (NAD).
Rationale: NAD molecules will absorb ultraviolet light; however, the production of NAD is not used in this reaction methodology.
E. Uridine diphosphate (UDP) glucuronyltransferase.
Rationale: UDP glucuronyltransferase is the enzyme that conjugates bilirubin to glucuronic acid. It is not directly measured in this assay.

34b. A. UDP glucuronyltransferase.
Rationale: UDP glucuronyltransferase is the enzyme that conjugates bilirubin to glucuronic acid. It is not directly measured in this assay.
B. Albumin.
Rationale: Albumin levels are not measured with this technique. A bromocresol green assay is commonly used to measure albumin.
C. Unconjugated bilirubin only.
Rationale: Unconjugated bilirubin is detected with this assay; however, conjugated bilirubin present in the sample will also react.
D. Conjugated bilirubin only.
Rationale: Conjugated bilirubin is detected with this assay; however, because of the presence of the accelerators, unconjugated bilirubin present in the sample will also react.
E. Total bilirubin.
Rationale: The addition of accelerants facilitates the measurement of unconjugated and conjugated bilirubin at the same time, yielding a total bilirubin value.

Major points of discussion
- Bilirubin is commonly measured using the diazo method, which results in azobilirubin production. Azobilirubin production is then measured spectrophotometrically because the compound absorbs light at 540 nm.
- Conjugated bilirubin (direct) can be measured using the diazo technique without accelerators. Direct bilirubin reacts more quickly than indirect bilirubin.

- When accelerators such as caffeine are added to the diazo method, both direct and indirect bilirubin will react. This reaction will give a total bilirubin value.
- Indirect bilirubin is calculated by subtracting direct from total bilirubin.
- UDP glucuronyltransferase is the enzyme that conjugates bilirubin to glucuronic acid. Conjugated bilirubin is water soluble and can be filtered by the kidney glomerulus.

35. A. Plasma hemoglobin levels.
Rationale: Plasma hemoglobin is increased by in vitro hemolysis and can be increased in intravascular hemolysis when hemoglobin levels exceed the clearing capacity of the haptoglobin/phagocytic system (about 100 to 200 mg/dL). With in vitro hemolysis, plasma hemoglobin levels become visible at about 20 to 50 mg/dL (corresponding to about 0.1% to 0.5% hemolysis).
B. Plasma potassium levels.
Rationale: Potassium can transiently increase in severe acute intravascular hemolysis, but homeostatic mechanisms including renal excretion will rapidly lead to normal levels.
C. Plasma AST levels.
Rationale: AST is significantly more abundant than ALT in erythrocytes and other blood cells and therefore will increase more than ALT both in vitro and in vivo hemolysis.
D. Plasma LDH levels.
Rationale: LDH is a major intracellular component in blood cells and will increase with both in vivo and in vitro hemolysis. Typically, expect about a 1% increase in LDH for each 1 mg/dL of plasma hemoglobin with in vitro hemolysis.
E. Plasma haptoglobin levels.
Rationale: Hemoglobin released in circulation from intravascular hemolysis will quickly bind to haptoglobin, and the haptoglobin-hemoglobin complexes are rapidly cleared by the phagocytic system. Therefore, a decrease in haptoglobin levels is consistent with in vivo hemolysis. Because there is no significant endocytosis of haptoglobin-hemoglobin complexes in an anticoagulated blood sample in vitro, plasma haptoglobin levels are unchanged by in vitro hemolysis.

Major points of discussion
- *Clostridium perfringens* sepsis is a cause of acute intravascular hemolysis, in part owing to production of a hemolysin by this anaerobic gram-positive bacillus. Hemolysis can be severe, with visible hemoglobinemia, hemoglobinuria, and jaundice. Blood smears often show pancytopenia, with spherocytosis and ghost cells, and toxic changes in neutrophils. Mortality is very high.
- Distinguishing in vitro from in vivo hemolysis is essential for proper diagnosis of the patient's condition, as well as for correct interpretation of laboratory values.
- Hemoglobinuria, decreased haptoglobin, increased unconjugated bilirubin and urinary urobilinogen, and reticulocytosis can occur only with in vivo hemolysis and are not seen with artifactual in vitro hemolysis.
- Conversely, false elevations of potassium and, to a lesser extent, phosphate, magnesium, and other intracellular electrolytes, are more often observed with in vitro

hemolysis because physiologic homeostatic mechanisms tend to strictly control electrolyte levels in vivo.

- Significant elevations of AST and LDH without ALT elevations are consistent with hemolysis because ALT is not significantly present in red blood cells.
- Whereas a haptoglobin decrease is a sensitive marker for intravascular and, to a lesser extent, extravascular hemolysis, it suffers from the caveat that haptoglobin is an acute-phase reactant and increases in conditions such as stress, infection, acute inflammation, and tissue necrosis. A normal C-reactive protein level can help rule out an acute-phase reaction.
- Other caveats of using haptoglobin for the diagnosis of hemolysis include the fact that it decreases with estrogen and liver disease and increases with corticosteroids and androgens. Situations of phagocytic system blockade, such as viral infections and infiltrative disorders of lipid or glycogen metabolism, may also result in impaired clearing of haptoglobin-hemoglobin complexes.[4,18,21]

36. A. Hemolytic anemia.

Rationale: Both hemolytic anemia (increased bilirubin production) and conjugation defects (such as *UGT1A1* defects and liver cirrhosis) result in mildly increased unconjugated bilirubin, as in this case. However, with increased heme catabolism, the liver is able to increase bilirubin conjugation and excretion, leading to higher levels of urobilinogen production and ultimately positive urine urobilinogen. In contrast, with conjugation defects, as well as with cirrhosis and extrahepatic cholestasis, urobilinogen levels are decreased because conjugated bilirubin excretion into the intestines is impaired.

B. Gilbert syndrome.

C. Crigler-Najjar syndrome.

Rationale: Urobilinogen levels are decreased because conjugated bilirubin excretion into the intestines is impaired.

D. Liver cirrhosis.

Rationale: When cirrhosis is accompanied by jaundice, it is predominantly associated with increased direct bilirubin, resulting from intrahepatic cholestasis, typically with negative urine urobilinogen and possibly positive urine bilirubin.

E. Extrahepatic cholestasis.

Rationale: Extrahepatic cholestasis typically results in increased conjugated (direct) bilirubin in plasma, predominating over unconjugated bilirubin. Urine bilirubin can be elevated, and urine urobilinogen is negative.

Major points of discussion

- Bilirubin derives from the catabolism of hemoglobin, more specifically from its heme moiety. With intravascular or extravascular hemolysis, the phagocytic system converts increased amounts of heme to bilirubin, which then is released into circulation, mostly in a noncovalent complex with albumin (unconjugated or "indirect" bilirubin). This high-molecular-weight complex does not typically appear in urine if glomerular function is intact.
- The liver then conjugates bilirubin to glucuronic acid, a reaction catalyzed by the UDP glucuronyltransferase

enzyme coded by the *UGT1A1* gene. Congenital defects in this gene lead to forms of Gilbert and Crigler-Najjar syndromes of hyper-unconjugated bilirubinemia.

- Excretion of conjugated bilirubin occurs through the biliary system into the intestines, where 95% is reabsorbed into the portal circulation and re-excreted by the liver. Very little conjugated bilirubin (measured as "direct" bilirubin) is present in the systemic circulation in the absence of intrahepatic or extrahepatic cholestasis.
- About 5% of intestinal bilirubin is further metabolized to urobilinogen by intestinal bacteria. About 80% of the urobilinogen is excreted in the stool, whereas 20% is reabsorbed into the circulation. Both urobilinogen and conjugated bilirubin are soluble in the plasma and can be excreted by the kidneys.
- Unconjugated bilirubin elevations can result from increased production (increased heme catabolism), such as in hemolysis and inefficient erythropoiesis, and from conjugation defects, such as severe liver insufficiency, genetic defects in *UGT1A1* (Crigler-Najjar and Gilbert syndromes), and inhibition of *UGT1A1* (e.g., anti-HIV protease inhibitors, oral contraceptives, hyperthyroidism).
- Severe hemolysis can be a cause of jaundice when the hepatic capacity to handle increased bilirubin production is exceeded. With preserved liver function, the degree of total bilirubin elevation in hemolysis is mild, rarely exceeding 5 mg/dL. All of the elevation is attributable to unconjugated (indirect) bilirubin.
- Urine urobilinogen is a sensitive marker for hemolysis, often elevated when total bilirubin is normal, because the liver increases bilirubin conjugation and biliary/intestinal excretion.[9,10]

37. A. ALT of 10,500 U/L (reference range, <45) and AST of 8500 U/L (reference range, <35).

Rationale: This pattern is more suggestive of acute viral hepatitis. An AST/ALT ratio greater than 1 is suggestive of progression of cirrhosis.

B. ALP of 650 U/L (reference range, 110 to 390) and GGT of 35 U/L (reference range, 7 to 49).

Rationale: Elevated ALP with normal GGT is more suggestive of bone disease. In alcoholic patients, GGT is usually elevated.

C. Albumin of 3.2 g/dL (reference range, 3.4 to 4.8) and total protein of 10.4 g/dL (reference range, 6.4 to 8.3).

Rationale: Severe cirrhosis is associated with hypoalbuminemia and polyclonal hypergammaglobulinemia, suggested by the elevated levels of total protein and globulin (total protein albumin).

D. Total bilirubin of 4.3 mg/dL (reference range, 0.2 to 1.1) and direct bilirubin of 3.2 mg/dL (reference range, <0.2).

Rationale: Elevation of bilirubin consisting predominantly of conjugated (direct) bilirubin is more suggestive of cholestasis. Bilirubin elevations associated with advanced cirrhosis typically are composed of unconjugated hyperbilirubinemia, resulting from hepatic insufficiency, and conjugated hyperbilirubinemia, reflecting intrahepatic cholestasis.

E. Prothrombin time of 12.2 seconds (reference range, 12.0 to 14.3) and platelet count of 350×10^9/L (reference range, 150 to 400).

Rationale: Hepatic insufficiency associated with advanced cirrhosis will lead to insufficient production of clotting factors and prolongation of the prothrombin time. Thrombocytopenia is also a common finding in liver cirrhosis.

Major points of discussion

■ Liver cirrhosis is characterized by replacement of the liver parenchyma with fibrous tissue and regenerative nodules, leading to loss of normal architecture and impaired liver function.

■ Chronic alcoholics are at risk for liver cirrhosis. Various contributory factors include chronic hepatic damage resulting from consistent alcoholic intake (usually >60 g/day for more than 10 years), malnutrition, genetic factors, oxidative stress, immunologic mechanisms, and hepatic comorbidities.

■ True tests of liver function include prothrombin time, which measures clotting factor synthetic capacity; the ratio of unconjugated bilirubin to conjugated bilirubin, which measures the hepatic ability to conjugate bilirubin; and albumin levels, which reflect the balance of liver synthesis, intravascular volume, and excretion. In cirrhosis, hypoalbuminemia contributes to low intravascular oncotic pressure. In addition, there is systemic vasodilation, lower renal perfusion, water retention associated with elevated levels of antidiuretic hormone, and hyponatremia. All of these factors result in expansion of the extravascular volume resulting in ascites and edema.

■ ALT and AST are markers of liver damage. In cirrhosis, elevations of aminotransferases are usually mild or absent. Because ALT is more susceptible to liver synthetic deficiency than AST, which is widely expressed in other tissues, the AST/ALT ratio tends to be more than 2 in liver cirrhosis with chronic hepatic insufficiency. Oxidative mitochondrial damage may also contribute to higher levels of AST.

■ Polyclonal hypergammaglobulinemia is common in cirrhosis. Contributory factors include impaired clearing of enteric bacterial organisms and antigens by the liver, chronic inflammation, and possibly loss of B-cell inhibitory regulation. Serum protein electrophoresis typically shows a broad increase in the β and γ regions, the so-called β-γ bridge. Often chronic liver disease also shows a decrease in the α_1-, α_2-, and β-globulins because of hepatic synthetic insufficiency.

■ A common finding with severe liver insufficiency is hepatic encephalopathy. Manifestations include disturbed sleep, altered consciousness, defects in higher mental functions and personality, flapping tremors, rigidity, and hyperreflexia. The pathogenesis has been attributed to high levels of ammonia associated with chronic liver disease. Normally the liver converts ammonia to urea by the Krebs urea cycle, or alternatively couples ammonia to glutamic acid to form glutamine, and liver insufficiency together with portosystemic shunting can result in high levels of ammonia. However, not all patients with high ammonia levels have encephalopathy, and conversely, normal levels of ammonia are seen in about 10% of the patients with hepatic encephalopathy, suggesting that other intestinal compounds cleared by the liver may play a role. There is no correlation between the degree of hyperammonemia and the severity of the encephalopathy; therefore, it is of little value to measure ammonia levels in these patients, with the possible exception of diagnostically unclear situations.

■ To diagnose progression to cirrhosis, particularly in chronic viral hepatitis, various investigators have attempted to estimate the degree of liver fibrosis with laboratory tests, frequently using combinations such as the AST/platelet ratio index (APRI), fibroindex (derived from platelet count, AST, and γ-globulins), and a variety of markers of collagen synthesis, including procollagen type III N-terminal peptide, triple-helix domain of type IV collagen, prolyl hydroxylase, and hyaluronic acid. A popular index (FibroTest or FibroSURE) uses a combination of α_2-macroglobulin, haptoglobin, apolipoprotein A1, GGT, and bilirubin to derive a value predictive of liver fibrosis and necroinflammatory activity.[15,20,37]

38. A. Total bilirubin.
Rationale: Hyperbilirubinemia can be a feature of primary biliary cirrhosis; however, this test is not specific for this disease.
B. Anti-SMAs.
Rationale: Anti-SMAs are associated with classic autoimmune hepatitis.
C. ALP.
Rationale: High levels of ALP can be seen in patients with primary biliary cirrhosis; however, this analyte is not specific for this disease.
D. Immunoglobulin M (IgM).
Rationale: Elevated levels of IgM can be seen in patients with primary biliary cirrhosis; however, this finding is not specific for this disease.
E. Antimitochondrial antibodies.
Rationale: An antimitochondrial antibody titer greater than 1:160 is highly predictive of primary biliary cirrhosis.

Major points of discussion

■ Primary biliary cirrhosis (PBC) is a cholestatic disorder of unknown etiology. The disease is characterized by inflammation and progressive destruction of the bile ducts within the liver.

■ The most sensitive diagnostic marker for PBC is the presence of antimitochondrial antibodies.

■ Antinuclear autoantibodies are a heterogeneous group of antibodies detected in a variety of autoimmune disorders, including autoimmune hepatitis and PBC.

■ Antimitochondrial antibodies are detected using indirect immunofluorescence microscopy.

■ The most common mitochondrial antigen in PBC is the M2 antigen.

39. A. Gilbert syndrome.
Rationale: Hyperbilirubinemia in Gilbert syndrome can be precipitated by dehydration, fasting, sepsis, and other causes of stress. However, the hyperbilirubinemia is mild and composed of unconjugated bilirubin.
B. Persistent intrahepatic cholestasis.
Rationale: Sepsis can be associated with intrahepatic cholestasis as illustrated in this patient during the acute phase. However, persistently elevated direct bilirubin in the absence of elevation in other markers of cholestasis, such as ALP and GGT, is unlikely to be caused by cholestasis.

C. Persistent hemolysis.
Rationale: Although intravascular hemolysis can rarely be associated with *S. aureus* sepsis, it will cause mild elevations of unconjugated bilirubin, not direct bilirubin.
D. Delayed clearing of albumin-bound bilirubin (delta fraction).
Rationale: In patients with prolonged cholestasis and elevated bilirubin, formation of a covalent complex of albumin and bilirubin (δ-bilirubin) can lead to persistent elevation of direct reacting bilirubin, whereas other bilirubin fractions quickly normalize after removal of the cholestasis. Although the unconjugated and glucuronide-conjugated bilirubin fractions have half-lives of minutes in circulation, δ-bilirubin has the half-life of albumin, about 2 to 3 weeks. In contrast to conjugated bilirubin, which can be excreted by the kidney and cause positive bilirubin urinalysis, δ-bilirubin, because of albumin conjugation, does not appear in the urine of patients with healthy renal glomeruli.
E. Heterophilic antibody interference with bilirubin assay.
Rationale: Bilirubin is assayed by a chemical method. There are no described instances of interference by antibodies.

Major points of discussion
- Intrahepatic cholestasis can accompany bacterial sepsis in 1% to 6% of adults and a slightly higher percentage of neonates. Gram-negative rods such as *Escherichia coli* and *Klebsiella* species are more common causes, whereas *Staphylococcus* and *Streptococcus* species sepsis can also cause jaundice. Congestion, hypoxia, bacterial products, and proinflammatory cytokines may be contributors to hepatic injury leading to cholestasis.
- Although usually mild, sepsis-associated jaundice can be intense, particularly in patients with preexisting hepatobiliary disease, and may divert attention from the diagnosis of underlying sepsis.
- Fractionation of bilirubin, for example, by liquid chromatography, shows the presence of four fractions:
  - Unconjugated bilirubin, loosely bound to albumin (α-bilirubin)
  - Bilirubin monoglucuronide (β-bilirubin)
  - Bilirubin diglucuronide (γ-bilirubin)
  - Bilirubin covalently conjugated to albumin (δ-bilirubin)
- Bilirubin is usually assayed by a colorimetric chemical method derived from the diazo reaction first described by Erlich in 1883. Most current methods use caffeine benzoate to displace unconjugated bilirubin from albumin and accelerate its reaction with a diazotized chromogen. In the presence of the accelerator, both conjugated and unconjugated bilirubin react quickly with the diazo dye, and the result is labeled total bilirubin.
- When the accelerator is omitted, unconjugated bilirubin reacts very slowly, whereas the other fractions react quickly but incompletely. The result is labeled as direct bilirubin. Unconjugated bilirubin can then be estimated by subtraction of total bilirubin minus direct bilirubin. However, accuracy of this estimation is hampered by the fact that between 1% and 10% of the unconjugated bilirubin can be measured as direct bilirubin.
- δ-Bilirubin is present in significant amounts in patients with persistent cholestasis and conjugated hyperbilirubinemia, probably as a result of displacement of glucuronide by albumin. Because δ-bilirubin can be variably measured as direct bilirubin, elevated δ-bilirubin

can result in overestimation of the levels of conjugated bilirubin and underestimation of unconjugated bilirubin. Moreover, in patients recovering from cholestasis, persistent elevation of bilirubin can be misconstrued as failure to recover from the disease.
- Alternative methods for bilirubin determination using dry-slide chemistry can discriminate conjugated (β and γ-bilirubin (Bc) from unconjugated (α) bilirubin (Bu) by spectrophotometric scanning in the present of a cationic mordant. In this method, δ-bilirubin is not measured at all. When used in conjunction with a total bilirubin method, δ-bilirubin can be calculated as the difference of total bilirubin − Bc − Bu.[12,38]

40. A. Antinuclear antibodies (ANAs) with a diffuse pattern.
Rationale: ANAs can be seen in PBC. The pattern is usually a nuclear rim pattern, indicating autoantibodies against the nuclear envelope, or a nuclear dot pattern. Antibodies showing a nuclear rim pattern include antinuclear pore glycoprotein 210, present in about one fourth of patients with PBC, and nuclear protein p62, present in about 30% to 55% of the cases. Both gp210 and p62 autoantibodies are highly specific (>97%) for PBC and good predictors of advanced disease, hepatic failure, and poor prognosis. Antibodies showing a nuclear dot pattern include sp100 proteins, promyelocytic leukemia protein, NDP52, and sp140 proteins. Of these, sp140 proteins are highly specific for PBC and present in about 15% of the cases.
B. Anti-SMA.
Rationale: Anti-SMAs, directed against antigens such as smooth muscle actin, myosin, tropomyosin, and troponin, can be present in PBC in up to 25% of cases but are typically associated with autoimmune hepatitis type III and may indicate the concurrent presence of this disease in the setting of PBC.
C. ANCA.
Rationale: ANCAs are primarily associated with systemic vasculitides but can be present in a minority (2% to 26%) of PBC patients.
D. Anti–pyruvate dehydrogenase (PDC-M2) antibodies.
Rationale: Antimitochondrial antibodies directed against the pyruvate dehydrogenase complex (labeled as M2 antibodies) are the predominant antibodies in PBC, present in 90% to 95% of the cases.
E. Anti–glutamic acid decarboxylase antibodies (GADA).
Rationale: Anti-GADAs are associated with type 1 diabetes and rarely (<5%) are present in PBC.

Major points of discussion
- PBC is an autoimmune disorder characterized by progressive destruction of small and medium-sized intrahepatic bile ducts, portal inflammation, and progressive liver fibrosis leading to cirrhosis and hepatic failure.
- PBC primarily affects middle-aged women and can present with cholestasis (e.g., jaundice, pruritus, xanthomas), hepatomegaly, and cirrhosis with portal hypertension, ascites, and gastrointestinal bleeding. PBC is often associated with other autoimmune disorders such as Sjögren syndrome, arthropathy, CREST syndrome (calcinosis, Raynaud's phenomenon, esophageal dysmotility, sclerodactyly, and telangiectasia), and autoimmune thyroiditis.
- In developed countries, most cases are asymptomatic at presentation and detected by abnormal LFT results. Most

commonly, markers of cholestasis, such as elevation of ALP and GGT, are seen. Less commonly, the patient presents with jaundice and conjugated hyperbilirubinemia. When the disease progresses to marked liver fibrosis and cirrhosis, markers of hepatocyte damage, such as mildly elevated aminotransferases, can be detected. With the development of hepatic insufficiency, hypoalbuminemia, prolonged prothrombin time, and elevated conjugated and unconjugated bilirubin can be seen. Hyperbilirubinemia is a sign of advanced or severe disease and an indicator for the possibility of liver transplantation.

- Antimitochondrial antibodies (M2, M4, M8, M9) are present in all patients with PBC and remain a pathognomonic hallmark of the diagnosis. Anti-M2 antibodies are directed against the pyruvate decarboxylase complex (PDC) in the inner mitochondrial membrane, and M4, M8, and M9 bind to the outer membrane. In 90% to 95% of cases, autoantibodies directed against the lipoyl domain of the E2 subunit of mitochondrial PDC are present. Anti-M2 antibodies can also be directed against other members of the PDC complex, including the E2 subunit of the branched-chain 2-oxoacid dehydrogenase complex, the E2 subunit of the 2-oxoglutarate dehydrogenase complex, E1t α-subunits of PDC, and E3-binding protein (protein X). Other mitochondrial targets of autoantibodies present in PBC include the β- and γ-subunits of F1F0 adenosine triphosphatase and sulfite oxidase (M4).
- Although antimitochondrial antibodies are very sensitive for the diagnosis of PBC, they are not entirely specific. First, they can present many years in advance of significant hepatic disease, although in this case they can serve as a predictor for development of PBC. Second, they can be present in other autoimmune disorders, including Sjögren syndrome, scleroderma, autoimmune hepatitis, and infectious diseases such as viral hepatitis and tuberculosis.
- The pathogenesis of PBC implicates liver-infiltrating autoreactive T cells against the dominant PDC-E2 autoantigen. Levels of antimitochondrial antibodies reflect the B-cell response and do not correlate with the severity of disease.
- Antinuclear antibodies, directed against pore glycoprotein 210, nuclear protein p62, sp100 proteins, promyelocytic leukemia protein, NDP52, and sp140 proteins, can be positive in about 50% of the minority of patients (5% to 10%) without detectable antimitochondrial antibodies.[14,17,24]

41. A. No reflex test is needed.
Rationale: A positive result on the anti-HAV total assay indicates the presence of antibodies, and it should be determined whether they are immunoglobulin M (IgM) (as in acute infection) or immunoglobulin G (IgG) (as in chronic/past infection).
B. Hepatitis A IgM testing.
Rationale: Anti-HAV IgM indicates an acute infection and is the appropriate reflex test if an assay for total anti-HAV antibodies is used as the initial screen for HAV. If the anti-

HAV IgM test result is negative, one can assume that anti-HAV IgG is positive, which is indicative of a past/chronic infection.
C. Hepatitis A IgA testing.
Rationale: There is not a routinely used or available test.
D. Hepatitis D IgG testing.
Rationale: Hepatitis D is associated with hepatitis B infection, not hepatitis A.
E. Hepatitis A nucleic acid testing.
Rationale: Nucleic acid testing for HAV is *not* approved by the U.S. Food and Drug Administration (FDA) for diagnostic purposes.

Major points of discussion
- There are three serologic assays for anti-HAV antibodies available:
  Total antibodies to HAV
  Only immunoglobulin G (IgG) antibodies to HAV
  Only immunoglobulin M (IgM) antibodies to HAV
  A combination of all or some of these three assays can be used for the laboratory workup of HAV infection.
- In the laboratory diagnosis of HAV infection, one possible algorithm uses a two-step procedure. The first step entails testing for the presence of total (IgG+IgM) anti-HAV antibodies; and if positive, the second step entails testing for the presence of IgM anti-HAV antibodies (indicating acute infection). If the IgM testing is negative, it is assumed that the patient's positive result on the screening test was caused by a chronic or past infection.
- A second possible method for testing uses two separate tests for IgG and for IgM. If this method is used, the test for IgG assesses chronic/past infection, whereas the IgM-based assay is used to assess acute infection.
- HAV is an RNA-based virus. It is transmitted through the fecal-oral route, usually through contaminated food or water or by direct contact with an infected individual. The incubation time is 2 to 6 weeks.
- The diagnosis and detection of HAV infection are routinely performed in the clinical laboratory using only serologic assays, *not* molecular assays. A reverse-transcriptase polymerase chain reaction (RT-PCR)-based approach has been successfully demonstrated in the scientific literature, but is not used in routine clinical practice. This is not the case for HBV and HCV, for which molecular assays are important in the management of infected patients.

42. A. Hepatitis B surface antigen.
Rationale: Hepatitis B surface antigen is the first-line diagnostic test for active HBV infection.
B. Anti–hepatitis B core total antibodies (IgG+IgM).
Rationale: This test indicates current or prior infection.
C. Anti–hepatitis B surface antibodies.
Rationale: This test indicates immunity after infection or vaccination.
D. Anti–hepatitis Be antibody.
Rationale: This test can be used to assess treatment response.
E. Hepatitis B genotyping.
Rationale: Genotyping of the hepatitis viruses is useful for epidemiologic and prognostic purposes.

Major points of discussion

- Hepatitis B virus (HBV) is a DNA-based virus. It is transmitted through contact with blood, semen, and other body fluids. The incubation period is 45 to 160 days.
- The appropriate serologic tests for hepatitis B infection include (1) hepatitis B surface antigen, (2) anti–hepatitis B core protein antibodies, (3) total anti-HBV antibodies, (4) anti–hepatitis B envelope protein antibodies, and (5) anti–hepatitis B core protein immunoglobulin M (IgM) antibodies.
- The first-line diagnostic for acute infection is the detection of hepatitis B surface antigen. A second test useful for assessing acute infection is IgM-based testing for anti–hepatitis B core.
- Several molecular tests are available for hepatitis B. These include tests used for monitoring response, predicting response, detecting mutation, and genotyping for epidemiologic and prognostic purposes.
- Hepatitis D infection is usually associated with hepatitis B infection. Coinfection of the two viruses can result in an unusually aggressive disease characterized by fulminant hepatic failure.

43. A. Recombinant immunoblot assay (RIBA) test for HCV.
Rationale: This is the confirmation test that should be performed after an initial positive screening.
B. HCV genotyping.
Rationale: This test is used to predict the likelihood of a therapeutic response.
C. Anti-HCV immunoglobulin M (IgM) antibodies.
Rationale: This test is not clinically used.

D. Anti-HCV immunoglobulin G (IgG) antibodies.
Rationale: This is the first-line screening test for acute and chronic HCV infection.
E. Hepatitis C surface antigen.
Rationale: There is no such antigen or test available.

Major points of discussion

- HCV is an RNA-based virus that is transmitted primarily through intravenous drug use (in the developed world) and through blood transfusions and unsafe medical procedures (in the developing world). The incubation period has a wide range of 14 to 180 days.
- The first-line screening test for HCV includes anti-HCV antibody testing.
- The Centers for Disease Control and Prevention (CDC) recommend one-time testing for HCV in anyone born between 1945 and 1965, using an HCV antibody test. Those with positive test results should be tested with a molecular test to determine whether an active infection is present.
- In HCV infection, elevated ALT levels, along with positive viral load, are sufficient for treatment initiation.
- Molecular assays for HCV include genotyping assays that are useful for predicting response and/or duration of treatment, and viral load assays. The latter are useful for highly sensitive quantitation, can confirm active infection, can predict response, and can be used for monitoring.

References

1. Alaedini A, Green PH. Autoantibodies in celiac disease. Autoimmunity 2008;41:19–26.
2. Annibale B, Lahner E, Fave GD. Diagnosis and management of pernicious anemia. Curr Gastroenterol Rep 2011;13:518–524.
3. Antunes DM, da Costa JP, Campos SM, et al. The serum D-xylose test as a useful tool to identify malabsorption in rats with antigen specific gut inflammatory reaction. Int J Exp Pathol 2009;90:141–147.
4. Baumann MA, Hanson GA, Reed KD, et al. Massive intravascular hemolysis without serum haptoglobin depletion. Hum Pathol 1985;16:1275–1277.
5. Carroccio A, Verghi F, Santini B, et al. Diagnostic accuracy of fecal elastase 1 assay in patients with pancreatic maldigestion or intestinal malabsorption: a collaborative study of the Italian Society of Pediatric Gastroenterology and Hepatology. Dig Dis Sci 2001;46:1335.
6. Castro-Rodríguez JA, Salazar-Lindo E, León-Barúa R. Differentiation of osmotic and secretory diarrhoea by stool carbohydrate and osmolar gap measurements. Arch Dis Child 1997;77:201–205.
7. Chang JWY, Chung CH. Diagnosing acute pancreatitis: amylase or lipase? Hong Kong J Emerg Med 2011;18:20.
8. Dunn W, Angulo P, Sanderson S, et al. Utility of a new model to diagnose an alcohol basis for steatohepatitis. Gastroenterology 2006;131:1057–1063.
9. Ellis E, Wagner M, Lammert F, et al. Successful treatment of severe unconjugated hyperbilirubinemia via induction of UGT1A1 by rifampicin. J Hepatol 2006;44:243–245.
10. Fabris L, Cadamuro M, Okolicsanyi L. The patient presenting with isolated hyperbilirubinemia. Digest Liver Dis 2009;41: 375–381.
11. Hahn JU, Kerner W, Maisonneuve P, et al. Low fecal elastase 1 levels do not indicate exocrine pancreatic insufficiency in type-1 diabetes mellitus. Pancreas 2008;36:274.
12. Hakeem MJ, ML, Bhattacharyya DN. Acute osteomyelitis presenting as cholestatic jaundice. Scot Med J 2006;51:57.
13. Harrington LK, Mayberry JF. A re-appraisal of lactose intolerance. Int J Clin Pract 2008;62:1541–1546.
14. Hu CJ, Zhang FC, Li YZ, et al. Primary biliary cirrhosis: what do autoantibodies tell us? World J Gastroenterol 2010;16:3616–3629.
15. Imbert-Bismut F, Messous D, Thibault V, et al. Intra-laboratory analytical variability of biochemical markers of fibrosis (Fibrotest) and activity (Actitest) and references ranges in healthy blood donors. Clin Chem Lab Med 2004;42:323–333.
16. Lamers CG, Van Tongeren JH. Comparative study of the value of the calcium, secretin, and meal stimulated increase in serum gastrin to the diagnosis of the Zollinger-Ellison syndrome. Gut 1977;18:128–135.
17. Leuschner U. Primary biliary cirrhosis: presentation and diagnosis. Clin Liver Dis 2003;7:741–758.
18. Lippi G, Plebani M, Di Somma S, et al. Hemolyzed specimens: a major challenge for emergency departments and clinical laboratories. Crit Rev Clin Lab Sci 2011;48:143–153.
19. Lippi G, Valentino M, Cervellin G. Laboratory diagnosis of acute pancreatitis: in search of the Holy Grail. Crit Rev Clin Lab Sci 2012;49:18–31.
20. Luo JC, Hwang SJ, Chang FY, et al. Simple blood tests can predict compensated liver cirrhosis in patients with chronic hepatitis C. Hepatogastroenterology 2002;49:478–481.
21. McArthur HL, Dalai BI, Kollmannsberger C. Intravascular hemolysis as a complication of *Clostridium perfringens* sepsis. J Clin Oncol 2006;24:2387–2388.

22. McRury JM, Barry RC. A modified Apt test: a new look at an old test. Pediatr Emerg Care 1994;10:189–191.

23. Miki K, Morita M, Sasajima M, et al. Usefulness of gastric cancer screening using the serum pepsinogen test method. Am J Gastroenterol 2003;98:735–739.

24. Miyachi K, Hankins RW, Matsushima H, et al. Profile and clinical significance of anti-nuclear envelope antibodies found in patients with primary biliary cirrhosis: a multicenter study. J Autoimmun 2003;20:247–254.

25. Newcomer AD, Hofmann AF, DiMagno EP, et al. Triolein breath test: a sensitive and specific test for fat malabsorption. Gastroenterology 1979;76:6–13.

26. Nyblom H, Berggren U, Balldin J, et al. High AST/ALT ratio may indicate advanced alcoholic liver disease rather than heavy drinking. Alcohol Alcoholism 2004;39:336–339.

27. Pavlidis TE, Pavlidis ET, Sakantamis AK. Advances in prognostic factors in acute pancreatitis: a mini-review. Hepatobiliary Pancreat Dis Int 2010;9:482–486.

28. Ranson JH, Rifkind KM, Roses DF, et al. Prognostic signs and the role of operative management in acute pancreatitis. Surg Gynecol Obstet 1974;139:69.

29. Ren Z, Pang G, Batey R, et al. Non-urease producing in chronic gastritis. Aust N Z J Med 2000;30:578–584.

30. Roberts E, Schilsky M. Diagnosis and treatment of Wilson disease: an update. Hepatology 2008;47:2089–2111.

31. Sepulveda JL. Protein markers for digestive tract tumors. In Sepulveda AR, Lynch JP, editors: *Molecular Pathology of Gastrointestinal Neoplasia*, New York: Springer, 2013, pp 131–148.

32. Sepulveda JL. Challenges in routine clinical chemistry: proteins and enzymes. In Dasgupta A, Sepulveda JL, editors: *Accurate Results in the Clinical Laboratory: A Guide to Error Detection and Correction*, San Diego: Elsevier, 2013, pp 131–148.

33. Strimpakos AS, Cunningham D, Mikropoulos C, et al. The impact of carcinoembryonic antigen flare in patients with advanced colorectal cancer receiving first-line chemotherapy. Ann Oncol 2010;21:1013–1019.

34. Sturgeon CM, Duffy MJ, Stenman UH, et al. National Academy of Clinical Biochemistry laboratory medicine practice guidelines for use of tumor markers in testicular, prostate, colorectal, breast, and ovarian cancers. Clin Chem 2008;54:e11–79.

35. Taupenot L, Harper KL, O'Connor DT. The chromogranin-secretogranin family. N Engl J Med 2003;348:1134–1149.

36. U.S. Preventive Services Task Force: Screening for Colorectal Cancer. Available at www.uspreventiveservicestaskforce.org/uspstf/uspscolo.htm.

37. Udell JA, Wang CS, Tinmouth J, et al. Does this patient with liver disease have cirrhosis? JAMA 2012;307:832–842.

38. Weiss JS, Gautam A, Lauff JJ, et al. The clinical importance of a protein-bound fraction of serum bilirubin in patients with hyperbilirubinemia. N Engl J Med 1983;309:147–150.

39. Wiwanitkit V. Faecal elastase-1 (EL-1) in pediatric patients with cystic fibrosis. J Pediatr 2011;87:273.

CHAPTER 6

CLINICAL CHEMISTRY: Toxicology and Therapeutic Drug Monitoring

Serge Cremers

QUESTIONS

1. A 5-year-old child is admitted to the hospital with hypertension, tachycardia, pruritus, poor muscle tone, and a desquamating, erythematous rash of the palms and soles. Plasma norepinephrine (NE) = 1250 pg/mL (reference range, 85 to 1252 pg/mL); urine NE = 360 nmol/mmol creatinine (Cr) (reference range, <59 nmol/mmol Cr); urine epinephrine = 110 nmol/mmol Cr (reference range, <22 nmol/mmol Cr). Chest radiography and ultrasound show no tumor, and iodine-131 scan shows normal adrenal glands and no extrarenal pheochromocytoma. Which one of the following might have caused the symptoms in this child?
   A. Acute iron poisoning.
   B. Acute arsenic poisoning.
   C. Acute mercury poisoning.
   D. Acute lead poisoning.

2. A 16-year-old female patient with borderline personality disorder presented to the emergency department at 6 AM, claiming she took "a lot of acetaminophen pills" the night before. Acetaminophen concentration in a plasma sample collected immediately after admission is 210 µg/mL with normal liver function tests (Figure 6-1). She denies chronic use of alcohol or acetaminophen. Which one of the following courses of treatment would you advise?
   A. Do nothing at this time; repeat acetaminophen measurement after a few hours and monitor serum levels of liver function tests.
   B. Do nothing at this time; patients with borderline personality often present after taking approximately ten 500-mg tablets of acetaminophen.
   C. Confirm the acetaminophen serum level by mass spectrometry.
   D. Immediately start treatment with N-acetylcysteine (i.e., Mucomyst).
   E. Immediately start treatment with fomepizole (Antizol).

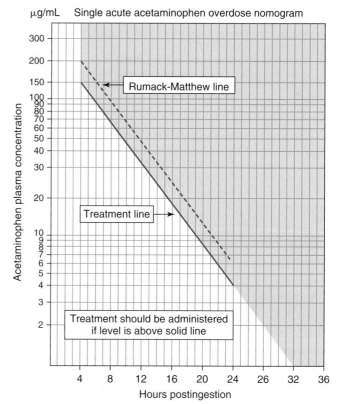

µg/mL   Single acute acetaminophen overdose nomogram

Acetaminophen plasma concentration

Rumack-Matthew line

Treatment line

Treatment should be administered if level is above solid line

Hours postingestion

Figure 6-1 Rumack-Matthew nomogram. A semi-logarithmic plot of serum acetaminophen concentration versus time after a single acute ingestion. The nomogram has been developed to estimate the probability of whether a plasma acetaminophen concentration in relation to the interval after ingestion will result in hepatotoxicity and, therefore, whether acetylcystine therapy should be administered. Cautions when using this chart: (1) Time coordinates refer to time after ingestion. (2) The graph relates only to plasma concentrations after a single, acute overdose ingestion. (3) The treatment line is plotted 25% below the Rumack-Matthew line to allow for potential errors in plasma acetaminophen assays and estimated time from ingestion of an overdose. (From Ford M, Delaney KA, Ling L, et al. *Clinical Toxicology.* Philadelphia, WB Saunders, 2001, pp 265–274.)

Table 6-1

	Result	Reference Range	Units
pH	7.14	7.35-7.45	
P_{CO_2}	16	32-45	mm Hg
P_{O_2}	120	72-104	mm Hg
HCO_3	10	32-45	mmol/L
Ca	9.2	8.7-10.2	mg/dL
Na	140	136-146	mmol/L
K	4.3	3.5-5.0	mmol/L
Cl	102	102-109	mmol/L
Cr	1.2	0.6-1.2	mg/dL
BUN	12	7-20	mg/dL
Glucose	75	75-115	mg/dL
Osmolality	354	275-295	mOsm/kg
Albumin	4.5	3.5-4.5	mg/dL
AST	25	12-38	U/L
ALT	30	7-41	U/L
Total bilirubin	0.8	0.1-0.4	mg/dL
CK	600	51-294	U/L

ALT, alanine aminotransferase; AST, aspartate aminotransferase; BUN, blood urea nitrogen; CK, creatine kinase.

3. A 52-year-old man with a history of alcohol use is brought into the emergency department in a coma (Glasgow Coma Scale score of 6). His cleaning lady found him on the kitchen floor in his home that morning. He has no history of psychiatric illness. He has difficulty breathing and a blood pressure of 120/60 mm Hg. Urinalysis is normal. A tier I toxicology screen is negative. His blood ethanol level is 250 mg/dL. Other laboratory results are provided in Table 6-1. Which one of the following is the most likely diagnosis?
  A. Ethanol intoxication.
  B. Combined ethanol and methanol intoxication.
  C. Ethylene glycol intoxication.
  D. Isopropanol intoxication.
  E. Combined ethanol and isopropanol intoxication.

4. A 48-year-old man (body weight, 80 kg) is treated once daily with intravenous gentamicin, 400 mg in a 30-minute infusion. After 3 days, the peak gentamicin concentration (1 hour after the start of the infusion) is 25 mg/L, and the trough concentration (30 minutes before the start of the infusion) is 1.5 mg/L. The target ranges are 15 to 20 mg/L for the peak level and 0.5 to 1 mg/L for the trough levels. What would be a once-daily dose regimen for this patient to achieve peak and trough levels within the target range?
  A. 400 mg once daily.
  B. 350 mg once daily.
  C. 300 mg once daily.
  D. 250 mg once daily.

5. A 50-year-old schizophrenic patient is treated with aripiprazole, 20 mg orally once daily. After several weeks, a predose blood sample is collected and aripiprazole and dehydroaripiprazole serum concentrations are measured as 200 µg/L and 76 µg/L, respectively. During a subsequent apparent manic episode, his psychiatrist decides to add oxazepam, 10 mg three times daily, and carbamazepine, 100 mg three times daily, as additional therapy. Aripiprazole and dehydroaripiprazole levels are then measured as 74 and 24 µg/L, respectively. Which one of the following best explains the altered antipsychotic drug levels?

  A. A metabolic interaction with oxazepam.
  B. A metabolic interaction with carbamazepine.
  C. Altered protein binding.
  D. CYP2D6 polymorphism (i.e., rapid metabolizer).
  E. CYP3A4 polymorphism (i.e., rapid metabolizer).

6. A urine sample of a 34-year-old female patient is examined by gas chromatography–mass spectrometry (GC-MS) after deglucuronidation, liquid/liquid extraction, and derivatization (Table 6-2 and Figure 6-2). Which one of the following compounds was definitely present in this patient's urine?
  A. Morphine.
  B. Fentanyl.
  C. THC-COOH (tetrahydrocannabinol carboxylic acid).
  D. Benzoylecgonine (BEG).
  E. Methadone.

Table 6-2

Substance	r_t (min)	Characteristic Ions (m/z)	LLOD (ng/mL)	LLOQ (ng/mL)
Cocaine-D3	3.596	185, 201, 306	—	—
EDDP-TMS	3.201	277, 262, 220, 200	100	200
Methadone	3.445	72, 165, 223, 294	10	25
Pentazocine-TMS	3.734	274, 289, 342, 357	10	25
Cocaine	3.613	182, 198, 272, 303	10	25
Cocaethylene	3.758	196, 82, 317	10	25
BEG-D3-TMS	3.775	243, 259, 364	—	—
BEG-TMS	3.784	240, 361, 256	25	50
Morphine-D3-2TMS	4.351	432, 404, 417	—	—
Codeine-TMS	4.236	178, 196, 234, 371	10	25
Morphine-2TMS	4.360	429, 236, 414, 401	10	25
O-6-MAM-TMS	4.499	399, 287, 340, 355	10	25
Norbuprenorphine-2TMS	5.627	468, 500, 510, 524, 557	2	5
Buprenorphine-TMS	6.065	450, 482, 506, 524, 539	2	5
THC-COOH-D3-2TMS	4.770	374, 476, 491	—	—
THC-COOH-2TMS	4.777	371, 473, 488	5	10
Fentanyl-D5	4.798	250, 194	—	—
Norfentanyl-TMS	3.230	155, 154, 247, 289, 304	10	25
Fentanyl	4.800	245, 146, 189, 202	5	10
Sufentanyl	4.927	289, 140, 187, 238, 289	2	5
Alfentanyl	5.185	289, 222, 268, 359	5	10

From Strano-Rossi S, Bermejo AM, de la Torre X, Botrè F. Fast GC-MS method for the simultaneous screening of THC-COOH, cocaine, opiates and analogues including buprenorphine and fentanyl, and their metabolites in urine. *Anal Bioanal Chem* 2011;399:1623–1630.
LLOD, lower limit of detection; LLOQ, lower limit of quantification.

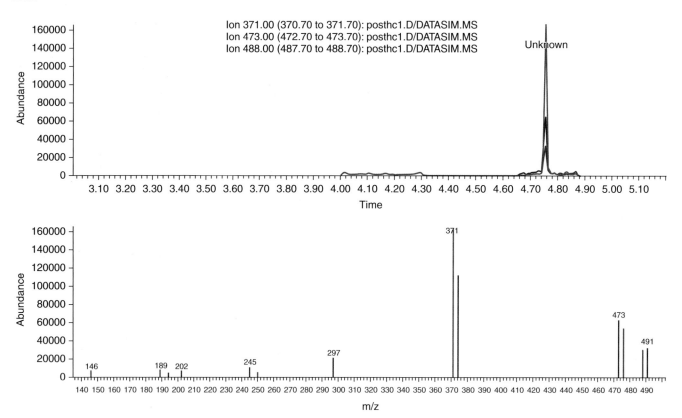

Figure 6-2 Compound table and gas chromatography–mass spectrometry chromatogram (GC-MS). Extracted ion GC-MS chromatogram. (From Strano-Rossi S, Bermejo AM, de la Torre X, Botrè F. Fast GC-MS method for the simultaneous screening of THC-COOH, cocaine, opiates and analogues including buprenorphine and fentanyl, and their metabolites in urine. *Anal Bioanal Chem* 2011;399:1623–1630).

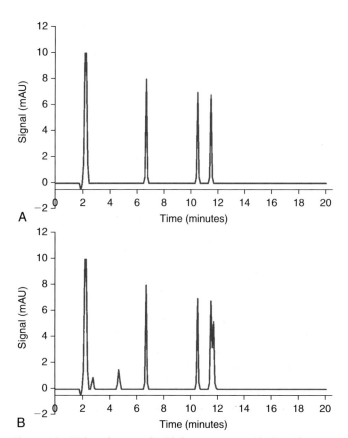

Figure 6-3 High-performance liquid chromatograms with ultraviolet detection (at 254 nm) of amitriptyline ($t_r = 11.5$ min), nortriptyline ($t_r = 10.5$ min), and the internal standard clovoxamine ($t_r = 6.7$ min). **A,** Control run; **B,** Evaluation of the patient sample. t_r, Retention time.

7. Amitriptyline and its desmethyl metabolite, nortriptyline, were measured in the plasma of a 42-year-old white woman with depression who had been taking amitriptyline tablets for 1 week. The blood sample was collected before the next dose. A high-performance liquid chromatography (HPLC) chromatogram of a calibrator with amitriptyline and nortriptyline plasma concentrations of 100 ng/mL is shown in panel A of Figure 6-3. The HPLC chromatogram of the patient sample is shown in panel B. Which one of the following is the cause for the difference in the shape of the amitriptyline peak when comparing panels A and B?

A. A deteriorating ultraviolet (UV) light detector.
B. The presence of an unknown interfering compound.
C. A deteriorating HPLC column.
D. The presence of an amitriptyline enantiomer.
E. Evaporation of solvent.

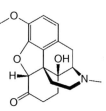

Figure 6-4 Chemical structure of an unknown compound.

8. The compound depicted in Figure 6-4 is which one of the following?
   A. A barbiturate.
   B. A benzodiazepine.
   C. A tricyclic antidepressant.
   D. An opioid.
   E. A selective serotonin reuptake inhibitor (SSRI).

9. Which one of the following drugs will most likely be detected in urine by automated immunoassay (i.e., tier I testing)?
   A. Lysergic acid diethylamide (LSD).
   B. γ-Hydroxybutyrate (GHB).
   C. Hydromorphone.
   D. Oxycodone.
   E. Mephedrone.

10. Tier I toxicology testing for drugs of abuse is usually performed by automated immunoassays. Which one of the following is the most common method currently used for tier II confirmatory testing?
    A. Quadrupole time of flight–liquid chromatography–mass spectrometry (qTOF-LC-MS).
    B. High-performance liquid chromatography with diode-array detection (HPLC-DAD).
    C. Liquid chromatography–mass spectrometry/mass spectrometry (LC-MS/MS).
    D. Gas chromatography with single quadrupole mass spectrometry (GC-MS).
    E. Gas chromatography with nitrogen-phosphorus detection (GC-NPD).

11. A 62-year-old male patient has been on amiodarone therapy (300 mg per day) for several months. His plasma amiodarone and desethylamiodarone concentrations measured by liquid chromatography–tandem mass spectrometry (LC-MS/MS) are 1.5 and 0.8 mg/L, respectively (reference ranges, 1.0 to 2.5 mg/L for amiodarone and 1 to 4 mg/L for amiodarone and desethylamiodarone together). To improve control of the patient's cholesterol levels, his physician accidentally prescribed simvastatin, despite the increased risk for myopathies resulting from this combination of drugs. However, because the prescribing physician remembered a potential interaction between simvastatin and amiodarone, he again checked the patient's amiodarone level 3 days after starting simvastatin. At that time, the plasma concentrations of amiodarone and desethylamiodarone were 1.6 and 0.9 mg/L, respectively. Which one of the following is the best explanation of the patient's most recent amiodarone and desethylamiodarone levels?
    A. Amiodarone and desethylamiodarone are within the reference range; therefore, the amiodarone dosage does not need to be adjusted.
    B. The desethylamiodarone concentration is within the reference range; therefore, the risk of developing amiodarone-induced pulmonary toxicity is minimal.
    C. Simvastatin inhibits biliary excretion of amiodarone.
    D. Simvastatin inhibits the metabolism of amiodarone.
    E. The blood sample was collected too soon after starting simvastatin to make any definitive conclusions regarding potential interactions between these drugs.

12. A 42-year-old man with manic depression was traveling in Malaysia for the past several weeks and is brought to the emergency department after he was found by his sister in his apartment. He is comatose (Glasgow Coma Scale score of 6) with blood pressure of 124/76 mm Hg, heart rate of 92 beats/min, temperature of 38°C, and respiratory rate of 4 breaths/min. His skin is dry and he has dilated pupils. The electrocardiogram shows normal sinus rhythm with a QRS of 148 msec (normal, <0.1 msec). His regular medications include lithium, amitriptyline, and oxazepam, which he has been taking for more than 1 year. Relevant laboratory results, including a tricyclic antidepressant level measured by immunoassay, are as shown in Tables 6-3, 6-4, and 6-5.

Table 6-3

	Result	Reference Range	Units
pH	7.22	7.35-7.45	
P_{CO_2}	61	32-45	mm Hg
Na	139	136-146	mmol/L
K	4.8	3.5-5.0	mmol/L
Cl	105	102-109	mmol/L
HCO_3	24.6	32-45	mmol/L
Creatinine	0.8	0.6-1.2	mg/dL
Glucose	80	75-115	mg/dL

Table 6-4

	Result
Ethanol	Negative
Benzodiazepines	Positive
Barbiturates	Negative
Opiates	Negative
Cocaine	Negative
Tetrahydrocannibinol	Negative

Table 6-5

	Result	Therapeutic Range	Units
Acetaminophen	Negative	10-30	µg/mL
Amitriptyline +nortriptyline	250	95-250	ng/mL
Acetylsalicylic acid	Negative	2-30	mg/dL
Lithium	0.72	0.6-1.2	mmol/L

Testing for tricyclic antidepressants other than amitriptyline was negative. Assuming there has not been a sample mix-up, which one of the following would be of the most benefit to this patient at this moment?
A. A pseudocholinesterase assay.
B. Toxicologic screening by GC-MS.
C. A methanol assay by gas chromatography (GC).
D. Toxicologic screening for amphetamines.
E. No additional testing is needed at this time.

13. A 28-year-old man with no prior history of psychosis was brought to the emergency department after his roommate reported he was standing on his bed screaming that there were snakes everywhere. The roommate also reported that the patient had "snorted a couple of lines of bath salts." The patient was tachycardic with a heart rate of 144 beats/min. An electrocardiogram showed occasional premature ventricular contractions and a corrected QT interval (QTc) of 430 msec (normal male, <430 msec; female, <450 msec). His temperature was 100.8°F and his pupils were dilated. Standard hematology, chemistry, and liver function tests were normal. Serum levels of acetaminophen and salicylate were negative. A blood alcohol level was also negative. A tier I urine screening test for drugs of abuse (DOA) was negative. Which one of the following best explains why the tier I urine screening test was negative?

  A. The bath salts contained cocaine, which is not detected by tier I DOA screening assays.

  B. The bath salts contained methamphetamine, which is not detected by tier I DOA screening assays.

  C. The bath salts contained oxycodone, which is not detected by tier I DOA screening assays.

  D. The bath salts contained 3,4-methylenedioxymethamphetamine (MDMA), which is not detected by tier I DOA screening assays.

  E. The bath salts contain mephedrone, which is not detected by tier I DOA screening assays.

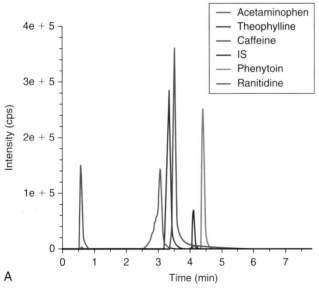

A

Figure 6-5 Chromatograms and a calibration line for caffeine. **A.** Chromatogram for acetaminophen, theophylline, caffeine, an internal standard *(IS)*, phenytoin, and ranitidine (all contained in a methanol solution containing 500 ng/mL of each analyte).

Continued

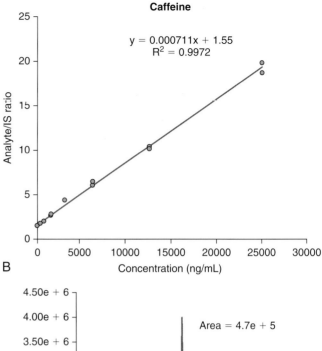

B

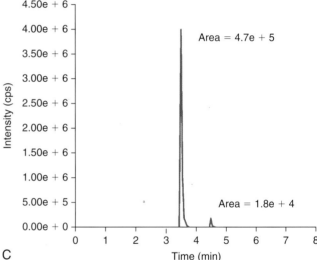

C

Figure 6-5, cont'd   B, Calibration line for caffeine. **C,** Chromatogram of the patient's serum sample.

14. A 1625-g white male baby was delivered by cesarean section at a gestational age of 34 weeks. The neonate showed signs of respiratory insufficiency necessitating artificial ventilation for 5 days. Apnea was treated with caffeine (10 mg/kg as a loading dose followed by a dose of 2.5 mg/kg once daily). On the seventh day after birth, he was transferred to another hospital. There were no changes in therapy, but 2 days after admission to the new hospital, the infant's condition deteriorated. Tachypnea, tachycardia, compromised circulation, vomiting, and convulsions were seen. A serum level of caffeine was determined by LC-MS/MS. The therapeutic range is 5 to 20 mg/L. Which one of the following represents the best explanation for this patient's symptoms and the accompanying data (Figure 6-5)?

  A. Caffeine intoxication.

  B. Subtherapeutic caffeine level.

  C. Acetaminophen intoxication.

  D. Phenytoin intoxication.

  E. Theophylline intoxication.

15. A 43-year-old depressed male farmer is brought to the emergency department by his wife after she found him in the barn 2 hours earlier. His symptoms included chest pain, dyspnea, and cough, accompanied by abundant secretion, blurred vision, constricted pupils, sweating, hypersalivation, hypotension, bradycardia, and fasciculations. A basic metabolic panel, liver function tests, and blood gases were all normal. Toxicologic screening for tricyclic antidepressants, acetaminophen, salicylate, barbiturates, benzodiazepines, and others drugs of abuse is negative. Despite these negative results, intoxication is still suspected. Which one of the following toxicology tests would you recommend performing with the highest priority?
   A. Serum screening by GC-MS.
   B. A serum butyrylcholinesterase activity assay.
   C. A serum strychnine assay.
   D. A serum clenbuterol assay.
   E. A serum cyanide assay.

16. A 30-year-old schizophrenic patient, who was discharged on olanzapine (15 mg per day) and lorazepam (8 mg per day), was readmitted to a psychiatric ward 10 days later for recurrence of auditory hallucinations and delusions of reference as well as aggressive behavior. His family actively monitors his drug compliance. The patient does not take caffeine-containing liquids or tablets and does not take St. John's wort or activated charcoal. On initial discharge from the hospital, the olanzapine plasma concentration measured by LC-MS/MS was 51.2 ng/mL. On readmission, this level was 15.6 ng/mL, which is below the suggested minimum threshold for therapeutic efficacy of 23.2 ng/mL. Which one of the following is the most likely reason for this fluctuation in this patient's plasma concentration of olanzapine?
   A. His inpatient diet differs from his outpatient diet.
   B. Olanzapine is metabolized by CYP1A2, and he is a slow metabolizer of olanzapine.
   C. Outside the hospital, he takes over-the-counter medication that interacts with olanzapine.
   D. Outside the hospital, he is more mobile, leading to decreased drug levels.
   E. Differences in smoking restrictions inside and outside the hospital lead to differences in drug levels.

Table 6-6

	Result	Reference Range	Units
Na	139	136-146	mmol/L
K	8.1	3.5-5.0	mmol/L
Cl	103	102-109	mmol/L
HCO₃	21	32-45	mmol/L
Creatinine	7.9	0.6-1.2	mg/dL
BUN	118	7-20	mg/dL
Glucose	146	75-115	mg/dL
pH	7.33	7.35-7.45	
Pco₂	35	32-45	mm Hg
Po₂	48	72-104	mm Hg

17. A 65-year-old woman presents to the emergency department with a chief complaint of weakness. She has an approximately 1-week history of increasing shortness of breath and several days of confusion, hallucinations, and minimal urine output. She is afebrile, but in moderate respiratory distress. She is also lethargic but oriented to person and place.

Chest examination revealed bilateral rales, and cardiovascular examination revealed a grade III/VI systolic ejection murmur at the left sternal border, radiating to the left axilla. Her past medical history is significant for adult-onset diabetes, peripheral vascular disease, congestive heart failure, neuropathy, nephropathy, anemia, and osteomyelitis. Her current medications include insulin NPH, 40 IU in the evening; glipizide, 10 mg in the morning; furosemide, 80 mg/day; and enalapril, digoxin, hydralazine, amitriptyline, and temazepam, all in unknown doses. Initial vital signs are blood pressure: 96/60 mm Hg; heart rate: 50 beats/min; respiratory rate: 20 breaths/min; and body weight: 80 kg. Laboratory values are shown in Table 6-6. An electrocardiogram showed wide-complex bradycardia without P waves. Toxicology screen results are: digoxin: 3.8 ng/mL (therapeutic range, 0.8 to 2.0 ng/mL); amitriptyline+nortriptyline: 256 ng/mL (therapeutic range, 95 to 250 ng/mL); and benzodiazepines positive on a urine screen. Which one of the following is the best explanation for her symptoms?
   A. Hyperkalemia resulting from amitriptyline toxicity.
   B. Hypokalemia and nortriptyline toxicity resulting from renal insufficiency.
   C. Hyperglycemia and respiratory acidosis resulting from benzodiazepine intoxication.
   D. Hyperglycemia resulting from insulin toxicity.
   E. Hyperkalemia and digoxin toxicity resulting from renal insufficiency.

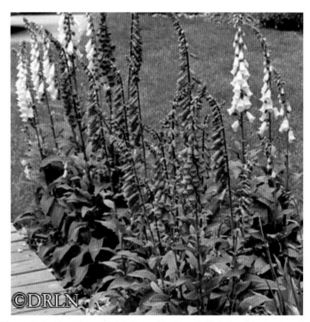

Figure 6-6 Plant from which the patient made "tea."

18. A 6-year-old girl is brought into the emergency department with nausea, vomiting, sinus bradycardia, and a blood pressure of 140/80 mm Hg. She drank "tea" that she made from some leaves she picked in the garden. The plants are shown in Figure 6-6. An assay for which one of the following compounds would most likely be positive in this patient?
   A. Phencyclidine (PCP).
   B. Salicylate.
   C. Cannabis.
   D. Digoxin.
   E. Opiates.

Table 6-7

	Result	Reference Range	Units
Na	128	136-146	mmol/L
K	4.3	3.5-5.0	mmol/L
Cl	105	102-109	mmol/L
HCO_3	28	32-45	mmol/L
Creatinine	1.0	0.6-1.2	mg/dL
BUN	14	7-20	mg/dL
Glucose	105	75-115	mg/dL
Albumin	4.3	3.5-5.5	g/dL
Calcium	9.3	9-10.0	mg/dL
ALT	22	0-35	U/L
AST	20	0-35	U/L
Total bilirubin	0.8	0.3-1.0	mg/dL
Creatine kinase	400	25-90 males	U/L
Lactate	20	5-15	mg/dL
pH	7.35	7.35-7.45	

Table 6-8

	Result	Reference Range	Units
Na	145	136-146	mmol/L
K	5.1	3.5-5.0	mmol/L
Cl	118	102-109	mmol/L
HCO_3	19	32-45	mEq/L
Creatinine	1.5	0.6-1.2	mg/dL
BUN	17	7-20	mg/dL
Glucose	215	75-115	mg/dL
Calcium	9.4	9-10.5	mg/dL
Lactate	42.3	5-15	mg/dL
pH	7.11	7.35-7.45	
P_{CO_2}	6	32-45	mm Hg
P_{O_2}	145	80-100	mm Hg
Lactate dehydrogenase	983	100-190	U/L
Creatine kinase	1515	25-90 in males	U/L
Osmol gap	16	−10 to +10	mOsm/kg
Urinary protein	30	<150	mg/dL

19. At midnight, a 21-year-old man is brought into the emergency department in a coma (Glasgow Coma Scale score of 8) after attending a dance party. On initial evaluation, he had the following vital signs: blood pressure: 85/60 mm Hg; temperature: 38.7°C. Laboratory results are shown in Table 6-7. Serum assays for acetaminophen, salicylate, and alcohol and urine screening for tier I DOA were negative except for the presence of amphetamines. Ingestion of which one of the following party drugs most likely caused the current condition of this patient?
    - A. Cannabis.
    - B. Magic mushrooms.
    - C. GHB.
    - D. Cocaine.
    - E. MDMA (Ecstasy).

20. An adult patient with manic depression is on sustained-release lithium carbonate therapy. She usually has a serum lithium concentration of approximately 0.6 mmol/L (therapeutic range, 0.6 to 1.2 mmol/L). You are consulted for your advice regarding a single recent lithium level of 2.1 mmol/L. The patient has not changed her dose regimen, nor were her other medications changed. The results of her basic metabolic panel were normal. The patient did not have any neurologic or gastrointestinal symptoms. The quality controls for the atomic absorption spectroscopy (AAS) assay performed in your clinical laboratory for lithium were within range. Which one of the following is the best explanation for this isolated elevated lithium level?
    - A. This assay gives higher values than normal.
    - B. This level was elevated because of hyperkalemia.
    - C. This level was elevated because of decreased metabolism of lithium.
    - D. This level was elevated because of decreased renal clearance of lithium.
    - E. This sample was collected in a green-top tube.

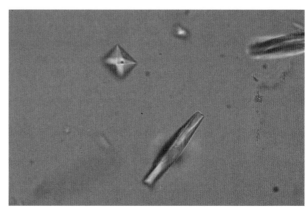

Figure 6-7 Envelope- and needle-shaped crystals. (From Jacobsen D, Hewlett TP, Webb R, et al. Ethylene glycol intoxication: evaluation of kinetics and crystalluria. *Am J Med* 1988;84:150.)

21. A 29-year-old man with a history of psychiatric illness and substance and alcohol abuse presented to the emergency department in a confused state. His routine medications included haloperidol and oxazepam at unknown doses. Initial vital signs were body temperature: 36.1°C; blood pressure: 180/100 mm Hg; heart rate: 110 beats/min; respiratory rate: 50 breaths/min; oxygen saturation: 98%. His pupils were equal, round, and reactive to light. Physical examination revealed a diffusely tender abdomen and hypoactive bowel sounds. Glasgow Coma Scale score was 11. His laboratory results are shown in Table 6-8. Figure 6-7 shows the crystals found in his urine. Which one of the following is the most likely toxicologic explanation for this patient's symptoms?
    - A. Aspirin intoxication.
    - B. Methanol intoxication.
    - C. Combined ingestion of disulfiram and ethanol.
    - D. Isopropanol intoxication.
    - E. Ethylene glycol intoxication.

22. Because of a planned elective surgery and a risk for delayed wound healing, the immunosuppressive regimen of a 47-year-old female kidney transplant recipient (3 years after transplantation) was changed from sirolimus+mycophenolate

mofetil + low-dose prednisolone to tacrolimus + low-dose prednisolone. Her sirolimus trough levels had always ranged between 5 and 8 ng/mL. Her mycophenolate mofetil levels were not monitored. In addition, her serum creatinine is 0.9 mg/dL (reference range, 0.6 to 1.2 mg/dL), and her hemoglobin level is 12 g/dL (reference range, 13.3 to 16.2 g/dL). After 6 days on tacrolimus (3 mg every 12 hours), the trough level measured by the antibody-conjugated magnetic immunoassay (ACMIA) technique run on a Dimension RxL (Siemens, Deerfield, IL) was 6.9 ng/mL. However, after 1 month of treatment, the trough level was 61 ng/mL. A follow-up level the next day was 51 ng/mL. Two days after stopping tacrolimus (the patient remained on low-dose prednisolone), the level decreased to 26 ng/mL. During the next 2 weeks, tacrolimus levels ranged between 19 and 27 ng/mL. Throughout this period, the patient's creatinine and hemoglobin levels remained unchanged. In addition, her liver function tests were normal. At this point, which one of the following is the best recommendation?

A. The patient should remain off tacrolimus until these levels have reached 5 to 10 ng/mL.
B. Tacrolimus should be discontinued, and a different immunosuppressive drug should be started when tacrolimus levels become undetectable.
C. The patient should immediately be started on a different immunosuppressive drug along with prednisolone.
D. The patient should be genotyped for CYP3A4/3A5 polymorphisms.
E. The samples should be retested for tacrolimus using another method.

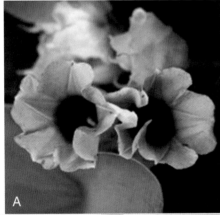
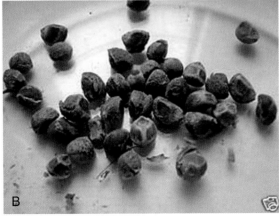

Figure 6-8 **A** and **B**, The Hawaiian baby woodrose plant (*Argyreia nervosa*) and its seeds.

23. You are provided with the urine sample of a 25-year-old man who was a regular cannabis user. He had soaked Hawaiian baby woodrose seeds (Figure 6-8) in water for approximately 3 hours and ingested six of them; he did not smoke marijuana that day. Approximately 40 minutes after ingesting the seeds, he started experiencing a sense of well-being as well as losing track of time. The urine sample was collected 9 hours after ingestion. His friend, a 29-year-old man, also ingested an unknown number of seeds; approximately 3 hours after ingestion, he became severely agitated and jumped out of a window, falling four floors. He was pronounced dead on arrival at the emergency department. Full tier I drug screening (i.e., opiates, cocaine, PCP, LSD, cannabinoids, barbiturates, benzodiazepines, and methadone) was performed on the β-glucuronidase/arylsulfatase–treated urine sample that you received. This was positive for cannabinoids and LSD. Which one of the following reasons best explains the positive results for cannabis and LSD on this urine drug screen?

A. Cannabis was used within the prior 3 weeks, and the seeds contain sufficient amounts of LSD to cause these symptoms and be detectable in urine.
B. Cannabis was used within the prior 3 weeks, and the seeds contain sufficient amounts of LSA (lysergamide), which cross-reacts with some immunoassays for LSD, to cause these symptoms and be detectable in urine.
C. Cannabis was used within the prior 3 weeks, and the seeds contain sufficient amounts of fentanyl, which cross-reacts with some immunoassays for LSD, to cause these symptoms and be detectable in urine.
D. Hawaiian baby woodrose seeds contain sufficient amounts of cannabinoids and fentanyl, which cross-react with some immunoassays for LSD, to cause these symptoms and be detectable in urine.
E. Hawaiian baby woodrose seeds contain sufficient amounts of fentanyl, which cross-reacts with some immunoassays for LSD and cannabis, to cause these symptoms and be detectable in urine.

24. A urine sample from a patient whose mother is suspected of having Munchausen syndrome by proxy is presented for stimulant laxative screening. The urine is from an 8-year-old boy with diarrhea who is otherwise healthy, but who took acetaminophen earlier that day for a headache. His mother, who is a smoker, has a long psychiatric history. There is suspicion of intoxication with Senokot, a senna-containing laxative. The urine sample was collected at the emergency department under observation by the treating physician and arrives in the laboratory a few hours later. The specimen is then sent to a reference laboratory that screens for stimulant laxatives by high-performance thin-layer chromatography (HP-TLC). The HP-TLC results come back as negative. A new sample is collected, again under observation by a physician, and is sent directly to a different reference laboratory that screens for stimulant laxatives by GC-MS. Rhein, the metabolite of senna, is found in this sample. Which one of the following is the best explanation for the negative result using the first sample, assuming that the alleged administration of a laxative has not changed?

A. HP-TLC is an outdated method that is prone to technical errors.
B. Cotinine from second-hand smoke interferes with the HP-TLC method, but not with the GC-MS method.

C. Rhein rapidly degrades in urine, within a few hours, when the sample is kept at room temperature.

D. The senna alkaloids in Senokot are not metabolized to rhein in this patient.

E. The acetaminophen taken for a headache interfered with the detection of rhein by HP-TLC.

25. A 70-year-old woman (body weight, 60 kg) with a history of Waldenström's lymphoma presented with mucosal bleeding. Her bone marrow was 95% replaced by malignant lymphoma cells. She is pancytopenic and febrile (38.5°C). Her white blood cell count is 0.39×10^9/L (reference range, 3.04 to 9.06×10^9/L), hematocrit is 25% (reference range, 38.8 to 46.6%), platelet count is 21×10^9/L (reference range, 165 to 415×10^9/L), relative serum viscosity of 2.3 cP (reference range, 1.4 to 1.8 cP), blood urea nitrogen is 18 mg/dL (reference range, 7 to 20 mg/dL), serum creatinine is 0.7 mg/dL (reference range, 0.6 to 1.2 mg/dL). In addition, an immunoglobulin M-κ monoclonal spike is present on serum protein electrophoresis with a concentration of 42.8 g/L. The patient was started on vancomycin, 1 g intravenously every 12 hours; ceftazidime, 2 g intravenously every 8 hours; and chemotherapy. The volume of distribution and half-life of ceftazidime are 0.23 L/kg of body weight and 1.6 hours, respectively. Ceftazidime shows first-order, one-compartment pharmacokinetics. On day 3, vancomycin and ceftazidime trough concentrations were measured by turbidimetric immunoassay and LC-MS/MS, respectively. The results were as follows: vancomycin, <0.1 mg/L (target trough level, 5 to 10 mg/L); ceftazidime, 4.8 mg/L (peak levels, 159 to 186 mg/L; trough levels not well established). Which one of the following statements best explains these drug levels and identifies which test(s) should follow?

A. Medication errors were made; the patient did not receive either vancomycin or ceftazidime. No additional laboratory tests are indicated.

B. There is a potential interference for the vancomycin assay. Ceftazidime levels are as expected. Recovery experiments should be performed for the vancomycin assay, and this level should be determined by another assay.

C. The sample tube for the vancomycin and ceftazidime assays was mixed up with another tube. A new blood sample should be collected and reevaluated with this assay.

D. The chemotherapeutic agents interfere with the vancomycin turbidimetric immunoassay. Therefore,

dilution and recovery experiments should be performed for the vancomycin assay, and this level should be determined by another assay.

E. The chemotherapeutic agents interfere with the ceftazidime assay. Therefore, dilution and recovery experiments should be performed for the ceftazidime assay, and this level should be determined by another assay.

Table 6-9

	Result	Reference Range	Units
Na	151	136-146	mmol/L
K	4.0	3.5-5.0	mmol/L
Cl	105	102-109	mmol/L
HCO$_3$	25	32-45	mmol/L
Creatinine	1.0	0.6-1.2	mg/dL
BUN	12	7-20	mg/dL
Glucose	90	75-115	mg/dL
ALT	25	0-35	U/L
AST	24	0-35	U/L

26. A 45-year-old woman with manic depression has been receiving haloperidol 5 mg daily, lithium carbonate 800 mg daily, and oxazepam 10 mg twice daily. Several days into a heat wave, her psychiatrist decides to add carbamazepine 200 mg twice daily as a mood stabilizer. Two days later, the patient develops drowsiness, tremors, and muscle weakness. Laboratory values are shown in Table 6-9 Serum chemistry results are carbamazepine = 8 mg/L by immunoassay (therapeutic range, 6 to 12 mg/L), lithium, 1.6 mmol/L by atomic absorption spectroscopy (AAS, therapeutic range, 0.6 to 1.2 mmol/L), haloperidol, 10 ng/mL by LC-MS/MS (therapeutic range, 2.0 to 15 ng/mL). Which one of the following answers best explains the patient's symptoms and represents the most appropriate therapeutic intervention?

A. The patient is a slow metabolizer of carbamazepine. The carbamazepine dose should be reduced.

B. The patient is dehydrated, leading to toxic lithium levels. The lithium dose should be reduced.

C. Carbamazepine induces the metabolism of haloperidol. The haloperidol dose should be reduced.

D. Oxazepam inhibits the metabolism of carbamazepine. The carbamazepine dose should be reduced.

E. Carbamazepine inhibits the metabolism of lithium. The lithium dose should be reduced.

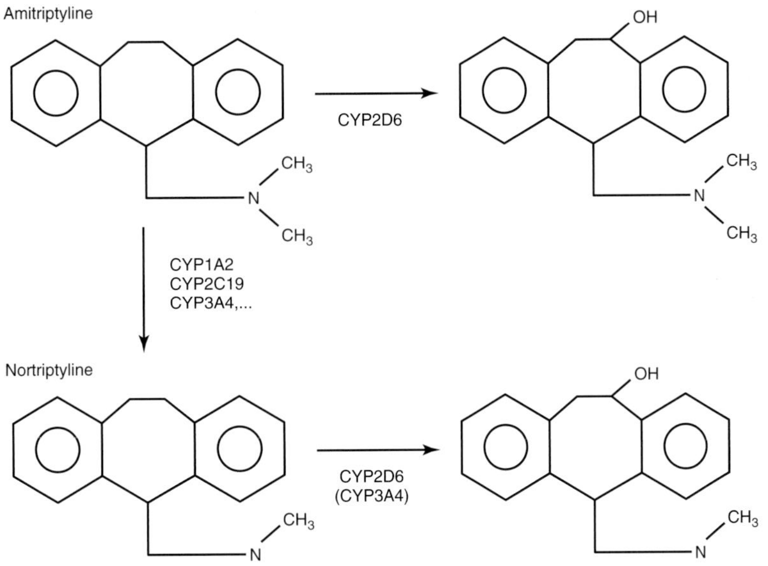

Figure 6-9 Metabolic pathway of amitriptyline and nortriptyline. (Modified from Franssen EJF, Kunst PWA, Bet PM, et al. Toxicokinetics of nortriptyline and amitriptyline: two case reports. *Ther Drug Monitor* 2003;25:248-251.)

27. A 58-year-old man with endogenous depression has been treated with amitriptyline for 3 years. His dose has been 50 mg 3 times per day. He also takes oxazepam (10 mg 3 times per day) and ranitidine (10 mg 2 times per day). Recently, his physician prescribed acetaminophen (500 mg 4 times per day) for back pain. Before treatment with acetaminophen, his amitriptyline and nortriptyline serum levels, as measured by LC-MS/MS, were 125 and 62 ng/mL, respectively (therapeutic range amitriptyline, 120 to 250 ng/mL; amitriptyline +nortriptyline, 150 to 300 ng/mL; Figure 6-9). However, serum concentrations of amitriptyline and its metabolite became subtherapeutic, at 74 and 25 ng/mL, respectively, 1 week after starting acetaminophen therapy. Which one of the following is the best reason for the low serum levels of these tricyclic antidepressants?

    A. Acetaminophen induces increased metabolism of amitriptyline.
    B. Acetaminophen inhibits the metabolism of oxazepam, which then induces increased metabolism of amitriptyline.
    C. Autoinduction of amitriptyline metabolism.
    D. The patient's blood sample was collected in a serum separator tube, rather than in a red-top tube (i.e., without gel).
    E. Acetaminophen displaces amitriptyline from serum albumin.

28. A 42-year-old man with alcoholism (body weight, 72 kg) is brought to the emergency department by ambulance. The patient is suspected to have drunk spiritus saponatus (spirit of soap). GS-MS analysis shows that his blood level of methanol is 495 mg/L. In addition, his blood alcohol level is 800 mg/L. The emergency department has run out of fomepizole, and you advise them to start intravenous ethanol therapy. Using the following information, which one of the following provides the best advice regarding the loading dose and maintenance dose for ethanol (i.e., the D_L and the D_M, respectively)?

$$D_L = V_d \times BW(C_e - C)$$
$$D_M = C_e \times Vmax/(Km + C_e)$$

where D_L=loading dose (mg); V_d=volume of distribution (=0.7 L/kg); BW=body weight (kg); C_e=the target concentration of ethanol (mg/L; the target is 1000 to 1500 mg/L); C=the measured concentration of ethanol; D_M=maintenance dose (mg/hour); Vmax=the maximum enzyme capacity (75 mg/kg/hr for nonalcoholic individuals and 175 mg/kg/hr for alcoholic individuals); Km=the Michaelis-Menten constant (138 mg/L in this case).

    A. D_L=23,000 mg and D_M=11,500 mg/hr.
    B. D_L=23,000 mg and D_M=157 mg/hr.
    C. D_L=11,500 mg and D_M=11,500 mg/hr.
    D. D_L=2,300 mg and D_M=157 mg/hr.
    E. D_L=46,000 mg and D_M=23,000 mg/hr.

29. A 17-year-old girl receives chemotherapy for osteosarcoma. The chemotherapeutic regimen includes high-dose methotrexate (MTX) at 12 g/m^2 in a 4-hour infusion. MTX is measured in plasma by a fluorescence-polarization immunoassay (FPIA) method in samples collected at 24 and 48 hours after completion of the infusion; these concentrations were 15 and 1.8 μmol/L, respectively (toxic level >0.5 μmol/L at 48 hours). Based on these levels, leucovorin is given at a dose of 50 to 100 mg/m^2 every 6 hours. The patient's serum creatinine is normal. According to protocol, a third plasma sample will be collected at 72 hours after completion of the infusion, and leucovorin will need to be continued at the same dose if the MTX plasma concentration at 72 hours is 0.1 to 0.9 μmol/L. Lower concentrations would lead to discontinuation of leucovorin; higher concentrations would lead to a higher dose of the leucovorin. Based on these numbers, which one of the following statements is correct?

    A. At 72 hours, the MTX plasma concentration will be 0.23 μmol/L, and leucovorin treatment will be continued at the same dose.

B. At 72 hours, the MTX plasma concentration will be 1.0 µmol/L, and leucovorin treatment will be continued at the same dose.

C. At 72 hours, the MTX plasma concentration will be 1.0 µmol/L, and leucovorin treatment can be stopped.

D. It is impossible to predict the MTX plasma concentration at 72 hours from knowing the earlier concentrations.

E. At 72 hours, the MTX plasma concentration will be 0.05 µmol/L, and leucovorin treatment can be stopped.

30. Your laboratory measures MTX plasma levels by an FPIA method. You receive a sample from a patient who received high-dose MTX as part of a chemotherapy regimen for lymphoma. Because of a potentially very high MTX concentration in the 96-hour postinfusion sample, it is diluted tenfold and 100-fold. Correcting for the dilutions, the MTX level in the tenfold diluted sample measures as 9.6 µmol/L, whereas the concentration in the 100-fold diluted sample measures as 50 µmol/L (toxic level > 0.5 µmol/L at 48 hours). At the time of the MTX infusion, the patient did not receive any other chemotherapeutic agents. However, the patient's serum creatinine level had risen from a preinfusion level of 0.8 mg/dL (reference range, 0.6 to 1.2 mg/dL) to its current level of 6.8 mg/dL. The patient was hydrated and alkalinized and also received leucovorin and glucarpidase to minimize the side effects of the high-dose MTX therapy. Which one of the following provides the best explanation for the discrepancy in the MTX concentration measured in the two serially diluted plasma samples and the best action to take?

A. FPIA is not an adequate method to measure MTX in samples obtained 96 hours after MTX infusions. Another method should be used.

B. Diluting plasma samples always leads to higher concentrations using an FPIA method. Another method should be used.

C. Leucovorin interferes with measurement of MTX levels by FPIA. Another method should be used.

D. Alkalinization with bicarbonate leads to higher MTX levels after dilution. The pH of the plasma sample should be adjusted before using this FPIA method.

E. Glucarpidase leads to the production of an inactive metabolite of MTX, which produces concentration-dependent cross-reactivity in the FPIA method. Another method should be used.

Table 6-10

	Patient	Reference Range	Units
Na	140	136-146	mmol/L
K	4.3	3.5-5.0	mmol/L
Cl	103	102-109	mmol/L
CO_2	24	22-30	mmol/L
BUN	14	7-20	mg/dL
Cr	6.8	0.6-1.2	mg/dL
Glucose	110	65-95	mg/dL
AST	27	12-38	U/L
ALT	22	7-41	U/L
Total bilirubin	0.9	0.1-0.4	mg/dL

31. A 57-year-old man (body weight, 70 kg) was mechanically ventilated and sedated for 3 days in the intensive care unit with a continuous infusion of midazolam (5 mg/hr). Five days after stopping the infusion, the patient was still comatose. The patient was roused by flumazenil, 0.4 mg. Blood samples were obtained at that time, and his laboratory values are shown in Table 6-10. Analysis of a serum sample by HPLC, which was collected 5 days after stopping the midazolam infusion, showed that midazolam (therapeutic range, 50 to 600 ng/mL) and α-hydroxymidazolam levels were both less than 1 ng/mL. Which one of the following statements best explains these observations?

A. A 5 mg/hr intravenous midazolam infusion for 3 days is, by definition, an overdose.

B. The patient has a single-nucleotide polymorphism in CYP3A5.

C. Pharmacologically active midazolam conjugates accumulate because of renal dysfunction.

D. The hydroxymetabolite of midazolam accumulates because of hepatic dysfunction.

E. Midazolam and its metabolites need to be monitored using samples of whole blood rather than serum.

32. An 8-year-old Hispanic boy (height, 4 feet, 3 inches; body weight, 103 pounds) receives intravenous gentamicin therapy at a dose of 2.5 mg/kg every 8 hours. Peak and trough levels are determined at the third dose, as measured by automated immunoassay. The results are C_{peak} of 12.5 mg/L (therapeutic range, 4 to 12 mg/L) and C_{trough} of 1.1 mg/L (therapeutic range, 1 to 2 mg/L). Serum creatinine and liver enzyme levels are normal. The patient is not in an intensive care unit, nor is he receiving any medications known to affect the pharmacokinetics of gentamicin. Which one of the following is the best explanation for these levels, and what is the best dose recommendation?

A. The patient is obese (BMI = 27.8 kg/m²). In obese patients, gentamicin dosing should be based on lean body mass (LBM), rather than actual body mass. Therefore, 1.5 mg/kg every 8 hours would be a better dose.

B. The current regimen (2.5 mg/kg every 8 hours) is, by definition, an overdose for any individual. Therefore, the dose should be lowered to 1.5 mg/kg every 8 hours.

C. Because the patient is obese, gentamicin is eliminated faster than normally. Therefore, the dose should be raised to 3.5 mg/kg every 8 hours.

D. Glomerular filtration is lower in obese patients, leading to decreased clearance of the drug and increased circulating levels. Therefore, the dose should be reduced to 1.5 mg/kg every 8 hours.

E. Single-nucleotide polymorphisms in the enzyme responsible for metabolizing gentamicin are prevalent in the Hispanic population and result in increased drug levels. Therefore, the dose should be reduced to 1.5 mg/kg every 8 hours.

33. A 20-year-old female kidney transplantation recipient, currently on tacrolimus, mycophenolate mofetil, and prednisone, now receives oral posaconazole (200 mg every 8 hours) for preventing invasive fungal infections. Posaconazole is measured by LC-MS/MS, and a serum trough sample is collected after 1 week of treatment. The posaconazole peak (701.3 > 683.2) in the sample has an intensity of 1.6E9. The internal standard (IS = cyanoimipramine, 306.2 > 218.0) has an intensity of 9.0E9. The calibration line is posaconazole/IS ratio = 0.0110 + 0.422 × Conc (mg/L). Posaconazole has a relatively long half-life (i.e., 31 hours), with a flat concentration time profile. Posaconazole exhibits saturable absorption with difficulties in increasing systemic drug exposure in a linear manner with progressive dosage escalation beyond 800 mg/day. This has been attributed to both the relatively poor solubility of

posaconazole and the action of P-glycoprotein, which continuously pumps the drug from the bloodstream into the gut. Given a target concentration for posaconazole of 0.7 mg/L, which one of the following is the best recommendation for treating this patient?

A. Decrease the dose to 200 mg every 12 hours and monitor the posaconazole level again after 1 week.

B. Decrease the dose to 200 mg every 24 hours and monitor the posaconazole level again after 1 week.

C. Decrease the dose to 200 mg every 12 hours and monitor the posaconazole level again the next day.

D. Increase the dose to 400 mg every 12 hours and monitor the posaconazole level again the next day.

E. Increase the dose to 400 mg every 8 hours and monitor the posaconazole level again after 1 week.

Table 6-11

	Result	Reference Range	Units
Na	148	136-146	mmol/L
K	7.2	3.5-5.0	mmol/L
Cl	107	102-109	mmol/L
HCO₃	11	32-45	mmol/L
Creatinine	0.8	0.6-1.2	mg/dL
BUN	15	7-20	mg/dL
Glucose	87	75-115	mg/dL
Lactate	20	5-15	mg/dL
pH	7.3	7.35-7.45	
Pco₂	20	32-45	mm Hg
Lactate	5.2	5-15	mg/dL
Plasma osmolality	282	285-295	mOsm/kg

34. A mother finds her otherwise healthy 12-year-old daughter in the morning alone in her room. The girl left a farewell note mentioning that the stress at school had become simply unbearable. A medicine bottle is found next to her with no label. The bottle is empty but has some white powder remaining in it and smells somewhat like vinegar. The patient is lethargic but arousable. The patient is hyperventilating (respiratory rate, 70 breaths/min), with a blood pressure of 90/70 mm Hg, a heart rate of 140 beats/min, and a body temperature of 40.2°C. Her laboratory test results in the emergency department are shown in Table 6-11.Which one of the following serum and/or urine assays is most likely to be positive?

A. Salicylate in serum.

B. Opiates in urine.

C. Acetaminophen in serum.

D. Benzodiazepines in serum.

E. Amphetamines in serum.

Table 6-12

	Result	Reference Range	Units
Na	139	136-146	mmol/L
K	4.3	3.5-5.0	mmol/L
Cl	105	102-109	mmol/L
HCO₃	38	32-45	mEq/L
Creatinine	0.8	0.6-1.2	mg/dL
BUN	10	7-20	mg/dL
Glucose	95	75-115	mg/dL
Calcium	8.9	9-10.5	mg/dL
Phosphorus	2.1	3-4.5	mg/dL
Serum protein	7.2	5.5-8.0	g/dL
Albumin	4.5	3.5-5.5	g/dL
ALT	30	0-35	U/L
AST	25	0-35	U/L
Hemoglobin	12.1	12-16 females	g/dL
Platelet count	250	130-400	×10⁹/L
Prothrombin time (PT)	145	12-15.5	seconds
International normalized ratio (INR)	19		
Activated partial thromboplastin time (aPTT)	80	24-35	seconds
Fibrinogen	289	200-400	mg/dL

35. A 48-year-old woman is admitted to the hospital because of recurrent periods of bruising, epistaxis, and hematochezia. The patient denies injury and is not on any medication. There is no personal or family history of abnormal bleeding. Initial laboratory values are as shown in Table 6-12. Platelet aggregation studies were normal. The patient's international normalized ratio (INR) and activated partial thromboplastin time (aPTT) were normalized by treatment with fresh frozen plasma and vitamin K (30 mg IV/day). After discharge, the patient redeveloped episodes of bleeding that successfully responded to fresh frozen plasma and vitamin K. During the daily infusion of 20 mg of vitamin K, her INR was 2.5 with an aPTT of 40 seconds. A temporary halt of the vitamin K therapy to enable evaluation of a possible hemorrhagic coagulopathy resulted in an increase of her INR and aPTT to 6.7 and 52 seconds, respectively, in 2 days. Coagulation tests revealed the following factor levels (reference range for each is 50% to 150%): FII=22.3%, FVII=8.0%, FX=4.4%, FV=130.5%, FIX=28.3%, FVII=15.5%. Protein C was 32.8% and free protein S was 25.8%. There was a prompt correction in vitro of her INR and aPTT after mixing patient and control plasma in a 1:1 ratio. Oral vitamin K (100 mg/day) completely corrected her INR and aPTT. Which one of the following intoxications best explains this clinical picture?

A. Rodenticide.

B. Acetylsalicylic acid.

C. Clopidogrel.

D. Warfarin.

E. Lithium.

36. An 18-month-old child with myelodysplastic syndrome is receiving a preparative chemotherapy-based regimen in preparation for hematopoietic stem cell transplantation. The regimen consists of busulfan, cyclophosphamide, and melphalan. Busulfan is given intravenously once daily for 4 days at a dose of 32 mg (80 mg/m²) per day. Therapeutic drug monitoring, using four blood samples collected on the first day

of the regimen, during which no clinical toxicity is observed, reveals an area under the serum concentration time curve (AUC_{0-24h}) for busulfan of 50 hours × mg/L. An optimal AUC_{0-24h} for busulfan in children is 74 to 82 hours × mg/L. The relationship between AUC_{0-24h} and busulfan dose is known to be linear. Which one of the following is the best recommendation with respect to the subsequent busulfan dosing based on these results?

A. The dose regimen should not be changed for the remaining 3 days.

B. The dose regimen needs to be decreased to 24 mg once daily for the remaining 3 days.

C. The dose regimen needs to be increased to 52 mg once daily for the remaining 3 days.

D. The dose regimen needs to be increased to 80 mg once daily for the remaining three days.

E. Given the risk for clinical toxicity, the busulfan should be stopped immediately.

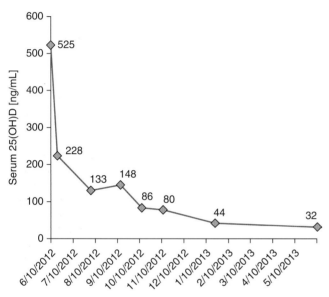

Figure 6-10   Change in 25-OH-vitamin D serum concentrations over time in a 51-year-old man.

37. A 51-year-old man of Dominican origin with newly diagnosed human immunodeficiency virus (HIV) infection was admitted to the hospital with a 3-month history of weight loss, fevers, night sweats, malaise, and a productive cough. Physical examination showed tachycardia, temporal wasting, and diffuse lymphadenopathy. The serum calcium concentration was 15.3 mg/dL (reference range, 9 to 10.5 g/dL), albumin was 3.1 g/dL (reference range, 3.5 to 5.5 mg/dL), and creatinine was 3.5 mg/dL (reference range, <1.5 mg/dL). The patient was found to have active pulmonary infection with *Mycobacterium bovis,* with multiple opacities on chest radiograph. Serum levels of parathyroid hormone (PTH) and parathyroid hormone–related peptide (PTHrP) were undetectable, 25-OH-vitamin D was 85 ng/mL (reference ranges: summer, 15 to 80 ng/mL; winter, 14 to 42 ng/mL), and 1,25-OH-vitamin D was 162 pg/mL (reference range, 25 to 45 pg/mL). After a course of antimycobacterial therapy, intravenous fluids, and glucocorticoids, the patient's serum calcium level stabilized to 11 mg/dL. He was readmitted 18 months later with recurrent *M. bovis* infection. At that time, his serum calcium was 17.1 mg/dL, PTH and PTHrP were again

undetectable, 25-OH-vitamin D was markedly elevated at 525 ng/mL, and 1,25-OH-vitamin D was greater than 180 pg/mL. These results and the temporal changes seen during this admission are shown in Figure 6-10. Which one of the following is the most likely reason for this patient's hypercalcemia and markedly elevated 25-OH-vitamin D levels?

A. HIV infection.

B. *M. bovis* infection.

C. Over-the-counter use of illegal vitamin D supplements.

D. Antiretroviral medications.

E. Antimycobacterial therapy.

38. An HIV-positive man is prescribed lamivudine-zidovudine (Combivir, 300/150 mg) and efavirenz (Stocrin, 600 mg) once daily. One month later, he develops an invasive ocular infection with *Aspergillus fumigatus,* for which he is treated with oral voriconazole, 400 mg twice daily for 1 day and then 200 mg twice daily. After 3 days, 12-hour levels of efavirenz and voriconazole are determined by LC-MS/MS; the concentrations are 4.5 mg/L and 0.11 mg/L, respectively. The therapeutic ranges for these drugs are voriconazole (12 hours after intake), 2 to 6 mg/L; efavirenz (>8 hours after intake), 1 to 4 mg/L. Which one of the following is the best recommendation?

A. Voriconazole inhibits efavirenz metabolism. Therefore, the efavirenz dose should be increased to 900 mg/day.

B. Voriconazole induces efavirenz metabolism. Therefore, the efavirenz dose should be decreased to 300 mg/day.

C. Efavirenz induces voriconazole metabolism. Therefore, the voriconazole dose should be decreased to 100 mg twice daily.

D. Efavirenz inhibits voriconazole metabolism. Therefore, the voriconazole dose should be increased to 400 mg twice daily.

E. Voriconazole inhibits efavirenz metabolism, and efavirenz induces voriconazole metabolism. Therefore, the efavirenz and voriconazole doses should be decreased and increased, respectively.

39. Recently, a local water company installed a new water distribution pipe to a dialysis center. The dialysis center uses high-flux dialysis, which makes dialysis fluid online from tap water. For some reason, the quality of the tap water was not adequately checked after installation of the new water pipe. In addition, several conductivity alarms from the dialysis instruments were misinterpreted as being caused by bubbles. Shortly after the renovation, the patients who underwent dialysis in this center started to show symptoms of "hard water syndrome" and had elevated serum calcium levels. The patients were treated for this syndrome and temporarily underwent dialysis at a different center. However, despite normalization of serum calcium levels, some patients developed transfusion-dependent microcytic anemia. In addition, some patients were admitted to the hospital because of severe neurologic symptoms (e.g., disorientation, myoclonus, convulsions, and coma) after a delay of several days to up to 3 weeks after their last dialysis at the implicated dialysis center. Which one of the following represents the best way to confirm the clinical diagnosis of acute aluminum intoxication?

A. Measure serum aluminum concentrations by HPLC-UV.

B. Measure serum aluminum concentrations by LC-MS.

C. Measure serum aluminum concentrations by AAS.

D. Measure serum aluminum concentrations by isotope ratio mass spectrometry.

E. Measure serum aluminum concentrations by GC-MS.

40. A neonate weighing 845 g is currently receiving intravenous amikacin (15 mg every 24 hours). Trough (therapeutic range, 4.0 to 8.0 mg/L) and peak (therapeutic range, 20 to 30 mg/L) levels collected before and shortly after the second dose are measured by automated immunoassay and are 15 and 48 mg/L, respectively. Given these levels, which one of the following recommendations regarding dosing is best?

A. Do not change the dose regimen.

B. Change the dose regimen to 10 mg every 24 hours.

C. Change the dose regimen to 10 mg every 36 hours.

D. Change the dose regimen to 20 mg every 24 hours.

E. Change the dose regimen to 30 mg every 36 hours.

41. A 43 year-old man suffering from refractory schizophrenia is currently taking the following medications: oxazepam (10 mg three times daily), fluvoxamine (50 mg three times daily), and clozapine (50 mg once daily). The clozapine and fluvoxamine serum concentrations measured by high-performance liquid chromatography with ultraviolet detection (HPLC-UV) are 324 and 108 ng/mL, respectively (therapeutic ranges: clozapine, 200 to 350 ng/mL; fluvoxamine, 50 to 250 ng/mL). The patient is 6 feet, 4 inches tall and weighs 187 pounds. Laboratory tests of liver function and renal function are all normal. In an attempt to simplify the drug therapy, his psychiatrist decides to change his SSRI to paroxetine (20 mg once daily), an event that increases the patient's smoking habit to 12 cigarettes per day instead of his usual 10 per day. Several weeks later, the patient finds that he is experiencing substantially more delusions and hallucinations. The clozapine and paroxetine serum concentrations are 98 and 48 ng/mL, respectively (the therapeutic range for paroxetine is 20 to 200 ng/mL). Which one of the following best explains these clinical events?

A. The patient has subtherapeutic paroxetine serum concentrations because of a drug-drug interaction with oxazepam.

B. The patient has subtherapeutic clozapine serum concentrations because of smoking an increased number of cigarettes.

C. The patient has subtherapeutic clozapine serum concentrations because of a drug-drug interaction with fluvoxamine.

D. The patient has subtherapeutic clozapine serum concentrations because of a drug-drug interaction with paroxetine.

E. The patient has subtherapeutic fluvoxamine serum concentrations because of a drug-drug interaction with oxazepam.

42. A 28-year-old man takes 30 mg of codeine as an analgesic. He is also taking omeprazole and acetaminophen. The patient complains of a lack of analgesic effect of the codeine. A blood sample is therefore obtained 2 hours after codeine intake to measure codeine and its metabolites by a validated LC-MS/MS method. The codeine plasma concentration was within the therapeutic range (34 ng/mL), but the concentrations of its metabolites (i.e., morphine, morphine-3-glucuronide, and morphine-6-glucuronide) were all less than 1 ng/mL. Typically, the levels of these compounds should be approximately 1.5, 45, and 12 ng/mL, respectively. Which one of the following is the best explanation for these observations?

A. LC-MS/MS is not a good method to measure drugs and their metabolites simultaneously.

B. Morphine and its metabolites are not stable in plasma.

C. Omeprazole inhibits the metabolism of codeine to morphine.

D. Acetaminophen inhibits the metabolism of codeine to morphine.

E. The patient is a poor metabolizer of codeine (CYP450 CYP2D6).

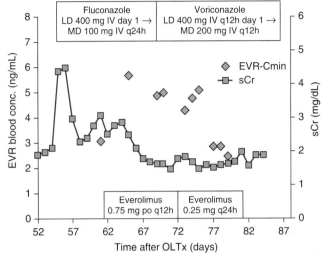

Figure 6-11 Trough blood concentrations of everolimus *(EVL)* and serum creatinine *(SCr)* during cotreatment with fluconazole and voriconazole in a patient after orthotopic liver transplantation *(OLTx)*. LD, Loading dose; MD, maintenance dose.

43. An orthotopic liver transplant (OLTx) recipient, who was previously taking cyclosporine and mycophenolate mofetil, was readmitted on post-transplantation day 55 with severe sepsis and acute renal failure. Empirical wide-spectrum antimicrobial therapy with piperacillin-tazobactam, teicoplanin, and fluconazole was started, and immunosuppressant therapy was temporarily withdrawn. After partial recovery, everolimus was started. Concomitant treatments included ranitidine, heparin, methylprednisolone, octreotide, insulin, and furosemide. In the absence of any published data on appropriate dosing of everolimus during cotreatment with fluconazole, a moderately reduced starting dosage of everolimus (0.75 mg every 12 hours orally) was used, which is a 25% to 50% reduction from the usual dose of 1 to 1.5 mg every 12 hours. Therapeutic drug monitoring of everolimus, measured by FPIA, was planned to maintain the whole blood minimum concentration (C_{min}) within the desired range of 3 to 8 ng/mL. On day 70, the patient was transferred to another hospital. On day 72, antifungal therapy was switched to voriconazole (intravenous loading dose of 400 mg every 12 hours for two doses, followed by maintenance doses of 200 mg every 12 hours) to treat invasive pulmonary aspergillosis. The everolimus dose was reduced to 0.25 mg every 24 hours. The everolimus C_{min}, now measured by LC-MS/MS, was within the range of 3 to 8 ng/mL (Figure 6-11). Which one of the following reasons best explains the relatively higher C_{min} of everolimus during voriconazole treatment?

A. Voriconazole is a stronger CYP3A4 inhibitor than fluconazole.

B. The LC-MS/MS method has a positive bias, yielding higher concentrations than FPIA.

C. Voriconazole displaces everolimus from albumin.

D. The patient had a decline in renal function, decreasing elimination of everolimus.

E. Voriconazole inhibits the enterohepatic cycle of everolimus metabolism.

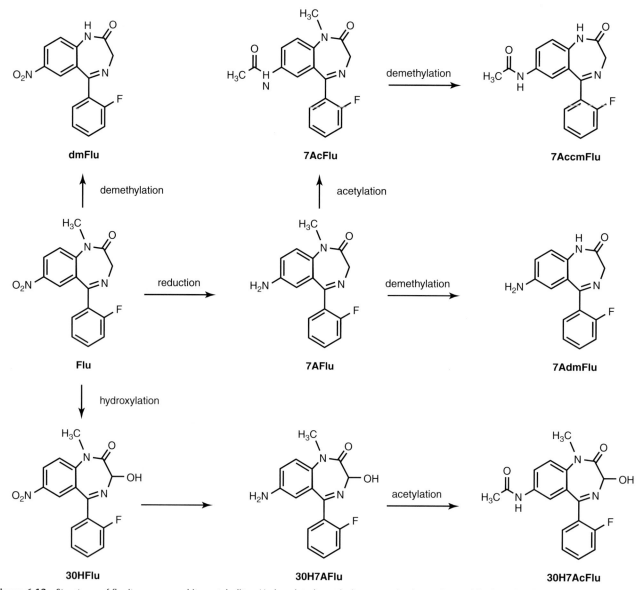

Figure 6-12 Structures of flunitrazepam and its metabolites. Hydroxylated metabolites may also be conjugated further. Flu, flunitrazepam; dmFlu, N-desmethylflunitrazepam; 7AFlu, 7-aminoflunitrazepam; 7Adm-Flu, 7-aminodesmethylflunitrazepam; 7AcFlu, 7-acetamidoflunitrazepam; 7AcdmFlu: 7-acetamidodesmethylflunitrazepam; 3OHFlu, 3-hydroxyflunitrazepam; 3OH7AFlu, 3-hydroxy-7-aminoflunitrazepam; 3OH7-AcFlu, 3-hydroxy-7-acetamidoflunitrazepam. (From Forsman M, Nystrom I, Roman M, et al. Urinary detection times and excretion patterns of flunitrazepam and its metabolites after a single oral dose. *J Anal Toxicol* 2009;33:491–501.)

44. A 28-year-old woman who does not take any medications or drugs awoke in her hotel room a few hours after eating a cookie that was offered to her by a gentleman she met earlier that day. Although she felt fine, her belongings were stolen. After a police investigation, she was taken to the emergency department, where a urine sample was collected approximately 12 hours after the patient ate the cookie. Urine screening for benzodiazepines (with a cutoff 300 µg/L) was negative. Because of a suspected "roofie" intoxication, the sample was treated with β-glucuronidase and reanalyzed by LC-MS/MS; the following concentrations were found: flunitrazepam less than 0.25 ng/mL, 7-aminoflunitrazepam 46 ng/mL, 7-aminodesmethylflunitrazepam 30 ng/mL (Figure 6-12). Based on these results, the best conclusion is that the patient was drugged with which one of the following?

A. Flunitrazepam.
B. Flurazepam.
C. Oxazepam.
D. The patient was not drugged because flunitrazepam was not detectable.
E. The patient was not drugged because the immunoassay was negative.

Table 6-13

	Result	Therapeutic Range	Units
Ibuprofen	17	Not established; peak plasma levels range from 1 to 50 µg/mL	µg/mL
Acetaminophen	18	10-30	µg/mL
Lithium	0.6	0.6-1.2	mEq/L
Lamotrigine	41.4	3-14	µg/mL
Amoxicillin	Undetectable	Not established*	

*Peak plasma levels range from 3.5 to 7.5 µg/mL.

45. A 17-year-old girl with bipolar disorder is transferred to your hospital after a probable suicide attempt in the psychiatric institution where she resides. In the patient's room, empty bottles and strips of lamotrigine, ibuprofen, acetaminophen, amoxicillin, and lithium carbonate were found. She was last observed by a staff member at 5:00 PM and was later found in her room at 8:00 PM unconscious (Glasgow Coma Scale score of 6) with uncontrolled movement of her limbs, dilated pupils, and a normal respiratory rate. She had vomited several times. On arrival in the hospital at 10:00 PM, her vital signs were stable. Laboratory results were as follows: O_2 saturation, 97% (reference range, 97% to 99%); normal P_{O_2} and P_{CO_2}; pH, 7.43 (reference range, 7.35 to 7.45); and base excess, -1.9 mEq/L (reference range, -2 to 2 mEq/L). Electrolytes, liver function tests, and serum creatinine were all normal. On a blood sample, comprehensive toxicologic screening and quantification by LC-MS/MS yielded the drug levels shown in Table 6-13. A blood alcohol level test result was negative. Which one of the following is the best recommendation?
A. Because her symptoms are not explained by any of these levels, do not initiate treatment yet. Because no comprehensive method detects 100% of all possible intoxicants, a comprehensive screen with another method should be initiated.
B. Begin immediate treatment for ibuprofen intoxication.
C. Begin immediate treatment for lithium intoxication.
D. Begin immediate treatment for acetaminophen intoxication.
E. Begin immediate treatment for lamotrigine intoxication.

46. A 52-year-old woman works in a stable at the racetrack. She was thirsty and reached out for a bottle of water and drank about 100 mL at 12:00 noon. She noticed that the water was bitter and was not actually water but, rather, a lead acetate–containing solution used to treat dermatologic afflictions of horses. She then was transported by emergency services to the local hospital. She was asymptomatic at the time of presentation, and a preliminary examination revealed no signs of lead intoxication. Radiographs of the abdomen did not reveal any opacity. A venous blood sample was taken at 1:37 PM on that day. Blood was collected in a lithium heparin Vacutainer tube. The blood lead concentration measured by inductively coupled plasma mass spectrometry (ICP-MS) was 244.7 ng/mL. Which one of the following represents the best course of action?
A. Lead levels measured by ICP-MS are not reliable. The measurement should be repeated by AAS.
B. Lithium heparin Vacutainer tubes can cause artificial increases in blood lead. A new sample should be collected in a different tube.

C. Given that the blood level is already decreasing, no follow-up sample or specific therapy is necessary.
D. Treatment with dimercaptopropane sulfonate sodium (250 mg every 4 hours) should be initiated.
E. Given that the patient is asymptomatic, specific treatment for lead intoxication should be withheld.

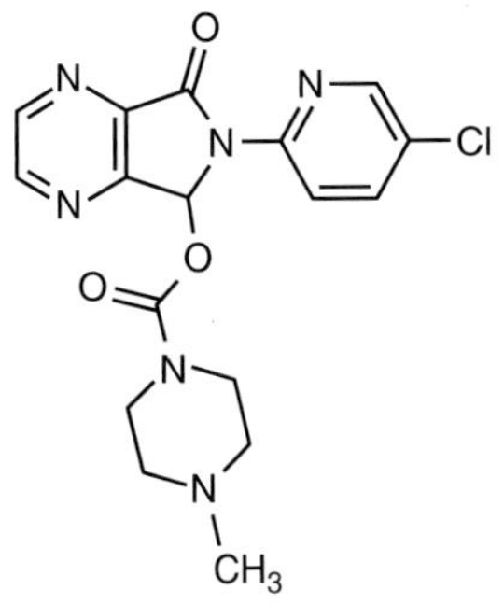

Figure 6-13 Chemical structure of zopiclone, the active ingredient in Lunesta.

47. A 78-year-old woman with osteoporosis takes the following on a daily basis: metoprolol, enalapril, furosemide, alendronate, and zopiclone (Lunesta; Figure 6-13). Which one of the following best explains why a urine benzodiazepine screening immunoassay performed on this patient is negative?
A. Metoprolol interferes with immunoassays for benzodiazepines.
B. Urine samples should be treated with β-glucuronidase before performing an immunoassay for benzodiazepines.
C. Furosemide interferes with the immunoassays for benzodiazepines.
D. None of this patient's medications is a benzodiazepine hypnotic, nor do any of the drugs show cross-reactivity with the immunoassay.
E. Zopiclone acts as a benzodiazepine.

48. A blood sample from a kidney transplant recipient was collected at a random time and sent to the laboratory. Twelve months after transplantation, the patient is on a stable regimen of tacrolimus, prednisolone, and mycophenolate mofetil (MMF). A week previously, the mycophenolic acid (MPA) trough level, as measured by LC-MS/MS, was 2.9 mg/L. The MPA serum concentration, as measured by the same LC-MS/MS method, is now 10 mg/L on the current sample. Which one of the following is the best explanation for this relatively high concentration?
A. MPA was measured in serum but should be measured in whole blood.
B. The current specimen is a randomly collected sample, rather than a trough level.
C. Tacrolimus increases MPA concentrations.
D. Intrapatient variability in MPA pharmacokinetics.
E. Lack of precision of the MPA assay.

49. An ethylenediaminetetraacetic acid (EDTA) blood sample is sent to your reference laboratory for MPA analysis in plasma. The trough sample was collected in a doctor's office, and the sample was sent to you at ambient temperature. The time between sample collection and sample processing is 4 days. The patient's medications include cyclosporine, MMF, and prednisolone. The MPA plasma concentration measured by LC-MS/MS is 5.3 mg/L (reference range, 1 to 3.5 mg/L). Which one of the following is the best recommendation in this case?
    A. Reduce the MMF dose.
    B. Reduce the cyclosporine dose.
    C. Increase the cyclosporine dose.
    D. Rerun this sample.
    E. Collect a new sample from the patient.

50. A 52-year-old female Asian patient (body weight, 57 kg) is receiving intravenous voriconazole (4 mg/kg every 12 hours) to treat a *Candida* species lung infection. A serum trough level collected after 3 days (target range, 2 to 6 mg/L) is measured using a validated and published LC-MS/MS method for azole drugs. The chemical structures of the azole drugs and an example chromatogram are shown in Figures 6-14 and 6-15, respectively. Using this approach, the serum voriconazole concentration is determined to be 0.07 mg/L. The pharmacy and the nurse records show that the patient did indeed receive the intravenous voriconazole at the prescribed dose. In addition, the external quality controls for the LC-MS/MS assay are within range. Which one of the following is the best explanation for this low serum concentration of voriconazole?
    A. Individuals of Asian descent generally have a very large volume of distribution of voriconazole.
    B. Many individuals of Asian descent are ultrarapid extensive metabolizers of voriconazole.
    C. Many individuals of Asian descent are slow metabolizers of voriconazole.
    D. Ion enhancement of the voriconazole signal by unknown compounds in the patient's serum can lead to artificially low measurements of voriconazole concentrations.
    E. Ion suppression of the voriconazole signal by unknown compounds in the patient's serum can lead to artificially low measurements of voriconazole concentrations.

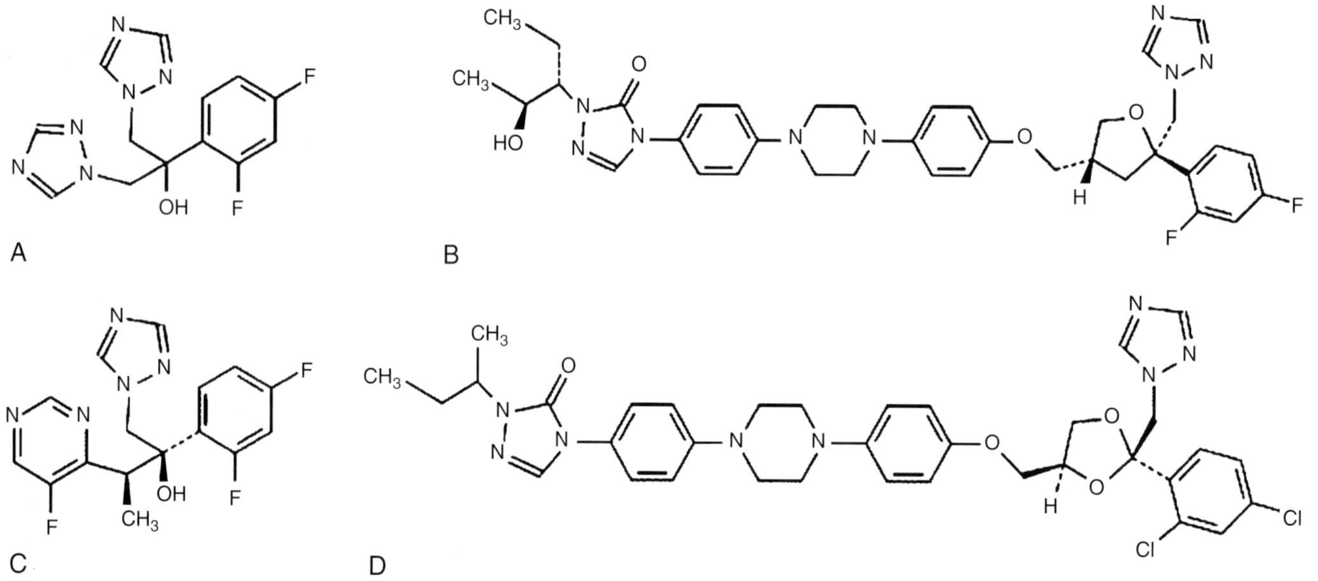

Figure 6-14 Chemical structures of azoles: *a*, fluconazole; *b*, posaconazole; *c*, voriconazole; *d*, itraconazole.

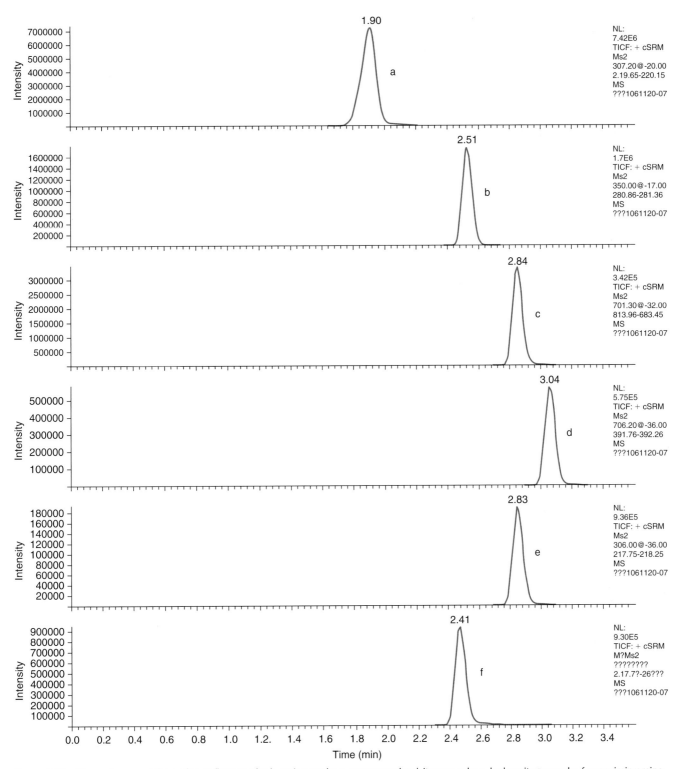

Figure 6-15 Chromatogram of the azoles: *a,* fluconazole; *b,* voriconazole; *c,* posaconazole; *d,* itraconazole; *e,* hydroxyitraconazole; *f,* cyanoimipramine (internal standard).

ANSWERS

1. A. Acute iron poisoning.
Rationale: The symptoms of acute iron poisoning are different from this presentation.
B. Acute arsenic poisoning.
Rationale: The symptoms of acute arsenic poisoning are different from this presentation.
C. Acute mercury poisoning.
Rationale: Mercury poisoning can masquerade as a pheochromocytoma.
D. Acute lead poisoning.
Rationale: The symptoms of acute lead toxicity poisoning are different from this presentation.

Major points of discussion
- Acute ingestion of more than 0.5 g of iron can produce severe irritation of the epithelial lining of the gastrointestinal tract and result in hemosiderosis, which may develop into hepatic cirrhosis. Acute iron poisoning can be confirmed by the detection of excessive iron levels in serum and urine.
- Clinical manifestations of acute arsenic intoxication are predominantly gastrointestinal, cardiovascular, neurologic, and renal in nature. A garlic-like odor on the breath or in perspiration is suggestive of arsenic poisoning.
- Mercury inhibits catechol-*O*-methyltransferase, a major enzyme in the metabolism of catecholamines, resulting in hypertension, tachycardia, and sweating. Thus, mercury can masquerade as a pheochromocytoma, which should be ruled out by performing 24-hour urine catecholamine determination and imaging. Mercury can also be measured in blood or urine (reference range, <10 µg/L), but this is of little use because mercury has a short half-life.
- Mercury poisoning (acrodynia or pink disease) has become a rare symptom complex, which can be recognized easily in the fully developed form. In children, apparently low exposure to mercury may lead to overt mercury poisoning through inhalation of mercury vapor, such as from a broken thermometer. Urinary levels of mercury can be "normal" even in case of overt acrodynia.
- Anemia and encephalopathy may occur in cases of acute exposure to massive levels of lead.[40,97,101]

2. A. Do nothing at this time; repeat acetaminophen measurement after a few hours and monitor serum levels of liver function tests.
Rationale: An acetaminophen level of 210 µg/mL should elicit a different response.
B. Do nothing at this time; patients with borderline personality often present after taking approximately ten 500-mg tablets of acetaminophen.
Rationale: The current acetaminophen concentration of 210 µg/mL is sufficiently high to dismiss this possibility.
C. Confirm the acetaminophen serum level by mass spectrometry.
Rationale: There is no need for confirmation at this time.
D. Immediately start treatment with *N*-acetylcysteine (i.e., Mucomyst).
Rationale: The current acetaminophen serum concentration is higher than 200 µg/mL, and it is very likely that the tablets were taken more than 4 hours before collecting the sample.
E. Immediately start treatment with fomepizole (Antizol).
Rationale: Fomepizole is not an antidote for acetaminophen intoxication but rather is used in cases of suspected methanol or ethylene glycol intoxication.

Major points of discussion
- In cases of acetaminophen intoxication, liver function tests should be monitored over time to evaluate hepatotoxicity. Hepatic necrosis typically begins 24 to 36 hours after a toxic ingestion and becomes severe by 72 to 96 hours after ingestion.
- Acetaminophen levels can be monitored to evaluate clearance of the drug (or indicate possible continuing absorption). The half-life of acetaminophen can also be a predictor of outcome, with hepatotoxicity being more probable when the half-life is more than 4 hours and hepatic coma more probable when the half-life is more than 12 hours.
- Gas chromatography–mass spectrometry (GC-MS), liquid chromatography–mass spectrometry (LC-MS), and/or liquid chromatography–mass spectrometry/mass spectrometry (LC-MS/MS) can be used to confirm that acetaminophen was the cause of the overdose. Depending on the assay used, various analytical interferences may occur.
- *N*-acetylcysteine therapy (intravenous and oral) has relatively minor side effects, so therapy can be initiated easily.
- In this case, the acetaminophen serum concentration is higher than 200 mg/L, and it is very likely that the tablets were taken more than 4 hours before collecting the sample. Therefore, according to the Rumack-Matthew nomogram (see Figure 6-1), it is very probable that hepatotoxicity will occur despite normal initial liver function tests. Hepatic necrosis typically begins 24 to 36 hours after a toxic ingestion and becomes severe by 72 to 96 hours after ingestion. Initiation of treatment with *N*-acetylcysteine is indicated. This therapy is most effective when administered well before hepatic injury occurs, as signified by elevations of serum levels of aspartate aminotransferase (AST) and alanine aminotransferase (ALT).[86]

3. A. Ethanol intoxication.
B. Combined ethanol and methanol intoxication.
Rationale: The patient has an osmol gap and a metabolic acidosis with an anion gap and a negative urinalysis. This is most consistent with combined ethanol and methanol intoxication.
C. Ethylene glycol intoxication.
Rationale: The patient has an osmol gap and metabolic acidosis with an anion gap. The absence of oxalate crystals in the urine suggests that ethylene glycol intoxication did not occur.
D. Isopropanol intoxication.
Rationale: Isopropanol generally does not lead to a metabolic acidosis.

E. Combined ethanol and isopropanol intoxication.
Rationale for A and E: This patient has an osmol gap that is not completely accounted for by his blood alcohol level; he also has metabolic acidosis with an anion gap. The latter cannot be accounted for by isopropanol ingestion.

Major points of discussion

- The patient presents with an osmol gap (Measured – Calculated = $354 - \{[1.86 \times 140] + 75/18 + 12/2.8\} = 67$ mOsm/kg) and a metabolic acidosis with an anion gap (Anion gap = $140 - [102 + 10] = 28$ mmol/L), which suggests a methanol or ethylene glycol intoxication.
  - Osmol gap = Measured osmol – Calculated osmol
  - Serum osmolality = [Serum Na (mEq/L) $\times$ 1.86] + [Glucose (mg/dL)/18] + [Urea (mg/dL)/2.8]
  - Anion gap = $Na^+ - (Cl^- + HCO_3^-)$
- The blood alcohol level indicates the presence of ethanol, and the patient's symptoms may be caused by an ethanol-induced coma.
- This patient has a history of alcohol abuse, but the osmol gap cannot be explained entirely by the ethanol levels. Only 54 mOsm/kg (i.e., 250/4.6) is explained by the ethanol level. A methanol level might therefore be close to $(67 - 54) \times 4.6 = 60$ mg/dL.
- Because his urinalysis is normal, the absence of urinary oxalate crystals indicates methanol, rather than ethylene glycol, intoxication.
- A blood sample should be analyzed by GC-MS to confirm the diagnosis.
- The presence of acetone in serum would indicate isopropanol intoxication.
- The patient should be treated for methanol intoxication when the ethanol level decreases below 150 mg/dL. Treatment for methanol intoxication includes fomepizole (Antizol), as well as intravenous ethanol (with a target concentration of 100 to 150 mg/dL).

4. A. 400 mg once daily.
Rationale: Peak concentration = $400/16 = 25$ mg/L (too high); trough concentration = $25 \times e^{-0.128 \times 22.5} = 1.5$ mg/L (too high).
B. 350 mg once daily.
Rationale: Peak concentration = $350/16 = 21.88$ mg/L (too high); trough concentration = $21.88 \times e^{-0.128 \times 22.5} = 1.23$ mg/L (too high).
C. 300 mg once daily.
Rationale: Peak concentration = $300/16 = 18.75$ mg/L (correct); trough concentration = $18.75 \times e^{-0.128 \times 22.5} = 1.05$ mg/L (too high).
D. 250 mg once daily.
Rationale: Peak concentration = $250/16 = 15.625$ mg/L (correct); trough concentration = $15.625 \times e^{-0.128 \times 22.5} = 0.88$ mg/L (correct).

Major points of discussion

- Volume (V) = Dose/Concentration (C) = $400/25 = 16$ L.
- $Ln(C_t) = Ln(C_0) - k*t = Ln(25) - k*22.5 = Ln(1.5) \rightarrow k = 0.125$ 1/h $\rightarrow t_{1/2} = 5.54$ hr.
- Peak concentration (C_{peak}) = Dose/V.
- Trough concentration (C_{trough}) = $C_{peak} \times e^{-k \times t}$.
- Gentamicin shows one-compartment pharmacokinetics. In one compartment pharmacokinetics, it is assumed

that the drug distributes evenly among all body fluids and tissues instantaneously. In two-compartment pharmacokinetics, the drug distributes rapidly to some tissues/fluids of the body and then more slowly to other tissues/fluids.
- Peak and trough concentrations are targeted to the therapeutic range to minimize nephrotoxicity and ototoxicity and to optimize antibacterial efficacy.

5. A. A metabolic interaction with oxazepam.
Rationale: Oxazepam is not an enzyme inducer.
B. A metabolic interaction with carbamazepine.
Rationale: Aripiprazole is metabolized in the liver by CYP3A4 and CYP2D6. Carbamazepine induces CYP3A4, which leads to decreased levels of aripiprazole.
C. Altered protein binding.
Rationale: Although aripiprazole and its metabolite are highly bound to proteins in serum, it is unlikely that a change in protein binding would cause the observed decrease in the total drug levels.
D. CYP2D6 polymorphism (i.e., rapid metabolizer).
E. CYP3A4 polymorphism (i.e., rapid metabolizer).
Rationale: A polymorphism with a rapid metabolizer phenotype should lead to a relatively low drug level in the first sample, and the levels would not further decrease after the start of additional drugs.

Major points of discussion

- Aripiprazole and its metabolite are more than 99% bound to serum proteins, predominantly albumin. Binding might, theoretically, be altered by other albumin-bound drugs, such as carbamazepine.
- Most assays quantify total drug concentrations in serum or plasma. Free (unbound) concentrations can be determined by using ultracentrifugation or equilibrium dialysis before the assay. Free drug levels are not always easily interpretable.
- Aripiprazole is metabolized in the liver by CYP3A4 and CYP2D6 to dehydroaripiprazole. Less than 1% is excreted unchanged in the urine. Dehydroaripiprazole is further metabolized by CYP3A4 and CYP2D6 to inactive metabolites. Carbamazepine induces CYP3A4, which leads to decreased levels of aripiprazole.
- Aripiprazole and dehydroaripiprazole can be measured in plasma by LC-MS/MS.
- The therapeutic range of aripiprazole and dehydroaripiprazole is 100 to 300 µg/L. The levels of the active metabolite (dehydroaripiprazole) are usually 30 to 110 µg/L. Toxicity consists of exaggerated side effects such as parkinsonism, orthostatic hypotension, QT prolongation, lethargy, tremor, and reflex tachycardia.[15]

6. A. Morphine.
Rationale: The retention time of the only compound detected in this case is 4.76 minutes. The retention time of the derivatized version of morphine (morphine-D3-2TMS) is 4.351.
B. Fentanyl.
Rationale: The retention time of fentanyl is 4.800; therefore, this answer could be correct. However, the mass spectrum does not confirm the presence of fentanyl because it does not shows major peaks at m/z 245, 146, 189, and 202.

C. THC-COOH (tetrahydrocannabinol carboxylic acid).
Rationale: The retention time of THC-COOH-2TMS, which is the product of THC-COOH after derivatization, is 4.777 minutes The mass spectrum also confirms the presence of THC-COOH-2TMS with significant peaks at m/z 371, 473, and 488..
D. Benzoylecgonine (BEG).
Rationale: The retention time of the derivatized version of BEG (i.e. BEG-TMS) is 3.784.
E. Methadone.
Rationale: The retention time of methadone is 3.445.

Major points of discussion

- Urine screens by GC-MS are usually preceded by immunoassay screenings.
- Confirmation by GC-MS is based on a combination of retention time and the mass spectrum.
- The mass spectrum shows peaks at varying m/z (mass-to-charge ratios) and is fairly unique for certain molecules.
- Many drugs are excreted into urine as glucuronides.
- Glucuronides are usually deglucuronidated before GC-MS.
- Most compounds need to be derivatized before GC-MS analysis in order to be retained.
- Mass spectra are derivatization specific.[93]

7. A. A deteriorating ultraviolet (UV) light detector.
Rationale: A deteriorating UV light detector can result in loss of signal and increased noise in the system but generally does not result in additional peaks or peak separation.
B. The presence of an unknown interfering compound.
Rationale: The additional peak is most likely the result of the presence of an unknown compound in the patient's plasma.
C. A deteriorating HPLC column.
Rationale: If the additional peak was caused by a deteriorating HPLC column, other peaks, such as the nortriptyline peak, would most likely also show peak separation.
D. The presence of an amitriptyline enantiomer.
Rationale: Although enantiomers can show small differences in retention times by routine HPLC, amitriptyline enantiomers do not exist.
E. Evaporation of solvent.
Rationale: Evaporation of solvent generally leads to a more polar solvent and, consequently, to a shift in the retention time of all the peaks.

Major points of discussion

- Many compounds absorb UV light of a wavelength of 254 nm, and without additional information, it is impossible to say from which compound this new peak originates.
- Part of the validation process for this assay consists of investigating potential interferences, which might be helpful in explaining this new peak.
- Because the amitriptyline peak is not completely separated from the contaminant peak, interpretation of the quantitative results should be done with caution.
- In this case, one may consider measuring amitriptyline and nortriptyline by another method, such as an alternative HPLC/UV method or by LC-MS/MS.
- For therapeutic drug monitoring of amitriptyline, the sum of amitriptyline and its metabolite, nortriptyline, is used. The target is usually 100 to 300 µg/L, with amitriptyline more than 50 µg/L and nortriptyline at 50 to 150 µg/L.

8. A. A barbiturate.
B. A benzodiazepine.
C. A tricyclic antidepressant.
Rationale: These have a different molecular structure.
D. An opioid.
Rationale: The molecular structure shown is oxycodone, an opioid. For illustrative purposes, morphine is shown in Figure 6-16, *D*.
E. A selective serotonin reuptake inhibitor (SSRI).
Rationale: SSRIs have different molecular structures (Figure 6-16, *E*).

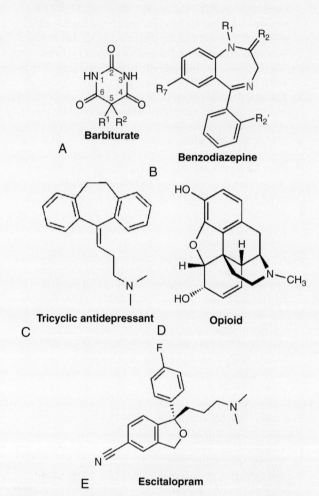

Figure 6-16 Chemical structures. **A**, Barbiturate. **B**, Benzodiazepine. **C**, Tricyclic antidepressant. **D**, Opioid. **E**, Selective serotonin reuptake inhibitor.

Major points of discussion

- Various classes of DOA have a basic chemical structure.
- Classes of drugs of abuse include opiates, barbiturates, benzodiazepines, and amphetamines.
- Other drugs also have a basic chemical structure, such as tricyclic antidepressants.
- The similarities between the molecular structures are useful for detecting classes of drugs by immunoassays.
- Knowledge of the chemical structure of drug classes can also help when considering the identity of other drugs and metabolites.
- Knowledge of the chemical structure of drug classes can also help interpret results obtained by mass spectrometry.

9. A. Lysergic acid diethylamide (LSD).
Rationale: LSD is not detected on automated urine immunoassay.
B. γ-Hydroxybutyrate (GHB).
Rationale: GHB is not detected on automated urine immunoassay.
C. Hydromorphone.
Rationale: Hydromorphone is adequately detected by most automated immunoassays.
D. Oxycodone.
Rationale: Although one of the most prescribed (and abused) opiates, oxycodone is not adequately detected by most automated immunoassays.
E. Mephedrone.
Rationale: Mephedrone, or bath salts, is often not detected on automated urine immunoassays.

Major points of discussion

- Tricyclic antidepressants, barbiturates, most amphetamines, methamphetamine, cocaine, cannabinoids, PCP, morphine, heroin, codeine, methadone, and ethyl alcohol are adequately detected by most automated immunoassays.
- Benzodiazepines are adequately detected by most automated immunoassays. Urine screens might be preceded by a preparation step of deglucuronidation.
- From a 2008 investigation using the College of American Pathologists Urine Drug Testing Surveys, it became clear that most laboratories correctly report that samples are positive for the following:
  - Tricyclic antidepressants, when challenged with urine samples that contained amitriptyline at a concentration of 1300 ng/mL, using a cutoff of 1000 ng/mL.
  - Benzodiazepines, when challenged with urine samples that contained lorazepam at a concentration of 750 ng/mL, using a cutoff of 300 ng/mL.
  - Opiates, when challenged with urine samples that contained hydromorphone at a concentration of 1000 ng/mL, using a cutoff of 300 ng/mL.
- Only 17% of laboratories correctly report that samples are positive for opiates when challenged with urine samples that contained oxycodone at a concentration of 7500 ng/mL, using a cutoff of 300 ng/mL. This percentage was even lower (i.e., 2.5%) when challenged with samples that contained oxycodone at a concentration of 1500 ng/mL. These failures result from differences in immunologic cross-reactivity for various opioids. A similar problem exists when testing for amphetamines.
- Immunoassays that are used to detect DOA rely on cross-reactivity with other compounds of the same class. This approach works better for some classes of drugs than for others.[68,103]

10. A. Quadrupole time of flight–liquid chromatography–mass spectrometry (qTOF-LC-MS).
Rationale: qTOF-LC-MS is increasingly being used in toxicology laboratories because of its specificity, but it is not the most commonly used method.
B. High-performance liquid chromatography with diode-array detection (HPLC-DAD).
Rationale: HPLC-DAD is a useful tool for confirmatory testing. Compounds are identified based on retention time and ultraviolet light spectrum, which are matched against a library of compounds. This method was, and still is, used in a number of toxicology laboratories for confirmatory testing and screening, but it is not the most commonly used method.
C. Liquid chromatography–mass spectrometry/mass spectrometry (LC-MS/MS).
Rationale: Liquid chromatography methods (HPLC or ultra-performance liquid chromatography) combined with tandem mass spectrometry (LC-MS/MS) are used in a growing number of toxicology laboratories. Compounds are identified based on retention time and the tandem mass spectrum, which are matched against a library of compounds. Currently, it is not the most commonly used method.
D. Gas chromatography with single quadrupole mass spectrometry (GC-MS).
Rationale: GC-MS is the most widely used method for confirmatory testing. Compounds are identified based on retention time and mass spectrum, which are matched against a library of compounds.
E. Gas chromatography with nitrogen phosphorus detection (GC-NPD).
Rationale: GC-NPD was used extensively before the advent of HPLC-DAD and GC-MS. It is still used in some laboratories, especially in combination with a mass spectrometer (i.e., GC-MS/NPD).

Major points of discussion

- Several methods are used for extensive screening in toxicology; all of them are chromatography based. None of these can identify 100% of the drugs or their metabolites that are potentially present in patient samples.
- Chromatography-based assays all take at least 1 hour to complete, which is the reason they are part of tier II testing. Ideally, the turnaround time for tier I testing is 1 hour.
- GC-MS is currently the method of choice for most laboratories, but the number of laboratories using a qTOF-LC-MS method is growing rapidly.
- Ingested compounds can be present in patient samples as the parent compound as well as its metabolites.
- In the case of intoxications, toxicokinetics, rather than pharmacokinetics, should be taken into account. For example, half-lives of the ingested compounds can be substantially longer because of saturation.[83]

11. A. Amiodarone and desethylamiodarone are within the reference range; therefore, the amiodarone dosage does not need to be adjusted.
B. The desethylamiodarone concentration is within the reference range; therefore, the risk of developing amiodarone-induced pulmonary toxicity is minimal.
Rationale: The concentration is within the reference range now, but over the next several weeks the circulating level may increase.
C. Simvastatin inhibits biliary excretion of amiodarone.
Rationale: Simvastatin does not inhibit the biliary excretion of amiodarone.
D. Simvastatin inhibits the metabolism of amiodarone.
Rationale: Although simvastatin is likely to inhibit the metabolism of amiodarone in this patient, any changes

resulting from decreased metabolism of amiodarone are likely to occur over the course of several weeks rather than 3 days.

E. The blood sample was collected too soon after starting simvastatin to make any definitive conclusions regarding potential interactions between these drugs.
Rationale: Because of the long half-life of any amiodarone already circulating in this patient, any changes in amiodarone levels because of decreased metabolism of amiodarone are likely to occur over the course of several weeks rather than 3 days. Therefore, the physician should wait longer before obtaining a blood sample to evaluate this issue.

Major points of discussion

- Oral bioavailability of amiodarone is 22% to 86%. The volume of distribution is 9 to 17 L/kg. Clearance is 0.1 to 0.2 L/kg/hr. Half-life is 40 to 55 days. Protein binding is 96%.
- Amiodarone and its metabolite both contribute to the therapeutic efficacy of amiodarone, which is a class III antiarrhythmic drug.
- Given the very long half-life of the drug, timing of blood collections is not relevant. However, repeat measurements of amiodarone and desethylamiodarone within a period of 1 month may not be useful because of their long half-life. In the case of decreased elimination, such as that resulting from enzyme inhibition by simvastatin, this period is probably even longer because the time to reach steady-state depends on the half-life of the drug, which in case of the combination of amiodarone and simvastatin is probably even longer than 40 to 55 days.
- Patients with higher amiodarone levels (>2.5 mg/L) are at increased risk for neurologic side effects (e.g., tremor, ataxia, paresthesias, and nightmares), as well as hepatic and neuromuscular side effects. Amiodarone-induced pulmonary toxicity seems to be associated with higher desethylamiodarone levels. Other side effects are gastrointestinal and ocular. Thyroid dysfunction (i.e., hypothyroidism and hyperthyroidism) is described in approximately 6% of patients on long-term therapy.
- Amiodarone is extensively metabolized by the CYP3A4 system.
- Amiodarone is also a strong CYP3A4 inhibitor and inhibits the metabolism of simvastatin, which leads to a significant risk for severe rhabdomyolysis. When a statin needs to be prescribed for a patient on amiodarone, preference should be given to pravastatin, rosuvastatin, or fluvastatin because these are not metabolized by the CYP3A4 system.
- Amiodarone and its metabolite can be measured by high-performance liquid chromatography with ultraviolet detection (HPLC-UV) and LC-MS/MS.[56,85,95]

12. A. A pseudocholinesterase assay.
Rationale: This is used as to test for organophosphate drugs. The symptoms seen in this patient do not suggest this possibility. This test, if offered, has a relatively long turnaround time.
B. Toxicologic screening by gas GC-MS.
Rationale: The initial drug screen was negative. Screening for unknown compounds by GC-MS could be indicated.

However, screening by GC-MS has a relatively long turnaround time.
C. A methanol assay by gas chromatography (GC).
Rationale: The absence of an anion gap suggests that this patient's presentation is not likely due to methanol intoxication. Measurements by GC-MS have a relatively long turnaround time.
D. Toxicologic screening for amphetamines.
Rationale: Given the patient's symptoms, intoxication with amphetamines cannot be entirely excluded at this time. Given the rapid turnaround time for these assays, one should screen for amphetamines, even though the symptoms are not entirely consistent with amphetamine intoxication.
E. No additional testing is needed at this time.
Rationale: The symptoms in the patient suggest a cholinergic syndrome, which could be related to amitriptyline intoxication. The serum level of tricyclic antidepressants in this case, as measured by an immunoassay, is not consistent with an overdose; therefore, the symptoms are not entirely explained by the current laboratory results.

Major points of discussion

- The symptoms in this patient can be caused by multiple drugs, including tricyclic antidepressants (TCAs). This patient was on amitriptyline, a TCA, but the serum concentration determined by immunoassay was at the upper end of the therapeutic range. Thus, this is not entirely consistent with TCA intoxication. Most immunoassays for TCAs are calibrated using nortriptyline, the desmethyl metabolite of amitriptyline, and show good cross-reactivity with the parent drug. A serum concentration of 250 ng/mL, representing the sum of amitriptyline and nortriptyline, is at the upper end of the therapeutic range.
- Some of the patient's symptoms can also be caused by other substances, including amphetamines.
- Screening for unknown substances by GC-MS is an excellent step in managing this patient, but it is characterized by a relatively long turnaround time. Therefore, even if available, it is advisable to initiate GC-MS screening in conjunction with a more rapid screening test, such as that for amphetamines.
- Screening for amphetamines by immunoassay has a very short turnaround time and, therefore, should be performed at this time in the patient's hospital course.
- An overdose with TCAs can cause coma, anticholinergic symptoms, QRS prolongation, and respiratory acidosis.
- Sample mix-up can happen in the performance of toxicologic screening and must always be considered.
- Symptoms from amphetamine intoxication depend on which amphetamine was ingested but can include dilated pupils, hyperthermia, hypertension or hypotension, cardiac arrhythmias, and coma.[19,36,95]

13. A. The bath salts contained cocaine, which is not detected by tier I DOA screening assays.
Rationale: Cocaine (benzylecgonine) is detected by all assays for cocaine and its metabolites.
B. The bath salts contained methamphetamine, which is not detected by tier I DOA screening assays.
Rationale: Methamphetamine is detected by tier I drugs of abuse screening assays.

C. The bath salts contained oxycodone, which is not detected by tier I DOA screening assays.
Rationale: The patient's symptoms are not suggestive of oxycodone use.
D. The bath salts contained 3,4-methylenedioxymethamphetamine (MDMA), which is not detected by tier I DOA screening assays.
Rationale: The use of MDMA would have led to a positive amphetamine result in this urine screening assay.
E. The bath salts contain mephedrone, which is not detected by tier I DOA screening assays.
Rationale: Mephedrone, a synthetic derivative of cathinone and a β-keto analog of amphetamine, is not detected by most immunoassays that test for amphetamines.

Major points of discussion
- There has been a recent surge in the sale, consumption, and abuse of synthetic stimulants packaged and sold as bath salts, which have been found to contain the stimulant compound mephedrone (i.e., 4-methyl-methcathinone).
- Mephedrone is among several synthetic derivatives of cathinones, a Schedule I stimulant substance found in the khat plant grown in east Africa.
- These β-keto analogs of amphetamines share psychoactive properties similar to cocaine, amphetamines, and MDMA and are known to produce a profound deliriogenic toxidrome, generating intense agitation and hallucinations.
- The β-keto analogs are not detected by routine assays that screen for amphetamines. However, they may possibly cause a false-positive test result for PCP.
- GC/MS and LC/MS-MS assays have been described that identify synthetic derivatives of cathinones.[52,91]

14. A. Caffeine intoxication.
Rationale: The peak seen at the mass transition of caffeine has a retention time similar to the caffeine standard. The ratio of this peak and the peak of the internal standard (area or height) suggests a caffeine concentration greater than 20 mg/L. Taken together with the patient's symptoms, this indicates caffeine intoxication.
B. Subtherapeutic caffeine level.
Rationale: A subtherapeutic caffeine level is less than 5 mg/L.
C. Acetaminophen intoxication.
Rationale: At the mass transition for acetaminophen, no peak is observed at acetaminophen's retention time.
D. Phenytoin intoxication
Rationale: At the mass transition for phenytoin, no peak is observed at phenytoin's retention time.
E. Theophylline intoxication.
Rationale: At the mass transition for theophylline, no peak is observed at theophylline's retention time.

Major points of discussion
- Caffeine is used in the treatment of neonatal apnea in premature infants.
- Caffeine can be measured in serum by HPLC-UV and by LC-MS/MS.
- Therapeutic serum levels of caffeine are 5 to 20 mg/L.
- Caffeine formulations for neonates are frequently compounded extemporaneously by pharmacists, which sometimes can lead to formulation errors.

- The combination of mass transition and retention time can be used to identify compounds in LC-MS/MS.
- With mass spectrometry–based quantitative assays, serum concentrations are often determined using calibration lines. The serum concentration is on the *x*-axis of the calibration line, and the signal of the compound of interest, or the ratio of the signal of the compound of interest relative to the signal of the internal standard, is on the *y*-axis.[30,99,104]

15. A. Serum screening by GC-MS.
Rationale: Serum screening by GC-MS would find many compounds that are not detected by initial drug screening and should be ordered. However, this is not the highest-priority test because it has a long turnaround time and another test can provide more specific information more rapidly in this clinical setting.
B. A serum butyrylcholinesterase activity assay.
Rationale: The patient clearly shows symptoms of a cholinergic syndrome, which is consistent with organophosphate or carbamate poisoning. Some farmers still use these compounds as insecticides. Measuring serum butyrylcholinesterase activity is a rapid test that strongly suggests the presence of these compounds; therefore, this should be the test with the highest priority.
C. A serum strychnine assay.
Rationale: The clinical symptoms of strychnine poisoning are not consistent with this patient's presentation. Symptoms include generalized tonic-clonic seizures and respiratory problems.
D. A serum clenbuterol assay.
Rationale: Clenbuterol is a long-acting β2-agonist primarily used in veterinary medicine in the United States. It is sometimes abused by humans for its anabolic properties.
E. A serum cyanide assay.
Rationale: Cyanide intoxication is usually characterized by flushing, headache, tachypnea, dizziness, and respiratory depression, which progresses rapidly to coma, seizure, complete heart block, and death with sufficiently large doses.

Major points of discussion
- Farmers use various compounds as insecticides. Exposure to these by ingestion, inhalation, or other mechanisms may lead to serious, life-threatening intoxications.
- Some insecticides are cholinesterase inhibitors, such as the organophosphates (e.g., malathion, parathion, diazinon, Dursban) and carbamates (e.g., Sevin, Furadan). Ingestion of these substances may lead to a cholinergic syndrome.
- Organophosphates phosphorylate and carbamates carbamylate the active-site serine hydroxyl group in cholinesterases.
- Treatment primarily involves the use of atropine. In addition, pralidoxime and, in some countries, obidoxime may be administered to reactivate the phosphorylated cholinesterase. The latter is mostly effective if "aging" of the phosphorylated enzyme complex has not yet occurred.
- Measurement of pseudocholinesterase or butyrylcholinesterase is an excellent test for identifying the presence and activity of organophosphates and carbamates.

■ The most definitive means of identifying organophosphates and carbamates is by measuring their urinary metabolites, usually by GC-MS or LC-MS/MS, but these assays have relatively long turnaround times.[16,26,94]

16. A. His inpatient diet differs from his outpatient diet.
Rationale: There is no direct influence of diet on the pharmacokinetics of olanzapine.
B. Olanzapine is metabolized by CYP1A2, and he is a slow metabolizer of olanzapine.
Rationale: The patient's genetic predisposition does not change and therefore does not explain the observed fluctuation in olanzapine levels.
C. Outside the hospital, he takes over-the-counter medication that interacts with olanzapine.
Rationale: St. John's wort is known to induce CYP1A2, and activated charcoal can decrease the absorption of olanzapine, both leading to decreased circulating levels of this medication. Other than these, little is known about potential pharmacokinetic interactions with other over-the-counter medications. Given the other possible answers provided, this explanation, although not impossible, is unlikely.
D. Outside the hospital, he is more mobile, leading to decreased drug levels.
Rationale: Mobility has not been shown to alter the levels of olanzapine within a 10-day time frame.
E. Differences in smoking restrictions inside and outside the hospital lead to differences in drug levels.
Rationale: There are clear differences in smoking policies between inpatient and outpatient settings. Smoking dose-dependently induces CYP1A2, decreasing circulating olanzapine concentrations, which may explain the fluctuation in the plasma concentration of olanzapine.

Major points of discussion
■ Olanzapine is metabolized to 4'-*N*-demethylolanzapine by the cytochrome P450 CYP1A2 isoenzyme. It is also metabolized to olanzapine *N*-oxide by the flavin-containing monooxygenase system. Metabolism to 2-hydroxymethylolanzapine by CYP2D6 is a minor pathway. Phase 2 reactions include glucuronidation of these metabolites.
■ LC-MS/MS is highly specific and, in most cases, does not show cross-reactivity with metabolites.
■ Smoking induces CYP1A2, leading to increased metabolism of olanzapine, increased clearance of the drug, and decreased plasma concentrations.
■ There are over-the-counter medications, such as St. John's wort, that induce CYP1A2.
■ Activated charcoal is an over-the-counter medication that can substantially decrease the absorption of various drugs, including olanzapine.
■ A minimum plasma concentration of 23.2 ng/mL has been suggested to be necessary for the therapeutic benefit of olanzapine.
■ The metabolisms of caffeine and theophylline strongly depend on CYP1A2.
■ CYP1A2 activity may be inhibited by fluvoxamine, ciprofloxacin, and oral contraceptives.[13,79]

17. A. Hyperkalemia resulting from amitriptyline toxicity.
Rationale: Although cardiotoxicity is part of amitriptyline intoxication, the combined amitriptyline and nortriptyline levels are within the therapeutic range.

B. Hypokalemia and nortriptyline toxicity resulting from renal insufficiency.
Rationale: The patient has hyperkalemia and renal insufficiency, and the combined amitriptyline and nortriptyline levels are within the therapeutic range.
C. Hyperglycemia and respiratory acidosis resulting from benzodiazepine intoxication.
Rationale: Benzodiazepines can cause respiratory suppression. However, her remaining symptoms and laboratory results suggest other causes.
D. Hyperglycemia resulting from insulin toxicity.
Rationale: The patient is slightly hyperglycemic, but this would not be caused by insulin toxicity and does not explain all the symptoms.
E. Hyperkalemia and digoxin toxicity resulting from renal insufficiency.
Rationale: The symptoms and laboratory values strongly suggest digoxin toxicity and hyperkalemia from renal dysfunction.

Major points of discussion
■ Hyperkalemia is a well-known result of digoxin toxicity and is most likely related to inhibition by digoxin of the Na/K ATPase, thereby inhibiting cellular sodium efflux and potassium influx.
■ Hypokalemia is known to increase digoxin's effects.
■ Most digoxin (i.e., 50% to 70%) is excreted unchanged or in the form of digoxigenin monosaccharides in the urine. Doses may need to be adjusted in the setting of renal impairment.
■ Digoxin is metabolized by CYP450 and is transported out of cells by P-glycoprotein (Pg), which explains the decreased clearance of digoxin when coadminstered with drugs such as cyclosporine, ritonavir, quinidine, sirolimus, tacrolimus, and verapamil.
■ Most assays for digoxin are nonisotopic immunoassays. The therapeutic range is 0.8 to 2.0 ng/mL, although some suggest a therapeutic range of 0.5 to 0.8 ng/mL.
■ Standard approaches can be used to treat hyperkalemia resulting from digoxin intoxication, including hemodialysis. In addition, antidigoxin antibodies can be administered.[17,33,65,100]

18. A. Phencyclidine (PCP).
Rationale: PCP is not found in plants.
B. Salicylate.
Rationale: Although salicylates are found in nature (i.e., in the bark of the white willow tree), this is not the plant shown in the picture.
C. Cannabis.
Rationale: Although cannabis is derived from plants, the plants shown in the figure do not contain cannabinoids.
D. Digoxin.
Rationale: The plants shown in the picture are *Digitalis purpurea* (purple foxglove), which contains digitoxin as an active compound and can be measured in digoxin assays.
E. Opiates.
Rationale: Although opiates are derived from plants, the plants shown in the picture do not contain opiates.

Major points of discussion
■ *D. purpurea* contains several potent and highly cardiotoxic cardenolide glycosides and their metabolites, including latanoside C, digitoxin, gitoxin, digitoxigenin,

digitoxigenin monodigitoxoside, and digitoxigenin bisdigitoxoside.

- Because of the cross-sensitivity of digoxin immunoassays and the serum concentrations reached by the glycosides and their metabolites, the digoxin immunoassay can become positive after intoxication with foxglove extracts.
- The exact glycosides and metabolites circulating in the patient's serum can be identified and quantified using liquid chromatography–electrospray mass spectrometry.
- Symptoms of digitalis intoxication include gastrointestinal distress (e.g., nausea, vomiting, abdominal pain, and anorexia) and cardiovascular dysfunction (e.g., hypotension, bradycardia, heart block, ventricular arrhythmias). Other known side effects include neurosensorial symptoms (e.g., headache, dizziness, blurred vision) and altered mental status (e.g., confusion, delirium).
- Ingesting only a few grams of *D. purpurea* leaves can be lethal.
- Cardenolides are a type of steroid found in plants, many of which are found in a form of cardiac glycosides.[58] *Digitalis lanata* and *Nerium oleander* are two other plants that contain cardenolide glycosides.

19. A. Cannabis.
Rationale: The urine screening test for tier I drugs of abuse includes tetrahydrocannabinol and should have been positive if this were the case.
B. Magic mushrooms.
Rationale: Hallucinogenic and other compounds from magic mushrooms (such as *Psilocybe semilanceata*) are not detected by urine screening test for tier I drugs of abuse. However, the symptoms seen with magic mushroom intoxication are different from those described in this case.
C. GHB.
Rationale: GHB is not detected by urine screening test for tier I DOA. However, the symptoms and laboratory results described in this case do not suggest intoxication with GHB.
D. Cocaine.
Rationale: Benzoylecgonine, the major metabolite of cocaine, is part of urine screening for tier I drugs of abuse.
E. MDMA (Ecstasy).
Rationale: MDMA (or Ecstasy) is an amphetamine. Amphetamines were detected in the urine of this patient. Therefore, the patient most likely took MDMA at the dance party.

Major points of discussion
- Testing for tier I DOA does not include all substances that can be abused in the party scene.
- Immunoassays for amphetamines, which are mostly used for tier I DOA testing, are not able to differentiate between different specific types of amphetamines.
- Severe MDMA (Ecstasy) intoxications are characterized by coma, hyperthermia, hypertension or hypotension, hyponatremia, and rhabdomyolysis.
- GHB, which is not detected by tier I DOA testing, is often used in combination with Ecstasy and may mask some of its effects. The rapid elimination of GHB within a few hours can coincide with the symptoms of a delayed full-blown Ecstasy intoxication.
- The active substances found in hallucinogenic mushrooms are not detected by tier I DOA testing.

- Clinical chemistry results help to identify likely intoxicants.
- Ecstasy tablets can contain other pharmacologically active compounds, such as atropine.[80,103]

20. A. This assay gives higher values than normal.
Rationale: In this case, the results with the quality-control samples would have been outside the reference range.
B. This level was elevated because of hyperkalemia.
Rationale: Because the results of the basic metabolic panel were normal, hyperkalemia was absent.
C. This level was elevated because of a decreased metabolism of lithium.
Rationale: Lithium is mostly excreted by the kidney, and the results of the basic metabolic panel were normal.
D. This level was elevated because of decreased renal clearance of lithium.
Rationale: Because the results of the basic metabolic panel were normal, the creatinine level was within the reference range; therefore, renal function was probably normal in this patient.
E. This sample was collected in a green-top tube.
Rationale: Green-top tubes contain lithium heparin as the anticoagulant, which lead to artificially elevated lithium levels.

Major points of discussion
- The use of incorrect sample collection tubes can lead to erroneous results. Standard operating procedures should be in place to prevent the use of incorrect sample collection tubes.
- Although it does not happen often, elevated lithium levels could be related to the use of sample collection tubes containing lithium heparin as the anticoagulant. This may contribute as much as 4 mmol/L to the lithium level in tubes that are not completely filled.
- More than 5000 lithium poisonings were reported to U.S. Poison Control Centers in 2003.
- There are several methods to measure lithium, including ion selective electrodes, AAS, and ICP-MS.
- Higher lithium levels as a result of overdose are usually accompanied by gastrointestinal and neurologic symptoms and/or by alterations in the basic metabolic panel.
- Most lithium (i.e., 88% to 98%) is excreted unchanged in the urine. The renal clearance of lithium depends greatly on the renal function of the patient.[59,74,102]

21. A. Aspirin intoxication.
Rationale: Metabolic acidosis and a large anion gap are signs of salicylate intoxication, but salicylates were not found in this patient's toxicology screen.
B. Methanol intoxication.
Rationale: This would lead to an osmolar gap and metabolic acidosis; however, this would not lead to the presence of oxalate crystals in the patient's urine.
C. Combined ingestion of disulfiram and ethanol.
Rationale: Disulfiram (Antabuse) inhibits acetaldehyde dehydrogenase, leading to increased acetaldehyde levels after alcohol intake; it is used to treat alcoholism. Oxalate crystals are not found in the urine of patients ingesting this combination of substances.
D. Isopropanol intoxication.

Rationale: This would lead to an osmolar gap, but not metabolic acidosis. In addition, these patients would not have oxalate crystals in their urine.

E. Ethylene glycol intoxication.

Rationale: The combination of an osmolar gap and metabolic acidosis, along with the presence of oxalate crystals in this patient's urine, are consistent with the diagnosis of ethylene glycol intoxication.

Major points of discussion

- GC-MS is the gold standard method for measuring ethylene glycol.
- An enzymatic assay for measuring ethylene glycol is also available.
- Laboratory findings of ethylene glycol poisoning often include a large anion gap and metabolic acidosis, an osmolar gap of more than 10 mOsm/kg, leukocytosis, and hypocalcemia. The findings identified by urinalysis often include calcium oxalate crystals, low specific gravity, proteinuria, and microscopic hematuria.
- The combined use of tests for osmolar gap, blood gas, anion gap, serum acetone, and urine oxalate allows for an initial differentiation between intoxication with ethanol, methanol, isopropanol, or ethylene glycol.
- Because of the toxicokinetics of ethylene glycol, the anion gap progressively increases with time, whereas the osmolar gap decreases as ethylene glycol is metabolized and its concentration decreases.
- The toxicity of ethylene glycol is caused by accumulation of its toxic metabolites (e.g., glycoaldehyde, glycolic acid, glyoxylic acid, oxalic acid). Measurements of glycolic acid can be helpful in the (postmortem) diagnosis of death from ethylene glycol intoxication.
- The toxicity of ethylene glycol is primarily neurologic, cardiopulmonary, and renal.[17,47,82,87]

22. A. The patient should remain off tacrolimus until these levels have reached 5 to 10 ng/mL.
B. Tacrolimus should be discontinued, and a different immunosuppressive drug should be started when tacrolimus levels become undetectable.
C. The patient should immediately be started on a different immunosuppressive drug along with prednisolone.
Rationale: It is unlikely that the tacrolimus levels would decrease further. Rather, falsely elevated tacrolimus levels should be suspected. However, before the patient is started on a different drug, or even on tacrolimus itself, this suspicion should be investigated.
D. The patient should be genotyped for CYP3A4/3A5 polymorphisms.
Rationale: The observed data are not explained by slow or ultrarapid extensive metabolizers.
E. The samples should be retested for tacrolimus using another method.
Rationale: Falsely elevated tacrolimus levels should be suspected at this time. This can be investigated with a different analytical technique such as the enzyme-multiplied immunoassay technique (EMIT) or LC-MS/MS.

Major points of discussion

- Tacrolimus is monitored closely because of its relatively narrow therapeutic range and variable pharmacokinetics.

- Most assays for tacrolimus, such as the microparticle enzyme immunoassay (MEIA) and LC-MS/MS in whole blood require a manual sample pretreatment step. The antibody-conjugated magnetic immunoassay (ACMIA) run on the Dimension instrument does not require such a pretreatment step.
- Because of the very elevated tacrolimus levels seen in this patient and the stabilization of these levels for 2 weeks despite stopping treatment, combined with the apparent absence of symptoms and laboratory results indicating nephrotoxicity, falsely elevated tacrolimus levels should be suspected. Not reacting to this concern could jeopardize the patient's renal function.
- The correct action in this case at this point is to confirm or reject the elevated tacrolimus levels. This can be done by measuring the drug with a different technique, such as MEIA, EMIT, chemiluminescence microparticle immunoassay (CMIA), or LC-MS/MS.
- Several factors can lead to falsely elevated tacrolimus levels. These are usually assay specific. In this case, the antibodies used in the ACMIA method might be suspected to be the cause.[84]

23. A. Cannabis was used within the prior 3 weeks, and the seeds contain sufficient amounts of LSD to cause these symptoms and be detectable in urine.
Rationale: Cannabis use can be detected in urine for up to 3 weeks after intake. Hawaiian baby woodrose seeds do not contain LSD.
B. Cannabis was used within the prior 3 weeks, and the seeds contain sufficient amounts of LSA (lysergamide), which cross-reacts with some immunoassays for LSD, to cause these symptoms and be detectable in urine.
Rationale: Hawaiian baby woodrose seeds contain LSA, which cross-reacts with some immunoassays for LSD and is present at high concentrations in urine after ingestion.
C. Cannabis was used within the prior 3 weeks, and the seeds contain sufficient amounts of fentanyl, which cross-reacts with some immunoassays for LSD, to cause these symptoms and be detectable in urine.
D. Hawaiian baby woodrose seeds contain sufficient amounts of cannabinoids and fentanyl, which cross-react with some immunoassays for LSD, to cause these symptoms and be detectable in urine.
E. Hawaiian baby woodrose seeds contain sufficient amounts of fentanyl, which cross-reacts with some immunoassays for LSD and cannabis, to cause these symptoms and be detectable in urine.
Rationale: Hawaiian baby woodrose seeds do not contain cannabinoids or fentanyl. However, fentanyl does cause false-positive reactions in some immunoassays for LSD. Fentanyl does not cause false-positive reactions in immunoassays for cannabinoids.

Major points of discussion

- Cannabinoid metabolites can be detected in urine for up to 3 weeks after chronic use of cannabis.
- Lysergamide (LSA), also known as lysergic acid amide (LSA) or ergine, is the nonalkylated amide analog of the potent and widely known hallucinogenic LSD. It is an ergot alkaloid found in the seeds of Convolvulaceae family members, including *Argyreia nervosa* (Hawaiian

baby woodrose), *Ipomoea violacea* (morning glory), and *Rivea corymbosa* (ololiuqui).

■ A small number (e.g., 5 to 10) of seeds of Hawaiian baby woodrose, which contain 2 to 5 mg of LSA, generate a 4- to 8-hour intoxication that reportedly has quantitative as well as qualitative differences from LSD intoxication.

■ A concentration of LSA in urine 9 hours after administration of 6 Hawaiian baby woodrose seeds has been determined to be 0.5 mg/L.

■ Immunoassays for LSD cross-react with other compounds, such as lysergic acid and fentanyl.[8,9,37,55]

24. A. HP-TLC is an outdated method that is prone to technical errors.

Rationale: Although HP-TLC is an older method, it is readily able to detect stimulant laxatives and has been used in clinical laboratories for years. However, a substantial number of false-negative results have been described; the sensitivity of GC-MS and LC-MS/MS methods is better.
B. Cotinine from second-hand smoke interferes with the HP-TLC method, but not with the GC-MS method.
Rationale: Cotinine does not interfere with the detection of stimulant laxatives by HP-TLC.
C. Rhein rapidly degrades in urine, within a few hours, when the sample is kept at room temperature.
Rationale: Rhein is stable for a relatively short period of time in urine maintained at room temperature.
D. The senna alkaloids in Senokot are not metabolized to rhein in this patient.
Rationale: Senna alkaloids are metabolized to rhein. If it were not metabolized to rhein, which is very unlikely, then rhein would also not have been detected by GC-MS in the second urine sample.
E. The acetaminophen taken for a headache interfered with the detection of rhein by HP-TLC.
Rationale: Acetaminophen does not interfere with the detection of rhein by HP-TLC.

Major points of discussion

■ Abuse of stimulant laxatives should be suspected in cases of idiopathic chronic diarrhea.

■ The two most frequently used stimulant laxatives are of the diphenol type, such as bisacodyl (the active ingredient of Ex-Lax, Correctol, and Dulcolax), and anthraquinones, such as senna (the active ingredient in Senokot, Castoria, and Black Draught).

■ Bisacodyl is found in the stool, whereas urine contains only its metabolic products (mainly dihydroxy compounds). Rhein, the metabolite of senna, is not found in stool but is found in urine.

■ HP-TLC testing for bisacodyl-induced diarrhea by a central reference laboratory revealed a sensitivity of 73% and a specificity of 73% when urine was tested and a sensitivity and specificity of 91% and 96%, respectively when stool was analyzed. HP-TLC by the same reference laboratory revealed 0% sensitivity. These results, which spurred the development of more modern GC-MS and LC-MS/MS methods for screening of stimulant laxatives in urine, are most likely related to a technical problem with the performance of the HP-TLC method, such as failure to use the appropriate standard (i.e., rhein) or failure to pretreat samples adequately with β-glucuronidase.

■ Other frequently used stimulant laxatives contain diphenols (i.e., phenolphthalein or sodium picosulfate).

■ Other anthraquinone compounds include aloin, cascara, frangula, and other plant-derived extracts.

■ Rhein can also be detected in urine after use of traditional Chinese medicine formulations such as Yin Chen Hao Tang, which is used for jaundice and liver disorders.

■ Anthraquinone laxatives are glycosides and, being resistant to digestion, reach the colon where bacterial β-glucuronidases release the active aglycones. The metabolites of senna, aloe, cascara, and frangula are rhein, aloe-emodin, and emodin, which are absorbed from the colon and excreted mainly in the urine.[7,27,63,88]

25. A. Medication errors were made; the patient did not receive either vancomycin or ceftazidime. No additional laboratory tests are indicated.
Rationale: Although not receiving vancomycin might explain the low level measured, these tests indicate that patient did receive ceftazidime.
B. There is a potential interference for the vancomycin assay. Ceftazidime levels are as expected. Recovery experiments should be performed for the vancomycin assay, and this level should be determined by another assay.
Rationale: High concentrations of monoclonal immunoglobulins may interfere with turbidimetric immunoassays. This can be investigated by performing dilution and recovery tests with the turbidimetric assay, as well as rerunning the sample with another method.
C. The sample tube for the vancomycin and ceftazidime assays was mixed up with another tube. A new blood sample should be collected and reevaluated with this assay.
Rationale: Although theoretically possible, the presence of ceftazidime in the sample suggests that the correct sample collection tube was used.
D. The chemotherapeutic agents interfere with the vancomycin turbidimetric immunoassay. Therefore, dilution and recovery experiments should be performed for the vancomycin assay, and this level should be determined by another assay.
Rationale: Chemotherapeutic agents do not interfere with the vancomycin turbidimetric immunoassay.
E. The chemotherapeutic agents interfere with the ceftazidime assay. Therefore, dilution and recovery experiments should be performed for the ceftazidime assay, and this level should be determined by another assay.
Rationale: The ceftazidime level is as expected. There is no need for any additional test.

Major points of discussion

■ All assays are prone to interferences, which can derive from endogenous compounds or xenobiotic compounds, such as drugs.

■ High concentrations of immunoglobulins, also known as paraproteins, can cause interference in turbidimetric immunoassays. Paraproteins can promote aggregation by nonspecific mechanisms (e.g., aggregation not mediated by antivancomycin antibodies), which can lead to falsely low results.

■ Potential interferences can be investigated by diluting a known standard or serum sample with either a serum pool or the suspected serum sample. The measurement of a concentration substantially different from the mean of the two specimens suggests the presence of an interfering factor, in this case of a nonspecific aggregating factor.

■ To confirm the interference and determine the concentration of the drug, the sample should also be run with another method, such as HPLC, LC-MS/MS, or another immunoassay.

■ Therapeutic drug monitoring is considered by many as useful to optimize therapy with intravenous vancomycin. Trough levels are typically targeted at 5 to 10 mg/L.

■ Therapeutic drug monitoring of ceftazidime is less common but might also be useful to optimize therapy. Using the given volume of distribution and the given half-life of ceftazidime, the dose, and the body weight of the patient, the trough level can be calculated ($[D/V] \times e^{-k \times t}$), such that 4.8 mg/L is a realistic trough level of ceftazidime.[89]

26. A. The patient is a slow metabolizer of carbamazepine. The carbamazepine dose should be reduced.
Rationale: The symptoms and the carbamazepine level do not suggest carbamazepine intoxication.
B. The patient is dehydrated, leading to toxic lithium levels. The lithium dose should be reduced.
Rationale: Increased proximal tubular reabsorption of lithium in dehydration leads to increased blood concentrations of lithium.
C. Carbamazepine induces the metabolism of haloperidol. The haloperidol dose should be reduced.
Rationale: Carbamazepine can induce the metabolism of haloperidol, but this would lead to lower levels of this antipsychotic drug. Clinical symptoms do not suggest subtherapeutic levels of haloperidol.
D. Oxazepam inhibits the metabolism of carbamazepine. The carbamazepine dose should be reduced.
Rationale: Oxazepam does not inhibit the metabolism of carbamazepine.
E. Carbamazepine inhibits the metabolism of lithium. The lithium dose should be reduced.
Rationale: Lithium is not metabolized; it is almost entirely excreted into the urine.

Major points of discussion
■ Carbamazepine and haloperidol are metabolized by the CYP3A4 isoenzyme, which has genetic polymorphisms in humans.
■ Lithium excretion parallels that of sodium. In dehydration, the proximal tubular reabsorption of sodium (and lithium) is increased, leading to decreased clearance of lithium and increased blood levels.
■ Lithium can be measured in serum, plasma, and urine by ion-selective electrode, flame emission photometry, AAS, or ICP-MS.
■ Therapeutic 12-hour serum levels of lithium are 0.6 to 1.2 mmol/L. Higher levels, especially more than 1.5 mmol/L, are associated with a significant risk for intoxication.
■ There are three types of lithium poisoning: acute, acute on chronic, and chronic.
■ Symptoms of mild lithium poisoning include lethargy, drowsiness, coarse hand tremor, muscle weakness, nausea, vomiting, and diarrhea. Moderate toxicity is associated with confusion, dysarthria, nystagmus, ataxia, myoclonic twitches, and electrocardiographic changes.

Severe, life-threatening toxicity is associated with grossly impaired consciousness, increased deep tendon reflexes, seizures, syncope, renal insufficiency, coma, and death.[17,96]

27. A. Acetaminophen induces increased metabolism of amitriptyline.
Rationale: Acetaminophen does increase the metabolism of amitriptyline.
B. Acetaminophen inhibits the metabolism of oxazepam, which then induces increased metabolism of amitriptyline.
Rationale: Acetaminophen does not inhibit the metabolism of oxazepam, nor does oxazepam affect the metabolism of amitriptyline.
C. Autoinduction of amitriptyline metabolism.
Rationale: Amitriptyline metabolism does not show autoinduction.
D. The patient's blood sample was collected in a serum separator tube, rather than in a red-top tube (i.e., without gel).
Rationale: The gel in certain serum separator tubes adsorbs certain drugs, which can then lead to decreased concentrations as measured in the resulting serum.
E. Acetaminophen displaces amitriptyline from serum albumin.
Rationale: Acetaminophen does not displace amitriptyline from serum albumin.

Major points of discussion
■ Serum separator tubes are used extensively to collect serum samples from patients. They contain a gel that can adsorb certain drugs, which may lead to lower concentrations measured in the resulting serum. The extent to which this artifact takes place depends on the manufacturer of the tubes, the drugs to be measured and their metabolites, and the time between specimen collection and processing. Standardization of collection and processing procedures may prevent this type of preanalytical error from happening.
■ The major pharmacologically active metabolite of amitriptyline is nortriptyline (or, equivalently, desmethyl-amitriptyline). The therapeutic range is defined as the sum of the amitriptyline and nortriptyline concentrations and is 150 to 300 ng/mL.
■ Amitriptyline is metabolized by CYP2D6. Major phase I metabolites include desmethyl-amitriptyline and a hydroxylated metabolite. Phase II metabolites include glucuronide and sulfate conjugates (see Figure 6-9).
■ Amitriptyline is 90% to 95% bound to serum proteins. Plasma protein binding of acetaminophen is approximately 25%. Protein-binding interactions, which have not been described for amitriptyline and acetaminophen, differ from drug to drug, and protein to protein, and are difficult to interpret.
■ Oxazepam is approximately 86% bound to plasma proteins. Its major metabolite is oxazepam-glucuronide, and no pharmacokinetic interaction has been described for this compound with amitriptyline.
■ Drugs can be adsorbed not only to the gel in serum separator tubes but also to other tube materials, such as glass or rubber stoppers. It is important to consider these possibilities when inexplicably low drug levels are found in serum, plasma, blood, cerebrospinal fluid, or urine samples.[24,36]

28. **A. $D_L = 23,000$ mg and $D_M = 11,500$ mg/hr.**
Rationale: This will yield an initial C_e (the target concentration of ethanol [mg/L; the target is 1000 to 1500 mg/L]) of approximately 1250 mg/L and a final C_e of approximately 1250 mg/L.
B. $D_L = 23,000$ mg and $D_M = 157$ mg/hr.
Rationale: This will yield an initial C_e of approximately 1250 mg/L but a final C_e of less than 1000 mg/L.
C. $D_L = 11,500$ mg and $D_M = 11,500$ mg/hr.
Rationale: This will yield an initial C_e of less than 1000 mg/L and a final C_e of approximately 1250 mg/L.
D. $D_L = 2,300$ mg and $D_M = 157$ mg/hr.
Rationale: This will yield an initial C_e of less than 1000 mg/L and a final C_e of less than 1000 mg/L.
E. $D_L = 46,000$ mg and $D_M = 23,000$ mg/hr.
Rationale: This will yield an initial C_e of more than 1250 mg/L and a final C_e of more than 1500 mg/L.

Major points of discussion
- Methanol intoxications can be treated with ethanol.
- The metabolism of ethanol in alcoholic individuals is faster than in nonalcoholic individuals.
- Equations can be used to calculate the loading dose and maintenance dose of intravenous ethanol.
- Methanol is usually measured by GC-MS. Its concentration can also be estimated from the osmolar gap and the blood ethanol level.
- The calculated loading and maintenance doses need to be translated into the values used for ethanol infusions, which are often given as a percentage (e.g., 10%).[17,44]

29. **A. At 72 hours, the MTX plasma concentration will be 0.23 μmol/L, and leucovorin treatment will be continued at the same dose.**
Rationale: See Major Points of Discussion.
B. At 72 hours, the MTX plasma concentration will be 1.0 μmol/L, and leucovorin treatment will be continued at the same dose.
C. At 72 hours, the MTX plasma concentration will be 1.0 μmol/L, and leucovorin treatment can be stopped.
Rationale: The MTX plasma concentration will be 0.23 μmol/L, not 1.0 μmol/L. In addition, if the concentration were 1.0 μmol/L, then the dose of leucovorin would need to be increased.
D. It is impossible to predict the MTX plasma concentration at 72 hours from knowing the earlier concentrations.
Rationale: Therapeutic drug monitoring is effective in this setting, and the MTX plasma concentrations can be predicted.
E. At 72 hours, the MTX plasma concentration will be 0.05 μmol/L, and leucovorin treatment can be stopped.
Rationale: At 72 hours, the MTX plasma concentration will be 1.0 μmol/L; therefore, leucovorin treatment cannot be stopped.

Major points of discussion
- High-dose MTX therapy can have severe side effects, such as nephrotoxicity and myelosuppression.
- Alkalinization, hydration, and leucovorin therapy can help minimize the side effects of MTX.[3,31,32,92]
- Therapeutic drug monitoring after high-dose MTX administration is warranted to minimize the side effects. The administration of leucovorin and its dose regimen can be guided by the MTX plasma levels.

- MTX can be monitored in plasma using automated immunoassays with a short turnaround time.
- The pharmacokinetics of MTX after infusion are triphasic, with a relatively short initial half-life (0.75 hours) reflecting distribution, a longer second half-life (3.5 hours) predominantly determined by renal clearance, followed by a third, longer half-life, which is thought to determine the seriousness of the hematologic and gastrointestinal side effects.
- The terminal half-life and the MTX plasma level at 72 hours can be estimated from the MTX plasma concentrations at 24 and 48 hours using the following equation:

$$LnC_{48h} = LnC_{24h} - k_{elm} \times 24; t_{1/2} = 0.693/k_{elm}; C_{72h}$$
$$= C_{48h} \times e^{-k_{elm} \times t}$$

- For the patient in the case described in this question, the half-life is 8 hours, and the concentration at 72 hours will be 0.23 μmol/L.
- It is always useful to confirm predictive estimations of MTX levels by measuring the MTX plasma concentration at 72 hours after completing the infusion.[32,92]

30. A. FPIA is not an adequate method to measure MTX in samples obtained 96 hours after MTX infusions. Another method should be used.
Rationale: Normally, the FPIA method is adequate for measuring MTX samples obtained 96 hours after infusion.
B. Diluting plasma samples always leads to higher concentrations using an FPIA method. Another method should be used.
Rationale: Diluting plasma samples does not lead to higher concentrations with FPIA. In contrast, it should yield the same result (after correction for the dilution).
C. Leucovorin interferes with measurement of MTX levels by FPIA. Another method should be used.
Rationale: Leucovorin does not interfere with the MTX FPIA.
D. Alkalinization with bicarbonate leads to higher MTX levels after dilution. The pH of the plasma sample should be adjusted before using this FPIA method.
Rationale: Alkalinization of the patient with bicarbonate does not interfere with the MTX FPIA.
E. Glucarpidase leads to the production of an inactive metabolite of MTX, which produces concentration-dependent cross-reactivity in the FPIA method. Another method should be used.
Rationale: Glucarpidase leads to the formation of the inactive metabolite of MTX (i.e., 2,4-diamino-N10-methylpteroic acid [DAMPA]), which interferes with MTX measurements by FPIA in a concentration-dependent manner. Another method to measure MTX, such as HPLC LC-MS/MS, should be used.

Major points of discussion
- Hydration, alkalinization, and leucovorin are all used to minimize side effects from high-dose MTX treatment. Leucovorin restores intracellular folate concentrations, and the dose is guided by MTX levels in plasma samples collected 24, 48, and 72 hours after infusion of MTX. Hemodialysis has also been used for MTX removal.
- Prolonged exposure to high levels of MTX can cause life-threatening nephrotoxicity, especially acute renal failure,

because of tubular obstruction by crystal deposits of MTX and its main metabolite, 7-hydroxy-MTX. In cases of life-threatening MTX-induced toxicity caused by high MTX levels, the use of glucarpidase (GPDG2) allows hydrolysis of MTX and 7-OH-MTX into nontoxic metabolites, including DAMPA, 7-OH-DAMPA, and glutamate.

- DAMPA is normally a minor metabolite of MTX, and its concentrations are usually very low after high-dose MTX infusions. GPDG2 administration decreases plasma MTX levels by 95% to 99% within 15 minutes in patients with MTX-induced toxicity. It also leads to high DAMPA levels. DAMPA is known to interfere with measurements of MTX by FPIA, causing marked overestimates of MTX concentrations when high DAMPA levels are present. Therefore, FPIA is not suitable for therapeutic monitoring of MTX levels after GPDG2 treatment.
- MTX can be measured with other assays. These include HPLC and LC-MS/MS methods. These typically do not show interference by DAMPA.
- When very high levels of MTX are identified by assays in the clinical laboratory, it is important to know how the patient has been treated for potential side effects of MTX.

31. A. A 5 mg/hr intravenous midazolam infusion for 3 days is, by definition, an overdose.
Rationale: This dose is correct for this clinical setting.
B. The patient has a single-nucleotide polymorphism in CYP3A5.
Rationale: Midazolam is metabolized by CYP3A4/3A5 isoenzymes.
C. Pharmacologically active midazolam conjugates accumulate because of renal dysfunction.
Rationale: Midazolam is metabolized to pharmacologically active conjugates (such as the hydroxyl-glucuronide), which accumulate in cases of renal dysfunction. However, this metabolite was not measured by the HPLC assay. This would explain these observations. In this case, the serum concentration of the glucuronide metabolite was 2000 ng/mL in the sample collected 5 days after stopping the infusion.
D. The hydroxymetabolite of midazolam accumulates because of hepatic dysfunction.
Rationale: This patient's laboratory results are not consistent with hepatic dysfunction.
E. Midazolam and its metabolites need to be monitored using samples of whole blood rather than serum.
Rationale: Midazolam and its metabolites are usually measured in serum or plasma, not in whole blood.

Major points of discussion
- Midazolam is used as an intravenous anesthetic. A normal dose regimen for sedation in the intensive care unit setting is 0.03 to 0.2 mg/kg/hr, which, in this case, would translate into a dosage of 2.1 to 14 mg/kg/hr.
- Midazolam is metabolized in the liver by CYP3A4/3A5 to α-hydroxymidazolam, which is quantitatively less relevant, but is, in turn, glucuronidated by uridine diphosphate glucuronyltransferase (UDPGT); the latter is excreted by the kidney through glomerular filtration and active tubular secretion.
- Dose corrections of midazolam are warranted in cases of hepatic or renal impairment.[5,67,75]

- To explain the effects of midazolam administration in a patient with renal impairment, it is important to measure serum concentrations of the drug and its active metabolites, especially hydroxymidazolam-glucuronide. Sedation is achieved at midazolam serum concentrations of 100 to 1000 ng/mL, with wide interpatient variability in concentration–effect relationships. Although the potency of hydroxymidazolam-glucuronide is less than that of midazolam, high levels can contribute to the sedative effects of midazolam therapy.
- The terminal half-life of midazolam is approximately 3 hours and shows considerable interpatient variability. This half-life is prolonged to approximately 13 hours in patients with acute renal failure. The half-life of the glucuronide is also significantly prolonged in patients with renal impairment.

32. **A. The patient is obese (BMI = 27.8 kg/m^2). In obese patients, gentamicin dosing should be based on lean body mass (LBM), rather than actual body mass. Therefore, 1.5 mg/kg every 8 hours would be a better dose.**
Rationale: Gentamicin predominantly distributes in the extracellular fluid. In obesity, the extracellular fluid and, therefore, the volume of distribution of gentamicin more closely relate to the LBM than to the actual body mass. Thus, the half-life of gentamicin is not substantially affected by obesity. A dose regimen of 1.5 mg/kg every 8 hours would lead to a C_{peak} of 7.7 mg/L and a C_{trough} of 7.7 mg/L.
B. The current regimen (2.5 mg/kg every 8 hours) is, by definition, an overdose for any individual. Therefore, the dose should be lowered to 1.5 mg/kg every 8 hours.
Rationale: Using 2.5 mg/kg every 8 hours is the correct dose regimen for normal-weight children 10 years of age.
C. Because the patient is obese, gentamicin is eliminated faster than normally. Therefore, the dose should be raised to 3.5 mg/kg every 8 hours.
Rationale: The half-life of the gentamicin in this patient is approximately 2.3 hours, which is normal. The proposed dose would lead to even higher levels, with an increased risk for toxicity.
D. Glomerular filtration is lower in obese patients, leading to decreased clearance of the drug and increased circulating levels. Therefore, the dose should be reduced to 1.5 mg/kg every 8 hours.
Rationale: Regardless of the effect of obesity on renal function, the half-life of the gentamicin in this patient is approximately 2.3 hours, which is normal. The proposed dose reduction would make sense.
E. Single-nucleotide polymorphisms in the enzyme responsible for metabolizing gentamicin are prevalent in the Hispanic population and result in increased drug levels. Therefore, the dose should be reduced to 1.5 mg/kg every 8 hours.
Rationale: Gentamicin is excreted by the kidney but is minimally metabolized. The proposed dose reduction would make sense.

Major points of discussion
- Aminoglycoside pharmacokinetics are influenced by various factors, including renal function, body weight, and body composition.
- Clearance of gentamicin is affected by renal function, which leads to altered trough levels of the drug.

- The volume of distribution of gentamicin is affected by body weight and body composition, which leads to altered peak levels of the drug.
- Aminoglycosides (including gentamicin) distribute predominantly in the extracellular fluid. Therefore, the volume of distribution is relatively larger in neonates and in patients with edema, ascites, sepsis, fever, and/or severe burn wounds. In obese patients, the extracellular fluid volume and, therefore, the volume of distribution of aminoglycosides are relatively smaller. In obese patients, the amount of extracellular fluid correlates better with LBM than with actual body mass. The volume of distribution of aminoglycosides also correlates better with LBM in obese patients. The volume of distribution determines the dose needed to reach certain target levels of gentamicin, and therefore, the dose of the drug also correlates better with LBM. Initial dosing of aminoglycosides in (pediatric and adult) obese patients should be based on LBM.
- Therapeutic drug monitoring of gentamicin helps further optimize the dose regimen of this drug.
- From C_{peak} and C_{trough} drug levels, the volume of distribution and half-life can be calculated. These results can then be translated into an improved dose regimen to achieve the desired values for C_{peak} and C_{trough}.
- LBM can be calculated as LBM (kg) $= 0.9 \times$ length (cm) $- 87$ for males, and LBM (kg) $= 0.9 \times$ length (cm) $- 91.5$ for females. For this patient, the LBM would be $(0.9 \times 129.5) - 87 = 29.6$ kg. A dose of 2.5 mg/kg (LBM) every 8 hours $= 74$ mg every 8 hours, which is close to the 1.5 mg/kg body weight every 8 hours (i.e., 70 mg every 8 hours) dose derived from the therapeutic drug monitoring data.[14,73,76]

33. A. Decrease the dose to 200 mg every 12 hours and monitor the posaconazole level again after 1 week.
B. Decrease the dose to 200 mg every 24 hours and monitor the posaconazole level again after 1 week.
C. Decrease the dose to 200 mg every 12 hours and monitor the posaconazole level again the next day.
Rationale: The posaconazole serum concentration is 0.4 mg/L at the current dose. Decreasing the dosage regimen would not lead to a target level of 0.7 mg/L.
D. Increase the dose to 400 mg every 12 hours and monitor the posaconazole level again the next day.
Rationale: Increasing the dosage regimen might lead to a target level of 0.7 mg/L. However, it takes longer than one day to see if this level has been reached.
E. **Increase the dose to 400 mg every 8 hours and monitor the posaconazole level again after 1 week.**
Rationale: Increasing the dosage regimen to 400 mg/day might lead to a target of 0.7 mg/L. Monitoring after 1 week will provide enough time to show if the target level has been reached.

Major points of discussion
- Therapeutic drug monitoring can optimize the prophylactic and therapeutic use of posaconazole.
- The exact therapeutic target levels of posaconazole are still subject of debate. Potential targets for prophylaxis and treatment of invasive aspergillosis are 0.7 and 1.25 mg/L, respectively.

- Posaconazole can be measured LC-MS/MS and will often be part of an azole panel.
- For quantification by LC-MS/MS, an internal standard is often used. Typically, this will be a deuterated version of the compound of interest. However, sometimes other compounds can also be used as internal standards, especially when the compound of interest is part of a panel.
- Mass transitions at which compounds are detected by tandem mass spectrometry are shown as follows: mass to charge (first quadrupole) greater than mass to charge (second quadrupole).
- Calibration lines are part of the quantification of compounds by LC-MS/MS.
- The drug's half-life and, therefore, the time it takes to achieve steady state should be taken into consideration when retesting a drug level.[2,43,48]

34. **A. Salicylate in serum.**
Rationale: Metabolic acidosis, combined with an anion gap and a normal osmolality, is consistent with salicylate intoxication. The smell of vinegar from the bottle strengthens this suspicion because it represents acetic acid resulting from degraded aspirin.
B. Opiates in urine.
Rationale: Opiates induce respiratory suppression, not hyperventilation
C. Acetaminophen in serum.
Rationale: Although a screen for acetaminophen should be performed, given this patient's symptoms and initial laboratory test results, salicylate intoxication is more likely.
D. Benzodiazepines in serum.
Rationale: Benzodiazepines induce respiratory suppression, not hyperventilation.
E. Amphetamines in serum.
Rationale: The patient's symptoms and initial laboratory test results do not strongly suggest amphetamine use.

Major points of discussion
- Salicylate is the active metabolite of acetylsalicylic acid (i.e., aspirin). During storage of aspirin, acetic acid can be formed, which smells like vinegar. Although bottles and strips found near patients can be helpful for a diagnosis, they might also be misleading.
- Salicylate is formed very quickly from acetylsalicylate ($t\frac{1}{2} = 15$ min). At therapeutic doses, salicylate has a half-life of 2 to 3 hours, but because of saturation of the pathways required for its metabolism, this half-life becomes much longer in cases of toxic doses (i.e., 15 to 30 hours). At high concentrations of salicylate, a higher portion of the dose is excreted into the urine as salicylate.
- The symptoms of salicylate intoxication include tinnitus, diaphoresis, hyperthermia, hyperventilation, nausea, vomiting, and acid-base disturbances. Neurologic effects include lethargy, disorientation, and, in severe cases, coma and seizures.
- The acid-base disturbance depends on the patient's age and the severity of the intoxication.
- Metabolic acidosis with an increased anion gap, but without an osmolar gap, should lead to a suspicion of salicylate intoxication.
- Most assays for salicylate are based on the Trinder method (i.e., Fe^{3+} and salicylate; measured at 540 nm),

which can also give false-positive results. Other methods are available.

- Therapeutic serum levels of salicylate are less than 300 mg/L. Tinnitus may be seen at serum levels of more than 200 mg/L. More serious side effects are seen at serum levels of more than 300 mg/L.
- Treatment is focused on decreasing further absorption (e.g., using active charcoal) and increasing elimination by alkaline diuresis and hemodialysis (in cases in which salicylate levels are >1000 mg/L). Bicarbonate is used to treat the metabolic acidosis.[18,38,70]

35. A. Rodenticide.
Rationale: Several rodenticides contain one or more "superwarfarins," which are long-acting, potent anticoagulants that act like warfarin but are much more potent and have a much longer half-life. The clinical symptoms, including the longer action of the intoxicant, as illustrated by increasing PT, INR, and aPTT after stopping vitamin K, strongly suggest a intoxication with a superwarfarin.
B. Acetylsalicylic acid.
Rationale: The coagulation abnormalities seen in salicylate intoxication are different. Thus, the PT, INR, and aPTT would not change, but platelet aggregation would be abnormal. Aggregation studies would show no aggregation in response to arachidonic acid, primary wave aggregation only in response to adenosine diphosphate (ADP), and decreased or absent aggregation in response to collagen.
C. Clopidogrel.
Rationale: Clopidogrel intoxication can result in bleeding. However, the PT, INR, and aPTT would not change; rather, platelet aggregation would be abnormal. ADP-induced platelet aggregation would typically be less than 65%.
D. Warfarin.
Rationale: This patient's symptoms, coagulation abnormalities, and response to therapy might be caused by warfarin intoxication. However, this patient is not receiving warfarin as a medication. In addition, the relative resistance to therapy in this patient suggests intoxication with a superwarfarin rather than with warfarin itself.
E. Lithium.
Rationale: Both acute and chronic lithium intoxication induce more gastrointestinal and neurologic symptoms than are described in this patient.

Major points of discussion
- PT, INR, and aPTT are altered by coumarins, such as warfarin and the superwarfarins. These levels are not altered by aspirin or clopidogrel.
- There are several types of rodenticides; some contain strychnine, and others contain metal phosphides, calciferols, or coumarins—the latter are usually superwarfarin compounds.
- Superwarfarin compounds include the long-acting coumarin derivatives brodifacoum, bromadiolone, and difenacoum. Similar to warfarin, they inhibit the synthesis of functional vitamin K–dependent coagulation factors by interfering with γ-carboxylation of the glutamic acid residues on these proteins. Superwarfarins are about 100 times more potent than warfarin. They accumulate in the liver, have large volumes of distribution, and have extremely long half-lives (i.e., 24 to 180 days).

- Symptoms of salicylate intoxication include gastrointestinal distress, tinnitus, tachypnea, and respiratory alkalosis. Symptoms of severe overdose may include metabolic acidosis, hyperpnea, diaphoresis, fever, altered mental status, seizures, coma, cerebral edema, pulmonary edema, and death. Chronic overdose may consist primarily of neurologic manifestations, such as confusion, delirium, and agitation. Coagulopathy, hepatic injury, and dysrhythmias are rare complications of a severe salicylate overdose.
- Superwarfarins can be measured in serum, plasma, and blood by HPLC, GC-MS, and LC-MS/MS. Warfarin and superwarfarins can be detected by certain extensive drug screens.[50,57,105]

36. A. The dose regimen should not be changed for the remaining 3 days.
Rationale: The dose regimen needs to be altered to achieve an optimal balance between toxicity and efficacy.
B. The dose regimen needs to be decreased to 24 mg once daily for the remaining 3 days.
Rationale: The dose regimen needs to be increased, instead of decreased, to achieve an optimal balance between toxicity and efficacy.
C. The dose regimen needs to be increased to 52 mg once daily for the remaining 3 days.
Rationale: With this change in dosing, the AUC_{0-24h} will become $(52/32) \times 50 = 81$ hours $\times$ mg/L, which is within the therapeutic window.
D. The dose regimen needs to be increased to 80 mg once daily for the remaining three days.
Rationale: This change in dosing would result in an area under the AUC_{0-24h} outside the therapeutic window, which would increase the risk of toxicity.
E. Given the risk for clinical toxicity, busulfan should be stopped immediately.
Rationale: This approach will lead to significant underexposure to busulfan, resulting in a lack of efficacy.

Major points of discussion
- Busulfan is widely used in preparative chemotherapy-based regimens as an alternative to total body irradiation in adult and pediatric patients undergoing subsequent hematopoietic stem cell transplantation.
- Busulfan was previously given orally four times per day. Intravenous formulations are now available and can be given either four times per day or as a once-daily dose regimen for 4 consecutive days.
- Depending on the indication and other factors, such as age, busulfan is given with other chemotherapeutic agents, which together determine toxicity and efficacy. A combination of busulfan, cyclophosphamide, and melphalan is common.
- Intravenous busulfan shows large interpatient variability in circulating drug levels.
- High exposure to busulfan predicts toxicity (e.g., veno-occlusive disease) as well as acute graft-versus-host disease. In contrast, low exposure to busulfan predicts graft rejection and disease relapse.
- Busulfan has a narrow therapeutic window.
- Busulfan can be measured in serum and plasma by HPLC with ultraviolet detection (HPLC-UV) and by LC-MS/MS.

- By measuring serum drug concentrations at multiple time points, the area under the curve (AUC) can be calculated using the trapezoidal rule (when there are sufficient numbers of samples) or using limited sampling models.
- When linear pharmacokinetics are relevant, dose adjustments can be calculated using the ratio of the AUCs.[4,20,53,90]

37. A. HIV infection.
Rationale: Serum 25-OH-vitamin D and calcium concentrations are typically low in patients with HIV.
B. *M. bovis* infection.
Rationale: Hypercalcemia has been described in patients with mycobacterial infections but is accompanied by low levels of 25-OH-vitamin D and 1,25-OH-vitamin D.
C. Over-the-counter use of illegal vitamin D supplements.
Rationale: Over-the-counter vitamin preparations, such as Soladek, which are readily available in the Dominican Republic and in predominantly Dominican neighborhoods in the United States, can contain large amounts of vitamin D (e.g., >800,000 units in the cholecalciferol form).
D. Antiretroviral medications.
Rationale: Antiretroviral medications can alter vitamin D metabolite levels, but these changes are relatively small.
E. Antimycobacterial therapy.
Rationale: Antimycobacterial drugs can alter vitamin D metabolite levels, but these changes are relatively small.

Major points of discussion
- The differential diagnosis of hypercalcemia includes hyperparathyroidism, malignancies, secondary hyperparathyroidism, the use of thiazide diuretics, and vitamin D intoxication. Measurements of parathyroid hormone (PTH), 25-OH-vitamin D, and 1,25-OH-vitamin D are used to identify the cause of the hypercalcemia.
- Several diseases and medications can influence serum levels of calcium, 25-OH-vitamin D, 1,25-OH-vitamin D, and PTH.
- In contrast to earlier reports, HIV infection does not appear to be associated with lower or higher levels of 25-OH-vitamin D.
- Antimycobacterial medications, such as rifampicin and isoniazid, can alter cytochrome P450 isoenzymes, including 25-hydroxylase, 1-α-hydroxylase, and 24-hydroxylase activities, and, therefore, serum calcium levels.
- Antiretroviral medications, especially protease inhibitors and certain non-nucleoside reverse transcriptase inhibitors, can lead to changes in serum levels of 25-OH-vitamin D and 1,25-OH-vitamin D.
- After discontinuing the use of Soladek supplements, the 25-OH-vitamin D serum concentrations in this patient normalized within a few months (see Figure 6-10).[10,35,62,72]

38. A. Voriconazole inhibits efavirenz metabolism. Therefore, the efavirenz dose should be increased to 900 mg/day.
Rationale: Voriconazole inhibits efavirenz metabolism, as reflected in the relatively high efavirenz levels. Therefore, the efavirenz dose should be decreased.
B. Voriconazole induces efavirenz metabolism. Therefore, the efavirenz dose should be decreased to 300 mg/day.

Rationale: Voriconazole inhibits, rather than induces, efavirenz metabolism. However, it is correct that the efavirenz dose should be decreased.
C. Efavirenz induces voriconazole metabolism. Therefore, the voriconazole dose should be decreased to 100 mg twice daily.
D. Efavirenz inhibits voriconazole metabolism. Therefore, the voriconazole dose should be increased to 400 mg twice daily.
Rationale: Efavirenz induces, rather than inhibits, voriconazole metabolism as reflected in the voriconazole trough level. However, it is correct that the voriconazole dose should be increased rather than decreased.
E. Voriconazole inhibits efavirenz metabolism, and efavirenz induces voriconazole metabolism. Therefore, the efavirenz and voriconazole doses should be decreased and increased, respectively.
Rationale: As reflected in the levels of both drugs, voriconazole inhibits efavirenz metabolism, and efavirenz induces voriconazole metabolism. The efavirenz and voriconazole doses should, therefore, be decreased and increased, respectively.

Major points of discussion
- Therapeutically effective voriconazole trough levels are 1 to 6 mg/L when used for cases of pulmonary aspergillosis, and 2 to 6 mg/L for aspergillosis infections in areas that are more difficult for voriconazole to penetrate, such as cerebral or sinus infections. Drug toxicity (most likely at levels >6 mg/L) primarily consists of neurologic symptoms (e.g., hallucinations, altered perception of color) and increased levels of standard liver function tests.
- Therapeutically effective efavirenz concentrations, collected more than 8 hours after drug intake, are 1 to 4 mg/L. Drug toxicity (most likely at levels >4 mg/L) are mainly neurologic, such as persistent sleeping disorders.
- Efavirenz is primarily metabolized by CYP2B6 and CYP3A4 isoenzymes and interacts in a complex manner with CYP450 enzymes, both inhibiting and inducing CYP3A4, CYP2C19, and CYP2C9.
- Voriconazole is both a substrate and inhibitor of CYP2C9, CYP3A4, and CYP2C19 isoenzymes.
- The prescribed combination leads to induction and inhibition of the metabolism of these two drugs. Therapeutic drug monitoring can help to optimize the dose regimen for these types of patients.
- Both of these drugs can be measured in plasma and serum by HPLC-UV as well as the more sensitive LC-MS/MS.[23,46,77]

39. A. Measure serum aluminum concentrations by HPLC-UV.
B. Measure serum aluminum concentrations by LC-MS.
C. Measure serum aluminum concentrations by AAS.
Rationale: Aluminum can be measured in serum by this method.
D. Measure serum aluminum concentrations by isotope ratio mass spectrometry.
E. Measure serum aluminum concentrations by GC-MS.
Rationale for A, B, D, and E: Aluminum is not measured in serum by these methods.

Major points of discussion
- Chronic aluminum intoxication can occur in dialysis patients, causing several syndromes such as bone disease and encephalopathy.

- Acute aluminum intoxication is characterized by a neurologic syndrome, which includes seizures, myoclonus, obtundation, and coma. Microcytic anemia can also occur.
- Aluminum can be measured in serum. However, special blood collection tubes are required for aluminum testing because aluminum eluted from the rubber stoppers of normal blood collection tubes can lead to artificially elevated levels of this analyte, typically up to 20 to 60 μg/L of aluminum.
- Aluminum can be measured in serum by ICP-MS and AAS.
- Reference ranges for serum aluminum are less than 7 μg/L in patients not on dialysis. For dialysis patients, aluminum levels should be interpreted in conjunction with parathyroid hormone levels.
- Epidemic forms of acute aluminum intoxication have been described after the use of water severely contaminated with this metal. This can be prevented by following adequate quality control and quality assurance procedures for water and dialysis fluids in dialysis units.
- The elevated aluminum (and calcium) levels in the case described were caused by leaching of aluminum and calcium from the cement mortar coating of the water distribution pipe into the water. The serum aluminum levels of patients who survived this episode were 113 to 490 μg/L. However, several patients did not survive; they had serum aluminum levels of 359 to 1189 μg/L.[6,41,66]

40. A. Do not change the dose regimen.
Rationale: The measured peak and trough levels are already too high.
B. Change the dose regimen to 10 mg every 24 hours.
Rationale: This will lead to peak and trough levels that will still be too high.
C. Change the dose regimen to 10 mg every 36 hours.
Rationale: This change will lead to peak and trough levels that will be in the therapeutic range.
D. Change the dose regimen to 20 mg every 24 hours.
E. Change the dose regimen to 30 mg every 36 hours.
Rationale: The measured peak and trough levels are already too high.

Major points of discussion
- Peak and trough levels of amikacin during different dose regimens can be predicted based on previous measurements. First, the volume of distribution, the elimination rate constant, and the half-life are calculated. Using these parameters, new peak and trough levels can be calculated. During multiple-dose administrations, serum concentrations of the drug will accumulate. Using the earlier calculated pharmacokinetic parameters, this accumulation can easily be calculated. There are several assumptions for these predictions. One of these is that the pharmacokinetics in this setting (such as clearance of the drug) does not change.
- Dose regimens can be adjusted in terms of both the amount that is administered and the dose (D) interval.
- In this case, volume of distribution = D/(Conc[peak] − Conc[trough]) = 15 (mg)/(48 − 15) (mg/L) = 0.455 L.
- $LnC_t = LnC_{0h} - k \times t = Ln(15) = Ln(48) - k \times 24$ implies that $k = (3.871 - 2.708)/24 = 0.0485/hr$.
$t\frac{1}{2} = 0.693/k = 0.693/0.0485/hr = 14.3$ hours.

- Based on the calculated pharmacokinetic parameters in this case, 10 mg of drug administered every 36 hours will lead to the following accumulation (if there is no prior amikacin):
  - C_{peak} at 0 hours = 10/0.455 = 22 mg/L
  - C_{trough} at 24 hours = $22 \times e^{-0.0485 \times 36} = 22 \times 0.174 = 3.8$ mg/L
  - C_{peak} at 24 hours = 22 + 3.8 = 25.8 mg/L
  - C_{trough} at 48 hours = 25.8 × 0.174 = 4.5 mg/L
  - C_{peak} at 48 hours = 22 + 4.5 = 26.5 mg/L
  - C_{trough} at 72 hours = 26.5 × 0.174 = 4.6 mg/L
- Following the institution of dose adjustments in a particular case, new drug levels should be measured to confirm the expected results.

41. A. The patient has subtherapeutic paroxetine serum concentrations because of a drug-drug interaction with oxazepam.
Rationale: The paroxetine serum concentration is within the therapeutic range.
B. The patient has subtherapeutic clozapine serum concentrations because of smoking an increased number of cigarettes.
Rationale: Although cigarette smoking induces clozapine metabolism, it is unlikely that an increase from 10 to 12 cigarettes per day further induces an already induced metabolism of this drug.
C. The patient has subtherapeutic clozapine serum concentrations because of a drug-drug interaction with fluvoxamine.
Rationale: Fluvoxamine inhibits the metabolism of clozapine. Discontinuing fluvoxamine and replacing it with an SSRI that does not inhibit CYP1A2 can lead to decreased and, therefore, subtherapeutic clozapine levels with clinical consequences.
D. The patient has subtherapeutic clozapine serum concentrations because of a drug-drug interaction with paroxetine.
Rationale: Although there may be a pharmacokinetic interaction between paroxetine and clozapine, it would lead to increased clozapine levels.
E. The patient has subtherapeutic fluvoxamine serum concentrations because of a drug-drug interaction with oxazepam.
Rationale: There is no pharmacokinetic interaction between fluvoxamine and oxazepam. The fluvoxamine concentrations are within the therapeutic range.

Major points of discussion
- The antipsychotic drug clozapine and its metabolites (e.g., desmethyl and *N*-oxide) can be measured in serum with HPLC-UV and LC-MS/MS. Although pharmacologically active, the metabolites are less potent and shorter acting. The therapeutic range for clozapine is only for the parent compound.
- Demethylation of clozapine is mediated by CYP450 1A2. Additional metabolism is mediated by CYP450 3A4 and 2D6.
- Smoking induces CYP450 1A2-mediated metabolism of clozapine. Therefore, serum concentrations of clozapine are relatively lower in smokers.
- Fluvoxamine inhibits the CYP450 1A2-mediated metabolism of clozapine. Therefore, concomitant use of

fluvoxamine can increase clozapine serum concentrations by a factor of 10. Discontinuing fluvoxamine treatment will lead to decreasing serum concentrations of clozapine.

■ Subtherapeutic levels (i.e., <200 ng/mL), but also concentrations greater than 700 ng/mL, of the antipsychotic drug are associated with increased clinical symptoms of schizophrenia.

■ Side effects of clozapine include agranulocytosis and cardiomyopathy, both of which should lead to cessation of treatment with this drug. High serum concentrations of clozapine (e.g., >600 ng/mL) have been associated with an increased risk for seizures.

■ Fever and infection are also associated with high clozapine serum concentrations.[29,51,60]

42. A. LC-MS/MS is not a good method to measure drugs and their metabolites simultaneously.
Rationale: LC-MS/MS is an excellent method to measure drugs and their metabolites simultaneously.
B. Morphine and its metabolites are not stable in plasma.[1,21,54]
Rationale: The LC-MS/MS method was validated; method validation should entail characterization of analyte stability in the relevant type of sample.
C. Omeprazole inhibits the metabolism of codeine to morphine.
Rationale: Omeprazole inhibits CYP450 2C19, which is not involved in the metabolism of codeine to morphine.
D. Acetaminophen inhibits the metabolism of codeine to morphine.
Rationale: Acetaminophen does not inhibit the metabolism of codeine to morphine.
E. The patient is a poor metabolizer of CYP450 CYP2D6.
Rationale: In poor metabolizers of CYP450 CYP2D6, little or no morphine is produced; therefore, little or none of its glucuronides are subsequently formed.

Major points of discussion

■ Most circulating codeine is metabolized by CYP3A4 and UGT2B7 to norcodeine and codeine-6-glucuronide. *O*-demethylation of codeine to morphine accounts for less than 10% of codeine clearance but is regarded as the bioactivation reaction essential for the analgesic activity of codeine.

■ There is significant genetic polymorphism in the CYP450 2D6 enzyme. Although most patients have the extensive metabolizer (EM) genotype, some patients can also have a genotype associated with either ultrarapid metabolism (UM) or poor metabolism (PM) activity of the CYP450 2D6 enzyme.

■ Codeine administration to CYP450 2D6 UM patients results in relatively high concentrations of morphine and its metabolites, which may be associated with enhanced analgesic activity and increased side effects.

■ Codeine administration to CYP450 2D6 PM patients results in normal codeine concentrations but relatively low concentrations of morphine and its metabolites, which may result in a lack of analgesic activity.

■ Codeine, morphine, morphine-3-glucuronide, and morphine-6-glucuronide can be quantified simultaneously in plasma using LC-MS/MS.

■ Morphine and its metabolites are stable in plasma.

43. **A. Voriconazole is a stronger CYP3A4 inhibitor than fluconazole.**
Rationale: Everolimus is metabolized by CYP3A4. Voriconazole is a stronger inhibitor of CYP3A4 than fluconazole. Therefore, the C_{min} of everolimus is relatively higher during voriconazole treatment.
B. The LC-MS/MS method has a positive bias, yielding higher concentrations than FPIA.
Rationale: Everolimus concentrations measured with FPIA are, on average, approximately 20% higher than concentrations quantified in the same samples by LC-MS/MS.
C. Voriconazole displaces everolimus from albumin.
Rationale: Everolimus is measured in whole blood. Approximately 75% of everolimus is partitioned into red blood cells, and approximately 75% of the remaining plasma fraction is protein bound. It is unlikely that any potential displacement of everolimus from albumin by voriconazole leads to such large relative increases in whole blood everolimus levels.
D. The patient had a decline in renal function, decreasing elimination of everolimus.
Rationale: Changes in renal function do not substantially affect the elimination of everolimus. Only 2% of everolimus (and its metabolites) is eliminated in urine.
E. Voriconazole inhibits the enterohepatic cycle of everolimus metabolism.
Rationale: Although approximately 98% of everolimus is excreted as metabolites in the bile, everolimus does not undergo enterohepatic recycling.

Major points of discussion

■ Everolimus is metabolized in the gut and the liver by cytochromes CYP3A4, 3A5, and 2C8. Hydroxylation and demethylation appear to be the major pathways of metabolism. At least 11 metabolites have been identified to date.

■ A large number of drugs inhibit CYP3A-mediated metabolism, including several antifungal drugs. Some of these (e.g., fluconazole) are stronger inhibitors than others (e.g., ketoconazole, voriconazole) and will more substantially decrease the metabolic clearance of a drug such as everolimus.

■ Everolimus is primarily excreted in the bile as its metabolites. Renal excretion is minor. The metabolites of some drugs that are excreted into bile are subject to an enterohepatic circulation.

■ Biliary excretion of some drugs is mediated by Pg. Therefore, Pg inhibitors can lead to higher circulating levels of those drugs. Some drugs can both inhibit CYP3A and Pg.

■ Several assays are available to measure everolimus levels in whole blood. FPIA yields results that are approximately 20% higher than those obtained on the same samples by LC-MS/MS. This is most commonly caused by cross-reactivity of the immunoassay with several metabolites of everolimus.[71,78]

44. **A. Flunitrazepam.**
Rationale: The patient's symptoms and the LC-MS/MS results indicate that flunitrazepam was ingested.
B. Flurazepam.
C. Oxazepam.

Rationale: Neither the immunoassay nor the LC-MS/MS results suggest ingestion of flurazepam or oxazepam.

D. The patient was not drugged because flunitrazepam was not detectable.

Rationale: This is not true because flunitrazepam metabolites were detected by LC-MS/MS.

E. The patient was not drugged because the immunoassay was negative.

Rationale: This is not true because the immunoassay could yield a false-negative result.

Major points of discussion

- Flunitrazepam (Rohypnol), also known as a "roofie," is often used for drug-facilitated sexual assault or robbery. It is added to drinks (i.e., by "drink spiking"), but it can also be eaten in cookies laced with flunitrazepam. Police investigations are often made difficult because of the anterograde amnesia in the victims caused by the drug.

- Flunitrazepam is absorbed quickly with a T_{max} of 20 to 30 minutes and a half-life of 13 to 19 hours. The sedative effect varies between 4 and 8 hours. The drug is metabolized extensively by the liver, and many metabolites have been identified in plasma and urine. The primary urinary metabolites are 7-aminoflunitrazepam and 7-aminodesmethylaminoflunitrazepam.

- Because of cross-reactivity, immunoassays for benzodiazepines can also detect flunitrazepam and its metabolites in the urine, especially after deglucuronidation. However, different immunoassays have different cross-sensitivities toward flunitrazepam and its metabolites. Therefore, some assays yield positive results for a particular sample, whereas other assays will be negative. Higher doses of the drug (e.g., 2 mg) are more likely to yield a positive result compared with lower doses of the drug (e.g., 0.5 mg).

- After intake of the drug, there is a time course for flunitrazepam and its metabolites in urine, with maximal values of 7-aminoflunitrazepam at approximately 24 hours after intake and an increasing ratio of 7-amonidesmethylflunitrazepam to 7-aminoflunitrazepam over time (Figure 6-17). The ratio of the two, which can be determined by LC-MS/MS, can be used to determine the approximate time of intake.

- This is a forensic case, and care must be taken regarding maintaining a careful chain of evidence.[22,28,34]

45. A. Because her symptoms are not explained by any of these levels, do not initiate treatment yet. Because no comprehensive method detects 100% of all possible intoxicants, a comprehensive screen with another method should be initiated.

Rationale: Indeed, no method detects 100% of all possible intoxicants. However, in this case, her symptoms are explained by the lamotrigine serum concentration.

B. Begin immediate treatment for ibuprofen intoxication.

Rationale: Her ibuprofen serum concentration is within the therapeutic range.

C. Begin immediate treatment for lithium intoxication.

Rationale: Her lithium serum concentration is within the therapeutic range.

D. Begin immediate treatment for acetaminophen intoxication.

Rationale: An acetaminophen level of 18 µg/mL at approximately 4 hours after administration indicates that there is no risk for hepatotoxicity.

E. Begin immediate treatment for lamotrigine intoxication.

Rationale: The therapeutic range for lamotrigine in serum is 3 to 14 µg/mL.

Major points of discussion

- Lamotrigine (Lamictal) is an antiepileptic drug. Like many other antiepileptic drugs, it is also used in psychiatry as a mood stabilizer.

- The reference range for lamotrigine trough serum concentrations is 3 to 14 µg/mL. At steady state, there is little fluctuation in the serum concentrations. A serum concentration of 41.4 µg/mL, although measured in a sample collected approximately 4 hours after drug intake, strongly suggests drug intoxication.

- The symptoms of this patient also correspond with the high lamotrigine serum concentration. The most commonly reported clinical effects of lamotrigine overdose are drowsiness/lethargy, vomiting, nausea, ataxia, dizziness, vertigo, and tachycardia. Major clinical effects also include coma, seizures, and respiratory suppression.

- Treatment is symptomatic, and to date, no deaths from lamotrigine overdose have been reported.

- Lamotrigine levels are also influenced by the concomitant intake of metabolism inducers, such as phenobarbital, phenytoin, and carbamazepine, and inhibitors, such as valproic acid. Lamotrigine levels are also influenced by polymorphisms in the Pg-encoding gene *ABCB1*.

- No comprehensive drug screening method detects 100% of all possible intoxicants. Combining several methods improves the chance of detecting a possible intoxicant.[61,64,81,83]

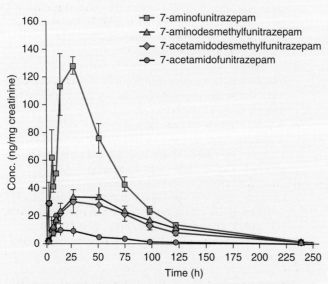

Figure 6-17 Mean metabolite excretion profiles after a 2.0-mg single dose of flunitrazepam, corrected for creatinine concentration (*n* = 8). (From Forsman M, Nystrom I, Roman M, et al. Urinary detection times and excretion patterns of flunitrazepam and its metabolites after a single oral dose. *J Anal Toxicol* 2009;33:491–501.)

46. A. Lead levels measured by ICP-MS are not reliable. The measurement should be repeated by AAS.
Rationale: Measurements of lead levels by ICP-MS are highly reliable.
B. Lithium heparin Vacutainer tubes can cause artificial increases in blood lead. A new sample should be collected in a different tube.
Rationale: The lithium heparin-containing Vacutainer tubes do not cause artificial increases in blood lead concentrations.
C. Given that the blood level is already decreasing, no follow-up sample or specific therapy is necessary.
Rationale: From this one sample, 1.5 hours after ingestion, it is not known whether the concentration is increasing or decreasing.
D. Treatment with dimercaptopropane sulfonate sodium (250 mg every 4 hours) should be initiated.
Rationale: Chelation therapy is indicated given this blood lead level.
E. Given that the patient is asymptomatic, specific treatment for lead intoxication should be withheld.
Rationale: The blood lead level and the patient's story suggest that treatment might be beneficial.

Major points of discussion

- Lead intoxications can be either chronic or acute. Acute intoxications can lead to gastrointestinal and renal symptoms. In addition to these symptoms, chronic intoxications have cardiovascular, endocrine, developmental, and neurologic effects.
- In blood, 99% of lead is bound to erythrocytes, which is one of the reasons lead levels are measured in whole blood samples. The bioavailability of lead after oral administration is approximately 20%. Lead is distributed in blood (2%), soft tissue (3%), and mineralized tissue, such as bone (95%), where it is sequestered and then slowly released. The elimination of lead is multiphasic, with half-lives of 36 days and 4 years.
- Blood collection tubes containing EDTA should not be used for whole blood assays because EDTA can chelate lead and cause low readings when a flame AAS method is used.
- The most common methods used to measure lead are flame AAS, graphite furnace atomic absorption spectrometry, anode stripping voltammetry, inductively coupled plasma–atomic emission spectroscopy, and ICP-MS.
- Normal ranges for blood lead are less than 100 to 200 ng/mL. In this clinical case, a potentially increasing, already elevated, blood lead level indicates that chelation therapy is necessary, despite the absence of symptoms. In this patient, a second lead level measured in a sample collected 9.5 hours after the acute intoxication was 412.9 ng/mL, confirming that the initiation of chelation therapy was the correct approach.
- Several intravenous and oral chelators are available, such as dimercaptopropane sulfonate sodium, EDTA, and succimer.
- Several markers of the effects of lead can also be determined to support blood lead measurements. These include measuring δ-aminolevulinic acid (ALA) excretion and δ-aminolevulinic acid dehydratase (ALA-D) enzymatic activity.[39,42,45]

47. A. Metoprolol interferes with immunoassays for benzodiazepines.
Rationale: Metoprolol does not interfere in these types of assays.
B. Urine samples should be treated with β-glucuronidase before performing an immunoassay for benzodiazepines.
Rationale: This is not the reason the screen is negative in this sample.
C. Furosemide interferes with the immunoassays for benzodiazepines.
Rationale: Furosemide does not interfere in these types of assays.
D. None of this patient's medications is a benzodiazepine hypnotic, nor do any of the drugs show cross-reactivity with the immunoassay.
Rationale: Zopiclone is often mistaken for a benzodiazepine but is not one. This patient's other medications are also not benzodiazepines, and none of them cross-reacts with immunoassays for benzodiazepines.
E. Zopiclone acts as a benzodiazepine.
Rationale: The effects of zopiclone (Lunesta) are similar to a benzodiazepine, but this is not the reason the screen is negative.

Major points of discussion

- Immunoassays for benzodiazepines are an essential part of tier I drug screenings.
- Many metabolites of benzodiazepines are excreted into urine as glucuronides, and treatment with β-glucuronidase increases the probability of detecting benzodiazepines in urine samples.
- Benzodiazepine assays are often calibrated with nordiazepam, but they can be used to measure most other benzodiazepines because of cross-reactivity with the benzodiazepine moiety.
- Zolpidem and zopiclone are often regarded as benzodiazepines because they are also hypnotics and act on the same pathway as benzodiazepines. However, their chemical structure and exact mechanism of action differ from those of the benzodiazepines.
- Because of their different chemical structures, zopiclone and zolpidem are usually not detected by benzodiazepine immunoassays.
- Exact cross-reactivity of immunoassays with other drugs differs from assay to assay. The assay-specific information for any particular assay can be found in the package insert provided by the manufacturer.

48. A. MPA was measured in serum but should be measured in whole blood.
Rationale: MPA is measured in serum, not in whole blood.
B. The current specimen is a randomly collected sample, rather than a trough level.
Rationale: After MMF drug intake, even at steady state, MPA serum concentrations increase and decrease, with an additional increase and decrease because of enterohepatic recycling.

C. Tacrolimus increases MPA concentrations.
Rationale: The regimen was stable; therefore, any interaction would also have been relevant regarding the prior sample.
D. Intrapatient variability in MPA pharmacokinetics.
Rationale: Although there is significant intrapatient variability, serum trough levels of MPA do not vary much in a stable patient.
E. Lack of precision of the MPA assay.
Rationale: The coefficient of variation (CV) of interassay precision for this type of assay is typically less than 20%.

Major points of discussion

- Blood samples for therapeutic drug monitoring (TDM) are usually collected before the next dose; these are called "trough levels." Sometimes blood sampling will occur soon after drug intake, leading to higher drug levels than expected.

- Mycophenolate mofetil is a prodrug, which is rapidly hydrolyzed to its active compound, MPA. MPA can be further metabolized, and its most predominant metabolite is the glucuronide (MPAG). MPAG is excreted into urine but also into the bile. After biliary secretion and deglucuronidation, free MPA can be taken up again, thereby forming an enterohepatic cycle, which contributes significantly to circulating levels of MPA. The enterohepatic cycle also causes a second peak in the MPA serum concentration time profile. This peak, which takes place approximately 8 hours after drug intake, is observed in most, but not all, patients.

- Although many immunosuppressive drugs, such as cyclosporine, tacrolimus, everolimus, and sirolimus, are measured in whole blood, MPA is measured in serum or plasma.

- The necessity for TDM of MPA is a subject of ongoing debate. However, TDM could provide the clinician with certainty about the systemic exposure to MPA, which shows significant interpatient variability.

- Some amount of the variability in drug levels is also caused by the imprecision of the assay.[11,12]

49. A. Reduce the MMF dose.
Rationale: Because of the delay in receiving and testing the sample, the MPA plasma level is not reliable. Therefore, any action based on this level might be incorrect.
B. Reduce the cyclosporine dose.
Rationale: A dose reduction of cyclosporine A will increase the MPA plasma concentration.
C. Increase the cyclosporine dose.
Rationale: A dose increase of cyclosporine will decrease the MPA plasma concentration.
D. Rerun this sample.
Rationale: The LC-MS/MS assays used to measure MPA typically have a CV of interassay of less than 20%.
E. Collect a new sample from the patient.
Rationale: MPA plasma concentrations are known to be artificially elevated when the blood sample is kept at ambient temperature for longer periods of time.

Major points of discussion

- MPAG and the acyl glucuronide, AcMPAG, may be deglucuronidated to MPA. This can take place ex vivo in whole blood and plasma and is time and temperature dependent.

- Stability of analytes should be considered when defining sample transport conditions.

- Samples should be rejected when requirements for transport conditions have not been met.

- The stability of glucuronides has also been a problem with certain LC-MS/MS methods for measuring MPA.[49,98]

50. A. Individuals of Asian descent generally have a very large volume of distribution of voriconazole.
Rationale: Individuals of Asian descent do not typically have a large volume of distribution of any drug.
B. Many individuals of Asian descent are ultrarapid extensive metabolizers of voriconazole.
Rationale: Not many individuals of Asian descent are ultrarapid extensive metabolizers of voriconazole.
C. Many individuals of Asian descent are slow metabolizers of voriconazole.
Rationale: The poor metabolizer phenotype of CYP2C19 is most commonly seen in individuals of Asian descent, with a frequency ranging from 13% to 23%. However, this leads to high voriconazole levels.
D. Ion enhancement of the voriconazole signal by unknown compounds in the patient's serum can lead to artificially low measurements of voriconazole concentrations.
Rationale: With the use of an internal standard with a retention time different from that of voriconazole, ion enhancement by unknown compounds could take place. However, this would lead to a higher signal of voriconazole and, therefore, higher voriconazole levels.
E. Ion suppression of the voriconazole signal by unknown compounds in the patient's serum can lead to artificially low measurements of voriconazole concentrations.
Rationale: With the use of an internal standard with a retention time different from that of voriconazole, ion suppression by unknown compounds could take place. Ion suppression would lead to a lower signal of voriconazole and, therefore, lower voriconazole levels.

Major points of discussion

- Voriconazole's metabolism is predominantly hepatic, through the CYP 450 system, with the primary pathways being CYP2C19 and, to a lesser extent, CYP2C9 and CYP3A4. This metabolism is saturable and nonlinear.

- Additionally, CYP2C19, the most predominant of the enzymatic pathways, exhibits significant genetic polymorphism, which essentially results in three phenotypes: ultrarapid extensive metabolizers (homozygous), extensive metabolizers (heterozygous), and poor metabolizers.

- The distribution of these phenotypes varies among populations. For example, the poor metabolizer phenotype of CYP2C19 is most commonly seen in individuals of Asian descent, with a frequency ranging from 13% to 23%. The poor metabolizer phenotype is most commonly associated with CYP2C19*2 and CYP2C19*3. Among whites, the frequency of the poor metabolizer phenotype is typically 3% to 5%. Multiple studies assessing the impact of this phenotype on voriconazole concentrations have shown a threefold to fourfold increase in concentration in patients with the poor metabolizer phenotype compared with ultrarapid extensive metabolizers and a twofold increase in concentration compared with extensive metabolizers.

■ LC-MS and LC-MS/MS methods are subject to interference from ion suppression (and enhancement), as well as metabolites producing isobaric ions.

■ Ion suppression takes place at the early stage of ionization when a component of the matrix coelutes from the chromatographic column with the compound of interest and suppresses the ionization of the analyte.

■ If both the compound of interest and its internal standard elute from the chromatographic column at the same time (e.g., when using a hexadeuterated version of the compound of interest as internal standard), both signals are suppressed, which is not optimal but may not affect the ratio of the two signals.

■ If the compound of interest elutes from the chromatographic column at a different time compared with the internal standard (which is the case for the method used for voriconazole), the signal of the compound of interest might be suppressed, whereas the internal standard signal is not. This will lead to a lower signal.

■ Various strategies exist to minimize the risk for ion suppression (or enhancement), as follows:
  ● Full validation of the method
  ● Substantial retention of both the internal standard and the compound of interest
  ● Use of a stable isotope version of the compound of interest as an internal standard (such as deuterated voriconazole in this case)

However, it is not possible to entirely prevent the risk for ion suppression and enhancement; therefore, it should always be considered, especially in the case of unexpected results.[2,25,69]

References

1. Ahsman MJ, van der Nagel BC, Mathot RA. Quantification of midazolam, morphine and metabolites in plasma using 96-well solid-phase extraction and ultra-performance liquid chromatography–tandem mass spectrometry. Biomed Chromatogr 2010;24:969–976.

2. Alffenaar JW, Wessels AM, van Hateren K, et al. Method for therapeutic drug monitoring of azole antifungal drugs in human serum using LC/MS/MS. J Chromatogr B Analyt Technol Biomed Life Sci 2010;878:39–44.

3. Al-Turkmani MR, Law T, Narla A, et al. Difficulty measuring methotrexate in a patient with high-dose methotrexate-induced nephrotoxicity. Clin Chem 2010;56:1792–1796.

4. Bartelink IH, Bredius RGM, Belitser S, et al. Association between busulfan exposure and outcome in children receiving intravenous busulfan before hematologic stem cell transplantation. Biol Blood Marrow Transplant 2009;15:231–241.

5. Bauer TM, Ritz R, Haberthur C, et al. Prolonged sedation due to accumulation of conjugated metabolites of midazolam. Lancet 1995;346:145–147.

6. Berend K, van der Voet G, Boer WH. Acute aluminum encephalopathy in a dialysis center caused by a cement mortar water distribution pipe. Kidney Int 2001;59:746–753.

7. Beyer J, Peters FT, Maurer HH. Screening procedure for detection of stimulant laxatives and/or their metabolites in human urine using gas chromatography-mass spectrometry after enzymatic cleavage of conjugates and extractive methylation. Ther Drug Monit 2005;27:151–157.

8. Bjornstad K, Hulten P, Beck O, et al. Bioanalytical and clinical evaluation of 103 suspected cases of intoxications with psychoactive plant materials. Clin Toxicol 2009;47:566–572.

9. Borsutzky M, Passie T, Paetzold W, et al. Hawaiian baby woodrose: (Psycho-)Pharmacological effects of the seeds of *Argyreia nervosa*. A case-orientated demonstration (in German). Nervenarzt 2002;73:892–896.

10. Brown TT, McComsey GA. Association between initiation of antiretroviral therapy with efavirenz and decreases in 25-hydroxyvitamin D. Antivir Ther 2010;15:425–429.

11. Bullingham R, Monroe S, Nicholls A, et al. Pharmacokinetics and bioavailability of mycophenolate mofetil in healthy subjects after single-dose oral and intravenous administration. J Clin Pharmacol 1996;36:315–324.

12. Bullingham R, Shah J, Goldblum R, et al. Effects of food and antacid on the pharmacokinetics of single doses of mycophenolate mofetil in rheumatoid arthritis patients. Br J Clin Pharmacol 1996;41:513–516.

13. Chiu C-C, Lu M-L, Huang M-C, et al. Heavy smoking, reduced olanzapine levels and treatment effects. Ther Drug Monitor 2004;26:579–581.

14. Choi JJ, Moffett BS, McDade EJ, et al. Altered gentamicin serum concentrations in obese pediatric patients. Pediatr Infect Disease J 2011;30:347–349.

15. Citrome L, Macher JP, Salazar DE, et al. Pharmacokinetics of aripiprazole and concomitant carbamazepine. J Clin Psychopharmacol 2007;27:279–283.

16. Burtis CA, Shaw LM, et al. Clinical toxicology. In Burtis CA, Ashwood ER, Bruns DE, *Tietz Textbook of Clinical Chemistry and Molecular Diagnosis*, 4th ed. St. Louis: Elsevier, 2005, 1315–1371.

17. Burtis CA, Shaw LM, et al. Clinical toxicology. In Burtis CA, Ashwood ER, Bruns DE, *Tietz Textbook of Clinical Chemistry and Molecular Diagnosis*, 4th ed. St. Louis: Elsevier, 2005, 1287–1369.

18. Burtis CA, Shaw LM, et al. Clinical toxicology. In Burtis CA, Ashwood ER, Bruns DE, *Tietz Textbook of Clinical Chemistry and Molecular Diagnosis*, 4th ed. St. Louis: Elsevier, 2005, pp 1306–1308.

19. Cohen Smith J, Curry SC. Prolonged toxicity after amitriptyline overdose in a patient deficient in CYP2D6 activity. J Med Toxicol 2011;7:220–223.

20. Cremers S, Schoemaker R, Bredius R, et al. Pharmacokinetics of intravenous busulfan in children prior to stem cell transplantation. Br J Clin Pharmacol 2002;53:386–389.

21. Crews KR, Gaedigk A, Dunnenberger HM, et al. Clinical pharmacogenetics implementation consortium (CPIC) guidelines for codeine therapy in the context of cytochrome P450 2D6 (CYP2D6) genotype. Clin Pharmacol Ther 2012;91:321–326.

22. Daderman AM, Strindlund H, Wiklund N, et al. The importance of a urine sample in persons intoxicated with flunitrazepam-legal issues in a forensic psychiatric case study of a serial murderer. Forensic Sci Int 2003;137:21–27.

23. Damle B, LaBadie R, Rownover P, et al. Pharmacokinetic interactions of efavirenz and voriconazole in healthy volunteers. Br J Clin Pharmacol 2008;65:523–530.

24. Dasgupta A, Yared MA, Wells A. Time-dependent absorption of therapeutic drugs by the gel of the Greiner Vacuette blood collection tube. Ther Drug Monitor 2000;22:427–431.

25. Dasgupta A. Impact of interferences including metabolite crossreactivity on therapeutic drug monitoring results. Ther Drug Monit 2012;34:496–506.

26. Daubert GP, Mabasa VH, Leung VWY, et al. Acute clenbuterol overdose resulting in supraventricular tachycardia and atrial fibrillation. J Med Toxicol 2007;3:56–60.

27. Duncan A. Screening for surreptitious laxative abuse. Ann Clin Biochem 2000;37:1–8.

28. Elliott SP, Burgess V. Clinical urinalysis of drugs and alcohol in instances of suspected surreptitious administration ("spiked drinks"). Sci Justice 2005;45:129–134.

29. Epnes KA, Heimdal KE, Spigset O. A puzzling case of increased serum clozapine levels in a patient with inflammation and infection. Ther Drug Monit 2012;34:489–492.

30. Ergenekon E, Dalgic N, Aksoy E, et al. Caffeine intoxication in a premature neonate. Paediatr Anaesth 2001;11:737–739.

31. Esteve MA, Devictor-Pierre B, Galy G, et al. Severe acute toxicity associated with high-dose methotrexate (MTX) therapy: use of therapeutic drug monitoring and test-dose to guide carboxypeptidase G2 rescue and MTX continuation. Eur J Clin Pharmacol 2007;63:39–42.

32. Evans WE, Pratt CB, Taylor RH, et al. Pharmacokinetic monitoring of high-dose methotrexate therap. Early recognition of high-risk patients. Cancer Chemother Pharmacol 1979;3:161–166.

33. Fenton F, Smally AJ, Laut J. Hyperkalemia and digoxin toxicity in a patient with kidney failure. Ann Emerg Med 1996;28:440–441.

34. Forsman M, Nystrom I, Roman M, et al. Urinary detection times and excretion patterns of flunitrazepam and its metabolites after a single oral dose. J Anal Toxicol 2009;33:491–501.

35. Fox J, Peters B, Prakash M, et al. Improvement in vitamin D deficiency following antiretroviral regime change: results from the MONET trial. AIDS Res Human Retrovir 2011;27:29–34.

36. Franssen EJM, Kunst PWA, Bet PM, et al. Toxicokinetics of nortriptyline and amitriptyline: two case reports. Ther Drug Monitor 2003;25:248–251.

37. Gagajewski A, Davis GK, Kloss J, et al. False-positive lysergic acid diethylamide immunoassay screen associated with fentanyl medication. Clin Chem 2002;48:205–206.

38. Galbois A, Ait-Oufella H, Baudel J-L, et al. An adult can still die of salicylate poisoning in France in 2008. Intensive Care Med 2009;35:1999.

39. Graziano JH. Validity of lead exposure markers in diagnosis and surveillance. Clin Chem 1994;40:1387–1390.

40. Henningsson C, Hoffmann S, McGonigle L, et al. Acute mercury poisoning (acrodynia) mimicking pheochromocytoma in an adolescent. J Pediatrics 1993;122:252–253.

41. Hernandez JD, Wesseling K, Salusky IB. Role of parathyroid hormone and therapy with active vitamin D sterols in renal osteodystrophy. Semin Dial 2005;18:290–295.

42. Ho G, Keutgens A, Schoofs R, et al. Blood, urine, and hair analysis following an acute lead intoxication. J Anal Toxicol 2011;35:60–64.

43. Howard SJ, Felton TW, Gomez-Lopez A, et al. Posaconazole: the case for therapeutic drug monitoring. Ther Drug Monit 2012;34:72–76.

44. AACC. Updates and Case Studies in Volatile Alcohols, Glycols, and Clinical Alcohol Testing. Available at www.aacc.org/events/online_progs/pages/clintox_alcohols.aspx.

45. Agency for Toxic Substances and Disease Registry. Available at www.atsdr.cdc.gov.

46. KKGT. First Round Discussion of the Patient Case of the International Interlaboratory Quality Control Program for Antifungal Drugs. Available at www.kkgt.nl/antifcase08.htm.

47. Jacobsen D, Hewlett TP, Webb R, et al. Ethylene glycol intoxication: evaluation of kinetics and crystalluria. Am J Med 1988;84:145–152.

48. Jang SH, Colangelo PM, Gobburu JV. Exposure-response of posaconazole used for prophylaxis against invasive fungal infections: evaluating the need to adjust doses based on drug concentrations in plasma. Clin Pharmacol Ther 2010;88:115–119.

49. Jeong H, Kaplan B. Therapeutic drug monitoring of mycophenolate mofetil. Clin J Am Soc Nephrol 2007;2:184–191.

50. Jim MC, Ouyang XK, Chen XH. High-performance liquid chromatography coupled with electrospray ionization tandem mass spectrometry for the determination of flocoumafen and brodifacoum in whole blood. J Appl Toxicol 2007;27:18–24.

51. Joos AA, König F, Frank UG, et al. Dose-dependent pharmacokinetic interaction of clozapine and paroxetine in an extensive metabolizer. Pharmacopsychiatry 1997;30:266–270.

52. Kasick DP, McKnight CA, Klisovic E. "Bath salt" ingestion leading to severe intoxication delirium: two cases and a brief review of the emergence of mephedrone use. Am J Drug Alcohol Abuse 2012;38:176–180.

53. Kellogg MD, Law T, Sakamoto M, et al. Tandem mass spectrometry for the quantification of serum busulfan. Ther Drug Monit 2005;27:625–629.

54. Kirchheiner J, Schmidt H, Tzvetkov M, et al. Pharmacokinetics of codeine and its metabolite morphine in ultra-rapid metabolizers due to CYP2D6 duplication. Pharmacogenomics J 2007;7:257–265.

55. Klinke HB, Muller IB, Steffenrud S, et al. Two cases of lysergamide intoxication by ingestion of seeds from Hawaiian baby woodrose. Forensic Sci Int 2010;197:e1–e5.

56. Kuhn J, Götting C, Kleesiek K. Simultaneous measurement of amiodarone and desethylamiodarone in human plasma and serum by stable isotope dilution liquid chromatography-tandem mass spectrometry assay. J Pharm Biomed Anal 2010;51:210–216.

57. Kuipers EA, den Hartigh J, Saverlkoul TJ, et al. A method for the simultaneous identification and quantitation of five superwarfarin rodenticides in human serum. J Anal Toxicol 1995;19:557–562.

58. Lacassie E, Marquet P, Martin-Dupont S, et al. A non-fatal case of intoxication with foxglove, documented by means of liquid chromatography-electrospray-mass spectrometry. J Forens Sc 2000;45:1154–1158.

59. Lee DC, Klachko MN. Falsely elevated lithium levels in plasma samples obtained in lithium containing tubes. J Toxicol Clin Toxicol 1996;34:467–469.

60. Liu H-C, Chang WH, Wei FC, et al. Monitoring of plasma clozapine levels and its metabolites in refractory schizophrenic patients. Ther Drug Monit 1996;18:200–207.

61. Lovric M, Bozina N, Hajnsek S, et al. Association between lamotrigine concentrations and ABCB1 polymorphisms in patients with epilepsy. Ther Drug Monit 2012;34:518–525.

62. Lowe H, Cusano N, Binkley N, et al. Vitamin D toxicity due to a commonly available "over the counter" remedy from the Dominican Republic. J Clin Endocrinol Metab 2011;96:291–295.

63. Lv H, Sun H, Wang X, et al. Simultaneous determination by UPLC-ESI-MS of scoparone, capillarisin, rhein, and emodin in rat urine after oral administration of Yin Chen Hao Tang preparation. J Sep Sci 2008;31:659–666.

64. Mallaysamy S, Johnson MG, Rao PGM, et al. Population pharmacokinetics of lamotrigine in Indian epileptic patients. Eur J Clin Pharmacol 2013;69:43–52.

65. Manini AF, Nelson LS, Hoffman RS. Prognostic utility of serum potassium in chronic digoxin toxicity: a case-control study. Am J Cardiovasc Drugs 2011;11:173–178.

66. McCarthy JT, Milliner DS, Kurtz SB, et al. Interpretation of serum aluminum values in dialysis patients. Am J Clin Pathol 1986;86:629–636.

67. McKenzie CA, McKinnon W, Naughton DP, et al. Differentiating midazolam over-sedation from neurological damage in the intensive care unit. Crit Care 2005;9:R32–R36.

68. Melanson SEF, Baskin L, Magnani B, et al. Interpretation and utility of drug of abuse immunoassays: lessons from laboratory drug testing surveys. Arch Pathol Lab Med 2010;134:735–739.

69. Meletiadis J, Chanock S, Walsh TJ. Human pharmacogenomic variations and their implications for antifungal efficacy. Clin Microbiol Rev 2006;19:763–787.

70. Minns AB, Cantrell FL, Clark R. Death due to salicylate intoxication despite dialysis. J Emerg Med 2011;40:515–517.

71. Moes DJAR, Press RR, de Fijter JW, et al. Liquid chromatography-tandem mass spectrometry outperforms fluorescence polarization immunoassay in monitoring everolimus therapy in renal transplantation. Ther Drug Monit 2010;32:413–419.

72. Nansera D, Graziano FM, Friedman DJ, et al. Vitamin D and calcium levels in Ugandan adults with human immunodeficiency virus and tuberculosis. Int J Tuberc Lung Dis 2011;15:1522–1527.

73. Ng PK. Determining aminoglycoside dosage and blood levels using a programmable calculator. Am J Hosp Pharm 1980;37:225–231.

74. Nordt SP, Cantrell FL. Elevated lithium level: a case a brief overview of lithium poisoning. Psychosom Med 1999;61:564–565.

75. Oldenhof H, de Jong M, Steenhoek A, et al. Clinical pharmacokinetics of midazolam in intensive care patients, a wide interpatient variability? Clin Pharmacol Ther 1988;43:263–269.

76. Pai MP, Nafziger AN, Bertino JS. Simplified estimation of aminoglycoside pharmacokinetics in underweight and obese adult patients. Antimicrob Agents Chemother 2011;55:4006–4011.

77. Pascual A, Calandra T, Bolay S, et al. Voriconazole therapeutic drug monitoring in patients with invasive mycoses improves therapeutic efficacy and safety outcomes. Clin Infect Dis 2008;46:201–211.

78. Pea F, Baccarini U, Tavio M, et al. Pharmacokinetic interaction between everolimus and antifungal triazoles in a liver transplant patient. Ann Pharmacother 2008;42:1711–1716.

79. Perry PJ, Lund BC, Sanger T, et al. Olanzapine plasma concentrations and clinical response: acute phase results of the North American Olanzapine Trial. J Clin Psychopharmacol 2001;21:14–20.

80. Ramcharan S, Meenhorst PL, Otten JMMB, et al. Survival after massive ecstasy overdose. Clin Toxicol 1998;36(7):727–731.

81. Reimers A, Reinholt G. Acute lamotrigine overdose in an adolescent. Ther Drug Monit 2007;29:669–670.

82. Rosano TG, Swift TA, Kranick CJ, et al. Ethylene glycol and glycolic acid in postmortem blood from fatal poisonings. J Anal Toxicol 2009;33:508–513.

83. Rosano TG, Wood M, Swift TA. Postmortem drug screening by non-targeted and targeted ultra-performance liquid chromatography-mass spectrometry technology. J Anal Toxicol 2011;35:411–423.

84. Rostaing L, Cointault O, Marquet P, et al. Falsely elevated whole-blood tacrolimus concentrations in a kidney-transplant patient: potential hazards. Transplant Int 2010;23:227–230.

85. Roten L, Schoenenberger RA, Krähenbühl S, et al. Rhabdomyolysis in association with simvastatin and amiodarone. Ann Pharmacother 2004;38:978–981.

86. Rumack BH, Matthew H. Acetaminophen poisoning and toxicity. Pediatrics 1975;55:871–876.

87. Sandberg Y, Rood PPM, Russcher H, et al. Falsely elevated lactate in severe ethylene glycol intoxication. Neth J Med 2010;68:320–323.

88. Shelton JH, Santa Ana CA, Thompson DR, et al. Factitious diarrhea induced by stimulant laxatives: accuracy of diagnosis by a clinical reference laboratory using thin layer chromatography. Clin Chem 2007;53:85–90.

89. Simons SA, Molinelli AR, Sobhani K, et al. Two cases with unusual vancomycin measurements. Clin Chem 2009;55:578–582.

90. Slattery JT, Sanders JE, Buckner CD, et al. Graft-rejection and toxicity following bone marrow transplantation in relation to busulfan pharmacokinetics. Bone Marrow Transplant 1995;16:31–42.

91. Sorensen LK. Determination of cathinones and related ephedrines in forensic whole-blood samples by liquid-chromatography-electrospray tandem mass spectrometry. J Chromatogr B 2011;879:727–736.

92. Stoller G, Hande KR, Jacobs SA, et al. Use of plasma pharmacokinetics to predict and prevent methotrexate toxicity. N Engl J Med 1977;297:630–634.

93. Strano-Rossi S, Bermejo AM, de la Torre X, et al. Fast GC-MS method for the simultaneous screening of THC-COOH, cocaine, opiates and analogues including buprenorphine and fentanyl, and their metabolites in urine. Anal Bioanal Chem 2011;399:1623–1630.

94. Tarbah FA, Kardel B, Pier O, et al. Acute poisoning with phosphamidon: determination of dimethyl phosphate (DMP) as a stable metabolite in a case of organophosphate insecticide intoxication. J Anal Toxicol 2004;28:198–203.

95. Burtis A, et al. Therapeutic drugs and their management. In Burtis CA, Ashwood ER, Bruns DE, eds. *Tietz Textbook of Clinical Chemistry and Molecular Diagnostics*, 4 ed. St Louis: Elsevier, 2005, pp 1256.

96. Timmer RT, Sands JM. Lithium intoxication. J Am Soc Nephrol 1999;10:666–674.

97. Tournel GL, Houssaye C, Humbert L, et al. Acute arsenic poisoning: clinical, toxicological, histopathological, and forensic features. J Forensic Sci 2011;56:S275–S279.

98. Tracey J, Brown NW, Tredger JM. Optimal storage temperature and matrix before analyzing mycophenolic acid. Ther Drug Monit 2012;34:148–152.

99. Van den Anker J, Jongejan HTM, Sauer PJJ. Severe caffeine intoxication in a preterm neonate. Eur J Pediatr 1992;151:466–468.

100. Van Deusen SK, Birkhahn RH, Gaeta TJ. Treatment of hyperkalemia in a patient with unrecognized digitalis toxicity. J Toxicol Clin Toxicol 2003;41:373–376.

101. Velzeboer SC, Frankel J, de Wolff FA. A hypertensive toddler. Lancet 1997;349:1810.

102. Wills BK, Mycyk MB, Mazor S, et al. Factitious lithium toxicity secondary to lithium heparin-containing blood tubes. J Med Toxicol 2006;2:61–63.

103. Wu AHB, McKay C, Broussard LA, et al. National Academy of Clinical Biochemistry. Recommendations for the use of laboratory tests to support poisoned patients who present to the emergency department. Clin Chem 2003;49:357–379.

104. Zhang Y, Mehrota N, Budha N, et al. A tandem mass spectrometry assay for the simultaneous determination of acetaminophen, caffeine, phenytoin, ranitidine, and theophylline in small volume pediatric plasma specimens. Clin Chim Acta 2008;398:105–112.

105. Zolcinski M, Padjas A, Musial J. Intoxication with three different superwarfarin compounds in an adult woman. Thromb Haemost 2008;100:156–157.

CHAPTER 7

CLINICAL CHEMISTRY:
Lipids and Glycoproteins

Tilla S. Worgall, Steven L. Spitalnik, Jeffrey S. Jhang

QUESTIONS

1. Lipoproteins are large macromolecular complexes. They transport hydrophobic lipids through body fluids. The lipoprotein core contains hydrophobic lipids. The core is surrounded by more hydrophilic lipids and proteins. Which one of the following constitutes the main lipid components of the lipoprotein core?
   A. Free cholesterol and triglycerides (TGs).
   B. Cholesteryl esters and TGs.
   C. Free cholesterol and cholesteryl esters.
   D. Phospholipids and TGs.
   E. Free cholesterol and phospholipids.

2. The National Cholesterol Education Program Expert Panel (NCEP), Adult Treatment Panel III (ATP III), recommends that patients achieve which one of the following values for total cholesterol?
   A. <100 mg/dL.
   B. <150 mg/dL.
   C. <200 mg/dL.
   D. <239 mg/dL.
   E. <240 mg/dL.

3. Plasma lipoproteins are divided into five major classes. These lipoprotein classes contain different concentrations of TGs, free cholesterol, esterified cholesterol, phospholipids, and apoproteins. Classification is based on their density, which ranges from less than 0.95 g/mL to about 1.20 g/mL. Which one of the following best describes the relationship between density and diameter?
   A. Density and diameter are directly proportional: High-density particles are the largest lipoproteins.
   B. Density and diameter are inversely proportional: High-density particles are the smallest lipoproteins.
   C. There is no relationship between density and diameter.

4. Most plasma cholesterol is carried as cholesteryl esters in which one of the following types of lipoprotein particle?
   A. Chylomicrons.
   B. Very-low-density lipoprotein (VLDL).
   C. Low-density lipoprotein (LDL).
   D. Intermediate-density lipoprotein (IDL).
   E. High-density lipoprotein (HDL).

5. Which one of the following statements regarding genetically determined hyperlipidemias is true?
   A. Increased chylomicrons are characteristic of type I hyperlipidemia.
   B. Defective LDL receptor binding results in low plasma cholesterol levels and high TG levels.
   C. Type III hyperlipidemia is associated with homozygosity for the ApoE E4/E4 genotype and results in equally increased cholesterol and TG levels.
   D. Type IIb hyperlipidemia is associated with increased LDL and HDL levels.
   E. Type V hyperlipidemia, or mixed hyperlipidemia, is associated with increased VLDL and LDL levels.

6. Which one of the following correctly describes the origin of plasma LDL?
   A. LDL originates directly from dietary uptake of cholesterol.
   B. LDL is synthesized by intestinal epithelium.
   C. LDL is secreted by the liver.
   D. LDL originates from chylomicron hydrolysis.
   E. LDL originates from VLDL hydrolysis.

7. Based on the 2001 recommendations of the NCEP ATP III, patients should be tested initially for which one of the following groups of parameters?
   A. Total cholesterol and HDL cholesterol.
   B. Total cholesterol, LDL cholesterol, HDL cholesterol, and TGs.
   C. Total cholesterol, LDL cholesterol, HDL cholesterol, TGs, and chylomicrons.
   D. Total cholesterol, HDL cholesterol, and LDL subfractions (i.e., small dense LDL particles).
   E. Total cholesterol, LDL cholesterol, HDL cholesterol, and chylomicrons.

8. Statin (3-hydroxy-3-methyl-glutaryl-CoA [HMG-CoA] reductase inhibitor) therapy lowers plasma cholesterol levels by which one of the following mechanisms?
   A. Increased upregulation of liver LDL receptors.
   B. Decreased uptake of cholesterol by enterocytes.
   C. Increased synthesis of anticholesterol particles.
   D. Increased secretion of cholesterol into bile.
   E. Decreased synthesis of apoprotein B.

9. A 10-year-old girl presents to her pediatrician with elevated orange-yellow xanthomas present superficially over her knees, wrists, and interdigital webs. These physical findings are characteristic for which one of the following conditions?
   A. Abetalipoproteinemia.
   B. Hepatic lipase deficiency.
   C. Diabetic dyslipidemia.
   D. Familial hypercholesterolemia.
   E. Metachromatic leukodystrophy.

10. Cholesteryl ester transfer protein (CETP) is a potential therapeutic target to decrease atherosclerotic disease. Which one of the following statements best describes the effect of CETP?
   A. CETP transfers cholesteryl esters from chylomicrons to HDL, thereby producing VLDL particles.
   B. CETP transfers cholesteryl esters from LDL to HDL particles, which are then cleared by the HDL receptor.
   C. CETP increases cholesteryl ester content in VLDL particles. The cholesteryl esters in the circulation are then cleared by the liver through VLDL receptors.
   D. CETP increases cholesteryl ester content in HDL particles. The cholesteryl esters in the circulation are then cleared by the liver through HDL receptors.
   E. CETP transfers TGs from apolipoprotein B (ApoB)-containing lipoproteins to HDL in exchange for cholesteryl esters. The cholesteryl esters in the circulation are then cleared by the liver through LDL receptors.

11. Which one of the following statements best describes the finding(s) in a patient with ABCA1 deficiency (i.e., Tangier disease)?
   A. Increased ApoA1 on plasma LDL particles.
   B. Absence of LDL particles in plasma.
   C. Very low plasma HDL cholesterol levels accompanied by lipid accumulation in peripheral cells.
   D. Fasting TG levels of more than 100 mg/dL, which may rise to more than 10,000 mg/dL postprandially.
   E. Milky plasma characterized by increased circulating levels of chylomicrons.

12. Which one of the following findings best characterizes lecithin cholesterol acyltransferase (LCAT) deficiency?
   A. Large chylomicrons and VLDL with very high TG levels.
   B. Decreased HDL levels.

C. Elevated LDL levels.
D. Increased LDL receptors expressed on the cell surface.
E. Increased lysolecithin.

13. Which one of the following best describes the changes associated with activation of the LDL receptor pathway?
   A. Decreased HMG-CoA reductase activity, increased acetyl-coenzyme A acetyltransferase (ACAT) activity, and decreased expression of LDL receptors.
   B. Increased HMG-CoA reductase activity, decreased ACAT activity, and decreased expression of LDL receptors.
   C. Decreased HMG-CoA reductase activity, decreased ACAT activity, and decreased expression of LDL receptors.
   D. Decreased HMG-CoA reductase activity, decreased ACAT activity, and increased expression of LDL receptors.
   E. Increased HMG-CoA reductase activity, increased ACAT activity, and increased expression of LDL receptors.

14. Which one of the following is the intraindividual physiologic variation in serum cholesterol?
   A. 1%.
   B. 6.5%.
   C. 8%.
   D. 20%.
   E. 50%.

15a. Which one of the following is the goal value for LDL cholesterol in patients with coronary heart disease (CHD) or CHD risk equivalent according to the recommendations made by the NCEP ATP guidelines?
   A. <40 mg/dL.
   B. <65 mg/dL.
   C. <100 mg/dL.
   D. <160 mg/dL.
   E. <200 mg/dL.

15b. Which one of the following is the cutoff value for a "high" HDL cholesterol according to the recommendations made by the NCEP ATP?
   A. <40 mg/dL.
   B. >40 mg/dL.
   C. <60 mg/dL.
   D. >60 mg/dL.
   E. <100 mg/dL.

ANSWERS

1. A. Free cholesterol and triglycerides (TGs).
   B. Cholesterol esters and TGs.
   Rationale: These components are highly hydrophobic and represent the bulk of the lipids in the lipoprotein core.
   C. Free cholesterol and cholesteryl esters.
   Rationale for A and C: Free cholesterol is too polar to exist in the lipoprotein core.
   D. Phospholipids and TGs.
   Rationale: Phospholipids typically contain polar head groups and, as such, are too polar to exist in the lipoprotein core.
   E. Free cholesterol and phospholipids.
   Rationale: Free cholesterol and phospholipids are too polar to exist in the lipoprotein core.

Major points of discussion
- The main task of lipoproteins is TG transport. In a normal adult human consuming an average diet, as much as 100 to 150 g of TGs is transported each day. Of this total, 70 to 100 g come from the diet and 30 to 60 g from endogenous synthesis in the liver.
- Free cholesterol is a component of phospholipid membranes.
- Cholesteryl esters are the storage form of cholesterol. The ester bond between the carboxylate group of a fatty acid (primarily linoleic acid or oleic acid) and the hydroxyl group of cholesterol is formed by the enzyme acyl-CoA cholesteryl acyltransferase (ACAT). Cholesteryl esters are more hydrophobic than cholesterol.

- Phospholipids are mainly found on the surface of the lipoprotein particle.
- TGs are esters, each composed of glycerol and three fatty acids. These fatty acids can be saturated or unsaturated. The fatty acids of most naturally occurring TGs contain 16, 18, or 20 carbon chains.

2. A. <100 mg/dL.
   B. <150 mg/dL.
   C. <200 mg/dL.
   D. <239 mg/dL.
   E. <240 mg/dL.
   Rationale: The NCEP ATP III guidelines recommend a total cholesterol of less than 200 mg/dL.

Major points of discussion

- The NCEP ATP III guidelines from 2002 identify major risk factors for CHD that modify the goal for LDL cholesterol. NCEP guidelines have shifted the focus from recognizing abnormal and normal cholesterol values to assessing overall cardiovascular risk based on cutoffs for cholesterol, TGs, HDL cholesterol, and LDL cholesterol (Table 7-1).
- The ATP III guidelines introduced several new concepts for the evaluation of hyperlipidemia. Diabetes mellitus is now considered a risk equivalent because it confers a high risk for new CHD within 10 years. This means that for evaluation of elevated cholesterol levels, diabetic patients are treated like patients who already have CHD. Also, ATP III recognized patients with metabolic syndrome and patients with a high 10-year risk for CHD based on the Framingham risk projections as candidates for intensive intervention and therapy.
- Risk status in persons without clinically manifested CHD or other clinical forms of atherosclerotic disease is determined by a two-step procedure. First, the number of risk factors is counted. Second, for persons with multiple (2+) risk factors, 10-year risk assessment is carried out with Framingham scoring to identify individuals whose short-term (10-year) risk warrants consideration of intensive treatment. Estimation of the 10-year CHD risk

adds a step to risk assessment beyond risk factor counting, but this step is warranted because it allows better targeting of intensive treatment to people who will benefit from it.[3]

3. A. Density and diameter are directly proportional: High-density particles are the largest lipoproteins.
   Rationale: Density correlates inversely with diameter. (HDL particles are the lipoprotein fraction with the smallest approximately 6 to 12 nm in diameter. The density is determined by the amount of lipid per particle.
   B. Density and diameter are inversely proportional: High-density particles are the smallest lipoproteins.
   C. There is no relationship between density and diameter.
   Rationale: Density correlates inversely with diameter. HDL particles (density, 1.063 to 1.1210 g/mL) are the lipoprotein fraction with the smallest diameter (~6 to 12 nm). Chylomicrons (density, <0.93 g/mL) are the lipoproteins with the highest diameter (80 to 1200 nm). The density is determined by the amount of lipid per particle.

Major points of discussion

- Because lipoproteins share common lipid and apolipoprotein components, the central problem in lipoprotein analysis is the separation of different lipoprotein classes from one another. Many methods have been applied to lipoprotein separation, including ultracentrifugation, adsorption, gel filtration, affinity chromatography, electrophoresis in various media, polyanion and alcohol precipitation, immunochemical procedures, and various combinations of these methods.
- Density correlates inversely with diameter. HDL particles (density, 1.063 to 1.1210 g/mL) are the lipoprotein fraction with the smallest diameter (~6 to 12 nm). Chylomicrons (density, <0.93 g/mL) are the lipoproteins with the highest diameter (80 to 1200 nm). The density is determined by the amount of lipid per particle.
- Cholesterol accounts for almost all of the sterol in plasma. It exists as a mixture of unesterified (30% to 40%) and esterified (60% to 70%) forms; the proportion of the two forms is fairly constant among normal individuals. Enzymatic methods of cholesterol quantification have virtually replaced the chemical methods that were used for most clinical and research purposes. Enzymatic methods measure total cholesterol directly in plasma or serum through a series of reactions in which cholesteryl esters are hydrolyzed. The 3-OH group of free cholesterol is then oxidized, and hydrogen peroxide, one of the reaction products, is quantified enzymatically.
- Currently, homogeneous assays are the most popular method for measuring HDL cholesterol. Unlike precipitation methods, these fully automated two-reagent procedures do not require off-line pretreatment and separation (hence the term *homogeneous*) and can be adapted to most chemistry analyzers. Thus, they reduce hands-on time and overall assay costs. Test kits distributed in the United States are based on various methods. Usually, the first reagent forms a stable complex with non-HDL lipoproteins, preventing them from participating in the reaction, and the second reagent releases HDL-cholesterol that is then measured enzymatically. According to surveys of the College of American Pathologists, the most common method uses a synthetic polymer together with a polyanion to block non-HDL

Table 7-1

Level	ATP III Classification
LDL Cholesterol	
<100	Optimal
100-129	Near optimal/above optimal
130-159	Borderline high
160-189	High
>190	Very high
Total Cholesterol	
<200	Desirable
200-239	Borderline high
≥240	High
HDL Cholesterol	
<40	Low
≥60	High
Triglycerides	
<150	Normal
150-199	Borderline high
200-499	High
≥500	Very high

lipoproteins, followed by a selective detergent to release HDL cholesterol (Genzyme Diagnostics, Cambridge, MA; Beckman Coulter, Inc Brea, CA). Other methods use polyethylene glycol–modified enzyme (Roche Diagnostics, Indianapolis), or immunoinhibition (Wako Chemicals USA, Inc., Richmond, VA) to block non-HDL lipoproteins. A fourth method (Polymedco Inc., Cortland Manor, NY) uses a special reagent to selectively eliminate cholesterol in non-HDL lipoproteins, followed by a second reagent that releases cholesterol from HDL (Denka Seiken Co., Niigata, Japan). These methods generally are not affected by high TGs, bilirubin, and globulins.

■ LDL cholesterol plays a causal role in the development of atherosclerosis. An LDL cholesterol level of more than 160 mg/dL with no other risk factors is an indication for therapy. With two or more CHD risk factors, the upper limit is lowered to 130 mg/dL for initiation of therapy. Several methods have been used to measure LDL cholesterol. The first, a reference laboratory procedure, involves ultracentrifugation to separate LDL from other lipoproteins, followed by analysis as described previously, to measure cholesterol. A much more common second method uses the Friedewald formula to calculate LDL cholesterol. Finally, more recently developed homogeneous methods for measuring LDL cholesterol are now available.

■ LDL cholesterol can be determined by using the Friedewald formula, originally described by Friedewald, Levy, and Fredrickson in 1972. Generally, in fasting plasma samples, LDL contains the cholesterol that is not present in HDL or VLDL. Thus, LDL cholesterol can be determined by the following equation:

$$\text{LDL cholesterol} = \text{Total cholesterol} - \text{HDL cholesterol} - \text{TGs}/5.0 \; (\text{mg/dL})$$

■ The last term in the equation is used to represent VLDL cholesterol.

4. A. Chylomicrons.
Rationale: Chylomicrons, which are not present in normal fasting subjects, carry very little cholesterol.
B. Very-low density lipoprotein (VLDL).
Rationale: VLDL particles primarily carry TGs, with relatively little cholesterol.
C. Low-density lipoprotein (LDL).
Rationale: LDL particles carry 60% to 70% of total plasma cholesterol in normal human subjects.
D. Intermediate-density lipoprotein (IDL).
Rationale: IDL particles are degradation products of VLDL and, as such, carry relatively little cholesterol.
E. High-density lipoprotein (HDL).
Rationale: HDL particles are small and dense and carry less cholesterol than LDL particles.

Major points of discussion
■ Chylomicrons (density, <0.95 g/mL; size, 80 to 1200 nm) are formed in the intestine during absorption of exogenous fat. Chylomicrons are the largest and lightest lipoproteins. Chylomicrons contain mainly TGs (90% to 96%), phospholipids (2% to 8%), free cholesterol (1%), cholesteryl esters (1% to 3%), and proteins (1% to 2%). After a 12-hour fast, chylomicrons are absent from the plasma. During fasting, the intestine releases small

amounts of small chylomicrons similar in size, density, and lipid composition to VLDL particles. Chylomicrons also carry fat-soluble vitamins absorbed from the diet.
■ VLDL is synthesized in the liver (density, 0.95 to 1.006 g/mL; size, 30 to 80 nm). Nascent VLDL contains cholesterol, cholesteryl esters, and TGs. Mature VLDL contains predominantly TGs (50% to 65%), phospholipids (12% to 18%), cholesteryl esters (8% to 14%), free cholesterol (5% to 8%), and proteins (6% to 10%).
■ LDL (density, 1.019 to 1.063 g/mL; size, 19 to 25 nm) originates from VLDL lipolysis. LDL particles carry 60% to 70% of total plasma cholesterol in healthy humans. The main components of LDL are cholesteryl esters (35% to 45%), phospholipids (20% to 25%), proteins (20% to 25%), TGs (6% to 12%), and free cholesterol (6% to 10%). Apoprotein B (ApoB) is the only apoprotein found in LDL particles.
■ High-density lipoprotein (HDL) (density, 1.063 to 1.210 g/mL; size, 6 to 11 nm) is the smallest lipoprotein. The liver and the intestine produce nascent lipid-poor HDL particles. Free cholesterol is acquired from macrophages and other cells and esterified by lecithin-cholesterol acyltransferase (LCAT) to generate mature HDL.
■ HDL particles can be separated further into HDL2 and HDL3, which differ by size. HDL3 is the smallest fraction (density, >1.125 g/mL, size 6 to 9 nm). The components are proteins (35% to 55%), phospholipids (25% to 40%), cholesteryl esters (8% to 20%), free cholesterol (1% to 6%), and TGs (3% to 6%). Apoprotein A-1 is the main apoprotein in HDL.

5. A. Increased chylomicrons are characteristic of type I hyperlipidemia.
Rationale: Increased circulating chylomicrons are characteristic of type I hyperlipidemia, resulting, for example, from lipoprotein lipase deficiency.
B. Defective LDL receptor binding results in low plasma cholesterol levels and high TG levels.
Rationale: Type IIa hyperlipidemia (or familial hypercholes-terolemia) is due to decreased LDL uptake as a result of defective LDL receptor (LDLR) function. It is associated with very high circulating cholesterol levels.
C. Type III hyperlipidemia is associated with homozygosity for the *ApoE E4/E4* genotype and results in equally increased cholesterol and TG levels.
Rationale: Type III hyperlipidemia is associate with the *ApoE E4/E4* genotype. Individuals with the *ApoE E4/E4* genotype are at increased risk for Alzheimer disease.
D. Type IIb hyperlipidemia is associated with increased LDL and HDL levels.
Rationale: Type IIb hyperlipidemia is associated with increased VLDL levels.
E. Type V hyperlipidemia, or mixed hyperlipidemia is associated with increased VLDL and LDL levels.
Rationale: Type V hyperlipidemia is associated with increased chylomicrons and VLDL.

Major points of discussion
■ Four major lipoprotein classes have been identified: chylomicrons, VLDLs, LDLs, and HDLs. The classification is based on the buoyant density of the particles. Several minor lipoproteins have also been identified, including IDL and lipoprotein(a) (Lp[a]).

- Lipoprotein lipase deficiency is a rare, autosomal recessive disorder that presents in childhood with abdominal pain and pancreatitis. Defective or absent lipoprotein lipase creates an inability to clear chylomicrons, creating the classic type I chylomicronemia syndrome. Fasting TG levels may be more than 100 mg/dL and may rise to more than 10,000 mg/dL postprandially. Patients with lipoprotein lipase deficiency do not develop premature coronary artery disease (CAD), implying that chylomicrons themselves are not atherogenic. Treatment with a low-fat diet to reduce chylomicron input is effective; fat-soluble vitamins should be supplemented, and drug therapy can be considered to lower endogenous VLDL production. Heterozygotes have 50% lipoprotein lipase activity and occur in the general population at a frequency of 1 in 500.
- Familial hypercholesterolemia is an autosomal dominant disorder caused by one of several mutations in the *LDLR* gene on chromosome 19. The resulting defective receptors cannot bind or clear LDL from the circulation. This disorder is characterized by xanthelasma, tendon xanthomas, premature coronary disease, and autosomal dominant familial inheritance.
- Type III hyperlipoproteinemias are due to high circulating levels of chylomicrons and IDL particles. The most common cause is the presence of the *ApoE ~~E4/E4~~ E2/E2* genotype.
- ApoE occurs as three common isoforms: apoE2, apoE3, and apoE4. This genetic variation is associated with different plasma lipoprotein levels, different responses to diet and lipid-lowering therapy, and a variable risk for cardiovascular disease and Alzheimer disease. Homozygosity for ApoE E2 causes type III hyperlipidemia. This disorder is associated with peripheral and CAD.

6. A. LDL originates directly from dietary uptake of cholesterol.
Rationale: Dietary cholesterol is packaged, after esterification into cholesteryl esters by the enterocyte, into chylomicrons.
B. LDL is synthesized by intestinal epithelium.
Rationale: LDL is derived from hydrolysis of VLDL. The intestinal epithelium is involved in the esterification of dietary cholesterol to synthesize cholesteryl esters.
C. LDL is secreted by the liver.
Rationale: The liver synthesizes VLDL, not LDL. LDL is derived from VLDL in the circulation by the action of lipoprotein lipase.
D. LDL originates from chylomicron hydrolysis.
Rationale: LDL is derived from VLDL in the circulation by the action of lipoprotein lipase.
E. LDL originates from VLDL hydrolysis.
Rationale: After synthesis by the liver, secreted VLDL is hydrolyzed by lipoprotein lipase on endothelial cell surfaces, leading to the production of LDL.

Major points of discussion
- The liver synthesizes VLDL. VLDL particles contain roughly equal amounts of cholesteryl esters and TGs. The TGs in VLDL originate from esterification of long-chain fatty acids in the liver. After secretion by the liver, VLDL is hydrolyzed by lipoprotein lipase, leading to the production of LDL. Lipoprotein lipase is anchored to the luminal

surface of endothelial cells. Lipoprotein lipase is found in high concentrations in muscle, heart, and fat. The VLDL remnants are called IDL particles, which are removed by the liver by binding of ApoE to the LDL receptor. Hepatic lipase (HL) remodels IDL to form LDL particles. LDL particles contain only ApoB. All other apoproteins that were found in VLDL (i.e., ApoC-I, ApoC-II, ApoC-III) or IDL (ApoE) are transferred to other lipoprotein particles.
- LDL particles carry the highest concentration of cholesteryl esters of all lipoproteins. LDL particles are taken up by binding to the LDL receptor. Statins (i.e., the HMG-CoA reductase inhibitor class of hypocholesterolemic drugs) increase LDLR expression, resulting in decreased plasma LDL concentrations.
- LDL is the primary target of therapy for hypercholesterolemia. The NCEP issues guidelines on the detection, evaluation, and treatment of high blood cholesterol levels in adults. The guidelines described by the ATP III call for intensive LDL-lowering therapy in certain settings, including primary prevention in individuals with multiple risk factors.
- Chylomicrons carry exogenous lipids. LDL transports endogenous lipids that are secreted by the liver as VLDL and result in LDL after VLDL hydrolysis.
- Dietary cholesterol is packaged, after esterification into cholesteryl esters by the enterocyte, into chylomicrons.

7. A. Total cholesterol and HDL cholesterol.
B. Total cholesterol, LDL cholesterol, HDL cholesterol, and TGs.
C. Total cholesterol, LDL cholesterol, HDL cholesterol, TGs, and chylomicrons.
D. Total cholesterol, HDL cholesterol, and LDL subfractions (i.e., small dense LDL particles).
E. Total cholesterol, LDL cholesterol, HDL cholesterol, and chylomicrons.
Rationale: The NCEP ATP III guidelines recommend that initial laboratory testing should focus on total cholesterol, LDL cholesterol, HDL cholesterol, and TGs.

Major points of discussion
- The NCEP ATP III guidelines identify major risk factors for CHD that modify the goal for LDL cholesterol (Table 7-2).
- CHD risk equivalents include the following:
  - Other clinical forms of atherosclerotic disease (e.g., peripheral arterial disease, abdominal aortic aneurysm, and symptomatic carotid artery disease)
  - Diabetes
  - Multiple risk factors that confer a 10-year risk for CHD of >20%
- The risk factors are:
  - Cigarette smoking
  - Hypertension (>140/90 mm Hg or use of an antihypertensive medication)

Table 7-2

Risk Category	LDL Goal (mg/dL)
CHD and CHD risk equivalents	<100
Multiple (2+) risk factors	<130
0 or 1 risk factor	<160

- Low HDL cholesterol (<40 mg/dL) (Note: HDL cholesterol >60 mg/dL is a negative risk factor; its presence removes one risk factor from the total count)
  - Family history of premature CHD (CHD in male first-degree relative <55 years; CHD in female first-degree relative <65 years)
  - Age (men, >45 years; women, >55 years)
- Risk assessment in individuals without clinically evident CHD or other forms of atherosclerotic disease is a two-step procedure. First, the number of risk factors is counted. Second, for individuals with multiple (i.e., ≥2) risk factors, a 10-year risk assessment is performed with Framingham scoring to identify individuals whose short-term (i.e., 10-year) risk warrants consideration of intensive treatment. Estimation of the 10-year CHD risk adds a step to risk assessment beyond risk factor counting but is warranted because it allows better targeting of intensive treatment to people who will benefit. When 0 or 1 risk factor is present, Framingham scoring is not necessary because the 10-year risk rarely reaches levels requiring intensive intervention; a very high LDL level in such a person may nevertheless warrant consideration of drug therapy to reduce long-term risk.
- Risk factors in Framingham scoring include age, total cholesterol, HDL cholesterol, blood pressure, and cigarette smoking. Total cholesterol is used for 10-year risk assessment because of a larger and more robust Framingham database for total than for LDL cholesterol, but LDL cholesterol is the primary target of therapy. Framingham scoring divides persons with multiple risk factors into those with 10-year risks for CHD of more than 20%, 10% to 20%, and less than 10%.
- According to NCEP ATP III guidelines, CHD risk is also influenced by other factors beside the major risk factors, including life-habit risk factors and emerging risk factors. The former include obesity, physical inactivity, and atherogenic diet; the latter include lipoprotein(a) and homocysteine levels, prothrombotic and proinflammatory factors, impaired fasting glucose, and evidence of subclinical atherosclerotic disease. The presence of these additional risk factors can modify clinical judgment and therapeutic decisions.[1]

8. A. Increased upregulation of liver receptors.
Rationale: Statins inhibit HMG-CoA reductase, leading to decreased cholesterol synthesis. When cholesterol levels decrease, the production of LDL receptors increases.
B. Decreased uptake of cholesterol by enterocytes.
Rationale: Decreased uptake of cholesterol by enterocytes characterizes the effect of bile acid sequestering agents, such as cholestyramine.
C. Increased synthesis of anticholesterol particles.
Rationale: Anticholesterol particles do not exist.
D. Increased secretion of cholesterol into bile.
Rationale: This is a characteristic result of using bile acid sequestering agents, such as cholestyramine.
E. Decreased synthesis of apoprotein B.
Rationale: Apoprotein B is the characteristic apolipoprotein in chylomicrons and LDL; its synthesis is not directly affected by statins.

Major points of discussion
- Statins inhibit HMG-CoA reductase in the cholesterol synthesis pathway. Inhibition of HMG-CoA reductase decreases cholesterol synthesis. When cholesterol levels decrease, the production of LDL receptors increases. This regulatory response is mediated by sterol regulatory element binding protein (SREBP) transcription factors. SREBP-mediated regulation of LDL receptors is essential for the action of statin drugs in lowering plasma LDL cholesterol levels in individuals at risk for CHD.
- SREBPs also increase HMG-CoA reductase levels, but this does not increase cholesterol synthesis because the enzyme is inhibited by the statin.
- The newly produced LDL receptors remove LDL particles from the blood by receptor-mediated endocytosis. The internalized LDL is digested, and its released cholesterol becomes available for metabolic purposes. The net effect is that the amount of cholesterol in the liver is maintained at a normal level and plasma levels of LDL cholesterol are simultaneously kept low.
- Bile acid sequestering agents, such as cholestyramine, decrease plasma cholesterol by increasing secretion of cholesterol into the bile.
- The mechanisms explaining how fibric acid derivatives (i.e., fibrates) decrease plasma cholesterol levels are not clearly defined. They may decrease HDL catabolism, increase lipoprotein lipase activity, and/or inhibit hepatic VLDL synthesis.

9. A. Abetalipoproteinemia.
Rationale: This rare autosomal recessive disorder results in the inability to synthesize apoB-containing lipoproteins. Therefore, one manifestation of this disorder is the inability to absorb fat-soluble vitamins from the diet, leading to associated vitamin deficiencies. Xanthomas are not seen in this disorder.
B. Hepatic lipase deficiency.
Rationale: This rare genetic disorder leads to significantly elevated circulating levels of TGs and total cholesterol. These patients typically present with palmar and tuberoeruptive xanthomas, not tendinous xanthomas.
C. Diabetic dyslipidemia.
Rationale: This is an atherogenic dyslipidemia seen in patients with type 2 diabetes but does not present with xanthomas.
D. Familial hypercholesterolemia. dominant
Rationale: This autosomal ~~recessive~~ disorder is due to defective function of LDL receptors, leading to very high circulating levels of LDL cholesterol, even in childhood. These patients can present with premature myocardial infarction and with tendinous xanthomas.
E. Metachromatic leukodystrophy.
Rationale: This autosomal recessive disorder is a sphingolipidosis (i.e., arylsulfatase A deficiency), not a hyperlipoproteinemia, and is not associated with xanthomas.

Major points of discussion
- Familial hypercholesterolemia (FH) is an autosomal dominant disorder caused by one of several mutations in the LDL receptor gene on chromosome 19. The resulting defective receptors cannot bind or clear LDL from the circulation.

■ Patients with homozygous FH present in childhood with LDL cholesterol levels higher than 400 mg/dL. Vascular deposition of lipid results in premature symptomatic CAD. Large cholesterol deposits can produce pathology in the coronary arteries, adjacent to heart valves, and in the cornea, in addition to producing tendinous xanthomas and xanthelasma. These signs generally develop in early childhood in homozygotes and by adulthood in heterozygotes. Statins, which inhibit HMG-CoA reductase, may be effective; however, because statins act indirectly by increasing LDLR activity, not all heterozygous patients will normalize their LDL cholesterol levels, despite receiving maximum doses of the drug. In homozygous patients with two abnormal LDLR genes, statin drugs are generally ineffective unless combined with therapeutic apheresis.

■ Elevated orange-yellow xanthomas are present superficially over the knees, wrists, and interdigital webs. These are due to the deposition of plasma LDL cholesterol in skin macrophages. A similar deposition of LDL-derived cholesterol occurred in the coronary arteries of the patient described in this question, producing arterial wall atheromas, which led to her first myocardial infarction at 8 years of age.

■ Hepatic lipase (HL) deficiency generally results from mutations of the HL gene. This rare disorder is associated with combined hyperlipidemia characterized by total cholesterol levels of 250 to 1500 mg/dL and TG levels of 400 to 8000 mg/dL. HDL cholesterol levels are normal or increased. Physical signs include palmar and tuberoeruptive xanthomas.

■ Diabetic dyslipidemia, which occurs in patients with type 2 diabetes, consists of an atherogenic dyslipidemia with high circulating levels of TGs, low HDL cholesterol levels, and small dense LDL particles. Although cholesterol levels may be within the "normal" range, treatment is often directed at decreasing LDL cholesterol because diabetes is viewed as a CAD risk equivalent, and guidelines thus recommend a lower than normal target cholesterol value.

10. A. CETP transfers cholesteryl esters from chylomicrons to HDL, thereby producing VLDL particles.
B. CETP transfers cholesteryl esters from LDL to HDL particles, which are then cleared by the HDL receptor.
C. CETP increases cholesteryl ester content in VLDL particles. The cholesteryl esters in the circulation are then cleared by the liver through VLDL receptors.
D. CETP increases cholesteryl ester content in HDL particles. The cholesteryl esters in the circulation are then cleared by the liver through HDL receptors.
Rationale: CETP transfers TG from VLDL and LDL to HDL in exchange for cholesteryl esters. The cholesteryl esters are then cleared by the liver by LDL receptor – mediated endocytosis of LDL particles.
E. CETP transfers TGs from apolipoprotein B (ApoB)-containing lipoproteins to HDL in exchange for cholesteryl esters. The cholesteryl esters in the circulation are then cleared by the liver through LDL receptors.
Rationale: See Major Points of Discussion.

Major points of discussion
■ CETP catalyzes the transfer of cholesterol esters to ApoB-100–containing particles in exchange for TGs. Phospholipid transfer protein (PLTP) facilitates the transfer of phospholipids from other lipoproteins HDL, allowing the particle to grow by acquiring surface phospholipid because it also accumulates esterified cholesterol and TG in its core. Once formed, HDL delivers excess lipids, especially cholesterol, to the liver and other tissues.

■ HDL is involved in the reverse transport of cholesterol from peripheral tissues to the liver. An important step in this process involves CETP, the plasma protein that facilitates the transfer of cholesteryl esters from HDL to ApoB-100–rich proteins (VLDL and LDL) in exchange for TGs.

■ CETP deficiency is an autosomal recessive disorder in which the transfer of cholesterol esters is inhibited. As a result, HDL particles are large and laden with cholesterol ester, and ApoA1 is increased, as are circulating HDL cholesterol levels (typically >100 mg/dL).

■ Individuals who are heterozygous for CETP deficiency have moderately increased HDL cholesterol levels.

■ Inhibition of CETP is an active area of pharmacologic research given the potential to raise HDL cholesterol levels.

11. A. Increased ApoA1 on plasma LDL particles.
Rationale: ApoA1 is found on HDL particles, whereas ApoB is found on LDL particles.
B. Absence of LDL particles in plasma.
Rationale: This is not a known phenotype in Tangier disease.
C. Very low plasma HDL cholesterol levels accompanied by lipid accumulation in peripheral cells.
Rationale: These findings are commonly seen in Tangier disease.
D. Fasting TG levels of more than 100 mg/dL, which may rise to more than 10,000 mg/dL postprandially.
Rationale: This phenotype is characteristic of lipoprotein lipase deficiency, which produces type I hyperlipidemia.
E. Milky plasma characterized by increased circulating levels of chylomicrons.
Rationale: This is characteristic of type I hyperlipidemia produced by lipoprotein lipase deficiency.

Major points of discussion
■ Tangier disease is a rare autosomal recessive disorder characterized by complete absence of HDL due to a mutation in the *ABCA1* gene on chromosome 9. This prevents the transfer of cholesterol and phospholipids in cells onto nascent ApoA1 proteins, resulting in increased cholesterol levels in cells. In the homozygous state, patients present with low or undetectable levels of plasma HDL cholesterol, hepatosplenomegaly, peripheral neuropathy, orange tonsils, and premature coronary disease.

■ In normal cells, the ABCA1 protein enables cholesterol to exit the cell, upon which it combines with ApoA1 to form HDL particles. The small amount of HDL that is present in patients with this disorder differs qualitatively from normal HDL.

■ ApoA1 is found on HDL particles, and ApoB is found on VLDL and LDL particles.
■ Lipoprotein lipase deficiency is a rare, autosomal recessive disorder that presents in childhood with abdominal pain and pancreatitis. Defective or absent lipoprotein lipase creates an inability to clear chylomicrons, creating the classic type 1 chylomicronemia syndrome.
■ Patients with lipoprotein lipase deficiency do not develop premature CAD, implying that chylomicrons themselves are not atherogenic. Treatment with a low-fat diet to reduce chylomicron input is effective, fat-soluble vitamins should be supplemented, and drug therapy can be considered to lower endogenous VLDL production.

12. A. Large chylomicrons and VLDL with very high TG levels.
Rationale: Large chylomicrons and VLDL with very high TG levels characterizes lipoprotein lipase (LPL) deficiency.
B. Decreased HDL levels.
Rationale: LCAT deficiency results in low HDL cholesterol concentrations.
C. Elevated LDL levels.
Rationale: Elevated LDL is characteristic for mutations in the LDLR and familial hypercholesterolemia.
D. Increased LDL receptors expressed on the cell surface.
Rationale: Gain-of-function mutations in *PCSK9* lead to more LDL in plasma.
E. Increased lysolecithin.
Rationale: Lysolecithin is decreased in LCAT deficiency.

Major points of discussion
■ Large chylomicrons and VLDL with very high TG levels characterizes LPL deficiency.
■ LCAT deficiency results in decreased HDL cholesterol concentrations. LCAT catalyzes the esterification of cholesterol, especially in HDL, by promoting transfer of fatty acids from lecithin to cholesterol. It enables HDL to accumulate cholesterol as cholesteryl ester. LCAT is activated by ApoA1.
■ Elevated LDL is characteristic of mutations in the LDLR and familial hypercholesterolemia.
■ Mutations in *PCSK9* affect the number of LDL receptors expressed on the cell surface. Depending on the mutation—either gain of function or loss of function—the presence of *PCSK9* affects availability of LDLR on the cell surface and, consequently, the levels of LDL in plasma. Gain of function leads to more LDL in plasma; loss of function associates with increased LDLR expression and thus less LDL in plasma.
■ Familial LCAT deficiency is due to deficiency in plasma LCAT (complete LCAT deficiency). Fish-eye disease is characterized by absence of LCAT activity toward HDL only.

13. **A. Decreased HMG-CoA reductase activity, increased acetyl-coenzyme A acetyltransferase (ACAT) activity, and decreased expression of LDL receptors.**
Rationale: After binding to the LDL receptor, LDL cholesterol undergoes receptor-mediated internalization, degradation by lysosomal hydrolases, and generation of LDL-derived cholesterol, which regulates the cell's cholesterol content by suppressing the activity of HMG-CoA reductase, activating a cholesterol-esterifying ACAT, and inhibiting transcription of the LDLR gene.
B. Increased HMG-CoA reductase activity, decreased ACAT activity, and decreased expression of LDL receptors.
Rationale: ACAT activity is increased in response to increased intracellular cholesterol; HMG-CoA reductase is decreased in response to increased intracellular cholesterol content.
C. Decreased HMG-CoA reductase activity, decreased ACAT activity, and decreased expression of LDL receptors.
Rationale: ACAT activity is increased in response to increased intracellular cholesterol.
D. Decreased HMG-CoA reductase activity, decreased ACAT activity, and increased expression of LDL receptors.
Rationale: ACAT activity is increased in response to increased intracellular cholesterol. LDLR expression is decreased in response to increased cholesterol content.
E. Increased HMG-CoA reductase activity, increased ACAT activity, and increased expression of LDL receptors.
Rationale: LDLR expression is decreased in response to increased cholesterol content.

Major points of discussion
■ The LDLR mediates the endocytosis of cholesterol-rich LDL.
■ After binding to the LDLR, LDL cholesterol undergoes receptor-mediated internalization, degradation by lysosomal hydrolases, and generation of LDL-derived cholesterol.
■ Increased intracellular cholesterol inhibits de novo synthesis of cholesterol by suppressing the activity of HMG-CoA reductase, the rate-limiting enzyme.
■ Increased intracellular cholesterol activates a cholesterol-esterifying enzyme (increased ACAT) to generate cholesteryl esters. Increased concentrations of free intracellular cholesterol are toxic. Cholesteryl esters are not toxic and can be stored.
■ Increased intracellular cholesterol inhibits the transcription of the LDLR gene. The sterol-regulatory element binding protein is the major transcriptional regulator of the LDLR gene. It is inhibited by cholesterol and polyunsaturated fatty acids.[2]

14. A. 1%.
Rationale: There are no lipoproteins that vary at this low percentage.
B. 6.5%.
Rationale: The coefficient of physiologic variation for cholesterol within an individual averages about 6.5%, but it can be higher in certain individuals. Cholesterol levels rise with age, starting in early adulthood, for both men and women. Although fasting has little effect on total cholesterol and HDL cholesterol levels, patients ideally should fast for 12 hours before venipuncture.
C. 8%.
Rationale: This physiologic variation characterizes determination of LDL cholesterol.
D. 20%.
Rationale: This physiologic variation characterizes determination of TGs. TG concentrations are increased in nonfasting samples. *Chylomicrons* are almost absent within 6 to 9 hours, and their presence after a 12-hour fast is

abnormal. Fasting has little effect on total cholesterol and HDL cholesterol levels.

E. 50%.

Rationale: There are no lipoproteins that vary to such a high percentage.

Major points of discussion

- The physiologic variation of TG determination is about 20%. TG concentrations are increased in nonfasting samples.
- The coefficient of physiologic variation for cholesterol within an individual averages about 6.5%, but it can be higher in certain individuals. Cholesterol levels rise with age, starting in early adulthood, in both genders.
- Fasting has little effect on total cholesterol and HDL cholesterol levels.
- The physiologic variation of LDL cholesterol is 8%.
- Chylomicrons are almost absent within 6 to 9 hours, and their presence after a 12-hour fast is abnormal.

15a. A. <40 mg/dL.

Rationale: An HDL level of less than 40 is considered a risk factor for CHD. An HDL level of 60 or greater decreases an individual's risk for CHD.

B. <65 mg/dL.

Rationale: CHD in a first-degree female relative when younger than 65 years is a risk factor for CHD.

C. <100 mg/dL.

Rationale: An LDL level of less than 100 mg/dL is the goal LDL for a patient with CHD or CHD equivalent.

D. <160 mg/dL.

Rationale: An LDL level of less than 160 mg/dL is the goal LDL for a patient with 0 to 1 risk factors for CHD.

E. <200 mg/dL.

Rationale: Total cholesterol of less than 200 mg/dL is a desirable target.

15b. A. <40 mg/dL.

B. >40 mg/dL.

C. <60 mg/dL.

Rationale: An HDL level of less than 40 mg/dL is considered a low HDL and is a risk factor for CHD.

D. >60 mg/dL.

Rationale: An HDL level of greater than 60 mg/dL is considered a high HDL and decreases CHD risk by one risk factor.

E. <100 mg/dL.

Rationale: The optimal LDL goal for a patient with CHD or CHD risk equivalent is less than 100 mg/dL.

Major points of discussion

- The NCEP ATP III guidelines identify major risk factors for CHD that modify the goal for LDL cholesterol. Diabetes mellitus is now considered a risk equivalent because it confers a high risk for new CHD within 10 years. This means that for evaluation of elevated cholesterol levels, diabetic patients are treated like patients who already have CHD. Also, ATP III recognized patients with metabolic syndrome and patients with a high 10-year risk for CHD based on the Framingham risk projections as candidates for intensive intervention and therapy.[3]

References

1. Expert Panel on Detection, Evaluation, and Treatment of High Blood Cholesterol in Adults. Executive summary of the third report of the National Cholesterol Education Program (NCEP) expert panel on detection, evaluation, and treatment of high blood cholesterol in adults (Adult Treatment Panel III). JAMA 2001;285: 2486–2497.

2. Goldstein JL, Brown MS. The LDL receptor. *Arterioscler Thromb Vasc Biol* 2009;29:431–438.

3. National Cholesterol Education Program Expert Panel. Third report of the National Cholesterol Education Program (NCEP) Expert Panel on Detection, Evaluation, and Treatment of High Blood Cholesterol in Adults (Adult Treatment Panel III): final report. *Circulation* 2002;106:3143–3421.

CHAPTER 8

CLINICAL CHEMISTRY: Cardiac, Cancer, and Other Biomarkers

Alex J. Rai, Michael A. Pesce, Tilla S. Worgall

QUESTIONS

1. A 72-year-old man presents to his physician with complaints of trouble urinating and discomfort in the pelvic area. His physician orders a serum prostate-specific antigen (PSA) test, with a subsequent result of 6 ng/mL (reference range ≤4 ng/mL). Which one of the following would be the best next step in the diagnostic workup for prostate cancer?
   A. Biopsy with subsequent staging/grading.
   B. Percent free PSA.
   C. Imaging studies to determine prostate volume and density.
   D. Digital rectal exam (DRE).
   E. No further action.

2. A patient has recently been diagnosed with ovarian cancer and will be starting a cisplatin-based chemotherapy regimen. Which one of the following is the best serum tumor marker to determine whether her treatment is effective?
   A. Carcinoembryonic antigen (CEA).
   B. Carbohydrate antigen 19-9 (CA-19-9).
   C. Cancer antigen 125 (CA-125).
   D. Alpha fetoprotein (AFP).
   E. Human chorionic gonadotropin (hCG) subunits.

3. Which one of the following tumor markers is approved by the Food and Drug Administration (FDA) for screening purposes?
   A. PSA with DRE for prostate cancer.
   B. CA-125 and ultrasound imaging for breast cancer.
   C. CEA for lung cancer in a patient with a history of smoking.
   D. AFP for hepatocellular carcinoma (HCC) in a patient with elevated levels of aspartate and alanine aminotransferase.
   E. Serial hCG measurements for breast cancer.

4. Which one of the following best describes the biological active forms of the natriuretic peptides that are found in serum?
   A. Brain natriuretic peptide (BNP) and N-terminal-prohormone of BNP (NT-ProBNP).
   B. BNP and pre-prohormone of BNP.
   C. Atrial natriuretic peptide (ANP) and BNP.
   D. Urodilatin and BNP.
   E. ANP and NT-prohormone of BNP.

5. Which one of the following best describes the clinical utility of BNP and NT-proBNP?
   A. Elevated BNP or NT-proBNP levels can be used to detect an acute myocardial infarction.
   B. Elevated BNP or NT-proBNP levels can be used to detect unstable angina.
   C. Elevated BNP or NT-proBNP levels can be used to detect cardiac ischemia.
   D. Elevated BNP or NT-proBNP levels can be used to screen for congestive heart failure in asymptomatic individuals.
   E. Normal BNP or NT-proBNP levels can be used to rule out congestive heart failure.

6. Which one of the following explains why creatine kinase (CK)-MB can be used to detect myocardial necrosis?
   A. CK-MB is detected in the blood before myoglobin after acute myocardial infarction.
   B. CK-MB is found only in cardiac muscle.
   C. CK-MB is detected in blood before troponin I or troponin T after an acute myocardial infarction.
   D. CK-MB is known to rise and fall predictably after an acute myocardial infarction.
   E. CK-MB is a better predictor than troponin I or T for risk stratification of patients with acute myocardial infarctions.

7. Which one of the following best describes the structure of CK-MB isoforms (i.e., CK-MB1 and CK-MB2)?
   A. Macromolecular complexes consisting of CK-MB bound to IgG.
   B. CK mitochondrial complexes.
   C. Artifactual forms of CK caused by binding of CK to albumin.
   D. Posttranslational modification of CK-MB.
   E. CK complexes consisting of CK-MB bound to immunoglobulin A (IgA).

8. Which one of the following serum proteins is most useful in determining whether an acute-phase response is due to a bacterial infection?
   A. C3.
   B. C4.
   C. Albumin.
   D. C-reactive protein (CRP).
   E. Transferrin.

9. Which one of the following is consistent with the European Society of Cardiology–American College of Cardiology established criteria for detection of an acute myocardial infarction?
   A. Measurement of troponin, myoglobin, and CK-MB.

B. Measurement of CK-MB and troponin.

C. Measurement of myoglobin and troponin.

D. Measurement of the rise and fall of troponin.

E. Measurement of CK-MB isoforms and troponin.

10. Which one of the following tests can be used as an early predictor of coronary artery disease in asymptomatic individuals?

A. Troponin I.

B. Ischemia modified albumin.

C. High-sensitivity CRP (hsCRP).

D. BNP.

E. CK-MB.

11. Which one of the following combinations of biomarkers best detects cardiac ischemia?

A. Ischemia-modified albumin (IMA) and glycogen phosphorylase isoenzyme BB.

B. IMA and troponin.

C. IMA and free fatty acid binding protein.

D. IMA and BNP.

E. IMA and myosin light chain.

12. Serum levels of lactate dehydrogenase (LDH) isoenzymes and haptoglobin were measured in a patient with liver disease. The LDH-1 fraction was greater than the LDH-2 fraction and haptoglobin was undetectable. Which one of the following interpretations is compatible with these laboratory results?

A. Concurrent cardiac ischemia.

B. Concurrent congestive heart failure.

C. Concurrent unstable angina.

D. Artifact due to hemolysis.

E. Increasing liver dysfunction.

13. Which one of the following reasons best explains how serum myoglobin levels can be used as a cardiac marker for patients admitted to the emergency department 4 hours after the onset of chest pain?

A. Elevated circulating myoglobin levels are diagnostic for an acute myocardial infarction.

B. Circulating myoglobin levels are elevated for days after an acute myocardial infarction.

C. Circulating myoglobin levels become elevated after troponin I or troponin T after an acute myocardial infarction.

D. Circulating myoglobin levels peak after CK-MB levels rise after an acute myocardial infarction.

E. Normal circulating myoglobin levels can be used to rule out an acute myocardial infarction.

14. The troponin complex is composed of which one of the following components?

A. Troponin T, calcium, and actin.

B. Troponin C, myoglobin, and actin.

C. Troponin I, actin, and tropomyosin.

D. Troponin I, troponin T, and troponin C.

E. Troponin T, tropomyosin, and calcium.

15. An external proficiency test survey sample to evaluate troponin I was sent to laboratories across the United States. The results of this interlaboratory survey for this sample showed up to a tenfold difference in troponin I levels among the laboratories. Which one of the following reasons represents the most likely cause of this variability?

A. Some troponin I methods are not accurate or precise.

B. Some troponin I methods cross-react with troponin T.

C. Some troponin I methods are standardized.

D. Some troponin I methods cross-react with troponin C.

E. Some troponin I methods measure different molecular forms of troponin I.

16. Which one of the following best describes the major advantage of using either troponin I or troponin T, rather than CK-MB, for detecting an acute myocardial infarction?

A. The troponin complex consists of cardiac troponin T, I, and C subunits that are structurally distinct from their skeletal muscle counterparts.

B. The troponin complex is not found in the cytosolic pool.

C. Troponin is released early into blood after an acute myocardial infarction because of degradation of the contractile apparatus.

D. Troponin is part of the thick filament (myosin) of muscle.

E. Cardiac troponin T and I subunits are distinctly different from their skeletal muscle counterparts.

17. Troponin I is used to evaluate infants with cardiac disease. Which one of the following best explains why troponin T cannot be used to evaluate cardiac injury in infants?

A. Bilirubin interferes with the troponin T method.

B. Skeletal muscle troponin T found in newborns cross-reacts with troponin T.

C. Precision of the troponin T method in newborns has not been established.

D. The troponin T method requires a large sample volume and is not suitable for use in newborn testing.

E. The analytical sensitivity of the troponin T method is not high enough and therefore cannot be used for newborn testing.

18. Troponin T and troponin I are the most frequently used biomarkers for the detection of an acute myocardial infarction. Although the measured troponin I results from different hospitals can be significantly different, there is usually no significant difference in troponin T results obtained from different hospitals. Which one of the following best explains the low interlaboratory variability for troponin T?

A. The troponin T method can detect more patients with an acute myocardial infarction than the troponin I method.

B. Troponin T is more stable in blood than troponin I.

C. The troponin T method is more precise than the troponin I method.

D. Only one method is available to measure troponin T.

E. Only one molecular form of troponin T is found in blood.

19. A 23-year-old pregnant woman, near the end of her first trimester, has a quantitative pregnancy test performed. Surprisingly, her hCG is 350 IU/mL, which is a value much less than would be expected based on her gestational age. Which one of the following is the best explanation for a falsely low serum level of hCG?

A. Heterophilic antibodies in the sample.

B. Imprecision of the assay.

C. Calibration using a sigmoidal curve.

D. Multiplex enzyme-linked immunosorbent assay (ELISA) used to perform this assay.

E. Presence of the hook effect.

20. A 70-year-old man presents to his physician with generalized bone pain, a recently broken hip, weight loss, nausea, and constipation. Which one of the following serum protein electrophoresis test results would be diagnostic of multiple myeloma?
   A. Presence of a band in the beta globulin fraction at a concentration of 0.2 g/dL.
   B. Presence of a band in the gamma globulin fraction at a concentration of 3 g/dL.
   C. Decreased level of a band in the albumin fraction to a concentration of 0.2 g/dL.
   D. Increased levels of bands in the alpha-1 and alpha-2 globulin fractions at a concentration of 0.2 g/dL each.
   E. Presence of a band in the prealbumin fraction at a concentration of 0.5 g/dL.

21. Which one of the following serum protein electrophoresis patterns best suggests an acute inflammatory response?
   A. Increased albumin; increased alpha-1, alpha-2, and beta globulins; and normal gamma globulins.
   B. Decreased albumin, increased alpha-1 and alpha-2 globulins, and normal beta and gamma globulins.
   C. Decreased albumin, decreased alpha-1 and alpha-2 globulins, and normal beta and gamma globulins.
   D. Increased albumin, decreased alpha-1 and alpha-2 globulins, normal beta globulins, and increased gamma globulins.
   E. Normal albumin; increased alpha-1, alpha-2, and beta globulins; and normal gamma globulins.

22. AFP is a major embryonic protein. After 12 weeks of gestation, which one of the following statements best describes the predominant site(s) of AFP synthesis?
   A. The yolk sac.
   B. The fetal pancreas.
   C. The yolk sac and fetal liver.
   D. The fetal liver.
   E. The fetal kidney.

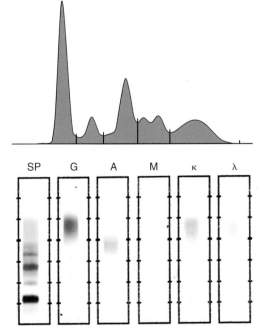

Figure 8-1 Serum protein electrophoresis (upper panel) and immunofixation electrophoresis (lower panel).

Table 8-1 Protein Fractions Determined by Serum Protein Electrophoresis

Protein Fractions	Patient Results (g/dL)	Reference Range (g/dL)
Albumin	2.2	3.6-4.8
Alpha-1	0.5	0.2-0.4
Alpha-2	1.4	0.6-0.9
Beta	0.9	0.6-1.0
Gamma	1.2	0.8-1.8
Total protein	6.2	6.7-8.6

23. The serum protein and immunofixation electrophoresis (IFE) patterns shown in Figure 8-1 and Table 8-1 were determined for a 55-year-old man with type 1 diabetes. The protein fractions are shown below. Which one of the following represents the best interpretation of these protein patterns?
   A. This is the serum protein electrophoresis pattern that is seen in severe liver disease.
   B. This is the serum IFE pattern for a monoclonal protein.
   C. This is the serum protein electrophoresis pattern that is usually seen in nephrosis.
   D. This is the serum protein electrophoresis pattern that is seen in iron deficiency anemia.
   E. This is the serum protein electrophoresis pattern that is seen in alpha-1 antitrypsin deficiency.

You have identified a biomarker signature composed of three proteins in plasma that appears to be useful in the management of patients with prostate cancer. This signature is found in virtually 100% of this population. Use this scenario to answer the following five questions.

24a. Which one of the following performance characteristics for this test is high?
   A. Sensitivity.
   B. Specificity.
   C. Precision.
   D. Negative predictive value.
   E. Accuracy.

24b. The biomarker signature is found only in prostate cancer patients and is not detected in other patient populations, such as patients with other types of cancer, or in healthy volunteers, Which one of the following performance characteristics is high?
   A. Sensitivity.
   B. Specificity.
   C. Positive predictive value.
   D. Negative predictive value
   E. Accuracy.

24c. Assume that this new biomarker signature has a low specificity and, therefore, is not useful for population-based screening for prostate cancer. Which one of the following performance characteristics can be improved by using it only in a high-risk clinic setting that serves only patients with a family history of this disease?
   A. Sensitivity.
   B. Precision.
   C. Positive predictive value.
   D. Reference interval.
   E. Accuracy.

24d. This novel biomarker signature is *not* detectable in a cohort of patients who are free of prostate cancer. The inability to detect this signature in such a population would produce a high value for which one of the following characteristics?
- **A.** Sensitivity.
- **B.** Precision.
- **C.** Positive predictive value.
- **D.** Negative predictive value.
- **E.** Accuracy.

24e. This newly discovered biomarker signature correlates well with the existing gold standard methodology, which is immunohistochemical analysis of prostate biopsy tissue. Which one of the following performance characteristics is high?
- **A.** Sensitivity.
- **B.** Specificity.
- **C.** Positive predictive value.
- **D.** Negative predictive value.
- **E.** Accuracy.

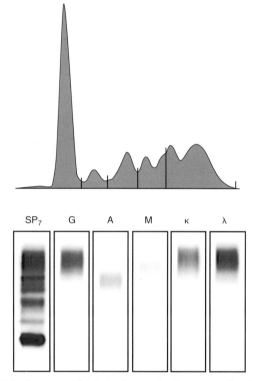

Figure 8-2 Serum protein electrophoresis densitometry tracing (upper panel) and immunofixation electrophoresis (lower panel).

Table 8-2 Protein Fractions Determined by Serum Protein Electrophoresis

Protein Fractions	Results (g/dL)	Reference Range (g/dL)
Albumin	2.9	3.6-4.8
Alpha-1	0.3	0.2-0.4
Alpha-2	0.7	0.6-0.9
Beta	0.9	0.6-1.0
Gamma	2.2	0.8-1.8
Total protein	7.0	6.7-8.6

25. Serum protein and IFE patterns were obtained for a 65-year-old man with a chronic history of fatigue and back pain. Protein fractions are shown in Figure 8-2 and Table 8-2. Which one of the following represents the best interpretation of these patterns?

A. Serum protein electrophoresis (SPEP) showed low albumin and slightly elevated gamma globulin levels and the possibility of a monoclonal protein in the gamma globulin region, which was identified by IFE as a monoclonal IgG lambda protein.

B. SPEP showed low albumin and slightly elevated gamma globulin levels and the possibility of a monoclonal protein in the gamma globulin region, which was identified by IFE as a free lambda light chain.

C. SPEP showed low albumin and slightly elevated polyclonal gamma globulin levels. No monoclonal protein was detected by IFE.

D. SPEP showed low albumin and slightly elevated gamma globulin levels and the possibility of a monoclonal protein in the gamma globulin region. No monoclonal protein was detected by IFE. The narrow band in the SPEP pattern is probably due to fibrinogen.

E. SPEP showed low albumin and slightly elevated gamma globulin levels and the possibility of a monoclonal protein in the gamma globulin region, which was identified by IFE as a monoclonal IgA lambda protein.

The epidermal growth factor receptor (EGFR) serves an important role in the transmission of growth signals from the plasma membrane to the nucleus. In recent years, multiple somatic mutations in EGFR have been characterized in tumor tissue derived from patients with non–small cell lung cancer (NSCLC). Use this scenario to answer the following four questions.

26a. Which one of the following best describes the significance of the L858R mutation in EGFR for patients with NSCLC?
- **A.** Acquisition of this mutation marks the transition from low-grade to high-grade cancer.
- **B.** Acquisition of this mutation marks the transition from early-stage to late-stage disease.
- **C.** This mutation correlates with sensitivity to chemotherapy using tyrosine kinase inhibitors.
- **D.** This mutation correlates with resistance to chemotherapy using tyrosine kinase inhibitors.
- **E.** This mutation portends a favorable outcome (i.e., is an indicator of good prognosis).

26b. Which one of the following best describes the significance of the T790M mutation in EGFR?
- **A.** Acquisition of this mutation marks the transition from low-grade to high-grade cancer.
- **B.** Acquisition of this mutation marks the transition from early-stage to late-stage disease.
- **C.** This mutation correlates with sensitivity to chemotherapy using tyrosine kinase inhibitors.
- **D.** This mutation correlates with resistance to chemotherapy using tyrosine kinase inhibitors.
- **E.** This mutation portends a favorable outcome (i.e., is an indicator of good prognosis).

26c. Which one of the following is the best serological tumor marker to monitor treatment for this patient with lung cancer?
- **A.** CA-15.3.
- **B.** PSA.
- **C.** AFP.
- **D.** hCG.
- **E.** CEA.

26d. The assay to measure CEA levels in blood is not useful for population-based cancer screening. Which one of the following answers best describes why this is true?
A. CEA has poor sensitivity for the diagnosis of lung cancer; only 20% of lung cancers are diagnosed using this marker.
B. CEA has poor specificity for lung cancer; there are multiple nonmalignant conditions resulting in elevated CEA levels.
C. The dynamic range of this assay is limited and not suitable for patients with late-stage or metastatic disease.
D. The analytical sensitivity of this assay does not meet the needs for early detection.
E. The assay is imprecise (i.e., the coefficient of variation is >20%).

27. Which one of the following statements best describes the setting(s) in which maternal serum measurements of AFP are most useful?
A. Anencephaly and myelomeningocele.
B. Anencephaly, myelomeningocele, and closed spina bifida.
C. Anencephaly and closed spina bifida.
D. Trisomy 21.
E. Trisomy 18.

28. Which one of the following pairs consists only of "negative" acute-phase proteins?
A. Albumin and alpha-1-antitrypsin.
B. Albumin and alpha-2-macroglobulin.
C. Haptoglobin and CRP.
D. Albumin and transferrin.
E. Transferrin and C3.

29. Which one of the following represents the currently recommended optimal approach for first-trimester maternal screening for the presence of Down syndrome?
A. Nuchal translucency (NT), free beta-hCG, and AFP.
B. NT, free beta-hCG, and pregnancy-associated plasma protein A (PAPP-A).
C. NT, free beta-hCG, and inhibin A.
D. NT, free beta-hCG, and unconjugated estriol (uE3).
E. NT, PAPP-A, and inhibin A.

30. The prevalence of neural tube defects (NTDs) in the general population of the United States significantly decreased when foods were supplemented with which one of the following nutrients?
A. Vitamin A.
B. Folic acid.
C. Vitamin D.
D. Vitamin K.
E. Vitamin E.

31. Maternal serum alpha-fetoprotein (MSAFP) levels are used to screen for fetal NTDs in pregnant women. The risk of NTDs for each patient is calculated by using the multiple of the medians (MOM), which is determined by obtaining a median MSAFP value in unaffected pregnancies for each gestational week and dividing the patient's MSAFP value by the median MSAFP value for the relevant gestational week. The cutoff for predicting a fetal NTD is a value of 2.5 or higher MOM. In addition, MSAFP levels increase with increasing gestational age. Therefore, the correct gestational age is extremely important in calculating the risk of a fetal NTD. If the risk of a fetal NTD is calculated based on the MOM obtained at a gestational age of 19 weeks,

but the true gestational age is 15 weeks, which one of the following best explains the risk of a fetal NTD?
A. Increased, because the MOM will be higher than expected.
B. Increased, because the MOM will be lower than expected.
C. Decreased, because the MOM will be lower than expected.
D. Decreased, because the MOM will be higher than expected.
E. Cannot be determined; therefore, another sample should be drawn to repeat the MSAFP determination.

32. Amniotic fluid alpha-fetoprotein (AFAFP) levels are used to help in the diagnosis of NTDs. The risk of a fetal NTD for each patient is calculated by using the MOM, which is determined by obtaining a median AFP level in unaffected pregnancies for each gestational week and dividing the patient's AFP value by the median AFP value for the relevant gestational week. The cutoff for diagnosing an NTD is a value of 2.0 or higher MOM. In addition, AFAFP concentrations decrease with increasing gestational age. Therefore, the correct gestational age is extremely important in calculating the risk of NTD. If the risk of a fetal NTD is calculated based on the MOM obtained at a gestational age of 20 weeks, but the true gestational age is 15 weeks, then which one of the following statements best describes the actual risk of a fetal NTD in this case?
A. Increased, because the actual MOM is higher than the calculated MOM.
B. Increased, because the actual MOM is lower than the calculated MOM.
C. Decreased, because the actual MOM is lower than the calculated MOM.
D. Decreased, because the MOM is higher than the calculated MOM.
E. Slightly decreased, but will not significantly affect the NTD risk calculation.

33. MSAFP levels are used during pregnancy to calculate the risk of fetal NTDs. MSAFP levels are affected by maternal weight. The weight correction for MSAFP levels is performed by comparing the weight of the patient with the weight that is used in a reference population (which is 140 lb) to calculate the risk of NTD. Therefore, which one of the following profiles would a 195-lb woman have if the weight correction was not performed?
A. Increased serum MSAFP level and increased risk of NTDs.
B. Increased serum MSAFP level and decreased risk of NTDs.
C. Decreased serum MSAFP level and increased risk of NTDs.
D. Decreased serum MSAFP level and decreased risk of NTDs.
E. No change in the risk for NTDs.

34. When a serum sample is placed in an electric field connected to a buffer at a pH of 8.6, which one of the following statements is correct regarding the electrophoretic migration of the proteins?
A. Proteins have a positive charge and migrate toward the anode.
B. Proteins have a positive charge and migrate toward the cathode.
C. Proteins have a negative charge and migrate toward the anode.
D. Proteins have a negative charge and migrate toward the cathode.
E. Proteins all have the same isoelectric point.

35. Screening for Down syndrome in the second trimester can be performed with the following four serum biomarkers (i.e., the quadratic screen): AFP, uE3, hCG, and inhibin A. Which one of the following patterns is most consistent with a high risk of Down syndrome?
    A. Elevated AFP, hCG, and inhibin A; low uE3.
    B. Elevated inhibin A; low AFP, hCG, and uE3.
    C. Elevated AFP; low or normal uE3, hCG, and inhibin A.
    D. Elevated inhibin A and uE3; low AFP and hCG.
    E. Elevated hCG and inhibin A; low AFP and uE3.

36. In the context of maternal serum screening in the second trimester to detect fetal Down syndrome, which one of the following statements provides the best explanation of the advantage of the quadratic screen (i.e., AFP, uE3, hCG, and inhibin A) over the triple screen (i.e., AFP, uE3, and hCG)?
    A. All cases of fetal Down syndrome are detected.
    B. There is an increase in the detection rate of fetal Down syndrome.
    C. The reagent cost is significantly reduced.
    D. Fetal trisomy 18 cases can be detected.
    E. The analytical method is automated.

37. Screening for a fetus with Edwards syndrome (i.e., trisomy 18) is performed in the second trimester by measuring maternal serum levels of AFP, uE3, and hCG. Which one of the following patterns best identifies a fetus with trisomy 18?
    A. AFP is elevated; uE3 and hCG are normal.
    B. AFP is very elevated; uE3 and hCG are low.
    C. uE3 and hCG are elevated; AFP is low.
    D. AFP, uE3, and hCG are all low.
    E. hCG is elevated; AFP and uE3 are low.

You are a clinical laboratory director at a cancer center charged with the selection, design, and validation of new tumor marker assays. Use this scenario to answer the following four questions.

38a. Which one of the following performance characteristics would best serve to implement an assay to measure AFP levels in both the general population and in a population of patients with cancer?
    A. Wide dynamic range.
    B. Analytical sensitivity at the low end.
    C. High precision.
    D. Minimal analytical interferences from drugs.
    E. Standardized results between different assays.

38b. Which one of the following performance characteristics would best serve to implement an assay for detecting recurrent prostate cancer in patients who have undergone radical prostatectomy?
    A. Wide dynamic range.
    B. Analytical sensitivity at the low end.
    C. High precision.
    D. Minimal analytical interferences from drugs.
    E. Standardized results between different assays.

38c. Your laboratory receives and analyzes proficiency test samples. In this case, 50 different laboratories in the United States (including yours) are provided with the same proficiency test sample and asked to measure the level of the CA-19.9 tumor marker. Half (i.e., 25) of the laboratories use assay No. 1 and obtain a mean of 36.5 (with a standard deviation [SD] of 4), whereas the other 25 laboratories use assay No. 2 and obtain a mean of 175.3 (SD 14). Which one of the following is the best

explanation for the differences in performance between assay No. 1 and assay No. 2?
    A. Wide dynamic range.
    B. Analytical sensitivity at the low end.
    C. High precision.
    D. Minimal analytical interferences from drugs.
    E. Lack of standardization among different assays.

38d. You are asked to implement an assay to measure CA-15.3. For monitoring the effectiveness of chemotherapy (i.e., for comparing pre- and posttreatment results) in an individual breast cancer patient, which one of the following performance characteristics for the CA-15.3 assay would be most important?
    A. Wide dynamic range.
    B. Analytical sensitivity at the low end.
    C. High precision.
    D. Minimal analytical interferences from drugs.
    E. Lack of standardization among different assays.

39. Which one of the following statements best describes type II cryoglobulinemia?
    A. Detection of a monoclonal protein in the cryoprecipitate.
    B. Detection of albumin and a monoclonal protein in the cryoprecipitate.
    C. Detection of alpha-1, alpha-2, and beta globulins in the cryoprecipitate.
    D. Detection of polyclonal immunoglobulins in the cryoprecipitate.
    E. Detection of a monoclonal protein and polyclonal immunoglobulins in the cryoprecipitate.

40. Which one of the following laboratory results would be characteristic in a patient with Wilson disease?
    A. Low serum ceruloplasmin and low urinary copper concentrations.
    B. Low serum ceruloplasmin and elevated urinary copper concentrations.
    C. Elevated serum ceruloplasmin and low urinary copper concentrations.
    D. Elevated serum ceruloplasmin and elevated urinary copper concentrations.
    E. Normal serum ceruloplasmin and low urinary copper concentrations.

41. Which one of the following tumor markers is best for monitoring patients with breast cancer when used in conjunction with imaging studies?
    A. CA-125.
    B. BRCA1/2.
    C. BRCA1 only.
    D. CA-15.3.
    E. EGFR genotyping.

42. Which one of the following tumor markers is best for monitoring patients with ovarian cancer when used in conjunction with imaging studies?
    A. CA-125.
    B. HE4.
    C. BRCA1/2.
    D. CA-15.3.
    E. EGFR genotyping.

43. Which one of the following two tumor markers (and/or diagnostic modalities) is best for monitoring patients with prostate cancer?
    A. PSA combined with DRE.
    B. PSA density combined with PC3.

C. PSA combined with PC3.

D. PSA combined with circulating tumor cells (CTCs).

E. No two modalities together; PSA alone is best.

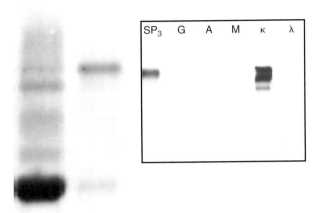

1   2

Figure 8-3 *Left panel:* Protein electrophoresis pattern of concentrated urine. An unremarkable protein electrophoresis pattern is seen in lane 1. The presence of a monoclonal protein in the gamma region is seen in lane 2. *Right panel:* IFE of the abnormal specimen (from left panel, lane 2) demonstrates the presence of monoclonal kappa proteins (i.e., kappa Bence-Jones proteins).

44. Which one of the following statements is correct regarding Figure 8-3?

A. Urine protein electrophoresis is not required to assess patients with hypogammaglobulinemia.

B. Urine protein electrophoresis should not be performed using an aliquot from a random urine collection.

C. Bence-Jones proteinuria is a diagnostic marker for multiple myeloma.

D. The monoclonal light chains are found in concentrated urine in very small amounts and cannot be quantified as an M-spike by protein electrophoresis.

E. Determination of serum free light chains is sufficient to diagnose Bence-Jones proteinuria.

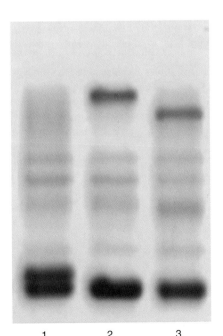

1   2   3

Figure 8-4 Serum protein electrophoresis gel.

45. Which one of the following answers best describes the findings seen in the three lanes in this serum protein electrophoresis gel shown in Figure 8-4?

A. Hypergammaglobulinemia in lane 1; increased albumin in lanes 2 and 3.

B. No abnormalities in lane 1; IgG kappa in lane 2; IgA lambda in lane 3.

C. Bisalbuminemia in lane 1; abnormal band in the gamma region in lanes 2 and 3.

D. Hypogammaglobulinemia in lane 1; hypergammaglobulinemia in lanes 2 and 3.

E. No abnormalities in lane 1; IgA lambda in lane 2; IgG kappa in lane 3.

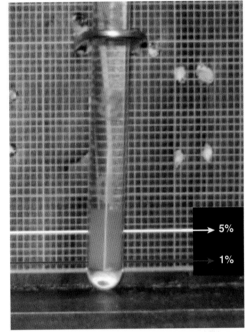

Figure 8-5 Cryoprecipitate obtained after incubation of serum at 4°C for 7 days. This serum contains an approximately 7% cryoprecipitate (i.e., the "cryocrit"). Cryoglobulinemia is divided into three types depending on the type of immunoglobulins composing the precipitate. Type I, monoclonal immunoglobulins; type II, monoclonal and polyclonal immunoglobulins; type III, polyclonal immunoglobulins. Identification of the cryoglobulins composing the cryoprecipitate requires performance of IFE.

46. Which one of the following represents the most likely clinical scenario for a patient presenting with the "cryocrit" shown in Figure 8-5?

A. A 22-year-old woman after a normal vaginal delivery.

B. A 45-year-old patient with diabetes mellitus.

C. A 45-year-old patient with hepatitis A.

D. A 45-year-old patient with hepatitis C.

E. A 5-year-old child with paroxysmal cold hemoglobinuria.

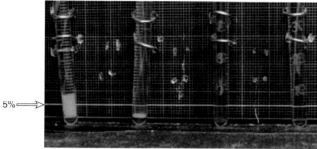

Figure 8-6   Cryoprecipitates in Wintrobe tubes. Lane 1, cryocrit of 8%; lane 2, cryocrit of 2%; lane 3, cryocrit of 1% (this precipitate is red because of sedimentation of erythrocytes in a hemolytic sample); lane 4, no cryoprecipitate.

47. Which one of the following is the correct statement about the transport and processing of a sample for the determination of the "cryocrit" shown in Figure 8-6?
   A. Transport at room temperature and incubate at room temperature.
   B. Transport at 37°C and incubate at 4°C.
   C. Transport at room temperature and incubate at 4°C.
   D. Transport at 4°C and incubate at 37°C.
   E. Transport at 4°C and incubate at 4°C.

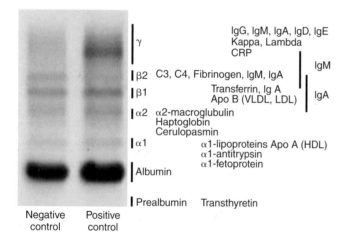

Figure 8-7   Separation of serum proteins can resolve six different major fractions. Immunoglobulins migrate primarily in the gamma fraction. IgM and IgA molecules are also found in the alpha-2, beta-1, and beta-2 fractions.

48. Monoclonal IgG proteins are most likely found in which one of the following fractions shown in Figure 8-7?
   A. Albumin fraction.
   B. Beta fraction.
   C. Gamma fraction.
   D. Alpha-1 fraction.
   E. Alpha-2 fraction.

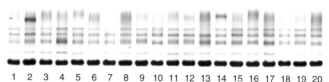

Figure 8-8   SPEP in a cellulose acetate gel. Lane 1 is the normal control. Lane 2 is the abnormal control. This gel demonstrates the serum protein electrophoresis results of 18 patients (lanes 3-20).

49. Which one of the following is the best diagnosis determined by analyzing the serum protein electrophoresis results shown in Figure 8-8?
   A. Lane 7 demonstrates the presence of hypogammaglobulinemia.
   B. Lane 14 demonstrates the presence of increased amounts of polyclonal immunoglobulins.
   C. Lane 12 demonstrates a band in the gamma region that represents fibrinogen.
   D. Lane 18 demonstrates the presence of polyclonal hypergammaglobulinemia.
   E. Lane 20 demonstrates hypoalbuminemia.

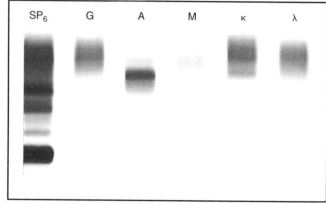

Figure 8-9   Immunofixation protein electrophoresis.

50. Which one of the following statements about monoclonal immunoglobulins is true about Figure 8-9?
   A. At very low concentrations, they can significantly increase the viscosity of blood, leading to problems with organ perfusion.
   B. The circulating concentration can be so high that the precipitating complexes by IFE will not stain properly.
   C. Quantitative monitoring clearly differentiates a benign from a malignant condition in the majority of cases.
   D. They are routinely detected using mass spectrometry methods.
   E. Identification of the constituent heavy chain and light chain types can be determined by IFE.

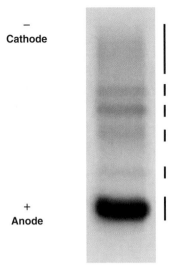

Figure 8-10 Serum protein fractions on a cellulose acetate gel separation of serum proteins on a cellulose acetate serum protein gel at a pH of 8.8.

51. The fractions seen on a serum protein electrophoresis gel are separated from the anode (positive pole) to the cathode (negative pole). Which one of the following best represents this order of separation in Figure 8-10?
   A. 1. Albumin; 2. gamma fraction; 3. alpha-1; 4. alpha-2; 5. beta-1; 6. beta-2.
   B. 1. Gamma fraction; 2. alpha-1; 3. alpha-2; 4. beta-1; 5. beta-2; 6. albumin.
   C. 1. Albumin; 2. alpha-1; 3. alpha-2; 4. beta-1; 5. beta-2; 6. gamma fraction.
   D. 1. Alpha-1; 2. alpha-2; 3. beta-1; 4. beta-2; 5. gamma fraction; 6. albumin.
   E. 1. Gamma fraction; 2. alpha-1; 3. alpha-2; 4. beta-1; 5. albumin; 6. beta-2.

52. Which one of the following best describes rheumatoid factor (RF)?
   A. RF is an antigen that is used as a biomarker for the detection of rheumatoid arthritis.
   B. RF consists of antigens that are bound to the Fc portion of IgG.
   C. RF can cause a false-positive result with some immunochemical assays that measure hormones and drugs.
   D. The diagnostic specificity of RF for the detection of rheumatoid arthritis is greater than anti-cyclic citrullinated peptide (anti-CCP).
   E. Elevated serum RF levels are seen in most patients with rheumatoid arthritis.

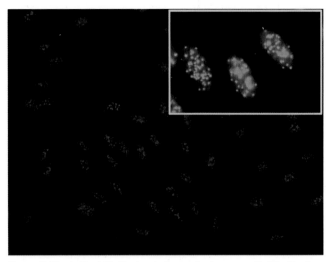

Figure 8-11 Indirect IF after incubating patient serum with HEp-2 cells.

53. Which disease is most commonly associated with the anti-nuclear antibody (ANA) staining pattern shown in Figure 8-11?
   A. Myositis.
   B. Systemic sclerosis/CREST syndrome (calcinosis, Raynaud phenomenon, esophageal dysmotility, sclerodactyly, and telangiectasia).
   C. Systemic lupus erythematosus (SLE).
   D. Drug-induced (procainamide and/or hydralazine) lupus-like syndrome.
   E. Chronic active hepatitis.

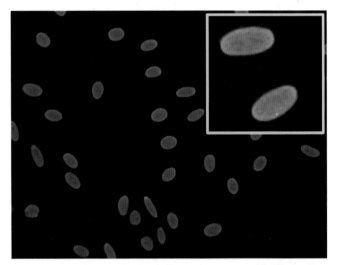

Figure 8-12 Indirect IF after incubating patient serum with HEp-2 cells.

54. Which one of the following diseases can be associated with the ANA staining pattern shown in Figure 8-12?
   A. Sjögren syndrome.
   B. Systemic sclerosis/CREST syndrome (calcinosis, Raynaud phenomenon, esophageal dysmotility, sclerodactyly, and telangiectasia).
   C. SLE.
   D. Asthma.
   E. Chronic active hepatitis.

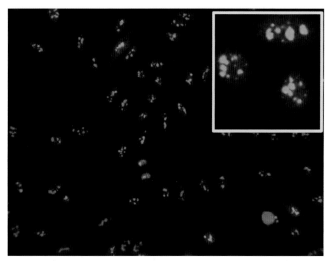

Figure 8-13 Indirect IF after incubating patient serum with HEp-2 cells.

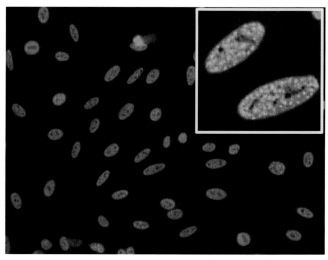

Figure 8-14 Indirect IF after incubating patient serum with HEp-2 cells.

55. Which disease is most commonly associated with the ANA staining pattern shown in Figure 8-13?
   A. Myositis.
   B. Systemic sclerosis/CREST syndrome (calcinosis, Raynaud phenomenon, esophageal dysmotility, sclerodactyly, and telangiectasia).
   C. SLE.
   D. Drug-induced (procainamide and/or hydralazine) lupus-like syndrome.
   E. Sjögren syndrome.

56. Which disease is most commonly associated with the ANA staining pattern shown in Figure 8-14?
   A. Sjögren syndrome.
   B. Systemic sclerosis/CREST syndrome (calcinosis, Raynaud phenomenon, esophageal dysmotility, sclerodactyly, and telangiectasia).
   C. SLE.
   D. Drug-induced (procainamide and/or hydralazine) lupus-like syndrome.
   E. Many antigens and connective tissue diseases.

ANSWERS

1. A. Biopsy with subsequent staging/grading.
Rationale: Although biopsy is the gold standard, it is an invasive procedure and should not be used until other noninvasive methods are exhausted.
B. Percent free PSA.
Rationale: Percent free PSA should be measured when PSA values are measured between 4 and 10 ng/mL.
C. Imaging studies to determine prostate volume and density.
Rationale: Although useful in the diagnostic workup, imaging studies would not be the next step.
D. Digital rectal exam (DRE).
Rationale: A digital rectal exam is usually part of the initial screen, not a follow-up procedure.
E. No further action.
Rationale: This is incorrect. The reference range indicates that 95% of the nondiseased population has PSA less than 4 ng/mL.

Major points of discussion
- A PSA value of 4 to 10 ng/mL is considered to be in the diagnostic gray zone. A value greater than 10 ng/mL is highly suspicious for prostate cancer and the patient should undergo biopsy.
- Biopsy of prostate tissue is the gold standard for the diagnosis of prostate cancer.
- PSA is a protease that circulates in the blood bound to protease inhibitors, and free PSA levels refer to the portion of PSA that is not bound to such proteins.

- Prostatic volume can be determined through imaging studies, and density measurements can be obtained using imaging and measurement of PSA levels.
- The measurement of PSA, along with digital rectal exam (DRE), is approved by the FDA for prostate cancer screening.

2. A. Carcinoembryonic antigen (CEA).
Rationale: CEA measurement in serum is useful in the management of patients with gastrointestinal and pancreatic cancers.
B. Carbohydrate antigen 19-9 (CA-19-9).
Rationale: CA 19-9 is useful in the management of patients with pancreatic cancer.
C. Cancer antigen 125 (CA-125).
Rationale: CA-125 is useful in the management of patients with ovarian cancer.
D. Alpha fetoprotein (AFP).
Rationale: AFP is useful in the management of patients with germ cell tumors or hepatocellular carcinoma (HCC).
E. Human chorionic gonadotropin (hCG) subunits.
Rationale: hCG subunits are useful in the management of patients with endocrine pancreatic tumors.

Major points of discussion
- The CA-125 epitope is an external fragment of a glycoprotein expressed on ovarian epithelial cells.

- CEA is a large glycoprotein, and its measurement in serum is useful in the management of patients with gastrointestinal and pancreatic cancers. It can also be elevated in smoking and other benign conditions.
- CA-19-9 is most useful in the management of patients with adenocarcinoma of the pancreas. It has been found *not* to be useful in patients with colon cancer.
- AFP is an oncodevelopmental antigen that was one of the first tumor markers used in clinical practice. It is expressed in the fetus and is elevated in the serum of patients with HCC.
- hCG is the "pregnancy hormone," but it is also elevated in germ cell and pancreatic cancers.

3. A. PSA with DRE for prostate cancer.
Rationale: PSA, with DRE, is FDA approved in the United States for screening of prostate cancer.
B. CA-125 and ultrasound imaging for breast cancer.
Rationale: CA-125 is useful in ovarian cancer, not breast cancer.
C. CEA for lung cancer in a patient with a history of smoking.
Rationale: CEA can be elevated above the reference range in smokers.
D. AFP, for HCC in a patient with elevated levels of aspartate and alanine aminotransferase.
Rationale: Although this combination may be elevated in HCC, other noncancerous conditions may also show elevation in these markers.
E. Serial hCG measurements for breast cancer.
Rationale: hCG has *not* been shown to be useful in the management of patients with breast cancer.

Major points of discussion
- Most biochemical tumor markers lack the sensitivity and/or specificity to be useful for screening purposes.
- Mammography is recommended for breast cancer screening.
- Testing for *BRCA1/BRCA2* mutations is recommended in individuals with a family history of breast and ovarian cancers.
- The majority of tumor markers are useful in monitoring therapy because they serve as surrogate markers of tumor burden.
- AFP-L3 is a glycosylated form of AFP and is useful in the monitoring of therapy for HCC.

4. A. Brain natriuretic peptide (BNP) and N-terminal-prohormone BNP (NT-ProBNP).
B. BNP and pre-prohormone of BNP.
C. Atrial natriuretic peptide (ANP) and BNP.
Rationale: Both are biologically active.
D. Urodilatin and BNP.
Rationale: Urodilatin is not biologically active.
E. ANP and N-terminal-prohormone BNP.
Rationale A, B, and E: NT-ProBNP and pre-proBNP are not biologically active.

Major points of discussion
- ANP is a 28–amino acid peptide found in the atria of the heart. BNP is a 32–amino acid that was isolated from porcine brain tissue, which explains the name of this peptide.

- Urodilatin is a 36–amino acid peptide likely produced in the kidney. It regulates water and sodium reabsorption in the kidneys. It is not detected in blood.
- BNP and NT-ProBNP are formed when the 134–amino acid pre-proBNP hormone is cleaved in myocytes to form the 108–amino acid proBNP molecule, along with the 26–amino acid signal peptide.
- ProBNP is cleaved by the enzyme corin to form two polypeptides: an inactive 76–amino acid, NT-ProBNP, and the bioactive 32–amino acid, BNP. NT-ProBNP is a linear molecule, whereas BNP is horseshoe shaped. The ring structure is essential for the biological activity of the natriuretic peptides.
- Both BNP and ANP are biologically active. ANP is usually not measured in serum because of its short half-life. BNP has a circulating half-life of 20 minutes, and NT-ProBNP has a circulating half-life of 1 to 2 hours. Circulating levels of NT-ProBNP are higher than those of BNP, and the values are not interchangeable.[19,25]

5. A. Elevated BNP or NT-ProBNP levels can be used to detect an acute myocardial infarction.
B. Elevated BNP or NT-ProBNP levels can be used to detect unstable angina.
C. Elevated BNP or NT-ProBNP levels can be used to detect cardiac ischemia.
Rationale A, B, and C: BNP and NT-ProBNP are not used to detect an acute myocardial infarction, unstable angina, or cardiac ischemia.
D. Elevated BNP or NT-ProBNP levels can be used to screen for congestive heart failure in asymptomatic individuals.
Rationale: BNP and NT-ProBNP are not used as screening tests for asymptomatic congestive heart failure.
E. Normal BNP or NT-ProBNP levels can be used to rule out congestive heart failure.
Rationale: A normal BNP or NT-ProBNP level is a good negative predictor for congestive heart failure.

Major points of discussion
- Heart failure is a serious and common disease in the United States. Heart failure in the United States affects approximately 5 million people with roughly 550,000 new cases per year. The projected deaths from heart failure are approximately 600,000 per year. It is the most frequent cause of hospitalization in those aged 65 and older.
- BNP and NT-ProBNP levels are used to rule out heart failure and are extremely helpful when the cause of dyspnea is not clear.
- Individuals with higher BNP or NT-ProBNP levels on admission to the hospital have a worse prognosis than those with lower BNP or NT-ProBNP levels.
- A significant reduction in BNP or NT-ProBNP levels during hospitalization predicts a better outcome. However, the change needed to improve prognosis must be between 50% and 80% because of the large biological variation in BNP and NT-ProBNP levels.
- Congestive heart failure can be ruled out if the BNP or NT-ProBNP levels are normal.
- BNP and NT-ProBNP are elevated in noncardiac disorders, such as acute or chronic renal failure, sepsis, liver cirrhosis with ascites, and Cushing syndrome.[19,25]

6. A. CK-MB is detected in the blood before myoglobin after acute myocardial infarction.
Rationale: After an acute myocardial infarction, myoglobin appears in the blood before CK-MB.
B. CK-MB is found only in cardiac muscle.
Rationale: CK-MB is found in both cardiac and skeletal muscle.
C. CK-MB is detected in blood before troponin I or troponin T after an acute myocardial infarction.
Rationale: After an acute myocardial infarction, CK-MB and troponin are detected in the blood at approximately the same time.
D. CK-MB is known to rise and fall predictably after an acute myocardial infarction.
Rationale: In the 1980s, CK-MB was the gold standard for detecting an acute myocardial infarction.
E. CK-MB is a better predictor than troponin I or T for risk stratification of patients with acute myocardial infarctions.
Rationale: Troponin is used for risk stratification in cardiac patients.

Major points of discussion
- CK is a dimer composed of two monomers, M (43,000 Da) and B (44,500 Da), which results in three isoenzymes: CK-MM, CK-MB, and CK-BB.
- CK is essential for cellular metabolism and is found in all tissues. The highest CK activity is found in skeletal muscle because of its physiological role in maintaining the ATP levels required for muscle contraction.
- CK-MM is the predominant isoenzyme in skeletal muscle, and CK-MB is the predominant isoenzyme in cardiac muscle. However, small amounts of CK-MB are detected in the red fibers, such as those in the soleus and intercostal muscles. Although the amount of CK-MB in skeletal muscle is small, CK-MB will be released when there is skeletal muscle damage; this may result in elevated CK-MB levels that incorrectly suggest cardiac damage.
- The kinetics of circulating CK-MB levels after an acute myocardial infarction are as follows: CK-MB levels in blood increase at 4 to 6 hours, peak at 10 to 24 hours, and return to baseline levels at 48 to 72 hours. Serial determinations of CK-MB enhance its efficiency for the diagnosis of acute myocardial infarction. CK-MB levels are usually measured at 4- to 6-hour intervals.
- Elevated circulating CK-MB levels can be observed following skeletal muscle trauma such as that seen in Duchenne muscular dystrophy, polymyositis, alcoholic myopathy, and marathon runners after a race. Therefore, CK-MB is not a completely specific biomarker for cardiac damage.[10,18]

7. A. Macromolecular complexes consisting of CK-MB bound to IgG.
B. CK mitochondrial complexes.
Rationale: They are not mitochondrial isoenzymes.
C. Artifactual forms of CK caused by binding of CK to albumin.
Rationale: They are not bound to albumin.
D. Posttranslational modification of CK-MB.
Rationale: A lysine residue is removed from the CK-M subunit of CK-MB, which yields the two CK-MB isoforms.
E. CK complexes consisting of CK-MB bound to immunoglobulin A (IgA).
Rationale A and E: Immunoglobulins are not part of the CK isoforms.

Major points of discussion
- After an acute myocardial infarction, CK-MB2 (the cardiac form of CK-MB) is released into the circulation and the C-terminal lysine residue is removed from the M subunit of CK-MB2 by the enzyme carboxypeptidase to form CK-MB1.
- In an acute myocardial infarction, the ratio of CK-MB2 to CK-MB1 in serum exceeds 1.5 within 6 hours after the onset of symptoms.
- The advantage of measuring CK-MB isoforms is that an acute myocardial infarction can be detected earlier by this approach, compared with measuring CK-MB alone.
- The disadvantage of measuring CK-MB isoforms to diagnose an acute myocardial infarction is that they have the same specificity as CK-MB and can be elevated in skeletal muscle disease.
- CK-MB isoforms are measured by a high-resolution electrophoresis procedure. This method is labor intensive and may not be able to detect small changes in CK-MB isoform concentrations. It also requires careful interpretation of the CK-MB isoform pattern.
- An immunochemical procedure for measuring CK-MB isoforms was developed, but there was cross-reactivity with CK-MM.[24]

8. A. C3.
Rationale: There is a small to moderate increase in C3 in bacterial infections.
B. C4.
Rationale: There is a small increase in C4 in bacterial infections.
C. Albumin.
Rationale: Albumin is a negative acute-phase protein.
D. C-reactive protein (CRP).
Rationale: There is a substantial increase in CRP after a bacterial infection.
E. Transferrin.
Rationale: Transferrin is a negative acute-phase protein.

Major points of discussion
- CRP is an acute-phase response protein. In response to acute inflammation, such as occurs during infection, trauma, or surgery, a significant increase in CRP, by as much as 100 to 1000 times over baseline levels, can occur.
- CRP begins to increase at approximately 6 to 12 hours after the onset of a bacterial infection and usually peaks at 48 hours. CRP concentrations are usually higher in bacterial than in viral infections. CRP is used in the assessment of inflammatory disease, such as rheumatoid arthritis, neonatal sepsis and meningitis, malignancy, and trauma.
- The magnitude of the increase in CRP levels is related to the severity of the inflammation and is the result of increased cytokine production, especially interleukin (IL)-6, which increases CRP synthesis.
- CRP levels in serum are used to monitor a patient's response to antibiotic treatment for bacterial infection.
- Measurement of CRP levels is also used as an indicator of risk for cardiovascular disease.[13]

9. A. Measurement of troponin, myoglobin, and CK-MB.
B. Measurement of CK-MB and troponin.

Rationale: Measurement of both biomarkers is not recommended in this setting.

C. Measurement of myoglobin and troponin.

Rationale for A and C: Measurement of myoglobin is not recommended in this setting.

D. Measurement of the rise and fall of troponin.

Rationale: This is the recommended biomarker for acute myocardial infarction.

E. Measurement of CK-MB isoforms and troponin.

Rationale: Measurement of CK-MB isoforms is not recommended in this setting.

Major points of discussion

- In 2007, the European Society of Cardiology and the American College of Cardiology updated their criteria for determining an acute myocardial infarction with the following recommendation: detection of the rise and fall of cardiac biomarkers, preferably troponin I or T. The troponin level should be above the 99th percentile of the upper reference limit together with one of the following four findings:
  1. Symptoms of ischemia.
  2. Changes on an electrocardiogram consistent with new ischemia, new ST-segment/T-wave changes, or new left bundle branch block.
  3. Development of new pathologic Q waves on the electrocardiogram.
  4. Imaging evidence of a new loss of viable myocardium or of a new regional wall motion abnormality.
- If troponin is not available, CK-MB can be used as the biomarker.[32]

10. A. Troponin I.

B. Ischemia modified albumin.

Rationale: This marker is used to rule out ischemia.

C. High-sensitivity CRP (hsCRP).

Rationale: This marker can be used to predict the risk of future cardiac events.

D. BNP.

Rationale: This is a marker of congestive heart failure.

E. CK-MB.

Rationale for A and E: These are the markers of myocardial necrosis.

Major points of discussion

- CRP is an indicator of acute or chronic inflammation and is a key component in the prediction of cardiovascular disease.
- The JUPITER study tested the hypothesis that daily treatment with a statin (20 mg of rosuvastatin) compared with placebo would decrease the rate of the first major cardiovascular event in individuals who had signs of a low-grade inflammatory response indicated by an hsCRP level of greater than 2 mg/L and a low-density lipoprotein cholesterol (LDL-C) level of less than 130 mg/dL, which is below the current treatment threshold for a statin.
- The JUPITER study was conducted in 17,802 apparently healthy persons from 1315 sites in 26 countries. The main baseline data showed an average LDL-C level of 108 mg/dL and an hsCRP level of 4.2 mg/L.
- In the JUPITER study, rosuvastatin reduced LDL-C levels by 50% and hsCRP levels by 39%. The occurrence of an adverse cardiovascular event was reduced by 44%

compared with placebo. The occurrence of myocardial infarction was reduced by 54% and that of unstable angina by 47%.

- The JUPITER study demonstrated that asymptomatic individuals without hyperlipidemia, but with hsCRP levels greater than 2 mg/L, benefited from statin therapy. Because of this study, there has been a significant increase in CRP testing in clinical laboratories.[26]

11. A. Ischemia-modified albumin (IMA) and glycogen phosphorylase BB.

Rationale: These are the markers that can be used to identify cardiac ischemia.

B. IMA and troponin.

Rationale: Troponin is used to identify myocardial necrosis, not cardiac ischemia.

C. IMA and free fatty acid binding protein.

Rationale: Fatty acid binding protein is a marker of myocardial necrosis.

D. IMA and BNP.

Rationale: BNP is a marker of congestive heart failure, not cardiac ischemia.

E. IMA and myosin light chain.

Rationale: Myosin light chain is a marker of myocardial necrosis, not cardiac ischemia.

Major points of discussion

- IMA is an FDA-approved test for cardiac ischemia. Glycogen phosphorylase BB is not currently approved by the FDA.
- Although both IMA and glycogen phosphorylase BB can be used to identify cardiac ischemia, IMA is the most frequently used biomarker for this purpose.
- During cardiac ischemia, the N-terminus of albumin is altered, probably through a series of chemical reactions involving free radical damage to albumin. As a result, IMA is not able to bind metals such as cobalt. When albumin circulating in the blood comes in contact with ischemic tissue in the heart, some of it is converted into IMA.
- IMA is produced continually during ischemia. IMA levels in blood rise quickly and remain elevated during an ischemic event. Ischemic patients have proportionally more IMA than do nonischemic patients.
- IMA is not completely specific for cardiac ischemia. Elevated IMA levels can be obtained in any type of ischemia—for example, in brain ischemia and gastrointestinal ischemia. IMA is a marker for any ischemic event.
- A normal IMA level has a high negative predictive value for patients who are being evaluated for acute coronary syndrome.[4]

12. A. Concurrent cardiac ischemia.

B. Concurrent congestive heart failure.

C. Concurrent unstable angina.

Rationale: LDH-1 is usually not elevated in ischemia, congestive heart failure, or unstable angina.

D. Artifact due to hemolysis.

Rationale: A low to absent haptoglobin level and a high LDH-1 fraction usually indicate hemolysis.

E. Increasing liver dysfunction.

Rationale: LD4 and LD5 are the isoenzymes associated with liver function.

Major points of discussion

- LDH has a molecular mass of about 135,000 Da and is a tetramer composed of heart (H) and muscle (M) subunits, which give rise to five isoenzymes. The LDH-1 (H4) isoenzyme is found mainly in heart, brain, and erythrocytes; the LDH-2 (H3M) is found in myocardium; and the LDH-5 isoenzyme predominates in the liver and skeletal muscle.
- In normal serum, LDH-2 is the most common isoenzyme, and the LDH-1/LDH-2 ratio is usually less than 1. The LDH-1 fraction will be greater than the LDH-2 fraction (i.e., "a flipped LDH-1/LDH-2 pattern") if (1) hemolysis is present or (2) it has been several days since an acute myocardial infarction.
- Haptoglobin is an acute-phase protein. Haptoglobin levels are decreased when there is hemolysis because the released hemoglobin binds haptoglobin and is rapidly cleared from the circulation.
- During hemolysis, significant amounts of LDH-1 isoenzyme are released from the erythrocytes, resulting in a flipped LDH-1/LDH-2 pattern.
- A flipped LDH-1/LDH-2 pattern is not a specific marker for myocardial necrosis.[8,27]

13. A. Elevated circulating myoglobin levels are diagnostic for an acute myocardial infarction.
Rationale: Myoglobin is not a specific cardiac marker.
B. Circulating myoglobin levels are elevated for days after an acute myocardial infarction.
Rationale: Myoglobin is an early cardiac marker.
C. Circulating myoglobin levels become elevated after troponin I or troponin T after an acute myocardial infarction.
Rationale: Myoglobin is elevated before troponin.
D. Circulating myoglobin levels peak after CK-MB levels rise after an acute myocardial infarction.
Rationale: Myoglobin is elevated before CK-MB.
E. Normal circulating myoglobin levels can be used to rule out an acute myocardial infarction.
Rationale: In an acute myocardial infarction, myoglobin would be elevated 4 hours after the onset of chest pain.

Major points of discussion

- Myoglobin is a relatively small (17.8 kDa) heme-containing protein. The primary function of myoglobin is to store oxygen in striated muscle for release during times of oxygen deprivation.
- Myoglobin is present in both cardiac and skeletal muscle and, therefore, is not a specific cardiac marker. Because of its low molecular weight, myoglobin is rapidly released by cells into the circulation and is the first marker to be elevated after an acute myocardial infarction.
- After an acute myocardial infarction, the serum levels of myoglobin increase between 1 and 4 hours, peak between 5 and 9 hours, and return to baseline levels between 24 and 36 hours. Serial determinations of myoglobin improve the predictive value of using a single myoglobin measurement to identify cardiac muscle injury.
- The advantages of measuring myoglobin are that it is elevated in serum before other cardiac markers and that myoglobin serum concentration is dependent on the amount of cardiac damage.
- The disadvantage of measuring myoglobin in the setting of a suspected acute myocardial infarction is that

myoglobin is not a specific marker for cardiac necrosis; it is also increased in any condition where there is skeletal muscle damage (e.g., after cardiopulmonary resuscitation) and in renal failure.
- A normal serum myoglobin value has a strong negative predictive value for an acute myocardial infarction in a patient admitted to the emergency department 6 hours after the onset of chest pain.[12]

14. A. Troponin T, calcium, and actin.
B. Troponin C, myoglobin, and actin.
C. Troponin I, actin, and tropomyosin.
D. Troponin I, troponin T, and troponin C.
Rationale: The troponin complex consists of troponins I, C, and T.
E. Troponin T, tropomyosin, and calcium.
Rationale for A, B, C, and E: Calcium, actin, tropomyosin, and myoglobin are not part of the troponin complex.

Major points of discussion

- The troponin complex consists of three proteins (i.e., troponin C, troponin I, and troponin T). The complex regulates the calcium-mediated contractile process of striated muscle.
- Troponin C is an 18-kDa protein that binds calcium.
- Troponin I is a 26.5-kDa actomyosin-ATP–inhibiting protein.
- Troponin T is a 39-kDa protein that binds tropomyosin.
- Troponin I and troponin T are present in the cytosolic pool at levels of 2% to 4% and 6% to 8%, respectively.[17]

15. A. Some troponin I methods are not accurate or precise.
Rationale: The currently available troponin I methods are very accurate and precise.
B. Some troponin I methods cross-react with troponin T.
C. Some troponin I methods are standardized.
Rationale: There is no standardization for troponin assays.
D. Some troponin I methods cross-react with troponin C.
Rationale for B and D: There is no cross-reactivity with troponin T or troponin C.
E. Some troponin I methods measure different molecular forms of troponin I.
Rationale: Many different immunochemical methods are used to measure troponin I, using different sets of antibodies, resulting in different analytical results.

Major points of discussion

- There are many immunochemical assays that are used to measure troponin I. Each method uses a different set of antibodies to measure troponin I.
- There at least seven different molecular forms of troponin I that are present in blood. Each immunochemical method uses different antibodies to measure each of the different molecular forms of troponin I. This results in significantly different troponin I results when comparing different methods.
- Some of the molecular forms of troponin I that have been detected in blood are free troponin I, troponin I–troponin C complex, troponin I–troponin C–troponin T complex, reduced and oxidized forms of troponin I, and phosphorylated and nonphosphorylated forms of troponin I.

- Each troponin I method has a different cutoff level for detecting an acute myocardial infarction.
- The sensitivity and specificity of the troponin I methods for detecting an acute myocardial infarction are each approximately 98%.[16]

16. A. The troponin complex consists of cardiac troponin T, I, and C subunits that are structurally distinct from their skeletal muscle counterparts.
Rationale: The cardiac troponin C and skeletal troponin C molecules have the same structure.
B. The troponin complex is not found in the cytosolic pool.
Rationale: There is some troponin in the cytosol.
C. Troponin is released early into blood after an acute myocardial infarction because of degradation of the contractile apparatus.
Rationale: Early release of troponin from the cytosolic pool is the reason why troponin is detected early after an acute myocardial infarction.
D. Troponin is part of the thick filament (myosin) of muscle.
Rationale: Troponin is bound to the myofibril structure.
E. Cardiac troponin T and I subunits are distinctly different from their skeletal muscle counterparts.
Rationale: Troponin I and troponin T are specific cardiac biomarkers, which are useful for detecting cardiac damage.

Major points of discussion

- The amino acid sequence for cardiac-derived troponin C is the same as that for skeletal muscle–derived troponin C. Therefore, troponin C cannot be used to distinguish between cardiac and skeletal muscle damage.
- The amino acid sequences of cardiac troponins I and T differ from those of skeletal muscle troponins I and T, respectively. Therefore, immunochemical methods can be developed that use antibodies to the cardiac-specific portions of the troponin I and troponin T molecules.
- Elevated troponin I and troponin T levels are detected in serum 4 to 6 hours after an acute myocardial infarction and can remain elevated up to 4 to 7 days afterward.
- There is a small amount of troponin I and troponin T in the cytosolic pool, which is released after an acute myocardial infarction as a result of cellular damage; this is responsible for the elevated troponin levels detected in blood 4 to 6 hours after an acute myocardial infarction.
- Troponins I and T are slowly released from the myofibril after an acute myocardial infarction; this is responsible for the sustained, elevated troponin levels seen for several days after an acute myocardial infarction.
- CK-MB is not completely cardiac specific and can also be detected in blood after skeletal muscle injury.[3]

17. A. Bilirubin interferes with the troponin T method.
Rationale: There is no interference from bilirubin with the troponin T method.
B. Skeletal muscle troponin T found in newborns cross-reacts with troponin T.
Rationale: Fetal skeletal muscle contains some cardiac troponin T, which cross-reacts with the troponin T detection method.
C. Precision of the troponin T method in newborns has not been established.
Rationale: The precision of the troponin T method is known.

D. The troponin T method requires a large sample volume and is not suitable for use in newborn testing.
Rationale: The sample volume for measuring troponin T is small, less than 50 μL.
E. The analytical sensitivity of the troponin T method is not high enough and therefore cannot be used for newborn testing.
Rationale: A high-sensitivity method is available for measuring troponin T.

Major points of discussion

- During fetal development, cardiac troponin T is also expressed in fetal skeletal muscle. Therefore, troponin T methods will provide erroneously high troponin T results if troponin T is measured in newborns.
- Troponin I is not expressed in fetal skeletal muscle.
- Reference ranges for troponin T have not been established for newborns.
- Reference ranges for troponin I have been established in newborns.
- Cardiac troponin I has an additional 31 amino acids at the N-terminal end of the molecule compared with skeletal muscle troponin I. Troponin I has complete cardiac specificity and, therefore, this assay is used to determine if there is cardiac damage in newborns.[5,6]

18. A. The troponin T method can detect more patients with an acute myocardial infarction than the troponin I method.
Rationale: There is no significant difference in the detection of an acute myocardial infarction using either the troponin I or troponin T methods.
B. Troponin T is more stable in blood than troponin I.
Rationale: There is no difference in stability between troponin I and troponin T in blood.
C. The troponin T method is more precise than the troponin I method.
Rationale: There is no significant difference in precision between the troponin I and troponin T methods.
D. Only one method is available to measure troponin T.
Rationale: There is only one immunochemical method from one vendor available to measure troponin T. In contrast, there are multiple methods for measuring troponin I.
E. Only one molecular form of troponin T is found in blood.
Rationale: Many molecular forms of troponin T are found in blood.

Major points of discussion

- The molecular forms of troponin T in blood are free troponin T, a troponin I–troponin T complex, and a troponin I–troponin C–troponin T complex.
- Although there are many molecular forms of troponin T in blood, only one immunochemical method, which uses one set of antibodies, is currently available to measure troponin T. Therefore, the troponin T results from different hospitals should be essentially the same because the same species of troponin T is being measured.
- The general protocol used for evaluating patients admitted to the emergency department with chest pain is to measure troponin T on admission and at 3- to 6-hour intervals.
- Elevated levels of troponin T are usually detected in serum by 4 to 6 hours after an acute myocardial infarction.

■ The sensitivity of the troponin T assay for detecting an acute myocardial infarction is approximately 98%. The specificity of the troponin T assay for detecting an acute myocardial infarction is approximately 95%.[2]

19. A. Heterophilic antibodies in the sample.
Rationale: Although heterophilic antibodies can produce a falsely depressed value, this type of response is likely to be an all-or-none phenomenon. Thus, this is not the best answer to this question.
B. Imprecision of the assay.
Rationale: Imprecision would not necessarily result in a falsely low value; it would manifest as a lack of reproducibility of the assay when measuring samples.
C. Calibration using a sigmoidal curve.
Rationale: The use of a sigmoidal calibration curve depends on the calibrators that are used for the assay. This feature of immunoassays has no bearing on producing false low (or high) values.
D. Multiplex enzyme-linked immunosorbent assay (ELISA) used to perform this assay.
Rationale: Multiplex assays allow for the measurement of more than one analyte simultaneously. They do not necessarily result in interferences between the analytes.
E. Presence of the hook effect.
Rationale: The hook effect occurs when the analyte of interest is present in very high concentrations, such that antigen molecules (i.e., the analyte) are bound to both the capture and detection antibodies. In such a scenario, a proportional signal cannot be generated and the resulting signal will be falsely low.

Major points of discussion
■ The hook effect is seen in immunoassays measuring analytes, such as hCG or other tumor markers, where antigen (i.e., analyte) levels can be very high.
■ Imprecise assays exhibit a high coefficient of variation (CV) and lack reproducibility.
■ Heterophilic antibodies are human xenoantibodies produced against a different species of animal (e.g., mice; human anti-mouse antibodies [HAMA]). They can cause interference in immunoassays that use antibodies from that particular animal species for capture and/or detection.
■ A multiplex ELISA is not a standard methodology for quantification of analytes in clinical laboratory assays, although they have been developed and are used in research settings.
■ A "sandwich immunoassay" refers to the use of both capture and detection antibodies, which sandwich the antigen of interest.

20. A. Presence of a band in the beta globulin fraction at a concentration of 0.2 g/dL.
Rationale: The beta fraction contains proteins such as transferrin and complement components C3 and C4.
B. Presence of a band in the gamma globulin fraction at a concentration of 3 g/dL.
Rationale: The gamma globulin fraction contains immunoglobulins, which are elevated as a monoclonal spike(s) in multiple myeloma.
C. Decreased level of a band in the albumin fraction to a concentration of 0.2 g/dL.

Rationale: The albumin fraction contains albumin, the most abundant protein in serum. The condition associated with a decrease in this fraction is referred to as hypoalbuminemia.
D. Increased levels of bands in the alpha-1 and alpha-2 globulin fractions at a concentration of 0.2 g/dL each.
Rationale: The alpha fractions contain proteins such as haptoglobin, which are acute-phase reactants, and which can increase in the setting of inflammation or infection.
E. Presence of a band in the prealbumin fraction at a concentration of 0.5 g/dL.
Rationale: The prealbumin fraction contains one protein (prealbumin or, equivalently, transthyretin), which is unrelated to multiple myeloma.

Major points of discussion
■ Albumin can constitute 50% of amount of total protein by weight in serum. It is the single most abundant protein in serum.
■ The monoclonal spike (i.e., the M-spike) is a sharp peak, typically present in the gamma globulin fraction of serum after separation by protein electrophoresis, and is indicative of a single species of immunoglobulin molecule. Its presence at this concentration is diagnostic for multiple myeloma.
■ CRP is a positive acute-phase reactant that can increase more than 100-fold above its normal levels in the setting of inflammation or infection. It migrates in the alpha globulin fraction of serum after separation via protein electrophoresis.
■ "Prealbumin," another name for the serum protein transthyretin, is not otherwise related to albumin. Prealbumin migrates ahead of the albumin peak in conventional agarose gel electrophoresis; therefore, this is how it was named.
■ Microalbumin refers to low concentrations of albumin that are present in urine. It is elevated in patients with kidney injury and kidney disease.

21. A. Increased albumin; increased alpha-1, alpha-2, and beta globulins; and normal gamma globulins.
B. Decreased albumin, increased alpha-1 and alpha-2 globulins, and normal beta and gamma globulins.
C. Decreased albumin, decreased alpha-1 and alpha-2 globulins, and normal beta and gamma globulins.
D. Increased albumin, decreased alpha-1 and alpha-2 globulins, normal beta globulins, and increased gamma globulins.
E. Normal albumin; increased alpha-1, alpha-2, and beta globulins; and normal gamma globulins.
Rationale: In acute inflammation, albumin is usually decreased, alpha-1 and alpha-2 globulins are increased, and beta and gamma globulins are normal.

Major points of discussion
■ Acute inflammation is characterized by increased production of acute-phase proteins.
■ In acute inflammation, alpha-1-antitrypsin is the major protein that is responsible for the increase in the alpha-1 region of the serum protein electrophoresis pattern. Alpha-1-acid glycoprotein is also an acute-phase protein, increased levels of which may be seen in the alpha-1 region in patients with sepsis.
■ In acute inflammation, haptoglobin is the major protein that is responsible for the increase in the alpha-2 region

of the serum protein electrophoresis pattern. Ceruloplasmin is also an acute-phase protein, increased levels of which may be seen in the alpha-2 region in patients with severe liver disease.
- CRP is increased in acute inflammation, but its concentration is usually too low to be detected by serum protein electrophoresis.[7]
- Albumin is decreased in acute inflammation because of increased production of IL-6, which decreases albumin synthesis in the liver.
- In acute inflammation, the beta and gamma globulin fractions in the serum protein electrophoresis pattern are usually normal.[14]

22. A. The yolk sac.
Rationale: This is the major site for AFP synthesis up to approximately 10 weeks of gestation.
B. The fetal pancreas.
Rationale: AFP is not synthesized in the fetal pancreas.
C. The yolk sac and fetal liver.
Rationale: AFP is not synthesized in the yolk sac after 12 weeks of gestation.
D. The fetal liver.
Rationale: This is the major site of AFP synthesis after 12 weeks of gestation.
E. The fetal kidney.
Rationale: AFP is not synthesized in the fetal kidney.

Major points of discussion
- AFP is initially synthesized in the yolk sac and fetal liver. At approximately 10 weeks of gestation, there is degeneration of the yolk sac and the fetal liver becomes the main source of AFP.
- Neural tube defects (NTDs) result from failure of the neural tube to close spontaneously between the third and fourth week of in utero development. NTDs usually occur before a woman knows she is pregnant.
- The concentration of AFP in the fetal blood is highest at about 10 to 13 weeks of gestation and is in the mg/mL range. The concentration of maternal serum AFP levels is normally in the ng/mL range.
- In open spina bifida and anencephaly, AFP levels are elevated because fetal blood, which contains high concentrations of AFP, is excreted into the amniotic fluid, where it is in contact with the maternal circulation. The result is an increase in maternal serum AFP levels.
- Only maternal serum and amniotic fluid AFP levels are used to screen for NTDs.

23. A. This is the serum protein electrophoresis pattern that is seen in severe liver disease.
Rationale: In liver disease, the gamma globulin fraction is usually elevated.
B. This is the serum IFE pattern for a monoclonal protein.
Rationale: The IFE pattern shows the presence of polyclonal immunoglobulins.
C. This is the serum protein electrophoresis pattern that is usually seen in nephrosis.
Rationale: This is a serum protein electrophoresis pattern with a low albumin, elevated alpha-2 globulin, a normal or decreased gamma globulin fraction, and a low total protein concentration is usually indicative of nephrosis.

D. This is the serum protein electrophoresis pattern that is seen in iron deficiency anemia.
Rationale: In iron deficiency anemia, the total protein concentration and the proteins in the alpha-2 region are usually normal.
E. This is the serum protein electrophoresis pattern that is seen in alpha-1 antitrypsin deficiency.
Rationale: It is not alpha-1 antitrypsin deficiency, because the proteins in the alpha-1 region are actually increased in concentration.

Major points of discussion
- The major proteins found in the alpha-2 region of the serum protein electrophoresis pattern are alpha-2-macroglobulin and haptoglobin. Ceruloplasmin, antithrombin III, and fibronectin are present at low concentrations and do not significantly contribute to the protein pattern.
- The elevated protein band in the alpha-2 region is most likely due to alpha-2-macroglobulin.
- Alpha-2-macroglobulin is a large protein with a molecular weight of 725 kDa that is not excreted into the urine. Alpha-2-macroglobulin is a protease inhibitor.
- A serum protein electrophoresis pattern with a low albumin, elevated alpha-2 globulin, a normal or decreased gamma globulin fraction, and a low total protein concentration is usually indicative of nephrosis.
- In nephrosis, albumin and other low molecular weight proteins are excreted into the urine and the hepatic synthesis of alpha-2-macroglobulin is increased to compensate for the decreased oncotic pressure. As a result, high levels of alpha-2-macroglobulin are observed in nephrosis.
- Although a monoclonal protein can be detected in the alpha-2 region, it is a rare occurrence.[30]

24a. A. Sensitivity.
B. Specificity.
C. Precision.
D. Negative predictive value.
E. Accuracy.
Rationale: See Major Points of Discussion.

24b. A. Sensitivity.
B. Specificity.
C. Positive predictive value.
D. Negative predictive value
E. Accuracy.
Rationale: See Major Points of Discussion.

24c. A. Sensitivity.
B. Precision.
C. Positive predictive value.
D. Reference interval.
E. Accuracy.
Rationale: See Major Points of Discussion.

24d. A. Sensitivity.
B. Precision.
C. Positive predictive value.
D. Negative predictive value.
E. Accuracy.
Rationale: See Major Points of Discussion.

24e. A. Sensitivity.
B. Specificity.
C. Positive predictive value.
D. Negative predictive value.
E. Accuracy.
Rationale: See Major Points of Discussion.

Major points of discussion

- Accuracy is the closeness of the result obtained by the assay to the true value, as measured by a gold standard method.
- Precision is an assessment of the repeatability (i.e., reproducibility) of an assay. It is measured by calculation of the CV. It is important to measure the interassay and intra-assay CV to determine precision.
- Predictive values (positive predictive value and negative predictive value) are characteristics that are dependent on the prevalence of the disease in the population being tested.
- Reference intervals are typically established using 120 samples from a nondiseased cohort and taking the range of values from the central 95% of this population—that is, excluding three samples from each extreme.
- Negative predictive value is the likelihood that a negative test result excludes disease.
- Sensitivity is the ability to detect true positives in a cohort of patients.
- The CV is determined by taking replicate measurements of a control sample and then dividing the standard deviation of those results by their mean. It is expressed as a percentage.

25. A. Serum protein electrophoresis (SPEP) showed low albumin and slightly elevated gamma globulin levels and the possibility of a monoclonal protein in the gamma globulin region, which was identified by IFE as a monoclonal IgG lambda protein.
B. SPEP showed low albumin and slightly elevated gamma globulin levels and the possibility of a monoclonal protein in the gamma globulin region, which was identified by IFE as a free lambda light chain.
Rationale: A monoclonal protein is not seen by IFE.
C. SPEP showed low albumin and slightly elevated polyclonal gamma globulin levels. No monoclonal protein was detected by IFE.
Rationale: SPEP showed the possibility of a monoclonal protein in the gamma globulin region.
D. SPEP showed low albumin and slightly elevated gamma globulin levels and the possibility of a monoclonal protein in the gamma globulin region. No monoclonal protein was detected by IFE. The narrow band in the SPEP pattern is probably due to fibrinogen.
Rationale: This is the correct interpretation.
E. SPEP showed low albumin and slightly elevated gamma globulin levels and the possibility of a monoclonal protein in the gamma globulin region, which was identified by IFE as a monoclonal IgA lambda protein.
Rationale: A monoclonal IgA lambda protein is not seen by IFE.

Major points of discussion

- A narrow band (i.e., a spike) in the SPEP may not be due to a monoclonal protein. Fibrinogen will migrate in the beta-gamma region and appear as a monoclonal protein in the SPEP. If IFE is performed on this sample and a monoclonal protein is not detected, protein electrophoresis should be repeated using another serum sample.
- Fibrinogen may be present in the "serum" sample if the blood has not been allowed to clot for a sufficient amount of time. If the patient is receiving an anticoagulant that prevents complete clotting, the sample is collected in a tube that contains an anticoagulant.
- A narrow band in the SPEP can be confirmed to be fibrinogen by performing IFE using antibodies to fibrinogen or by treating the sample with thrombin followed by serum protein electrophoresis; in the latter case, the band will disappear.
- At very high concentrations of CRP, a small band may appear in the gamma globulin region of the SPEP.
- A narrow band may appear at the application point and in all lanes on the IFE gel because of the presence of pentameric IgM aggregates or from polymerized IgA. This sample can be treated with 2-mercaptoethanol to break up these polymers. An IFE on the treated sample will then determine whether a monoclonal protein is present.
- In cases of severe hemolysis, formation of a hemoglobin-haptoglobin complex may appear as a monoclonal band in the beta globulin region of the SPEP. Visual inspection of the specimen will reveal gross hemolysis.[29]

26a. A. Acquisition of this mutation marks the transition from low-grade to high-grade cancer.
B. Acquisition of this mutation marks the transition from early-stage to late-stage disease.
Rationale: No such marker currently exists that can accurately characterize this transition.
C. This mutation correlates with sensitivity to chemotherapy using tyrosine kinase inhibitors.
D. This mutation correlates with resistance to chemotherapy using tyrosine kinase inhibitors.
Rationale: The T790M mutation has been identified in tumors that have developed resistance to tyrosine kinase inhibitors.
E. This mutation portends a favorable outcome (i.e., is an indicator of good prognosis).
Rationale for C and E: The L858R mutation was initially found to be an indicator of a poor prognosis. It was later found that tumors harboring this mutation were sensitive to tyrosine kinase inhibitors.

26b. A. Acquisition of this mutation marks the transition from low-grade to high-grade cancer.
B. Acquisition of this mutation marks the transition from early-stage to late-stage disease.
Rationale: No such marker currently exists that can accurately characterize this transition.
C. This mutation correlates with sensitivity to chemotherapy using tyrosine kinase inhibitors.
D. This mutation correlates with resistance to chemotherapy using tyrosine kinase inhibitors.
Rationale: The T790M mutation was identified in tumors that developed resistance to tyrosine kinase inhibitors.
E. This mutation portends a favorable outcome (i.e., is an indicator of good prognosis).

Rationale for C and E: The L858R mutation was initially found to be an indicator of a poor prognosis. It was later found that tumors harboring this mutation were sensitive to tyrosine kinase inhibitors.

26c. A. CA-15.3.
Rationale: CA-15.3 is FDA approved for breast cancer monitoring.
B. PSA.
Rationale: PSA is FDA approved for prostate cancer monitoring.
C. AFP.
Rationale: AFP is used in monitoring patients with HCC and for patients with germ cell tumors.
D. hCG.
Rationale: hCG is primarily used in monitoring patients with germ cell tumors.
E. CEA.
Rationale: CEA is used to monitor disease in patients with lung cancer.

26d. A. CEA has poor sensitivity for the diagnosis of lung cancer; only 20% of lung cancers are diagnosed using this marker.
Rationale: CEA is not useful for diagnostic purposes but is an important tumor marker for monitoring patients with lung cancer.
B. CEA has poor specificity for lung cancer; there are multiple nonmalignant conditions resulting in elevated CEA levels.
Rationale: Smoking and multiple inflammatory conditions are characterized by elevated circulating levels of CEA.
C. The dynamic range of this assay is limited and not suitable for patients with late-stage or metastatic disease.
Rationale: The dynamic range of an assay should not affect screening for disease.
D. The analytical sensitivity of this assay does not meet the needs for early detection.
Rationale: Although analytical sensitivity may impact early detection, this is not related to the problems related to population-based screening.
E. The assay is imprecise (i.e., the coefficient of variation is >20%).
Rationale: Assay (im)precision does not directly affect population-based screening.

Major points of discussion
- Most (i.e., ~80%) lung cancers are classified as NSCLCs; the remaining approximately 20% are small cell lung cancers.
- Several tumor markers have been used for lung cancer, but none are ideal. The markers used include CEA, neuron-specific enolase (NSE), cytokeratin-19 fragments (CYFRA 21-1), progastrin-releasing peptide (ProGRP), squamous cell carcinoma antigen (SCCA), and chromogranin A.
- The tumor markers listed above are primarily useful for differential diagnosis, prognosis, postoperative surveillance, monitoring therapy, and recurrence detection.
- In recent years, the EGFR has been well characterized at the molecular level. Several genetic aberrations have been identified in patients with NSCLC, including the L858R and T790M mutations.
- The most widely used tumor marker used for managing patients with lung cancer is CEA. However, it suffers from a lack of specificity because it can be elevated in many non–lung cancer conditions.

27. **A. Anencephaly and myelomeningocele.**
Rationale: Maternal serum AFP levels are usually elevated in anencephaly and myelomeningocele.
B. Anencephaly, myelomeningocele, and closed spina bifida.
C. Anencephaly and closed spina bifida.
Rationale: Screening for closed spina bifida using maternal serum AFP levels is not possible because the maternal serum AFP level is not elevated.
D. Trisomy 21.
E. Trisomy 18.
Rationale: A single biomarker is not used to screen for trisomy 21 or trisomy 18.

Major points of discussion
- Maternal screening for NTDs is usually performed at 14 to 21 or 15 to 20 weeks of gestation. A positive NTD result is followed up with a high intensity ultrasound and with measurement of amniotic fluid AFP levels.
- Patients with anencephaly have very elevated AFP levels. False-negative results are rare because there is usually no overlap in AFP values between anencephaly and patients with AFP values in the reference range.
- False-negative results for NTDs can be obtained in patients with open spina bifida.
- Patients with closed spina bifida usually have AFP values that are in the reference range, because AFP does not leak from the fetal blood into the maternal circulation in this setting.
- False-positive screening results for NTDs can be obtained in multiple disorders, including intrauterine fetal demise, intrauterine growth retardation, gastroschisis, oligohydramnios, omphalocele, and congenital nephrosis.
- Approximately 95% of patients with an NTD have no family history of NTDs.
- The incidence of open NTDs in the United States is approximately 1:1000 live births.[11]

28. A. Albumin and alpha-1-antitrypsin.
Rationale: Alpha-1-antitrypsin is a positive acute-phase protein, the concentration of which increases in the setting of inflammation.
B. Albumin and alpha-2-macroglobulin.
Rationale: Alpha-2-macroglobulin is a protease inhibitor and is a positive acute-phase protein.
C. Haptoglobin and CRP.
Rationale: Haptoglobin and CRP are positive acute-phase proteins, the concentrations of which increase in the setting of inflammation.
D. Albumin and transferrin.
Rationale: These are both negative acute-phase proteins, the concentrations of which decrease in the setting of inflammation.

E. Transferrin and C3.
Rationale: C3, a component of the complement system, is a positive acute-phase protein, the concentration of which increases in the setting of inflammation.

Major points of discussion

- Alpha-1-antitrypsin migrates in the alpha-1 region of the SPEP pattern. It is a positive acute-phase protein that is increased in pregnancy, liver disease, and malignancy.
- Transferrin, the major iron-binding protein in serum, migrates in the beta-1 region of the serum protein electrophoresis pattern. It is a negative acute-phase protein. In acute inflammation, transferrin synthesis by the liver is decreased, resulting in low transferrin levels.
- Albumin is the most abundant protein in normal serum. It is a negative acute-phase protein. In chronic infections and acute inflammation, decreased albumin levels are usually seen because of increased production of IL-6, which decreases albumin synthesis by the liver.
- Haptoglobin migrates in the alpha-2 region of the SPEP pattern. It is a positive acute-phase protein that is increased in pregnancy and cirrhosis.
- C3, a component of the complement system, migrates in the beta-2 region of the SPEP pattern. It is a positive acute-phase protein that is increased during inflammation.
- Transthyretin and retinol-binding protein are also negative acute-phase proteins, but their concentration in serum is too low to be detected by routine SPEP.

29. A. Nuchal translucency (NT), free beta-hCG, and AFP.
Rationale: AFP is not used in the first trimester to screen for fetal Down syndrome.
B. NT, free beta-hCG, and pregnancy-associated protein A (PAPP-A).
Rationale: These are the markers that are used to screen for fetal Down syndrome in the first trimester.
C. NT, free beta-hCG, and inhibin A.
D. NT, free beta-hCG, and unconjugated estradiol (uE3).
Rationale: uE3 is not used in the first trimester to screen for fetal Down syndrome.
E. NT, PAPP-A, and inhibin A.
Rationale for C and E: Inhibin A is not used in the first trimester to screen for fetal Down syndrome.

Major points of discussion

- First-trimester maternal screening for fetal Down syndrome is performed between 10 and 13 weeks of gestation.
- Patients with a high risk for fetal Down syndrome have a low PAPP-A level, a high free beta-hCG level, and a high NT measurement.
- First-trimester maternal screening for fetal Down syndrome is usually followed by measuring maternal serum AFP levels in the second trimester to test for the presence of fetal NTDs.
- First-trimester maternal screening has improved the detection rate for fetal Down syndrome. With a false-positive rate of 5%, the detection rate for fetal Down syndrome is 86%.
- Integrated testing uses the maternal screening results of the first and second trimesters to calculate the risk of fetal Down syndrome. First-trimester maternal screening followed by the maternal quadratic screen in the second

trimester increases the detection rate for fetal Down syndrome to 95%, with a false-positive rate of 5%.
- PAPP-A is a zinc-containing metalloproteinase glycoprotein that is produced by the trophoblast. PAPP-A interacts with insulin-like growth factor binding proteins to release insulin-like growth factors, which promote fetal growth and development.[20]

30. A. Vitamin A.
Rationale: Vitamin A is not associated with NTDs. Vitamin A promotes vision and plays a role in humoral immunity.
B. Folic acid.
Rationale: The introduction of folic acid into foods in 1998 significantly decreased the occurrence of NTDs in the United States.
C. Vitamin D.
Rationale: Vitamin D is not associated with NTDs. Vitamin D is needed for bone growth and development.
D. Vitamin K.
Rationale: Vitamin K is not associated with NTDs. Vitamin K is important in the synthesis of proteins required for blood clotting.
E. Vitamin E.
Rationale: Vitamin E is not associated with NTDs. Vitamin E is an antioxidant that functions as a free radical scavenger.

Major points of discussion

- Folic acid deficiency is associated with an increased risk of NTDs.
- In 1998, the U.S. Public Health Service required that folic acid be added to breakfast cereals, infant formulas, pasta, rice, flour, and cornmeal.
- After the fortification of foods with folic acid, the prevalence of NTDs in the United States decreased by 36%, from 10.8 per 10,000 population during 1995–1996 to 6.9 at the end of 2006.
- Fortification of foods with folic acid is effective in preventing NTDs, because folic acid is accessible to all women of childbearing age without requiring any behavioral changes.
- The Centers for Disease Control and Prevention recommends that all women of childbearing age take a multivitamin with 0.4 mg of folic acid per day. Women with a previous history of NTDs should take 4.0 mg of folic acid per day.[9]

31. A. Increased, because the MOM will be higher than expected.
B. Increased, because the MOM will be lower than expected.
Rationale: The MOM calculated using the median MSAFP value at 19 weeks of gestation would be lower than expected when the true gestational age is 15 weeks, because MSAFP levels increase with increasing gestational age.
C. Decreased, because the MOM will be lower than expected.
Rationale: Overestimation of gestational age would decrease both the MOM and risk of an NTD.
D. Decreased, because the MOM will be higher than expected.
Rationale: The MOM would be lower than expected, because MSAFP levels increase with increasing gestational age.
E. Cannot be determined; therefore, another sample should be drawn to repeat the MSAFP determination.

Rationale: Another sample should not be drawn. The risk for a fetal NTD can be recalculated from the original MSAFP result by using the correct gestational age.

Major points of discussion

- An incorrect gestational age is a common cause for an erroneous calculation of fetal NTD risk.
- Calculation of the gestational age based on the last menstrual period is not always accurate and is the major reason physicians call the laboratory to ask for a recalculation of NTD risk based on a different gestational age.
- Calculation of gestational age based on ultrasound is the preferred method.
- Overestimation of gestational age will result in a lower calculated risk for a fetal NTD.
- Underestimation of gestational age will result in a higher calculated risk for a fetal NTD.
- MSAFP levels can increase by approximately sevenfold in anencephaly and approximately fourfold in open spina bifida.

32. A. Increased, because the actual MOM is higher than the calculated MOM.
B. Increased, because the actual MOM is lower than the calculated MOM.
C. Decreased, because the actual MOM is lower than the calculated MOM.
D. Decreased, because the MOM is higher than the calculated MOM.
Rationale: The MOM calculated using the median AFP value at 20 weeks of gestation would be higher than expected when the true gestational age is 15 weeks, because the AFAFP levels decrease with increasing gestational age. Therefore, the actual risk is lower than the calculated risk using the incorrect gestational age.
E. Slightly decreased, but will not significantly affect the NTD risk calculation.
Rationale: The NTD risk at 15 and 20 weeks of gestation is significantly different because of the change in AFP levels between 15 and 20 weeks of gestation.

Major points of discussion

- A positive serum AFP result is a common reason for measuring an amniotic fluid AFP (AFAFP) level to rule out or confirm the diagnosis of a fetal NTD.
- A positive AFAFP result is confirmed by measuring fetal hemoglobin levels and acetylcholinesterase in the amniotic fluid.
- Detection of fetal hemoglobin in amniotic fluid as a result of amniocentesis can correlate with elevated AFAFP levels, because AFP is present in fetal blood at high concentrations.
- Cerebrospinal fluid contains the enzyme acetylcholinesterase, which is specific to neural tissue but normally absent from amniotic fluid. In a case of open spina bifida, acetylcholinesterase leaks into the amniotic fluid. Detection of acetylcholinesterase in amniotic fluid is most likely the result of a fetal NTD.
- In normal pregnancies, AFAFP levels decrease with increasing gestational age. Inaccurate estimation of gestational age will hinder the provision of an accurate risk of a fetal NTD.[22]

33. A. Increased serum MSAFP level and increased risk of NTDs.
B. Increased serum MSAFP level and decreased risk of NTDs.
Rationale: The serum MSAFP levels are lower in overweight women, because of an increase in maternal plasma volume.
C. Decreased serum MSAFP level and increased risk of NTDs.
Rationale: The risk of NTDs is lower when MSAFP levels are decreased.
D. Decreased serum MSAFP level and decreased risk of NTDs.
Rationale: The maternal plasma volume is higher in overweight patients, resulting in lower than expected serum MSAFP levels. Therefore, a lower than expected risk for NTDs would be obtained if the weight correction were not performed.
E. No change in the risk for NTDs.
Rationale: Any change in the MSAFP levels affects the risk for NTDs.

Major points of discussion

- There is an inverse relationship between MSAFP levels and maternal weight. The MSAFP levels decrease with increasing maternal weight, because the maternal plasma total volume is higher in overweight patients.
- Because the serum MSAFP level is lower than expected in overweight patients, this results in a lower risk for NTDs if the weight correction is not performed.
- The serum MSAFP levels increase with decreasing maternal weight because the maternal plasma volume is lower in underweight patients.
- Because the MSAFP level is higher than expected in underweight patients, this results in a higher risk for NTDs if the weight correction is not performed.
- In general, overweight women have an increased risk for open spina bifida.[34]

34. A. Proteins have a positive charge and migrate toward the anode.
B. Proteins have a positive charge and migrate toward the cathode.
C. Proteins have a negative charge and migrate toward the anode.
Rationale: Proteins have a negative charge at a pH of 8.6 and migrate toward the positively charged anode.
D. Proteins have a negative charge and migrate toward the cathode.
Rationale: At a pH of 8.6, proteins migrate toward the anode.
E. Proteins all have the same isoelectric point.
Rationale: Proteins have different isoelectric points.

Major points of discussion

- Proteins are amphoteric because of ionization of the acidic and basic side chains of amino acids.
- At a pH of 8.6, serum proteins are negatively charged and, when placed in an electric field, they migrate towards the anode (i.e., positive electrode).
- Albumin migrates the fastest and gamma globulins the slowest. The proteins in the alpha-1, alpha-2, and beta globulin regions migrate between albumin and the gamma globulins.

- Electrophoresis is the migration of charged particles in an electric field. The rate of migration of proteins depends on the charge of the molecule, the size and shape of the molecule, the applied voltage, the nature of the support medium, and the pH and ionic strength of the buffer.
- When the pH of a buffer solution equals the isoelectric point of the protein, the protein has no net charge and does not migrate in an applied electric field. When the pH of the solution is above the isoelectric point of the protein, the protein has a negative charge and migrates toward the anode.[15]

35. A. Elevated AFP, hCG, and inhibin A; low uE3.
Rationale: AFP is low in Down syndrome.
B. Elevated inhibin A; low AFP, hCG, and uE3.
Rationale: Low AFP, hCG, and uE3 levels are seen in trisomy 18. hCG is elevated in Down syndrome.
C. Elevated AFP; low or normal uE3, hCG, and inhibin A.
Rationale: This is the pattern that is seen in with fetal neural tube defects. hCG and inhibin A are elevated and AFP is low in Down syndrome.
D. Elevated inhibin A and uE3; low AFP and hCG.
Rationale: hCG is elevated in Down syndrome. uE3 is decreased in Down syndrome.
E. Elevated hCG and inhibin A; low AFP and uE3.
Rationale: Elevated hCG and inhibin A; low AFP and uE3 are seen in Down syndrome.

Major points of discussion

- In normal pregnancies, serum AFP and uE3 levels increase with increasing gestational age and hCG levels decrease with increasing gestational age. Inhibin A levels do not significantly change at 14 to 19 weeks of gestation. From 19 to 21 weeks of gestation, there is a small increase in inhibin A levels.
- When a fetus has Down syndrome, AFP and uE3 concentrations are low and hCG and inhibin A levels are high.
- An accurate gestational age is important in calculating the risk for Down syndrome, because overestimation of gestational age in a normal pregnancy can yield the same quadratic screening pattern that is seen when a fetus has Down syndrome.
- Although the serum biomarkers levels are corrected for maternal weight, the risk for Down syndrome is not significantly affected by maternal weight.
- The definitive test for detecting Down syndrome is chromosome analysis (e.g., cytogenetics).
- The unadjusted risk for Down syndrome at term is approximately 1:385.[11,20]

36. A. All cases of fetal Down syndrome are detected.
Rationale: False-negative results are obtained with both screening methods.
B. There is an increase in the detection rate of fetal Down syndrome.
Rationale: More cases of Down syndrome are detected using the quadratic screen.
C. The reagent cost is significantly reduced.
Rationale: The reagent cost is higher using the quadratic screen.
D. Fetal trisomy 18 cases can be detected.

Rationale: Both the quadratic screen and triple screen are used to detect cases of fetal trisomy 18.
E. The analytical method is automated.
Rationale: The quadratic screen and triple screen methods can both be automated.

Major points of discussion

- Using the triple screen (i.e., AFP, uE3, and hCG), the detection rate for fetal Down syndrome is 70%, with a false-positive rate of 5%.
- Using the quadratic screen (i.e., AFP, uE3, hCG, and inhibin A), the detection rate for fetal Down syndrome is 81% with a false-positive rate of 5%.
- Calculation of the correct gestational age is important for obtaining accurate risk assessments of Down syndrome. Ultrasound evaluation of the gestational age is now the standard approach.
- The age of the mother is important in calculating the risk of fetal Down syndrome; this risk increases with increasing maternal age.
- In women undergoing assisted reproduction, the age of the egg donor is used to calculate the risk of fetal Down syndrome.[11,20]

37. A. AFP is elevated; uE3 and hCG are normal.
Rationale: This pattern can be seen when a fetus has an NTD.
B. AFP is very elevated; uE3 and hCG are low.
Rationale: This pattern can be seen when a fetus has anencephaly.
C. uE3 and hCG are elevated; AFP is low.
Rationale: uE3 is not elevated in trisomy 18.
D. AFP, uE3, and hCG are all low.
Rationale: This is the pattern that is seen when a fetus has trisomy 18.
E. hCG is elevated; AFP and uE3 are low.
Rationale: This is the pattern that is seen when a fetus has trisomy 21.

Major points of discussion

- Screening programs for trisomy 21 (i.e., Down syndrome), using either the quadratic screen (i.e., maternal serum levels of AFP, uE3, hCG, and inhibin A) or the triple screen (AFP, uE3, and hCG) can also be used to screen for trisomy 18, because inhibin A levels are not used to calculate the risk for trisomy 18.
- The unadjusted incidence of trisomy 18 is approximately 1:8000 at term.
- Screening methods based on the quadratic screen can identify approximately 60% of affected pregnancies with a false-positive rate of less than 0.4%.
- More than 90% of infants born with trisomy 18 die within the first year of life.
- A significant number of pregnancies affected by trisomy 18 are lost between prenatal diagnosis and term. Approximately 72% of pregnancies diagnosed with trisomy 18 end in miscarriage or stillbirth.[23]

38a. A. **Wide dynamic range.**
Rationale: AFP levels can range from the ng/mL (in the general population) to the mg/mL range (in late-stage liver cancer patients). Thus, an assay with a wide dynamic range is important.
B. Analytical sensitivity at the low end.

Rationale: Analytical sensitivity at the low limit of detection would not be sufficient in this situation; the high end of the range is also important.
C. High precision.
D. Minimal analytical interferences from drugs.
Rationale: These are desirable but would not be specifically relevant for this scenario.
E. Standardized results between different assays.
Rationale: As long as the same assay is used to measure the values in the entire population, a lack of standardization between different assays measuring the same analyte is not relevant in this situation.

38b. A. Wide dynamic range.
B. Analytical sensitivity at the low end.
Rationale: Detection of recurrence after radical prostatectomy requires robust performance at the lower end of the analytical range.
C. High precision.
Rationale for A and C: Although this is an important parameter for all assays, it is not the most important characteristic for this situation. Detection of recurrence after radical prostatectomy requires robust performance at the lower end of the analytical range.
D. Minimal analytical interferences from drugs.
Rationale: Although this is important for any assay, it is not necessarily relevant for the current scenario.
E. Standardized results between different assays.
Rationale: As long as the same assay is used to measure the values when following any one individual patient, this attribute may not be necessary.

38c. A. Wide dynamic range.
Rationale: A wide dynamic range would not explain these differences in results between these two different assays.
B. Analytical sensitivity at the low end.
Rationale: Analytical sensitivity at the low end would help in measuring low levels of analyte near the lower limit of detection but does not explain the different results obtained using these two different assays.
C. High precision.
Rationale: High precision would help with the reproducibility on any one platform but does not explain the differences in results between these two assays.
D. Minimal analytical interferences from drugs.
Rationale: Minimal interference with drugs is important is important for any assay but does not explain the difference in results between these two different assays.
E. Lack of standardization among different assays.
Rationale: In this case, the assays are different and, for example, use different capture and detection antibodies, which measure slightly different epitopes. This results in different values being measured for this analyte with the two different assays.

38d. A. Wide dynamic range.
Rationale: Although a wide dynamic range may be generally important for tumor marker assays, it is not the most important characteristic for this situation.
B. Analytical sensitivity at the low end.

Rationale: This is not important in this situation, where analyte levels are being measured and compared in the elevated to higher end of the range, not the lower end of the range.
C. High precision.
Rationale: This is most critical for serial assessment of specific patients, as levels of the tumor marker can be compared before, during, and after completion of the treatment regimen.
D. Minimal analytical interferences from drugs.
Rationale: This is generally important for any assay, but not specifically for this scenario.
E. Lack of standardization among different assays.
Rationale: Standardization between different assays is not necessary for this scenario.

Major points of discussion
- A wide dynamic range is generally important for tumor marker assays, so that the same assay can be used for patients without disease, with early-stage disease, and with metastatic disease.
- An assay with high analytical sensitivity (i.e., low limit of detection) is important in situations where there is a need to measure low levels of the analyte of interest.
- Standardization among different assays for the same analyte is important when comparisons are made using results from the different assays. This does not necessarily apply to situations for comparison of results using just one assay.
- When monitoring a cancer patient with tumor marker(s), it is ideal to make such an assessment using pre- and posttreatment measurements with the same methodology/analyzer in the same laboratory.
- Some tumor markers can also be used for noncancer purposes; examples include hCG for detecting pregnancy and AFP for assessing fetal development in quadratic screening. The requirements in performance characteristics for these situations may differ based on the intended use of the analyte measurement.

39. A. Detection of a monoclonal protein in the cryoprecipitate.
Rationale: This is the definition of type I cryoglobulinemia.
B. Detection of albumin and a monoclonal protein in the cryoprecipitate.
Rationale: Albumin is not included in the definition of type II cryoglobulinemia.
C. Detection of alpha-1, alpha-2, and beta globulins in the cryoprecipitate.
Rationale: These proteins are not included in the definition of type II cryoglobulinemia.
D. Detection of polyclonal immunoglobulins in the cryoprecipitate.
Rationale: This is the definition of type III cryoglobulinemia.
E. Detection of a monoclonal protein and polyclonal immunoglobulins in the cryoprecipitate.
Rationale: See Major points of discussion.

Major points of discussion
- Cryoglobulins are immunoglobulins that precipitate at temperatures less than 37°C and dissolve when rewarmed to 37°C.

- Proper sample collection is important for detection of cryoglobulins. Blood samples should be collected in warm tubes, transported to the laboratory at 37°C, and immediately centrifuged. False-negative cryoglobulin results can be obtained if the blood sample is allowed to clot at temperatures less than 37°C.
- Analysis for cryoglobulins involves storing the serum for 7 days at 4°C and examining the sample for the presence of a cryoprecipitate. If present, the cryoprecipitate is washed several times and redissolved, and serum protein electrophoresis and IFE are performed.
- Type I cryoglobulinemia is defined as the presence of a monoclonal protein (usually IgG or IgM) in the cryoprecipitate, and is associated with multiple myeloma and Waldenström macroglobulinemia. Type I cryoglobulins occur in about 10% of all cryoprecipitates.
- Type II cryoglobulinemia is defined as the presence of a monoclonal protein (usually IgG or IgM) together with polyclonal immunoglobulins in the cryoprecipitate, and is associated with hepatitis C virus (HCV) infection, autoimmune diseases, and non-Hodgkin lymphoma.
- Type III cryoglobulinemia is defined as the presence of only polyclonal immunoglobulins (usually IgM and IgG) in the cryoprecipitate and is associated with rheumatoid arthritis, autoimmune diseases, and chronic infections.[28,33]

40. A. Low serum ceruloplasmin and low urinary copper concentrations.
Rationale: Urinary copper concentrations are elevated in Wilson disease.
B. Low serum ceruloplasmin and elevated urinary copper concentrations.
Rationale: Low serum ceruloplasmin and elevated urinary copper concentrations are characteristic of Wilson disease.
C. Elevated serum ceruloplasmin and low urinary copper concentrations.
D. Elevated serum ceruloplasmin and elevated urinary copper concentrations.
E. Normal serum ceruloplasmin and low urinary copper concentrations.
Rationale: Serum ceruloplasmin concentrations are low and urinary copper concentrations are elevated in Wilson disease.

Major points of discussion
- Wilson disease is an autosomal recessive disorder with an incidence of approximately 1:40,000. It is caused by mutations in the *ATP7B* gene, a copper-transporting ATPase.
- *ATP7B* is expressed in hepatocytes and is needed for biliary copper excretion and for copper incorporation into ceruloplasmin. Absence or malfunction of *ATP7B* results in copper overload and incorporation of copper into the brain, liver, and cornea.
- Ceruloplasmin is a copper-containing enzyme that transports about 95% of the copper from the gastrointestinal tract to peripheral tissues for synthesis of copper containing enzymes.
- In Wilson disease, serum ceruloplasmin levels are low; urinary copper levels are elevated; and Kayser-Fleischer rings may be seen in the cornea. An elevated hepatic copper level is the gold standard for diagnosis. In some patients with Wilson disease, normal serum

ceruloplasmin levels can be obtained because ceruloplasmin is an acute-phase protein and is increased in the setting of inflammation.
- Wilson disease may present as unexplained hepatitis, as cirrhosis, with acute hemolytic anemia, or as a neuropsychiatric disorder.[1]

41. A. CA-125.
Rationale: CA-125 is useful for monitoring ovarian cancer, not breast cancer.
B. *BRCA1/2*.
C. *BRCA1* only.
Rationale: Genotyping for *BRCA1* and *BRCA2* is useful to assess predisposition to breast and ovarian cancers.
D. CA-15.3.
Rationale: CA-15.3 is the best tumor marker for monitoring breast cancer patients.
E. EGFR genotyping.
Rationale: EGFR genotyping is useful to predict response to therapy in patients with NSCLC.

Major points of discussion
- CA-15.3 is approved by the FDA for monitoring patients with breast cancer. It is also useful in the detection of recurrence.
- CA-15.3 levels also correlate with tumor burden. Thus, they are generally higher with advanced-stage disease and as the tumor proliferates.
- The family of CA markers correspond to cancer antigens. Most are glycosylated proteins that were the target of monoclonal antibodies produced when mice were challenged after injection of tumor cells.
- The CA-15.3 and CA-27.29 assays measure different epitopes on the same protein.
- The CA-15.3 assay is available through different diagnostic companies. The assays report slightly different values. When following any one particular patient, it is important that the same assay be used for monitoring purposes. Results from different CA-15.3 assays should not be compared directly.

42. A. CA-125.
Rationale: CA-125 is the best tumor marker for monitoring ovarian cancer.
B. HE4.
Rationale: HE4 is a new biomarker for monitoring ovarian cancer but is not yet the standard of care for this disease.
C. *BRCA1/2*.
Rationale: Genotyping for *BRCA1* and *BRCA2* is useful to assess predisposition of breast and ovarian cancers.
D. CA-15.3.
Rationale: CA-15.3 is the best tumor marker for monitoring breast cancer patients but is not useful for evaluating patients with ovarian cancer.
E. EGFR genotyping.
Rationale: EGFR genotyping is useful to assess patients with NSCLC.

Major points of discussion
- CA-125 is approved by the FDA for monitoring ovarian cancer.
- Approximately 80% of ovarian cancers are of the serous epithelial type. The remaining 20% are a mixture of the

mucinous, clear cell, endometrioid, and undifferentiated subtypes.

- HE4 is a newly characterized biomarker that is useful in monitoring for recurrence and disease progression of serous epithelial ovarian cancer. When using this marker, a change is considered significant if this value increases or decreases by 25% or greater.
- Mesothelin (i.e., soluble mesothelin-related peptides) is also used as a tumor marker for serous types of epithelial ovarian cancer.
- ROMA (risk of ovarian malignancy algorithm) is a recently approved test to determine whether a biopsy sample is likely to show a malignancy. It is an index combining circulating HE4 and CA-125 levels, in conjunction with menopause status.

43. A. PSA combined with DRE.
Rationale: PSA combined with DRE is approved for screening purposes but may not necessarily be useful for monitoring.
B. PSA density combined with PC3.
Rationale: PSA density is obtained through imaging analysis and serum PSA measurement. PC3 is a new molecular-based prostate cancer biomarker measured in urine.
C. PSA combined with PC3.
Rationale: PC3, a new molecular-based prostate cancer biomarker measured in urine, has not yet been demonstrated to be useful in this setting.
D. PSA combined with circulating tumor cells (CTCs).
Rationale: Both markers are approved by the FDA for monitoring purposes.
E. No two modalities together; PSA alone is best.
Rationale: Although PSA alone is satisfactory, combining this test with CTCs is the best approach.

Major points of discussion
- PSA levels combined with a DRE is an FDA-approved modality for prostate cancer screening. It is one of the only examples where a tumor marker is recommended for screening purposes.
- PSA density is calculated after performing a transrectal ultrasound, calculating the prostate volume (length × width × height × 0.52), then dividing the serum PSA (in ng/mL) by this value. A value of 0.15 or greater is used to determine whether further workup (including biopsy) is required.
- PSA velocity refers to the rate of change of PSA. It evaluates the increase in PSA values over a defined period of time. A high PSA velocity may signify a more aggressive, rapidly growing tumor.
- The CTC assay involves counting the number of CTCs in whole blood, after a capture, detection, and imaging procedure.
- The CTC assay is FDA approved for monitoring patients with metastatic prostate cancer, as well as for monitoring patients with metastatic breast or colorectal cancer.

44. A. Urine protein electrophoresis is not required to assess patients with hypogammaglobulinemia.
Rationale: Hypogammaglobulinemia can be seen in patients who have a monoclonal light chain clone that suppresses the production of normal polyclonal immunoglobulins. The abnormal monoclonal light chain is usually not seen in plasma but can be detected in urine.

B. Urine protein electrophoresis should not be performed using an aliquot from a random urine collection.
Rationale: Urine protein electrophoresis can use either a random or a 24-hour collection to identify the presence of a monoclonal protein. However, a 24-hour urine collection is necessary to determine the total amount of protein secreted. Therefore, in the latter case, it is necessary to know the total amount of urine produced during a 24-hour period.
C. Bence-Jones proteinuria is a diagnostic marker for multiple myeloma.
Rationale: The detection of monoclonal light chains in the urine (i.e., Bence-Jones proteinuria) has been used as a diagnostic marker for multiple myeloma since the report by Dr. Henry Bence-Jones in 1847.
D. The monoclonal light chains are found in concentrated urine in very small amounts and cannot be quantified as an M-spike by protein electrophoresis.
Rationale: Serum free light chain determination is based on antibody binding to epitopes that are normally hidden by association with heavy chains. Light chains are normally synthesized in slight excess compared with heavy chains but are rapidly cleared from the circulation so that they do not accumulate in serum/plasma.
E. Determination of serum free light chains is sufficient to diagnose Bence-Jones proteinuria.
Rationale: Bence-Jones proteinuria is defined as the presence of monoclonal light chains in the urine.

Major points of discussion
- Current laboratory procedures use protein electrophoresis and IFE to identify and characterize urine monoclonal light chains. In addition, the monoclonal light chains may be present in sufficient amounts to allow quantification of an M-spike by protein electrophoresis. Measuring the electrophoretic M-spike is the recommended method of monitoring patients with various monoclonal gammopathies, such as multiple myeloma. Monitoring the urine M-spike is especially useful in patients with light chain multiple myeloma in whom the serum M-spike may be absent or present at very low concentrations, whereas the urine M-spike is present at easily detectable concentrations.
- Urine protein electrophoresis interpretation is challenging because it is often necessary to detect monoclonal immunoglobulins in the presence of significant proteinuria. Proteinuria is defined as more than 150 mg of urine protein in 24 hours; this is equivalent to a more than 0.15 protein/creatinine ratio in a random "spot" urine sample.
- To determine the amount of monoclonal protein produced, it is necessary to analyze an aliquot obtained from a 24-hour urine collection.
- Urine must be concentrated to identify its relevant protein fractions. The concentration of clinically relevant monoclonal light chains can be low in unfractionated urine. Therefore, urine must be concentrated up to 100-fold to visualize all protein fractions. The optimal concentration of protein in urine for appropriate visualization by electrophoresis is 25 to 50 mg protein/mL. Urine can be concentrated using solvent absorption devices, lyophilization, or protein spin columns.
- Monoclonal light chains can occasionally be seen in serum, even though their serum half-life is only 2 to 6 hours.

- Possible scenarios are as follows:
  - Production of large quantities of monoclonal protein by a light chain myeloma.
  - Monoclonal light chains can occasionally exist as homotetramers, which are then too large to be filtered through the glomerular basement membrane.
  - A reduced number of nephrons due to underlying renal disease, which reduces the clearance of monoclonal light chains.
  - Monoclonal light chains may bind to other serum proteins, which are then too large to be filtered through the glomerular basement membrane, and produce multiple bands by serum protein electrophoresis and IFE.

45. A. Hypergammaglobulinemia in lane 1; increased albumin in lanes 2 and 3.
B. No abnormalities in lane 1; IgG kappa in lane 2; IgA lambda in lane 3.
C. Bisalbuminemia in lane 1; abnormal band in the gamma region in lanes 2 and 3.
Rationale for B and C: A "split" albumin band is seen in lane 1. Although lanes 2 and 3 each show a monoclonal spike in the gamma region, it is not possible to determine the constituent heavy and light chains by standard serum protein electrophoresis; IFE is required for this purpose.
D. Hypogammaglobulinemia in lane 1; hypergammaglobulinemia in lanes 2 and 3.
Rationale for A and D: Gamma globulins migrate in the gamma region of the gel, which is most cathodal; the concentration of these proteins is not elevated in lane 1. Lanes 2 and 3 each show a monoclonal spike in the gamma region. A split albumin band is seen in lane 1.
E. No abnormalities in lane 1; IgA lambda in lane 2; IgG kappa in lane 3.
Rationale: A split albumin band is seen in lane 1. Although lanes 2 and 3 each show a monoclonal spike in the gamma region, it is not possible to determine the constituent heavy and light chains by standard serum protein electrophoresis; IFE is required for this purpose.

Major points of discussion
- A split albumin band (i.e., bisalbuminemia) is seen in lane 1. Bisalbuminemia is not a disease but a normal variation. It may affect binding of drugs. The incidence can be 1:1000 to 1:10,000 in Caucasians and Japanese. The incidence is very high (i.e., 1:100) in some Native American tribes.
- Homogeneous proteins are seen in the gamma region of both lanes 2 and 3. This finding strongly suggests the presence of a monoclonal protein. Immunofixation electrophoresis is required for identification of the abnormal proteins. It is not possible to know the type of immunoglobulin that constitutes the abnormal clone using only serum protein electrophoresis.
- A monoclonal band of immunoglobulins indicates that a clonal population of B cells or plasma cells exists, which has escaped normal regulation and might result in a plasma cell dyscrasia, such as multiple myeloma. In contrast, a polyclonal distribution of immunoglobulins generally indicates a reactive process of an otherwise normal immune system.

- Five different classes of antibody are known: immunoglobulin (Ig)M, IgG, IgA, IgD, and IgE, each with a distinct heavy chain. Two different light chain types have been identified: kappa and lambda. IgG is prevalent in blood and tissue fluids; IgM is found mainly in the blood; secretory IgA is found primarily on epithelial surfaces; IgD is mostly bound to the surface of B cells; and IgE is largely bound to the surface of basophils and mast cells.
- Monoclonal increases in immunoglobulins suggest the presence of a plasma cell dyscrasia. Polyclonal increases in immunoglobulins occur as part of the immune response and may be found in chronic disease.

46. A. A 22-year-old woman after a normal vaginal delivery.
Rationale: Cryoglobulinemia is not associated with normal childbirth.
B. A 45-year-old patient with diabetes mellitus.
Rationale: Cryoglobulinemia is not associated with diabetes.
C. A 45-year-old patient with hepatitis A.
Rationale: Cryoglobulinemia is not typically associated with hepatitis A.
D. A 45-year-old patient with hepatitis C.
Rationale: Hepatitis C is commonly associated with type II cryoglobulinemia and is seen in approximately 35% of such cases.
E. A 5-year-old child with paroxysmal cold hemoglobinuria.
Rationale: Cryoglobulinemia is not associated with paroxysmal cold hemoglobinuria. In this setting, the pathologic antibody binds to red blood cells at cold temperatures but does not precipitate in the cold.

Major points of discussion
- Accurate laboratory test results for patients with cryoglobulins are especially sensitive to improper preanalytic handling. Therefore, clinicians must be aware of specimen temperature requirements when ordering these studies to avoid false-negative results. Serum must not cool below 37°C after collection before reaching the laboratory testing site, because the precipitating cryoglobulins (if present) would be lost when the sample tube is centrifuged to obtain the serum for testing. The warm serum must be centrifuged while the sample tube is still warm, and the resulting serum is then incubated for up to 7 days at 4°C in graduated, calibrated Wintrobe tubes. After centrifugation, the volume of the cryoprecipitate is read; this is referred to as the "cryocrit."
- To determine the type of cryoglobulinemia (i.e., types I, II, III), the cryoprecipitate is washed to remove any contaminating liquid serum remaining. The goal is to wash off all proteins that are not part of the precipitate. Washing up to 5 times with NaCl 0.9% is necessary to achieve a satisfactory result. The resulting pellet is then resolubilized and processed for IFE.
- Type I cryoglobulins typically form a relatively large volume of cryoprecipitate (e.g., a cryocrit of up to 10%, or even 20%). Upon IFE, type I cryoglobulins exhibit a single heavy chain and a single light chain type. Type I cryoglobulinemia is associated with monoclonal gammopathy of undetermined significance, macroglobulinemia, or multiple myeloma.
- Type II cryoglobulins typically show only a small amount of cryoprecipitate (i.e., less than 1% of the serum volume). Quantifying the cryocrit is not analytically

valid for serial measurements to monitor this type of patient's progress. IFE most often shows a monoclonal IgM band plus polyclonal IgG. Type II cryoglobulinemia is associated with autoimmune disorders, such as vasculitis, glomerulonephritis, systemic lupus erythematosus, rheumatoid arthritis, and Sjögren syndrome. It may be seen in infections such as hepatitis, infectious mononucleosis, cytomegalovirus, and toxoplasmosis. Type II cryoglobulinemia may also be "essential"; this is, it may occur in the absence of an underlying disease.

- In type III cryoglobulinemia, IFE demonstrates both polyclonal IgM and polyclonal IgG. Type III cryoglobulinemia usually presents with only trace levels of cryoprecipitate, which may take up to 7 days to appear, and is associated with the same disease spectrum as type II cryoglobulinemia.
- Potential causes for cryoglobulinemia:
  - Infection
  - Hepatitis C
  - Autoimmune disease
    ○ Lupus
    ○ Polyarteritis nodosa
    ○ Rheumatoid arthritis
  - Other
    ○ Thyroid disease
    ○ Kidney disease
  - Hematological malignancies
    ○ Multiple myeloma
    ○ Leukemia
  - Unknown cause in approximately 10% of cases

47. A. Transport at room temperature and incubate at room temperature.
    B. Transport at 37°C and incubate at 4°C.
    C. Transport at room temperature and incubate at 4°C.
    D. Transport at 4°C and incubate at 37°C.
    E. Transport at 4°C and incubate at 4°C.
    Rationale: To obtain accurate results regarding the presence or absence of a cryoprecipitate, the patient's blood sample must be maintained at 37°C before reaching the performing laboratory. Once in the laboratory, the sample is centrifuged at 37°C, and then the resulting serum is incubated at 4°C.

Major points of discussion

- Cryoglobulins are immunoglobulins that precipitate when cooled and redissolve when warmed. Because these proteins precipitate when cooled, patients may experience symptoms when exposed to cold ambient temperatures.
- Common causes of cryoglobulinemia are given in the Major Points of Discussion for Question 46.
- Warm (37° to 40°C) serum samples are required for proper determination of cryoglobulinemia. If a patient's blood sample is not maintained at this temperature before reaching the performing laboratory, the cryoglobulins may precipitate and settle on top of the red blood cell layer. Therefore, when the tube is centrifuged to separate the serum, the cryoglobulins form a sediment with the coagulated/cellular fraction. Rewarming the initial whole blood tube does not correct this preanalytical error because cryoglobulins that were trapped in the coagulated layer cannot be mobilized.

- To achieve appropriate results, the blood sample obtained from the patient can be kept warm by wrapping the tube in a "heel warmer," or the tube can be transported in a warm water bath. Failure to follow the relevant specimen-handling instructions may cause false-negative results.
- The presence of albumin in a cryoprecipitate IFE gel indicates insufficient washing of the precipitate. Albumin is the major protein constituent in serum. If serum contamination is present, it is not clear whether visualized polyclonal immunoglobulins that define type II (mixed-type) and type III (polyclonal) cryoglobulinemia originate from the contaminating serum component or from the cryoprecipitate itself.
- Testing for cryoglobulinemia is not useful for general population screening without a clinical suspicion of cryoglobulinemia.

48. A. Albumin fraction.
    Rationale: Albumin is the most abundant, and most anodal, fraction on the gel.
    B. Beta fraction.
    C. Gamma fraction.
    Rationale: This fraction is most cathodal. Most immunoglobulins migrate in the gamma fraction. There are almost no other proteins that migrate in this fraction.
    D. Alpha-1 fraction.
    E. Alpha-2 fraction.
    Rationale for B, D, and E: Most immunoglobulins migrate in the gamma fraction.

Major points of discussion

- Albumin is the most abundant protein. It runs in the anodal region of the cellulose acetate gel. It may be depressed owing to decreased synthesis (e.g., malnutrition, malabsorption, liver failure, diversion to synthesis of other proteins) or increased loss (e.g., proteinuria, accumulation of ascites fluid, enteropathy). Immunoglobulins are primarily found in the cathodal region of the gel. Polyclonal immunoglobulins may be elevated owing to increased synthesis of many different proteins as part of acute or chronic reactions to disease.
- Apo A1 (mainly found on high density lipoproteins), alpha-1 fetoprotein, and alpha-1 antitrypsin migrate in the alpha-1 fraction of a standard SPEP gel.
- Alpha-2 macroglobulin, haptoglobin, and ceruloplasmin migrate in the alpha-2 region of a standard SPEP gel.
- Fibrinogen and complement factors C3 and C4 migrate in the beta-2 region of a standard SPEP gel. The presence of fibrinogen in a sample can result in the false-positive detection of a band in the beta-2 region.
- Haptoglobulin migrates in the alpha-2 region of a standard SPEP gel. In sera from patients with hemolytic anemia or other forms of hemolysis, some haptoglobin-hemoglobin complexes may be seen.

49. A. Lane 7 demonstrates the presence of **hypogammaglobulinemia.**
    Rationale: This finding can be seen in a patient with a monoclonal light chain disorder. A monoclonal light chain disorder can result from the replacement of normal plasma cells, which produce polyclonal immunoglobulins, by a

malignant clone(s). Monoclonal free light chains are cleared rapidly and SPEP is typically not sensitive enough to detect these. Therefore, urine should be evaluated for the presence of monoclonal free light chains (i.e., Bence-Jones proteins).

B. Lane 14 demonstrates the presence of increased amounts of polyclonal immunoglobulins.

Rationale: This lane shows the presence of a sharp band consistent with a monoclonal spike, not the presence of increased amounts of polyclonal immunoglobulins. Polyclonal increases in immunoglobulins have been associated with (Job syndrome), Wiskott-Aldrich syndrome, and AIDS.

C. Lane 12 demonstrates a band in the gamma region that represents fibrinogen.

Rationale: Although there should be no fibrinogen remaining in serum, remnants of fibrinogen due to incomplete clotting can result in the false-positive interpretation of a monoclonal band. The band in this lane represents a low concentration of a monoclonal spike.

D. Lane 18 demonstrates the presence of polyclonal hypergammaglobulinemia.

Rationale: The protein concentration in the gamma globulin region is actually decreased. Nonetheless, polyclonal increases in immunoglobulins have been associated with many diseases. These include immunodeficiency diseases such as hyperimmunoglobulin E (Job syndrome), Wiskott-Aldrich syndrome, and AIDS.

E. Lane 20 demonstrates hypoalbuminemia.

Rationale: Albumin is the fastest band migrating toward the anode (at the bottom of the figure); the albumin level appears to be normal in this case.

Major points of discussion

■ Polyclonal increases in immunoglobulins have been associated with many diseases. These include immunodeficiency diseases, such as hyperimmunoglobulin E (Job syndrome), Wiskott-Aldrich syndrome, and AIDS.

■ Hypergammaglobulinemia can also be seen in infections, liver diseases (acute and chronic hepatitis, biliary cirrhosis, lupoid hepatitis), pulmonary disorders (sarcoidosis, berylliosis, pulmonary hypersensitivity syndrome), Down syndrome, amyloidosis, narcotic addiction, and renal tubular disease.

■ Monoclonal immunoglobulins or fragments of immunoglobulins have been associated with multiple disease conditions. These include:
  ● Multiple myeloma
  ● Waldenström macroglobulinemia
  ● Chronic lymphocytic leukemia
  ● Other leukemias
  ● Lymphomas
  ● "Benign" monoclonal gammopathy
  ● Systemic capillary leak syndrome
  ● Amyloidosis
  ● Chronic liver disease, such as chronic active hepatitis and primary biliary cirrhosis
  ● Autoimmune disorders, including rheumatoid arthritis, systemic lupus erythematosus, thyroiditis, pernicious anemia, polyarteritis nodosa, Sjögren syndrome
  ● Gaucher disease
  ● Malignancies of various types

  ● Hereditary spherocytosis
  ● HIV infection, including AIDS

■ The term *monoclonal gammopathy of undetermined significance* (MGUS) categorizes individuals in whom a monoclonal component is demonstrated in the serum but who lack other key features for diagnosing a malignant condition. As many as 3% of individuals over the age of 70 have MGUS. Subjects with MGUS may have as many as 10% plasma cells in their bone marrow. The risk of progression to multiple myeloma in patients with MGUS is approximately 1% per year, even after 25 years of a stable condition. It is recommended that such patients be followed up with SPEP every 6 to 12 months to determine whether the process is progressing or regressing.

■ False-positive interpretations of monoclonal bands can occur owing to the presence of fibrinogen from an incompletely clotted specimen or when hemolysis occurs as the result of improper specimen collection. Confirmation that a faint band is a monoclonal paraprotein is typically done by using IFE.

50. A. At very low concentrations, they can significantly increase the viscosity of blood, leading to problems with organ perfusion.

Rationale: The hyperviscosity syndrome can be seen in the setting of multiple myeloma or Waldenström macroglobulinemia.

B. The circulating concentration can be so high that the precipitating complexes by IFE will not stain properly.

Rationale: The circulating concentration can be so high that there is not enough reagent antibody to form precipitating complexes on IFE. This is analogous to the "hook effect" in clinical chemistry or the "pro-zone effect" in immunohematology.

C. Quantitative monitoring clearly differentiates a benign from a malignant condition in the majority of cases.

Rationale: This approach is important in differentiating multiple myeloma from MGUS. However, it is helpful, but not diagnostic.

D. They are routinely detected using mass spectrometry methods.

Rationale: Clinical laboratories do not routinely use mass spectrometry approaches to measure large molecules, such as antibodies.

E. Identification of the constituent heavy chain and light chain types can be determined by IFE.

Rationale: To identify the type of immunoglobulin, monospecific antisera are applied directly to the separated serum proteins. The gel is washed, and the protein-antibody conjugates are stained and read directly.

Major points of discussion

■ IFE is performed using replicate samples of patient serum. These are separated by electrophoresis. To identify the type of immunoglobulin, monospecific antisera are applied directly to the separated serum proteins. The gel is washed, and the protein-antibody conjugates are stained and read directly.

■ Requests to examine sera for the presence of a monoclonal protein usually are generated by a physician who recognizes that a patient has clinical symptoms and signs consistent with such a disorder. Alternatively, this is determined when laboratory examination of a SPEP gel suggests the presence of a monoclonal protein. Many times, the physician's suspicion of a plasma cell dyscrasia is triggered by findings of anemia (with one or more cytopenias), elevated total serum protein with elevated globulins, and proteinuria; other findings may include hyperuricemia, hypercalcemia, elevated alkaline phosphatase, bone pain, or lytic lesions of bone on radiography.

- If monoclonal proteins are detected by SPEP and IFE, it is then recommended to quantify the immunoglobulins.
- Quantitative immunoglobulins are useful in monitoring the course of the disease and its treatment and may be helpful in separating a benign from a malignant condition. Monoclonal IgG levels of 2 g/dL, or IgA levels of 1 g/dL or greater, suggest a malignant condition. In many malignant immunocytopathies, the concentration of nonmonoclonal immunoglobulins is reduced. Thus, a deficiency of polyclonal immunoglobulins is also suggestive of malignancy.
- Immunoglobulins at very high concentrations can significantly increase the viscosity of blood, leading to problems with organ perfusion (e.g., headache, visual disturbances, renal dysfunction).

51. A. 1. Albumin; 2. gamma fraction; 3. alpha-1; 4. alpha-2; 5. beta-1; 6. beta-2.
B. 1. Gamma fraction; 2. alpha-1; 3. alpha-2; 4. beta-1; 5. beta-2; 6. albumin.
C. 1. Albumin; 2. alpha-1; 3. alpha-2; 4. beta-1; 5. beta-2; 6. gamma fraction.
D. 1. Alpha-1; 2. alpha-2; 3. beta-1; 4. beta-2; 5. gamma fraction; 6.albumin.
E. 1. Gamma fraction; 2. alpha-1; 3. alpha-2; 4. beta-1; 5. albumin; 6. beta-2.
Rationale: The correct electrophoretic migration order from anode to cathode is: albumin, followed by alpha-1, followed by alpha-2, followed by beta-1, followed by beta-2, followed by the gamma fraction.

Major points of discussion

- Modern understanding of the protein composition of serum and plasma derives from the electrophoretic techniques introduced by Arne Wilhelm Kaurin Tiselius (1902–1971), a Swedish biochemist who won the Nobel Prize in Chemistry in 1948. He separated proteins dissolved in an electrolyte solution by application of an electric current through a U-shaped quartz tube that held the protein solution. At a pH of 7.6, four serum protein fractions, designated albumin, alpha, beta, and gamma, were identified and quantified optically by change in refractive index at the boundaries among these bands.
- Current approaches separate proteins at a pH of 8.6 on solid support media such as cellulose acetate membranes, agarose gels, starch gels, and polyacrylamide gels that can separate up to five fractions: albumin, alpha-1, alpha-2, beta, and gamma proteins. The beta fraction can also be subdivided into beta-1 and beta-2 fractions.
- Proteins are large molecules composed of covalently linked amino acids. Depending on electron distributions resulting from covalent or ionic bonding of structural subgroups, proteins have different electrical charges at a given pH. Protein separation occurs due to size and charge.
- A voltage is applied between the electrodes, generating a current that passes through the gel, usually for a period of approximately 30 minutes, to achieve the desired resolution. The ionic strength of the buffer determines the amount of current and the movement of the proteins for a fixed voltage. If ionic strength is low, relatively more current is carried by the charged proteins. If ionic strength is high, less current is carried by the proteins, which move a shorter distance. Through manipulations of buffer salt composition, endosmotic properties of the medium, and means of sample application, commercially available agarose plates now achieve consistently high-resolution quality that allows routine separation of all major serum protein species.
- Albumin is the most abundant serum protein. It is found at the anodal (the positive pole) end of the gel. Immunoglobulins are found in the gamma fraction, which is most cathodal (the negative pole).
- Proteins are negatively charged at a pH of 8.6 and migrate toward the anode. Exceptions include gamma globulins and some beta globulins, which migrate toward the cathode. The movement of cationic buffer ions toward the cathode pulls weaker charged proteins along; this process is called endosmosis.

52. A. RF is an antigen that is used as a biomarker for the detection of rheumatoid arthritis.
B. RF consists of antigens that are bound to the Fc portion of IgG.
Rationale: RFs are autoantibodies that bind to the Fc portion of IgG.
C. RF can cause a false-positive result with some immunochemical assays that measure hormones and drugs.
Rationale: See Major points of discussion.
D. The diagnostic specificity of RF for the detection of rheumatoid arthritis is greater than anti-cyclic citrullinated peptide (anti-CCP).
Rationale: Anti-CCP is a more specific biomarker than RF for the detection of rheumatoid arthritis.
E. Elevated serum RF levels are seen in most patients with rheumatoid arthritis.
Rationale: RF levels can be in the reference range in the early stages of rheumatoid arthritis.

Major points of discussion

- RF is not a specific biomarker for rheumatoid arthritis. It can be detected in other autoimmune diseases, such as systemic lupus erythematosus, mixed connective tissue disease, and Sjögren syndrome. It can also occur in viral infections, such as chronic active hepatitis, inflammatory bowel disease, and sarcoidosis. RF can also be present in the serum of healthy elderly individuals.
- RF is an autoantibody directed against the Fc region of IgG. Although IgM is the most common isotype of RFs, RF reactivity can also be detected in the IgA, IgG, and IgD subclasses.
- The diagnostic specificity of anti-CCP is better than RF for the detection of rheumatoid arthritis. The combination of RF and anti-CCP has been proposed for detecting rheumatoid arthritis.

- The most common methods for measuring RF are automated nephelometric or turbidimetric procedures. In these assays, polystyrene beads are coated with an immune complex consisting of human gamma globulin and sheep anti-human IgG. Agglutination occurs when a specimen containing RF is added to these beads. The amount of turbidity that is formed is determined by the intensity of the light scattered in nephelometric assays or by the amount of light absorbed in turbidimetric assays.
- High levels of circulating RF can cause positive interferences with some free T_4, thyroid-stimulating hormone (TSH), troponin I, and tacrolimus immunochemical assays. Thus, RF can bind to both the capture and labeled antibodies and produces a signal independent of the analyte that is being measured. This interference can be eliminated by adding animal immunoglobulins to the reagents, thereby preventing RF binding to the capture antibody. This is the same type of interference that can be caused by human anti-animal antibodies (i.e., HAAAs).[21,31]

53. A. Myositis.
Rationale: Patients with myositis rarely exhibit a centromeric staining pattern.
B. Systemic sclerosis/CREST syndrome (calcinosis, Raynaud phenomenon, esophageal dysmotility, sclerodactyly, and telangiectasia).
Rationale: Anti-centromeric antibodies are common (44% to 98%) in patients with scleroderma, specifically CREST.
C. Systemic lupus erythematosus (SLE).
Rationale: SLE patients exhibit positivity to double-stranded DNA (dsDNA), which reveals a homogeneous staining pattern.
D. Drug-induced (procainamide and/or hydralazine) lupus-like syndrome.
Rationale: This condition usually results in a homogeneous pattern.
E. Chronic active hepatitis.
Rationale: Patients with hepatitis rarely exhibit a centromeric staining pattern.

Major points of discussion
- Antinuclear antibody (ANA) testing provides a screening test for connective tissue diseases, including SLE, drug-induced lupus-like syndrome, mixed connective tissue disease, Sjögren syndrome, scleroderma, CREST syndrome, polymyositis-dermatomyositis, and rheumatoid arthritis. The figure shows a centromeric staining pattern.
- The standard method for ANA testing in the United States uses IFE analysis of HEp-2 cells. Mouse liver cells can also be used, but they are less sensitive than Hep-2 cells. Nondiseased individuals may exhibit ANA titers as high as 1:80 when HEp-2 cells are used.
- ELISA-based methods can be used for screening purposes. However, the disadvantage of using such an approach is that this methodology cannot provide information on IF patterns, which have been the gold standard for decades.
- There are three antibodies commonly associated with systemic scleroderma: (1) anti-topoisomerase I, (2) anti-RNA polymerase, and (3) anti-centromere. Thus, a speckled or nucleolar pattern may be observed.

- Anti-centromeric antibodies are common (44% to 98%) in patients with CREST syndrome (a subset of scleroderma patients). CREST patients suffer from skin changes that are not systemic but are limited to the hands and face.

54. A. Sjögren syndrome.
Rationale: Sjögren syndrome patients usually exhibit a nucleolar staining pattern.
B. Systemic sclerosis/CREST syndrome (calcinosis, Raynaud phenomenon, esophageal dysmotility, sclerodactyly, and telangiectasia).
Rationale: Patients with CREST usually exhibit a centromeric staining pattern.
C. SLE.
Rationale: Patients with SLE can exhibit a homogeneous (or peripheral) staining pattern.
D. Asthma.
Rationale: Asthma is not necessarily characterized by homogeneous staining patterns.
E. Chronic active hepatitis.
Rationale: Chronic active hepatitis is not necessarily characterized by homogeneous staining patterns.

Major points of discussion
- Absence of ANAs essentially rules out SLE, where more than 96% of patients are positive for ANAs when HEp-2 cells are used. The figure shows a homogeneous ANA staining pattern.
- Results from anti-dsDNA antibody testing are elevated in a majority of patients with SLE (approximately 70% in one study and up to 90% at some point during the course of disease). dsDNA positivity usually produces a homogeneous or peripheral staining pattern in ANA testing.
- The homogeneous (diffuse) pattern corresponds to specific nuclear antigens associated with chromatin, histones, and also DNA.
- SLE patients usually exhibit a peripheral pattern, although homogeneous and sometimes speckled patterns have also been observed.
- A homogeneous pattern is also observed in more than 90% of patients with drug-induced lupus-like syndrome (precipitated by procainamide or hydralazine). An important caveat to this testing is that multiple drugs can result in a false-positive ANA result.

55. A. Myositis.
Rationale: Patients with myositis do not commonly exhibit a nucleolar pattern.
B. Systemic sclerosis/CREST syndrome (calcinosis, Raynaud phenomenon, esophageal dysmotility, sclerodactyly, and telangiectasia).
Rationale: These patients usually exhibit a centromeric staining pattern.
C. SLE.
Rationale: Patients with SLE will usually exhibit a peripheral or homogeneous staining pattern.
D. Drug-induced (procainamide and/or hydralazine) lupus-like syndrome.
Rationale: This will usually exhibit a homogeneous staining pattern.
E. Sjögren syndrome.

Rationale: A majority of patients with Sjögren syndrome usually exhibit a nucleolar pattern.

Major points of discussion

- One algorithm for ANA testing uses IFE slides in both the screening and titration steps. Those samples that screen positive are subject to titration to end point, with both the titer and pattern being reported. Titers alone can be used to monitor therapy for patients. Alternatively, ELISA-based testing for the specific autoantigens of interest can also be performed, and quantitative values can be used to monitor patients. A nucleolar ANA staining pattern is shown in the figure.
- There are four basic staining patterns: (1) homogeneous (diffuse), (2) peripheral, (3) speckled, and (4) nucleolar. Each is characteristic of a different set of autoantigens that can produce ANAs.
- It is important to note that the presence of any one pattern does *not* correlate 100% with any one connective tissue disease. However, reasonable generalizations can be made to classify groups of antigens based on the observed patterns.
- The nucleolar pattern corresponds to proteins of the nucleolus including RNA polymerase.
- Patients with Sjögren syndrome or scleroderma usually exhibit a nucleolar pattern with ANA testing.

56. A. Sjögren syndrome.
Rationale: Patients with Sjögren syndrome commonly exhibit a nucleolar pattern.
B. Systemic sclerosis/CREST syndrome (calcinosis, Raynaud phenomenon, esophageal dysmotility, sclerodactyly, and telangiectasia).
Rationale: This usually exhibits a centromeric staining pattern.
C. SLE.
Rationale: This usually exhibits a peripheral or homogeneous staining pattern.

D. Drug-induced (procainamide and/or hydralazine) lupus-like syndrome.
Rationale: This usually exhibits a homogeneous staining pattern.
E. Many antigens and connective tissue diseases.
Rationale: Of all the IF patterns observed in ANA testing, the speckled pattern is the most nonspecific and is observed in multiple conditions.

Major points of discussion

- In recent years, a "reverse algorithm" has been developed for laboratory analysis of ANA testing. This procedure uses an immunoassay-based technique for anti-dsDNA as the first line screen. Samples that are positive are then subject to an IF staining procedure, where titer and pattern are reported.
- The advantages of a reverse algorithm approach for ANA testing include that it (1) reduces labor (technologist time) required for screening *all* samples by IF and (2) provides for a quantitative and objective (vs. subjective) means to identify the positive samples that require further workup.
- A speckled ANA pattern is shown in the figure. Although there are four basic staining patterns (homogeneous, peripheral, speckled, and nucleolar) revealed through IF analysis of ANA, it is important to note that the presence of any one pattern does not correspond 100% to any one disease group; only generalizations can be made to correlate distinct antigens with specific diseases.
- The speckled pattern observed in ANA testing corresponds to non-DNA nuclear constituents, such as RNPs (ribonuclear proteins) or the Sm, SS-A, and SS-B antigens.
- Of all the patterns, the speckled pattern is least specific. It has been observed with multiple connective tissue diseases.

References

1. Ala A, Walker A, Ashkan K, et al. Wilson's disease. Lancet 2007;369:397–408.
2. Apple FS. A new season for cardiac troponin assay: it's time to keep a scorecard. Clin Chem 2009;55:1303–1306.
3. Apple FS. Tissue specificity of cardiac troponin I, cardiac troponin T, and creatine kinase MB. Clin Chim Acta 1999;282:151–159.
4. Aslan D, Apple FS. Ischemia modified albumin measured by the albumin cobalt binding test: a clinical and analytical review. Lab Med 2004;35:44–47.
5. Bodor GS, Porterfield D, Voss EM, et al. Cardiac troponin I is not expressed in fetal and adult human skeletal muscle tissue. Clin Chem 1992;41:1710–1714.
6. Bodor GS, Survant L, Voss EM, et al. Cardiac troponin T composition in normal and regenerating human skeletal muscle. Clin Chem 1997;43:476–484.
7. Bologa RM, Levine DM, Parker TS, et al. Interleukin-6 predicts hypoalbuminemia, hypocholesterolemia, and mortality in hemodialysis patients. Am J Kidney Dis 1998;32:107–114.
8. Bruns DE, Emerson JC, Intemann S, et al. Lactate dehydrogenase isoenzyme 1: changes in the first day after acute myocardial infarction. Clin Chem 1981;27:1821–1823.
9. Centers for Disease Control, Prevention. Grand Rounds: Additional opportunities to prevent neural tube defects with folic acid fortification. MMWR Morbid Mortal Wkly Rep 2010;59:980–984.
10. Chan KM, Ladenson JH, Pierce G, Jaffe AS. Increased creatine kinase MB in the absence of acute myocardial infarction. Clin Chem 1986;32:2044–2051.
11. Dugoff L, Hobbins JC, Malone FD, et al. Quad screen as a predicator of adverse pregnancy outcome. Obstet Gynecol 2005;106:260–267.
12. Eggers KM, Oldgren J, Nordenskjold A, et al. Diagnostic value of cardiac markers in patients with chest pain: limited value of adding myoglobin to troponin I for exclusion of myocardial infarction. Am Heart J 2004;148:574–581.
13. Ehl S, Gering B, Bartmann P, et al. C-reactive protein is a useful marker for guiding duration of antibiotic therapy in suspected neonatal bacterial infection. Pediatrics 1997;99:216–221.
14. Gabay C, Kushner I. Acute-phase proteins and other systemic responses to inflammation. N Engl J Med 1999;340:448–454.
15. Jeppsson J-O, Laurell C-B, Franzen B. Agarose gel electrophoresis. Clin Chem 1979;25:629–638.
16. Katrukha AG, Bereznikova AV, Eskova TV, et al. Troponin I is released in bloodstream of patients with acute myocardial infarction not in free form but as a complex. Clin Chem 1997;43:1379–1385.

17. Katus HA, Scheffold T, Remppis A, et al. Proteins of the troponin complex. Lab Med 1992;23:311–317.

18. Lee TH, Weisberg MC, Cook EF, et al. Evaluation of creatine kinase and creatine kinase MB for diagnosing myocardial infarction. Arch Intern Med 1987;147:115–121.

19. Maisel AS, Krishnaswamt P, Nowak RM, et al. Rapid measurement of B-type natriuretic peptide in the emergency diagnosis of heart failure. N Engl J Med 2002;347:161–167.

20. Malone FD, Canick JA, Ball RH, et al. First-trimester or second-trimester screening, or both, for Down's syndrome. N Engl J Med 2005;353:2001–2011.

21. Martin BB, Marquet P, Ferrer JM, et al. Rheumatoid factor interference in a tacrolimus immunoassay. Ther Drug Monit 2009;31(6): 743–745.

22. Muller F. Prenatal biochemical screening for neural tube defects. Childs Nerv Syst 2003;19:433–435.

23. Palomaki GE, Haddow JE, Knight GJ, et al. Risk-based prenatal screening for trisomy 18 using alpha-fetoprotein, unconjugated oestriol and human chorionic gonadotropin. Prenat Diagn 1995; 15(8):713–723.

24. Puelo PR, Meyer D, Wathen C, et al. Use of a rapid assay of subforms of creatine kinase–MB to diagnose or rule out acute myocardial infarction. N Engl J Med 1994;331:561–566.

25. Rehman SU, Martinez-Rumayor A, Mueller T, Januzzi JL Jr. Independent and incremental prognostic value of multimarker testing in acute dyspnea: results from the ProBNP Investigation of Dyspnea in the Emergency Department (PRIDE) Study. Clin Chim Acta 2008;392:41–45.

26. Ridker PM, Danielson E, Fonesca FAH, et al. Rosuvastatin to prevent vascular events in men and women with elevated C-reactive protein. N Engl J Med 2008;359:2195–2207.

27. Rotenberg Z, Seif R, Wolfe LA, et al. Flipped patterns of lactate dehydrogenase isoenzymes in serum of elite basketball players. Clin Chem 1988;34:2351–2354.

28. Shihabi ZK. Review: cryoglobulins: an important but neglected clinical test. Ann Clin Lab Sci 2006;36:395–408.

29. Strobel SL. The incidence and significance of pseudoparaproteins in a community hospital. Ann Clin Lab Sci 2000;30:289–294.

30. Tate J, Caldwell G, Daly J, et al. Recommendations for standardized reporting of protein electrophoresis in Australia and New Zealand. Ann Clin Biochem 2012;49:242–256.

31. Taylor P, Gartemann J, Hsieh J, et al. A systematic review of serum biomarkers anti-cyclic citrullinated peptide and rheumatoid factor as tests for rheumatoid arthritis. *Autoimmune Dis* 2012:734069, 2012.

32. Thygesen K, Alpert JS, White HD. Universal definition of myocardial infarction. Eur Heart J 2007;28:2525–2538.

33. Vermeersch P, Gijbels K, Marien G, et al. A critical appraisal of current practice in the detection, analysis, and reporting of cryoglobulins. Clin Chem 2008;54:39–43.

34. Wald NJ, Cuckle HS, Densem JW, et al. Maternal serum screening for Down syndrome: the effect of routine ultrasound scan determination of gestational age and adjustment for maternal weight. Br J Obstet Gynaecol 1992;99:144–149.

CHAPTER 9

CLINICAL CHEMISTRY: Electrolytes, Blood Gases, Renal Function

Michael A. Pesce, Alex J. Rai, Jorge L. Sepulveda, Serge Cremers

QUESTIONS

1. A 22-year-old woman with a history of type 1 diabetes mellitus and poor medication compliance presents to the emergency department obtunded. As part of her workup, serum electrolytes show a sodium level of 127 mEq/L (reference range, 137 to 145 mEq/L). Reference ranges are as follows:
   - Glucose: 75 to 115 mg/dL
   - Potassium: 3.5 to 5.0 mEq/L
   - pH: 7.38 to 7.44
   - Na_{urine}: 10 to 26 mEq/L

   Which one of the following choices most likely represents her additional lab findings?
   A. Glucose = 100 mg/dL; K = 3.2 mEq/L; pH = 7.3; Na_{urine} = 30 meq/L.
   B. Glucose = 500 mg/dL; K = 6.9 mEq/L; pH = 7.1; Na_{urine} = 30 meq/L.
   C. Glucose = 100 mg/dL; K = 2.9 mEq/L; pH = 7.1; Na_{urine} = 55 meq/L.
   D. Glucose = 180 mg/dL; K = 3.2 mEq/L; pH = 7.3; Na_{urine} = 55 meq/L.
   E. Glucose = 40 mg/dL; K = 4.0 mEq/L; pH = 7.3; Na_{urine} = 30 mEq/L.

2. An 18-month-old child with a history of respiratory infections had a sweat chloride result of 52 mmol/L. According to the Cystic Fibrosis Foundation, a sweat chloride level of 60 mmol/L or higher is suggestive of cystic fibrosis; a chloride level between 40 and 59 mmol/L is an intermediate level; and a chloride level of 39 mmol/L or less is considered normal. Based on this test result in this patient, which one of the following is the most appropriate next step in the workup?
   A. Diagnose cystic fibrosis based on this chloride level and clinical symptoms.
   B. Measure immunoreactive trypsinogen levels in the blood to confirm the diagnosis of cystic fibrosis.
   C. Diagnose this individual as a cystic fibrosis carrier with a mutated cystic fibrosis transmembrane conductance regulator (CFTR) gene.
   D. Collect another sweat sample and repeat the chloride measurement.
   E. Measure serum sodium and chloride levels to confirm the diagnosis of cystic fibrosis.

3. Which one of the following is the most common quantitative method used to measure sweat chloride concentrations in patients suspected of having cystic fibrosis?
   A. Ion-selective electrode (ISE) with a potentiometric end point.
   B. Mercuric ferric thiocyanate-colorimetric method.
   C. Enzymatic measurement.
   D. Coulometric titration procedure.
   E. Isotopic dilution mass spectrometry method.

4. Which one of the following tests is used to diagnose cystic fibrosis?
   A. Measurement of sweat osmolality.
   B. Measurement of immunoreactive trypsinogen.
   C. Measurement of sweat chloride.
   D. Measurement of sweat conductivity.
   E. Measurement of serum chloride.

5. Arterial blood gas measurements should be performed as soon as possible after the blood sample is obtained from the patient. Which one of the following will occur as a result of glycolysis if the blood is kept in the syringe at room temperature for 1 hour?
   A. Increased pH, Po_2, and Pco_2.
   B. Decreased pH and increased Po_2 and Pco_2.
   C. Decreased pH and Pco_2 and increased Po_2.
   D. Decreased pH and Po_2 and increased Pco_2.
   E. Decreased pH, Po_2, and Pco_2.

6. An arterial blood gas sample, collected in a heparinized syringe from a patient who was not receiving oxygen therapy, was sent to the laboratory on ice but was exposed to room air for approximately 30 minutes. Which one of the following sets of changes in the blood gas measurements will occur?
   A. Increased Po_2, pH, and Pco_2.
   B. Decreased Po_2, pH, and Pco_2.
   C. Increased Po_2 and pH and decreased Pco_2.
   D. Unchanged Po_2 and decreased Pco_2 and pH.
   E. Decreased Po_2 and pH and increased Pco_2.

7. Which one of the following techniques is used to correct for interferences in the automated Jaffe reaction?
   A. Online dialysis to remove proteins.
   B. Fluorescence measurement of the color produced.
   C. Spectrophotometric measurement of the color produced at two different wavelengths.
   D. Spectrophotometric measurement of the color produced after the reaction has gone to completion.
   E. Kinetic assay, where the reaction rate is measured between 20 and 60 seconds.

8. Which one of the following combinations of the concentration of urea (in both mg/dL and mmol/L) is equivalent to a serum blood urea nitrogen (BUN) concentration of 15 mg/dL?
   ■ Urea: NH_2CONH
   ■ Atomic weights: N=14, C=12, O=16, H=1.
   A. 32 mg/dL and 11.4 mmol/L.
   B. 32 mg/dL and 5.3 mmol/L.
   C. 7 mg/dL and 5.3 mmol/L.
   D. 7 mg/dL and 11.4 mmol/L.
   E. 64 mg/dL and 15 mmol/L.

9. A physician orders multiple tests for her patient in the intensive care unit. Postprandial samples are collected in a blood gas syringe and in a serum separator tube (SST). Electrolytes are measured on both sample types and a discrepancy is noted in the sodium concentration (i.e., $[Na^+]$) when comparing the results obtained with the blood gas analyzer (syringe) and the automated laboratory analyzer (SST). Which one of the following is the most likely explanation for this discrepancy?
   A. Higher imprecision using the blood gas analyzer.
   B. Wider dynamic range with the automated laboratory analyzer.
   C. Lower coefficient of variation with the automated laboratory analyzer.
   D. Different methods are used for this analysis on these two instruments.
   E. Greater accuracy using the automated laboratory analyzer.

10a. Which one of the following sets of laboratory results on a serum sample is most consistent with primary hypoparathyroidism?
   A. Decreased intact parathyroid hormone (PTH), increased calcium.
   B. Increased intact PTH, increased calcium.
   C. Decreased intact PTH, decreased calcium.
   D. Increased intact PTH, decreased calcium.
   E. Increased intact PTH, calcium within the normal range.

10b. Which one of the following sets of laboratory results on a serum sample is most consistent with the presence of malignancy?
   A. Decreased intact PTH, increased calcium.
   B. Increased intact PTH, increased calcium.
   C. Decreased intact PTH, decreased calcium.
   D. Increased intact PTH, decreased calcium.
   E. Increased intact PTH, calcium within the normal range.

10c. Which one of the following sets of laboratory results on a serum sample is most consistent with primary hyperparathyroidism?
   A. Decreased intact PTH, increased calcium.
   B. Increased intact PTH, increased calcium.

C. Decreased intact PTH, decreased calcium.
D. Increased intact PTH, decreased calcium.
E. Decreased intact PTH, calcium within the normal range.

10d. Which one of the following sets of laboratory results on a serum sample is most consistent with secondary hyperparathyroidism due to renal failure?
   A. Decreased intact PTH, increased calcium.
   B. Increased intact PTH, increased calcium.
   C. Decreased intact PTH, decreased calcium.
   D. Increased intact PTH, decreased calcium.
   E. Decreased intact PTH, calcium within the normal range.

11. The fractional hemoglobin saturation (i.e., Fo_2Hb) refers to the percentage of total hemoglobin that is saturated with oxygen. If the oxygen saturation (So_2) is known, which one of the following choices identifies the two additional parameters necessary for calculating the Fo_2Hb?
   A. Carboxyhemoglobin and deoxyhemoglobin.
   B. Deoxyhemoglobin and methemoglobin.
   C. Sickle hemoglobin and methemoglobin.
   D. Sickle hemoglobin and deoxyhemoglobin.
   E. Carboxyhemoglobin and methemoglobin.

12. Which one of the following patterns is most likely to be observed in patients with primary hyperparathyroidism?
   A. Elevated serum and urine levels of calcium and inorganic phosphate.
   B. Elevated levels of serum calcium and inorganic phosphate, elevated levels of urine calcium, and low levels of urine inorganic phosphate.
   C. Elevated levels of serum and urine calcium and low levels of serum and urine inorganic phosphate.
   D. Elevated levels of serum calcium, low levels of serum inorganic phosphate, low levels of urine calcium, and elevated levels of urine inorganic phosphate.
   E. Elevated levels of serum and urine calcium, low levels of serum inorganic phosphate, and elevated levels of urine inorganic phosphate.

13. In assessing hyponatremia, which one of the following analytes is least important?
   A. Plasma potassium.
   B. Plasma sodium.
   C. Urine sodium.
   D. Plasma calcium.
   E. Plasma glucose.

14. Which one of the following settings will lead to a falsely decreased plasma sodium concentration when measured by an indirect ISE method?
   A. Elevated circulating chloride and glucose levels.
   B. Elevated circulating protein and lipid levels.
   C. Decreased circulating protein and lipid levels.
   D. Decreased circulating protein and glucose levels.
   E. Decreased circulating protein and chloride levels.

15. Which one of the following is the most likely cause of a low BUN/creatinine ratio?
   A. Congestive heart failure.
   B. A high-protein diet.
   C. Acute tubular necrosis.
   D. Acute glomerular injury.
   E. Severe liver disease.

16. Which one of the following best describes the use of the Modification of Diet in Renal Disease (MDRD) equation for estimating the glomerular filtration rate (GFR)?
    A. The calculation requires the serum creatinine and urine creatinine levels along with patient age, gender, and race.
    B. The calculation requires the serum creatinine and BUN levels along with patient age, gender, and race.
    C. The calculation requires the serum creatinine and cystatin C levels along with patient age, gender, and race.
    D. The calculation requires the serum and urine creatinine levels along with the volume of urine.
    E. The calculation uses the serum creatinine level along with patient age, gender, and race.

Table 9-1

Test	Patient	Reference Range	Units
Na	138	136-146	mmol/L
K	4.0	3.5-5.0	mmol/L
Cl	105	101-109	mmol/L
CO_2	12	22-29	mmol/L
pH	7.32	7.36-7.41	
P_{CO_2}	40	32-45	mm Hg

17. A patient has the laboratory results shown in Table 9-1. Which one of the following conditions is the most likely underlying cause of these results?
    A. Metabolic acidosis with an elevated anion gap.
    B. Metabolic acidosis with a normal anion gap.
    C. Respiratory acidosis with an elevated anion gap.
    D. Renal tubular acidosis (RTA).
    E. Respiratory acidosis with a normal anion gap.

18. Which one of the following would most likely be seen in a patient with severe diarrhea?
    A. Metabolic alkalosis with an elevated anion gap.
    B. Respiratory acidosis with an elevated anion gap.
    C. Metabolic acidosis with a normal anion gap.
    D. Metabolic acidosis with an elevated anion gap.
    E. RTA type 2 with an elevated anion gap.

Table 9-2

Test	Patient	Reference Range	Units
Na	141	136-146	mmol/L
K	4.0	3.5-5.0	mmol/L
Cl	88	101-109	mmol/L
CO_2	48	22-29	mmol/L
pH	7.48	7.36-7.41	
P_{CO_2}	47	32-45	mm Hg

19. A patient has the laboratory results shown in Table 9-2. Which one of the following is the most likely cause of these results?
    A. Metabolic acidosis.
    B. Respiratory acidosis.

C. Metabolic alkalosis.
D. Diabetic ketoacidosis (DKA).
E. Respiratory alkalosis.

20. Blood gas analysis was performed on a patient sample and the following results were obtained: pH = 7.40 (reference range, 7.36 to 7.41), P_{CO_2} = 55 mm Hg (reference range, 32 to 45 mm Hg), and HCO_3^- = 46 mmol/L (reference range, 22 to 29 mmol/L). Which one of the following conditions is the most likely underlying cause of these results?
    A. Metabolic alkalosis with respiratory compensation.
    B. Metabolic alkalosis.
    C. Metabolic acidosis.
    D. Respiratory acidosis.
    E. Respiratory alkalosis with metabolic compensation.

21. Which one of the following best describes the significance of microalbuminuria?
    A. Predicts glomerulonephritis.
    B. Contributes to multiple myeloma staging.
    C. Identifies the presence of end-stage renal disease.
    D. Predicts kidney transplant rejection.
    E. Predicts diabetic nephropathy.

22. Which one of the following answers best describes the most significant laboratory result(s) for identifying nephrotic syndrome?
    A. Increased serum BUN and creatinine concentrations.
    B. Increased serum cystatin C concentration.
    C. Increased serum cholesterol concentration.
    D. Microalbuminuria.
    E. Proteinuria of greater than 3.0 g/day.

A 58-year-old man who underwent colon resection was treated with an aminoglycoside for a surgical infection. A day and a half after beginning this therapy, his creatinine jumped from 0.8 mmol/L to 3.8 mmol/L (reference range, 0.6 to 1.2 mmol/L) with a BUN of 60 mg/dL (reference range, 7 to 20 mg/dL). Use this scenario to answer the following two questions.

23a. Which one of the following would be the next most helpful diagnostic test?
    A. Renal artery ultrasound.
    B. Serum and urine osmolality.
    C. Serum potassium.
    D. Plasma aminoglycoside levels.
    E. Renal biopsy.

23b. The patient's renal failure was determined to be of tubular etiology based on the diagnostic test you recommended above. Which one of the following is the most likely serum calcium, ionized calcium, and phosphate, respectively, that would be seen in this patient? Reference ranges are as follows:
    - Calcium (8.7 to 10.2 mg/dL)
    - Ionized calcium (4.5 to 5.3 mg/dL)
    - Phosphate (2.5 to 4.3 mg/dL)
    A. 6 g/dL, 0.99 g/dL, 4 g/dL.
    B. 6 g/dL, 0.89 g/dL, 6 g/dL.
    C. 9 g/dL, 0.89 g/dL, 6 g/dL.
    D. 9 g/dL, 0.99 g/dL, 4 g/dL.
    E. 6 g/dL, 0.99 g/dL, 2 g/dL.

Table 9-3

Test	Patient	Reference Range	Units
Na	138	136-146	mmol/L
K	4.3	3.5-5.0	mmol/L
Cl	90	101-109	mmol/L
CO_2	40	22-29	mmol/L
pH	7.32	7.36-7.41	
P_{CO_2}	78	32-45	mm Hg

24. A patient has the laboratory results shown in Table 9-3. Which one of the following conditions is the most likely underlying cause of these results?
    A. Metabolic acidosis with a normal anion gap.
    B. Metabolic acidosis with an elevated anion gap.
    C. Respiratory acidosis with an elevated anion gap.
    D. RTA with an elevated anion gap.
    E. Respiratory acidosis with a normal anion gap.

Table 9-4

Test	Patient	Reference Range	Units
Na	139	136-146	mmol/L
K	4.0	3.5-5.0	mmol/L
Cl	114	101-109	mmol/L
CO_2	17	22-29	mmol/L
pH	7.50	7.36-7.41	
P_{CO_2}	17	32-45	mm Hg

25. A patient has the laboratory results shown in Table 9-4. Which one of the following conditions is the most likely underlying cause of these results?
    A. Metabolic acidosis.
    B. Respiratory acidosis.
    C. Metabolic alkalosis.
    D. Respiratory alkalosis.
    E. DKA.

26. Which one of the following mechanisms physiologically compensates for a respiratory alkalosis?
    A. Renal regulation of P_{CO_2}.
    B. Renal regulation of HCO_3^-.
    C. Hyperventilation.
    D. Renal excretion of H^+.
    E. Renal excretion of organic acids.

27. Which one of the following serum patterns is most likely to be observed in children with rickets?
    A. Low levels of calcium, 25-hydroxyvitamin D, inorganic phosphate, and PTH.
    B. Low levels of calcium, 25-hydroxyvitamin D, and inorganic phosphate, and an elevated PTH level.
    C. Low levels of calcium and 25-hydroxyvitamin D, and elevated levels of inorganic phosphate and PTH.
    D. Low levels of calcium, 25-hydroxyvitamin D, and PTH, and an elevated inorganic phosphate level.
    E. Elevated levels of calcium and PTH and low levels of 25-hydroxyvitamin D and inorganic phosphate.

28. S_{O_2} refers to the percent of functional hemoglobin (Hb) that is saturated with oxygen. Which one of the following pairs identifies the two forms of Hb that are necessary for this calculation?
    A. Oxyhemoglobin and carboxyhemoglobin.
    B. Oxyhemoglobin and deoxyhemoglobin.
    C. Oxyhemoglobin and methemoglobin.
    D. Deoxyhemoglobin and carboxyhemoglobin.
    E. Deoxyhemoglobin and methemoglobin.

Table 9-5

Test	Patient	Reference Range	Units
Na	140	136-146	mmol/L
K	6.5	3.5-5.0	mmol/L
Cl	105	102-109	mmol/L
CO_2	24	22-30	mmol/L
Cr	0.7	0.6-1.2	mg/dL
Albumin	3.8	3.5-4.5	mg/dL
Calcium	4.2	8.7-10.2	mg/dL
Phosphate	4.0	2.5-4.8	mg/dL

29. A 35-year-old asymptomatic woman has the laboratory results shown in Table 9-5. Which one of the following is the most likely explanation for these results?
    A. Anticoagulant contamination.
    B. Chronic kidney failure.
    C. Renal tubular acidosis.
    D. Primary hyperaldosteronism.
    E. Congenital adrenal hyperplasia.

Table 9-6

Test	Patient	Reference Range	Units
Na	156	136-146	mmol/L
K	4.1	3.5-5.0	mmol/L
Cl	120	102-109	mmol/L
CO_2	24	22-30	mmol/L
BUN	39	7-20	mg/dL
Cr	1.4	0.6-1.2	mg/dL
Glucose	76	65-95	mg/dL

A 38-year-old woman presented for elective cholecystectomy with the preoperative laboratory values shown in Table 9-6. Use this scenario to answer the following three questions.

30a. A previous electrolyte profile performed 2 months ago showed similar results, except for sodium of 145 mmol/L, creatinine of 1.1 mg/dL, and BUN of 23 mg/dL. The patient reported that for the last 5 months she had increased dyspnea on exertion and ingested 5 to 6 cups of water a night, except the previous night, when she was fasting for the next day's operation. Which one of the following is the most likely diagnosis?
    A. Addison disease.
    B. Conn syndrome.
    C. Syndrome of inappropriate antidiuretic hormone secretion.
    D. Diabetes insipidus.
    E. Diabetes mellitus.

30b. On further testing, the chest radiograph revealed bilateral hilar adenopathy and fine reticular opacities; blood testing showed serum calcium 13.5 mg/dL (reference range, 8.7 to 10.2 mg/dL), phosphorus 5.7 mg/dL (reference range, 2.5 to 4.8 mg/dL), PTH 15 pg/mL (reference range, 50 to 330 pg/mL), 25-hydroxyvitamin D 25 ng/mL (reference range, 30 to 74 ng/mL), antidiuretic hormone (ADH) 12 pg/mL (reference range, 4 to 12 pg/mL) with serum osmolality 300 mOsm/kg (reference range, 285 to 295 mOsm/kg), and cortisol 6 mg/dL (reference range, 5 to 23 mg/dL). Urinalysis was unremarkable except for urine osmolality 80 mOsm/kg (>850 mOsm/kg with fluid restriction). Which one of the following clinical conditions best explains these results?

A. Ectopic adrenocorticotropic hormone (ACTH) production.

B. Lung cancer–producing ADH.

C. Nephrogenic diabetes insipidus.

D. Central diabetes insipidus.

E. Diabetic nephropathy.

30c. Clinical evaluation and elevated plasma angiotensin-converting enzyme levels confirmed a past history of pulmonary sarcoidosis. Which one of the following laboratory results is most consistent with the patient's diagnosis?

A. Unchanged cortisol after ACTH administration

B. Increased urine osmolality after water deprivation and ADH administration.

C. Elevated 1,25-dihydroxyvitamin D.

D. Elevated PTH-related peptide (PTHrP).

E. Elevated C-peptide after a standard meal.

31. A 65-year-old man with a history of chronic myeloid leukemia presented with a white cell count of 185×10^9/L (reference range, 3.04 to 9.06×10^9/L), with 54% blasts, 26% myeloid precursors, 15% neutrophils, 4% basophils, 1% eosinophils, platelet count 256×10^9/L (reference range, 165 to 415×10^9/L), hemoglobin 11.5 g/dL (reference range, 13.3 to 16.2 g/dL), and normal basic metabolic panel except for a glucose of 60 g/dL (reference range, 65 to 95 g/dL) and potassium of 2.5 mmol/L (reference range, 3.5 to 5.5 mmol/L). Vital signs, neurological examination, and electrocardiogram were normal. Which one of the following most likely accounts for these findings?

A. Rhabdomyolysis secondary to blood hyperviscosity.

B. Adrenal insufficiency due to leukemic infiltration.

C. Acute tubular necrosis of the kidney.

D. Pseudohypokalemia due to leukocytosis.

E. Lactic acidosis due to leukemic anaerobic metabolism.

32. A diabetic 56-year-old man with a history of type 2 diabetes presents to the emergency department with weakness, nausea, altered mental status, and the laboratory results shown in Table 9-7. Which one of the following statements most likely corresponds to the clinical situation?

A. The normal BUN/creatinine ratio is inconsistent with dehydration.

B. The hyponatremia is probably due to increased extracellular water content.

C. The hyperkalemia indicates excess total body potassium.

D. There is significant ketoacidosis due to insulin deficiency.

E. Effective plasma osmolality is consistent with a hyperosmolar hyperglycemic state.

Table 9-8

Test	Patient	Reference Range	Units
Na	155	136-146	mmol/L
↑K	5.2	3.5-5.0	mmol/L
Cl	165	102-109	mmol/L
CO_2	7	22-30	mmol/L
↑Glucose	482	65-95	mg/dL
↓pH	7.0	7.35-7.45	

33. A 13-month-old girl with consanguineous parents presented with polydipsia, diuresis, vomiting, and lethargy and showed signs of dehydration, deep sighing respiration, and smelled of ketones. Her lab results are shown in Table 9-8. Her urine was strongly positive for ketones and urine culture grew *Escherichia coli*. Levels of hemoglobin A1c were 5.3% (reference range, normal <5.7%), C-peptide was within normal range, and autoantibodies against glutamic acid decarboxylase and islet cells were not present. Urine organic acid analysis revealed elevated levels of methylmalonic acid. Plasma levels of vitamin B_{12}, folate, and homocysteine were normal. Plasma acylcarnitine analysis showed elevation in C3 carnitine esters. Plasma lactate was elevated (36 mg/dL; reference range, 5 to 15 mg/dL) with normal pyruvate. The patient gradually improved after treatment of the urinary tract infection, initiation of a low-protein diet, cyanocobalamin, and L-carnitine supplementation. Which one of the following is the best explanation for this patient's results?

A. Type 1 diabetes complicated by urinary tract infection.

B. Fatty acid oxidation defect.

C. Pyruvate dehydrogenase deficiency.

D. Malnutrition with chronic vitamin B_{12} deficiency.

E. Adenosylcobalamin synthesis defect.

34. Which one of the following statements is true regarding physiological preanalytical effects on electrolyte levels?

A. A standard meal will decrease plasma phosphate levels within 2 hours.

B. A shift from supine to upright position causes increases in plasma calcium.

C. Acute ethanol intoxication is frequently associated with metabolic alkalosis.

D. Vigorous exercise often leads to lower potassium levels.

E. Stress (e.g., during acute myocardial infarction) often causes hyperkalemia.

Table 9-7

Test	Patient	Reference Range	Units
↓Na	132	136-146	mmol/L
↑K	5.2	3.5-5.0	mmol/L
BUN	15	7-20	mg/dL
↑Cr	1.5	0.6-1.2	mg/dL
↑Glucose	1068	65-95	mg/dL
↓pH	7.33	7.35-7.45	
↓CO_2	19	22-30	mmol/L

35. A 25-year-old asymptomatic woman was hospitalized for persistent plasma hyperkalemia of approximately 7.0 mmol/L (reference range, 3.5 to 5.0 mmol/L), first identified during routine blood work. Physical examination and electrocardiogram were normal. Examination of the plasma supernatant showed no evidence of hemolysis. On a subsequent phlebotomy, both plasma and serum samples were measured, which showed potassium levels of 5.6 and 4.3 mmol/L, respectively. When a blood sample was collected and immediately centrifuged, the potassium levels were 4.3 mmol/L, but incubation at room temperature for 6 hours resulted in potassium levels of 7.5 mmol/L. Which one of the following is the best explanation for these results?
    A. Ethanol contamination during phlebotomy.
    B. Prolonged tourniquet time with fist clenching.
    C. Thrombocytosis.
    D. Leukocytosis.
    E. Familial pseudohyperkalemia.

Table 9-9

Test	Patient	Reference Range	Units
Na	143	136-146	mmol/L
K	3.3	3.5-5.0	mmol/L
Cl	121	102-109	mmol/L
CO_2	14	22-30	mmol/L
Cr	1.0	0.6-1.2	mg/dL
Glucose	65	65-95	mg/dL
Calcium	8.9	8.7-10.2	mg/dL
Phosphate	3.2	3.4-6.0	mg/dL
Albumin	3.7	3.5-4.5	mg/dL

A 26-month-old girl with mild developmental delay and at the 5th percentile for height has the laboratory results shown in Table 9-9. Urinalysis showed pH 5.0 and was positive for glucose without other abnormalities. Use this scenario to answer the following two questions.

36a. Which one of the following best explains the patient's presentation?
    A. Organic aciduria.
    B. Type 1 (distal) RTA.
    C. Type 2 (proximal) RTA.
    D. Hyporeninemic hypoaldosteronism.
    E. DKA.

36b. Which one of the following test results would most likely be found on confirmatory testing?
    A. High urinary levels of methylmalonic acid by gas chromatography–mass spectrometry.
    B. Increased urinary pH after NH_4Cl load.
    C. Elevated fractionary urinary excretion of HCO_3 after bicarbonate load.
    D. Decreased plasma aldosterone/renin ratio.
    E. High plasma levels of β-hydroxybutyrate.

Table 9-10

Test	Patient	Reference Range	Units
pH	7.43	7.35-7.45	
Pco_2	34	32-45	mm Hg
Po_2	95	72-104	mm Hg
HCO_3	26	22-30	mEq/L

37. A 19-year-old man presented with low-grade fever, coughing, sore throat, and conjunctivitis. Blood counts and a basic metabolic panel were within the reference ranges except for a total CO_2 of 15 mmol/L (reference range, 22 to 30 mmol/L). The physician was concerned about an acid-base disturbance, so an arterial blood gas analysis was performed (Table 9-10). Which one of the following best explains these findings?
    A. Respiratory acidosis.
    B. Respiratory alkalosis.
    C. Metabolic acidosis with respiratory compensation.
    D. Spuriously low venous bicarbonate due to hypotension.
    E. Spurious loss of CO_2 in the venous sample.

Table 9-11

Test	Patient	Reference Range	Units
Na	149	136-146	mmol/L
K	5.7	3.5-5.0	mmol/L
Cl	117	102-109	mmol/L
CO_2	15	22-30	mmol/L
BUN	8	7-20	mg/dL
Cr	1.2	0.6-1.2	mg/dL
Glucose	94	65-95	mg/dL
Lactate	6.9	8-15	mg/dL
Total bilirubin	9.1	0.3-1.3	mg/dL
Direct bilirubin	0.6	0.0-0.4	mg/dL
Ammonia	2165	170-341	μg/dL

38. A full-term boy was born after an uneventful pregnancy from consanguineous parents with 3.4-kg birth weight. Apgar scores (9 and 9) were normal. The next day after delivery, the baby presented with increased lethargy, jitteriness, and refusal to feed. During the admission, the baby developed respiratory failure and status epilepticus. Laboratory results are shown in Table 9-11. Plasma amino acid levels were normal except for plasma glutamine of 2870 nmol/mL (reference range, <1060 nmol/mL), alanine of 3800 nmol/mL (reference range, <820 nmol/mL), and undetectable citrulline. Orotic acid and reducing sugars were absent in the urine. Acylcarnitine profile was normal. Which one of the following enzymatic defects is most consistent with these findings?
    A. Carbamoyl phosphate synthase (CPS).
    B. Argininosuccinate lyase (ASL).
    C. Carnitine palmitoyltransferase II (CPT2).
    D. Aldolase B (ALDOB).
    E. Lysosomal beta-glycosidase (GBA).

39. Which one of the following combinations of laboratory findings is most likely to be observed in ethylene glycol intoxication?
    A. Decreased pH, increased serum osmolality and osmolal gap, decreased anion gap.
    B. Increased pH, decreased serum osmolality and osmolal gap, increased anion gap.
    C. Decreased pH, increased serum osmolality and osmolal gap, normal anion gap.
    D. Decreased pH, increased serum osmolality and osmolal gap, increased anion gap.
    E. Normal pH, increased serum osmolality and osmolal gap, increased anion gap.

ANSWERS

1. A. Glucose = 100 mg/dL; K = 3.2 mEq/L; pH = 7.3; Na$_{urine}$ = 30 mEq/L.
Rationale: These represent normal lab values.
B. Glucose = 500 mg/dL; K = 6.9 mEq/L; pH = 7.1; Na$_{urine}$ = 30 mEq/L.
Rationale: This is a classic presentation for DKA in a type 1 diabetic. The hyperosmolarity of the serum resulting from the high glucose causes efflux of cellular water that in turn dilutes the serum sodium. The hyperkalemia is a result of red cell buffering of the acidosis, which results from the hyperglycemia. Urine Na should be normal in this setting.
C. Glucose = 100 mg/dL; K = 2.9 mEq/L; pH = 7.1; Na$_{urine}$ = 55 mEq/L.
Rationale: These values would be seen in cases of loop diuretic abuse (note potassium wasting).
D. Glucose = 180 mg/dL; K = 3.2 mEq/L; pH = 7.3; Na$_{urine}$ = 55 mEq/L.
Rationale: These values would be seen in the setting of syndrome of inappropriate antidiuretic hormone secretion.
E. Glucose = 40 mg/dL; K = 4.0 mEq/L; pH = 7.3; Na$_{urine}$ = 30 mEq/L.
Rationale: These values would not be seen in DKA. The only abnormality seen here is hypoglycemia.

Major points of discussion

- DKA is characterized by hyperglycemia, metabolic acidosis, positive serum ketones, and an increased anion gap (>10-12 mEq/L).
- The high serum osmolality causes an efflux of cellular water, diluting the serum sodium.
- Hyperkalemia results from red cell buffering of the acidosis.
- Urine Na concentrations should be relatively normal in the setting of DKA, assuming renal function is uncompromised.
- "Pseudo" is used to describe the hyponatremia seen in DKA because total body sodium stores are normal in the setting of low serum sodium.

2. A. Diagnose cystic fibrosis based on this chloride level and clinical symptoms.
Rationale: This is an intermediate chloride level and is not diagnostic for cystic fibrosis.
B. Measure immunoreactive trypsinogen levels in the blood to confirm the diagnosis of cystic fibrosis.
Rationale: Immunoreactive trypsinogen is a screening test and cannot be used to diagnose cystic fibrosis.
C. Diagnose this individual as a cystic fibrosis carrier with a mutated cystic fibrosis transmembrane conductance regulator (*CFTR*) gene.
Rationale: An intermediate chloride level cannot be used to predict who is a carrier of cystic fibrosis.
D. Collect another sweat sample and repeat the chloride measurement.
Rationale: Intermediate sweat chloride levels require the collection of another sweat sample and measurement of chloride.
E. Measure serum sodium and chloride levels to confirm the diagnosis of cystic fibrosis.
Rationale: Serum sodium and chloride levels are not used to diagnose cystic fibrosis.

Major points of discussion

- According to the Cystic Fibrosis Foundation, a sweat chloride level of 60 mmol/L or greater is suggestive of cystic fibrosis; a chloride level between 40 and 59 mmol/L is an intermediate level; and a chloride level of 39 mmol/L or less is considered normal. For indeterminate chloride levels, another sweat sample is collected on the same day or on a different day and sweat chloride levels are remeasured. If values are still in the intermediate range, genetic testing is usually performed.
- In addition to cystic fibrosis, several disorders, such as anorexia nervosa, atopic dermatitis, and protein-calorie malnutrition, can cause an elevated sweat chloride result. Sweat chloride measured after treatment of these conditions usually results in a normal chloride level.
- A significant problem with sweat collection is that the amount of sweat collected may not be sufficient for chloride analysis. The Cystic Fibrosis Foundation recommends that if sweat is collected properly, 95% of the patients tested should have sufficient sweat for chloride analysis.
- Technical problems associated with the collection of sweat and determination of chloride include skin contamination by salt-containing compounds, evaporation of the sweat during collection, errors in chloride determination, and errors in the calculation of sweat chloride results.
- The collection of sweat and measurement of sweat chloride are manual procedures that are subject to technical errors. Only skilled technologists, who are trained in the collection of sweat and measurement of sweat chloride, should be used for these assays.
- Sweat collection is usually not performed in newborns less than 48 hours after birth because the chloride values can be transiently elevated.[7,40]

3. A. Ion-selective electrode (ISE) with a potentiometric end point.
Rationale: This is the most frequent method used to measure chloride levels in serum or plasma.
B. Mercuric ferric thiocyanate-colorimetric method.
Rationale: This method is seldom used to measure sweat chloride.
C. Enzymatic measurement.
Rationale: This method is not available.
D. Coulometric titration procedure.
Rationale: This is the most common method used to measure sweat chloride and is recommended by the Cystic Fibrosis Foundation.
E. Isotopic dilution mass spectrometry method.
Rationale: This method is used in research laboratories.

Major points of discussion

- The coulometric titration method involves the reaction of chloride ions in the sample with silver ions generated from a silver electrode to produce silver chloride. The end point in the titration is reached when there is a rapid increase in the concentration of silver ions that occurs when all of the chloride ions in the sample are consumed.

The time required to generate the excess silver ions is recorded and related to the concentration of chloride in the sample.

- The ISE method measures the potential that develops across a selective membrane. The low concentrations of chloride in sweat limit the use of the ISE method.
- The mercuric ferric thiocyanate spectrophotometric method is usually not used for sweat chloride analysis because it is not sensitive at low chloride concentrations.
- Isotopic dilution mass spectrometry is the ability to quantify a compound relative to an isotope species (in this case ^{37}Cl) of known concentration. This is a manual procedure that is time consuming and not used in the routine clinical laboratory.
- Measurement of sweat chloride levels is usually a manual procedure.[7,40]

4. A. Measurement of sweat osmolality.
Rationale: Sweat osmolality is a screening test for cystic fibrosis.
B. Measurement of immunoreactive trypsinogen.
Rationale: Immunoreactive trypsinogen is a screening test for cystic fibrosis.
C. Measurement of sweat chloride.
Rationale: Quantitative measurement of sweat chloride is used to *diagnose* cystic fibrosis.
D. Measurement of sweat conductivity.
Rationale: Sweat conductivity measurement is a screening test for cystic fibrosis.
E. Measurement of serum chloride.
Rationale: Serum chloride levels are not used to diagnose cystic fibrosis.

Major points of discussion

- Immunoreactive trypsinogen measurement, along with DNA testing, is used to screen newborns for cystic fibrosis. A positive result requires confirmation by sweat chloride testing.
- The Cystic Fibrosis Foundation requires quantitative sweat chloride measurements to be used to confirm the diagnosis of cystic fibrosis. A sweat chloride level of 60 mmol/L or greater is suggestive of cystic fibrosis. A chloride level between 40 and 59 mmol/L is an intermediate level, and a chloride level of 39 mmol/L or less is considered normal.
- The Cystic Fibrosis Foundation suggests that two positive sweat chloride results be obtained to confirm the diagnosis of cystic fibrosis. An initial positive sweat chloride result should trigger the collection of another sweat sample and measurement of sweat chloride.
- Almost all children with cystic fibrosis (99%) have elevated sweat chloride values.
- Serum chloride levels are usually normal in cystic fibrosis patients.[7,40]

5. A. Increased pH, Po_2, and Pco_2.
B. Decreased pH and increased Po_2 and Pco_2.
C. Decreased pH and Pco_2 and increased Po_2.
D. Decreased pH and Po_2 and increased Pco_2.
E. Decreased pH, Po_2, and Pco_2.
Rationale: Decreased pH and po_2 and increased Pco_2 will occur when glucose is metabolized to pyruvate and lactate.

Major points of discussion

- If the specimen is not chilled to 4 °C, glycolysis will occur and glucose will be metabolized by the Embden-Meyerhof pathway to pyruvate and lactate.
- The longer the specimen is kept at room temperature, the more lactate is produced, and the lower the pH will be.
- Glucose can be converted to CO_2 when pyruvate enters the tricarboxylic acid cycle and is metabolized to CO_2 and water. Leukocytes will metabolize oxygen and a falsely low Po_2 will be obtained.
- Because of glycolysis, a blood gas sample kept at 37 °C for 1 hour will result in a lower pH of approximately 0.04 to 0.08, a lower Po_2 of approximately 5 to 10 mm Hg, and an increased Pco_2 of approximately 5 mm Hg. Therefore, the sample should be placed on ice if analysis cannot be performed soon after obtaining the blood sample from the patient.
- If the white blood cell count is high, glycolysis and its effect on pH, Pco_2, and Po_2 will be significantly exacerbated.[31]

6. A. Increased Po_2, pH, and Pco_2.
B. Decreased Po_2, pH, and Pco_2.
C. Increased Po_2 and pH and decreased Pco_2.
D. Unchanged Po_2 and decreased Pco_2 and pH.
E. Decreased Po_2 and pH and increased Pco_2.
Rationale: An arterial blood sample exposed to air will lead to an increase in Po_2 and pH and a decrease in Pco_2.

Major points of discussion

- If blood is exposed to air or if there is an air bubble in the syringe, the Po_2 and pH levels will increase and the Pco_2 will decrease.
- Room air contains a Pco_2 of essentially zero and a Po_2 of approximately 150 mm Hg. Therefore, extraneous air in a blood sample will cause a diffusion of CO_2 out of the specimen and O_2 into the specimen (if the Po_2 in the patient sample is actually <150 mm Hg).
- If the Po_2 in the patient sample is actually greater than 150 mm Hg, which can occur in patients receiving oxygen therapy, the Po_2 will diffuse out of the specimen and a lower Po_2 will be obtained. The error will be greater as the amount of time the blood sample is exposed to room air increases.
- The Pco_2 of blood exposed to air will decrease and the pH, which is dependent on the $HCO_3^-/0.03$ Pco_2 ratio, will increase.
- If the Po_2 is greater than 110 mm Hg and the patient is not being given oxygen, air contamination of the sample should be considered. The reference range for Po_2 in an arterial blood sample is 80 to 100 mm Hg and, for a venous blood sample, it is 30 to 50 mm Hg.[24]

7. A. Online dialysis to remove proteins.
Rationale: Dialysis is not performed.
B. Fluorescence measurement of the color produced.
Rationale: Fluorescence is not used in the automated Jaffe reaction.
C. Spectrophotometric measurement of the color produced at two different wavelengths.
Rationale: Bichromatic measurements are not used in the automated Jaffe reaction.

D. Spectrophotometric measurement of the color produced after the reaction has gone to completion.
Rationale: The color is not measured at the end point of the reaction.
E. Kinetic assay, where the reaction rate is measured between 20 and 60 seconds.
Rationale: The method involves the reaction of picric acid with creatinine in an alkaline solution to form an orange-red complex that is measured spectrophotometrically at a wavelength of 520 nm.

Major points of discussion
- Creatinine is a waste product formed by muscles from the nonenzymatic dehydration of creatine. Serum creatinine concentration is a direct reflection of muscle mass; men typically have higher serum creatinine levels than women.
- The Jaffe method is used to measure creatinine. It was first described in 1886 and is the oldest clinical chemistry method routinely used in the clinical laboratory.
- Noncreatinine substances can also react with picric acid but produce color at a slower or faster rate than creatinine. A significant number of substances in serum, other than creatinine, react with picric acid, causing positive interference.
- The positive interferences from acetoacetate, pyruvate, acetone, protein, cephalosporins, glucose, uric acid, and ascorbic acid observed with the Jaffe reaction can be eliminated or significantly reduced using a kinetic rate procedure for measuring creatinine. Using this approach, these interfering analytes do not significantly react with picric acid during the 20- to 60-second time interval during which the measurements are taken.[41]

8. A. 32 mg/dL and 11.4 mmol/L.
   B. 32 mg/dL and 5.3 mmol/L.
   C. 7 mg/dL and 5.3 mmol/L.
   D. 7 mg/dL and 11.4 mmol/L.
   E. 64 mg/dL and 15 mmol/L.
   Rationale: The molecular weight of urea is 60. Urea contains 2 nitrogen atoms, with a combined molecular weight of 28. To convert from urea nitrogen in mg/dL to urea in mg/dL, divide 60 by 28 to obtain a factor of 2.14; therefore, 2.14 g of urea is equivalent to 1.0 g of urea nitrogen. If the urea nitrogen value of 15 mg/dL is multiplied by 2.14, one obtains a concentration of urea of 32 mg/dL. To convert the urea concentration of 32 mg/dL into mmol/L, one multiplies 32 by 10 and then divides by the molecular weight of urea (i.e., 60) to obtain 5.3 mmol/L.

Major points of discussion
- Historically, serum concentrations of urea have been expressed in terms of its nitrogen content. This occurred because, in the early years of clinical chemistry, the quantity of nitrogen in urea was compared with levels of other non-protein nitrogen–containing compounds.
- Traditionally, urea concentration is still calculated in terms of the urea nitrogen when expressed on a mass basis.
- However, in SI (International System) units, the urea nitrogen is expressed as mmol/L of the intact molecule.[19]

9. A. Higher imprecision using the blood gas analyzer.
   Rationale: This would not necessarily explain the discrepancy.

B. Wider dynamic range with the automated laboratory analyzer.
Rationale: This is an advantage but would not explain the discrepancy.
C. Lower coefficient of variation with the automated laboratory analyzer.
Rationale: This would result in improved precision but would not explain the discrepancy.
D. Different methods are used for this analysis on these two instruments.
Rationale: Indirect versus direct measurement methods are used on the two different instruments.
E. Greater accuracy using the automated laboratory analyzer.
Rationale: This is not definitive and would not necessarily explain the discrepancy.

Major points of discussion
- In "normal" situations, plasma consists of approximately 93% water and 7% proteins and lipids. Ions are confined to the water space, which is 93% of the volume in plasma.
- Samples that are high in protein and/or lipids are considered "abnormal" and may result in an interference of measurement when dilution of samples is required. This occurs in indirect methods.
- Indirect measurement methods typically require dilution of the sample before measurement. This is the most common method used with ion-specific electrodes on automated laboratory analyzers.
- Direct measurement methods, such as those used on blood gas analyzers, do not require sample dilution before introduction to the ion-specific electrode.
- A discrepancy can result between blood gas analyzers and automated analyzers if samples with high protein and/or high lipid levels are measured. This may cause confusion for ordering physicians who use this information for adjusting, initiating, and/or stopping fluid therapy.

10a. A. Decreased intact parathyroid hormone (PTH), increased calcium.
   B. Increased intact PTH, increased calcium.
   C. Decreased intact PTH, decreased calcium.
   D. Increased intact PTH, decreased calcium.
   E. Increased intact PTH, calcium within the normal range.
   Rationale: The circulating intact PTH and serum calcium levels should be low in primary hypoparathyroidism.

10b. **A. Decreased intact PTH, increased calcium.**
   B. Increased intact PTH, increased calcium.
   C. Decreased intact PTH, decreased calcium.
   D. Increased intact PTH, decreased calcium.
   E. Increased intact PTH, calcium within the normal range.
   Rationale: The circulating intact PTH level is usually low in malignant conditions. Serum calcium is expected to be high in malignant conditions.

10c. A. Decreased intact PTH, increased calcium.
   B. Increased intact PTH, increased calcium.
   C. Decreased intact PTH, decreased calcium.
   D. Increased intact PTH, decreased calcium.
   E. Decreased intact PTH, calcium within the normal range.
   Rationale: The circulating intact PTH level and the serum calcium level should be elevated in primary hyperparathyroidism.

10d. A. Decreased intact PTH, increased calcium.
B. Increased intact PTH, increased calcium.
C. Decreased intact PTH, decreased calcium.
D. Increased intact PTH, decreased calcium.
E. Decreased intact PTH, calcium within the normal range.
Rationale: The circulating intact PTH level should be elevated in secondary hyperparathyroidism resulting from renal failure. Serum calcium levels are usually low in secondary hyperparathyroidism caused by renal failure.

Major points of discussion
- In the assessment of physiological states of calcium homeostasis, simultaneous measurements of ionized calcium and PTH should be conducted.
- The PTH molecule is a short polypeptide composed of 84 amino acids and has a short half-life in blood of 5 minutes.
- Multiple assays are available for PTH. These include the intact PTH assay and separate assays for the biologically active amino-terminal portion of the molecule, internal PTH fragments, and the carboxyl-terminal portion of the molecule. It is important to know which assay is used for measurement of PTH.
- The intact PTH assay detects the entire molecule and is the preferred assay for measuring this molecule because it provides excellent overall sensitivity and specificity.
- The assays for PTH fragments provide improved sensitivity for the detection of disease but can be elevated under other conditions, including compromised kidney function.

11. A. Carboxyhemoglobin and deoxyhemoglobin.
Rationale: Because carboxyhemoglobin contains bound carbon monoxide, it is nonfunctional; however, deoxyhemoglobin is functional with regard to oxygen-binding capacity.
B. Deoxyhemoglobin and methemoglobin.
Rationale: Because methemoglobin contains iron in the ferric state, it is nonfunctional; however, deoxyhemoglobin is functional with regard to oxygen-binding capacity.
C. Sickle hemoglobin and methemoglobin.
D. Sickle hemoglobin and deoxyhemoglobin.
Rationale: The sickle cell hemoglobin level (HbS) is not relevant in these contexts.
E. Carboxyhemoglobin and methemoglobin.
Rationale: These two components correspond to nonfunctional forms of hemoglobin, which comprises the difference between So_2 and Fo_2.

Major points of discussion
- The total hemoglobin (Hb) level is composed of the oxy-, deoxy-, met-, and carboxy- forms of Hb.
- Oxy- and deoxy- forms of Hb are functional because they are able to bind oxygen and carbon dioxide.
- MetHb and carboxy Hb are nonfunctional with regard to oxygen-binding capacity.
- So_2 corresponds to the percentage of Hb that is bound to oxygen, relative to the amount of functional Hb (oxy +deoxy Hb).
- Fo_2 corresponds to the percentage of Hb that is bound to oxygen, relative to the amount of total Hb (functional +nonfunctional forms).

12. A. Elevated serum and urine levels of calcium and inorganic phosphate.
Rationale: Serum levels of phosphate are low in primary hyperparathyroidism.
B. Elevated levels of serum calcium and inorganic phosphate, elevated levels of urine calcium, and low levels of urine inorganic phosphate.
Rationale: Serum phosphate levels are low and urine phosphate levels are high in primary hyperparathyroidism.
C. Elevated levels of serum and urine calcium and low levels of serum and urine inorganic phosphate.
Rationale: Urine phosphate levels are high in primary hyperparathyroidism.
D. Elevated levels of serum calcium, low levels of serum inorganic phosphate, low levels of urine calcium, and elevated levels of urine inorganic phosphate.
Rationale: Urine calcium levels are elevated in primary hyperparathyroidism.
E. Elevated levels of serum and urine calcium, low levels of serum inorganic phosphate, and elevated levels of urine inorganic phosphate.
Rationale: Urine phosphate levels and urine calcium levels are high in primary hyperparathyroidism, and serum phosphate levels are low in primary hyperparathyroidism.

Major points of discussion
- Facts about primary hyperparathyroidism:
  - Defined as an increased secretion of PTH by abnormal parathyroid glands.
  - Incidence is 1:1000, with a female/male ratio of 3:1.
  - Peak incidence occurs at 30 to 60 years of age.
  - Symptoms are often vague and include the following:
    - Bone pain, osteoporosis, kidney stones, polyuria, vomiting, nausea constipation, fatigue, and depression.
  - In approximately 85% of the cases, it is caused by a single, benign, parathyroid adenoma.
    - The remaining are caused by multiple adenomas and/or diffuse enlargement of all the parathyroid glands.
- PTH is an 84–amino-acid polypeptide with a molecular mass of 9425 Da that is synthesized and secreted by the chief cells of the parathyroid gland. Calcium homoeostasis is maintained by the actions of PTH on the bone, kidney, and indirectly in the intestine.
  - In bone, PTH mobilizes calcium and phosphate to the extracellular fluid, increasing circulating calcium and phosphate concentrations.
  - In the kidney, PTH increases renal tubular reabsorption of calcium, decreases tubular reabsorption of phosphate, and increases the excretion of phosphate.
  - In the intestine, PTH increases the absorption of dietary calcium by increasing the renal synthesis of 1,25-dihydroxyvitamin D, which stimulates intestinal absorption of calcium and phosphate.
- Laboratory parameters in primary hyperparathyroidism
  - Elevated serum PTH levels resulting from increased secretion by the abnormal parathyroid glands.
  - Elevated serum calcium levels caused by the actions of PTH.

- Low serum inorganic phosphate levels caused by increased renal phosphate excretion.
- Increased urine levels of calcium and inorganic phosphate caused by increased secretion.

■ The treatment of primary hyperparathyroidism involves surgical removal of the hypersecreting parathyroid glands. Intraoperative PTH measurements are used to determine the success or failure of the procedure. The rationale for using PTH measurements to monitor parathyroid surgery is that PTH is produced only in the parathyroid glands. PTH has a short circulating half-life in patients with normal renal function; the intact PTH molecule has a half-life of less than 5 minutes. A rapid 50% decrease in PTH concentrations is observed if all hyperplastic/adenomatous parathyroid tissue has been removed. The secretion of PTH by the abnormal gland suppresses PTH secretion by the nearby normal parathyroid glands. After removal of the hyperplastic/adenomatous tissue, the normal glands begin to secrete PTH at appropriate levels.[2,20]

13. A. Plasma potassium.
Rationale: Potassium is an important cation and contributes to plasma osmolality.
B. Plasma sodium.
Rationale: Plasma sodium contributes greatly to osmolality; this factor alone can be used to estimate osmolality in plasma.
C. Urine sodium.
Rationale: Urine sodium is important in the differential diagnosis, helping to distinguish between various causes of hyponatremia.
D. Plasma calcium.
Rationale: Calcium does not contribute greatly to plasma osmolality.
E. Plasma glucose.
Rationale: Glucose is an important analyte that contributes to plasma osmolality.

Major points of discussion
■ The hypothalamus responds to changes in osmolality, which is mainly composed of sodium and associated anions.
■ Osmolality is regulated by changes in water balance, with hyperosmolality stimulating secretion of ADH.
■ Sodium levels are also regulated by blood volume, primarily through the renin-angiotensin-aldosterone system.
■ The osmolality of plasma (in mmol/L) can be estimated by the equation $2 \times [Na^+]$.
■ Approximately 75% of the NaCl in plasma is osmotically active. Therefore, 1 mole of NaCl dissociates into 0.75 mol $Na^+ + 0.75$ mol $Cl^- + 0.25$ mol NaCl.

14. A. Elevated circulating chloride and glucose levels.
Rationale: Elevated circulating chloride and glucose concentrations will not affect the indirect ISE assay.
B. Elevated circulating protein and lipid levels.
Rationale: Elevated circulating protein and lipid concentrations will lower sodium levels obtained by an indirect method.
C. Decreased circulating protein and lipid levels.
Rationale: Low circulating protein and lipid concentrations will not affect the indirect ISE assay.

D. Decreased circulating protein and glucose levels.
Rationale: Low circulating protein and glucose concentrations will not affect the indirect ISE assay.
E. Decreased circulating protein and chloride levels.
Rationale: Low circulating protein and chloride concentrations will not affect the indirect ISE assay.

Major points of discussion
■ ISE methods for measuring sodium use a glass ion-exchange membrane. Direct ISE methods measure sodium in an undiluted sample. Indirect ISE methods measure sodium in a prediluted sample.
■ The dilution-based ISE method determines the concentration of sodium in the total sample volume, which includes dissolved solids as well as water. However, the clinically relevant sodium value is the plasma water concentration, not the total plasma concentration.
■ In the dilution method, sodium is calculated based on the assumption that 93% of plasma is water. However, in cases of severe hyperlipidemia, or in patients with large amounts of monoclonal proteins or with polyclonal gammopathies, the dissolved solids will increase and the percentage of plasma water will decrease.
■ When there is a decrease in plasma water, the calculated plasma sodium concentration will decrease. For example, if the serum protein concentration is 8.0 g/dL and the triglyceride concentration is 6.0 g/dL, the dissolved solids will comprise 14 g of every 100 g of plasma; this is equivalent to 14%, resulting in a water content of 86%. In this case, the sodium concentration will be decreased by 86/93, or 8%. This condition is termed "pseudohyponatremia" and is observed in patients with hyperlipidemia or with elevated protein concentrations.
■ Specimens with elevated concentrations of lipids or proteins do not affect the direct ISE methods because they measure the sodium concentration directly in plasma and make no assumption about the water content.

15. A. Congestive heart failure.
Rationale: Prerenal azotemia will be observed in patients with congestive heart failure, resulting in a high BUN/creatinine ratio.
B. A high-protein diet.
Rationale: A high-protein diet will result in a high BUN/creatinine ratio.
C. Acute tubular necrosis.
Rationale: Acute tubular necrosis will result in increases in both BUN and creatinine, with variable effects on the BUN/creatinine ratio.
D. Acute glomerular injury.
Rationale: Acute glomerular injury leads to increases in both BUN and creatinine, resulting in either a normal or elevated BUN/creatinine ratio.
E. Severe liver disease.
Rationale: Liver disease will result in a low BUN/creatinine ratio. Malnutrition will lead to the same effect.

Major points of discussion
■ Urea is synthesized in the liver from the ammonia produced by the deamination of amino acids. Urea is the major excretion product of protein metabolism.

■ Although blood urea concentration increases as glomerular filtration declines, urea is a poor marker for kidney disease because urea production rates are not constant and depend on the activity of the urea cycle enzymes and the protein load.

■ Urea, as BUN, is usually measured along with creatinine. Therefore, the BUN/creatinine ratio may be used as a diagnostic tool. The normal serum or plasma BUN/creatinine ratio is 10 to 20. A low BUN/creatinine ratio is seen in patients following a low-protein diet and in severe liver disease because of the reduced synthesis of urea.

■ In a healthy individual, a high-protein diet will result in an increased synthesis of urea, resulting in a high BUN/creatinine ratio.

■ In renal tubular injury, the BUN and creatinine increase in parallel and a normal BUN/creatinine ratio is often maintained.[19]

16. A. The calculation requires the serum creatinine and urine creatinine levels along with patient age, gender, and race.
Rationale: Urine creatinine concentrations are not used to calculate the GFR using the MDRD equation.
B. The calculation requires the serum creatinine and BUN levels along with patient age, gender, and race.
Rationale: BUN concentrations are not used to calculate the GFR using the MDRD equation.
C. The calculation requires the serum creatinine and cystatin C levels along with patient age, gender, and race.
Rationale: Cystatin C concentrations are not used to calculate the GFR using the MDRD equation.
D. The calculation requires the serum and urine creatinine levels along with the volume of urine.
Rationale: Urine volume is not used to calculate the GFR using the MDRD equation.
E. The calculation uses the serum creatinine level along with patient age, gender, and race.
Rationale: The estimated GFR is calculated based on the serum creatinine level, age, gender, and race of the patient.

Major points of discussion

■ The GFR is calculated from the equation derived from the MDRD study. The estimated GFR is calculated based on the serum creatinine level, age, gender, and race of the patient. BUN and albumin were originally included in the calculation but were found to yield inaccurate results.

■ GFR is used to estimate kidney function. A decrease in GFR precedes kidney failure. A GFR value of more than 60 mL/min/1.73 m^2 is considered normal.

■ The MDRD equation was validated against an iothalamate reference method for estimating the GFR. The GFR calculated by the MDRD equation is more accurate than the GFR calculated from the creatinine clearance, and it is the most commonly used equation in the United States for estimating the GFR.

■ A limitation of the MDRD equation is that it shows a negative bias at high GFR values. Therefore, it has been recommended that the numerical value of the GFR calculated using the MDRD equation be reported only up to 60 mL/min/1.73 m^2.

■ An equation from the Chronic Kidney Disease Epidemiology Collaboration (CKD-EPI) study, which is based on the log serum creatinine concentration along with age, gender, and race, has also been used to calculate the GFR. The CKD-EPI equation more accurately

categorized the risk of kidney disease and mortality than the MDRD equation. Many other equations have been derived that estimate the GFR.

■ Serum creatinine level is not a perfect marker for GFR. Tubular secretion, diet, drugs, muscle mass, and analytical interferences affect the creatinine concentration.[22]

17. **A. Metabolic acidosis with an elevated anion gap.**
Rationale: The patient has a metabolic acidosis with an elevated anion gap.
B. Metabolic acidosis with a normal anion gap.
C. Respiratory acidosis with an elevated anion gap.
Rationale: The P_{CO_2} is elevated in respiratory acidosis.
D. Renal tubular acidosis (RTA).
Rationale: In renal tubular acidosis, the anion gap is normal.
E. Respiratory acidosis with a normal anion gap.
Rationale for B and E: In this patient, the anion gap is elevated.

Major points of discussion

■ Metabolic acidosis can be caused by an increase in the production of organic acids. In uncontrolled diabetes, acetoacetic acid and hydroxybutyric acid are produced by the oxidation of fatty acids. Lactic acidosis can be observed after extreme muscle excretion and in hypoxia, when there is decreased oxygen delivery to tissues.

■ In addition, ingestion of toxic compounds that are metabolized to acid metabolites (e.g., methanol is converted to formic acid; ethylene glycol is converted to oxalic acid) will also result in metabolic acidosis.

■ Metabolic organic acids react with plasma HCO_3^- to form carbonic acid, which is converted to CO_2 gas and is eliminated from the body by ventilation. In this setting, there is a decrease in HCO_3^- concentration with little or no loss of P_{CO_2}.

■ The anion gap is the difference between the measured cations and the measured anions. The anion gap is calculated as [measured cations (Na+K)] – [measured anions (Cl+HCO$_3$)]. The reference range is 7 to 16 mmol/L.

■ In the case described in this question, the anion gap is 25 mmol/L. An elevated anion gap is observed when organic acids cause the acidosis.

■ In metabolic acidosis, HCO_3^- is decreased and P_{CO_2} can be normal or slightly decreased. The $HCO_3^-/0.03\ P_{CO_2}$ ratio, which is used in the Henderson-Hasselbalch equation to calculate the pH, is decreased, thereby causing the low pH.

■ Compensation of metabolic acidosis is achieved by hyperventilation, which decreases the P_{CO_2} and increases the $HCO_3^-/0.03\ P_{CO_2}$ ratio, thereby helping to increase the pH.[25]

18. A. Metabolic alkalosis with an elevated anion gap.
B. Respiratory acidosis with an elevated anion gap.
C. Metabolic acidosis with a normal anion gap.
Rationale: In the setting of diarrhea, the metabolic acidosis occurs as the result of an increased loss of HCO_3^- through the gastrointestinal tract. The anion gap is normal in diarrhea.
D. Metabolic acidosis with an elevated anion gap.
Rationale for A, B, and D: The anion gap is normal in diarrhea.

E. RTA type 2 with an elevated anion gap.
Rationale: RTA type 2 is caused by decreased reabsorption of HCO_3^-. The anion gap is normal in renal tubular acidosis.

Major points of discussion

- In diarrhea, metabolic acidosis occurs as the result of an increased loss of HCO_3^- through the gastrointestinal tract. The pancreas produces large amounts of HCO_3^-, which is reabsorbed in the distal small bowel and colon. Patients with severe diarrhea can lose significant amounts of HCO_3^- in a short period of time.
- In severe diarrhea, in addition to HCO_3^-, there is a loss of Na^+ and K^+ as part of the watery stool. As HCO_3^- is lost, chloride ions are reabsorbed along with Na^+ or K^+ to maintain electrical neutrality. If the water, K^+, and HCO_3^- in the intestine are not reabsorbed, hypokalemia, along with a normal anion gap, will occur.
- The $HCO_3^-/0.03$ Pco_2 ratio, which is used in the Henderson-Hasselbalch equation to calculate the pH, is decreased resulting in a low pH.
- In diarrhea, although chloride ions may be elevated, the anion gap is in the normal range.
- In severe diarrhea, if there are no additional organic acids present (e.g., lactic acid and acetoacetic acid), the anion gap will be normal.[25]

19. A. Metabolic acidosis.
Rationale: The pH is low in metabolic acidosis.
B. Respiratory acidosis.
Rationale: The pH is low in respiratory acidosis.
C. Metabolic alkalosis.
Rationale: The pH is low [high] in metabolic alkalosis. Pco_2 is normal or slightly increased.
D. Diabetic ketoacidosis (DKA).
Rationale: The pH is low in DKA.
E. Respiratory alkalosis.
Rationale: The Pco_2 is low in respiratory alkalosis.

Major points of discussion

- Metabolic alkalosis can result, for example, from ingestion of large amounts of alkali antacids or aggressive intravenous treatment with bicarbonate solutions. Loss of gastric hydrochloric acid from the stomach caused by severe vomiting, or aspiration of gastric fluids, can also result in metabolic alkalosis.
- Hypovolemia (e.g., from severe vomiting) will result in reabsorption of Na^+ to restore volume, and the renal retention of HCO_3^- in the presence of low chloride concentrations to maintain electrical neutrality. The decrease of chloride in metabolic alkalosis is known as hypochloremic alkalosis.
- In addition, K^+ and H^+ are excreted in exchange for Na^+, which will increase the blood pH. The urine pH may be acidic in metabolic alkalosis.
- The anion gap is the difference between the measured cations and the measured anions. The anion gap is calculated as [measured cations (Na+K)] − [measured anions (Cl+HCO_3^-)]. The reference range is usually 7 to 16 mmol/L. In the case in this question, the anion gap was 9 mmol/L. A normal anion gap is usually observed in metabolic alkalosis.

- In metabolic alkalosis, HCO_3^- is increased, Pco_2 is normal or slightly increased, and the $HCO_3^-/0.03$ Pco_2 ratio, which is used in the Henderson-Hasselbalch equation to calculate the pH, is increased, which causes the elevated blood pH.[14,25]

20. **A. Metabolic alkalosis with respiratory compensation.**
Rationale: The pH is elevated in metabolic alkalosis, but it is near normal in this patient because of respiratory compensation (increased Pco_2).
B. Metabolic alkalosis.
Rationale: The pH is elevated in metabolic alkalosis.
C. Metabolic acidosis.
Rationale: The pH is low in metabolic acidosis.
D. Respiratory acidosis.
Rationale: The pH is low in respiratory acidosis.
E. Respiratory alkalosis with metabolic compensation.
Rationale: The Pco_2 is not elevated in respiratory alkalosis.

Major points of discussion

- In metabolic alkalosis, the $HCO_3^-/0.03$ Pco_2 ratio, which is used in the Henderson-Hasselbalch equation to calculate the pH, is increased.
- The increase in blood pH depresses the respiratory center. The physiological response to metabolic alkalosis is hypoventilation, which raises the Pco_2 (partial pressure of carbon dioxide) and HCO_3^- concentrations in the blood.
- The rise in Pco_2 is greater than the increase in HCO_3^-. As a result, the $HCO_3^-/0.03$ Pco_2 ratio is decreased, which lowers the pH. However, the actual concentrations of both HCO_3^- and Pco_2 remain elevated.
- The result of this physiological compensation is a pH level that is at, or close to, the reference range in the presence of an elevated HCO_3^- level.
- This physiological mechanism for adjusting the pH during metabolic alkalosis is termed compensatory respiratory acidosis.[25]

21. A. Predicts glomerulonephritis.
Rationale: Microalbuminuria is not used to predict glomerulonephritis.
B. Contributes to multiple myeloma staging.
Rationale: Beta-2 microglobulin is used in the staging of multiple myeloma.
C. Identifies the presence of end-stage renal disease.
Rationale: Microalbuminuria is not used to detect end-stage renal disease.
D. Predicts kidney transplant rejection.
Rationale: Microalbuminuria is not used to predict kidney rejection.
E. Predicts diabetic nephropathy.
Rationale: Microalbuminuria is an indicator of deteriorating renal function in diabetic patients and is the first abnormal biochemical marker to appear in diabetic nephropathy.

Major points of discussion

- Microalbuminuria is defined as the presence of low, but abnormal, levels of albumin in urine—low enough that they are not detectable by urine dipstick measurements. The term "microalbuminuria" is misleading because it suggests the presence of an abnormally low-molecular-weight albumin molecule. The albumin that is measured in urine is the same molecule as the albumin circulating in the blood

- Diabetic nephropathy is the leading cause of chronic renal failure in the United States. The number of patients with diabetic nephropathy reflects the increase in the prevalence of obesity, metabolic syndrome, and type 2 diabetes in the United States.
- Microalbuminuria is an indicator of deteriorating renal function in diabetic patients and is the first abnormal biochemical marker to appear in diabetic nephropathy. Microalbuminuria occurs because of structural changes in the glomerular filtration barrier, which cause leakage of albumin.
- Elevated levels of albumin in urine appear before there is a decrease in the glomerular filtration rate. In diabetic patients, microalbuminuria is also an important risk factor for predicting the development of cardiovascular disease.
- Patients with diabetes should have their microalbumin levels measured at least once per year. If an elevated microalbumin level is obtained, other risk factors (hypertension, obesity, and so forth) should be controlled to prevent or delay the onset of renal damage.[3,35]

22. A. Increased serum BUN and creatinine concentrations.
Rationale: BUN and creatinine are elevated in nephrotic syndrome, but they are not the major abnormalities in this setting.
B. Increased serum cystatin C concentration.
Rationale: Cystatin C is elevated in nephrotic syndrome but is not the major abnormality in this setting.
C. Increased serum cholesterol concentration.
Rationale: Cholesterol is elevated in nephrotic syndrome but is not the major abnormality in this setting.
D. Microalbuminuria.
Rationale: Significant proteinuria, much greater than that seen with microalbuminuria, is observed in nephrotic syndrome.
E. Proteinuria of greater than 3.0 g/day.
Rationale: Significant proteinuria is observed in the nephrotic syndrome.

Major points of discussion
- Nephrotic syndrome is defined as proteinuria of more than 3.0 g/day, hyperlipidemia, hypoalbuminemia, and edema. Proteinuria of more than 3.0 g/day is the most significant laboratory finding in nephrotic syndrome. Other laboratory findings seen include elevated serum BUN, creatinine, and α_2-macroglobulin concentrations, and an elevated urine albumin concentration.
- Nephrotic syndrome can be caused by primary kidney disease, such as focal segmental glomerulosclerosis and membranous nephropathy, or can result from secondary causes, such as diabetes mellitus and infections. Renal biopsy plays a major role in the evaluation of patients with nephrotic syndrome.
- The "nephrotic pattern" results from the loss of albumin and other low-molecular-weight serum proteins through the damaged nephron.
- Physiological attempts to compensate for nephrotic syndrome by restoring oncotic pressure include increasing the synthesis of large-molecular-weight proteins, such as α_2-macroglobulin and lipoproteins. Dyslipidemia results in an increase in total cholesterol

and low-density lipoprotein cholesterol, which contributes to an increase in cardiovascular mortality in these patients.
- The reduction of circulating levels of albumin caused by renal loss, accompanied by decreased urine output, ultimately leads to edema.[18,32]

23a. A. Renal artery ultrasound.
Rationale: Renal artery ultrasound is used when prerenal defects, such as would be implied by a BUN/creatinine ratio more than 20, are suspected.
B. Serum and urine osmolality.
Rationale: The most likely etiology of his renal failure is intrinsic renal disease because the patient's BUN/creatinine ratio is between 10 and 20, and he was recently exposed to nephrotoxic agents. To determine whether the damage is in the glomerular or tubular compartment of the kidney, examination of urine and serum osmolality during fluid restriction is informative. A normal ratio of urine to serum osmolality implies properly functioning tubules and suggests glomerular injury. A low ratio (<1.2 in a fluid-restricted sample) suggests the primary concentration mechanism localized in the tubules is defective.
C. Serum potassium.
Rationale: Serum potassium is elevated in acute renal failure but is not helpful in etiologic determinations.
D. Plasma aminoglycoside levels.
Rationale: Aminoglycoside levels may be informative after the presence of tubular injury is confirmed.
E. Renal biopsy.
Rationale: An invasive procedure such as a renal biopsy is not indicated at this time.

23b. A. 6 g/dL, 0.99 g/dL, 4 g/dL.
Rationale: This is a typical profile seen in hypoalbuminemic patients.
B. 6 g/dL, 0.89 g/dL, 6 g/dL.
Rationale: The classic finding in renal failure of tubular etiology is a low calcium level with a high phosphate level. In renal tubular disease, phosphate excretion is prevented because of nonresponsiveness to PTH. This hyperphosphatemia, along with defective vitamin D regulation, contributes to hypocalcemia. The ionized calcium is a reflection of the biologically available calcium and should also be low.
C. 9 g/dL, 0.89 g/dL, 6 g/dL.
Rationale: Total calcium, not just the ionized fraction, should be low in renal failure.
D. 9 g/dL, 0.99 g/dL, 4 g/dL.
Rationale: This is a normal profile.
E. 6 g/dL, 0.99 g/dL, 2 g/dL.
Rationale: This profile is not consistent with a renal tubular etiology.

Major points of discussion
- In renal tubular disease, phosphate excretion is prevented because of nonresponsiveness to PTH.
- This hyperphosphatemia, along with defective vitamin D regulation, contributes to hypocalcemia.
- The ionized calcium is a reflection of the biologically available calcium and should also be low.
- A normal ratio of urine to serum osmolality implies properly functioning tubules and suggests glomerular injury.

- A low urine/serum osmolality (<1.2 in a fluid restricted sample) suggests the primary concentration mechanism localized in the tubules is defective.

24. A. Metabolic acidosis with a normal anion gap.
B. Metabolic acidosis with an elevated anion gap.
Rationale: In metabolic acidosis, the P_{CO_2} is normal.
C. Respiratory acidosis with an elevated anion gap.
Rationale: In respiratory alkalosis, the anion gap is normal.
D. RTA with an elevated anion gap.
Rationale: In RTA, the anion gap is normal.
E. Respiratory acidosis with a normal anion gap.
Rationale: An elevated P_{CO_2} level characterizes all causes of respiratory acidosis.

Major points of discussion

- Respiratory acidosis is caused by disorders that interfere with the ability of the lungs to expel CO_2. Decreased ventilation, caused by mechanical failure, a depressed breathing center, or physical blockage of the airways, results in respiratory acidosis.
- An elevated P_{CO_2} level characterizes all causes of respiratory acidosis. The physiological response to respiratory acidosis includes renal excretion of acids and chloride and retention of sodium and HCO_3^-.
- The anion gap is the difference between the measured cations and the measured anions. The anion gap is calculated as [measured cations (Na+K)] – [measured anions ($Cl+HCO_3^-$)]. The reference range is 7 to 16 mmol/L.
- In the case described in this question, the anion gap was 12 mmol/L. A normal anion gap is usually observed in respiratory acidosis.
- In respiratory acidosis, there is an increase in both P_{CO_2} and HCO_3^-. However, the increase in HCO_3^- is less than the increase in P_{CO_2}, and the HCO_3^-/0.03 P_{CO_2} ratio, which is used in the Henderson-Hasselbalch equation to calculate the pH, is decreased, thereby leading to a low pH.[25]

25. A. Metabolic acidosis.
Rationale: The pH is low in metabolic acidosis.
B. Respiratory acidosis.
Rationale: The pH is low in respiratory acidosis.
C. Metabolic alkalosis.
Rationale: The P_{CO_2} is normal in metabolic alkalosis.
D. Respiratory alkalosis.
Rationale: Respiratory alkalosis is caused by hyperventilation, which decreases the P_{CO_2}.
E. DKA.
Rationale: The pH is low in DKA.

Major points of discussion

- Respiratory alkalosis is caused by hyperventilation, which decreases the P_{CO_2}. Respiratory alkalosis is the result of direct stimulation of the respiratory center either by nonpulmonary or pulmonary disorders.
- Respiratory alkalosis can be caused by pulmonary disorders such as pneumonia, pulmonary embolism, interstitial lung disease, and pulmonary fibrosis. Nonpulmonary causes of respiratory alkalosis include anxiety, hysteria, fever, hypoxia, and drugs.
- The anion gap is the difference between the measured cations and the measured anions. The anion gap is

calculated as [measured cations (Na+K)] – [measured anions ($Cl+HCO_3^-$)]. The reference range is 7 to 16 mmol/L. In the case described in this question, the anion gap was 12 mmol/L. A normal anion gap is usually observed in respiratory alkalosis.
- In respiratory alkalosis, the P_{CO_2} is decreased and the HCO_3^-/0.03 P_{CO_2} ratio, which is used in the Henderson-Hasselbalch equation to calculate the pH, is increased. Respiratory alkalosis is associated with a decreased P_{CO_2}, an increased pH, and a low HCO_3^- because of renal compensation.
- Individuals living at high altitudes chronically hyperventilate because of hypoxia and typically have a lower P_{CO_2} than individuals living at sea level.[25]

26. A. Renal regulation of P_{CO_2}.
B. Renal regulation of HCO_3^-.
Rationale: Renal compensation in respiratory alkalosis occurs when the kidneys excrete increased amounts of $HCO3^-$.
C. Hyperventilation.
Rationale: Hyperventilation would decrease the P_{CO_2} and increase the pH.
D. Renal excretion of H^+.
Rationale: Excretion of hydrogen ions would result in an increase in pH.
E. Renal excretion of organic acids.
Rationale: Excretion of organic acids occurs in metabolic acidosis, resulting in an increase in pH.

Major points of discussion

- Respiratory alkalosis is caused by hyperventilation, which decreases the P_{CO_2} level. This causes an increase in the HCO_3^-/0.03 P_{CO_2} ratio in the Henderson-Hasselbalch equation, thus increasing the pH.
- In respiratory alkalosis, two types of physiological compensation are typically used to lower the HCO_3^- concentration;:tissue buffering and renal compensation.
- Compensation by tissue buffering of HCO_3^- involves both erythrocytes and tissue buffers, which provide H^+ to react with HCO_3^- to produce carbonic acid, which is then converted to CO_2 and water. The CO_2 is removed by hyperventilation.
- Renal compensation in respiratory alkalosis occurs when the kidneys excrete increased amounts of HCO_3^-. The proximal tubules of the kidney also contribute to this effect by decreasing the reabsorption of HCO_3^-. The renal response to respiratory alkalosis is termed "compensatory metabolic acidosis."
- Metabolic compensation is very effective in respiratory alkalosis and, in some cases, the pH returns to a normal level. In respiratory alkalosis,[25] alkalinization of the urine may occur as a result of the increased circulating HCO_3^-.

27. A. Low levels of calcium, 25-hydroxyvitamin D, inorganic phosphate, and PTH.
Rationale: Serum PTH levels are elevated in rickets.
B. Low levels of calcium, 25-hydroxyvitamin D, and inorganic phosphate, and an elevated PTH level.
Rationale: Rickets is a childhood disease that is primarily caused by vitamin D deficiency.
C. Low levels of calcium and 25-hydroxyvitamin D, and elevated levels of inorganic phosphate and PTH.
Rationale: Serum phosphate levels are low in rickets.

D. Low levels of calcium, 25-hydroxyvitamin D, and PTH, and an elevated inorganic phosphate level.
Rationale: Serum PTH levels are elevated and serum phosphate levels are low in rickets.
E. Elevated levels of calcium and PTH and low levels of 25-hydroxyvitamin D and inorganic phosphate.
Rationale: Serum calcium levels are low in rickets.

Major points of discussion

■ Rickets is a childhood disease that is primarily caused by vitamin D deficiency. Vitamin D is a fat-soluble hormone that is needed for bone growth and development.

■ Vitamin D is synthesized in the skin when ultraviolet B (UVB) radiation from the sun reacts with 7-dehydrocholesterol to form vitamin D_3, which is metabolized in the liver to 25-hydroxyvitamin D_3 and in the kidney to the active metabolite 1,25-dihydroxyvitamin D_3. Vitamin D can also be obtained from foods, such as fatty fish, or from vitamin supplements.

■ Vitamin D is a hormone that increases the intestinal absorption of calcium and inorganic phosphate into the blood. Without sufficient levels of vitamin D, only approximately 10% of dietary calcium and 60% of dietary phosphate are released into the circulation by passive diffusion. The stimulation of active transport of calcium and phosphate from the intestine into the blood by vitamin D accounts for approximately 40% of dietary calcium and 80% of dietary phosphate absorption.

■ In rickets, low levels of serum calcium, phosphate, and 25-hydroxyvitamin D, and elevated levels of PTH are seen. The low serum calcium level triggers the release of PTH from the parathyroid glands. PTH acts on osteoclasts to release calcium and phosphate from bone to help maintain normal calcium levels. Therefore, in rickets, the bones are soft and weak, which results in the skeletal deformities seen in these children.

■ In the United States, fortification of foods with vitamin D has significantly reduced the incidence of rickets. However, rickets is commonly seen in developing countries when the mother is vitamin D deficient and breastfeeding is the major source of infant nutrition.[12,13]

28. A. Oxyhemoglobin and carboxyhemoglobin.
Rationale: Oxyhemoglobin is functional, but carboxyhemoglobin is bound to carbon monoxide and, therefore, is nonfunctional and cannot bind oxygen or carbon dioxide.
B. Oxyhemoglobin and deoxyhemoglobin.
Rationale: Both oxyhemoglobin and deoxyhemoglobin are functional.
C. Oxyhemoglobin and methemoglobin.
Rationale: Oxyhemoglobin is functional, but methemoglobin contains the ferric form of iron; therefore, it is not functional and cannot bind oxygen or carbon dioxide.
D. Deoxyhemoglobin and carboxyhemoglobin.
Rationale: Deoxyhemoglobin is able to bind to oxygen, but carboxyhemoglobin is bound to carbon monoxide; therefore, it is nonfunctional and cannot bind oxygen or carbon dioxide.
E. Deoxyhemoglobin and methemoglobin.

Rationale: Deoxyhemoglobin can readily accept oxygen, but methemoglobin contains the ferric form of iron; therefore, it is not functional and cannot bind oxygen or carbon dioxide.

Major points of discussion

■ So_2 can range from 0 to 100% and is mathematically calculated using the following formula:
$So_2 = oxyhemoglobin/(oxyhemoglobin + deoxyhemoglobin)$.

■ Although So_2 is a measurement of functional hemoglobin that is bound to O_2, Po_2 is more commonly used in assessing oxygen-binding capacity in the lungs.

■ Decreased Po_2 can be caused by decreased pulmonary ventilation, impaired gas exchange, or altered blood flow between the heart and lungs.

■ Carboxyhemoglobin contains carbon monoxide (CO) bound to hemoglobin; carbon monoxide has a much higher affinity for hemoglobin than O_2.

■ Methemoglobin contains iron in its ferric (Fe^{3+}), not ferrous (Fe^{2+}), state and, therefore, cannot bind oxygen or carbon dioxide.

29. **A. Anticoagulant contamination.**
Rationale: Contamination with potassium-ethylenediaminetetraacetic acid (EDTA) will cause spurious hyperkalemia and hypocalcemia.
B. Chronic kidney failure.
Rationale: Chronic kidney failure is commonly associated with hyperkalemia, hyperphosphatemia, and hypocalcemia. This is unlikely in this patient with normal creatinine and normal phosphatemia.
C. Renal tubular acidosis.
Rationale: RTA will cause hyperchloremic metabolic acidosis with low total CO_2. Proximal RTA can cause hypophosphatemia, whereas distal RTA typically is associated with hypokalemia and hypercalcemia.
D. Primary hyperaldosteronism.
Rationale: Excessive mineralocorticoid activity results in hypokalemia with metabolic alkalosis.
E. Congenital adrenal hyperplasia.
Rationale: Mineralocorticoid deficiency can cause hyperkalemia with metabolic acidosis. Calcium is usually normal.

Major points of discussion

■ Spurious hyperkalemia from potassium-EDTA contamination is common, especially when liquid K_3-EDTA is used as an anticoagulant. In commonly used purple top tubes, the amount of K_2-EDTA in the tube is about 17 nmol, which will increase the potassium concentration in 4 mL of blood by about 8 mmol/L and chelate all of the ionized calcium, magnesium, and zinc in the plasma. Therefore, even relatively minor contamination with the anticoagulant can cause spurious hyperkalemia, hypocalcemia, hypomagnesemia, and hypozincemia.

■ Potassium-EDTA contamination is common and may still result in normal levels of potassium, calcium, and magnesium. This could potentially mask dangerous hypokalemia. In this case, measurement of EDTA itself is critical to identify the source of spurious results.

- Mechanisms of contamination include backflow from vacuum tubes if EDTA tubes are used before others, decanting from EDTA tubes into others, and needle contamination when EDTA tubes are used first.
- Other examples of spurious hyperkalemia include contamination from intravenous potassium infusion, prolonged tourniquet time with fist clinching, in vitro hemolysis, release from leukocytes or platelets, and cold storage of the sample before serum separation.
- Causes of true hyperkalemia include decreased renal elimination (kidney insufficiency, hypoadrenalism, type 4 RTA, potassium-sparing diuretics, cardiac failure, cirrhosis), cell lysis (rhabdomyolysis, tumor lysis syndrome, massive blood transfusion), or excessive potassium administration (diet or intravenous, usually in combination with one of the above).[4,34,37]

30a. A. Addison disease.
Rationale: Hypoadrenalism leads to hypotension, hyperkalemia, and metabolic acidosis with decreased bicarbonate and elevated chloride.
B. Conn syndrome.
Rationale: Hyperaldosteronism causes renal loss of potassium and protons, resulting in hypokalemia and hypochloremic metabolic alkalosis.
C. Syndrome of inappropriate antidiuretic hormone secretion.
Rationale: Excessive secretion of ADH leads to increased water reabsorption and hyponatremia.
D. Diabetes insipidus.
Rationale: Lack of ADH or poor response to ADH leads to loss of water with resulting polydipsia and hypernatremia if water intake is restricted.
E. Diabetes mellitus.
Rationale: Osmotic diuresis caused by hyperglycemia can lead to dehydration and hypernatremia if water intake is restricted.

30b. A. Ectopic adrenocorticotropic hormone (ACTH) production.
Rationale: This would result in increased cortisol.
B. Lung cancer–producing ADH.
Rationale: ADH is high-normal but other results (hypernatremia) are inconsistent with excess ADH production.
C. Nephrogenic diabetes insipidus.
Rationale: Hypercalcemia can cause nephrogenic diabetes insipidus; ADH is normal or elevated in the presence of water losses.
D. Central diabetes insipidus.
Rationale: This condition results in decreased ADH.
E. Diabetic nephropathy.
Rationale: This condition causes proteinuria and progressive decline in the GFR; water reabsorption is usually preserved.

30c. A. Unchanged cortisol after ACTH administration.
Rationale: This would indicate adrenal insufficiency.
B. Increased urine osmolality after water deprivation and ADH administration.
Rationale: In central diabetes insipidus, urine remains dilute with water deprivation but normalizes after ADH

administration, while in nephrogenic diabetes insipidus urine osmolality does not respond to ADH.
C. Elevated 1,25-dihydroxyvitamin D.
Rationale: Macrophages in granulomatous tissue, such as in sarcoidosis, have high levels of CYP27B1 enzyme (25-hydroxyvitamin D-1α-hydroxylase), which converts 25-hydroxyvitamin D to 1,25-dihydroxyvitamin D, causing hypercalcemia.
D. Elevated PTH-related peptide (PTHrP).
Rationale: Increased PTHrP is a possible cause of malignancy-associated hypercalcemia; in this case, sarcoidosis with elevated 1,25-dihydroxyvitamin D is a more likely cause of hypercalcemia. Rarely, sarcoidosis has been associated with elevated PTHrP; however, in most cases, it is undetectable.
E. Elevated C-peptide after a standard meal.
Rationale: This is a rarely used test to help distinguish type 1 from type 2 diabetes.

Major points of discussion

- Diabetes insipidus is defined as polyuria (>3 L/24 hr) of dilute urine (<300 mOsm/kg), caused by insufficient secretion of ADH (central diabetes insipidus) or poor response of the renal tubules to ADH (nephrogenic diabetes insipidus).
- ADH or arginine-vasopressin (AVP) is synthesized in the supraoptic and paraventricular nuclei of the hypothalamus, packaged into neurosecretory granules, which then migrate to the posterior pituitary. Secretion occurs predominantly in response to higher plasma osmolality sensed by osmoreceptors in the hypothalamus. Central diabetes insipidus results from damage to the hypothalamic-pituitary axis (e.g., surgery, tumors, trauma, vascular malformations, infarction, infectious, granulomatous, and inflammatory diseases). In this patient, neurosarcoidosis should be investigated as a possible cause of central diabetes insipidus. In children, congenital defects in ADH synthesis, storage, and release can cause central diabetes insipidus.
- Nephrogenic diabetes insipidus results from a tubular defect in the response to ADH, which is mediated by the ADH receptor (AVPR2), a G protein–coupled receptor present in the basolateral membrane of the collecting duct. Binding of ADH to AVPR2 results in activation of GαS, adenylcyclase, protein kinase A, and transport of the water channel aquaporin 2 (AQP2) present in intracellular vesicles to the apical surface of the collecting ducts. Water reabsorption from the tubular lumen is initiated by flow to the intracellular space through AQP2, followed by exit to the basolateral side through AQP3 and AQP4.
- Mutations in either *AVPR2* or *AQP2* can cause congenital nephrogenic diabetes insipidus. Acquired defects include drugs (lithium, cisplatin, foscarnet), postacute tubular necrosis, postobstruction diuresis, osmotic diuresis, and electrolyte disturbances, including hypokalemia and hypercalcemia. High levels of calcium reduce the response to ADH in the tubule, perhaps by interfering with AQP2 expression and movement to the apical surface, in addition to causing polydipsia.
- Two other forms of diabetes insipidus include primary polydipsia, where psychogenic increases in water intake result in lower plasma osmolality and suppressed ADH

production, and gestational diabetes insipidus, resulting from excessive metabolism of ADH by placental enzymes.
- The various forms of diabetes insipidus can be distinguished by performing a water deprivation test, which should be performed with close supervision given the risk of dehydration and hypovolemia. Plasma and urine osmolality is measured hourly, and the test is stopped when the urine osmolality stops increasing or the plasma osmolality exceeds 300 mOsm/kg. ADH is administered to assess the ability of the kidneys to respond. In both central and nephrogenic diabetes insipidus, the urine does not concentrate more than plasma in response to water deprivation, in contrast to psychogenic polydipsia. After ADH administration, the urine osmolality does not increase by more than 10% in nephrogenic diabetes insipidus, but it will increase by more than 50% in central diabetes insipidus.
- Sarcoidosis can cause diabetes insipidus by infiltration of the hypothalamic pituitary axis or by production of 1,25-dihydroxyvitamin D (calcitriol) from granulomatous macrophages expressing *CYP27B1*. Excessive production of calcitriol will result in increased absorption and bone mobilization of calcium and phosphorus, with resulting suppression of PTH and PTHrP.[23,30,42]

31. A. Rhabdomyolysis secondary to blood hyperviscosity.
Rationale: Hyperviscosity due to leukocytosis is usually not seen with blast counts less than 100,000/μL. Rhabdomyolysis is not typically associated with chronic myelogenous leukemia and would more likely result in hyperkalemia due to cell lysis.
B. Adrenal insufficiency due to leukemic infiltration.
Rationale: This would likely result in hyperkalemia with metabolic acidosis.
C. Acute tubular necrosis of the kidney.
Rationale: Unlikely with normal creatinine and hypokalemia.
D. Pseudohypokalemia due to leukocytosis.
Rationale: Low glucose and potassium levels are due to the consumption of glucose and potassium by metabolically active leukocytes before serum separation.
E. Lactic acidosis due to leukemic anaerobic metabolism.
Rationale: This is a rare complication of acute leukemia, possibly due to anaerobic metabolism by leukemic cells, and would manifest as an increased anion gap acidosis with low total CO_2, often with hypoglycemia and normal or elevated potassium.

Major points of discussion
- Pseudohypokalemia is common in leukemia and other causes of leukocytosis. It is caused by active intracellular influx of potassium into the leukemic cells. Factors contributing to in vitro levels of potassium include total leukocyte count, blast count (blasts have increased expression of sodium/potassium exchangers), ambient temperature, time to separation, use of clotting versus anticoagulant tubes, and mechanical trauma to the sample (e.g., pneumatic tube).
- Pseudohypokalemia is seen with ambient temperatures higher than 30°C in samples when separation of plasma has been delayed. Seasonal variations in the proportion of hypokalemia have been reported, with frequency peaking in hot summer periods. With continued

metabolic activity at temperatures higher than 30°C, consumption of glucose can lead to cell death and release of potassium from leukocytes, potentially resulting in spurious hyperkalemia.
- In contrast, pseudohyperkalemia can be seen when whole blood is incubated at lower temperatures, which inhibit the cellular metabolism required for sodium/potassium exchange, resulting in a rise of about 0.2 to 0.3 mmol/L/hr at 4°C. It is also seen in cases of leukocytosis with fragile cells (e.g., chronic lymphocytic leukemia), particularly during clotting, resulting in potassium levels higher in serum than in plasma. In some cases, reverse pseudohyperkalemia is seen when heparin induces release of potassium from leukemic cells into the plasma.
- Given the potential for misleading potassium levels (hypokalemia and hyperkalemia) in patients with high leukocyte counts, it is recommended that whole blood samples be rapidly centrifuged with a gel separator. If centrifugation must be delayed, incubation on ice may prevent spurious hypokalemia but should not exceed 1 hour to avoid pseudohyperkalemia.
- In some patients with acute leukemia, true hypokalemia occurs as a result of leukemic nephritis with renal potassium wasting. Therefore, careful attention to preanalytical factors is essential for the correct management of these patients.[21,27,36]

32. A. The normal BUN/creatinine ratio is inconsistent with dehydration.
Rationale: With adequate water intake in the setting of severe hyperglycemia with osmotic diuresis, the BUN/creatinine ratio can be normal or low despite severe water and electrolyte losses and intracellular dehydration.
B. The hyponatremia is probably due to increased extracellular water content.
Rationale: Hyperglycemia causes osmotic expansion of the extravascular compartment and dilutional hyponatremia. Plasma sodium is corrected according to the following formula: Na (corrected) = Na (measured) + 0.016 × (glucose – 100), which gives a sodium level of 147 mmol/L in the absence of osmotic expansion.
C. The hyperkalemia indicates excess total body potassium.
Rationale: Although patients can present with hyperkalemia, mainly resulting from mild acidosis and decreased activity of the sodium-potassium-ATPase pump, leading to intracellular to extracellular shifts, patients with hyperosmolar hyperglycemia are truly potassium depleted as the result of osmotic diuresis and renal losses. Careful replenishment of potassium guided by plasma levels is critical to avoid arrhythmias, cardiac arrest, and respiratory muscle weakness.
D. There is significant ketoacidosis due to insulin deficiency.
Rationale: Typically, DKA is accompanied by severe metabolic acidosis characterized by pH less than 7.30 and bicarbonate less than 15 mmol/L.
E. Effective plasma osmolality is consistent with hyperosmolar hyperglycemic state.
Rationale: Plasma osmolality can be calculated by the following formula: 2 × Na + glucose/18 + BUN/2.8, giving a result of 329 mOsm/kg in this patient (reference range, 285 to 295). Effective osmolality does not include BUN as urea freely crosses cell membranes. This patient's effective

osmolality is 323 mOsm/kg, consistent with a hyperglycemic hyperosmolar state (>320 mOsm/kg according to American Diabetic Association guidelines).

Major points of discussion

■ This patient presented with a hyperosmolar hyperglycemic state (HHS), which can be a life-threatening event. Although it may overlap with DKA, HHS can be generally by distinguished in the laboratory by plasma glucose levels greater than 600 mg/dL, effective osmolality greater than 320 mOsm/kg, pH higher than 7.30, and bicarbonate greater than 15 mmol/L, with low or absent ketonemia.

■ Marked hyperglycemia induces fluid shifts to the extravascular compartment and osmotic diuresis, resulting in intracellular hyperosmolality and dehydration.

■ The BUN/creatinine ratio reflects production of urea and creatinine, as well as the GFR (reflected by creatinine levels) and the degree of urea reabsorption in the proximal tubule. With severe hyperglycemia, osmotic diuresis occurs with high urine flow and decreased urea reabsorption. With adequate water intake, the BUN/creatinine ratio can be normal or even low in situations of high osmotic diuresis, despite significant intracellular dehydration. While osmotic diuresis depletes the extracellular compartment of water, the BUN/creatinine ratio increases in proportion to the degree of dehydration. Most patients with HHS present with dehydration and an elevated BUN/creatinine ratio.

■ The measurement of sodium truly reflects its concentration in the extravascular fluid but it should be appropriately corrected by the degree of hyperglycemia to estimate total body sodium. This should not be confused with pseudohyponatremia caused by reduced plasma water (e.g., with hypertriglyceridemia, hyperproteinemia) when indirect ion-specific electrodes make these measurements.

■ The actual plasma sodium concentration reflects the balance of water distribution between the extracellular and intracellular compartments, as well as between water and sodium intake and losses. In HHS, the average sodium is 144 mmol/L, but it can be low (as in this patient) or elevated, especially because water losses tend to be higher than sodium losses as a result of osmotic diuresis. In virtually all cases of HHS, the total body sodium (and potassium) stores are depleted because of large renal losses, even when plasma concentrations are normal or high.[17]

33. A. Type 1 diabetes complicated by urinary tract infection.
Rationale: This presentation mimics DKA, but the lack of elevated hemoglobin A1c and autoantibodies associated with type 1 diabetes makes it less likely.
B. Fatty acid oxidation defect.
Rationale: Typically presents with hypoglycemia and low ketones.
C. Pyruvate dehydrogenase deficiency.
Rationale: Typically presents with lactic acidosis and elevated pyruvate.
D. Malnutrition with chronic vitamin B_{12} deficiency.
Rationale: Unlikely in the presence of normal levels of vitamin B_{12} and homocysteine.
E. Adenosylcobalamin synthesis defect.

Rationale: This condition causes accumulation of methylmalonic acid but not homocysteine, explaining the patient's condition.

Major points of discussion

■ This patient presented with a clinical picture similar to DKA, with dehydration, hyperglycemia, ketonuria, and high anion gap metabolic acidosis. In infants with severe metabolic decompensation, inconsistent laboratory findings (such as normal hemoglobin A1c and negative autoimmune antibodies), consanguineous parents and/or lack of response to conventional therapy should point to the possibility of an inborn error of metabolism (IEM).

■ The clinical presentation of ketoacidosis with high anion gap points to organic acidemia. The most important causes of organic acidemia resulting from an IEM are methylmalonic acidemia and the related propionyl acidemia. Propionyl-CoA is derived from the metabolism of isoleucine, valine, methionine, threonine, and thymine, as well as cholesterol and odd-chain fatty acids and is converted to methylmalonyl-CoA by propionyl-carboxylase.

■ Vitamin B_{12} is metabolized to methylcobalamin and adenosylcobalamin. Adenosylcobalamin is required for the mitochondrial enzyme methylmalonyl CoA mutase (MUT), which isomerizes methylmalonyl-CoA to succinyl-COA. Defects in MUT or adenosylcobalamin formation result in methylmalonic acid accumulation. Methylcobalamin is required for the cytoplasmic enzyme methionine synthase, which adds a methyl group to homocysteine to form methionine. In isolated deficiencies of methylcobalamin formation, levels of homocysteine would be increased. In deficiencies of cobalamin, such as pernicious anemia or nutritional vitamin B_{12} deficiency, both methylmalonic acid and homocysteine would be elevated.

■ Patients with methylmalonic or propionic acidemia typically present with hypoglycemia, possibly caused by inhibition of gluconeogenesis by propionate, methylmalonate, or their acyl-CoA derivatives. However, acute decompensation with severe ketoacidosis and hyperglycemia can be a rare presentation. In some of these cases, the hyperglycemia responds to insulin therapy and treatment of the underlying precipitating factor, such as infection. In other cases, lack of response to insulin treatment points to an IEM as a possible cause.

■ Measurement of C3-acylcarnitine (propionyl-carnitine) by tandem mass-spectrometry is used as a prenatal screening tool for propionyl or methylmalonyl acidemia. In these defects, backup flux leads to accumulation of propionyl-CoA and its conversion to propionyl-carnitine and expulsion from the mitochondria.

■ Secondary lactic acidosis results from depletion of succinyl-CoA, which leads to impaired oxidative phosphorylation and therefore increased anaerobic glycolysis with lactate accumulation. The lactate/pyruvate ratio increases in situations distal to pyruvate dehydrogenase, as is the case with impaired oxidative phosphorylation, while a normal ratio with increases in both pyruvate and lactate indicates a deficiency in pyruvate dehydrogenase or other steps of gluconeogenesis.[6,10,33]

34. A. A standard meal will decrease plasma phosphate levels within 2 hours.
Rationale: Release of intracellular phosphates from organic foods often results in increases in phosphatemia by 15% approximately 2 hours after a standard meal. Within 2 to 3 hours postprandial, insulin induces glucose and phosphate uptake by cells with gradual normalization of phosphate levels.
B. A shift from supine to upright position causes increases in plasma calcium.
Rationale: Increased total calcium parallels a 10% to 15% increase in albumin.
C. Acute ethanol intoxication is frequently associated with metabolic alkalosis.
Rationale: Metabolism of ethanol to acetate leads to metabolic acidosis, often compounded by associated ketoacidosis resulting from inhibition of glycolysis by alcohol.
D. Vigorous exercise often leads to lower potassium levels.
Rationale: Vigorous exercise can result in transient hyperkalemia, as high as 8 mmol/L in arterial blood, especially in poorly trained individuals. Well-trained athletes have a higher density of sodium-potassium exchangers in their muscles and much lower increases in potassium.
E. Stress (e.g., during acute myocardial infarction) often causes hyperkalemia.
Rationale: Catecholamines acting through β-adrenergic receptors induce intracellular influx and renal excretion of potassium. Hypokalemia is frequent in acute myocardial infarction and can predispose patients to severe arrhythmias.

Major points of discussion
- Interpretation of electrolyte measurements must take into consideration preanalytical variables affecting electrolyte concentrations. For example, posture, exercise, meals, drugs, and stress can cause transient changes in some electrolyte levels that are sufficient to confound interpretation of test results if those effects are not considered.
- Postural effects can affect plasma electrolyte levels. Compared with recumbency, the upright position causes increased intravascular pressure and a flow of fluid from the intravascular to the extravascular compartment, resulting in about an 8% to 15% decrease in plasma volume and corresponding increase in hematocrit. With normal permeability, substances larger than 4 nm in diameter (such as proteins) are retained in the intravascular space, while water and electrolytes flow into the extravascular space. While most electrolytes are not complexed and equilibrate rapidly between the two compartments, the portion of total calcium that is protein bound (around 40%) is retained in the intravascular compartment and its concentration can increase by about 5% to 10%. Only 25% to 30% of magnesium is complexed with albumin, and therefore, increases only by about 3% to 5%. In addition, posture induces changes in the renin-angiotensin-aldosterone axis with corresponding effects in renal excretion of sodium and potassium.
- Exercise can lead to increased release of intracellular ions such as potassium, phosphate, and magnesium.

Although total calcium does not change with exercise, lactate production during intense exercise may cause pH-induced dissociation of protein-bound calcium and transient increases in ionized calcium.
- Meals can cause transient increases in intracellular ions, particularly phosphate (up to 15%) and potassium (up to 5%), which are followed by insulin-stimulated intracellular influx and normalization within 2 to 3 hours.
- Many drugs affect plasma electrolyte concentrations, particularly those affecting renal and cardiovascular function such as diuretics and angiotensin-converting enzyme inhibitors.
- Ethanol intoxication can cause ketosis and metabolic acidosis. Excess protons in metabolic acidosis compete with potassium for intracellular influx and may result in hyperkalemia.
- In addition to mineralocorticoids, various hormones affect electrolyte levels. For example, insulin and catecholamines induce intracellular influx of potassium and phosphate.[15]

35. A. Ethanol contamination during phlebotomy.
Rationale: This will cause hemolysis and hyperkalemia in both plasma and serum.
B. Prolonged tourniquet time with fist clenching.
Rationale: This will cause release of potassium from muscle; however, both plasma and serum potassium should be elevated.
C. Thrombocytosis.
Rationale: Elevated platelet counts will cause release of potassium during clotting, with serum potassium higher than plasma (about 0.15 mmol/L per 100,000 platelets/μL).
D. Leukocytosis.
Rationale: Leukocytosis can cause mild pseudohyperkalemia in both serum and plasma samples caused by the release from leukocytes, particularly from fragile cells such as in chronic leukemias.
E. Familial pseudohyperkalemia.
Rationale: This condition is characterized by plasma potassium higher than serum and increases in plasma and serum potassium if cell separation is delayed.

Major points of discussion
- Spurious hyperkalemia is the artifactual increase in potassium levels in vitro and is one of the most common sources of misleading results in the clinical laboratory. "Pseudohyperkalemia" is strictly defined as serum potassium levels higher than plasma potassium by more than 0.4 mmol/L, whereas in "reverse pseudohyperkalemia" the plasma potassium is higher than serum potassium.
- Hemolysis is the most frequent cause of spurious hyperkalemia. Since the intracellular concentration of potassium is about 105 mmol/L in red cells, even a minor amount of hemolysis results in significant increases in plasma potassium. On average, potassium increases about 0.2 to 0.5 mmol/L per 0.1 g/dL of plasma hemoglobin. Hemolysis is typically visible with the naked eye when plasma hemoglobin is above 20 to 70 mg/dL. Potentially clinically significant spurious increases in potassium generally occur with hemoglobin levels above 100 mg/dL (corresponding

to lysis of about 0.7% of the red cells with a hematocrit of 45%).

- Causes of hemolysis include ethanol contamination, difficult phlebotomy, inappropriate needle diameter, collection with syringe and needle, inappropriate storage or transport temperature, transport via pneumatic tube, excessive centrifugation speed, and so on. A particular problem is spurious hyperkalemia during whole blood analysis, which does not benefit from visual or spectrometric detection of plasma hemoglobin.
- Additional causes of spurious hyperkalemia include contamination with intravenous fluids high in potassium and with anticoagulants containing potassium, most frequently K2-EDTA, which will also cause spurious hypocalcemia.
- In vitro release of potassium from other blood cells in the absence of hemolysis can also occur with thrombocytosis and leukocytosis, particularly with fragile leukocytes, such as in chronic lymphocytic and chronic myelomonocytic leukemia. The degree of spurious potassium elevation tends to be higher in serum than plasma because of cell lysis during clotting. However, in certain cases, reverse pseudohyperkalemia is seen, with heparin-induced lysis of leukemic cells and consequent higher levels in plasma than serum.
- Prolonged application of a tourniquet, especially when coupled with fist clenching, can result in release of potassium from muscle without signs of hemolysis. Prolonged incubation of unseparated blood at refrigerated temperatures inhibits the sodium-potassium ATPase that maintains high levels of intracellular potassium. Similarly, prolonged incubation at temperatures higher than 30°C can lead to consumption of glucose and dysfunction of the ATPase.
- Familial pseudohyperkalemia (FP) is caused by an autosomal dominant gene defect, leading to leakage of potassium at temperature less than 37°C. This defect is due to structural alterations in the red cell membrane that increases permeability at lower temperatures. Recent evidence implicates mutations in the ABCB6 transporter in FP. Similar defects with ion leakage are also seen in some hereditary stomatocytoses. Prompt separation of plasma from cells after blood collection is essential for accurate potassium measurements. This condition has no clinical significance other than erroneous interpretation of potassium levels, leading to inappropriate therapeutic intervention.[1,37]

36a. A. Organic aciduria.
Rationale: Congenital defects in organic acid metabolism can cause metabolic acidosis with increased anion gap.
B. Type 1 (distal) RTA.
Rationale: Characterized by failure to acidify urine (pH >5.3, usually ~6.5) in the presence of hyperchloremic metabolic acidosis.
C. Type 2 (proximal) RTA.
Rationale: This condition best explains hyperchloremic metabolic acidosis with proper urine acidification, glycosuria, and hypophosphatemia.
D. Hyporeninemic hypoaldosteronism.
Rationale: This condition (type IV renal tubular acidosis) would cause hyperkalemia and would not explain glycosuria and hypophosphatemia.

E. DKA.
Rationale: Ketoacidosis would cause increased anion gap metabolic acidosis with hyperglycemia.

36b. A. High urinary levels of methylmalonic acid by gas chromatography–mass spectrometry.
Rationale: This would be expected with organic aciduria due to defects in methylmalonic acid metabolism.
B. Increased urinary pH after NH_4Cl load.
Rationale: Failure to acidify urine after acid load is typical of type 1 RTA.
C. Elevated fractionary urinary excretion of HCO_3 after bicarbonate load.
Rationale: Losses of bicarbonate in the proximal renal tubule are characteristic of type 2 RTA.
D. Decreased plasma aldosterone/renin ratio.
Rationale: In hyporeninemic hypoaldosteronism the ratio may be normal, increased, or decreased, but both aldosterone and renin are low.
E. High plasma levels of β-hydroxybutyrate.
Rationale: This is one of the ketone bodies elevated in DKA.

Major points of discussion

- RTA is defined as hyperchloremic metabolic acidosis (normal anion gap) caused by urinary losses of acid as a result of tubular defects. It can be subclassified as type 1 (distal), 2 (proximal), and 4 (hyporeninemic hypoaldosteronism). Type 3 refers to a mixed proximal and distal condition and does not represent a distinct clinical entity.
- Type 1 RTA is caused by insufficient H^+ excretion at the distal tubule. Therefore, the kidney is unable to eliminate excessive acid and acidify the urine in situations of systemic acidosis. Causes include calcium-induced tubular damage, drugs (e.g., lithium, amphotericin B, nonsteroidal anti-inflammatory drugs), toxins (toluene), paraproteins, autoimmune disorders, and genetic defects in distal transporters (SLC4A1, ATP6V1B1, ATP6V0A4). Since acid excretion is reduced, sodium preferably exchanges with potassium at the distal tube, and hypokalemia can be present. In hyperkalemic type I RTA, the sodium load to the distal tube is reduced and therefore potassium secretion is impaired. This can result from any cause of marked volume depletion with enhanced proximal tubule reabsorption of sodium or from inhibition of distal sodium reabsorption with potassium-sparing diuretics, lithium, trimethoprim, sickle cell nephropathy, lupus nephritis, or urinary obstruction.
- Type 2 RTA is caused by failure of the proximal tubule to reabsorb bicarbonate. When the distal tubule is unable to reabsorb all the excessive bicarbonate lost by the proximal tubule, bicarbonaturia results with a consequent decrease in plasma bicarbonate (metabolic acidosis) and contraction of the plasma volume, leading to increases in aldosterone secretion and hypokalemia. Although the plasma bicarbonate stabilizes at a lower level and the distal tubule increases bicarbonate reabsorption and acid secretion, this is a self-limiting condition and acidosis can be resolved. Type 2 RTA can result from an isolated defect of bicarbonate

reabsorption, such as mutations in the NBC1 sodium/bicarbonate transporter or in carbonic anhydrase 2, or from a generalized impairment in the reabsorption of small molecules, including phosphate, glucose, uric acid, calcium, citrate, and amino acids. In generalized defects (Fanconi syndrome), the levels of these substances are reduced in the plasma. Causes include genetic defects, as well as proximal tubular damage or inhibition by nephrotic syndrome, amyloidosis, toxins, drugs, paraproteins, and biochemical defects (cystinosis, Wilson disease, methylmalonic acidemia, galactosemia, glycogen storage diseases, and so on).

- Type 4 RTA is due to defects in mineralocorticoid production or response and manifests by hyperkalemia with hyperchloremic metabolic acidosis, usually in the setting of renal failure (diabetic or hypertensive nephrosclerosis, tubulointerstitial disease, acquired immunodeficiency syndrome).

- NH_3 is secreted by the distal tubule to bind H^+ as NH_4^+, acidifying the urine. Ammonium can be indirectly estimated by calculating the urinary anion gap (UAG) = $urNa^+ + urK^+ - urCl^-$. With extrarenal causes of metabolic acidosis, the kidney is able to increase NH_4^+ production, and the UAG becomes negative (due to the compensatory increase in Cl^- excretion). In RTA, NH_4^+ production is reduced and the UAG is usually positive.

- The fractionary excretion of bicarbonate is calculated by the following formula:

$$\frac{\text{Urine } HCO_3^- \times \text{ plasma creatinine}}{\text{Plasma } HCO_3^- \times \text{ urine creatinine}}$$

which increases to greater than 15% after a bicarbonate load in proximal RTA but remains low (<5%) in distal and type 4 RTA.[9,26,29]

37. A. Respiratory acidosis.
B. Respiratory alkalosis.
C. Metabolic acidosis with respiratory compensation.
Rationale: Unlikely with normal arterial blood gas results.
D. Spuriously low venous bicarbonate due to hypotension.
Rationale: Poor perfusion can cause discrepancies between arterial and venous bicarbonate, with venous higher than arterial by more than 1 mmol/L.

E. Spurious loss of CO_2 in the venous sample.
Rationale: If the sample is left uncapped or the tube is incompletely filled, loss of CO_2 through diffusion results in low bicarbonate levels.

Major points of discussion
- "Total CO_2" or "CO_2 content" refers to the plasma content of carbon dioxide, which is transported in the form of dissolved gaseous CO_2, bicarbonate ion, and carbonic acid. The equilibrium between these forms is represented by the Henderson-Hasselbalch equation: $CO_2 + H_2O \rightleftharpoons H_2CO_3 \rightleftharpoons HCO_3^- + H^+$. At the physiologic pH of 7.40, about 4% of total CO_2 (1.2 mmol/L) is transported as dissolved gas (exerting a partial pressure of about 40 mm Hg), while most is transported as bicarbonate 21 to 28 mmol/L, and less than 0.1% as

carbonic acid. In addition, a small amount of CO_2 is transported loosely bound to plasma or red cell proteins.

- Measurement of total CO_2 is performed after conversion of all carbon dioxide to CO_2 by acidification of diluted plasma, or conversely, by conversion of all CO_2 to bicarbonate by addition of alkali. A Pco_2 electrode measures gaseous CO_2, while bicarbonate is detected by an enzymatic method, usually using phosphoenolpyruvate (PEP) carboxylase to convert PEP to oxaloacetate, which is then converted to malate by malate dehydrogenase, in the process generating reduced nicotinamide adenine dinucleotide (NADH), which can be measured spectrophotometrically.

- Blood gas analyzers do not measure bicarbonate or total CO_2 content directly due to the difficulties in alkalinizing or acidifying whole blood. Instead, they measure Pco_2 and pH by potentiometry and bicarbonate is calculated from the Henderson-Hasselbalch equilibrium.

- Loss of CO_2 occurs in uncapped tubes, resulting in total CO_2 decline at the approximate rate of 0.6 to 1 mmol/L/hr at room temperature, and this rate can increase at higher temperatures or decrease at lower temperatures. Even in capped tubes, if the amount of air space is increased because of underfilling, losses of CO_2 occur, about 0.5 mmol/L per extra milliliter of air in a 10-mL tube.

- In the absence of hypotension or other poor perfusion states, venous blood gas analysis can be used to reliably determine most acid-base disturbances with the knowledge that the venous pH is usually 0.02 to 0.05 pH units lower, the Pco_2 is 4 to 5 mm Hg higher, and the bicarbonate is only 1 to 2 mmol/L higher.[11,16,39]

38. **A. Carbamoyl phosphate synthase (CPS).**
Rationale: This is a typical presentation of a severe urea cycle disorder. They are usually accompanied by elevations in glutamine and alanine. In the case of ornithine transcarbamoylase or CPS deficiency, the downstream substrate citrulline will be reduced. They can be differentiated by elevated urine orotic acid in ornithine transcarbamylase deficiency but not CPS deficiency.
B. Argininosuccinate lyase (ASL).
Rationale: This urea cycle deficiency lies distal to citrulline synthesis and results in accumulation of argininosuccinate and citrulline.
C. Carnitine palmitoyltransferase II (CPT2).
Rationale: Defects in this enzyme prevent the transport of long-chain fatty acids into the mitochondria for beta-oxidation and manifest with nonketotic hypoglycemia, respiratory failure, seizures, hepatomegaly, and cardiomyopathy. It is characterized by elevated acylcarnitines centering on C16 and a high acylcarnitine/free carnitine ratio.
D. Aldolase B (ALDOB).
Rationale: ALDOB deficiency causes hereditary fructose intolerance, characterized by fructosuria with high reducing sugar test positivity. After introduction of fructose-containing foods (typically at 3 to 6 months), infants can show poor feeding, vomiting, neurologic damage, and hepatomegaly.
E. Lysosomal beta-glycosidase (GBA).

Rationale: Defects in lysosomal beta-glycosidase, which is also known as glucocerebrosidase, cause Gaucher disease. Gaucher disease usually manifests after 6 months of age with neurological symptoms and hepatosplenomegaly.

Major points of discussion

- Hyperammonemia in an infant can be due to several causes and it is critical to quickly make the appropriate diagnosis to start potential lifesaving therapy.
- Hyperammonemia presenting with respiratory distress at birth or in the first 24 to 36 hours can be due to transient hyperammonemia of the newborn, often in large premature infants with symptomatic pulmonary disease. Although the etiology is unknown, it can be treated with dialysis or hemofiltration and will not recur.
- Many IEMs can lead to hyperammonemia, usually manifested by respiratory distress and neurological symptoms 24 hours after delivery. The presence of hypoglycemia, severe acidosis, and ketosis points to a defect in organic acid metabolism, while urea cycle disorders manifest usually with normal or mildly decreased glycemia, mild acidosis (due to lactate), and absent ketonuria.
- The pattern of plasma amino acid levels is helpful to point to a particular urea cycle defect. Plasma citrulline is reduced or undetectable in defects proximal to citrulline synthesis (CPS and ornithine transcarbamylase [OTC]) and elevated in defects in argininosuccinate synthase and ASL. Argininosuccinate is markedly elevated in ASL deficiency. Plasma arginine is markedly elevated in the very rare arginase deficiency but usually normal or decreased in other urea cycle defects.
- Urine orotic acid, derived from excessive carbamoyl phosphate, is significantly elevated in people with defects or deficiencies of OTC and may be elevated in other urea cycle defects with the exception of CPS deficiency.
- Functional urea cycle deficiency can also occur in lysinuric protein intolerance as the result of a defect in the cationic amino acid transporter SLC7A7. Renal losses of cationic amino acids lysine, arginine, and ornithine lead to their plasma depletion and a decrease in the urea cycle from substrate depletion. Similarly, the hyperornithinemia-hyperammonemia-homocitru-llinuria syndrome, which is due to a deficiency in the mitochondrial ornithine transporter (ORNT1), results in a urea cycle syndrome characterized by marked elevations in plasma ornithine.[8,38]

39. A. Decreased pH, increased serum osmolality and osmolal gap, decreased anion gap.
   Rationale: The anion gap is increased in ethylene glycol toxicity.
   B. Increased pH, decreased serum osmolality and osmolal gap, increased anion gap.

Rationale: The pH is acidic, and the serum osmolality and osmolal gap are increased in ethylene glycol toxicity.
C. Decreased pH, increased serum osmolality and osmolal gap, normal anion gap.
Rationale: The anion gap is elevated in ethylene glycol toxicity.
D. Decreased pH, increased serum osmolality and osmolal gap, increased anion gap.
Rationale: In ethylene glycol toxicity, there is an increase in the anion gap, serum osmolality, and osmolal gap; the blood pH is decreased; and calcium oxalate crystals are detected in the urine.
E. Normal pH, increased serum osmolality and osmolal gap, increased anion gap.
Rationale: The pH is acidic in ethylene glycol toxicity.

Major points of discussion

- Osmolality is defined as the number of moles of dissolved particles per kilogram of water. The most common method used in the laboratory for measuring serum osmolality is freezing point depression.
- The osmolal gap is the difference between the measured osmolality and the calculated osmolality. There are many equations that can be used to calculate osmolality. The most common equation is osmolality $(mOsm/kg) = [2 \times Na \ (mEq/L)] + glucose \ (mg/dL)/18 + BUN \ (mg/dL)/2.8$.
- An increased osmolal gap indicates an increased concentration of unmeasured low-molecular-weight substances in the blood. As examples, when ethanol, methanol, isopropanol, ethylene glycol, or acetone is present at high concentrations, they will each increase the serum osmolality and the osmolal gap.
- In ethylene glycol toxicity, there is an increase in the anion gap, serum osmolality, and osmolal gap, the blood pH is decreased, and calcium oxalate crystals are detected in the urine. Calcium oxalate can also precipitate in the lungs and brain, thereby causing significant damage to these organs.
- Ethylene glycol is metabolized by alcohol dehydrogenase to glycoaldehyde. Aldehyde dehydrogenase converts glycoaldehyde to glycolic acid, which is the primary metabolite in serum and the cause of the metabolic acidosis observed in ethylene glycol toxicity. Glycolic acid is converted to glyoxylic acid and, finally, to oxalate as the end product of ethylene glycol metabolism.
- In the early stages of ethylene glycol toxicity, the serum osmolality and osmolal gap are elevated, but the anion gap may be normal because there is not enough time for ethylene glycol to be metabolized to its acid metabolites.
- In the late stages of ethylene glycol toxicity, the anion gap is increased, but the serum osmolality and osmolal gap may be normal because the acid metabolites of ethylene glycol do not contribute to the osmolal gap.[5,28]

References

1. Andolfo I, Alper SL, Delaunay J, et al. Missense mutations in the ABCB6 transporter cause dominant familial pseudohyperkalemia. Am J Hematol 2013;88:66–72.
2. Carter AB, Howanitz PJ. Intraoperative testing for parathyroid hormone. Arch Pathol Lab Med 2003;127:1424–1442.
3. Cerasola G, Cottone S, Mule G. The progressive pathway of microalbuminuria: from early marker of renal damage to strong cardiovascular risk predictor. J Hypertens 2010;28:2357–2769.
4. Cornes MP, Ford C, Gama R. Spurious hyperkalaemia due to EDTA contamination: common and not always easy to identify. Ann Clin Biochem 2008;45:601–603.

5. Coulter, Farquhar SE, Mcsherry CM, et al. Methanol and ethylene glycol poisonings—predictors of mortality. Clin Toxicol 2011;49:900–906.

6. de Seigneux S, Martin PY. Management of patients with nephrotic syndrome. Swiss Med Wkly 2009;139:416–422.

7. Dietzen DJ, Rinaldo P, Whitley RJ, et al. National Academy of Clinical Biochemistry Laboratory Medicine practice guidelines: follow-up testing for metabolic disease identified by expanded newborn screening using tandem mass spectrometry; executive summary. Clin Chem 2009;55:1615–1626.

8. Farrell PM, Rosenstein BJ, White TB, et al. Guidelines for diagnosis of cystic fibrosis in newborns through older adults: Cystic Fibrosis Foundation Consensus Report. J Pediatr 2008;153:S4–S14.

9. Ficicioglu C, Yudkoff M. Urea cycle: disease aspects. In: William JL, Lane MD, editors: Encyclopedia of Biological Chemistry, Waltham, MA: Academic Press, 2013, pp 494–501.

10. Golembiewska E, Ciechanowski K. Renal tubular acidosis—underrated problem? Acta Biochim Pol 2012;59:213–217.

11. Guven A, Cebeci N, Dursun A, et al. Methylmalonic acidemia mimicking diabetic ketoacidosis in an infant. Pediatr Diabetes 2012;13:e22–e25.

12. Herr RD, Swanson T. Pseudometabolic acidosis caused by underfill of Vacutainer tubes. Ann Emerg Med 1992;21:177–180.

13. Holick MF, Binkley NC, Heike A, et al. Evaluation, treatment, and prevention of vitamin D deficiency: an Endocrine Society Clinical Practice Guideline. J Clin Endocrinol Metab 2011;96:1911–1930.

14. Holick MF. Vitamin D, deficiency. N Engl J Med 2007;357:266–281.

15. Hood JL, Scott MG. Physiology and disorders of water, electrolyte and acid-base metabolism. In: Burtis CA, Ashwood ER, Bruns DE, editors: Tietz Textbook of Clinical Chemistry and Molecular Diagnostics, 5th ed. St. Louis: Elsevier, 2012, pp 1609–1635.

16. Jacob G, et al. Effect of standing on neurohumoral responses and plasma volume in healthy subjects. J Appl Physiol 1998;84:914–921.

17. Kirschbaum B. Loss of carbon dioxide from serum samples exposed to air. Effect on blood gas parameters and strong ions. Clin Chim Acta 2003;334:241–244.

18. Kitabchi AE, Umpierrez GE, Miles JM, et al. Hyperglycemic crises in adult patients with diabetes. Diabetes Care 2009;32:1335–1343.

19. Kodner C. Nephrotic syndrome in adults: diagnosis and management. Am Fam Physician 2009;80:1129–1134.

20. Lamb EJ, Price CP. Kidney function tests. In: Burtis CA, Ashwood ER, Bruns DE, editors: Tietz Textbook of Clinical Chemistry and Molecular Diagnostics, 5th ed. St. Louis: Elsevier, 2012, pp 669–707.

21. Marocci C, Cetani F. Clinical practice. Primary hyperparathyroidism. N Engl J Med 2011;365:2389–2397.

22. Masters PW, Lawson N, Marenah CB, et al. High ambient temperature: a spurious cause of hypokalaemia. BMJ 1996;312:1652–1653.

23. Matsushita K, Mahmoodi BK, Woodward M, et al. Comparison of risk prediction using the CKD-EPI equation and the MDRD study equation for estimated glomerular filtration rate. JAMA 2012;307:1941–1951.

24. Moeller HB, Rittig S, Fenton RA. Nephrogenic diabetes insipidus: essential insights into the molecular background and potential therapies for treatment. Endocr Rev 2013;34:278–301.

25. Biswas CK, Ramos JM, Agroyannis B, et al. Blood gas analysis: effects of air bubbles in syringe and delay in estimation. Br Med J (Clin Res Ed) 1982;284:923–927.

26. Park SH, An D, Chang YJ, et al. Development and validation of an arterial blood gas analysis interpretation algorithm for application in clinical laboratory services. Ann Clin Biochem 2011;48:130–135.

27. Pereira PC, Miranda DM, Oliveira EA, et al. Molecular pathophysiology of renal tubular acidosis. Curr Genom 2009;10:51–59.

28. Polak R, Huisman A, Sikma MA, et al. Spurious hypokalaemia and hypophosphataemia due to extreme hyperleukocytosis in a patient with a haematological malignancy. Ann Clin Biochem 2010;47(Pt 2):179–181.

29. Porter WH. Ethylene glycol poisoning: quintessential clinical toxicology; analytical conundrum. Clin Chim Acta 2012;413:365–377.

30. Reddy P. Clinical approach to renal tubular acidosis in adult patients. Int J Clin Pract 2011;65:350–360.

31. Sam R, Feizi I. Understanding hypernatremia. Am J Nephrol 2012;36:97–104.

32. Scott MG, LeGrys VA, Hood JL. Electrolytes and blood gases. In: Burtis CA, Ashwood ER, Bruns DE, editors: Tietz Textbook of Clinical Chemistry and Molecular Diagnostics, 5th ed. St. Louis: Elsevier, 2012, pp 829–830.

33. Sharda S, Angurana SK, Walia M, et al. Defect of cobalamin intracellular metabolism presenting as diabetic ketoacidosis: a rare manifestation. JIMD Rep 2013;11:43–47.

34. Sharratt CL, Gilbert CJ, Cornes MC, et al. EDTA sample contamination is common and often undetected, putting patients at unnecessary risk of harm. Int J Clin Pract 2009;63:1259–1262.

35. Singh A, Satchell SC. Microalbuminuria: causes and implications. Pediatr Nephrol 2011;26:1957–1965.

36. Sodi R, Davison AS, Holmes E, et al. The phenomenon of seasonal pseudohypokalemia: effects of ambient temperature, plasma glucose and role for sodium-potassium-exchanging-ATPase. Clin Biochem 2009;42:813–818.

37. Stankovic AK, Smith S. Elevated serum potassium values: the role of preanalytic variables. Am J Clin Pathol 2004;121(Suppl):S105–S112.

38. Steiner RD, Cederbaum SD. Laboratory evaluation of urea cycle disorders. J Pediatr 2001;138(1 Suppl):S21–S29.

39. Toftegaard M, Rees SE, Andreassen S. Correlation between acid-base parameters measured in arterial blood and venous blood sampled peripherally, from vena cavae superior, and from the pulmonary artery. Eur J Emerg Med 2008;15:86–91.

40. American College of Obstetricians and Gynecologists Committee on Genetics. ACOG Committee Opinion No. 486. Update on carrier screening for cystic fibrosis. Obstet Gynecol 2011;117:1028–1031.

41. Weber JA, van Zanten AP. Interferences in current methods for measurements of creatinine. Clin Chem 1991;37:695–700.

42. Zhang JT, Chan C, Kwun SY, et al. A case of severe 1,25-dihydroxyvitamin D-mediated hypercalcemia due to a granulomatous disorder. J Clin Endocrinol Metab 2012;97:2579–2583.

CHAPTER 10

HEMATOLOGY: Red Blood Cells

Jeffrey S. Jhang, Alexander Kratz, Patrice F. Spitalnik

QUESTIONS

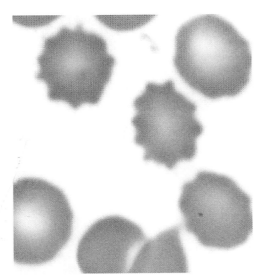

Figure 10-1 Blood smear showing Burr cells.

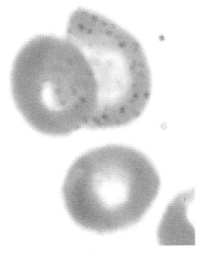

Figure 10-2 A red cell with basophilic stippling.

1. An example of the findings on a blood smear is shown in Figure 10-1. Which one of the following is the most likely explanation?
   A. Liver disease.
   B. Delay between blood draw and preparation of the blood smear.
   C. Hemoglobin C disease.
   D. Status postsplenectomy.
   E. Iron deficiency.

2. As part of an anemia workup, you review the hemoglobinopathy evaluation of a 4-year-old boy. Electrophoresis indicates no evidence of a structural hemoglobinopathy, and the levels of hemoglobin A2 and F are within normal limits. The mean corpuscular volume (MCV) is normal. A representative example of the findings on the blood smear is shown in Figure 10-2. Which one of the following is the best interpretation of these findings?
   A. β-Thalassemia trait.
   B. Anemia secondary to chronic renal failure.
   C. Hemoglobinopathy not detected by electrophoresis.
   D. Lead intoxication.
   E. Liver disease.

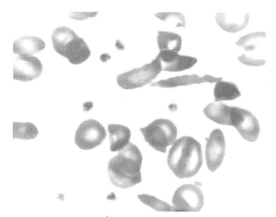

Figure 10-3 Blood smear from a patient.

3. A 25-year-old African-American woman is admitted to the hospital because of respiratory failure. She complains of pain in her back, thighs, and knees. Figure 10-3 shows a representative view of her blood smear. Which one of the following is the most likely diagnosis?
   A. Sickle cell disorder.
   B. Homozygous hemoglobin S.
   C. Lead poisoning.
   D. Thrombotic thrombocytopenic purpura.
   E. Hereditary elliptocytosis.

Table 10-1

	Patient	Reference Range	Units
WBC	8.4	3.04-9.06	×10⁹/L
RBC	5.96	4.3-5.6	×10¹²/L
Hemoglobin	15.6	13.3-16.2	g/dL
Hematocrit	44.9	38.8-46.4	%
MCV	75.3	79.0-93.3	fL
MCH	26.2	26.7-31.9	pg
MCHC	34.7	32.3-35.9	g/dL
RDW	13.8	<14	%
PLT	175	165-415	×10⁹/L
Ferritin	129	29-248	ng/mL

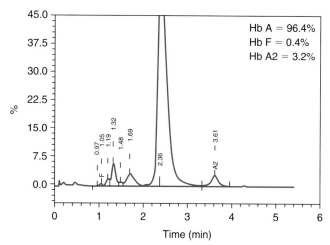

Hb A = 96.4%
Hb F = 0.4%
Hb A2 = 3.2%

Figure 10-4 Hemoglobin fractionation by HPLC (fraction percentages shown at upper right).

4. A 29-year-old man presents to his physician for partner screening. The complete blood cell count (CBC) and ferritin level are shown in Table 10-1. Figure 10-4 shows the hemoglobin fractions identified on high-performance liquid chromatography (HPLC). Which one of the following is the most likely diagnosis?
   A. α-Thalassemia trait.
   B. β-Thalassemia trait.
   C. δβ-Thalassemia trait.
   D. Hemoglobin E trait.
   E. Hemoglobin Lepore.

Table 10-2

	Patient	Reference Range	Units
WBC	8.5	3.04-9.06	×10⁹/L
RBC	5.14	4.3-5.6	×10¹²/L
Hemoglobin	10.9	13.3-16.2	g/dL
Hematocrit	33.2	38.8-46.4	%
MCV	64.6	79.0-93.3	fL
MCH	21.2	26.7-31.9	pg
MCHC	32.8	32.3-35.9	g/dL
RDW	13.8	<14	%
PLT	175	165-415	×10⁹/L
Ferritin	112	29-248	ng/mL

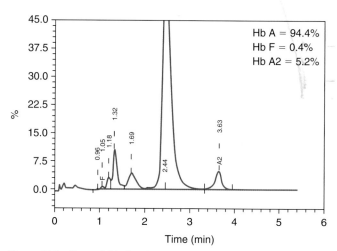

Hb A = 94.4%
Hb F = 0.4%
Hb A2 = 5.2%

Figure 10-5 Hemoglobin fractionation by HPLC (hemoglobin percentages shown at upper right).

5. A 23-year-old pregnant woman at 12 weeks' gestation presents to her obstetrician for prenatal screening. A CBC and a ferritin level are shown in Table 10-2. Figure 10-5 shows hemoglobin fractionation by HPLC. Which one of the following is the most likely diagnosis?
   A. α-Thalassemia trait.
   B. β-Thalassemia trait.
   C. δβ-Thalassemia trait.
   D. Hemoglobin E trait.
   E. Hemoglobin Constant Spring.

Table 10-3

	Patient	Reference Range	Units
WBC	8.5	3.04-9.06	$\times 10^9$/L
RBC	5.12	4.3-5.6	$\times 10^{12}$/L
Hemoglobin	12.8	13.3-16.2	g/dL
Hematocrit	39.9	38.8-46.4	%
MCV	77.9	79.0-93.3	fL
MCH	25.0	26.7-31.9	pg
MCHC	32.1	32.3-35.9	g/dL
RDW	13.8	<14	%
PLT	265	165-415	$\times 10^9$/L
Ferritin	112	29-248	ng/mL

Table 10-4

	Patient	Reference Range	Units
RBC	6.0	4.3-5.6	$\times 10^{12}$/L
Hemoglobin	14.5	13.3-16.2	g/dL
Hematocrit	43.5	38.8-46.4	%
MCV	71.1	79.0-93.3	fL
MCH	24.2	26.7-31.9	pg
MCHC	33.9	32.3-35.9	g/dL
RDW	15.6	<14	%

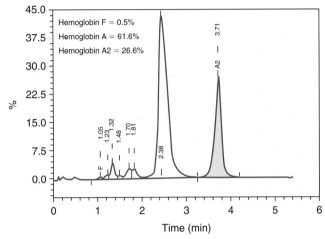

Figure 10-7 HPLC for hemoglobin fractionation (hemoglobin percentages on *y*-axis and retention time on *x*-axis).

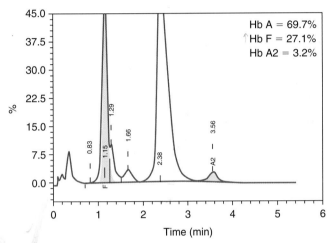

Figure 10-6 Hemoglobin fractionation by HPLC (relative hemoglobin percentages shown at upper right).

6. A 23-year-old woman who is 12 weeks pregnant presents to her obstetrician for prenatal screening. A CBC and a ferritin level are shown in Table 10-3. Figure 10-6 shows hemoglobin fractionation by HPLC. Which one of the following is the most likely diagnosis?
   A. α-Thalassemia trait.
   B. β-Thalassemia trait.
   C. δβ-Thalassemia trait.
   D. Hemoglobin E trait.
   E. Hemoglobin Constant Spring.

7. Which one of the following is the preferred anticoagulant for a CBC specimen?
   A. 3.2% sodium citrate.
   B. Hirudin.
   C. K_2EDTA (dipotassium ethylenediaminetetra-acetic acid).
   D. K_3EDTA (tripotassium ethylenediaminetetraacetic acid).
   E. Sodium heparin.

8. A 27-year-old Thai man with no significant medical history presents to a genetic counselor for partner testing. Which one of the following diagnoses is most consistent with the complete cell blood count in Table 10-4 and HPLC chromatogram (Figure 10-7)?
   A. β-Thalassemia trait.
   B. Hemoglobin C trait.
   C. Hemoglobin D–Los Angeles.
   D. Hemoglobin E trait.
   E. Hemoglobin S trait.

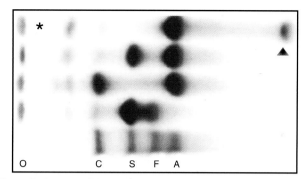

Figure 10-8 Hemoglobin electrophoresis at pH = 8.2. The origin (*O*) and hemoglobin controls (hemoglobins *A, F, S,* and *C*) are shown. The asterisk marks the lane for this patient.

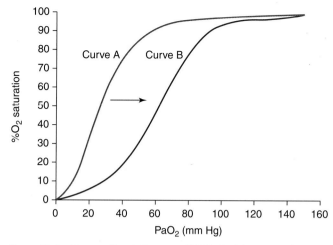

Figure 10-9 Oxygen dissociation curve (ODC). Partial pressure of oxygen is plotted on the *x*-axis, and the percent hemoglobin saturation is plotted on the *y*-axis. Curve A represents the ODC under normal physiologic conditions. Curve B represents the curve under conditions that shift it to the right.

Table 10-5

	Patient	Reference Range	Units
WBC	8.4	3.04-9.06	$\times 10^9$/L
RBC	4.83	4.3-5.6	$\times 10^{12}$/L
Hemoglobin	8.8	13.3-16.2	g/dL
Hematocrit	32.2	38.8-46.4	%
MCV	66.7	79.0-93.3	fL
MCH	18.2	26.7-31.9	pg
MCHC	27.3	32.3-35.9	g/dL
RDW	24.4	<14	%
PLT	255	165-415	$\times 10^9$/L
Ferritin	129	29-248	ng/mL

PLT, platelets.

A 69-year-old Vietnamese man with a past medical history of fatigue presented to his primary care physician with a painful, swollen joint and was found after a routine CBC to have anemia. Hemoglobin electrophoresis is shown in Figure 10-8, and the CBC is shown in Table 10-5. Use this scenario to answer the following three questions.

9a. Which one of the following is the most likely diagnosis?
   A. α-Thalassemia trait.
   B. Hemoglobin H disease.
   C. Hemoglobin Barts.
   D. Hemoglobin N–Baltimore trait.
   E. Hemoglobin J trait.

9b. Which one of the following hemoglobins represents the hemoglobin at the arrowhead shown in Figure 10-8?
   A. α_4.
   B. β_4.
   C. γ_4.
   D. $\zeta_2\varepsilon_2$.
   E. $\alpha_2\varepsilon_2$.

9c. Which one of the following clinical syndromes is associated with deletion of four α-globin genes?
   A. Hydrops fetalis.
   B. α-Thalassemia retardation syndrome.
   C. α-Thalassemia myelodysplasia syndrome.
   D. Cooley's anemia.
   E. Hemolytic disease of the fetus and newborn (HDFN).

10. Which one of the following conditions shifts the hemoglobin oxygenation curve to the right in Figure 10-9?
   A. Hypothermia.
   B. Acidosis.
   C. Decreased 2,3-diphosphoglycerate (DPG).
   D. CO_2 release by hemoglobin.
   E. High-affinity hemoglobin.

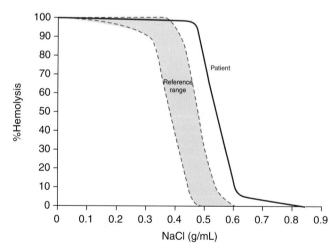

Figure 10-10 Immediate osmotic fragility test. The *y*-axis shows percent hemolysis with changes in concentration of sodium chloride on the *x*-axis (0 to 0.85% normal saline).

11. Which one of the following disorders is associated with the osmotic fragility test shown in Figure 10-10?
   A. Iron deficiency.
   B. Hereditary pyropoikylocytosis.
   C. β-Thalassemia trait.
   D. α-Thalassemia trait.
   E. Sickle cell anemia.

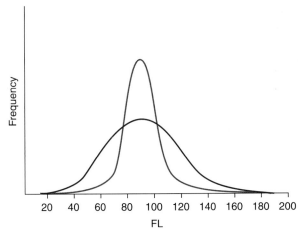

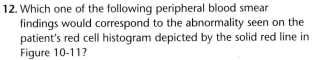

Figure 10-11 A normal red cell histogram (frequency distribution curve) is depicted by the blue curve with the number of cells counted on the *y*-axis and the size of the red cells in femtoliters (*FL*) on the *x*-axis. The red curve depicts the histogram.

12. Which one of the following peripheral blood smear findings would correspond to the abnormality seen on the patient's red cell histogram depicted by the solid red line in Figure 10-11?
    A. Anisocytosis.
    B. Hypochromia.
    C. Macrocytosis.
    D. Microcytosis, iron deficiency.
    E. Microcytosis, β-thalassemia trait.

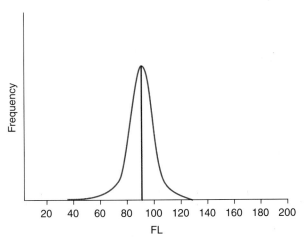

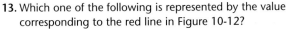

Figure 10-12 A red cell histogram generated by an automated hematology analyzer shows the number of red cells on the *y*-axis and the size of the red cells on the *x*-axis in femtoliters (*FL*).

13. Which one of the following is represented by the value corresponding to the red line in Figure 10-12?
    A. Red blood cell count (RBC).
    B. Hematocrit (HCT).
    C. Mean corpuscular volume (MCV).
    D. Mean corpuscular hemoglobin (MCH).
    E. Red cell distribution width (RDW).

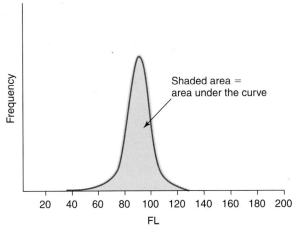

Figure 10-13 A red cell histogram generated by an automated hematology analyser shows the number of red cells on the y-axis and the size of the red cells on the x-axis in femtoliters (*FL*).

14. Which one of the following is represented by the value of the area under the curve in Figure 10-13?
    A. RBC
    B. HCT.
    C. MCV.
    D. MCH.
    E. RDW.

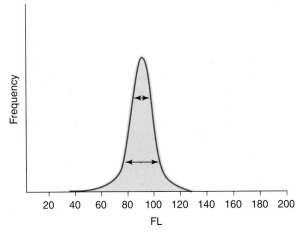

Figure 10-14 A red cell histogram generated by an automated hematology analyzer shows the number of red cells on the y-axis and the size of the red cells on the x-axis in femtoliters (*FL*).

15. Which one of the following is represented by the value corresponding to the distance between the arrowheads in Figure 10-14?
    A. RBC.
    B. HCT.
    C. MCV.
    D. MCH.
    E. RDW.

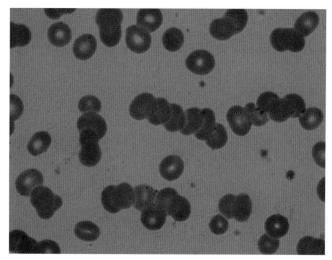

Figure 10-15 Wright-Giemsa–stained peripheral blood smear (×100).

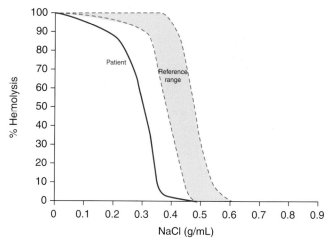

Figure 10-16 Immediate osmotic fragility test. The *y*-axis shows percent hemolysis with increasing concentration of sodium chloride (0 to 0.85% normal saline).

16. Which one of the following can be falsely decreased on an automated hematology analyzer by the finding shown in Figure 10-15?
    A. Hemoglobin.
    B. MCV.
    C. MCH.
    D. RBC.
    E. RDW.

17. Which one of the following disorders is most compatible with a normal zinc protoporphyrin (ZPP) level?
    A. α-Thalassemia trait.
    B. Anemia of chronic disease.
    C. Iron deficiency anemia.
    D. Lead poisoning.
    E. Sideroblastic anemia.

18a. Which one of the following spectrophotometer wavelengths does the cyanmethemoglobin colorimetric method use for measuring hemoglobin concentration?
    A. 260 nm.
    B. 340 nm.
    C. 450 nm.
    D. 540 nm.
    E. 1100 nm.

18b. Which one of the following is an advantage of the cyanmethemoglobin colorimetric method for determination of hemoglobin concentration?
    A. Measures all forms of hemoglobin.
    B. Reagents are very stable.
    C. Reagents are nontoxic.
    D. Method is not affected by lipemia.
    E. Completion of the reaction in 1 minute.

19. Which one of the following disorders is associated with the osmotic fragility test shown in Figure 10-16?
    A. Hereditary spherocytosis (HS).
    B. Hereditary pyropoikilocytosis.
    C. Hereditary elliptocytosis.
    D. α-Thalassemia trait.
    E. Warm autoimmune hemolytic anemia.

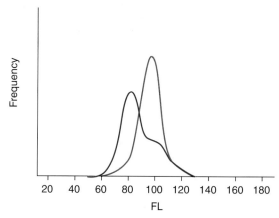

Figure 10-17 The size distribution of red cells is depicted in the figure by the red cell histogram. The number of cells is plotted on the *y*-axis and the size of the cells on the *x*-axis. The blue curve is a reference for a normal histogram. The red curve represents the curve referenced in Question 20.

20. Which one of the following most likely explains the findings shown by the red curve on the red cell histogram in Figure 10-17?
    A. β-Thalassemia trait.
    B. End-stage liver disease.
    C. Pseudothrombocytopenia.
    D. Treated B$_{12}$ deficiency.
    E. Treated iron deficiency anemia.

A 21-year-old woman with no past medical history sees her physician with complaints of fatigue and palpitations. Physical examination reveals conjunctival pallor. A CBC shows hemoglobin = 9 g/dL (12.0 to 15.8 g/dL), MCV = 73 fL (79.0 to 93.3 fL), and reticulocyte count = 1.3% (0.8% to 2.0%). Use this scenario to answer the following four questions.

21a. Which one of the following best characterizes this anemia?
- **A.** Normocytic, hyperproliferative anemia.
- **B.** Microcytic, hypoproliferative anemia.
- **C.** Macrocytic, hypoproliferative anemia.
- **D.** Microcytic, hyperproliferative anemia.

21b. The mean corpuscular hemoglobin concentration (MCHC) is 33.3 g/dL (32.2 to 35.9 g/dL), and the RDW is 17% (<14.5%). Which one of the following is the most informative diagnostic test the clinician could order?
- **A.** Manual differential.
- **B.** B_{12} and folate levels.
- **C.** Serum iron and ferritin.
- **D.** Bone marrow biopsy.

21c. The woman is treated appropriately, and her anemia resolves. On her follow-up visit a year later, she has a normal CBC. At that visit, it is discovered she is pregnant, and she gives birth 8 months later. Her labor was complicated by a massive obstetric hemorrhage requiring pressors and a brief stay in the intensive care unit. She survived and on a follow-up outpatient visit was found to have the following CBC parameters: hemoglobin = 9 g/dL (12.0 to 15.8 g/dL) and MCV = 103 fL (79.0 to 93.3 fL) consistent with a macrocytic anemia. A smear shows normal white cell morphology and macroovalocytes. Which one of the following tests would be the best test to order next?
- **A.** Iron panel.
- **B.** B_{12} and folate.
- **C.** Bone marrow biopsy.
- **D.** Thyroid-stimulating hormone (TSH) and free thyroxine (fT_4).

21d. In a patient with pituitary failure after obstetric hemorrhage, which one of the following patterns would the thyroid function tests typically show?
- **A.** Low TSH, low fT_4.
- **B.** High TSH, low fT_4.
- **C.** High TSH, high fT_4.
- **D.** Low TSH, high fT_4.

Table 10-6

	Patient	Reference Range	Units
WBC	5.8	3.04-9.06	×10⁹/L
RBC	3.7	4.3-5.6	×10¹²/L
Hemoglobin	10.9	13.3-16.2	g/dL
Hematocrit	30.6	38.8-46.4	%
MCV	81.0	79.0-93.3	fL
MCH	28.8	26.7-31.9	pg
MCHC	35.6	32.3-35.9	g/dL
RDW	13.3	<14	%
PLT	271	165-415	×10⁹/L

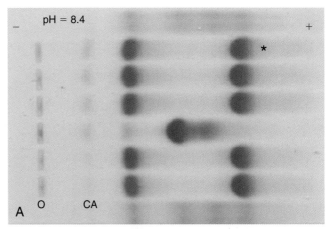

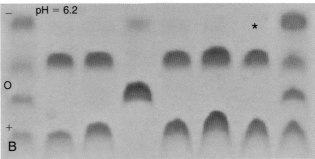

Figure 10-18 **A,** Alkaline hemoglobin electrophoresis. **B,** Acid hemoglobin electrophoresis. The asterisk indicates the lane with the patient sample. *O,* origin; *CA,* carbonic anhydrase.

22. A 23-year-old African-American woman is seen by her obstetrician for a routine prenatal visit. A CBC was performed and is shown in Table 10-6. Results of hemoglobin electrophoresis are shown in Figure 10-18. The sickle solubility test result was negative. Which one of the following is the best diagnosis based on these results?
- **A.** No hemoglobin variant or thalassemia.
- **B.** α-Chain variant.
- **C.** β-Chain variant.
- **D.** Unstable hemoglobin variant.
- **E.** Sickling hemoglobin variant.

23. A previously healthy 50-year-old man is seen at the dermatology office for removal of a mole on his left forearm. The dermatologist applied benzocaine topical anesthetic and then performed the procedure without complications. Before leaving the office, the patient complained of a headache and became progressively more confused and short of breath. The physician observed cyanotic lips and bluish tongue. The patient was transferred to the emergency department where the cyanosis did not respond to treatment with oxygen 15 L/min by nonrebreather mask. Co-oximetry showed a methemoglobin of 26% (reference range, <1%), and he was diagnosed with acquired methemoglobinemia. Which one of the following would be the best initial treatment for this patient?
- **A.** Ascorbic acid.
- **B.** Crystal violet.
- **C.** Gastric lavage.
- **D.** Methylene blue.
- **E.** Red cell exchange.

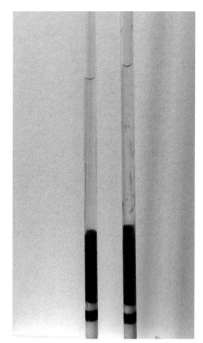

Figure 10-19 Microhematocrit capillary tubes from a whole blood sample run in duplicate (hematocrit, 30%).

24. A microhematocrit was run in duplicate on a K₂EDTA anticoagulated whole blood sample as shown in Figure 10-19. The packed cell volume, when run in duplicate, was 30% in both capillary tubes. Which one of the following factors can lead to a falsely low packed cell volume (PCV) determined by the microhematocrit method?
    A. Decreased time for centrifugation.
    B. β-Thalassemia trait.
    C. Sickle cell disease.
    D. Increased erythrocyte sedimentation rate.
    E. Decreased centrifugal force.

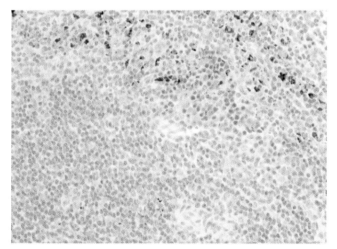

Figure 10-20 Prussian blue stain of paraffin-embedded spleen cells.

25. A 55-year-old woman with long-standing untreated rheumatoid arthritis is complaining of fatigue and found to have a normochromic, normocytic anemia. Figure 10-20

represents a Prussian blue iron stain of her spleen, suggesting accumulation of iron in red pulp macrophages. Which one of the following pairs best relates the expected serum hepcidin level with the patient's most likely type of anemia?
    A. Iron deficiency anemia; low serum hepcidin levels.
    B. Iron deficiency anemia; high serum hepcidin levels.
    C. Megaloblastic anemia; high serum hepcidin levels.
    D. Anemia of chronic disease; low serum hepcidin levels.
    E. Anemia of chronic disease; high serum hepcidin levels.

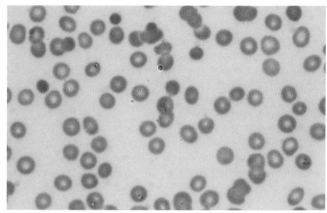

Figure 10-21 Wright-Giemsa–stained peripheral blood smear (×100).

26. A 54-year-old man with ulcerative colitis was recently being tapered off steroids. While traveling to New Haven, Conn., to drop his son off at college, he developed worsening of his abdominal pain and diarrhea. When he returned home, his physician increased his dose of prednisone to 40 mg per day. Five days later, the patient developed severe fatigue, dizziness, and shortness of breath. A CBC sample was sent to the laboratory. The peripheral blood film is shown in Figure 10-21. Which one of the following is the most likely cause of his symptoms?
    A. *Babesia microti.*
    B. *Borrelia burgdorferi.*
    C. *Leishmania donovani.*
    D. *Toxoplasma gondii.*
    E. *Trypanosoma cruzi.*

27. An asymptomatic 48-year-old patient was screened for *HFE* gene mutations after a sibling was discovered to have a homozygous mutation in this gene (C282Y/C282Y). The patient's ferritin level is currently 2200 ng/mL (12 to 300 ng/mL), and there is no evidence of inflammation (e.g., C-reactive protein levels within normal range). If serum hepcidin levels were measured, which one of the following choices is most correct for the expected hepcidin level?
    A. Low hepcidin level as seen in nutritional iron deficiency.
    B. High hepcidin level as seen in transfusion-induced iron overload.
    C. Normal hepcidin level as seen in an iron-replete male.
    D. Low hepcidin level as seen in transfusion-induced iron overload.
    E. High hepcidin level as seen in nutritional iron deficiency.

Table 10-7

	Patient	Reference Range	Units
WBC	6.2	3.5-9.1	$\times 10^9$/L
RBC	4.12	4.5-5.4	$\times 10^{12}$/L
Hemoglobin	11.1	13.0-16.0	g/dL
Hematocrit	29.3	37.0-48.0	%
MCV	71.1	80.0-94.0	fL
MCH	26.9	26.7-31.9	pg
MCHC	37.9	32.3-35.9	g/dL
RDW	16.3	<14	%
PLT	217	165-415	$\times 10^9$/L

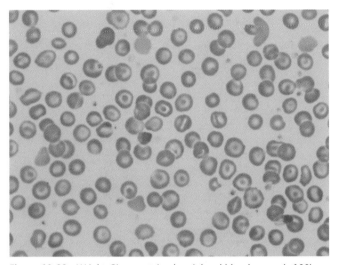

Figure 10-22 Wright-Giemsa–stained peripheral blood smear ($\times$100).

28. A 9-year-old boy comes into the emergency department complaining of headache, abdominal pain, and joint pain. His mother states that he has sickle cell disease. He has never had a transfusion in the past. The CBC is shown in Table 10-7, and the peripheral blood smear is shown in Figure 10-22. Based on these tests, which one of the following is the most likely disorder?
   A. Sickle cell trait.
   B. Sickle cell disease.
   C. Hemoglobin SC disease.
   D. β-Thalassemia trait.
   E. α-Thalassemia trait.

29. You are asked to review a peripheral blood smear showing 60% acanthocytes. Which one of the following conditions is associated with more than 10% acanthocytosis?
   A. Autoimmune hemolytic anemia.
   B. McLeod blood group phenotype.
   C. Microangiopathic hemolytic anemia.
   D. Sickle cell disease.
   E. Uremia.

30. Which one of the following porphyrias is *not* associated with photosensitivity?
   A. Acute intermittent porphyria.

   B. Hereditary coproporphyria.
   C. Erythropoietic protoporphyria.
   D. Congenital erythropoietic porphyria.
   E. Porphyria cutanea tarda.

31. Which one of the following statements about automated counting of reticulocytes is true?
   A. Automated methods to count reticulocytes often involve digital image analysis.
   B. Automated methods to count reticulocytes require specialized equipment dedicated to this assay only.
   C. Automated reticulocyte counts frequently require confirmation by manual slide review.
   D. Automated reticulocyte counts are more accurate and precise than manual counts.
   E. Automated reticulocyte counts are based on measurements of the size of reticulocytes compared with the size of mature red cells.

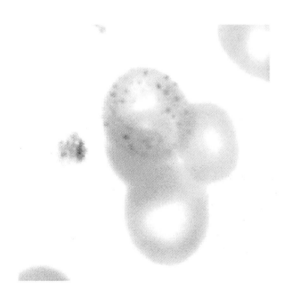

Figure 10-23 Wright-Giemsa–stained peripheral blood smear ($\times$100).

32a. The red cell in Figure 10-23 is most consistent with which one of the following?
   A. Malaria.
   B. Babesiosis.
   C. Sideroblastic granules (Pappenheimer bodies).
   D. Basophilic stippling.
   E. Howell-Jolly bodies.

32b. Basophilic stippling is most frequently observed in which one of the following?
   A. Iron overload.
   B. Malaria.
   C. Babesiosis.
   D. Thalassemias.
   E. Iron deficiency.

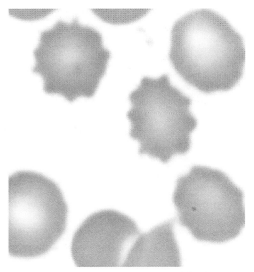

Figure 10-24 Wright-Giemsa–stained peripheral blood smear (×100).

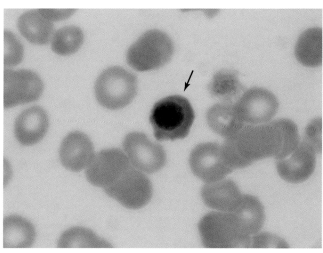

Figure 10-25 Wright-Giemsa–stained peripheral blood smear (×100).

33a. The red cells in Figure 10-24 are most consistent with which one of the following?
  A. Stomatocytes.
  B. Teardrop cells.
  C. Schistocytes.
  D. Acanthocytes.
  E. Burr cells (echinocytes).

33b. In which one of the following pathologic states are Burr cells most frequently seen?
  A. Uremia.
  B. Abnormalities of lipid metabolism.
  C. Infections.
  D. Hereditary abnormalities of red cell metabolism.
  E. Myelodysplastic syndrome.

33c. A medical student calls the laboratory and asks for the preparation of a slide from a CBC sample obtained 36 hours ago. Review of the blood smear shows a large number of Burr cells (echinocytes). A basic metabolic profile from a sample obtained at the same time as the CBC sample and analyzed within 4 hours of phlebotomy showed normal results. Which one of the following is the best explanation for these results?
  A. The Burr cells are an artifact caused by the long interval between phlebotomy and preparation of the blood film.
  B. The basic metabolic panel results are most likely wrong because Burr cells indicate the presence of uremia.
  C. The Burr cells may be caused by an abnormality in the patient's lipid metabolism.
  D. The Burr cells may be caused by a malignant process.
  E. The Burr cells may be caused by an infection.

34a. A K_2EDTA anticoagulated whole blood sample is sent to the laboratory for a CBC. A manual differential is performed because of an instrument flag. Which one of the following cells is indicated by the arrow in Figure 10-25?
  A. Apoptotic lymphocyte.
  B. Atypical lymphocyte.
  C. Giant platelet.
  D. Nucleated red cell.
  E. Plasma cell.

34b. The patient's white blood cell count (WBC) is 4.5×10^9/L (reference range 3.04-9.06), and the laboratory technologist reports 10 of the cells indicated by the arrow in Figure 10-25 for every 100 WBCs. Which one of the following is the correct WBC after correction for the cells indicated by the arrow?
  A. 0.5
  B. 4.1
  C. 4.5
  D. 4.6
  E. 5.0

35. A 17-year-old boy with erythropoietic protoporphyria (EPP) has photosensitivity and acute abdominal pain. He has fulminant liver failure and is awaiting liver transplantation. Which one of the following enzymes is deficient in this patient?
  A. Aminolevulinic acid (ALA) synthetase.
  B. Coproporphyrinogen oxidase.
  C. Ferrochelatase.
  D. Uroporphyrinogen III cosynthetase.
  E. Uroporphyrinogen decarboxylase.

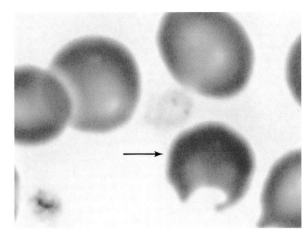

Figure 10-26 Wright-Giemsa–stained peripheral blood smear (×100).

36. Which one of the following disorders is associated with the cell indicated by the arrow in Figure 10-26?
   A. Glucose-6-phosphate dehydrogenase deficiency.
   B. Hereditary pyropoikilocytosis.
   C. Hereditary spherocytosis.
   D. Splenectomy.

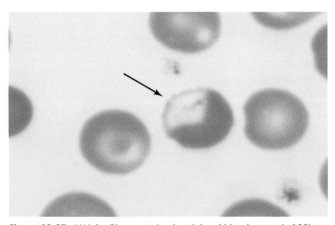

Figure 10-27 Wright-Giemsa–stained peripheral blood smear (×100).

37. Which one of the following mechanisms produces the cell indicated by the arrow in Figure 10-27?
   A. Crystallization.
   B. Heavy metal poisoning.
   C. Oxidative damage.
   D. Spectrin gene mutation.
   E. Splenectomy.

38. Which one of the following is associated with an elevated hemoglobin A2 level?
   A. α-Thalassemia trait.
   B. Antiretroviral therapy.
   C. $(\delta\beta)^0$-Thalassemia trait.
   D. Hypothyroidism.
   E. Sideroblastic anemia.

39. Hemoglobin Barts is a result of the formation of which one of the following hemoglobin tetramers?
   A. α_4.
   B. β_4.
   C. γ_4.
   D. δ_4.
   E. ζ_4.

40. Which one of the following promoters controls the transcription of the hemoglobin Lepore gene?
   A. α-Globin.
   B. γ-Globin.
   C. δ-Globin.
   D. β-Globin.
   E. ε-Globin.

41. An 18-year-old male student athlete undergoes hemoglobinopathy screening before playing football in his first year of college. He is found to have sickle cell trait. In which one of the following settings can this patient experience sickle cell formation leading to vascular occlusion?
   A. Local anesthesia.
   B. Renal medullary carcinoma.
   C. Severe hypothermia.
   D. Travel to New York City in autumn.
   E. Vigorous exercise.

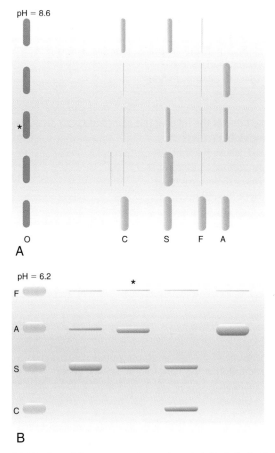

pH = 8.6

*

O   C   S   F   A

A

pH = 6.2

*

F

A

S

C

B

Figure 10-28 **A,** Cellulose acetate electrophoresis (pH=8.6). **B,** Citrate agar electrophoresis (pH=6.2). The origin (*O*) and hemoglobin controls (hemoglobins *A, F, S,* and *C*) are shown. The asterisk marks the lane for this patient.

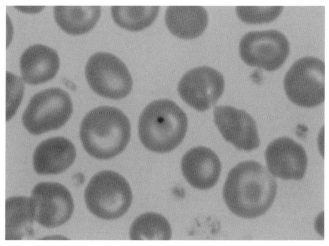

Figure 10-29 Wright-Giemsa–stained peripheral blood smear (×100).

43. You are asked to review a peripheral blood smear from a 19-year-old woman with sickle cell disease (homozygous hemoglobin S). An RBC inclusion is identified and is shown in Figure 10-29. The inclusion is composed of which one of the following constituents?
    A. Denatured hemoglobin.
    B. Denatured hemoglobin H.
    C. DNA.
    D. Iron.
    E. RNA.

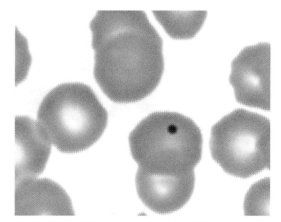

Figure 10-30 Wright-Giemsa–stained peripheral blood smear (×100).

42. A 34-year-old pregnant African American woman is seen in her obstetrician's office and undergoes hemoglobinopathy screening. The alkaline and acid hemoglobin electrophoreses are shown in Figure 10-28, *A* and *B,* respectively. The sickle solubility test is positive. Which one of the following would be most characteristic of the CBC?
    A. High MCV.
    B. Low hemoglobin (HGB) concentration.
    C. Low RBC.
    D. High MCH.
    E. Normal RDW.

44. The inclusion in the red cell in Figure 10-30 is most consistent with which one of the following?
    A. *Babsia microti.*
    B. Cabot's ring.
    C. Howell-Jolly body.
    D. Basophilic stippling.
    E. Pappenheimer body.

45. Which one of the following individuals would be expected to have the lowest MCV?
    A. 2-month-old, healthy boy.
    B. 32-year-old pregnant woman with sickle cell trait.
    C. 18-year-old man with sickle cell disease on hydroxyurea therapy.
    D. 6-month-old, healthy boy.
    E. 2-year-old boy with Fanconi's anemia.

46. Which one of the following statements about manual counting of reticulocytes is true?
    A. Manual counting of reticulocytes can be performed on a standard Wright-Giemsa–stained blood smear.
    B. Manual counting of reticulocytes is performed by counting 100 red cells.
    C. Manual counting of reticulocytes is highly reproducible.
    D. Manual counting is the only method available to quantify reticulocytes; no alternative methods are available.
    E. In most laboratories, manual counting of reticulocytes has been replaced by automated cell counters.

47. Which one of the following is the best method for the diagnosis of paroxysmal nocturnal hemoglobinuria (PNH)?
    A. A careful review of the blood smear.
    B. The sucrose lysis test.
    C. The acidified serum test (Ham's test).
    D. Flow cytometry.
    E. Genetic testing.

48. The acidified serum test (Ham's test) can be characterized as which one of the following?
    A. Gold standard for the definitive diagnosis of PNH.
    B. Requires highly specialized equipment.
    C. Requires mixing of treated patient and control blood to prove that the patient's hemolysis is caused by an increased susceptibility of his red cells to activated complement.
    D. Absence of lysis of the patient's red cells by his acidified serum excludes the diagnosis of PNH.
    E. Requires the mixing of patient blood and sucrose to prove that the patient's hemolysis is caused by an increased susceptibility of his red cells to activated complement.

49. Which one of the following statements about the sucrose lysis test is true?
    A. Allows a definite diagnosis of PNH.
    B. Must be carried out with a sample of whole blood anticoagulated with EDTA.
    C. Is a screening test for PNH.
    D. Requires expensive laboratory instrumentation.
    E. Is based on the lysis of white cells by complement in patients with PNH.

50. The rapid determination of a patient's hemoglobin level is important in surgical and intensive care settings. Which one of the following is the most commonly used method in handheld devices for point-of-care (POC) hemoglobin measurement?
    A. Impedance method.
    B. Flow cytometry–based method.
    C. Conductivity-based method.
    D. Centrifugation.
    E. Light-absorption–based method.

51. Which one of the following is a cause of polycythemia?
    A. Decreased 2,3-diphosphoglycerate (2,3-DPG or 2,3-BPG).
    B. Cobalamin poisoning.
    C. Familial decrease in erythropoietin synthesis.
    D. Low-affinity hemoglobin.
    E. After renal transplantation.

52. Which one of the following is the most common inherited enzyme deficiency of the glycolytic pathway?
    A. Aldolase.
    B. Glucose-6-phophate isomerase.
    C. Hexokinase.
    D. Phosphofructokinase.
    E. Pyruvate kinase.

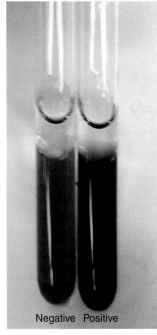

Figure 10-31 The tests tubes show a qualitative, colorimetric glucose-6-phosphate dehydrogenase (G6PD) activity assay. A false-negative test is shown on the left, and a G6PD-deficient patient sample is shown on the right.

53. A qualitative, colorimetric glucose-6-phosphate dehydrogenase (G6PD) activity assay is performed on two samples. The sample on the right side of Figure 10-31 is from a G6PD-deficient patient after 40 minutes of incubation, which suggests G6PD deficiency. The sample on the left is from another patient after 40 minutes of incubation. According to the qualitative test, the patient does not have G6PD deficiency. However, the patient undergoes further testing using a quantitative assay and is found to be G6PD deficient. Which one of the following circumstances can account for this false-negative result?
    A. Hemizygous male.
    B. Heterozygous woman.
    C. Hypergammaglobulinemia.
    D. Reticulocytopenia.
    E. Sickle cell trait.

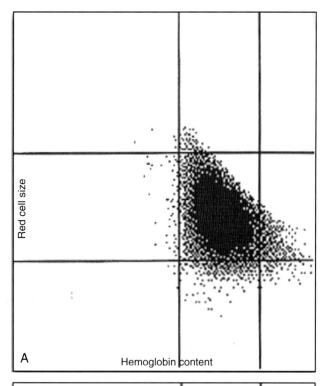

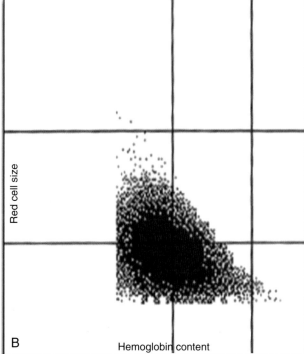

Figure 10-32 Red cell cytogram from an automated hematology analyser. Individual red cell volume (*y*-axis) is plotted against individual red cell hemoglobin content (*x*-axis). **A**, Red cell cytogram for a normal donor (normocytic, normochromic). **B**, Red cell cytogram for the patient.

Table 10-8

	Patient	Reference Range	Units
WBC	8.2	3.04-9.06	$\times 10^9/L$
RBC	1.88	4.3-5.6	$\times 10^{12}/L$
Hemoglobin	6.2	13.3-16.2	g/dL
Hematocrit	16.9	38.8-46.4	%
MCV	89.9	79.0-93.3	fL
MCH	33.0	26.7-31.9	pg
MCHC	36.7	32.3-35.9	g/dL
RDW	19.5	<14	%
PLT	136	165-415	$\times 10^9/L$
Reticulocytes	2.0	0-2.0	%

55. A 92-year-old man with a history of diabetes, hypertension, and atrial fibrillation (not anticoagulated) and a recent diagnosis of chronic lymphocytic leukemia presents to the emergency department with complaints of one week of fatigue, shortness of breath, and dizziness. His laboratory evaluation shows that he has a warm autoimmune hemolytic anemia. The CBC is shown in Table 10-8. Which one of the following is the reticulocyte index (RI)?
   A. 0.12
   B. 0.38
   C. 0.75
   D. 2.70
   E. 5.30

56. Which one of the following staining methods is recommended as the comparability method (i.e., gold standard) for enumerating reticulocytes?
   A. Auramine O.
   B. Ethidium bromide.
   C. Monoclonal antibodies (anti-CD71).
   D. New methylene blue (NMB).
   E. Thiazole orange.

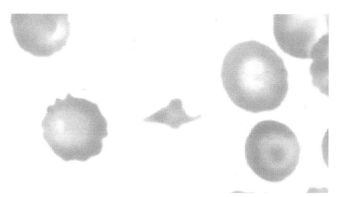

Figure 10-33 Wright-Giemsa–stained peripheral blood smear (×100).

54. Which one of the following disorders is most consistent with the red cell cytogram shown in Figure 10-32, *B*?
   A. β-Thalassemia trait.
   B. Congenital dyserythropoietic anemia.
   C. Iron deficiency anemia.
   D. Megaloblastic anemia.
   E. Sickle cell disease.

57a. The red cell in the center of Figure 10-33 is most consistent with which one of the following?
   A. Burr cell.
   B. Acanthocyte.
   C. Stomatocyte.
   D. Teardrop cell.
   E. Schistocyte.

57b. Schistocytes are found in which one of the following?
  A. Abnormalities of lipid metabolism.
  B. On blood smears prepared over 36 hours after phlebotomy.
  C. In blood smears from uremic patients.
  D. In blood smears from patients with lead poisoning.
  E. In blood smears from patients with microangiopathic hemolytic anemias.

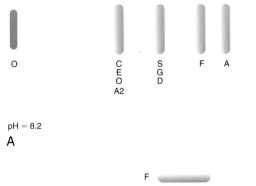

pH = 8.2

A

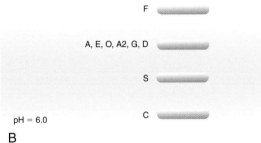

pH = 6.0

B

Figure 10-34 **A,** Alkaline hemoglobin electrophoresis. **B,** Acid hemoglobin electrophoresis. The bands represent the approximate position of the migrating hemoglobins. O, origin with hemoglobin fractions migrating from left to right (i.e., A runs faster than C).

58. Cellulose acetate electrophoresis (Figure 10-34) performed at pH 8.2 is a method used to separate which one of the following pairs of hemoglobins?
  A. Hemoglobins S and G-Philadelphia.
  B. Hemoglobins S and D-Punjab.
  C. Hemoglobins C and E.
  D. Hemoglobins C and A2.
  E. Hemoglobins O-Arab and D-Punjab.

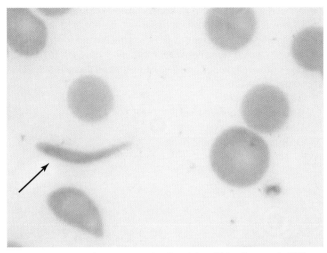

Figure 10-35 Wright-Giemsa–stained peripheral blood smear (×100).

59. Which one of the following disorders is associated with the cell indicated by the arrow in Figure 10-35?
  A. Hemoglobin C disease (homozygous hemoglobin C).
  B. Hemoglobin SD disease (double heterozygous hemoglobin S and hemoglobin D).
  C. Hereditary elliptocytosis.
  D. *Plasmodium falciparum.*
  E. Microangiopathic hemolytic anemia.

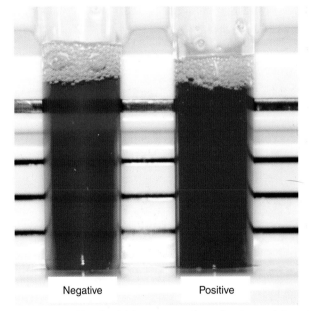

Negative   Positive

Figure 10-36 Sickle cell solubility test control samples. A normal donor is on the left, and a sample from a patient with sickle cell disease is on the right.

60. A sickle solubility test is performed by adding sodium hydrosulfite in a phosphate buffer to a hemolysate. If hemoglobin S is present, it will be reduced and form liquid crystals, which turn the solution cloudy (Figure 10-36). Which one of the following disorders can cause a false-positive sickle solubility test result?

A. Severe anemia.
B. Deglycerolized red cells.
C. Elevated hemoglobin F.
D. Hypergammaglobulinemia.
E. Newborn.

Table 10-9

	Patient	Reference Range	Units
WBC	7.9	3.04-9.06	$\times 10^9$/L
RBC	1.88	4.3-5.6	$\times 10^{12}$/L
Hemoglobin	6.2	13.3-16.2	g/dL
Hematocrit	16.9	38.8-46.4	%
MCV	89.9	79.0-93.3	fL
MCH	33.0	26.7-31.9	pg
MCHC	36.7	32.3-35.9	g/dL
RDW	21.5	<14	%
PLT	<10	165-415	$\times 10^9$/L
Reticulocytes	8.7	0-2.0	%
PT	13.4	12.7-15.4	seconds
aPTT	34.3	26.3-39.4	seconds
Fibrinogen	788	233-496	mg/dL
D-dimer	440	220-740	ng/mL FEU

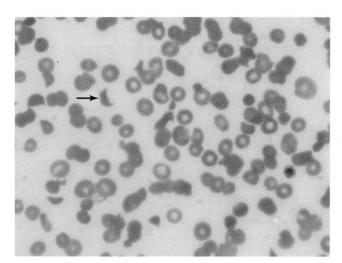

Figure 10-37 Wright-Giemsa–stained peripheral blood smear (×100).

A 17-year-old boy is seen in his primary care physician's office for nausea, abdominal pain, fatigue, and dyspnea on exertion. There is no evidence of bleeding, and no splenomegaly. The CBC, coagulation studies, and laboratory studies are shown in Table 10-9. The patient is type O+ with a negative red cell antibody screen and a negative direct antiglobulin test. The peripheral blood smear is shown in Figure 10-37. Use this scenario to answer the following three questions.

61a. Which one of the following laboratory tests would be expected to be below the reference range?

A. Creatinine.
B. Blood by urine dipstick.
C. Haptoglobin.
D. Lactate dehydrogenase.
E. Total bilirubin.

61b. Which one of the following cells is indicated by the arrow in Figure 10-37?

A. Acanthocyte.
B. Echinocyte.
C. Reticulocyte.
D. Schistocyte.
E. Spherocyte.

61c. Which one of the following would be the most appropriate treatment for this patient?

A. Eculizumab.
B. Plasma exchange.
C. Red cell exchange.
D. Rituximab.
E. Single-donor platelets.

62. Which one of the following results is *least* likely in a 45-year-old man presenting with macrocytic anemia?

A. Decreased plasma vitamin B_{12}.
B. Increased plasma methylmalonic acid.
C. Increased plasma homocysteine.
D. Decreased plasma folate.
E. Increased γ-glutamyl transpeptidase.

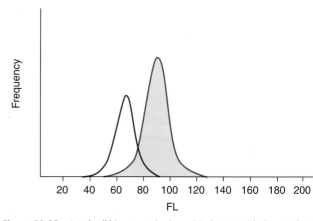

Figure 10-38 A red cell histogram (*red curve*) is shown, with the number of red cells on the y-axis and the size of the red cells on the x-axis. A normal red cell histogram (*blue curve*) is shown as a reference.

63. Which one of the following conditions is most consistent with the solid red line (red cell histogram) in Figure 10-38?

A. Zidovudine therapy.
B. Folate deficiency.
C. Hydroxyurea therapy.
D. Lead poisoning.
E. End-stage liver disease.

Answers

1. A. Liver disease.
   Rationale: Liver disease leads to target cells and acanthocytes, not to Burr cells seen in this patient.
   B. Delay between blood draw and preparation of the blood smear.
   Rationale: The delay between blood draw and preparation of a blood smear leads to the development of Burr cells, which are shown in the figure.
   C. Hemoglobin C disease.
   Rationale: Patients with hemoglobin C disease have hemoglobin C crystals and folded cells, not Burr cells, on their blood smear.
   D. Status postsplenectomy.
   Rationale: Asplenic patients have Howell-Jolly bodies on their blood smears, not Burr cells.
   E. Iron deficiency.
   Rationale: Iron-deficient patients have microcytic hypochromic red cells, teardrop cells, and elliptocytes, not Burr cells.

   ## Major points of discussion
   - Burr cells (echinocytes) are red blood cells with projections equally spaced over the entire cell surface.
   - They are most commonly seen on blood smears that were prepared more than 8 hours after phlebotomy.
   - They can also be seen in patients with uremia or burns and after a red cell transfusion.
   - Burr cells need to be distinguished from acanthocytes, which show irregularly spaced projections.
   - Burr cells are reversible; patients who have had transfusions will only have Burr cells within approximately 48 hours after transfusion.

2. A. β-Thalassemia trait.
   Rationale: Although basophilic stippling is present in patients with β-thalassemia, the normal MCV and hemoglobin A2 argue against this diagnosis.
   B. Anemia secondary to chronic renal failure.
   Rationale: Basophilic stippling is not present in patients with anemia of renal origin.
   C. Hemoglobinopathy not detected by electrophoresis.
   Rationale: Although basophilic stippling can be present in some hemoglobinopathies, the most likely explanation for the basophilic stippling in a child with anemia, normal hemoglobin electrophoresis, and normal hemoglobin A2 is lead poisoning.
   D. Lead intoxication.
   Rationale: Lead intoxication and thalassemia are frequent causes of basophilic stippling in children. In the absence of evidence of thalassemia, lead poisoning is the most probable explanation. Lead levels should be determined.
   E. Liver disease.
   Rationale: Basophilic stippling is not present in patients with liver disease.

   ## Major points of discussion
   - Basophilic stippling consists of evenly distributed granules that stain deep blue with Wright's stain.
   - The granules consist of ribonucleoproteins and mitochondrial remnants.
   - Basophilic stippling can be found in conditions that show defective or accelerated heme synthesis.
   - These conditions include lead intoxication, thalassemias, hemoglobinopathies, myelodysplasias, and megaloblastic anemia.
   - Unless there is evidence of thalassemia, lead levels should be determined in children with basophilic stippling.

3. **A. Sickle cell disorder.**
   Rationale: The patient's blood smear shows sickle cells and boat cells. The most likely diagnosis is a sickle cell disorder, such as hemoglobin SS, SC, hemoglobin S with β-thalassemia, or hemoglobin C–Harlem.
   B. Homozygous hemoglobin S.
   Rationale: Although the blood smear is fully consistent with hemoglobin SS, the patient could also have other sickling disorders, such as hemoglobin S with β-thalassemia.
   C. Lead poisoning.
   Rationale: Lead poisoning causes basophilic stippling on the blood smear, not the sickle cells and boat cells as shown in the figure.
   D. Thrombotic thrombocytopenic purpura.
   Rationale: Thrombotic thrombocytopenic purpura produces the schistocytes seen on the blood smear, not the sickle cells shown in the figure.
   E. Hereditary elliptocytosis.
   Rationale: Hereditary elliptocytosis causes elliptocytes on the blood smear. The cells shown in the figure are boat cells and sickle cells, not elliptocytes.

   ## Major points of discussion
   - Disorders associated with sickle cells include hemoglobin SS, hemoglobin SC, hemoglobin S with β-thalassemia trait, and hemoglobin C-Harlem.
   - The red cell deformation is caused by the formation of rodlike structures consisting of polymerized hemoglobin S.
   - Sickle cells are irreversibly deformed; boat cells are plumper than sickle cells, and their deformation is reversible.
   - Therapy for sickle cell disorders includes transfusion of red blood cells, red blood cell exchange, hydroxyurea, and bone marrow transplantation.
   - A leading cause of death in patients with sickle cell disorders is acute chest syndrome.

4. A. α-Thalassemia trait.
   Rationale: A presumptive diagnosis of α-thalassemia trait can be made when there is microcytosis, normal hemoglobin fractions (normal hemoglobin A2), and normal iron studies.
   B. β-Thalassemia trait.
   Rationale: β-Thalassemia trait presents with microcytosis and an elevated hemoglobin A2.
   C. δβ-Thalassemia trait.
   Rationale: δβ-Thalassemia trait presents with microcytosis, elevated hemoglobin F, and normal hemoglobin A2.
   D. Hemoglobin E trait.
   Rationale: Hemoglobin E trait can present with microcytosis. It shows as a peak eluting in the A2-window on HPLC.
   E. Hemoglobin Lepore.

Rationale: Hemoglobin Lepore can present with microcytosis. It shows as a peak eluting in the A2-window on HPLC.

Major points of discussion

■ There are four α-globin genes (two on each chromosome) with two α-globin genes in *cis* on each chromosome (α2, α1). α-Thalassemias are most commonly caused by deletion of one or more α-globin genes.

■ α-Thalassemia trait can be inherited as one α-globin gene deletion (-α/αα), two α-globin gene deletions in *trans* (-α/-α), or two α-globin genes deleted in *cis* (--/αα).

■ One α-globin gene deletion -α/αα) is usually clinically and hematologically silent but can show mild microcytosis and hypochromia.

■ α-Thalassemia trait caused by two gene deletions in *cis* or *trans* (--/αα or -α/-α, respectively) is hematologically mild; there may be a very mild anemia, but the hemoglobin can have overlap with the reference range; and an elevated RBC, a reduced MCV, and a reduced MCH are generally present.

■ A presumptive diagnosis of α-thalassemia trait can be made when there are red cell indices suggestive of thalassemia (i.e., elevated RBC; low MCV and MCH), a normal hemoglobin A2 and F, and normal iron studies.

5. A. α-Thalassemia trait.
Rationale: A presumptive diagnosis of α-thalassemia trait can be made in the presence of thalassemic red cell indices with normal hemoglobin A2, normal hemoglobin F, and normal iron studies.
B. β-Thalassemia trait.
Rationale: β-Thalassemia trait presents with microcytosis and an elevated hemoglobin A2.
C. δβ-Thalassemia trait.
Rationale: δβ-Thalassemia trait presents with microcytosis, elevated hemoglobin F, and normal hemoglobin A2.
D. Hemoglobin E trait.
Rationale: Hemoglobin E trait can present with microcytosis. It shows as a variant peak eluting in the A2-window on HPLC. No variants are present on the chromatogram shown in the figure.
E. Hemoglobin Constant Spring.
Rationale: Hemoglobin Constant Spring can present with microcytosis. It shows as late-eluting variant peaks caused by the instability of this hemoglobin variant. No variants are present on the chromatogram shown in the figure.

Major points of discussion

■ Individuals have two β-globin genes; one on each chromosome.

■ β-Thalassemia is caused by deletions or mutations that cause decreased (or absence) of β-globin synthesis. β⁺-Thalassemia denotes a gene that produces decreased amounts of globin compared with a normal β-globin gene. β⁰-Thalassemia denotes a gene that does not produce β-globin.

■ β-Thalassemia trait is caused by the inheritance of one abnormal β-thalassemia gene. Homozygosity or double heterozygosity for β-thalassemia can result in a clinically significant disorder, also known as β-thalassemia intermedia or β-thalassemia major.

■ β-Thalassemia minor is a clinical description, which genetically corresponds to β-thalassemia trait. It denotes a clinically asymptomatic condition that does not require chronic red cell transfusions.

■ β-Thalassemia major is a transfusion-dependent disorder caused by homozygous or double heterozygous β-thalassemia (e.g., β⁰/β⁰ or β⁰/β⁺).

■ β-Thalassemia intermedia is a disorder caused by homozygous or double heterozygous β-thalassemia in which the patient is not transfusion dependent but does require transfusion support during times of stress (e.g., β⁺/β⁺).

■ A presumptive diagnosis of β-thalassemia trait can be made in the presence of thalassemic red cell parameters (i.e., high RBC, low MCV, and low MCH with an elevated hemoglobin A2 on hemoglobin fractionation).

6. A. α-Thalassemia trait
Rationale: A presumptive diagnosis of α-thalassemia trait can be made in the presence of microcytosis with a normal hemoglobin A2, normal hemoglobin F, and normal iron studies.
B. β-Thalassemia trait.
Rationale: β-Thalassemia trait is associated with microcytosis and an elevated hemoglobin A2.
C. δβ-Thalassemia trait.
Rationale: δβ-Thalassemia trait is associated with microcytosis, elevated hemoglobin F, and normal hemoglobin A2.
D. Hemoglobin E trait.
Rationale: Hemoglobin E trait can be associated with microcytosis. It shows as a peak eluting in the A2-window on HPLC. No variant peak is present on HPLC in the figure.
E. Hemoglobin Constant Spring.
Rationale: Hemoglobin Constant Spring can present with microcytosis. It shows as late-eluting peaks caused by the instability of this hemoglobin variant. No variant peaks are present on HPLC in the figure.

Major points of discussion

■ The β-globin–like genes are located on chromosome 11. They are arranged in the order of expression from embryonic life to adulthood from 5′ to 3′: ε-^{G}γ-^{A}γ-δ-β.

■ Deletions of the β-globin–like genes can result in a thalassemic syndrome. Deletional β-thalassemias are less common than point mutations. (δβ)⁰-Thalassemia trait is caused by a deletion of both the δ and β genes, which are adjacent to one another on chromosome 11.

■ (δβ)⁰-Thalassemia trait is generally clinically silent but hematologically resembles β-thalassemia. The hemoglobin A2 is normal, but the hemoglobin F percentage is elevated in (δβ)⁰-thalassemia trait. The hemoglobin F can represent up to 20% of the total hemoglobin.

■ (δβ)⁰-Thalassemia trait should be considered when thalassemic red cell indices are present (i.e., high RBC, low MCV, and low MCH) with a normal hemoglobin A2 and elevated hemoglobin F.

■ Homozygotes for (δβ)⁰-thalassemia and double heterozygous (δβ)⁰-thalassemia and β-thalassemia usually present as β-thalassemia intermedia because almost all of the hemoglobin is hemoglobin F.

7. A. 3.2% sodium citrate.
Rationale: Sodium citrate is a liquid anticoagulant that dilutes the blood sample and can also shrink cells.
B. Hirudin.
Rationale: Hirudin has been studied as an anticoagulant for CBCs, but it is not used as an anticoagulant for blood sample collection.
C. K₂EDTA (dipotassium ethylenediamine tetra-acetic acid).
Rationale: K₂EDTA is the anticoagulant of choice.
D. K₃EDTA (tripotassium ethylenediaminetetra-acetic acid).
Rationale: K₃EDTA can cause cell shrinkage and slight dilution of the sample.
E. Sodium heparin.
Rationale: Sodium heparin can cause white cell clumping.

Major points of discussion
- Ethylenediamine tetra-acetic acid (EDTA) is the preferred anticoagulant for performance of the CBC.
- The International Council for Standardization in Hematology recommends the dipotassium EDTA (K₂EDTA) form of this salt.
- K₃EDTA can cause cell shrinkage, which can lead to lower MCV and HCT; slight dilution of the sample occurs because it is a liquid.
- 3.2% sodium citrate is a liquid anticoagulant that dilutes the sample. It can also shrink cells.
- Sodium heparin may cause white cell clumping and artifacts on peripheral blood smear.[1]

8. A. β-Thalassemia trait.
Rationale: Hemoglobin A2 in β-thalassemia trait is usually greater than 3.5%, but not greater than 5.0% to 6.0%.
B. Hemoglobin C trait.
Rationale: Hemoglobin C elutes at a retention time (C-window), which is later than hemoglobin A2 (A2-window); the proportion of hemoglobin C is generally 35% to 45% of the total hemoglobin; although microcytosis can be present, it is usually not present to this degree.
C. Hemoglobin D–Los Angeles.
Rationale: Hemoglobin D elutes at a retention time (D-window), which is later than hemoglobin A2 (A2-window). The proportion of hemoglobin D is generally 35%; microcytosis is not usually a feature of hemoglobin D trait.
D. Hemoglobin E trait.
Rationale: Hemoglobin E trait elutes at approximately the same retention time as hemoglobin A2 (A2-window) and is associated with thalassemic red cell parameters (low MCV, low MCH, high RBC).
E. Hemoglobin S trait.
Rationale: Hemoglobin S elutes in the S-window, which is later than hemoglobin A2 (A2-window). It is not associated with microcytosis unless a concomitant α-thalassemia is present; the percentage is 35% to 45% of the total hemoglobin.

Major points of discussion
- Hemoglobin E is found predominantly in patients from Southeast Asia.
- Hemoglobin E is caused by a point mutation $\beta^{26Glu \rightarrow Lys}$. This mutation leads to the gain of +2 charges and also leads to an alternate splice site causing an unstable mRNA. This causes not only a structural variant but also thalassemic red cell parameters.

- Hemoglobin E trait is associated with normal hemoglobin or mild anemia and may be associated with microcytosis. It is clinically asymptomatic. Homozygous hemoglobin E is clinically insignificant.
- It is important to identify hemoglobin E because it can cause a sickling disorder when coinherited with hemoglobin S. In addition, hemoglobin E/β-thalassemia is a severe thalassemic disorder (i.e., thalassemia major).
- Hemoglobin E runs in the C-position on alkaline electrophoresis but migrates to the A-position on acid electrophoresis.

9a. A. α-Thalassemia trait.
Rationale: A presumptive diagnosis of α-thalassemia trait can be made in the presence of microcytosis with a normal hemoglobin A2 and normal iron studies. The hemoglobin in α-thalassemia trait is either at the lower end of the reference range or slightly below it.
B. Hemoglobin H disease.
Rationale: Hemoglobin H is a fast-migrating hemoglobin that is produced in hemoglobin H disease, which is caused by the absence of three α-globin genes. It presents with a low to normal hemoglobin and severe microcytosis and hypochromia.
C. Hemoglobin Barts.
Rationale: Hemoglobin Barts is a fast-migrating hemoglobin formed from unpaired γ-globin tetramers. It results from the absence of all four α-globin genes. The affected fetuses will either die in utero or die shortly after birth.
D. Hemoglobin N–Baltimore trait.
Rationale: Hemoglobin N–Baltimore is a fast-migrating hemoglobin. It is a beta chain variant and composes approximately 45% of the total hemoglobin in heterozygous individuals. By itself, it is not associated with microcytosis or anemia.
E. Hemoglobin J trait.
Rationale: Hemoglobin J is a fast-migrating hemoglobin variant. It represents up to 45% of the total hemoglobin in heterozygous individuals. By itself, it is not associated with microcytosis or anemia.

9b. A. α_4.
Rationale: α-Globin tetramers are not formed in hemoglobin H disease.
B. β_4.
Rationale: Hemoglobin H, which is formed in hemoglobin H disease, is made up of β-globin tetramers.
C. γ_4.
Rationale: Hemoglobin Barts (γ_4) is composed of γ-globin tetramers. It is found in hemoglobin Barts disease, which is caused by the absence of four functioning α-globin genes. It is not compatible with life, and fetuses either die in utero or die shortly after birth.
D. $\zeta_2\varepsilon_2$.
Rationale: Hemoglobin Gower-1 is an embryonic hemoglobin that is not expressed in adulthood.
E. $\alpha_2\varepsilon_2$
Rationale: Hemoglobin Gower-2 is an embryonic hemoglobin that is not expressed in adulthood.

9c. **A. Hydrops fetalis.**
Rationale: Barts disease results from the deletion of four α-globin genes.

B. α-Thalassemia retardation syndrome.
Rationale: α-Thalassemia retardation syndrome can result from chromosome abnormality on chromosome 16 (ATR-16) or from a *trans* acting factor on the X chromosome (ATRX).
C. α-Thalassemia myelodysplasia syndrome.
Rationale: α-Thalassemia can be acquired from myelodysplasia and hematologic malignancies. It is not caused by deletion of four α-globin genes.
D. Cooley's anemia.
Rationale: β-Thalassemia major, also known as Cooley's anemia, is a result of inheritance of two β-thalassemia genes.
E. Hemolytic disease of the fetus and newborn (HDFN).
Rationale: HDFN can result in hydrops fetalis, as does Barts disease. However, HDFN is a result of maternal red cell alloantibodies that cross the placenta and cause hemolysis in the fetus.

Major points of discussion

- There are four α-globin genes (two on each chromosome) with two genes in *cis* on each chromosome (α2, α1). α-Thalassemias are most commonly caused by deletion of one or more α-globin genes.
- α-Thalassemia trait can be inherited as one α-globin gene deletion (-α/αα), two α-globin gene deletions in trans (-α/-α), or two α-globin genes deleted in cis (--/αα).
- One α-globin gene deletion (-α/αα) is usually clinically and hematologically silent but can show mild microcytosis and hypochromia.
- α-Thalassemia trait caused by two gene deletions in *cis* or *trans* (--/αα or -α/-α) is hematologically mild; there may be a very mild anemia, but the hemoglobin can have overlap with the reference range. There also may be an elevated RBC, a reduced MCV, and a reduced MCH. A presumptive diagnosis of α-thalassemia trait can be made when there are red cell indices suggestive of thalassemia (i.e., elevated RBC; low MCV and MCH) with a normal hemoglobin A2 and F.
- Presence of three α-globin deletions (-α/--) results in hemoglobin H disease, which results in chronic hemolysis that may go unnoticed or is clinically significant. There is significant hypochromia and microcytosis. The hemoglobin A2 may be normal or low. Unpaired β-globin chains form tetramers ($β_4$, hemoglobin H), which is a fast-migrating hemoglobin. H bodies are golf ball–sized red cell inclusions formed when oxidized.
- The absence of four α-globin genes results in Barts disease (hydrops fetalis). Unpaired γ-globin chains form hemoglobin Barts ($γ_4$). Hemoglobin Barts is a fatal disease that results in stillbirth or death shortly after birth.

10. A. Hypothermia.
Rationale: Fever shifts the curve to the right.
B. Acidosis.
Rationale: Acidosis shifts the curve to the right.
C. Decreased 2,3-diphosphoglycerate (DPG).
Rationale: Increased DPG shifts the curve to the right.
D. CO_2 release by hemoglobin.
Rationale: CO_2 binding by hemoglobin shifts the curve to the right.
E. High-affinity hemoglobin.
Rationale: High-affinity hemoglobins have decreased binding of DPG, which shifts the curve to the left.

Major points of discussion

- The hemoglobin oxygen dissociation curve (ODC) is constructed by plotting the oxygen saturation on the *y*-axis versus oxygen tension on the *x*-axis.
- The ODC is sigmoidal because of cooperativity. After one heme group binds oxygen, the molecular shape of the remaining heme groups are altered, which makes it easier for the other three heme groups to acquire oxygen.
- The p50 is the oxygen tension associated with 50% saturation of hemoglobin with oxygen. Hemoglobin has a p50 of 27 mm Hg.
- Different conditions alter the ODC and change the affinity of hemoglobin for oxygen.
- Shifts to the right leads to increased oxygen delivery to the tissues and shifts to the left decrease oxygen delivery to the tissues.
- Fever, acidosis, increased 2,3-DPG, and CO_2 binding to hemoglobin shift the curve to the right.
- Hypothermina, alkalosis, and decreased 2,3-DPG shift the curve to the left.
- Higher affinity hemoglobins, such as hemoglobin F and hemoglobin Chesapeake, shift the curve to the left.

11. A. Iron deficiency.
B. Hereditary pyropoikylocytosis.
Rationale: Increases osmotic fragility.
C. β-Thalassemia trait.
D. α-Thalassemia trait.
E. Sickle cell anemia.
Rationale for A, C, D, and E: These decrease osmotic fragility.

Major points of discussion

- An osmotic fragility test is performed by incubating patient red cells with decreasing concentrations of sodium chloride solution.
- The amount of hemolysis is determined by measuring free hemoglobin released into the supernatant using spectrophotometry at 540 nm.
- Normal donors will have 100% lysis by 0.3% NaCl concentration.
- Conditions that decrease the surface area/volume ratio lead to increased osmotic fragility. Complete hemolysis occurs at higher NaCl concentration than normal red cells.
- Spherocytes increase the surface/volume ratio. Spherocytes are often seen in hemolytic anemias, such as warm autoimmune hemolytic anemia and hereditary spherocytosis (HS).
- Increased osmotic fragility is a useful test for the diagnosis of HS, hereditary elliptocytosis (HE), and hereditary pyropoikylocytosis (a subtype of HE).
- However, warm autoimmune hemolytic anemia can also produce spherocytes and the osmotic fragility can be increased in the absence of HS and HE.

12. A. Anisocytosis.
Rationale: The RDW is a measure of anisocytosis (unequal red cell sizes) and is determined from the red cell histogram.
B. Hypochromia.
Rationale: The presence of hypochromia on a peripheral blood smear is represented by the MCH. The MCH is calculated as MCH = hemoglobin/RBC.
C. Macrocytosis.

Rationale: The presence of macrocytes on a peripheral blood smear is represented by an elevated MCV. The MCV is the mean of the red cell histogram and is reported in femtoliters.
D. Microcytosis, iron deficiency.
E. Microcytosis, β-thalassemia trait.
Rationale: The presence of microcytosis on peripheral blood smears is represented by an decreased MCV. The MCV is the mean of the red cell histogram and is reported in femtoliters. The RDW is classically within the reference range in β-thalassemia trait and increased in iron deficiency.

Major points of discussion
- The Coulter method is an impedance-based (electrical resistance) method. Cells are suspended in an electrolyte solution and passed through an aperture that has an electric field across it. As cells pass through the aperture, changes in impedance allow the number of cells to be counted and the size of the cell to be determined.
- The number of cells of a particular size that are counted by the analyzer can be shown graphically as a red cell histogram. The number of cells counted for each red cell size is plotted: size on the x-axis and the number on the y-axis.
- The RDW is a measure of the spread of the red cell histogram. An elevated RDW corresponds to anisocytosis on a peripheral blood smear. Anisocytosis describes the observation of a wide range of differing red cell sizes.
- The RDW can be measured in two ways from the red cell histogram. The RDW-SD (standard deviation) is determined by measuring the distance between the upward and downward slopes of the distribution at 20% of the height. The RDW-CV (coefficient of variation) is calculated as $RDW - CV = SD/MCV$, where SD is the standard deviation of the distribution and MCV is the mean corpuscular volume.
- Examples of conditions that lead to an elevated RDW include recent hemorrhage, iron deficiency anemia, treated iron deficiency anemia, sideroblastic anemia, reticulocytosis, B_{12} and folate deficiency, and others.

13. A. Red blood cell count (RBC).
Rationale: The area under the red cell histogram is the RBC.
B. Hematocrit (HCT).
Rationale: Some instruments can directly measure HCT, but it can also be a calculated value: $HCT = RBC \times MCV$, where RBC is the RBC and MCV is the mean corpuscular volume.
C. Mean corpuscular volume (MCV).
Rationale: MCV is the mean of the distribution shown in the red cell histogram.
D. Mean corpuscular hemoglobin (MCH).
Rationale: The mean cell hemoglobin can be measured directly or calculated: $MCH = HGB/RBC$, where is HGB is the hemoglobin and RBC is the RBC
E. Red cell distribution width (RDW).
Rationale: The RDW is determined by the standard deviation (RDW-SD) or coefficient of variation (RDW-CV) of the red cell histogram.

Major points of discussion
- The Coulter method is an impedance-based (electrical resistance) method. Cells are suspended in an electrolyte solution and passed through an aperture that has an electric field across it. As cells pass through the aperture,

changes in impedance allow the number of cells to be counted and the size of the cell to be determined.
- The number of cells corresponding to red cell size that are counted by the analyzer can be shown graphically as a red cell histogram. The number of cells counted for each red cell size is plotted: size on the x-axis and the number on the y-axis.
- The MCV is the average size of the red cells.
- If an automated instrument is not used, then a manual RBC (hemocytometer) and manual HCT (packed cell volume) can be used to calculate the MCV. $MCV = HCT \times 1000/RBC$, where HCT is the hematocrit and RBC is the red blood cell count.
- In automated hematology analyzers, the MCV is determined from the mean of the red cell histogram.
- An elevated MCV corresponds to macrocytosis, and a decreased MCV indicates microcytosis, which both can be seen on the peripheral blood smear.

14. **A. RBC.**
Rationale: The area under the red cell histogram is the RBC.
B. HCT.
Rationale: Some instruments can directly measure HCT, but it can also be a calculated value: $HCT = RBC \times MCV$, where RBC is the red blood cell count and MCV is the mean corpuscular volume.
C. MCV.
Rationale: MCV is the mean of the distribution shown in the red cell histogram.
D. MCH.
Rationale: The MCH can be measured directly or calculated: $MCH = HGB/RBC$, where HGB is the hemoglobin and RBC is the red blood cell count.
E. RDW.
Rationale: The RDW is determined by the standard deviation or coefficient of variation of the red cell histogram. It is a measure of anisocytosis.

Major points of discussion
- The Coulter method is an impedance-based (electrical resistance) method. Cells are suspended in an electrolyte solution and passed through an aperture that has an electric field across it. As cells pass through the aperture, changes in impedance allow the number of cells to be counted and the size of the cell to be determined.
- The number of cells of a particular size that are counted by the analyzer can be shown graphically as a red cell histogram. The number of cells counted for each red cell size is plotted: size on the x-axis and the number on the y-axis.
- The number of red cells can be counted manually by taking a sample, diluting it with an appropriate diluent, and then counting the number of cells in a given volume of the hemocytometer (usually 1 μL). Automated analyzers have replaced this method because it has a high variability and is time and labor intensive.
- The RBC on automated hematology analyzers can be determined by determining the area under the curve on the red cell histogram. It is expressed as the number of cells $\times 10^{12}/L$.
- The RBC is not a measure of red cell mass. For example, pregnant women have an increased total blood volume and a lower RBC. However, the total red cell mass is increased.

15. A. RBC.
Rationale: The area under the red cell histogram is the RBC.
B. HCT.
Rationale: Some instruments can directly measure HCT, but it can also be calculated: HCT = RBC × MCV, where RBC is the red blood cell count and MCV is the mean corpuscular volume.
C. MCV.
Rationale: MCV is the mean of the distribution shown in the red cell histogram.
D. MCH.
Rationale: The MCH can be measured directly or calculated: MCH = HGB/RBC, where HGB is the hemoglobin and RBC is the red blood cell count.
E. RDW.
Rationale: The RDW is determined by the standard deviation (RDW-SD) or coefficient of variation (RDW-CV) of the red cell histogram.

Major points of discussion

- The Coulter method is an electrical impedance-based (resistance) method. Cells are suspended in an electrolyte solution and passed through an aperture that has an electric field across it. As cells pass through the aperture, changes in impedance allow the number of cells to be counted and the size of the cell to be determined.
- The number of cells that are counted by the analyzer can be shown graphically as a histogram. The histogram corresponding to the range of red cell size is the red cell histogram. The number of cells counted for each red cell size is plotted: size on the *x*-axis (femtoliters) and the number on the *y*-axis.
- The RDW measures the range of the sizes of the red cells in the sample. The higher the RDW, the greater the spread of cell sizes.
- The RDW corresponds to the degree of anisocytosis on a manual peripheral blood smear review.
- The RDW can be determined by two methods. The RDW-SD is the distance between the points on the upward and downward sloping curves at 20% off the baseline. The RDW-CV is 1 standard deviation of the distribution divided by the mean corpuscular volume (SD/MCV).
- The RDW is useful in determining what kind of anemia is present. For example, iron deficiency and thalassemia are both microcytic, but iron deficiency tends to be accompanied by an elevated RDW and thalassemia a relatively normal one.

16. A. Hemoglobin.
Rationale: Hemoglobin is measured after lysing the red cells. Lysing agents can break up agglutinates and rouleaux.
B. MCV.
C. MCH.
Rationale: MCH = HGB/RBC, where HGB is the hemoglobin and RBC is the red blood cell count; hemoglobin is unchanged with rouleaux and the RBC is decreased. Therefore, the MCH is falsely elevated with rouleaux.
D. RBC.
Rationale for B and D: Red cells stick together in rouleaux, pass together though the analyzer aperture, and then appear as a single, very large cell. Therefore, the MCV would be falsely elevated and the RBC decreased.

E. RDW.
Rationale: The distribution of red cells becomes wider since rouleaux creates a population of what appears to be large cells.

Major points of discussion

- Rouleaux are present when four or more red cells are attached to each other with the length greater than the width. The red cells are arranged as a "stack of coins."
- Rouleaux are formed when there are elevated levels of γ-globulins or acute-phase proteins such as fibrinogen.
- Conditions associated with rouleaux include: lymphoproliferative disorders (e.g., multiple myeloma), chronic liver disease, and chronic inflammatory disorders.
- Rouleaux in vitro can lead to erroneous results on automated hematology analyzers. The red cells pass through the aperture as several cells together, which appear to the instrument as a single, large cell. This reduces the RBC and increases the MCV. The RDW is wide because the rouleaux create a population of what appear to be large red cells. The hemoglobin concentration (HGB) is generally unchanged because all of the cells are lysed before analysis and agglutinates and rouleaux are broken up. The MCH is increased because the RBC is decreased (MCH = HGB/RBC).
- Rouleaux should be differentiated from agglutination where the cells are stacked such that the width and length are approximately equal. Agglutination is seen in the presence of immunoglobulin M antibodies, as seen in cold agglutinin disease, Epstein-Barr virus infection, and mycoplasma infection. Paroxysmal cold hemoglobinuria can also cause agglutination.

17. **A. α-Thalassemia trait.**
Rationale: ZPP is normal in α-thalassemia trait.
B. Anemia of chronic disease.
Rationale: ZPP is increased in anemia of chronic disease.
C. Iron deficiency anemia.
Rationale: ZPP is increased in iron deficiency anemia.
D. Lead poisoning,
Rationale: ZPP is increased in lead poisoning.
E. Sideroblastic anemia.
Rationale: ZPP is increased in sideroblastic anemia.

Major points of discussion

- Iron is inserted into protoporphyrin IX to form heme. In the absence of iron, heme cannot be formed, and protoporphyrin IX increases.
- Zinc binds to protoporphyrin IX to form ZPP, which can be measured in serum.
- In iron deficiency or anemia of chronic disease, where iron is not available to form heme, ZPP levels increase. ZPP levels can also increase in lead poisoning, erythropoietic protoporphyria, and sideroblastic anemia.
- ZPP levels are normal in thalassemia.
- ZPP is measured using a fluorescent assay. Therefore, hyperbilirubinemia and increased riboflavin can falsely elevate ZPP.
- ZPP is not sensitive enough as a screening test for lead poisoning in children.

18a. A. 260 nm.
Rationale: Ribonucleic acid (RNA) can be measured at 260 nm.

B. 340 nm.

Rationale: 340 nm is used to measure G6PD activity by measuring reduced nicotinamide adenine dinucleotide phosphate production using a kinetic method.

C. 450 nm.

Rationale: Bilirubin can be measured in amniotic fluid (OD450) and plotted on a Liley curve to manage hemolytic disease of the newborn.

D. 540 nm.

Rationale: 540 nm is used to measure hemoglobin concentration in the cyanmethemoglobin method.

E. 1100 nm.

Rationale: Many of the currently available clinical spectrophotometers in the ultraviolet (UV)/visible range go up to 1100-nm wavelengths.

18b. A. Measures all forms of hemoglobin.

Rationale: All forms of hemoglobin *except* sulfhemoglobin are measured by the cyanmethemoglobin method.

B. Reagents are very stable.

Rationale: The reagents are considered to be generally stable.

C. Reagents are nontoxic.

Rationale: Cyanide is a known lethal chemical. Although the concentration in the reagent is low, it still must be handled with care and must be disposed of properly.

D. Method is not affected by lipemia.

Rationale: The method is spectrophotometric and is subject to interference by lipemia and high protein levels.

E. Completion of the reaction in 1 minute.

Rationale: The reaction time is rapid (10 minutes), but not as fast as 1 minute.

Major points of discussion

- The cyanmethemoglobin colorimetric method is recommended as the reference method for measuring hemoglobin concentration in a sample of blood.
- The reagent (Drabkin's reagent) contains ferricyanide and potassium cyanide. The ferricyanide converts hemoglobin to methemoglobin. (Fe^{2+} in hemoglobin is oxidized to Fe^{3+} to form methemoglobin). Cyanide then converts the methemoglobin into cyanmethemoglobin, which can be stably measured at 540 nm. The reaction is completed in about 10 minutes.
- Characteristics of the method:
  1. Relatively rapid (10 minutes).
  2. Reagents are stable.
  3. All forms of hemoglobin except sulfhemoglobin are measured.
  4. Reagents contain cyanide, which can be a lethal chemical.
- To measure hemoglobin concentration, a calibration curve is drawn by determining the absorption at 540 nm for varying concentration of hemoglobin (e.g., 0 to 80 g/dL). The absorbance from a patient sample is analyzed and read off the calibration curve.
- Errors include incomplete conversion to cyanmethemoglobin, lipemia, or hyperproteinemia, and being prone to pipetting errors.
- The important principles for clinical practice are outlined in the previous bullets. Nonetheless, review the Beer-Lambert law when studying spectrophotometry.

19. A. Hereditary spherocytosis (HS).

B. Hereditary pyropoikilocytosis.

C. Hereditary elliptocytosis.

D. α-Thalassemia trait.

Rationale: Decreased osmotic fragility.

E. Warm autoimmune hemolytic anemia.

Rationale for A, B, C, and E: Increased osmotic fragility.

Major points of discussion

- An osmotic fragility test is performed by incubating patient red cells with decreasing concentrations of sodium chloride solution (i.e., 0.85% normal saline to 0%).
- The amount of hemolysis is determined by measuring free hemoglobin released into the supernatant using spectrophotometry at 540 nm.
- Normal donors will have 100% lysis by 0.3% NaCl concentration.
- Conditions that increase the surface area/volume ratio lead to decreased osmotic fragility. Complete hemolysis occurs at lower NaCl concentration than normal red cells.
- Conditions that decrease osmotic fragility:
  - α- and β-thalassemia trait
  - Iron deficiency
  - Chronic liver disease
  - Hyponatremia
  - Sickle cell disease
  - Hemoglobin C (target cells)

20. A. β-Thalassemia trait.

Rationale: β-Thalassemia trait is microcytic with a uniform distribution of red cells.

B. End-stage liver disease.

Rationale: End-stage liver disease can show macrocytosis, but it would not explain the microcytic population of red cells.

C. Pseudothrombocytopenia.

Rationale: Platelet clumps can be counted as red cells on automated hematology analyzers, but usually they are smaller than the large distribution of microcytic cells shown in the histogram.

D. Treated B_{12} deficiency.

Rationale: Treated B_{12} deficiency should show macrocytosis. It does not account for the microcytic population of red cells.

E. Treated iron deficiency anemia.

Rationale: Iron deficiency anemia is a microcytic anemia. The population of normal to macrocytic red cells in treated iron deficiency represent the reticulocytosis that occurs. This leads to a dimorphic red cell population.

Major points of discussion

- The Coulter method is an electrical impedance-based (resistance) method. Cells are suspended in an electrolyte solution and passed through an aperture that has an electric field across it. As cells pass through the aperture, changes in impedance allow the number of cells to be counted and the size of the cell to be determined.
- The number of cells that are counted by the analyzer can be shown graphically as a histogram. The histogram corresponding to the range of red cell size is the red cell histogram. The number of cells counted for each red cell size is plotted: size on the *x*-axis (femtoliters) and the number on the *y*-axis.

- A dimorphic red cell histogram corresponds to the presence of two populations of red cells (or RBC-sized particles).
- Dimorphic red cell histograms can be caused by treated iron deficiency anemia (microcytic population) accompanied by a second population of normal to macrocytic red cells, which can represent transfused red cells or reticulocytes after iron replacement. Early iron deficiency can lead to an emerging population of microcytic cells among normal sized cells.
- Other causes of a dimorphic red cell histogram include treated megaloblastic anemia (B_{12} or folate deficiency), sideroblastic anemia, and hemolytic anemias (warm autoimmune, delayed hemolytic transfusion reactions, hereditary pyropoikilocytosis, and others).
- The red cell histogram is very informative because the MCV can be normal in the presence of a dimorphic population (average of microcytic and macrocytic populations).[4]

21a. A. Normocytic, hyperproliferative anemia.
Rationale: Normocytic anemias show a normal MCV. Hyperproliferative anemias have an elevated reticulocyte count relative to the degree of anemia (reticulocyte production index). This anemia is hypoproliferative.
B. Microcytic, hypoproliferative anemia.
Rationale: CBC shows a microcytic (MCV <80 fL) and hypoproliferative (low reticulocyte count relative to the degree of anemia) anemia.
C. Macrocytic, hypoproliferative anemia.
Rationale: Macrocytic anemias show an elevated MCV (>100 fL). The reticulocyte count is consistent with a hypoproliferative anemia (low reticulocyte count relative to the degree of anemia).
D. Microcytic, hyperproliferative anemia.
Rationale: This is a microcytic (MCV <80 fL) anemia. Hyperproliferative anemias have an elevated reticulocyte count relative to the degree of anemia (reticulocyte production index). This anemia is hypoproliferative.

21b. A. Manual differential.
Rationale: The manual differential may show additional pathology but is not the most informative in the diagnosis of an iron deficiency anemia.
B. B_{12} and folate levels.
Rationale: B_{12} and folate deficiencies are associated with macrocytosis, not microcytosis.
C. Serum iron and ferritin.
Rationale: The microcytic, hypoproliferative anemia can be caused by iron deficiency anemia, sideroblastic anemia, and anemia of chronic disease. Serum iron and serum ferritin are low in iron deficiency anemia.
D. Bone marrow biopsy.
Rationale: Bone marrow biopsy, which is an invasive procedure, may be indicated if serologic testing is not diagnostic.

21c. A. Iron panel.
Rationale: Iron deficiency anemia would present with microcytic anemia.
B. B_{12} and folate.
Rationale: Although B_{12} and folate deficiencies will cause macrocytosis, they will also cause hypersegmented neutrophils.

C. Bone marrow biopsy.
Rationale: A bone marrow biopsy might yield additional information in the diagnosis of causes of macrocytosis, but would not be the logical next step given the invasive nature of such a procedure.
D. Thyroid-stimulating hormone (TSH) and free thyroxine (fT_4).
Rationale: This patient's obstetric hemorrhage has left her with a hypofunctioning pituitary gland resulting in a hypothyroidism. One cause of a macrocytic anemia with normal white cell morphology is hypothyroidism.

21d. **A. Low TSH, low fT_4.**
Rationale: The patient would be expected to have a central or secondary hypothyroidism. This means the fT_4 would be low, but the TSH, normally from the pituitary, would also be low.
B. High TSH, low fT_4.
Rationale: Seen in primary hypothyroidism.
C. High TSH, high fT_4.
Rationale: Seen in secondary hyperthyroidism.
D. Low TSH, high fT_4.
Rationale: Seen in primary hyperthyroid states.

Major points of discussion

- The MCV is a measure of the mean red cell volume and can be calculated as HCT/red blood cell (HCT/RBC) when the RBC and HCT are measured manually, or it can be measured directly from the red cell distribution histogram in automated hematology analyzers. A normal MCV is between 80 and 100 fL.
- The reticulocyte production index (RPI) is a corrected reticulocyte count that corrects for the degree of anemia and should be more than 2 in anemic patients, reflecting corrective hyperproliferation in the marrow. If the RPI is less than 2, it is a hypoproliferative anemia.
- Iron deficiency anemia is a microcytic, hypochromic, hypoproliferative anemia; serum iron and serum ferritin should both be low. However, the CBC and iron studies may be difficult to interpret in early or treated iron deficiency anemia.
- Anemia of chronic disease also can have similar CBC parameters as iron deficiency anemia, but the iron panel is characterized by a normal to high ferritin.
- The diagnosis of anemia in a patient may begin with the CBC but encompasses many other areas of the clinical laboratory. For example, thyroid function tests may be necessary years after a severe obstetric bleed.

22. A. No hemoglobin variant or thalassemia.
Rationale: A hemoglobin variant is present and is migrating in the C position on alkaline and acid electrophoresis. In the absence of microcytosis, thalassemia is unlikely, but it is not ruled out completely.
B. α-Chain variant.
Rationale: An α-chain variant would be expected to comprise approximately 25% of the total hemoglobin (1 of 4 α genes affected). In addition, a hemoglobin A2 variant can also be present. The most common α-chain variant is hemoglobin G–Philadelphia.
C. β-Chain variant.
Rationale: The variant comprises approximately 35% to 45% of the total hemoglobin; it migrates in the C position on

alkaline and acid electrophoresis; the sickle solubility test is negative; the CBC is normal. These findings are consistent with hemoglobin C trait.
D. Unstable hemoglobin variant.
Rationale: Degradation products may be seen on electrophoresis in the presence of an unstable hemoglobin variant. The most common unstable hemoglobin variant is hemoglobin Köln.
E. Sickling hemoglobin variant.
Rationale: The sickle solubility test is negative. There are no bands in the S position for the lanes corresponding to the patient sample.

Major points of discussion

- Hemoglobin C is a β-chain hemoglobin variant that results from a mutation in the β-globin gene ($\beta^{6Glu \to Lys}$).
- Glutamate is a negatively charged amino acid and lysine is positively charged; which results in a +2 net gain of charge. Therefore, it migrates slower than hemoglobin A and hemoglobin S on alkaline electrophoresis.
- Hemoglobin C trait (hemoglobin A/hemoglobin C; $\beta\beta^C$) is a clinically asymptomatic hemoglobinopathy.
- It is important to identify the presence of hemoglobin C for genetic counseling and prenatal testing. When a child inherits hemoglobin C from one parent and hemoglobin S (β^S) from the other parent, the child will have the clinically significant sickling disorder hemoglobin SC disease.
- Hematologically, the hemoglobin is usually normal in hemoglobin C trait. The MCV and MCH can be normal or slightly below the reference range because of red cell dehydration. The peripheral blood smear is normal, or it can show hypochromia and microcytosis and/or target cells.

23. A. Ascorbic acid.
Rationale: Although ascorbic acid can decrease some of the cyanosis in chronic methemoglobinemia, it does not have a significant role in the initial management of acute methemoglobinemia.
B. Crystal violet.
Rationale: Crystal violet is a dye that is used in histology and inkjet printing. It is also used as an antibiotic. However, it is not used in the treatment of methemoglobinemia.
C. Gastric lavage.
Rationale: Gastric lavage can be used when an ingested agent incites the acquired methemoglobinemia. Gastric lavage would not be useful in this situation because the benzocaine was applied topically.
D. Methylene blue.
Rationale: Methylene blue can be used to stain RNA and DNA or as a redox indicator in chemistry. More important for this patient, it has reducing properties when administered at high doses and is the treatment of choice in symptomatic methemoglobinemia.
E. Red cell exchange.
Rationale: In life-threatening situations or in cases of refractoriness to methylene blue, red cell exchange can be used to treat methemoglobinemia, but it is not the initial treatment of choice.

Major points of discussion

- Methemoglobin is formed when the iron in hemoglobin is converted from the ferrous state (Fe^{2+}) to the ferric state (Fe^{3+}). The presence of methemoglobin gives blood a bluish or chocolate color.
- Methemoglobin has an increased affinity for oxygen compared with normal hemoglobin. Patients with elevated levels can become cyanotic and clinically symptomatic because the methemoglobin does not release the oxygen to the tissues.
- Methemoglobin is formed continuously in the normal state. However, NADH methemoglobin reductase (cytochrome b5 reductase) and, to a lesser extent, NADPH methemoglobin reductase, ascorbic acid, and the glutathione pathway, reduce the ferric iron back to ferrous iron. Therefore, most normal individuals will have less than 1% methemoglobin in the circulation.
- Inherited loss of NADH methemoglobin reductase and NADPH methemoglobin reductase can lead to methemoglobinemia. In addition, inheritance of hemoglobin variants, such as hemoglobin M, can also result in methemoglobinemia.
- There are many known causes of acquired methemoglobinemia. Exposure to certain antibiotics (e.g., dapsone), local anesthetics (e.g., benzocaine), nitrites, and many other drugs and chemicals can overwhelm the protective enzymes and lead to methemoglobin accumulation.
- Initial treatment should include oxygen therapy and, if clinically indicated, methylene blue can be administered. It should be noted that methylene blue treatment would not work if there were a concomitant G6PD deficiency because NADPH is required. In life-threatening or methylene blue–refractory methemoglobinemia, red cell exchange may be considered.

24. A. Decreased time for centrifugation.
Rationale: The PCV is increased because of excess plasma trapping.
B. β-Thalassemia trait.
C. Sickle cell disease.
Rationale: The PCV is increased by microcytosis, sickle cell disease, and other causes of decreased red cell deformability.
D. Increased erythrocyte sedimentation rate.
Rationale: Increased erythrocyte sedimentation rate is associated with decreased plasma trapping.
E. Decreased centrifugal force.
Rationale: The PCV is increased because of incomplete reduction of plasma trapping.

Major points of discussion

- The microhematocrit method determines the PCV (the percentage of red cells in whole blood) from a potassium EDTA anticoagulated whole blood sample. A small volume of blood is taken up by capillary action into a fixed-bore capillary tube.
- Plastic tubes are preferred because glass tubes can fracture and cause puncture injuries, potentially exposing the technologist to bloodborne pathogens.
- The end of the tube is heat sealed or sealed with clay and then centrifuged for 5 to 10 minutes at high rate. The sample separates into red cells, white cells and platelets, and plasma layer.
- The percentage of the column occupied by the red cells (linear distance) compared with the total column is the packed cell volume.

- Factors affecting the microhematocrit include centrifugation time, centrifugal force, red cell size and deformability, increased erythrocyte sedimentation rate, anticoagulant type, and deoxygenation of hemoglobin.
- The amount of time needed to centrifuge the sample can be determined by running several capillary tubes of the same sample at 30-second intervals. The minimum amount of time required is at the time when consecutive PCVs are the same.[9]

25. A. Iron deficiency anemia; low serum hepcidin levels.
Rationale: Iron deficiency anemia would not stain strongly with Prussian blue but would be expected to have low serum hepcidin levels.
B. Iron deficiency anemia; high serum hepcidin levels.
Rationale: Iron deficiency anemia would not stain strongly with Prussian blue and would not be expected to have high serum hepcidin levels.
C. Megaloblastic anemia; high serum hepcidin levels.
Rationale: The patient has a normocytic anemia; therefore, this is unlikely to be megaloblastic in which the MCV is elevated.
D. Anemia of chronic disease; low serum hepcidin levels.
Rationale: The hepcidin level is high in anemia of chronic disease.
E. Anemia of chronic disease; high serum hepcidin levels.
Rationale: The hepcidin level is high because of chronic inflammation in the anemia of chronic disease.

Major points of discussion
- Hepcidin is a 25–amino acid peptide hormone predominantly produced by the liver.
- In addition to being regulated by iron status, hepcidin is an acute-phase reactant and is upregulated by certain cytokines (e.g., interleukin-6). Thus, hepcidin is elevated in anemia of inflammation or anemia of chronic disease.
- Hepcidin results in degradation of the iron channel, ferroportin, on both macrophages and gut enterocytes. Thus, elevated hepcidin levels will trap iron inside macrophages because the iron cannot be released without ferroportin.
- Ferritin is an acute-phase reactant frequently used to estimate body iron stores; however, ferritin is inaccurate for this purpose in the setting of inflammation.
- Some cases of anemia of chronic disease manifest a microcytic, hypochromic anemia because the elevated levels of hepcidin impair normal iron delivery to bone marrow precursors.

26. A. *Babesia microti.*
Rationale: The smear shows intraerythrocytic ring forms. Although Maltese crosses are not present, there are cells containing multiple trophozoites.
B. *Borrelia burgdorferi.*
Rationale: Borrelia is a spirochete and would not present as intraerythrocytic ring forms.
C. *Leishmania donovani.*
Rationale: Leishmania promastigotes live in macrophages and neutrophils.
D. *Toxoplasma gondii.*
Rationale: Toxoplasma invades tissues, such as epithelial cells, but not erythrocytes.

E. *Trypanosoma cruzi.*
Rationale: Trypanosoma infects human tissues, most commonly the heart, colon, and peripheral nervous system.

Major points of discussion
- *B. microti* is a parasite transmitted to humans through bites of the *Ixodes* species of ticks. These ticks are the same vector for Lyme disease and ehrlichiosis. The intermediate hosts are deer and rodents.
- *Babesia* sporozoites are transferred while the tick is feeding. They invade erythrocytes and multiply. *Babesia* can also be transfusion-transmitted from a blood donor with a subclinical infection.
- Clinical symptoms can be mild and unnoticed, or they can be more severe, with fever, chills, and severe hemolytic anemia. Very young, elderly, and immunocompromised patients are more susceptible to severe infection.
- Peripheral blood smear shows intraerythrocytic rings forms. These forms can be mistaken for malaria. The appearance of Maltese crosses is essentially diagnostic for *Babesia*.
- Often, the clinical history is helpful in distinguishing malaria from *Babesia*. Malaria will be found in patients traveling to endemic malarial regions (e.g., sub-Saharan Africa, Asia), whereas patients with *Babesia* will more likely have a travel history to Long Island, New York, or Connecticut.
- The hemolytic anemia can be treated with antibiotics. If the parasitemia is very high and the patient has severe disease, red cell exchange can be performed.

27. A. **Low hepcidin level as seen in nutritional iron deficiency.**
Rationale: Although hemochromatosis is a disease of iron overload, hepcidin levels are low as if the patient were iron deficient.
B. High hepcidin level as seen in transfusion-induced iron overload.
Rationale: Although hepcidin is elevated in secondary iron overload syndromes, the primary cause of iron overload in hemochromatosis is low hepcidin.
C. Normal hepcidin level as seen in an iron-replete male.
Rationale: The patient has accumulated iron and likely has a mutation consistent with hemochromatosis; thus, his hepcidin level is not expected to be normal.
D. Low hepcidin level as see in transfusion-induced iron overload.
Rationale: The hepcidin level is expected to be high in transfusion-induced iron overload.
E. High hepcidin level as seen in nutritional iron deficiency.
Rationale: The hepcidin level is low in nutritional iron deficiency.

Major points of discussion
- The C282Y mutation in the *HFE* gene is the most common mutation causing hemochromatosis.
- About 1 in 200 northern Europeans carries the C282Y homozygous mutation. However, the disease has variable penetrance, so most cases are asymptomatic.
- Mature hepcidin is a 25–amino acid peptide hormone that regulates iron homeostasis by regulating the amount of iron that enters the circulation from gut enterocytes.

- Hepcidin causes degradation of the iron channel, ferroportin, which resides on the basolateral side of gut enterocytes. Thus, a high hepcidin level decreases iron absorption and a low level enhances iron absorption.
- Although the exact mechanism controlling hepcidin levels has yet to be determined, mutations in the *HFE* gene result in too low of a hepcidin level for the host's iron status.

28. A. Sickle cell trait.
Rationale: Sickle cell trait is clinically and hematologically silent except in rare circumstances such as high altitude, extreme exertion, anesthesia, and high fever.
B. Sickle cell disease.
Rationale: Sickle cell disease is a good choice, but hemoglobin SC is a better choice. The level of hemoglobin is higher than is usually found in hemoglobin SS, and microcytosis is not typically seen in hemoglobin SS unless accompanied by thalassemia. The peripheral blood smear does not typically show target cells or folded ("taco," "clam-shell") cells.
C. Hemoglobin SC disease.
Rationale: Hemoglobin concentration of more than 10 g/dL, microcytosis, and peripheral blood smear findings (target cells, taco cells) are characteristic of SC disease.
D. β-Thalassemia trait.
Rationale: The peripheral blood smear in β-thalassemia trait may show microcytosis and basophilic stippling, but taco cells and target cells are not usually seen. The hemoglobin can be at the lower end of normal or slightly below it. The hemoglobin in this case is a little low for β-thalassemia trait alone.
E. α-Thalassemia trait.
Rationale: The peripheral blood smear in α-thalassemia trait may show hypochromia and microcytosis, but taco cells and target cells are not usually seen. The hemoglobin can be at the lower end of normal or slightly below it. The hemoglobin in this case is a little low for α-thalassemia trait alone.

Major points of discussion
- Hemoglobin SC disease is an inherited sickling disorder in which a β^S is inherited from one parent and β^C is inherited from the other parent.
- Hemoglobin SC disease can have the same clinical presentation as sickle cell anemia (homozygous hemoglobin S), although the severity can be less in hemoglobin SC disease.
- The CBC characteristically shows a hemoglobin of more than 10 g/dL and an MCV at the lower end of the normal range or slightly below it.
- The peripheral blood smear characteristically shows folded cells (taco cells; clam-shell cells), boat cells, and target cells. Occasionally, hemoglobin C crystals can be seen.
- In the absence of hemoglobin fractionation, hemoglobin SC can be distinguished from hemoglobin SS by the higher hemoglobin, lower MCV, and peripheral blood smear findings.
- On hemoglobin electrophoresis, HPLC, or other hemoglobin fractionation method, hemoglobins S and C are usually easily separated.

29. A. Autoimmune hemolytic anemia.
Rationale: Autoimmune hemolytic anemia is associated with spherocytes and can be associated with less than 10% acanthocytes.

B. McLeod blood group phenotype.
Rationale: Acanthocytosis of more than 10% is associated with the McLeod blood group phenotype.
C. Microangiopathic hemolytic anemia.
Rationale: Microangiopathic hemolytic anemia is associated with schistocytes, spherocytes, and less than 10% acanthocytes.
D. Sickle cell disease.
Rationale: Sickle cell disease is associated with sickle cells, boat cells, Howell-Jolly bodies, and blister cells. Acanthocytes can be present in small numbers.
E. Uremia.
Rationale: Uremia and chronic renal disease is associated with echinocytes, which have short, evenly distributed projections.

Major points of discussion
- Acanthocytes are red cells that have irregularly distributed spicules of varying shapes and sizes.
- Changes in the lipid content of the red cell membrane leads to acanthocytosis.
- Acanthocytes are seen in many disease states, but only a few have more than 10% acanthocytes. These disorders include abetalipoproteinemia, homozygous hypobetaproteinemia, the McLeod blood group phenotype, and advanced liver disease.
- The absence of the Kx protein of the Kell blood group system leads to the McLeod phenotype, which is associated with more than 10% acanthocytosis. The McLeod phenotype is also associated with chronic granulomatous disease.
- Abetalipoproteinemia is a rare genetic disorder that results in the absence of abetalipoprotein B (apo B). Without apo B, triglycerides are not able to be absorbed through the gastrointestinal tract.

30. A. Acute intermittent porphyria.
Rationale: Acute intermittent porphyria is caused by a deficiency in uroporphyrinogen I synthetase. Patients are not photosensitive.
B. Hereditary coproporphyria.
Rationale: Hereditary coproporphyria is caused by coproporphyrinogen oxidase deficiency. Patients are photosensitive.
C. Erythropoietic protoporphyria.
Rationale: This is caused by a ferrochelatase deficiency. Patients are photosensitive.
D. Congenital erythropoietic porphyria.
Rationale: Congenital erythropoietic porphyria is caused by uroporphyrinogen III cosynthetase deficiency. Patients are photosensitive.
E. Porphyria cutanea tarda.
Rationale: Porphyria cutanea tarda is caused by uroporphyrinogen decarboxylase deficiency. Patients are photosensitive.

Major points of discussion
- There are eight steps in the synthesis of heme. The major sites of heme synthesis are the liver and erythrocyte precursors in the bone marrow.
- The first step in heme synthesis is the formation of δ-aminolevulinic acid (ALA) from succinyl–coenzyme A and glycine, which is catalyzed by ALA synthetase. ALA synthetase is inhibited by heme (i.e., end-product

inhibition). The last step in the formation of heme is the insertion of Fe^{2+} into the tetrapyrrole ring of protoporphyrin IX to form heme. This step is catalyzed by ferrochelatase.

- Porphyrias are inherited or acquired disorders of heme synthesis. Almost all inherited porphyrias are autosomal dominant.
- Patients with enzyme defects that lead to the accumulation of tetrapyrrole rings have photosensitivity. The following enzyme deficiencies lead to the accumulation of tetrapyrrole rings: coproporphyrinogen oxidase, ferrochelatase, uroporphyrinogen III cosynthetase, and uroporphyrinogen decarboxylase. They are all associated with photosensitivity.
- Acute intermittent porphyria is associated with neuropsychiatric symptoms. It is caused by a deficiency in the uroporphyrinogen I synthetase enzyme, which catalyzes the conversion of porphobilinogen to pre-uroporphyrinogen. This leads to the accumulation of ALA and porphobilinogen (one ring) so that it is not associated with photosensitivity.

31. A. Automated methods to count reticulocytes often involve digital image analysis.
B. Automated methods to count reticulocytes require specialized equipment that is dedicated to this assay only.
C. Automated reticulocyte counts frequently require confirmation by manual slide review.
D. Automated reticulocyte counts are more accurate and precise than manual counts.
E. Automated reticulocyte counts are based on measurements of the size of reticulocytes compared with the size of mature red cells.
Rationale: See Major Points of Discussion.

Major points of discussion
- Automated reticulocyte counts are based on the measurement of the RNA content of red cells.
- Automated methods to count reticulocytes generally involve absorption, impedance, light scatter, or fluorescence intensity.
- Automated counting of reticulocytes is generally performed on automated cell counters that also provide CBCs and white cell differentials.
- Automated reticulocyte counts almost never require confirmation by manual slide review.
- Automated reticulocyte counts are more accurate and precise than manual counts.[15]

32a. A. Malaria.
Rationale: Intracellular inclusions in malaria present as ring forms or schizonts, not as evenly distributed granules.
B. Babesiosis.
Rationale: Intracelluar inclusions in babesiosis present as ring forms, not as evenly distributed granules.
C. Sideroblastic granules (Pappenheimer bodies).
Rationale: Sideroblastic granules (Pappenheimer bodies) appear in clusters in the periphery of red cells, not evenly distributed over the red cell.
D. Basophilic stippling.
Rationale: This is correct. Basophilic stippling consists of evenly distributed granules of variable size and number that stain deep blue with Wright's stain.
E. Howell-Jolly bodies.

Rationale: Howell-Jolly bodies are usually single blue inclusions in red cells, *not* evenly distributed granules.

32b. A. Iron overload.
Rationale: In iron overload, sideroblastic granules (Pappenheimer bodies) can be present, not basophilic stippling.
B. Malaria.
Rationale: In malaria infection, intracellular ring forms and schizonts, not basophilic stippling, can be observed.
C. Babesiosis.
Rationale: In babesiosis, intracellular and extracellular ring forms and schizonts, not basophilic stippling, can be observed.
D. Thalassemias.
Rationale: This is correct. In thalassemias, basophilic stippling is a frequent finding.
E. Iron deficiency.
Rationale: Basophilic stippling is not seen in iron deficiency.

Major points of discussion
- Basophilic stippling in red cells consists of evenly distributed granules of variable size and number that stain deep blue with Wright's stain.
- The stippling consists of ribonucleoprotein and mitochondrial remnants.
- Basophilic stippling occurs in any condition showing defective or accelerated heme synthesis.
- Basophilic stippling is most frequently seen in patients with thalassemia or lead intoxication.
- Basophilic stippling can also be observed in patients with structural hemoglobinopathies, myelodysplasias, severe megaloblastic anemia, or congenital dyserythropoietic anemia.

33a. A. Stomatocytes.
Rationale: Stomatocytes ("mouth cells") have a slitlike central area of pallor, leading to a fish-mouth appearance.
B. Teardrop cells.
Rationale: Teardrop cells have one elongated side with a blunt or round tip.
C. Schistocytes.
Rationale: Schistocytes are split red blood cells, often showing a half-disk shape with two or three pointed extremities; they may be small, irregular fragments.
D. Acanthocytes.
Rationale: Acanthocytes are irregularly spiculated red blood cells with projections of varying length and position.
E. Burr cells (echinocytes).
Rationale: Burr cells (echinocytes) are spiculated red blood cells with short, evenly spaced projections over the entire surface.

33b. **A. Uremia.**
Rationale: Burr cells (echinocytes) are present in uremia.
B. Abnormalities of lipid metabolism.
Rationale: Burr cells (echinocytes) are present in uremia, not in abnormalities of lipid metabolism.
C. Infections.
Rationale: Burr cells (echinocytes) are present in uremia, not in infections.
D. Hereditary abnormalities of red cell metabolism.
Rationale: Burr cells (echinocytes) are present in uremia, not in hereditary abnormalities of red cell metabolism.

E. Myelodysplastic syndrome.
Rationale: Burr cells (echinocytes) are present in uremia, not in myelodysplastic syndrome.

33c. A. The Burr cells are an artifact caused by the long interval between phlebotomy and preparation of the blood film.
Rationale: Burr cells are very frequent artifacts, caused by long delays before preparation of a blood smear or improperly prepared smears.
B. The basic metabolic panel results are most likely wrong because Burr cells indicate the presence of uremia.
Rationale: It is more probable that the Burr cells were caused by the delay in sample preparation.
C. The Burr cells may be caused by an abnormality in the patient's lipid metabolism.
Rationale: Abnormalities in lipid metabolism generally do not cause Burr cells.
D. The Burr cells may be caused by a malignant process.
Rationale: A malignant process generally does not directly cause Burr cells.
E. The Burr cells may be caused by an infection.
Rationale: An infection generally does not cause Burr cells.

Major points of discussion
- Burr cells are spiculated red blood cells with short, evenly spaced projections over the entire surface.
- Burr cells do have central pallor.
- Burr cells are reversible.
- Burr cells can be found in patients with uremia and burns.
- The most frequent cause of Burr cells is prolonged storage of the blood before preparation of the blood smear.
- Patients who have received blood transfusions may also show Burr cells on their blood smear for up to 48 hours after transfusion.

34a. A. Apoptotic lymphocyte.
Rationale: Apoptotic bodies should have karyorrhectic nuclei.
B. Atypical lymphocytes.
Rationale: Atypical lymphocytes have bluish cytoplasm and a larger nucleus with open chromatin.
C. Giant platelets.
Rationale: Giant platelets are blue with granules throughout. They do not have a nucleus.
D. Nucleated red cells.
Rationale: Nucleated red cells have bluish-pink cytoplasm and a round nucleus.
E. Plasma cells.
Rationale: Plasma cells have blue cytoplasm, a perinuclear clearing, and a peripherally located nucleus containing a clock-face pattern.

34b. A. 0.5
Rationale: This would be a result of the incorrect formula of WBC/(NRBC/WBC).
B. 4.1
Rationale: The corrected count is: WBC/[1+(NRBC/WBC)] = 4.5/[1+(10/100)] = 4.5/1.1 = 4.1.
C. 4.5
Rationale: The WBC should be corrected for NRBC.
D. 4.6

Rationale: This is the WBC+0.1.
E. 5.0
Rationale: This would be a result of the incorrect formula WBC/[1 − (NRBC/WBC)].

Major points of discussion
- The sequence of red cell development (erythropoiesis) goes from proerythroblast→basophilic erythroblast→polychromatophilic→normoblast →reticulocyte→mature red blood cell. During development, the nucleus shrinks and then is extruded from the normoblast to become a reticulocyte. On Wright-Giemsa stain, the cytoplasm changes from basophilia (blue) because of the high ribosomal RNA content to eosinophilia (pink) because of the production of hemoglobin.
- The WBC should be adjusted for nucleated red cells on automated instruments. Many automated instruments now automatically make this adjustment or it can also be made within the laboratory information system.
- To correct the WBC, the following formula should be used:
  - WBC = WBC/[1+(NRBC/WBC)]
- If the WBC is 4.5 and 10 NRBCs are counted for every 100 WBCs:
  - WBC = 4.5/[1+(10/100)] = 4.1
- Elevated NRBCs are found when there is damage to the bone marrow or if there is extramedullary erythropoiesis.
- Conditions that can cause elevated normoblasts include, but are not limited to, hyposplenia or asplenia, stress erythropoiesis, hematologic malignancies, infiltrative disorders of bone marrow (e.g., histiocytosis), hypoxia, extramedullary erythropoiesis, and others.
- Cord blood can have NRBCs, but the NRBCs quickly disappear from neonates during the newborn period.[3]

35. A. Aminolevulinic acid (ALA) synthetase.
Rationale: ALA synthetase is decreased by hemin or heme (end-product inhibition). A deficiency does not cause EPP.
B. Coproporphyrinogen oxidase.
Rationale: Hereditary coproporphyria is caused by coproporphyrinogen oxidase deficiency. Patients are photosensitive.
C. Ferrochelatase.
Rationale: EPP is caused by ferrochelatase deficiency. Patients are photosensitive.
D. Uroporphyrinogen III cosynthetase.
Rationale: Congenital erythropoietic porphyria is caused by uroporphyrinogen III cosynthetase deficiency. Patients are photosensitive.
E. Uroporphyrinogen decarboxylase.
Rationale: Porphyria cutanea tarda is caused by uroporphyrinogen decarboxylase deficiency. Patients are photosensitive.

Major points of discussion
- There are eight steps in the synthesis of heme. The major sites of heme synthesis are the liver and erythrocyte precursors in the bone marrow.
- The first step in heme synthesis is the formation of δ-ALA from succinyl-coenzyme A and glycine, which is

catalyzed by ALA synthetase. ALA synthetase is inhibited by heme (i.e., end-product inhibition).

■ The last step in the formation of heme is the insertion of Fe^{2+} into the tetrapyrrole ring of protoporphyrin IX to form heme. This step is catalyzed by ferrochelatase.

■ Porphyrias are inherited or acquired disorders of heme synthesis. Almost all porphyrias are inherited in an autosomal dominant fashion.

■ The symptoms of porphyria include photosensitivity if the enzyme deficiency leads to the accumulation of tetrapyrrole rings.

■ EPP is caused by deficiency of the mitochondrial enzyme ferrochelatase. Protoporphyrin IX accumulates in the tissue and can lead to photosensitivity, abdominal pain, and liver failure.

36. **A. Glucose-6-phosphate dehydrogenase deficiency.**
Rationale: Bite cells are produced when macrophages take a "bite" out of sites of oxidant damage on red cells.
B. Hereditary pyropoikilocytosis.
Rationale: This is a severe form of hereditary elliptocytosis, and the peripheral blood smear looks as if it is from a patient with thermal burns.
C. Hereditary spherocytosis.
Rationale: HS is a hereditary red cell membrane disorder that has spherocytes on peripheral blood smear.
D. Splenectomy.
Rationale: Splenectomy can lead to the presence of Howell-Jolly bodies.

Major points of discussion
■ G6PD deficiency is an X-linked enzyme deficiency that is associated with a nonimmune hemolytic anemia when the patient is under oxidative stress.
■ G6PD is an enzyme in the pentose phosphate pathway, which is the major pathway to regenerate NADPH in red cells. Because NADPH is required to regenerate reduced glutathione, low NADPH levels can lead to decreased levels of reduced glutathione. Without this mechanism of reversing oxidative damage on red cells, hemolysis can occur under oxidative stress.
■ Oxidative stress can be in the form of infection or administration of medication, such as antimalarials (e.g., primaquine) and antibiotics (sulfas; dapsone). Oxidative stress is also associated with the ingestion of fava beans that can result in hemolysis ("favism").
■ Oxidative damage can be detected in red cells by observing Heinz body inclusions using a supravital stain. Staining with new methylene blue stains the inclusions a bluish color.
■ These inclusions and damaged membranes can be removed by macrophages leading to the formation of "bite cells."
■ Blister cells can also be seen in G6PD deficiency. Blister cells contain a vacuole within the red cells with a very thin membrane surrounding it.[2]

37. A. Crystallization.
Rationale: Hemoglobin C crystals can form in patients with hemoglobin CC, C/β^0, or SC.

B. Heavy metal poisoning.
Rationale: Heavy metal poisoning, such as lead poisoning, may show basophilic stippling on peripheral blood smear.
C. Oxidative damage.
Rationale: Oxidative damage of red cells can occur in disorders such as G6PD deficiency. Bite cells and blister cells are seen in this disorder and other disorders associated with red cell oxidative damage.
D. Spectrin gene mutation.
Rationale: Spectrin gene mutations are associated with hereditary spherocytosis.
E. Splenectomy.
Rationale: After splenectomy or autosplenectomy (e.g., sickle cell disease), patients can have Howell-Jolly bodies in red cells.

Major points of discussion
■ G6PD deficiency is an X-linked enzyme deficiency that is associated with a nonimmune hemolytic anemia when the patient is under oxidative stress.
■ G6PD is an enzyme in the pentose phosphate pathway, which is the major pathway to regenerate NADPH in red cells. Because NADPH is required to regenerate reduced glutathione, low NADPH levels can lead to decreased levels of reduced glutathione. Without this mechanism of reversing oxidative damage on red cells, hemolysis can occur under oxidative stress.
■ Oxidative stress can be in the form of infection or administration of medication, such as antimalarials (e.g., primaquine) and antibiotics (sulfas; dapsone). Oxidative stress is also associated with the ingestion of fava beans that can result in hemolysis ("favism").
■ Oxidative damage can be seen in red cells by observing Heinz body inclusions using a supravital stain. Staining with new methylene blue stains the inclusions a bluish color.
■ These inclusions and damaged membranes can be removed by macrophages, leading to the formation of bite cells.
■ Blister cells can also be seen in G6PD deficiency. Blister cells contain a vacuole within the red cells with a very thin membrane surrounding it.

38. A. α-Thalassemia trait.
Rationale: Associated with normal or decreased hemoglobin A2 (especially hemoglobin H disease)
B. Antiretroviral therapy.
Rationale: Results in an increased hemoglobin A2.
C. (δβ)^0-Thalassemia trait.
Rationale: Usually presents with a normal hemoglobin A2 and elevated hemoglobin F.
D. Hypothyroidism.
E. Sideroblastic anemia.
Rationale: Associated with a decreased hemoglobin A2.

Major points of discussion
■ Hemoglobin A2 is a minor hemoglobin fraction in adults that consists of two α chains and two δ chains ($\alpha_2\delta_2$). It has little influence on oxygen-carrying capacity but is very useful diagnostically.
■ Microcytosis + normal iron studies + normal hemoglobin fractionation pattern (no variants; hemoglobin A, A2, and F within the reference range) is a presumptive diagnosis of α-thalassemia trait.

- Microcytosis+normal iron studies+elevated hemoglobin A2 is a presumptive diagnosis of β-thalassemia trait.
- Causes of decreased hemoglobin A2 include α-thalassemia, iron deficiency, lead poisoning, sideroblastic anemia, hypothyroidism, and δ-chain variants.
- The most common δ-chain variant is hemoglobin A2′ (B2). It is present in 1% to 2% of African Americans and is hematologically and clinically silent. This variant is diagnostically important because the sum of hemoglobin A2 and hemoglobin A2′ must be used when ruling out β-thalassemia trait.
- Elevated hemoglobin A2 is most commonly associated with β-thalassemia. However, it can also be seen in B_{12} and folate deficiency, hyperthyroidism, and antiretroviral therapy.
- Hemoglobin E coelutes with hemoglobin A2 on HPLC. Therefore, hemoglobin A2 levels greater than 7% or 8% should be evaluated for the presence of a hemoglobin variant using an alternative method such as hemoglobin electrophoresis.

39. A. α_4.
Rationale: α-Globin tetramers are formed in β-thalassemia. They are not detected by traditional electrophoresis or HPLC.
B. β_4.
Rationale: Hemoglobin H is composed of four β-globin genes. It is a minor hemoglobin fraction in hemoglobin H disease, which is caused by three absent or nonfunctioning α-globin genes.
C. γ_4.
Rationale: Hemoglobin Barts is composed of four γ chains. It is the major hemoglobin when all four α-globin genes are absent or nonfunctional.
D. δ_4.
Rationale: Hemoglobin A2 is composed of two α-globin chains and two δ-globin chains. δ-Globin tetramers are not formed in hemoglobinopathies.
E. ζ_4.
Rationale: ζ Globin is an α-like globin chain expressed in embryonic life. ζ-Globin tetramers are not formed in hemoglobinopathies.

Major points of discussion
- α-Thalassemia is caused by the deletion of one or more of the four α-globin genes (two α-globin genes per chromosome 16; αα/αα).
- Deletion of one or two genes is referred to as α-thalassemia trait. Deletion of three genes results in hemoglobin H disease. Deletion of four genes results in hemoglobin Barts disease.
- One gene deletion is also referred to as heterozygous α⁺-thalassemia (-α/αα). Deletion of two genes in *trans* is referred to as homozygous α⁺-thalassemia (-α/-α). Deletion of two genes in *cis* is heterozygous α⁰-thalassemia (--/αα). Hemoglobin H disease is caused by three α-globin gene deletions: double heterozygous α⁺-thalassemia and α⁰-thalassemia (--/-α).
- Hemoglobin Barts results from deletion of all four α-globin genes (--/--) and is a result of the inheritance of two α⁰-thalassemia (--/) alleles.

- Fetuses with hemoglobin Barts disease develop hydrops fetalis and are either stillborn or die shortly after birth.
- Intrauterine transfusions can be a lifesaving treatment for fetuses with hemoglobin Barts disease and can lead to liveborn infants.
- Hemoglobin Barts is composed of four γ chains (γ_4) and represents most of the hemoglobin in hemoglobin Barts disease.
- Hemoglobin Barts is a fast-migrating hemoglobin on cellulose acetate (alkaline) hemoglobin electrophoresis and HPLC (retention time <1 minute).

40. A. α-Globin.
Rationale: Hemoglobin Lepore is located on the β-globin gene cluster.
B. γ-Globin.
Rationale: The hemoglobin Lepore fusion gene does not involve the γ-globin genes.
C. δ-Globin.
Rationale: Hemoglobin Lepore is a δ-β fusion gene that is under control of the δ-globin promoter.
D. β-Globin.
Rationale: The β-globin promoter does not control the fusion gene.
E. ε-Globin.
Rationale: The ε-globin promoter does not control the transcription of the fusion gene.

Major points of discussion
- Hemoglobin Lepore is a hemoglobin variant that is formed by the fusion of the δ- and β-globin genes (*HBB* and *HBD*) during a crossover event.
- The fusion gene is under the control of the δ-globin promoter, which is not efficient and leads to decreased production of hemoglobin Lepore. Therefore, hemoglobin Lepore is a thalassemic hemoglobin variant.
- In the heterozygous form, the imbalance between α and β globins leads to a β-thalassemia minor phenotype, and patients present with a mild hypochromic, microcytic anemia, which can be associated with a mild elevation of hemoglobin F.
- In the homozygous form, which is rare, patients present with a phenotype that ranges between β-thalassemia intermedia and β-thalassemia major.
- On hemoglobin electrophoresis, hemoglobin Lepore runs at the S-position on alkaline cellulose acetate and between hemoglobin A and A2 on cation exchange chromatography. Hemoglobin Lepore represents approximately 5% to 15% of the total hemoglobin in the heterozygous state.
- There are three major forms of hemoglobin Lepore: Lepore-Washington-Boston, Lepore-Baltimore, and Lepore-Hollandia.
- Hemoglobin Lepore can be coinherited with hemoglobin S, hemoglobin C, or β-thalassemia.[10]

41. A. Local anesthesia.
Rationale: General anesthesia is a risk factor for vasoocclusion in sickle cell trait.
B. Renal medullary carcinoma.
Rationale: Renal medullary carcinoma is associated with sickle cell trait, but it is not a risk factor for vasoocclusion.
C. Severe hypothermia.

Rationale: Fever is associated with vasoocclusion in sickle cell trait.

D. Travel to New York City in autumn.

Rationale: Travel to high-altitude locations (e.g., mountain climbing, flying, high-altitude cities such as Denver, CO) can cause vasoocclusive crisis.

E. Vigorous exercise.

Rationale: Vigorous exercise with dehydration, such as in competitive sports or military training, can lead to vasoocclusive crisis.

Major points of discussion

- Sickle cell trait (heterozygous hemoglobin S) is caused by a β-globin mutation $\beta^{6Glu\rightarrow Val}$. In the homozygous state, hemoglobin polymerization often leads to red cell sickling and vasoocclusive crises. However, in the heterozygous state, clinical symptoms are very rare.
- Sickle cell trait is generally considered a benign disorder both hematologically (normal CBC) and clinically.
- It is important to diagnose sickle cell trait for genetic counseling. A potential mother and father who are both sickle trait positive have a 25% chance of producing a child with sickle cell disease (hemoglobin S/S).
- Although sickle cell trait is generally not considered to be clinically significant, these patients may have vasoocclusive crises under certain conditions, such as fever, hypoxia (e.g., high-altitude travel, air travel, and mountain climbing), vigorous exercise, dehydration, and general anesthesia.
- In addition, sickle cell trait is associated with sudden death, isosthenuria, renal papillary necrosis, and renal medullary carcinoma.

42. A. High MCV.

Rationale: The MCV is normal in sickle cell trait. It can be decreased when coinherited with α-thalassemia.

B. Low hemoglobin (HGB) concentration.

Rationale: The HGB is normal in sickle cell trait.

C. Low RBC.

Rationale: The RBC is normal in sickle cell trait.

D. High MCH.

Rationale: The MCH is usually normal in sickle cell trait but may occasionally be low. It can also be decreased when coinherited with α-thalassemia trait.

E. Normal RDW.

Rationale: The RDW is normal in sickle cell trait.

Major points of discussion

- Sickle cell trait (heterozygous hemoglobin S) is caused by a β-globin mutation $\beta^{6Glu\rightarrow Val}$. In the homozygous state, hemoglobin polymerization leads to red cell sickling, which can cause vasoocclusive crises. However, in the heterozygous state, clinical symptoms are very rare.
- Sickle cell trait is generally considered a benign disorder both hematologically (normal CBC) and clinically.
- Sickle cell trait on hemoglobin electrophoresis is characterized by the identification of one band in the A-position and one band in the S-position on both alkaline cellulose acetate and acid electrophoresis. It can also be readily identified on cation exchange HPLC, isoelectric focusing, and capillary zone electrophoresis. The sickle solubility test is positive.

- Sickle cell trait is diagnosed by identifying the presence of hemoglobin A and hemoglobin S using two independent tests. In addition, hemoglobin A must be greater than hemoglobin S (usually 35% to 45% of total hemoglobin).
- The peripheral blood smear and CBC are usually completely normal in sickle cell trait. However, microcytosis and target cells may occasionally be seen. Sickle cells are generally not present.

43. A. Denatured hemoglobin.

Rationale: Heinz bodies are composed of denatured hemoglobin.

B. Denatured hemoglobin H.

Rationale: Hemoglobin H bodies are composed of denatured hemoglobin H.

C. DNA.

Rationale: Howell-Jolly bodies are composed of DNA.

D. Iron.

Rationale: Pappenheimer bodies are composed of iron.

E. RNA.

Rationale: Reticulocytes and platelets contain ribosomal RNA. Supravital stains can distinguish reticulocytes from mature red blood cells, which do not contain ribosomal RNA.

Major points of discussion

- Howell-Jolly bodies are usually present when there is asplenia or when hyposplenism is present.
- Howell-Jolly bodies are formed when erythrocytes do not extrude all of their DNA (nuclear extrusion) as they mature. Therefore, Howell-Jolly bodies are composed of DNA.
- The DNA appears as a small, round, basophilic inclusion on the erythrocyte.
- These inclusions are usually removed by macrophages in the spleen. However, if asplenia or hyposplenia is present, these remnants are not removed and are seen on circulating red cells as Howell-Jolly bodies.
- Asplenia is seen after splenectomy (e.g., after trauma), autosplenectomy (e.g., sickle cell disease), and splenic irradiation.

44. A. Babesia.

Rationale: Babesia parasites usually present as ring forms, not as single, round, blue inclusions.

B. Cabot's ring.

Rationale: Cabot's ring is usually a reddish ring or in a "figure of eight" conformation.

C. Howell-Jolly body.

Rationale: This is correct. Howell-Jolly bodies present as single or sometimes multiple blue inclusions in red cells.

D. Basophilic stippling.

Rationale: Basophilic stippling consists of evenly distributed granules of variable size, not of a single, round, blue inclusion.

E. Pappenheimer bodies.

Rationale: Pappenheimer bodies are small, irregular inclusions along the periphery of red blood cells that appear in clusters, not singly.

Major points of discussion

- Howell-Jolly bodies are nuclear remnants containing DNA.
- This nuclear material is normally removed by the spleen.

- Howell-Jolly bodies are, therefore, seen in patients with functional hyposplenia and following splenectomy.
- They can also be observed in patients with megaloblastic anemia, thalassemia, or hemolytic anemias.
- The absence of Howell-Jolly bodies after splenectomy can indicate the presence of an accessory spleen.

45. A. 2-month-old, healthy boy.
Rationale: Neonates to about 2 months of age have large red blood cells (mean MCV of 105 fL).
B. 32-year-old pregnant woman with sickle cell trait.
Rationale: The MCV increases slightly with pregnancy and should not change with sickle cell trait.
C. 18-year-old man with sickle cell disease on hydroxyurea therapy.
Rationale: Hydroxyurea therapy makes red cells macrocytic.
D. 6-month-old, healthy boy.
Rationale: By 6 months of age, the MCV decreases to a mean of 76 fL.
E. 2-year-old boy with Fanconi's anemia.
Rationale: Fanconi's anemia is associated with macrocytosis and reticulocytopenia.

Major points of discussion
- Age-related, gender-related, and physiologic changes must be considered when evaluating red cell indices.
- Red cells are large in neonates (mean MCV of 105 fL), and then the size decreases so that by 6 months of age, the red cells are smaller than adult red cells (mean MCV of 76 fL). Red cells remain small throughout childhood and then increase to adult levels.
- During pregnancy, red cell size increases slightly with the greatest change in the third trimester.
- Macrocytosis can be seen in numerous conditions and disorders, including megaloblastic anemia from B_{12} and folate deficiency; liver disease and chronic alcohol use; inherited and acquired anemias, such as Fanconi's anemia and aplastic anemia; medications, such as phenytoin and hydroxyurea (compliance with hydroxyurea therapy in sickle cell disease can be determined with red cell size).
- The MCV can be incorrectly elevated in the presence of cold agglutinins and with prolonged storage (red cells will swell with storage).[13]

46. A. Manual counting of reticulocytes can be performed on a standard Wright-Giemsa–stained blood smear.
B. Manual counting of reticulocytes is performed by counting 100 red cells.
C. Manual counting of reticulocytes is highly reproducible.
D. Manual counting is the only method available to quantitate reticulocytes; no alternative methods are available.
Rationale: See Major Points of Discussion.
E. In most laboratories, manual counting of reticulocytes has been replaced by automated cell counters.
Rationale: In most clinical laboratories, reticulocytes are quantified by automated cell counters, not by manual cell counting.

Major points of discussion
- Manual counting of reticulocytes is performed on slides stained with new methylene blue or brilliant cresyl blue.

- At least 1000 appropriately stained red cells must be counted for a manual reticulocyte count.
- Because of the small number of actual reticulocytes counted, manual reticulocyte counts are highly variable.
- Most clinical laboratories use automated cell counters, not manual counts, to quantify reticulocytes.[15]

47. A. A careful review of the blood smear.
Rationale: There are no characteristic findings on blood smear review that would allow a diagnosis of PNH.
B. The sucrose lysis test.
Rationale: The sucrose lysis test is a screening test for PNH; it is not used to make a definitive diagnosis.
C. The acidified serum test (Ham's test).
Rationale: The acidified serum test used to be the gold standard for the diagnosis of PNH; it has been replaced by the flow cytometric measurement of CD55 and CD59 levels on red blood cells.
D. Flow cytometry.
Rationale: Flow cytometric determination of decreased levels of CD55 and/or CD59 allows a definitive diagnosis of PNH.
E. Genetic testing.
Rationale: PNH is virtually always an acquired disorder; genetic testing is not used for diagnosis.

Major points of discussion
- PNH is virtually always an acquired stem cell disorder that leads to the production of abnormal red cells, white cells, and platelets.
- The red cell defect renders the cells more susceptible to complement-mediated hemolysis.
- The disease is diagnosed by flow cytometric determination of decreased levels of CD55 and/or CD59.[11]

48. A. Gold standard for the definitive diagnosis of PNH.
Rationale: Flow cytometric measurement of CD55 and CD59 has replaced the acidified serum test as the gold standard in the diagnosis of PNH.
B. Requires highly specialized equipment.
Rationale: The acidified serum test does not require highly specialized equipment.
C. Requires the mixing of treated patient and control blood to prove that the patient's hemolysis is caused by an increased susceptibility of his red cells to activated complement.
Rationale: In the acidified serum test, the patient's red cells and serum are mixed with control serum and red cells. Complement is inactivated by heat or activated by acidification, and it is shown that the patient's hemolysis is caused by an increased susceptibility of his red cells to complement.
D. Absence of lysis of the patient's red cells by his acidified serum excludes the diagnosis of PNH.
Rationale: Depending on the amount of residual complement in the patient's serum, his serum may or may not lyse his own red cells.
E. Requires the mixing of patient blood and sucrose to prove that the patient's hemolysis is caused by an increased susceptibility of his red cells to activated complement.
Rationale: The patient's blood is mixed with sucrose in the sucrose hemolysis test, not in the acidified serum test.

Major points of discussion
- PNH is virtually always an acquired stem cell disorder that leads to the production of abnormal red cells, white cells, and platelets.
- The red cell defect renders the cells more susceptible to complement-mediated hemolysis.
- Sometimes, the patient's own cells are not lysed by his own activated serum because the complement in the patient's serum has already been consumed.
- In the past, the acidified serum test was the gold standard for the diagnosis of PNH; it has been replaced by the flow cytometric measurement of CD55 and CD59 levels on blood cells.

49. A. Allows a definite diagnosis of PNH.
Rationale: The sucrose lysis test is a screening test for PNH; it does not allow a definitive diagnosis.
B. Must be carried out with a sample of whole blood anticoagulated with EDTA.
Rationale: EDTA blocks complement activation; samples that are anticoagulated with EDTA can, therefore, not be used for the sucrose lysis test.
C. Is a screening test for PNH.
Rationale: The sucrose lysis test is a simple screening test for PNH.
D. Requires expensive laboratory instrumentation.
Rationale: The sucrose lysis test does not require expensive laboratory instrumentation.
E. Is based on the lysis of white cells by complement in patients with PNH.
Rationale: The sucrose lysis test is based on the lysis of red cells, not white cells, by complement in patients with PNH.

Major points of discussion
- PNH is virtually always an acquired stem cell disorder that leads to the production of abnormal red cells, white cells, and platelets.
- The red cell defect renders the cells more susceptible to complement-mediated hemolysis.
- Sucrose provides a medium of low ionic strength that promotes the binding of complement to red cells.
- The acidified serum test used to be the gold standard for the diagnosis of PNH; it has been replaced by the flow cytometric measurement of CD55 and CD59 levels on red blood cells.[11]

50. A. Impedance method.
Rationale: The impedance method is used in automated cell counters that provide a CBC, not in handheld POC devices.
B. Flow cytometry–based methods.
Rationale: Flow cytometry–based methods are used in automated cell counters that provide a CBC, not in handheld POC devices.
C. Conductivity-based methods.
Rationale: This is correct. Most handheld POC devices use conductivity-based methods to determine hemoglobin levels.
D. Centrifugation.
Rationale: Centrifugation is not used in handheld POC devices to determine hemoglobin levels.
E. Light-absorption–based methods.
Rationale: Light-absorption–based methods are not used in handheld POC devices to determine hemoglobin levels.

Major points of discussion
- Most handheld POC devices that measure hemoglobin use conductivity-based methods.
- The method is based on the fact that the electrical conduction in plasma is reduced as the amount of cellular elements increases.
- Conductivity-based methods of hemoglobin and HCT determination can be significantly influenced by plasma composition, including electrolyte and protein concentrations.
- Manufacturers of POC instruments are aware of this problem and suggest that HCT measurements outside the normal plasma protein range be adjusted appropriately. This makes the use of HCT and hemoglobin measurements obtained with the conductivity method difficult in critically ill patients. Many hospitals have, therefore, disabled the HCT and hemoglobin function in intensive care units and operating rooms.
- Because most central laboratories use the optical method for hemoglobin measurement, results from the POC instruments will not always correlate with the central laboratory results.[5,7]

51. A. Decreased 2,3-diphosphoglycerate (2,3-DPG or 2,3-BPG).
Rationale: Increased 2,3-DPG leads to increased affinity for hemoglobin. Tissue perceives low oxygen delivery, and more red cells are produced.
B. Cobalamin poisoning.
Rationale: Cobalt poisoning is an acquired cause of polycythemia.
C. Familial decrease in erythropoietin synthesis.
Rationale: Familial increase in erythropoietin synthesis leads to increased red cell production.
D. Low-affinity hemoglobin.
Rationale: A high-affinity hemoglobin is associated with impaired release of oxygen with compensatory increase in red cell production.
E. After renal transplantation.
Rationale: Post-transplantation erythrocytosis is not an uncommon complication of renal transplantation, often requiring therapeutic phlebotomy.

Major points of discussion
- Polycythemia is an increase in the number of circulating red cells and often includes a rise in hemoglobin above the reference range for age and gender.
- However, the hemoglobin concentration and HCT can rise because of dehydration and would not be considered polycythemia or can be referred to as a relative polycythemia. An increase in the red cell count when the hemoglobin is normal (α- and β-thalassemia trait) would also not be considered polycythemia.
- Primary causes of polycythemia are caused by an intrinsic marrow disorder that increases red cell production. Therefore, normal feedback mechanisms lead to decreased erythropoietin production.
- Secondary causes of polycythemia are caused by a physiologic response to hypoxia or inappropriate production of erythropoietin.
- Examples of primary polycythemia:
  - Inherited: erythropoietin (EPO) receptor gene mutation causing increased EPO sensitivity
  - Acquired: polycythemia vera

■ Examples of secondary polycythemia:
  ● Inherited: high-affinity hemoglobin variants, hemoglobin M, inappropriate EPO synthesis
  ● Acquired: cyanotic heart disease, sleep apnea, carbon monoxide poisoning, renal tumors, after renal transplantation, EPO administered for performance enhancement, cobalt toxicity

52. A. Aldolase.
Rationale: Rare; associated with neurologic abnormalities.
B. Glucose-6-phophate isomerase.
Rationale: Rare.
C. Hexokinase.
Rationale: Rare.
D. Phosphofructokinase.
Rationale: These deficiencies are rare. Aldolase is associated with neurologic abnormalities, and phosphofructokinase is associated with myopathy.
E. Pyruvate kinase.
Rationale: Although seen infrequently, pyruvate kinase (PK) deficiency accounts for 90% of cases of hereditary nonspherocytic hemolytic anemia caused by an enzyme deficiency in the glycolytic pathway.

Major points of discussion
■ Deficiencies in enzymes of the glycolytic pathway can lead to hereditary nonspherocytic hemolytic anemia (HNSA). The lack of enzyme activity leads to the inability to produce adenosine triphosphate from the glycolytic pathway. The abnormal red cells then have decreased in vivo red cell survival.
■ The most common enzyme deficiency of the glycolytic pathway that causes HNSA is PK deficiency. It is less common than G6PD deficiency, which is the most common enzyme deficiency of the hexose monophosphate shunt.
■ Although PK deficiency is rare, the other glycolytic enzyme deficiencies are even rarer. These include hexokinase, aldolase, glucose phosphate isomerase, phosphofructokinase, and phosphoglycerate kinase deficiency.
■ PK deficiency is an autosomal recessive disorder that presents in infancy or childhood as a cause of jaundice or HNSA.
■ Most affected individuals do not require treatment, but patients with more severe disease may require red cell exchange transfusions or splenectomy.

53. A. Hemizygous male.
Rationale: A hemizygous male is an affected male and should have low activity by the qualitative and quantitative assay.
B. Heterozygous woman.
Rationale: A heterozygous woman should have approximately 50% G6PD activity depending on the degree of lyonization. Qualitative test results can be negative in this range of enzyme activity, especially if reticulocytosis is present.
C. Hypergammaglobulinemia.
Rationale: Hypergammaglobulinemia can lead to false-positive results in the sickle solubility test because of increased turbidity. However, it should not affect the colorimetric G6PD assay.

D. Reticulocytopenia.
Rationale: Reticulocytes from patients with G6PD deficiency have higher levels of G6PD than the patient's mature red cells. Testing during a hemolytic crisis when the reticulocyte count is high can lead to false-negative results. Reticulocytopenia would ~~not~~ cause a false-positive test result.
E. Sickle cell trait.
Rationale: Sickle cell trait is often coinherited with G6PD deficiency. It should not cause false-negative test results.

Major points of discussion
■ G6PD deficiency is caused by mutations that lead to decreased G6PD activity. G6PD is required to maintain normal NADPH levels. In turn, NADPH is required to regenerate reduced glutathione. In the absence of adequate levels of NADPH, red cell oxidative damage cannot be reversed, leading to red cell damage and increased red cell clearance.
■ G6PD activity can be measured by many different methods: colorimetric, fluorescent, and spectrophotometric.
■ The qualitative G6PD colorimetric assay is performed by adding glucose-6-phosphate and NADP to a whole blood sample. G6PD activity can be measured by adding a dye (dichlorophenolindophenol) that is cleared when NADPH is generated. Therefore, G6PD-deficient patients will have less NADPH and will take longer to clear the dye.
■ Heterozygous females should have activity levels of about 50% depending on the extent of lyonization. At this level, the qualitative test may give false-negative results, especially if there is reticulocytosis.
■ Reticulocytes cause false-negative results because younger red cells have higher levels of G6PD activity. If a patient is tested during an acute episode of hemolysis, there can be a brisk reticulocytosis, which can elevate the G6PD activity enough to produce a negative qualitative test result.

54. A. β-Thalassemia trait.
Rationale: β-Thalassemia trait shows microcytosis (downward shift), but the hemoglobin content per cell does not decrease (no leftward shift).
B. Congenital dyserythropoietic anemia.
Rationale: Congenital dyserythropoietic anemia is usually macrocytic (upward shift).
C. Iron deficiency anemia.
Rationale: The cytogram for iron deficiency anemia should show microcytosis (downward shift) and decreased hemoglobin content (leftward shift). This can be distinguished from β-thalassemia trait, which shows only a downward shift without a significant leftward shift.
D. Megaloblastic anemia.
Rationale: Megaloblastic anemia is usually macrocytic (upward shift).
E. Sickle cell disease.
Rationale: Sickle cell disease is usually a normochromic, normocytic anemia (no shift).

Major points of discussion
■ Automated hematology analyzers use different technologies to count and characterize red cells. One

method is to measure the size and the hemoglobin content of each red cell analyzed. The distribution of red cells can then be plotted on a two-dimensional red cell cytogram.

- If red cell size is plotted on the *y*-axis and the hemoglobin content of the cell is plotted on the *x*-axis for a normal donor, the red cell distribution falls around the center of the graph, which is normocytic, normochromic.
- If microcytosis is present, then the distribution will shift downward. If macrocytosis is present, then the distribution will shift upward. If anisocytosis is present, the distribution will show a greater spread vertically.
- Iron deficiency anemia is a microcytic, hypochromic anemia usually associated with an elevated RDW (anisocytosis). β-Thalassemia trait is microcytic, hypochromic, and is usually associated with a normal or slightly elevated RDW.
- However, on the red cell cytogram, the hemoglobin content per cell decreases in iron deficiency and remains approximately normal in β-thalassemia trait. Therefore, the cytogram can be used to distinguish between these two causes of microcytosis.

55. A. 0.12
Rationale: This is an incorrect calculation of the RI. RI does not equal reticulocytes/HCT.
B. 0.38
Rationale: This is the reticulocyte production index (RPI) = (reticulocytes × HCT)/(normal HCT × correction factor). RPI = 2 × 16.9/2 × 45.
C. 0.75
Rationale: This is the correct calculation of the RI; RI = reticulocytes × HCT/normal HCT.
RI = 2 × 16.9/45.
D. 2.70
Rationale: RI does not equal reticulocytes × normal HCT/ 2 × HCT.
E. 5.30
Rationale: RI does not equal reticulocytes × normal HCT/HCT.

Major points of discussion

- Reticulocytes are young red cells that have entered the peripheral blood circulation. They contain varying amounts of RNA, with the youngest cells containing the greatest amount. Therefore, it is a measure of the bone marrow's production of new red cells.
- Reticulocytes are expressed as a percentage of the total red cells counted.
- The reticulocyte count can be used to differentiate different types of anemia. Anemia can be caused by the destruction of red cells, bleeding, or decreased production of red cells. In the absence of red cell destruction or bleeding, anemia results when there is an inability for the marrow to produce red cells.
- Although the RI and RPI have been used to correct for varying factors in the production of red cells, they are not commonly used explicitly in clinical practice. However, the calculations are useful for the concepts on how to interpret the reticulocyte count in the context of anemia and the ability of the bone marrow to compensate for the anemia.
- The RI is a correction factor based on the HCT. Because reticulocytes are expressed as a percentage of red cells, the percentage of reticulocytes will not reflect the absolute

number of reticulocytes being produced by the bone marrow. RI = reticulocytes × HCT/normal HCT.
- Because erythropoietic stress releases reticulocytes earlier than under unstressed conditions, the reticulocytes exist in the peripheral circulation as reticulocytes for a longer period of time. An additional correction factor is added to the denominator to create the RPI. The correction factor can be retrieved from many available textbooks. RPI = (reticulocytes × HCT)/(normal HCT × correction factor).
- The following correction factors are generally used[8,12]:
  - \>35:1.0
  - 26 – 35:1.5
  - 16 – 25:2.0
  - <16:2.5

56. A. Auramine O.
Rationale: Auramine O is a fluorescent stain used for fluorescent detection in automated hematology analyzers. It is not considered the standard method for reticulocyte counting.
B. Ethidium bromide.
Rationale: Ethidium bromide is a fluorescent stain used for fluorescent detection in automated hematology analyzers. It is not considered the standard method for reticulocyte counting.
C. Monoclonal antibodies (anti-CD71).
Rationale: Fluorescently labeled monoclonal antibodies can be used in flow cytometry or in automated hematology instruments. It is not considered the standard method for reticulocyte counting.
D. New methylene blue (NMB).
Rationale: NMB is the stain of choice for standardization of reticulocyte counting. Analysis can be performed by automated instrumentation or by a manual counting procedure.
E. Thiazole orange.
Rationale: Thiazole orange is used as a fluorescent dye in automated hematology analyzers. It is not considered the standard method for reticulocyte counting.

Major points of discussion

- Reticulocytes are young red cells produced in the bone marrow that are then released into the peripheral blood circulation. They contain varying amounts of RNA, with the youngest cells containing the greatest amount (immature reticulocyte fraction).
- Reticulocytes are generally larger than mature red cells and contain more RNA. On Wright-Giemsa or Romanowsky stain, the red color of the hemoglobin and the blue color of the ribosomes/RNA give a red-blue color to the cytoplasm, which is called *polychromasia*.
- Reticulocytes can be identified by use of supravital dyes such as NMB or brilliant cresyl blue. It is important not to mistake Howell-Jolly bodies, Pappenheimer bodies, Heinz bodies, or hemoglobin H bodies for ribosomal RNA.
- Reticulocytes can also be identified by fluorescent stains for RNA such as thiazole orange, auramine O, and ethidium bromide, which are commonly used to count reticulocytes in automated analyzers.
- Reticulocytes are expressed as a percentage of total red cells counted. If the RBC is available, the absolute reticulocyte count can be provided.[8,12]

57a. A. Burr cell.
Rationale: Burr cells are spiculated red blood cells with short, evenly spaced projections over the entire surface.
B. Acanthocyte.
Rationale: Acanthocytes are irregularly spiculated red blood cells with projections of varying length and position.
C. Stomatocyte.
Rationale: Stomatocytes are red cells with a central area of pallor that is slitlike instead of round.
D. Teardrop cell.
Rationale: A teardrop cell has an elongation with a blunt or round tip; it may resemble a pear.
E. Schistocyte.
Rationale: This is correct. Schistocytes are split red cells, often showing a half-disk shape with two or three pointed extremities; it may be a small, irregular fragment.

57b. A. Abnormalities of lipid metabolism.
Rationale: Schistocytes are not found in abnormalities of lipid metabolism.
B. On blood smears prepared over 36 hours after phlebotomy.
Rationale: Burr cells and target cells are found on blood smears prepared over 36 hours after phlebotomy; schistocytes are not found in such samples.
C. In blood smears from uremic patients.
Rationale: Burr cells are found in blood smears from uremic patients; schistocytes are not found in such samples.
D. In blood smears from patients with lead poisoning.
Rationale: Basophilic stippling is found in blood smears from patients with lead poisoning; schistocytes are not found in such samples.
E. In blood smears from patients with microangiopathic hemolytic anemias.
Rationale: This is correct. Schistocytes are found in blood smears from patients with microangiopathic hemolytic anemias.

Major points of discussion
- Schistocytes are fragmented red blood cells, often showing a half-disk shape with two or three pointed extremities; they may be a small, irregular fragment.
- Schistocytes can be found in the microangiopathic hemolytic anemias, thrombotic thrombocytopenic purpura (TTP), and hemolytic uremic syndrome (HUS).
- Because TTP is lethal unless treated with plasmapheresis or plasma infusion, the correct reporting of schistocytes can be of utmost clinical importance.
- Schistocytes can also be seen in patients with disseminated intravascular coagulation.
- Other conditions in which schistocytes can be seen include severe burns, march hemoglobinuria, and heart valve hemolysis.

58. A. Hemoglobins S and G–Philadelphia.
Rationale: Hemoglobins S and G–Philadelphia comigrate on alkaline electrophoresis. They can be subsequently separated on acid electrophoresis.
B. Hemoglobins S and D–Punjab.
Rationale: Hemoglobins S and D–Punjab comigrate on alkaline electrophoresis. They can be subsequently separated on acid electrophoresis.
C. Hemoglobins C and E.

Rationale: Hemoglobins C and E comigrate on alkaline electrophoresis. They can be subsequently separated on acid electrophoresis.
D. Hemoglobins C and A2.
Rationale: Hemoglobins C and A2 comigrate on alkaline electrophoresis. They can be subsequently separated on acid electrophoresis.
E. Hemoglobins O-Arab and D-Punjab.
Rationale: Hemoglobins O–Arab migrates in the C-position, and D–Punjab migrates in the S-position on alkaline electrophoresis.

Major points of discussion
- On alkaline electrophoresis (cellulose acetate), hemoglobins C, E, O-Arab, and A2 comigrate in the C-position, hemoglobins F and A migrate in separate bands (see Figure 10-34, *A*).
- On alkaline electrophoresis, hemoglobins S, G–Philadelphia, and D–Punjab (D-Los Angeles) comigrate in the S-position.
- On alkaline electrophoresis, hemoglobin A runs ahead of hemoglobin F.
- Hemoglobin C can be separated from hemoglobins E and O–Arab on acid electrophoresis. Hemoglobin C migrates in the C-position, and hemoglobins E and O migrate in the A-position.
- Hemoglobin S can be separated from hemoglobins G and D (see Figure 10-34, *B*) on acid electrophoresis. Hemoglobin S migrates in the S-position, and hemoglobins G and D migrate in the A-position.

59. A. Hemoglobin C disease (homozygous hemoglobin C).
Rationale: The arrow indicates a sickle cell, not a hemoglobin C crystal, which is rhomboid in shape.
B. Hemoglobin SD disease (double heterozygous hemoglobin S and hemoglobin D).
Rationale: Hemoglobin SS, hemoglobin SC, hemoglobin SD, and hemoglobin S/β-thalassemia are sickling disorders in which sickle cells can be seen on peripheral blood smear.
C. Hereditary elliptocytosis.
Rationale: Elliptocytes have rounded rather than pointed ends.
D. *Plasmodium falciparum.*
Rationale: Falciparum gametocytes are crescent or banana shaped with central chromatin.
E. Microangiopathic hemolytic anemia.
Rationale: Schistocytes are small red cell fragments that are irregular in size and shape. They are seen in microangiopathic hemolytic anemias.

Major points of discussion
- Sickle hemoglobin is caused by a point mutation in the β-globin gene $β^{6Glu \rightarrow Val}$. In the homozygous state, sickle hemoglobin can polymerize under low oxygen tension, which then distorts the red cells into a sickle shape. Trapping of these rigid, elongated cells in the small vessels leads to vasoocclusion and tissue damage.
- The sickling hemoglobinopathies include hemoglobin SS, SC, SD, SO, and S/β-thalassemia. In most circumstances, a sickling disorder is not seen in individuals with hemoglobin S trait. Hemoglobin SG–Philadelphia behaves like sickle cell trait.

- Sickle cells are irreversibly damaged red cells that are crescent shaped with pointed ends. They are very dense and lack central pallor.
- Reversibly distorted cells, often referred to as *boat cells*, are also seen in sickling disorders. Reoxygenation can restore these red cells to their more discoid shape.
- Potential errors in misidentification include identification of these cells as elliptocytes or ovalocytes in hereditary elliptocytosis; schistocytes that are formed by fragmentation in microangiopathic hemolytic anemias (e.g., TTP); hemoglobin C crystals, which are also dense and long, but rhomboid in shape; *P. falciparum* gametocytes, which are also crescent shaped but contain chromatin.

60. A. Severe anemia.
Rationale: Severe anemia can cause false-negative sickle solubility test results.
B. Deglycerolized red cells.
Rationale: Sickle solubility tests should not be significantly affected by deglycerolization.
C. Elevated hemoglobin F.
Rationale: Elevated hemoglobin F levels can lead to false-negative test results. The hemoglobin F will interfere with sickling.
D. Hypergammaglobulinemia.
Rationale: Hypergammaglobulinemia can increase the turbidity of the solution, which can obscure the lines behind the tube. A cloudy solution from turbidity can lead to a false positive test result.
E. Newborn.
Rationale: Newborns with hemoglobin S can have a false-negative test result because hemoglobin F levels are high and hemoglobin S levels have not reached adult levels.

Major points of discussion
- The sickle solubility test is a qualitative screen for the presence of hemoglobin S. It cannot distinguish among hemoglobin S trait, hemoglobins SS, SC, SD, SG, SE, SO, S/β⁰, etc. Hemoglobin C–Harlem will give a positive sickle solubility test result.
- The sickle solubility test is performed by preparing a hemolysate by adding saponin to erythrocytes. A phosphate solution containing sodium hydrosulfite is added to the hemolysate. This reduces hemoglobin S, which then forms liquid hemoglobin crystals called *tactoids*. As the tactoids form, the solution becomes cloudy.
- To read a sickle solubility test, the tubes containing the hemolysate and sodium hydrosulfite solution are held up against a white background with black lines or against newspaper. If the lines can be read clearly behind the tube, then the test result is negative. If the lines cannot be read, then the test result is positive.
- False-negative results can occur in the presence of severe anemia or elevated levels of hemoglobin F. In addition, newborns who are homozygous for hemoglobin S have a low percentage of hemoglobin S and higher levels of hemoglobin F. This leads to false-negative test results. Therefore, sickle solubility testing should not be performed in patients younger than 6 months old.
- False-positive results are produced in settings of increased turbidity: high protein levels, hypergammaglobulinemia (e.g., multiple myeloma), cryoglobulinemia, and

hyperlipidemia. Polycythemia can also lead to false-positive test results.

61a. A. Creatinine.
Rationale: Renal failure is a part of the pentad of findings in TTP. The creatinine can be increased in TTP.
B. Blood by urine dipstick.
Rationale: Blood detected on a urine dipstick can be seen in TTP. Microscopic exam results should be negative for red cells (i.e., no hematuria) to confirm that the dipstick is detecting hemoglobinuria.
C. Haptoglobin.
Rationale: Haptoglobin is decreased and often undetectable in TTP.
D. Lactate dehydrogenase.
Rationale: Lactate dehydrogenase is increased in TTP because of red cell destruction and tissue damage.
E. Total bilirubin.
Rationale: Clearance of hemoglobin from the circulation leads to increased total bilirubin and indirect bilirubin.

61b. A. Acanthocyte.
Rationale: Acanthocytes are cells with "spikes" or "thorns" on the surface. Acanthocytosis is associated with abetalipoproteinemia, McLeod's syndrome, neuroacanthosis, and liver disease.
B. Echinocyte.
Rationale: Similar to acanthocytes, echinocytes have "spikes" or "thorns," but the projections are more irregularly spaced and are fewer in number. Echinocytes are also called *Burr cells* and are found in patients with uremia.
C. Reticulocyte.
Rationale: Reticulocytes are young red cells that have been released from the bone marrow. They are larger than more mature red cells and contain a greater amount of ribonucleoprotein, which gives the cell a bluish hue (i.e., polychromasia).
D. Schistocyte.
Rationale: The arrow points to a schistocyte, which is a red cell fragment. In TTP, red cells are fragmented in the microvasculature by fibrin strands. These schistocytes can have many forms and sizes depending on how the cell is sheared.
E. Spherocyte.
Rationale: Spherocytes, which are red cells that are smaller than normal red cells with loss of the central clearing, are present on this peripheral blood smear. However, it is not being pointed to by the arrow. Spherocytes can be seen in hereditary spherocytosis but can also be seen when there is red cell hemolysis. For example, spherocytes can be seen in TTP and warm autoimmune hemolytic anemia.

61c. A. Eculizumab.
Rationale: Eculizumab is a C5 inhibitor used for the treatment of PNH to prevent the complement-mediated lysis of red blood cells.
B. Plasma exchange.
Rationale: Plasma exchange is a lifesaving treatment in TTP. The procedure removes antibodies against ADAMTS13 and replaces normal ADAMTS13 present in donor plasma.
C. Red cell exchange.

Rationale: A red cell exchange would not be beneficial in TTP. Simple transfusion is sufficient to restore oxygen-carrying capacity.

D. Rituximab.

Rationale: Rituximab is an anti–B cell medication that can be used as a second-line treatment in patients with TTP who do not respond to steroids and plasmapheresis.

E. Single-donor platelets.

Rationale: Platelets are contraindicated in TTP. The fear is that giving platelets will increase the risk for thrombosis.

Major points of discussion

■ TTP is a microangiopathic hemolytic anemia that can result from a congenital or acquired deficiency of the enzyme ADAMTS13.

■ The normal function of ADAMTS13 is to cleave large von Willebrand factor (vWf) multimers into smaller multimers. A deficiency in ADAMTS13 leads to the presence of large vWf multimers that trap platelets in the microvasculature. Red cells become sheared in the microvasculature, which results in a hemolytic anemia.

■ TTP classically presents with the pentad of fever, thrombocytopenia, microangiopathic hemolytic anemia, renal failure, and mental status changes. Patients are at increased risk for arterial thrombosis (e.g., stroke).

■ Microangiopathic hemolytic anemia can be diagnosed by the findings of a hemolytic anemia (low hemoglobin, elevated reticulocytes, elevated lactate dehydrogenase, elevated total and indirect bilirubin, urine dipstick blood without red cells, and decreased haptoglobin). The peripheral blood smear should show decreased platelets, spherocytes, and schistocytes, which are red cell fragments produced by physical shearing of red cells while passing through the microvasculature. In this setting, evidence of disseminated intravascular coagulation is usually absent (e.g., normal D-dimer).

■ Treatment should be initiated as soon as possible because plasmapheresis with fresh frozen plasma replacement is lifesaving. Immunosuppression with steroids should also be initiated.

62. A. Decreased plasma vitamin B_{12}.

B. Increased plasma methylmalonic acid.

C. Increased plasma homocysteine.

Rationale: Likely in vitamin B_{12} deficiency,

D. Decreased plasma folate.

Rationale: Unlikely because of widespread folate supplementation.

E. Increased γ-glutamyltranspeptidase.

Rationale: Likely in chronic alcoholism, a frequent cause of macrocytosis.

Major points of discussion

■ Macrocytic anemias are defined by an MCV greater than 100 fL. The most common causes for macrocytic anemia include chronic alcoholism, possibly as a direct toxic effect of alcohol on erythropoiesis, liver, renal, or splenic diseases associated with codocyte or target cell formation, and the megaloblastic anemias, caused by defects in DNA synthesis that cause asynchronous maturation of the nucleus and cytoplasm in the

erythroblast. The latter group is also characterized by hypersegmented neutrophils and can be caused by deficiencies of vitamin B_{12}, folate, toxins, chemotherapy, and myelodysplasia.

■ Vitamin B_{12} deficiency remains prevalent and difficult to assess clinically (e.g., only 65% of B_{12}-deficient patients show macrocytosis). Measurement of plasma vitamin B_{12} levels is important in patients with unexplained macrocytosis or those at risk for vitamin B_{12} deficiency, for example, in autoimmune gastritis. Measurement of plasma methylmalonic acid levels is recommended to diagnose vitamin B_{12} deficiency in patients with borderline vitamin B_{12} levels.

■ In contrast, because of generalized grain fortification with folate since the late 1990s, the prevalence of folate deficiency is very low (<0.05%).

■ More than 90% of the patients with low folate levels are not anemic, and even in those patients, the etiology of the anemia is often unrelated to folate deficiency.

■ Serum folate testing is recommended only in the case of persistent macrocytosis after other common causes have been excluded, or in pregnant or preconception women who may be malnourished or have no access to or refuse folate supplementation. Routine bundling of vitamin B_{12} and folate testing should be discontinued.[1,14]

63. A. Zidovudine therapy.

Rationale: Zidovudine increases red cell size (i.e., elevated MCV).

B. Folate deficiency.

Rationale: Megaloblastic anemia classically presents with a macrocytic anemia (elevated MCV).

C. Hydroxyurea therapy.

Rationale: Hydroxyurea therapy is used in the treatment of sickle cell disease to increase hemoglobin F percentage. Red cell size increases (elevated MCV) after hydroxyurea therapy and can be used to monitor compliance.

D. Lead poisoning.

Rationale: Microcytosis (low MCV), hypochromia, and basophilic stippling can be seen in lead poisoning. The red cell histogram shows a low MCV.

E. End-stage liver disease.

Rationale: End-stage liver disease can be associated with increased red cell size (elevated MCV).

Major points of discussion

■ The Coulter method is an electrical impedance (resistance)-based method. Cells are suspended in an electrolyte solution and pass through an aperture with an electric field across it. As cells pass through the aperture, changes in impedance allow the number of cells, as well as the size of the cells, to be counted.

■ The number of cells counted by the analyzer can be shown graphically as a histogram. The red cell histogram graphically depicts the range of red cell sizes. The number of cells counted for each red cell size is plotted: size on the x-axis (in femtoliters) and the number on the y-axis.

- The mean of the red cell histogram is the MCV or the average of the red cell distribution. The normal MCV ranges from 80 to 100 fL.
- A low MCV corresponds to microcytosis that can be seen on the peripheral blood smear. The solid red line in the figure has an MCV of approximately 65 fL, which is microcytic.
- Microcytosis can be seen in iron deficiency anemia, sideroblastic anemia, anemia of chronic disease, and lead poisoning.

- The MCV can be misleading in microcytic anemias after correction or transfusion. The second population of transfused red cells or reticulocytes can "average out" the MCV such that it is normal. In this scenario, the RDW would be significantly widened and a dimorphic red cell population can be seen on the histogram.

REFERENCES

1. Berg RL, Shaw GR. Laboratory evaluation for vitamin B12 deficiency: the case for cascade testing. Clin Med Res 2013;11:7–15.
2. Capellini MD, Fiorelli G. Glucose-6-phosphate dehydrogenase deficiency. Lancet 2008;371:64–74.
3. Constantino BT, Cogionis B. Nucleated RBCs: significance in the peripheral blood film. Lab Med 2000;31:223–229.
4. Constantino BT. The red cell histogram and the dimorphic red cell population. Lab Med 2011;42:300–308.
5. Hopfer SM, Nadeau FL, Sundra M, et al: Effect of protein on hemoglobin and hematocrit assays with a conductivity-based point-of-care testing device: comparison with optical methods. Ann Clin Lab Sci 2004;34:75–82.
6. International Council for Standardization in Haematology: Expert Panel on Cytometry. Recommendations of the International Council for Standardization in Haematology for Ethylenediaminetetraacetic Acid Anticoagulation of Blood for Blood Cell Counting and Sizing. Am J Clin Pathol 1993;100:371–372.
7. Myers GJ, Browne J. Point of care hematocrit and hemoglobin in cardiac surgery: a review. Perfusion 2007;22:179–183.
8. National Committee for Clinical Laboratory Standards. Methods for Reticulocyte Counting: Approved Guideline. 2nd ed. Wayne, PA: NCCLS, 2004.
9. National Committee for Clinical Laboratory Standards. Procedure for Determining Packed Cell Volume by the Microhematocrit Method; Approved Standard. 3rd ed. Wayne, PA: NCCLS, 2000.
10. Ostertag W, Smith EW. Hemoglobin Lepore-Baltimore, a third type of a delta, beta crossover (delta 50, beta 86). Eur J Biochem 1969;10:371–376.
11. Perkins S. Paroxysmal nocturnal hemoglobinuria. In: Kjeldsberg CJ, editor: Practical Diagnosis of Hematologic Disorders, Chicago: American Society for Clinical Pathology: 2000, pp 171–181.
12. Riley RS, Ben-Ezra JM, Ann Tidwell MT. Reticulocyte enumeration: past and present. Lab Med 2001;10:599–608.
13. Saarinen UM, Siimes MA. Developmental changes in red blood cell counts and indices of infants after exclusion of iron deficiency by laboratory criteria and continuous iron supplementation. J Pediatr 1978;92:412–416.
14. Shojania AM, von Kuster K. Ordering folate assays is no longer justified for investigation of anemias, in folic acid fortified countries. BMC Res Notes 2010;3:22.
15. Vajpayee N, Graham SS, Bern S. Basic examination of blood and bone marrow. In McPherson RA, Pincus MR, editors: Henry's Clinical Diagnosis and Management by Laboratory Methods, 22nd ed. Philadelphia: Elsevier Saunders: 2011, pp 509–535.

CHAPTER 11

HEMATOLOGY: White Blood Cells, Lymph Nodes, and Flow Cytometry

Adriana I. Colovai, Mark D. Ewalt, Paul R. Hosking

QUESTIONS

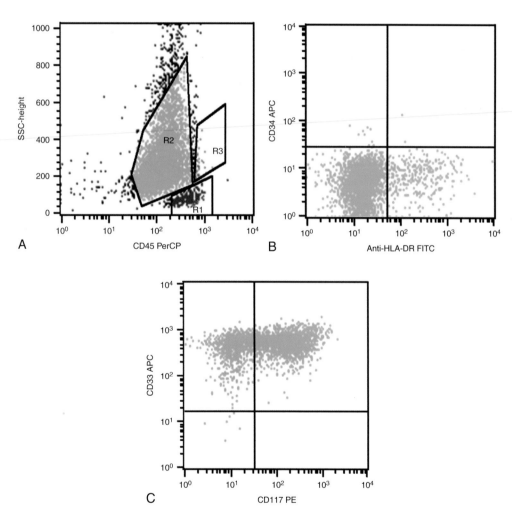

Figure 11-1 Flow cytometric analysis of a peripheral blood sample.

1. A peripheral blood sample obtained from a 78-year-old woman with a white blood cell (WBC) count of 266×10^9/L (reference range, 4.4 to 11.3×10^9/L) was submitted for flow cytometric analysis. In the dot plots shown in Figure 11-1, the cells of interest are highlighted in green. Which one of the following is the most likely diagnosis based on these findings?

A. Acute monoblastic leukemia.

B. Acute myelomonocytic leukemia.

C. Acute myeloid leukemia (AML) without maturation.

D. Acute promyelocytic leukemia (APL).

E. Acute T-cell leukemia.

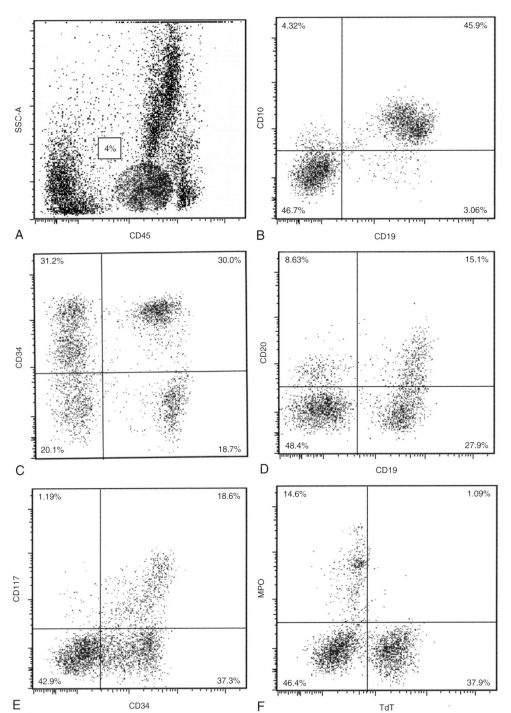

Figure 11-2 Flow cytometric analysis of a bone marrow aspirate sample.

2. A bone marrow aspirate sample obtained from a 3-year-old girl with a history of acute B-lymphoblastic leukemia (B-ALL) was submitted for flow cytometry and cytogenetic analysis as part of the end-of-treatment evaluation. Cytogenetic analysis indicated no abnormalities in the current bone marrow aspirate. The flow cytometry panel shown in Figure 11-2 illustrates the results obtained from the same specimen. CD45 dim/low side scatter cells (SSCs), which include hematopoietic precursors, represent 4% of all nucleated cells and are shown in red. Which one of the following is true based on these results?

A. There is clear evidence of acute B-ALL. Flow cytometry results are not in agreement with the cytogenetic findings.

B. There is no clear evidence of B-ALL. However, the findings are suggestive of myelodysplasia with an excess of blasts.

C. There is no clear evidence of B-ALL. Normal lymphoid and myeloid precursors in a regenerating marrow are observed.

D. There is no clear evidence of B-ALL. However, the flow cytometry findings are suggestive of a mature B-cell neoplasm.

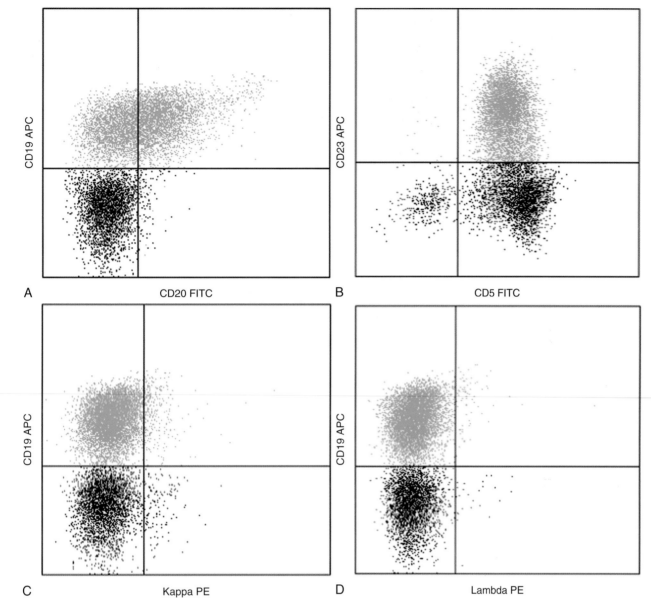

Figure 11-3 Flow cytometric analysis of a peripheral blood sample.

3. A peripheral blood sample from a 33-year-old woman with lymphocytosis and severe anemia was sent for flow cytometric analysis. The dot plots shown in Figure 11-3 illustrate the cell surface profile of the lymphocytes, with the cells of interest represented in green. Which one of the following is the most likely diagnosis?
   A. Chronic lymphocytic leukemia.
   B. Mantle cell lymphoma (MCL).
   C. Acute B-ALL.
   D. Normal B cells.
   E. Follicular lymphoma (FL).

4. Which one of the following best describes compensation in flow cytometric analysis?
   A. Adjustment of forward and side scatter signals.
   B. Adjustment of the instrument noise using nonfluorescent particles.
   C. Adjustment for signals from fluorochromes other than the specific fluorochrome in a single detector.
   D. Adjustment of the excitation and emission spectra of different fluorochromes.
   E. Excitation of a primary fluorochrome that transfers energy to a secondary fluorochrome.

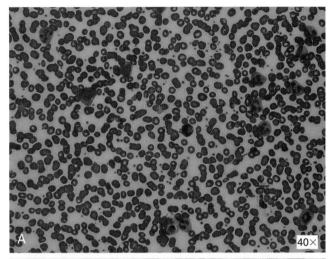

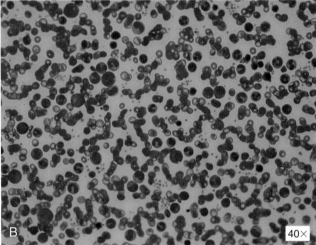

Figure 11-4 **A** and **B**, The patient's peripheral blood smear.

5a. A 62-year-old man presents to his primary care physician with 2 months of fatigue and a 5-lb weight loss. His physician orders a complete blood count with differential, and his peripheral blood smear is shown in Figure 11-4, *A*. Which one of the following genetic/karyotypic abnormalities is diagnostic of the disease from which this patient most likely suffers?
   A. JAK2 V617F.
   B. Translocation t(9;22)(q34;q11.2).
   C. Trisomy 8.
   D. Translocation t(9;14)(p13;q32).
   E. Deletion 5q.

5b. The patient is treated with targeted therapy for the genetic alteration noted above and enters clinical remission. After 5 years, the patient begins to feel fatigued again and notes abdominal fullness. When he returns to his primary care physician, he is found to have splenomegaly, and a complete blood cell count shows hemoglobin 10 g/dL (reference range, 13.3 to 15.2 g/dL), platelets 99×10^9/L (reference range, 165 to 415×10^9/L), and WBC count 53×10^9/L (reference range, 3.5 to 9.1×10^9/L) with 18% myeloblasts. Which one of the following is the patient's diagnosis at this time (Figure 11-4, *B*)?
   A. AML with recurrent genetic abnormalities.
   B. AML, therapy-related (t-AML).

C. Chronic myelogenous leukemia, accelerated phase (CML, AP).
   D. Myelodysplastic syndrome (MDS), refractory anemia with excess blasts II (MDS/RAEB-II).
   E. Blastic plasmacytoid dendritic cell neoplasm (BPDC).

5c. Which one of the following factors is most important in this patient's prognosis?
   A. Bone marrow blast count.
   B. Degree of bone marrow fibrosis.
   C. Presence of cytogenetic abnormalities.
   D. Response to targeted therapy.
   E. Transfusion dependence.

Table 11-1

Test	Result	Reference Range	Units
WBCs	4.5	3.5-9.1	$\times 10^9$/L
Neutrophils	51	40-70	%
Lymphocytes	37	20-50	%
Monocytes	10	4-8	%
Eosinophils	2	0-6	%
Basophils	1	0-2	%

6a. The differential blood count results shown in Table 11-1 are from a 44-year-old man with HIV. Flow cytometric analysis of the same blood sample showed that CD4$^+$ T cells represent 2% of all lymphocytes. Which one of the following is the CD4$^+$ T-cell count of this patient?
   A. 33×10^6/L.
   B. 740×10^6/L.
   C. 90×10^6/L.
   D. There is insufficient information to determine the CD4$^+$ T-cell count.

6b. Flow cytometric analysis of this patient's peripheral blood identified a subpopulation of CD3$^+$ CD4$^-$ CD8$^-$ T cells, which accounted for 10% of the lymphocytes. Which one of the following do these cells most likely represent?
   A. Natural killer (NK) cells.
   B. Helper T cells showing HIV-induced downregulation of CD4 expression.
   C. Gamma/delta T cells.
   D. Immature T cells.

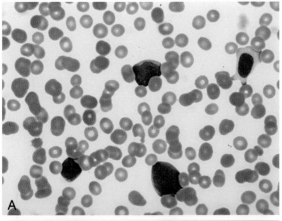

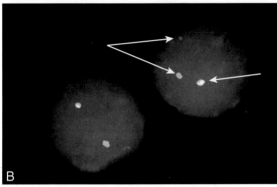

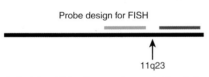

Probe design for FISH

11q23

Figure 11-5 **A**, Peripheral blood smear demonstrating lesional cells. **B**, FISH using break-apart probes.

A 4-year-old girl presents to the emergency department with multiple bruises on her limbs and recent weight loss of 4 lb. When asked, the patient's mother reports that the child has been progressively fatigued and seems to be weak. The patient's past medical history is significant for hemophagocytic lymphohistiocytosis, for which she was treated with etoposide, corticosteroids, cyclosporine, and intrathecal methotrexate. She then received a bone marrow transplantation. Her current complete blood cell count shows anemia, thrombocytopenia, and marked lymphocytosis with 88% blasts. The peripheral smear is shown in Figure 11-5, *A*. Use this scenario to answer the following three questions.

7a. Which one of the following statements regarding the phenotypic characteristics of acute leukemia is true?
- **A.** Terminal deoxynucleotidyl transferase (TdT) can be positive in a subset of AMLs.
- **B.** If the lesional cells express CD13, they must be of the myeloid lineage.
- **C.** CD19 expression is almost never observed in AML.
- **D.** CD117 is commonly seen in ALL.
- **E.** It is not uncommon to see the absence of CD19 on B-cell lymphoblastic leukemias.

7b. Flow cytometry demonstrates that the patient's neoplastic cells are of B-cell lineage. Results of the fluorescence in situ hybridization (FISH) studies are shown (Figure 11-5, *B*). Which one of the following is true?
- **A.** The patient's lesional cells will likely be CD10 positive.
- **B.** This particular cytogenetic finding is predictive of a good prognosis.
- **C.** Administration of methotrexate is a recognized risk factor for the development of this child's disease.
- **D.** This genetic defect causes promyelocytic differentiation in AML.
- **E.** FISH is required to identify this cytogenetic abnormality.

7c. Which one of the following statements regarding the molecular characteristics of B-ALL is true?
- **A.** The presence of greater than 52 chromosomes in the neoplastic cells is associated with a particularly poor prognosis.
- **B.** The BCR/ABL translocation that can occur in B-ALL is molecularly identical to the translocation seen in chronic myeloid leukemia (CML).
- **C.** A karyotype characterized by fewer than 40 chromosomes confers a favorable prognosis.
- **D.** The presence of the BCR/ABL translocation confers a distinctly poor prognosis.
- **E.** A translocation between chromosomes 12 and 21 is prognostically unfavorable.

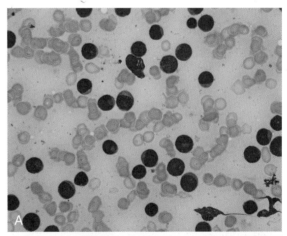

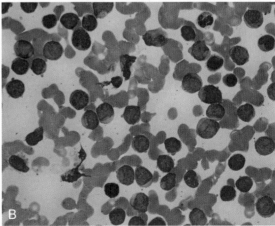

Figure 11-6 **A**, Wright-Giemsa–stained peripheral blood smear (×100). **B**, Wright-Giemsa–stained bone marrow aspirate smear (×100).

8. A 74-year-old woman with a new diagnosis of leukemia undergoes molecular testing to assess her prognosis. Which one of the following alterations associated with the blast morphology seen in Figure 11-6 has the worst prognosis?
   A. Core-binding factor β-subunit myosin heavy-chain 11 *(CBFB-MYH11)* fusion.
   B. *CEBPA* (CCAAT/enhancer-binding protein) mutation.
   C. *FLT3* mutation
   D. *NPM1* mutation.
   E. *RUNX1-RUNX1T1* fusion.

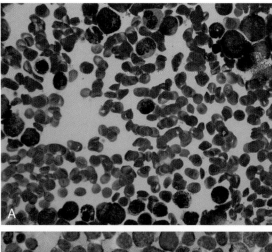

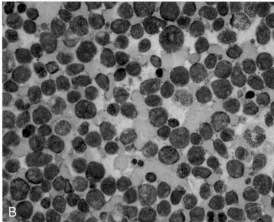

Figure 11-7 **A,** Wright-Giemsa–stained peripheral blood smear (×100). **B,** Wright-Giemsa–stained bone marrow aspirate smear (×100).

9. A 68-year-old man is diagnosed with leukemia. His peripheral blood and bone marrow aspirates smears are shown in Figure 11-7, *A* and *B,* respectively. Which one of the following good prognostic cytogenetic abnormalities is most likely present in this patient?
   A. inv(3).
   B. t(8;21).
   C. t(9;11).
   D. t(15;17).
   E. inv(16).

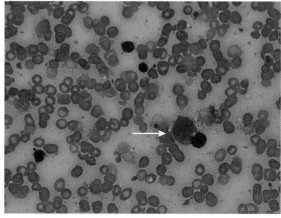

Figure 11-8 A bone marrow aspirate smear. The *arrow* indicates a representative blast cell identified in the differential count.

10. A 4-month-old infant girl is noted by her parents to be lethargic with abdominal distention. Physical examination by her physician reveals hepatomegaly and splenomegaly, and a complete blood cell count shows anemia (hemoglobin, 9.2 g/dL; reference range, 10.0 to 14.0 g/dL) and thrombocytopenia (76×10^9/L; reference range, 150 to 450×10^9/L). Bone marrow examination is performed and reveals 24% blasts. A representative blast is shown in Figure 11-8. Which one of the following genetic abnormalities does this patient most likely have?
   A. inv(3).
   B. t(8;21).
   C. t(15;17).
   D. inv(16).
   E. +21.

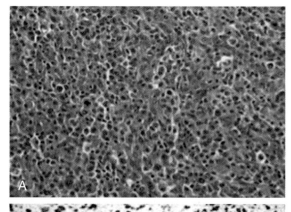

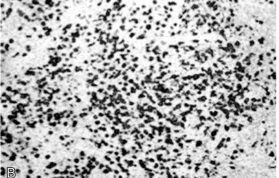

Figure 11-9 **A** and **B,** H&E-stained lymph node biopsy specimen with accompanying ALK immunohistochemistry.

11. A 7-year-old boy is taken to the pediatrician's office by his parents with swollen lymph nodes in his neck and axillae and persistent fever over the past several weeks. In addition, the child complains that he often wakes during the night to find his pillow soaking wet from sweat. A section from an excisional biopsy of a lymph node is shown in Figure 11-9. No B-cell markers are positive when immunohistochemistry is performed. Which one of the following statements is true?

   A. Because the lesional cells express anaplastic lymphoma kinase (ALK), the child's prognosis is poor.

   B. Immunohistochemistry for CD30 is expected to be negative.

   C. This disease is almost always driven by Epstein-Barr virus (EBV).

   D. IgH (immunoglobulin heavy locus) is almost always rearranged in this disease.

   E. The cells in this disease typically express epithelial membrane antigen (EMA).

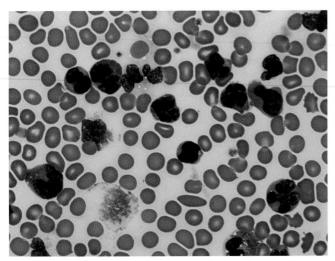

Figure 11-10 Peripheral blood smear.

12. A 42-year-old Jamaican woman presents to her physician with a persistent nonproductive cough, recent 8-lb weight loss, and night sweats. Her pulse and respiratory rate are elevated, and her oxygen saturation is measured at 86%. She is sent to the emergency department for evaluation. A chest radiograph demonstrates diffuse granular opacities consistent with *Pneumocystis jiroveci* pneumonia (PCP). A complete blood cell count with differential shows a WBC count of 23×10^9/L (reference range, 6.0 to 11.0×10^9/L) and absolute lymphocytosis with "many atypical cells." She is found to have splenomegaly and scattered nodules on her lower posterior trunk. The patient's family history reveals that her mother "can't use her legs at all." The patient's peripheral smear is shown in Figure 11-10. Which one of the following statements is true?

   A. The patient will likely have an elevated calcium level when serum chemistries are evaluated.

   B. With aggressive treatment and bone marrow transplantation, the patient's prognosis is good.

   C. The patient's disease is related to a chronic parasitic infection that is endemic in the Caribbean islands.

   D. The atypical cells will most likely be CD16 and CD56 positive.

   E. The patient is immunocompromised because her bone marrow is likely replaced by neoplastic cells.

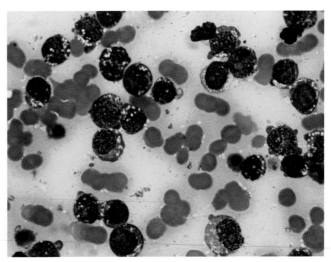

Figure 11-11 Peripheral blood smear.

13. A 16-year-old boy is taken to the emergency department with abdominal pain that has worsened over the past week. He complains of abdominal tenderness and reveals that he has not had a bowel movement for the past 4 days. The patient is sent for a computed tomography (CT) scan of the abdomen, which shows a large abdominal mass and dilated loops of bowel suggestive of obstruction. He is scheduled for exploratory laparotomy, and his preoperative peripheral smear is shown in Figure 11-11. Which one of the following is true regarding the patient's diagnosis?

   A. This disease is almost always associated with EBV in the Western world.

   B. Phenotypic analysis will likely show that these cells are CD10 negative.

   C. A histologic hallmark of this disease is the absence of tingible body macrophages.

   D. Despite aggressive treatment with chemotherapy, the long-term prognosis is poor.

   E. This disease usually involves the fusion of one of several genes to chromosome 8.

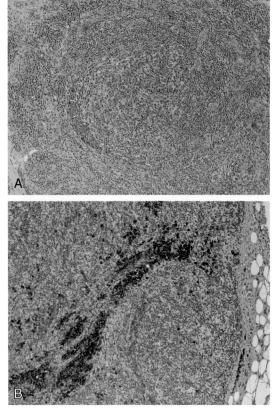

Figure 11-12 **A,** H&E-stained section of the patient's lymph node (×10). **B,** CD138 immunohistochemical stain of the same lymph node (×10).

14. A 32-year-old woman develops multiple enlarged cervical lymph nodes and presents to her physician. He decides to send her for an excisional biopsy of one of the nodes, as shown in Figure 11-12. Which one of the following infections is most often linked to this patient's adenopathy?
   A. Cytomegalovirus (CMV).
   B. EBV.
   C. Hepatitis C virus (HCV)
   D. Human herpesvirus 8 (HHV-8).
   E. Human T-lymphotropic virus 1 (HTLV-1).

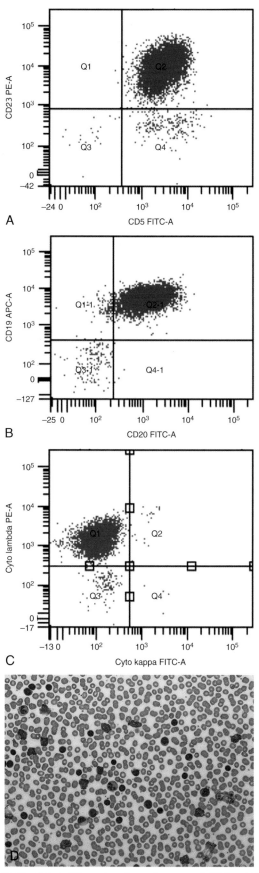

Figure 11-13 Selected flow cytometry scattergrams. **A,** CD5 and CD23. **B,** CD20 and CD19. **C,** κ and λ. **D,** Wright-Giemsa stain of peripheral blood smear (×40).

A 63-year-old woman with hypertension and hyperlipidemia presents to her primary care physician for a routine checkup. She feels well and has well-controlled blood pressure and lipid levels; however, a complete blood cell count shows mild leukocytosis (WBC count, 13.0×10^9/L; reference range, 3.54 to 9.06×10^9/L) with atypical lymphocytosis (60% neutrophils, 5% lymphocytes, 30% atypical lymphocytes, 3% monocytes, and 2% eosinophils; reference ranges, 40% to 70% neutrophils, 20% to 50% lymphocytes, 2% to 8% monocytes, 0% to 6% eosinophils, 1% to 2% basophils). Her physician chooses to send a sample for flow cytometry evaluation. Representative flow cytometry results are shown in Figure 11-13. Use this scenario to answer the following four questions.

15a. Which one of the following is the most appropriate diagnosis for this patient?
   A. B-cell prolymphocytic leukemia (B-PLL).
   B. Chronic lymphocytic leukemia (CLL).
   C. Hairy cell leukemia (HCL).
   D. Monoclonal B-cell lymphocytosis (MBL).
   E. Reactive lymphocytosis (RL).

15b. The patient receives appropriate therapy and follow-up for her diagnosis but returns over the following year with increasing leukocytosis (WBC count $\geq 52 \times 10^9$/L for 4 months; reference range, 3.54 to 9.06×10^9/L) and increasing atypical lymphocytosis (11% neutrophils, 12% lymphocytes, 74% atypical lymphocytes, 2% monocytes, and 1% eosinophils; reference ranges, 40% to 70% neutrophils, 20% to 50% lymphocytes, 2% to 8% monocytes, 0% to 6% eosinophils, 1% to 2% basophils). Flow cytometry shows the same immunoprofile noted previously. A peripheral blood smear at this time is shown (Figure 11-13, *D*). Which one of the following is the most appropriate diagnosis for this patient at this time?
   A. B-PLL.
   B. CLL.
   C. HCL.
   D. Large granular lymphocytic leukemia (LGL leukemia).
   E. MBL.

15c. Which one of the following factors is associated with the best prognosis in this disease?
   A. CD38 expression.
   B. Deletion 13q.
   C. Deletion 17p.
   D. Germline *IGHV* (immunoglobulin heavy variable cluster) gene.
   E. ZAP-70 (ζ-chain [T-cell receptor]-associated kinase 70) expression.

15d. Several years later, this patient's disease progresses again and she is noted to have several enlarged lymph nodes. Eight months after this development, the patient dies. Which one of the following is the most likely diagnosis for this patient's transformed disease?
   A. ALL.
   B. Classic Hodgkin's lymphoma (CHL).
   C. Diffuse large B-cell lymphoma (DLBCL).
   D. LGL leukemia.
   E. Small lymphocytic lymphoma (SLL).

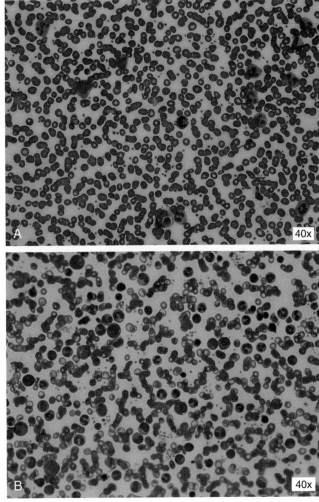

Figure 11-14 **A,** Peripheral blood smear. **B,** Bone marrow aspirate smear.

16a. A 62-year-old man presents to his primary care physician with 2 months of fatigue and a 5-lb weight loss. His physician orders a complete blood cell count with differential and a bone marrow biopsy. His peripheral blood smear and bone marrow aspirate are shown in Figure 11-14. Which one of the following genetic/karyotypic abnormalities is diagnostic of the disease from which this patient most likely suffers?
  A. JAK2 V617F.
  B. Translocation t(9;22)(q34;q11.2).
  C. Trisomy 8.
  D. Translocation t(9;14)(p13;q32).
  E. Deletion 5q.

16b. The patient is treated with targeted therapy for the genetic alteration noted previously and enters clinical remission. After 5 years, the patient begins to feel fatigued again and notes abdominal fullness. When he returns to his primary care physician, he is found to have splenomegaly and a complete cell blood count shows anemia (10.2 g/dL; reference range, 13.3 to 16.2 g/dL), thrombocytopenia (99×10^9/L; reference range, 165 to 415×10^9/L), and leukocytosis (53×10^9/L; reference range, 3.54 to 9.06×10^9/L), with a marked left shift (18% myeloblasts). Which one of the following is the patient's diagnosis at this time?
  A. AML with recurrent genetic abnormalities.
  B. t-AML.
  C. CML, AP.
  D. MDS/RAEB-II.
  E. BPDC.

16c. Which one of the following factors is most important in this patient's prognosis?
  A. Bone marrow blast count.
  B. Degree of bone marrow fibrosis.
  C. Presence of cytogenetic abnormalities.
  D. Response to targeted therapy.
  E. Transfusion dependence.

17. A 64-year-old man presents to his primary care physician with a rash that developed over the past several months. The rash is a generalized erythroderma that is intensely and persistently pruritic. Physical examination reveals hepatosplenomegaly and diffuse lymphadenopathy. The patient is sent for routine blood work, and he is referred to a dermatologist for further evaluation. An image from the patient's peripheral blood smear is shown in Figure 11-15. Which one of the following statements is true?
  A. A biopsy of this patient's rash will show epidermal involvement by the lesional cells.
  B. The lesional cells will have an NK phenotype.
  C. Peripheral blood involvement of cutaneous lesions of this type is a strong indication that the bone marrow will also be involved.
  D. Prognosis is affected by the degree of lymph node and/or peripheral blood involvement by the lesional cells.
  E. With aggressive treatment, this patient has an excellent prognosis.

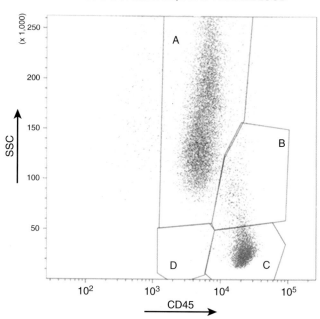

FLOW CYTOMETRY, PERIPHERAL BLOOD

Figure 11-16 Scatterplot (CD45 versus side scatter) on a peripheral blood sample from a healthy patient.

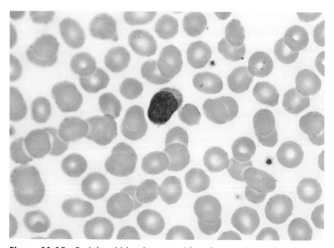

Figure 11-15 Peripheral blood smear with a characteristic cell from the disease described.

18. Blood is taken from a healthy patient and flow cytometry is performed on the sample shown in Figure 11-16. Which one of the following statements is true?
    A. Chloroacetate esterase (CAE) positivity is specific for the cells that are found in gate A.
    B. The cells in gate B will be negative when stained with naphthyl acetate esterase staining.
    C. The cells in gate C will stain positive with Sudan Black B.
    D. Myeloperoxidase staining is nearly 100% specific for the cells that are found in gate A.
    E. The cells in gate C will be reactive when treated with nitroblue-tetrazolium (NBT).

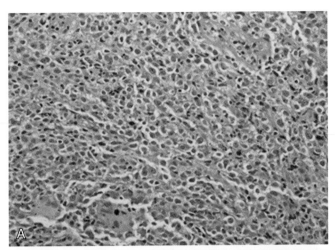

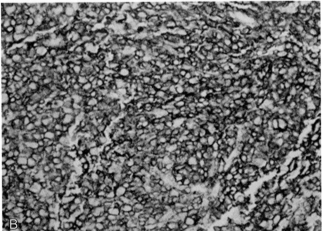

Figure 11-17 H&E-stained lymph node biopsy specimen with accompanying CD20 immunohistochemistry.

19. A 72-year-old woman sees her primary care doctor because she noticed a lump in her right axilla. She also complains of night sweats and fatigue over a period of 1 to 2 months. The mass is excised, and the biopsy specimen is shown in Figure 11-17. Which one of the following statements is true?
    A. Necrosis is an uncommon feature in lymph node biopsy of a patient with this disease.
    B. CD10- or bcl6-positivity is prognostically unfavorable.
    C. The bone marrow is almost always involved when this disease is diagnosed.
    D. A gene normally expressed in germinal centers is the most common cytogenetic abnormality.
    E. The proliferation index (assessed by Ki-67 positivity) is almost universally greater than 90%.

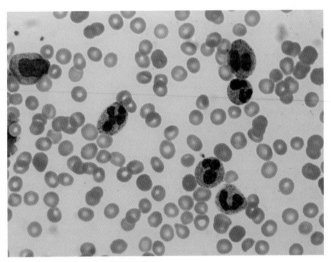

Figure 11-18 Peripheral blood smear.

20. A 23-year-old man is taken by ambulance to the trauma center with third-degree burns covering 30% of his body. His peripheral smear is shown in Figure 11-18. Which one of the following statements is true regarding the patient's neutrophilic inclusions?
    A. These inclusions are rarely seen in conjunction with toxic granulation.
    B. These inclusions demonstrate piled-up fragments of mitochondrial remnants on electron microscopy.
    C. These inclusions will be destroyed by treatment with ribonuclease.
    D. These inclusions are a sign of a relatively slow turnover of neutrophils compared with systemic demands.
    E. These inclusions are more likely to be identified evenly distributed through the cell as opposed to on the periphery.

Table 11-2

Test	Patient	Reference Range	Units
WBCs	1.9	4.5-13.5	$\times 10^9$/L
Red blood cells	2.2	3.9-5.3	$\times 10^{12}$/L
Hemoglobin	7.4	11.5-13.5	g/dL
Hematocrit	22.2	34.0-40.0	%
Mean corpuscular volume	82.1	75.0-90.0	fL
Mean corpuscular hemoglobin	31.6	26.7-31.9	pg
Mean corpuscular hemoglobin concentration	33.0	28.0-36.0	g/dL
Red cell distribution width	13.8	<14.5	%
Platelets	4	165-415	$\times 10^9$/L
Reticulocytes	0.2	0.8-2.3	%

21. A 6-year-old girl from South Africa presents to the emergency department with altered mental status. Neurologic examination reveals focal deficits including right limb paralysis. Skin examination reveals petechiae on the patient's truck and several bruises on the patient's limbs, in addition to café-au-lait spots. She is noted to be short for her age, and truncal dissymmetry suggestive of scoliosis is observed. Laboratory testing is performed, and her complete blood count with differential is shown in Table 11-2. Which one of the following is true about the patient's *most likely* diagnosis?
    A. If the patient has a sibling, there is a 50% chance that he or she will also have the same disease.
    B. Patients with this disease will have positive chromosome breakage studies.
    C. Most patients with this condition never experience aplastic anemia.
    D. Patients with this disorder are no more likely to develop a hematopoietic malignancy.
    E. A single gene is implicated in this disease.

22. A 68-year-old man sees his primary doctor after noticing a "lump in his armpit." On examination, he is found to have diffuse adenopathy. The patient is sent for laboratory testing and a CT scan of the head/neck and chest. You are the pathologist covering the hematology laboratory and are asked to review the patient's peripheral smear (Figure 11-19). Which one of the following statements is true regarding the patient's condition?
    A. The patient's flow cytometry will likely show a T-cell phenotype for the abnormal cells seen.
    B. Lymph node versus bone marrow grade discordance (high versus low) suggests a slightly better prognosis than high-grade concordance.
    C. The patient's disease is associated with a translocation involving a cell cycle regulator gene.
    D. Bone marrow involvement is commonly found in this patient's disease and is typically characterized by a diffuse pattern of infiltration.
    E. The expression of CD10 is stronger in higher-grade lesions of this type.

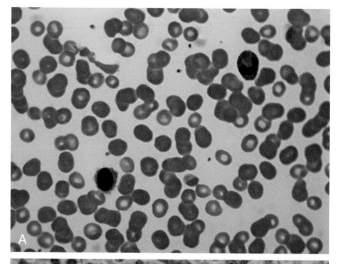

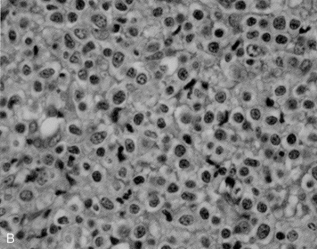

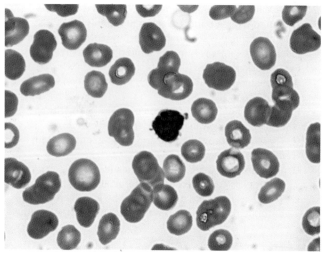

Figure 11-19 A peripheral blood smear demonstrating a characteristic lesional cell from the disease described.

Figure 11-20 Wright-Giemsa peripheral blood smear and bone marrow biopsy specimen.

23. A 68-year-old man goes to see his primary care doctor to be evaluated for progressive weakness and decreased exercise tolerance. Review of systems reveals that he is not eating as much as he normally does and that he feels full after eating only a small portion of the food on his plate. Physical examination shows splenomegaly, petechial bruises, and purpura on his lower limbs bilaterally. The patient is sent to have blood work and imaging studies. He is found to be pancytopenic. A bone marrow biopsy is subsequently performed. His peripheral smear and bone marrow biopsy are shown in Figure 11-20. Which one of the following statements is true?
    A. Cytogenetic studies play no role in prognosis in this disease.
    B. The villi that are seen on the lesional cells are characteristically polar.
    C. Marrow fibrosis is not a common feature in this disease.
    D. Monocytosis is a common feature in this disease.
    E. Diffuse adenopathy is usually present in patients with this disease.

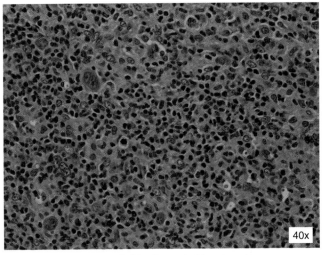

Figure 11-22 H&E-stained slide of a cervical lymph node.

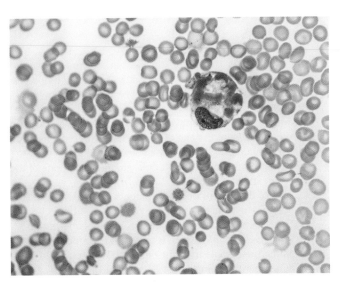

Figure 11-21 Bone marrow aspirate smear.

24. A 5-week-old newborn boy is taken to the emergency department with yellow skin and eyes and increasing somnolence. He has had intermittent fever over the past several days. On physical examination, the baby is found to have hepatosplenomegaly. A complete blood cell count shows profound anemia and thrombocytopenia. In addition, his serum aspartate aminotransferase (AST), alanine aminotransferase (ALT), and total and direct bilirubin are all found to be elevated. Further history reveals that the infant's parents are first cousins. The patient undergoes a bone marrow biopsy, and the Giemsa-Wright–stained aspirate is shown in Figure 11-21. Which one of the following statements is true?
    A. The main immunologic defect in this disease involves CD4$^+$ lymphocytes.
    B. Hypoferritinemia is characteristic in this disease.
    C. Hemophagocytosis is necessary and sufficient to make this diagnosis.
    D. High levels of soluble CD25 (sCD25) are highly specific for this disease.
    E. The quantity of CD16$^+$/CD56$^+$ cells is characteristically reduced in this disease.

25. A 40-year-old man presents to his physician with fevers and weight loss. Physical examination reveals cervical lymphadenopathy; the lymph node biopsy is shown in Figure 11-22. Which one of the following immunoprofiles is most consistent with the large cells in the above lymph node infiltrate and has the best overall prognosis?
    A. CD15$^+$ CD20$^-$ CD30$^+$ CD45$^-$ PAX5$^+$ LMP1$^+$.
    B. CD15$^-$ CD20$^+$ CD30$^+$ CD45$^+$ PAX5$^+$ LMP1$^+$.
    C. CD15$^-$ CD20$^+$ CD30$^-$ CD45$^+$ PAX5$^+$ LMP1$^-$.
    D. CD15$^-$ CD20$^-$ CD30$^+$ CD45$^+$ PAX5$^+$ LMP1$^+$.
    E. CD15$^-$ CD20$^+$ CD30$^-$ CD45$^-$ PAX5$^-$ LMP1$^-$.

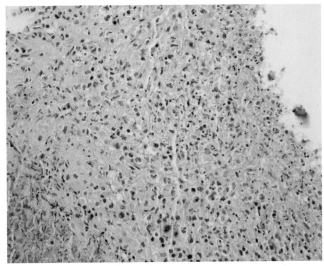

Figure 11-23 H&E-stained lymph node biopsy specimen.

26. A 19-year-old Japanese immigrant presents to her physician with unilateral posterior cervical lymphadenopathy that she initially noticed about 2 weeks before, along with intermittent fevers, chills, and myalgias. An autoimmune workup is negative. The lymph node is excised, and the hematoxylin and eosin (H&E)-stained slide is shown in Figure 11-23. Which one of the following statements is true?
   A. An abundance of plasma cells is expected to be identified in this biopsy.
   B. The absence of neutrophils is characteristic of this disease.
   C. This patient's clinical course will likely be characterized by lifelong intermittent disease.
   D. Human herpesvirus-6 (HHV-6) is the causative agent in this disease.
   E. CD4⁺ cells are the predominant cells in affected lymph nodes.

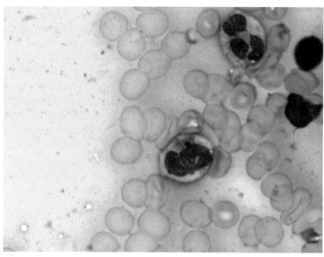

Figure 11-25 Neutrophil found in the peripheral blood smear.

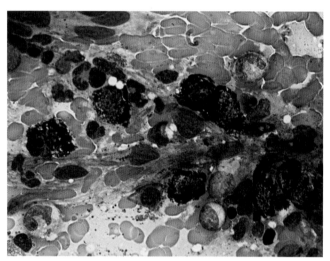

Figure 11-24 Giemsa-Wright–stained slide of bone marrow aspirate.

27. A 68-year-old man comes to his primary care physician for a routine checkup. The patient complains of a generalized pruritic rash and recent weight loss. In addition, he says that he often has hot flashes associated with facial redness. Physical examination reveals that a wheal develops when the affected skin is scratched with the wooden end of a cotton swab. Mild splenomegaly is noted; however, no lymphadenopathy or hepatomegaly is appreciated. Blood work reveals leukocytosis with eosinophila, mild anemia, and mild thrombocytosis. The patient is sent for a bone marrow biopsy; a Giemsa-Wright–stained slide of the aspirate is shown in Figure 11-24. Which one of the following statements is true?
   A. These findings are not associated with hematopoietic disease.
   B. CD117 positivity in the cells seen in the patient's bone marrow biopsy is evidence of neoplasia.
   C. Elevated histamine levels are highly specific for the patient's condition.
   D. Fibrosis is an uncommon feature in the bone marrow when this disease is identified.
   E. The patient's serum tryptase level will likely be elevated.

28. You are the clinical hematopathologist in the core laboratory facility, and you receive the preoperative complete blood cell count and accompanying peripheral blood smear shown in Figure 11-25. The patient is a 16-year-old deaf boy who is accompanied by his adoptive parents. He was initially found to have proteinuria at the age of 12 years, and his renal function has steadily declined over the past several years. He is now scheduled for a dialysis catheter placement. Which one of the following statements is true?
   A. Both of the patient's biologic parents are at least carriers of the genetic defect causing the patient's disorder.
   B. The patient has a defect in microtubule polymerization.
   C. When electron microscopy is performed, the inclusions seen within the cytoplasm of the neutrophils are enriched in degenerated organelles.
   D. The gene implicated in this patient's condition is implicated in numerous similar diseases.
   E. This patient has a lysosomal storage disease.

A 78-year-old woman presents to her physician with increasing fatigue. A complete blood cell count is ordered and is notable for pancytopenia. The peripheral smear is shown in Figure 11-26, *A*). In response to these findings, a bone marrow biopsy is performed; the aspirate smear is shown in Figure 11-26, *B*. Use this scenario to answer the following three questions.

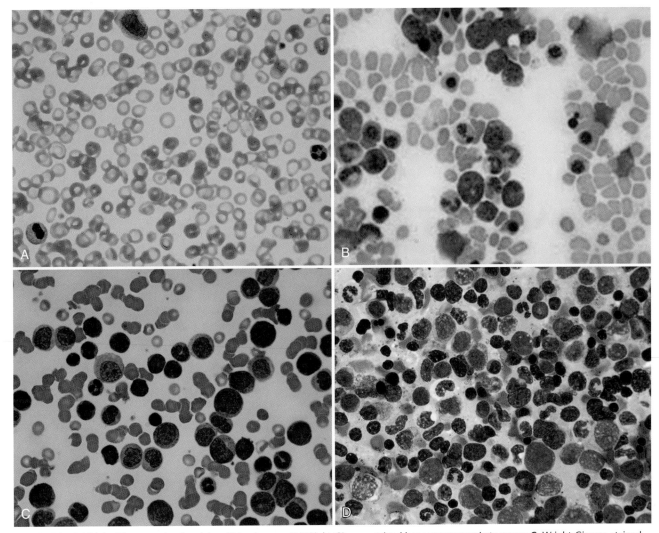

Figure 11-26 **A,** Wright-Giemsa–stained peripheral blood smear. **B,** Wright-Giemsa–stained bone marrow aspirate smear. **C,** Wright-Giemsa–stained peripheral blood smear. **D,** Wright-Giemsa–stained bone marrow aspirate smear.

29a. Which one of the following combinations of factors is most important in predicting the prognosis in this patient?
  A. Age, bone marrow blast percentage, cytopenias, FLT3 status.
  B. Age, bone marrow blast percentage, cytopenias, karyotype.
  C. Age, bone marrow blast percentage, FLT3 status, karyotype.
  D. Age, cytopenias, FLT3 status, karyotype.
  E. Bone marrow blast percentage, cytopenias, FLT3 status, karyotype.

29b. Which one of the following genetic changes is associated with the best prognosis in this patient?
  A. t(3;21).
  B. del(5q).
  C. del(7q).
  D. +8.
  E. i(17q).

29c. The patient is followed for 3 years and treated according to standard of care. At this point, she has required escalating intensity of intervention. A repeat bone marrow biopsy is performed; the aspirate is shown in Figure 11-26, *C* and *D*. Which one of the following is the most appropriate diagnosis for this patient at this point?
  A. Refractory anemia with excess blasts II (RAEB-2).
  B. Refractory anemia with ringed sideroblasts (RARS).
  C. Refractory cytopenia with multilineage dysplasia (RCMD).
  D. Refractory cytopenia with unilineage dysplasia.
  E. Refractory neutropenia (RN).

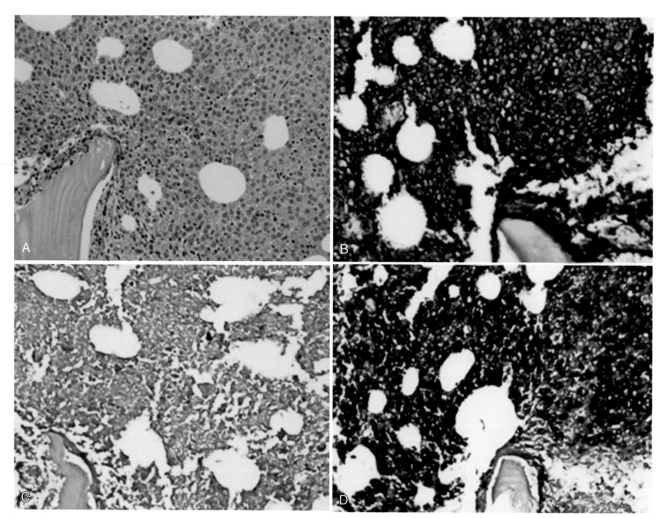

Figure 11-27 H&E-stained bone marrow biopsy specimen with accompanying CD138 immunohistochemistry and κ/λ in situ hybridization.

30a. A 72-year-old white man presents to his primary care doctor with complaints of increasing shortness of breath and fatigue. Further questioning reveals that the patient has been experiencing worsening pain in his mid and lower back. Laboratory workup demonstrates normocytic anemia, thrombocytopenia, and neutropenia. A bone marrow biopsy and immunohistochemical and in situ hybridization studies are shown in Figure 11-27. Which one of the following statements regarding the patient's biopsy is likely to be true?

A. Expression of CD56 by the lesional cells in the bone marrow biopsy favors a reactive condition.

B. A perivascular distribution of suspicious cells is the histologic hallmark of neoplasia in this setting.

C. Fibrosis is an uncommon feature in bone marrow biopsies in patients with this disease.

D. Sampling error in bone marrow biopsies can be problematic in this disease because the infiltrate is often patchy.

E. Cytoplasmic staining for immunoglobulin M (IgM) will likely be positive.

30b. Which one of the following is true regarding this patient's disease?

A. Primary amyloidosis occurs in a minority of cases and is usually associated with κ light chains.

B. In the United States, this disease is most commonly seen in African American men.

C. The presence of clonal plasma cells comprising less than 10% of nucleated marrow elements rules out this diagnosis.

D. Decreased β₂-microglobulin is prognostically unfavorable.

E. The absence of a paraprotein on serum protein electrophoresis indicates the patient likely has a nonsecretory form of the disease.

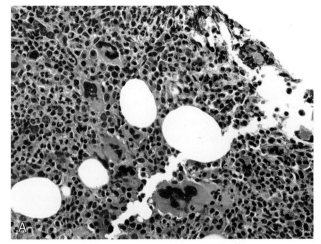

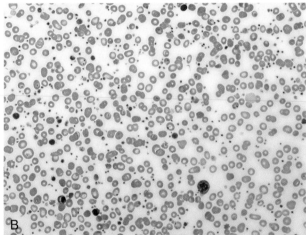

Figure 11-28 **A.** H&E-stained bone marrow trephine biopsy specimen (×40). **B,** Wright-Giemsa–stained peripheral blood smear (×40).

30c. Which one of the following statements is true regarding the cytogenetics of this patient's disease?
  A. Karyotypic analysis is usually sufficient to characterize the cytogenetic abnormalities in this disease.
  B. Cases with a hyperdiploid genotype characteristically contain gains in even-numbered chromosomes.
  C. The t(11;14) induces constitutive tyrosine kinase activity and unregulated cell proliferation.
  D. Cytogenetics is of limited use in providing clinically prognostic information.
  E. 17p13 deletion is prognostically unfavorable, with a median survival of about 1 year.

A 73-year-old woman presents to her physician with persistent headaches and dizziness. Her physical examination is notable for hypertension and splenomegaly. Her complete blood cell count is abnormal and a bone marrow biopsy is performed. A representative section of the bone marrow biopsy is shown in Figure 11-28, *A*. Use this scenario to answer the following three questions.

31a. Which one of the following sets of factors is most important to establish a definitive diagnosis for this patient?
  A. Age, bone marrow cell counts, bone marrow fibrosis, clinical presentation.
  B. Bone marrow cell counts, bone marrow fibrosis, duration of illness, mutation testing.
  C. Bone marrow fibrosis, duration of illness, mutation testing, peripheral blood counts.

  D. Bone marrow cell counts, duration of illness, mutation testing, peripheral blood counts.
  E. Age, bone marrow cell counts, mutation testing, peripheral blood counts.

31b. The patient also has a complete blood cell count performed, which is notable for elevated hemoglobin (hemoglobin, 17.3 g/dL; reference range, 12.0 to 15.8 g/dL) and elevated platelet count (platelets, 600×10^9/L; reference range, 165 to 415×10^9/L). Her smear is shown in Figure 11-28, *B*. Another peripheral blood sample is sent for genetic analysis. Which one of the following genetic alterations is most likely to be present?
  A. *BCR-ABL* translocation.
  B. *FGFR1* translocation.
  C. *JAK2* mutation.
  D. *MPL* mutation.
  E. *PDGFRA* translocation.

31c. The patient is managed conservatively and after 14 years, her hemoglobin and platelet counts drop and she is able to discontinue therapy. In addition, her peripheral blood smear is notable for 3% blasts and 2% nucleated red blood cells. Which one of the following is the most likely cause of this change?
  A. Development of pure red cell aplasia.
  B. Leukemic transformation.
  C. Progression to spent phase.
  D. Therapy-induced remission.
  E. Transformation to MDS.

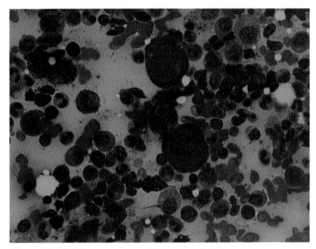

Figure 11-29 Bone marrow aspirate smear (×63).

32. A 6-year-old previously healthy boy acutely develops fever and headache. Within 2 days, he starts to feel fatigued and presents to his pediatrician. A complete blood cell count is notable for anemia (hemoglobin, 8.4 g/dL; reference range, 12.0 to 14.0 g/dL). In the following days, the patient develops a lacy malar rash and remains fatigued. A repeat complete blood cell count 2 weeks later reveals persistent anemia. He undergoes a bone marrow biopsy; the aspirate is shown in Figure 11-29. Which one of the following is the most likely cause of this patient's illness?
  A. CMV.
  B. EBV.
  C. HHV-6.
  D. HHV-8.
  E. Parvovirus B19.

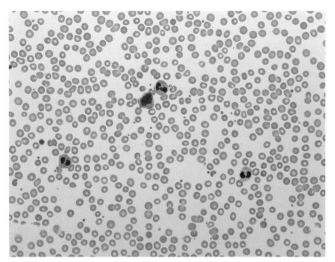

Figure 11-30 Representative field of a Wright-Giemsa–stained peripheral blood smear (×40).

33. A 2-year-old boy with developmental delay and epilepsy presents to his primary care doctor for a checkup. The physician orders a complete blood cell count with differential, and the technologists note the neutrophils shown (Figure 11-30). Which one of the following is the most likely diagnosis in this patient?
    A. Alder-Reilly anomaly.
    B. May-Hegglin anomaly.
    C. MDS.
    D. Myelokathexis.
    E. Pelger-Huët anomaly.

34. A 37-year-old African-American man presents with worsening bilateral cervical lymphadenopathy. He had been in his normal state of health until noticing the swollen lymph nodes. He feels well otherwise, and his review of systems is negative. An excisional biopsy is performed; representative sections stained with H&E, CD68, S100, and CD1a are shown in Figure 11-31. Which one of the following statements is true?
    A. An acid-fast bacillus causes this disease.
    B. Central nervous system involvement has not been reported for this disease.
    C. Plasmacytosis is infrequent in this disease.
    D. Expression of CD1a is concerning for malignancy.
    E. Hemophagocytosis is characteristic of this disease.

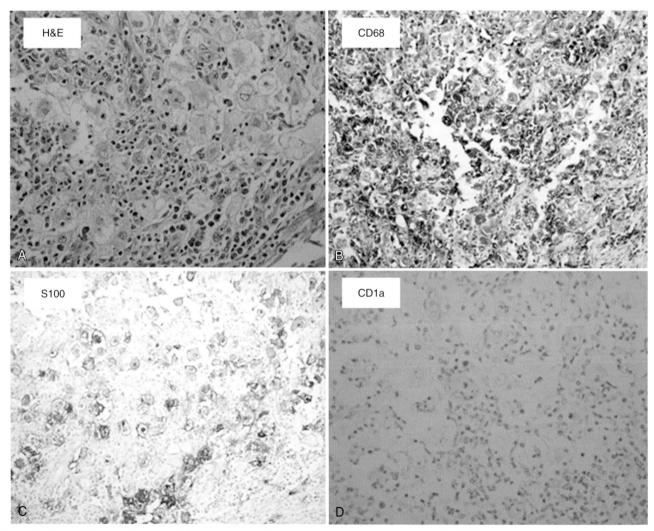

Figure 11-31 **A,** H&E-stained lymph node biopsy specimen. **B,** Lymph node biopsy specimen stained with CD68. **C,** Lymph node biopsy specimen stained with S100. **D,** Lymph node biopsy specimen stained with CD1a.

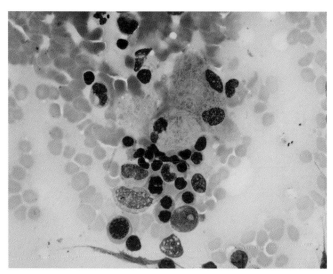

Figure 11-32 Wright-Giemsa–stained bone marrow aspirate smear.

35. A 36-month-old girl is taken to the emergency department after falling on her arm. According to the patient's parents, she tripped over the household cat and tumbled. She is appropriately sedated and evaluated. A humerus fracture and evidence of osteoporosis are seen on radiographic examination. On further examination, the patient is found to have marked splenomegaly and, to a lesser extent, hepatomegaly. Additionally, her height is less than the fifth percentile for her age and sex. Blood work demonstrates anemia and thrombocytopenia. A hematologist is also called, who recommends a bone marrow examination. Both of the patient's parents are of Ashkenazi Jewish descent. A Wright-Giemsa–stained aspirate from the patient's bone marrow is shown in Figure 11-32. Which one of the following statements is true?

A. The patient has a histiocytic neoplasm.

B. The histiocyte in the figure has accumulated heavy metal.

C. Histiocytes with this morphology are diagnostic of this patient's disease.

D. This patient likely has a de novo mutation.

E. Enzyme replacement therapy is available for this disease.

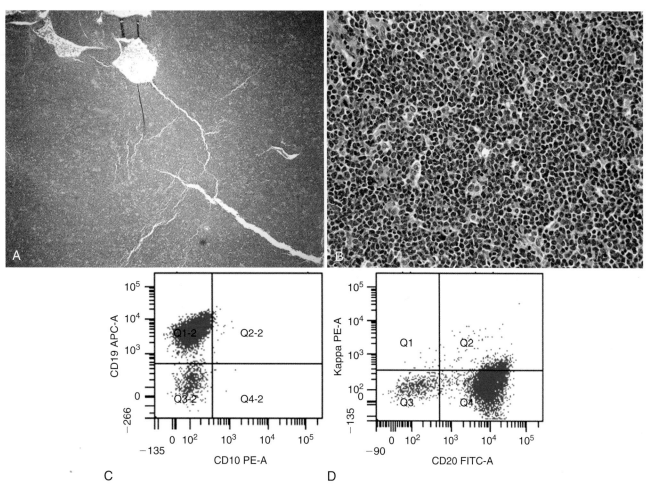

Figure 11-33 **A,** Lymph node morphology (×4). **B,** Lymph node morphology (×40). **C,** Flow cytometry scatterplot CD19 and CD10 staining. **D,** Flow cytometry scatterplot κ light-chain and CD20 staining.

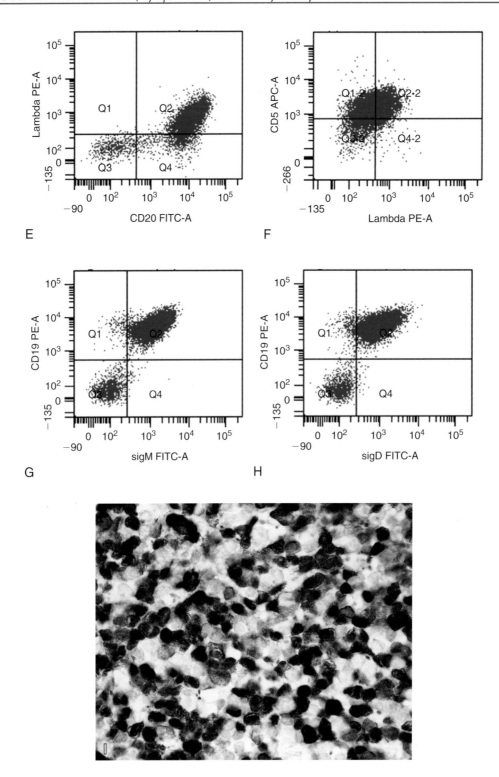

Figure 11-33—cont'd **E,** Flow cytometry scatterplot λ light-chain and CD20 staining, **F,** Flow cytometry scatterplot CD5 and λ light-chain staining. **G,** Flow cytometry scatterplot CD19 and surface immunoglobulin M (IgM) staining. **H,** Flow cytometry scatterplot CD19 and surface IgD staining. **I,** Diagnostic immunostain.

36. A 68-year-old man presents to his primary care physician complaining of a 20-lb unintentional weight loss, fevers, and feeling bloated. Physical examination reveals hepatosplenomegaly and prominent left groin lymphadenopathy. A complete blood cell count shows marked lymphocytosis, and a diagnostic excisional lymph node biopsy is performed on one of the inguinal nodes. The node is sent for permanent section and flow cytometry. Representative H&E sections of the lymph node and flow cytometry scatterplots are shown in

Figure 11-33. Which one of the following is the most common cytogenetic change accounting for the diagnostic immunostain shown in image I?

A. t(3;14)(q27;q32).

B. t(8;14)(q24;q32).

C. t(9;22)(q34;q11.2).

D. t(11;14)(q13;q32).

E. t(14;18)(q32;q21).

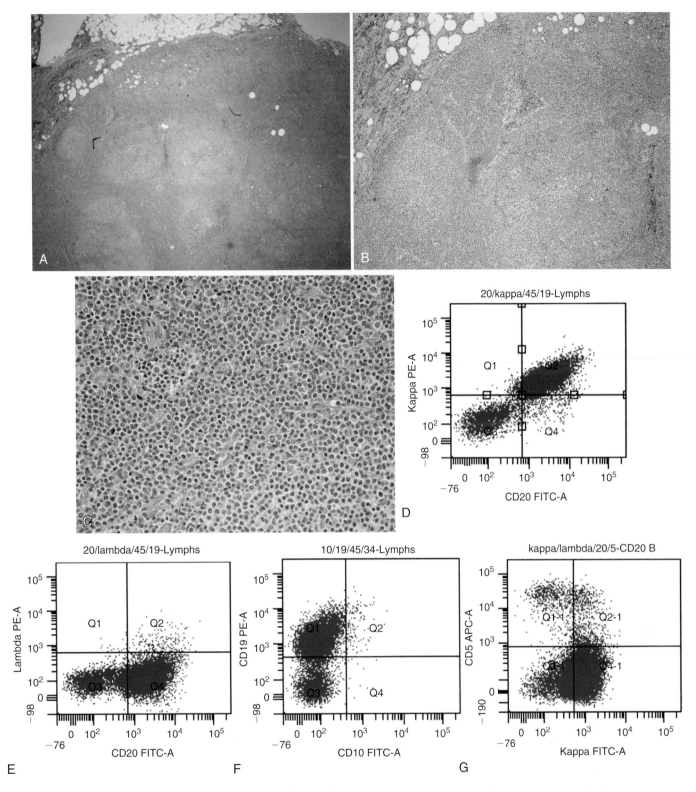

Figure 11-34 **A,** H&E stain, lymph node (×4). **B,** H&E stain, lymph node (×10). **C,** H&E stain, lymph node (×40). **D,** Flow cytometry scatterplot κ light-chain and CD20 staining. **E,** Flow cytometry scatterplot λ light-chain and CD20 staining. **F,** Flow cytometry scatterplot CD19 and CD10 staining. **G,** Flow cytometry scatterplot CD5 and κ light-chain staining.

37. A 63-year-old woman with a strong family history of breast cancer presents to her primary care physician with prominent axillary lymphadenopathy. She is referred for excisional biopsy, and frozen section results are negative for carcinoma. A portion of the lymph node is sent for flow cytometry, and the remaining tissue is sent for permanent section. Representative H&E sections of the lymph node and flow cytometry scatterplots are shown in Figure 11-34. Which one of the following is the most likely diagnosis in this patient?

A. FL.

B. Mantle cell lymphoma.

C. Marginal zone lymphoma.

D. Reactive lymph node.

E. SLL.

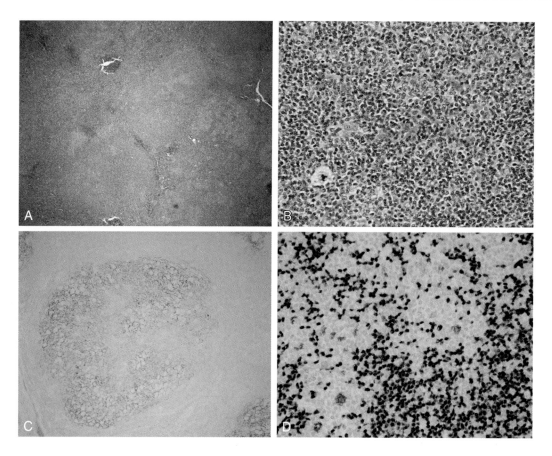

Figure 11-35   Stained sections of right inguinal lymph node. **A,** H&E stain (×4). **B,** H&E stain (×40). **C,** CD21 (×10). **D,** PAX5 (×40).

38. A 34-year-old man presents to his primary care physician with "lumps" in his right groin that have persisted for 4 months. Right inguinal lymphadenopathy without hepatosplenomegaly is noted on physical examination. Test results for sexually transmitted diseases are negative, and the patient undergoes an excisional biopsy. Representative sections of the lymph node are shown in Figure 11-35. The large cells show the following phenotype with immunohistochemical staining: CD15$^-$, CD20$^+$, CD30$^-$, and CD45$^+$. Which one of the following is the most likely diagnosis in this patient?

A. Lymphocyte-depleted Hodgkin lymphoma.
B. Lymphocyte-rich Hodgkin lymphoma (LRCHL).
C. Mixed-cellularity Hodgkin lymphoma.
D. Nodular lymphocyte-predominant Hodgkin lymphoma (NLPHL).
E. Nodular sclerosis Hodgkin lymphoma (NSCHL).

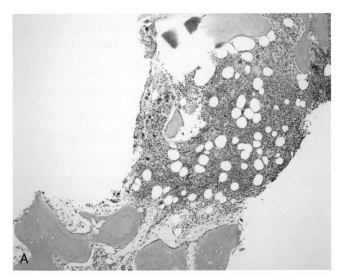

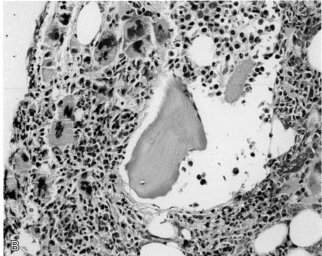

Figure 11-36 Sections of decalcified bone marrow. **A**, H&E stain × 10. **B**, H&E stain × 40.

39. The bone marrow biopsy specimen shown in Figure 11-36 is from a 68-year-old man with mild anemia (hemoglobin, 12 g/dL; reference range, 10.5 to 13.5 g/dL) with normal leukocyte (5.2 × 10⁹/L; reference range, 6.0 to 11.0 × 10⁹/L) and platelet counts (538 × 10⁹/L, reference range, 130 to 400 × 10⁹/L). Which one of the following is part of the major criteria for the diagnosis of primary myelofibrosis (PMF)?
   A. Anemia.
   B. Bone marrow fibrosis.
   C. Increased blast count.
   D. JAK2 V617F mutation.
   E. Splenomegaly.

Table 11-3

Analyte	Patient Result	Reference Range	Units
WBC counts	2.3	6.0-11.0	×10⁹/L
Hemoglobin	11.4	10.5-13.5	g/dL
Platelet count	105	150-440	×10⁹/L
Neutrophil %	9	40-70	%
Lymphocyte %	75	20-50	%
Atypical lymphocyte %	12	0	%
Monocyte %	4	4-8	%
Serum IgA	0.1	0.20-1.00	g/L
Serum IgM	0.1	0.19-1.46	g/L
Serum IgG	3.8	4.53-9.16	g/L

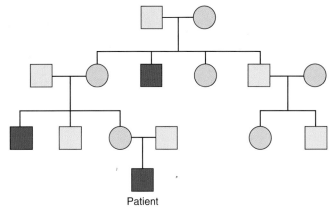

Figure 11-37 Family pedigree with affected individuals in dark blue. Males are denoted as squares and females as circles.

A previously healthy 14-month-old boy presents to his primary care doctor with 5 days of fever and lethargy. His vital signs were notable for a body temperature of 102.2°F and heart rate of 140 beats/min. Results of his laboratory testing are shown in Table 11-3. Several members of the patient's family have had a similar illness, and the family's pedigree is shown in Figure 11-37. Use this scenario to answer the following two questions.

40a. Which one of the following mutations is the most likely cause of the boy's illness?
   A. Bruton tyrosine kinase *(BTK)*.
   B. CD40 ligand *(CD40L)*.
   C. Inducible T-cell costimulator *(ICOS)*.
   D. Myosin 5A *(MYO5A)*.
   E. Signaling lymphocyte activation molecule *(SLAM)*.

40b. Which one of the following viral infections causes severe immune dysregulation in patients with this disease?
   A. CMV.
   B. EBV.
   C. HHV-8.
   D. HIV-1.
   E. HTVL-1.

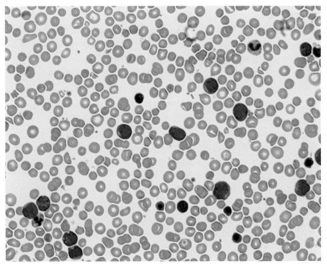

Figure 11-38 Giemsa-Wright–stained peripheral blood smear demonstrating the presence of circulating blasts.

41. A 3-week-old boy with trisomy 21 is taken to his pediatrician for a checkup. He has been a healthy and happy baby since birth. The parents have no concerns at this time. Routine blood work is done that shows marked leukocytosis and thrombocytopenia. The peripheral smear is shown in Figure 11-38. Which one of the following statements is true?

   A. This patient has acute leukemia and should be treated immediately with chemotherapy.

   B. The prognosis of AML in young children with this cytogenetic abnormality is worse than in patients in the same age group with normal cytogenetics.

   C. This condition will likely regress, and the patient will have no greater chance of developing acute leukemia than children with normal cytogenetics in his age group.

   D. Aside from leukocytosis, thrombocytopenia is the most prominent cytopenia is this clinical situation.

   E. The cells in the figure are expected to be of lymphoid lineage.

ANSWERS

1. A. Acute monoblastic leukemia.
Rationale: Expression of CD33 (bright) and CD117 by the abnormal cells is compatible with acute monoblastic leukemia. However, absent or low human leukocyte antigen (HLA)-DR expression is not characteristic for this AML subtype.
B. Acute myelomonocytic leukemia.
Rationale: Expression of CD33 and CD117 is compatible with acute myelomonocytic leukemia. However, absent or low expression of HLA-DR is not common in this type of AML.
C. Acute myeloid leukemia (AML) without maturation.
Rationale: Expression of CD33 and progenitor cell marker CD117 is compatible with AML without maturation. However, lack of CD34 and HLA-DR is not characteristic for this AML subtype.
D. Acute promyelocytic leukemia (APL).
Rationale: Expression of CD33 (bright) and CD117, absence of CD34, and absent or low expression of HLA-DR are characteristic for acute promyelocytic leukemia.
E. Acute T-cell leukemia.
Rationale: Expression of myeloid markers, such as CD33 and CD117, is seen in acute T-cell leukemia. However, lack of CD34 is not characteristic for this type of leukemia. Furthermore, no information about the expression of pan-T-cell markers is provided. Thus, these results cannot be interpreted as characteristic for acute leukemia involving the T-cell lineage.

Major points of discussion
- Phenotypic and cytogenetic features of APL:
  - APL with (t15:17)(q22;q12) represents a distinct AML category, which includes both hypergranular (typical) and hypogranular (microgranular) types.
  - A subset of cases shows variant translocations involving retinoic acid receptor-α (RARA).
  - Abnormal promyelocytes are characterized by low expression or absence of human leukocyte antigen (HLA)-DR and CD34, expression of CD117 and myeloperoxidase (MPO), bright expression of CD33, and variable expression of CD13.
- Differential diagnosis:
  - Hypogranular (atypical) APL and acute myelomonocytic leukemia may display similar morphology.
  - Specific cytogenetic and immunophenotypic features may help distinguish these two types of AML.
  - Typical and microgranular APL cases are frequently associated with disseminated intravascular coagulation (DIC).

- Prognosis and treatment of APL:
  - The prognosis of APL, treated appropriately, is more favorable than for any other AML cytogenetic subtype.
  - APL is sensitive to all-*trans*-retinoic acid (ATRA), which acts as a differentiation agent.

2. A. There is clear evidence of B-ALL. Flow cytometry results are not in agreement with the cytogenetic findings.
Rationale: There is no clear evidence of B-ALL. No maturation block is observed. Both CD34$^+$ and CD34$^-$ subpopulations are detected within CD19$^+$ CD10$^+$ cells.
B. There is no clear evidence of B-ALL. However, the findings are suggestive of myelodysplasia with an excess of blasts.
Rationale: Myeloid blasts, identified as CD34$^+$ CD117$^+$ precursor cells, are frequently detected after treatment, regenerating bone marrows. The myeloid precursors identified in this specimen are not in excess, accounting for less than 1% of all nucleated cells.
C. There is no clear evidence of B-ALL. Normal lymphoid and myeloid precursors in a regenerating marrow are observed.
Rationale: The cell markers displayed by the B-cell precursors detected in this specimen are characteristic for normal B-cell precursors in a regenerating bone marrow.
D. There is no clear evidence of B-ALL. However, the flow cytometry findings are suggestive of a mature B-cell neoplasm.
Rationale: The phenotype of the B cells observed in this sample is that of precursor B lymphocytes.

Major points of discussion
- Prognostic factors in B-ALL:
  - Age: B-ALL has a good prognosis in children and a less favorable prognosis in adults.
  - Slow response to initial therapy is a poor prognosis indicator.
  - The presence of minimal residual disease is a poor prognosis indicator.
  - Specific cytogenetic abnormalities.
- Detection of minimal residual disease (MRD) in B-ALL:
  - Significance: independent prognostic factor.
  - Performed by sensitive techniques, such as polymerase chain reaction (PCR) and flow cytometry.
  - Major difficulty: discrimination between normal B cell precursors (hematogones) and residual leukemic cells.[10,11]

3. A. Chronic lymphocytic leukemia.
Rationale: Expression of CD5, CD23, CD20 dim, and low or undetectable cell surface expression of immunoglobulin (Ig) light chains by CD19$^+$ B cells is characteristic for CLL.

B. Mantle cell lymphoma (MCL).
Rationale: Abnormal B cells from patients with MCL express CD5. However, CD23 expression is typically negative or weak, whereas expression of CD20 and Ig light chain (frequently lambda) is strongly positive.
C. Acute B-ALL.
Rationale: Dim expression of CD20 and lack of Ig light chain expression is characteristic for B-ALL. However, expression of CD5 and CD23 is not typical for B-ALL.
D. Normal B cells.
Rationale: The patient's B lymphocytes display several abnormal features: (1) They express CD5 and CD23. (2) They lack expression of Ig light chains. (3) They express dim levels of CD20. Thus, they cannot be considered normal.
E. Follicular lymphoma (FL).
Rationale: Expression of CD5 and lack of Ig light chain expression are not typical for follicular lymphoma.

Major points of discussion

- CLL is a mature B cell neoplasm of monomorphic small round lymphocytes with clumped chromatin and scant cytoplasm in the peripheral blood, bone marrow, and lymph nodes. Occasional prolymphocytes and para-immunoblasts may be seen.
- CLL predominantly affects older individuals with a median age of 65 years. Men are affected more commonly than woman, with a ratio of 2:1.
- Patients typically are asymptomatic and present with an elevated lymphocyte count (typically $>10 \times 10^9$/L). Infection, autoimmune hemolytic anemia, splenomegaly, hepatomegaly, and lymphadenopathy may also be present. Some patients may produce a monoclonal immunoglobulin or M-protein.
- The neoplastic cells are characteristically CD5 and CD23 positive. They are also positive for CD19, CD79a, CD43, surface IgM and/or IgD (weak), CD20 (weak), CD22 (weak), and CD11c (weak). They are typically negative for CD10, cyclin D1, FMC7, and CD79b.
- The clinical staging system, Rai and Binet, is the best predictor of survival. The median overall survival for CLL is about 7 years.
- Progression and transformation of CLL to high-grade lymphoma (Richter syndrome) has the associated morphologic features of increased cell size and proliferative activity and confluence of proliferation centers in lymph nodes and bone marrow.

4. A. Adjustment of forward and side scatter signals.
Rationale: Forward and side scatter signals are proportional to the size and internal complexity of the cells, respectively. The adjustment of these parameters does not involve adjustments of the fluorescence signals.
B. Adjustment of the instrument noise using nonfluorescent particles.
Rationale: Adjustment of the flow cytometer noise using nonfluorescent particles is an important part of the daily quality control operations. It is different from compensation.
C. Adjustment for signals from fluorochromes other than the specific fluorochrome in a single detector.
Rationale: Compensation is the process by which the fluorescence of a specific fluorochrome is determined by

subtracting the portion of the signals contributed by other fluorochromes in a single detector.
D. Adjustment of the excitation and emission spectra of different fluorochromes.
Rationale: Excitation and emission spectra of various fluorochromes are dictated by their chemical structures and cannot be adjusted during flow cytometric analysis.
E. Excitation of a primary fluorochrome that transfers energy to a secondary fluorochrome.
Rationale: This process is used for the design of tandem fluorochromes and is different from the compensation process.

Major points of discussion

- Flow cytometry is a laser-based technology that can be used to count cells and detect expression of specific cell markers to help diagnose disease.
- A heterogeneous mixture of cells can be sorted or differentiated based on size (forward scatter), granularity or complexity (side scatter), and expression of specific proteins.
- Fluorescently labeled antibodies are used to detect the expression of specific cell markers by the population of cells being studied.
- Essential quality control operations in the flow cytometry laboratory:
  - Adjustment of the instrument noise using nonfluorescent particles.
  - Adjustment of the fluorescent signals and compensation using fluorescent particles.
  - Testing of signal linearity.
  - Testing of fluorescent monoclonal antibodies.
  - Design and testing of antibody panels.
  - Optimization of cell analysis.

5a. A. JAK2 V617F.
Rationale: The JAK2 V617F (Janus kinase 2 V617F) mutation is associated with other myeloproliferative neoplasms (polycythemia vera, primary myelofibrosis, and essential thrombocytosis) but not with CML.
B. Translocation t(9;22)(q34;q11.2).
Rationale: The diagnosis of CML requires the presence of the breakpoint cluster region-Abelson (BCR-ABL) fusion protein resulting from the translocation of chromosomes 9 and 22. This translocation can be identified in 90% to 95% of cases by routine karyotyping, whereas the remaining cases have variant or cryptic translocations resulting in this fusion protein.
C. Trisomy 8.
Rationale: Trisomy 8 can be found in other myeloproliferative/myelodysplastic neoplasms, MDSs, and AML but is not specific for or diagnostic of CML.
D. Translocation t(9;14)(p13;q32).
Rationale: Translocation t(9;14)(p13;q32) is associated with lymphoplasmacytic lymphoma but not with CML.
E. Deletion 5q.
Rationale: Deletion 5q is associated with various myeloid disorders. In patients with MDS, the presence of an isolated deletion 5q confers a good prognosis.

5b. A. AML with recurrent genetic abnormalities.
B. AML, therapy-related (t-AML).
Rationale: The diagnosis of AML requires a blast count of at least 20% in either the peripheral blood or bone marrow.

C. Chronic myelogenous leukemia, accelerated phase (CML, AP).
Rationale: In the natural course of CML progression, patients may enter an accelerated phase (AP) when their course worsens and becomes unresponsive to therapy. When the blast count in the periphery reaches 20%, a diagnosis of blast phase (BP) or AML can be made.
D. Myelodysplastic syndrome, refractory anemia with excess blasts II (MDS/RAEB-II).
Rationale: Patients with refractory anemia with excess blasts II (RAEB-II) do have peripheral blast counts of 6% to 19% or bone marrow blast counts of 10% to 19%; however, CML does not progress to MDS/RAEB-II.
E. Blastic plasmacytoid dendritic cell neoplasm (BPDC).
Rationale: BPDC is a rare hematopoietic neoplasm characterized by skin lesions and frequent adenopathy; however, it is unrelated to CML.

5c. A. Bone marrow blast count.
B. Degree of bone marrow fibrosis.
C. Presence of cytogenetic abnormalities.
D. Response to targeted therapy.
E. Transfusion dependence.
Rationale: In the modern era, response to targeted (protein tyrosine kinase inhibitor) therapy is the most important prognostic factor. This is an important prognostic factor in other myeloid neoplasms, including MDS and AML.

Major points of discussion
- CML is a myeloproliferative neoplasm characterized by proliferation of all myeloid elements with preserved maturation.
- Smears from patients with CML show full-spectrum maturation of all myeloid elements. The presence of basophils is often helpful in making the diagnosis on a peripheral blood or bone marrow aspirate smear.
- The presence of the BCR-ABL fusion protein due to a t(9;22)(q34;q11.2) translocation is required for the diagnosis of CML.
- The JAK2 V617F mutation is seen in many myeloproliferative neoplasms, particularly polycythemia vera; however, it is not specific for or diagnostic for CML.
- In the modern era, CML is treated with imatinib (Gleevec), which is a tyrosine kinase inhibitor with activity against the BCR-ABL fusion protein. This has significantly improved survival.
- Failure of therapy in patients with CML is characteristic of progression to accelerated AP or BP of disease.
- Response to therapy with tyrosine kinase inhibitors is the most important prognostic factor in CML.[8]

6a. **A. 33×10^6/L.**
Rationale: The CD4$^+$ T-cell count is calculated as follows: %CD4$^+$ T cells $\times$ %lymphocytes $\times$ WBC count. This is the correct result.
B. 740×10^6/L.
Rationale: The calculation used the lymphocyte percentage instead of the lymphocyte count.
C. 90×10^6/L.
Rationale: The lymphocyte percentage was not correctly used in the calculation.
D. There is insufficient information to determine the CD4$^+$ T-cell count.

Rationale: The CD4$^+$ T-cell percentage, lymphocyte percentage, and WBC count are sufficient to determine the CD4$^+$ T-cell count.

6b. A. Natural killer (NK) cells.
Rationale: NK cells are CD4$^+$ and CD8$^-$. However, NK cells do not have a complete T-cell receptor complex and are negative for surface CD3. NK cells may be positive for cytoplasmic CD3 because they usually express part of the T-cell receptor complex. The key marker for NK cells is CD56, which functions in cell adhesion.
B. Helper T cells showing HIV-induced downregulation of CD4 expression.
Rationale: HIV infection causes a decline of the number of CD4$^+$ T cells, but it does not cause significant downregulation of the CD4 antigen on helper T-cell surfaces.
C. Gamma/delta T cells.
Rationale: Gamma/delta T cells are CD3$^+$ CD4$^-$ CD8$^-$ and are present in peripheral blood.
D. Immature T cells.
Rationale: Immature T cells, such as pro- and pre-T cells, lack expression of CD4 and CD8. However, these precursors are surface CD3 negative and are rarely found in circulation. They may be detected by flow cytometry in patients with acute T-lymphoblastic leukemia.

Major points of discussion
- The significance of CD4$^+$ T-cell (helper) counts in monitoring progression to AIDS and response to highly active antiretroviral therapy (HAART) in patients with HIV:
  - HIV-1 and HIV-2 retroviruses are cytotropic for CD4$^+$ T lymphocytes (and other cells, such as macrophages, monocytes, and central nervous system microglial cells) and are responsible for direct killing of infected cells and indirect killing of bystander cells.
  - Progression to AIDS is accompanied by a marked decrease in the number of helper T cells and an imbalance of CD4$^+$ helper/CD8$^+$ T-cytotoxic cells.
- Applications of the lymphocyte subset analysis using flow cytometry:
  - Detection of immunodeficiency diseases. Abnormal percentages and absolute values of lymphocyte subsets can be seen in patients with immunodeficiency diseases, such as DiGeorge syndrome, major histocompatibility complex (MHC) class II deficiency, and ζ-chain–associated protein kinase 70 (ZAP-70) deficiency.
  - Monitoring of the effect of lymphocyte-depleting agents, such as thymoglobulin, alemtuzumab (Campath), and rituximab, in transplant recipients and patients with hematologic malignancies.
  - Immune reconstitution studies after stem cell transplantation.

7a. **A. Terminal deoxynucleotidyl transferase (TdT) can be positive in a subset of AMLs.**
Rationale: Lymphoid markers can be expressed in myeloid leukemias.
B. If the lesional cells express CD13, they must be of the myeloid lineage.
Rationale: Myeloid markers can be expressed in lymphoid leukemias.
C. CD19 expression is almost never observed in AML.

Rationale: CD19 is not uncommonly seen in AML and is associated with t(8;21).

D. CD117 is commonly seen in ALL.

Rationale: CD117 is almost 100% specific for the myeloid lineage, as opposed to CD13 and CD33, which can be expressed in a subset of lymphoblastic leukemias.

E. It is not uncommon to see the absence of CD19 on B-cell lymphoblastic leukemias.

Rationale: B-cell markers such as CD19, cytoplasmic CD79a, and cytoplasmic CD22 are almost always expressed in B-lymphoblastic leukemia.

7b. A. The patient's lesional cells will likely be CD10 positive.

Rationale: This patient's FISH study is consistent with mixed lineage leukemia (MLL) gene translocation. These cells are typically CD10 negative and CD15 positive and often have weak B-cell markers such as CD79a or CD22.

B. This particular cytogenetic finding is predictive of a good prognosis.

Rationale: The MLL translocation is associated with a poor prognosis.

C. Administration of methotrexate is a recognized risk factor for the development of this child's disease.

Rationale: Topoisomerase II inhibitors (i.e., etoposide) are associated with MLL rearrangement, not methotrexate. Methotrexate is often used to treat MLL leukemia.

D. This genetic defect causes promyelocytic differentiation in AML.

Rationale: The cells with MLL rearrangement in AML typically have monoblastic differentiation and thus tend to express CD4, CD14, CD64, and CD11b. APL is associated with t(15;17).

E. FISH is required to identify this cytogenetic abnormality.

Rationale: Not all anomalies in the 11q23 involve the MLL gene locus. An MLL break-apart probe is required for confirmation of translocation.

7c. A. The presence of greater than 52 chromosomes in the neoplastic cells is associated with a particularly poor prognosis.

Rationale: A high-hyperdiploid karyotype (>52 chromosomes) is associated with a favorable prognosis.

B. The BCR/ABL translocation that can occur in B-ALL is molecularly identical to the translocation seen in chronic myeloid leukemia (CML).

Rationale: The BCR-ABL translocation in acute B-ALL is that of the minor breakpoint rearrangement versus the major breakpoint rearrangement found in CML (190 kDa versus 210 kDa).

C. A karyotype characterized by fewer than 40 chromosomes confers a favorable prognosis.

Rationale: Hypodiploidy (<50 chromosomes) is associated with a poor prognosis.

D. The presence of the BCR/ABL translocation confers a distinctly poor prognosis.

Rationale: This cytogenetic feature confers a poor prognosis.

E. A translocation between chromosomes 12 and 21 is prognostically unfavorable.

Rationale: The TEL/AML translocation is favorable.

Major points of discussion

- CD117 is highly specific for myeloid leukemias compared with CD13 and CD33. CD79a, CD10, CD2, and CD3 are almost never present with a pure myeloid lineage leukemia.
- A B-cell phenotype is more commonly expected when the presentation is mostly a leukemic process, and a T-cell phenotype is more common in the lymphomatous equivalent.
- Certain translocations are associated with phenotypic characteristics in B-ALL. The MLL translocation typically confers CD10 negativity and CD15 positivity, and ALL with t(1;19) is typically positive for CD19, CD10, and CD9 and negative for CD34 and CD20.
- MLL translocation is associated with a clinicopathologically distinct form of B-ALL characterized by a particular phenotype (CD10$^-$, CD15$^+$), poor prognosis, and association with topoisomerase inhibitors. MLL translocations can occur in AML as well.
- There is a molecular difference between the BCR-ABL translocations identified in B-ALL and CML. CML is associated with a translocation in the major breakpoint cluster region t(9;22)(q34;q11), which produces a fusion protein that is 210 kDa or the p210 isoform. ALL is associated with a translocation in the minor breakpoint cluster region, which produces a fusion protein that is 190 kDa or the p190 isoform.[7]
- Table 11-4 shows the cytogenic findings that confer a favorable or poor prognosis in AML.

Table 11-4

Favorable Prognosis	Poor Prognosis
TEL/AML rearrangement: t(12;21)	BCR/ABL rearrangement: t(9;22)
High hyperdiploidy	MLL rearrangement (11q23) Hypodiploidy

8. A. *CBFB-MYH11* fusion.

Rationale: The CBFB-MYH11 fusion protein is associated with inv(16) and a good prognosis in AML.

B. *CEBPA* (CCAAT/enhancer-binding protein) mutation.

Rationale: The *CEBPA* mutation is associated with a good prognosis in AML.

C. *FLT3* mutation.

Rationale: FLT3 (fms-related tyrosine kinase 3) mutations are associated with a poor prognosis and decreased event-free and overall survival in AML patients.

D. *NPM1* mutation.

Rationale: The *NPM1* mutation is associated with a good prognosis in AML.

E. *RUNX1-RUNX1T1* fusion.

Rationale: The *RUNX1-RUNX1T1* fusion is associated with t(8;21) and a good prognosis in AML.

Major points of discussion

- AML displays a wide spectrum of phenotypes, many of which are associated with specific cytogenetic changes.
- AML can be categorized into four major categories as defined by the World Health Association:
  - AML with recurrent genetic abnormalities.
  - AML with multilineage dysplasia.

- t-AML (usually alkylating agents).
- AML, not otherwise categorized.
- AML with recurrent genetic abnormalities generally occurs in younger patients and has a favorable prognosis.
- AML with multilineage dysplasia generally occurs in older patients and has a less favorable prognosis.
- Prognosis in AML is often related to specific genetic alterations.
- *FLT3* mutations, either internal tandem duplication *(FLT3-ITD)* or *FLT3* tyrosine kinase domain *(FLT3-TKD)* mutations, are both associated with worse prognosis and shorter disease-free and overall survival. The severity increases as patients lose expression of wild-type FLT3.
- AML with *FLT3* mutations have been described as being associated with undifferentiated myeloblasts with cuplike nuclear inclusions.
- *CEBPA* mutations in AML convey a good prognosis.
- *NPM1* mutations in AML convey a good prognosis.
- CBFB-MYH11 fusion protein is generated from inv(16) and is associated with AML with eosinophilia (formerly M4 Eo in the FAB classification). This entity has a good prognosis.
- RUNX1-RUNX1T1 fusion protein is generated from t(8;21) and is associated with AML with myeloblasts with prominent granulations (formerly M2 in the FAB classification). This entity has a good prognosis. Large blasts with Auer rods, abnormal granulation, and basophilic cytoplasm are seen. These cells are CD13, CD33, CD117, CD19, and CD34 positive.

9. A. inv(3).
Rationale: AML with inv(3) is associated with ribophorin-1–ecotropic viral integration site-1 *(RPN1-EVI1)* fusion and prominent dysplasia.
B. t(8;21).
Rationale: AML with t(8;21) is associated with *RUNX1-RUNX1T1* fusion and differentiating myeloblasts (FAB classification AML M2).
C. t(9;11).
Rationale: AML with t(9;21) is associated with myeloid/lymphoid or mixed lineage leukemia; translocated to 3-mixed lineage leukemia (MLLT3-MLL) and a monocytic phenotype.
D. t(15;17).
Rationale: AML with t(15;17) is associated with promyelocytic leukemia–retinoic acid receptor-α (PML-RARA) and is classified as APL.
E. inv(16).
Rationale: AML with inv(16) is associated with CBFB-MYH11, abnormal marrow eosinophils (FAB AML M4 Eo), and a good prognosis.

Major points of discussion

- A diagnosis of AML requires 20% blasts in either the bone marrow or the peripheral blood.
- Myeloblasts are typically positive for MPO, CD13, CD33, and CD117.
- AML with prominent eosinophils (formerly FAB AML M4 Eo) is associated with inv(16) and the CBFB-MYH11 fusion protein. Blasts with both monocytic and neutrophilic differentiation are seen. The blasts are CD13, CD33, CD14, CD4, and CD64 positive. AML with inv(16) has a good prognosis.

- AML with inv(3) is associated with the RPN1-EVI1 fusion protein and marked marrow dysplasia and may be associated with AML arising from an MDS.
- AML with t(9;11) is associated with the MLLT3-MLL fusion protein and is associated with a monocytic phenotype. These cells are positive for CD13, CD33, CD34, CD57, and sometimes CD56. If monocytic differentiation is present, the cells will be positive for CD14, CD4, and CD36. The prognosis is less favorable compared with other types of AML.
- AML with t(15;17) is associated with the PML-RARA fusion protein and is classified as APL. Promyelocytes with azurophilic granules and Auer rods are seen. This disease has a good prognosis if it is responsive to ATRA.

10. A. inv(3).
Rationale: AML with inv(3) is associated with normal to high platelet counts and marrow dysplasia. It also tends to present in adults. It is related to activation of the oncogene ecotropic virus integration site-1 *(EVI1)*.
B. t(8;21).
Rationale: AML with t(8;21) is associated with neutrophilic differentiation and is associated with myeloid sarcomas at presentation. It is related to RUNX1-RUNX1T1–driven transformation.
C. t(15;17).
Rationale: AML with t(15;17) is also known as APL and is associated with fusion of the *PML-RARA* genes.
D. inv(16).
Rationale: AML with inv(16) is associated with monocytic and granulocytic differentiation and abnormal bone marrow eosinophilia. It is related to the CBFB-MYH11 fusion protein.
E. +21.
Rationale: The image shows a megakaryoblast, and AML with megakaryoblastic features is most commonly seen in infants and young children with trisomy 21 (Down syndrome). It is associated with the ribonucleic acid–binding motif protein-15–megakaryoblastic leukemia-1 (RBM15-MKL1) fusion protein. It is also associated with anemia and thrombocytopenia at presentation.

Major points of discussion

- AML is often associated with recurrent genetic abnormalities.
- AML with inv(3) is associated with a normal to high platelet count and marrow dysplasia and is related to activation of the oncogene *EVI1*.
- AML with t(8;21) is associated with neutrophilic differentiation and is associated with myeloid sarcomas at presentation. It is related to RUNX1-RUNX1T1–driven transformation.
- AML with t(15;17) is also known as APL and is associated with fusion of the *PML-RARA* genes.
- AML with inv(16) is associated with monocytic and granulocytic differentiation and abnormal bone marrow eosinophilia. It is related to the CBFB-MYH11 fusion protein.
- AML with megakaryoblastic features is most commonly seen in infants and young children with trisomy 21 (Down syndrome). It is associated with the RBM15-MKL1 fusion protein.
- AML with multilineage dysplasia may be de novo or occur from MDS. This disease is typically seen in older individuals and has a poor prognosis. These patients

must meet the basic criteria for AML with 20% blasts in the bone marrow or peripheral blood; however, greater than 50% dysplasia in cells in two or more lineages must be present.

- Patients with AML with multilineage dysplasia may present with cytogenetic abnormalities typically seen in MDS, such as 3q–, –5, –7, 7q–, 12p–, –18, and +21.
- t-AML may be associated with alkylating agents or topoisomerase inhibitors. AML associated with alkylating agents has a poor prognosis. The prognosis for patients with AML secondary to topoisomerase inhibitors may be similar to other types of de novo AML. More data are needed to predict the long-term survival of these patients.
- AML not otherwise categorized includes cases that do not meet the criteria for one of the other categories.

11. A. Because the lesional cells express anaplastic lymphoma kinase (ALK), the child's prognosis is poor.
Rationale: ALK positivity is prognostically favorable with a 5-year survival rate approaching 80%.
B. Immunohistochemistry for CD30 is expected to be negative.
Rationale: Membranous and Golgi staining for CD30 is characteristic of anaplastic large cell lymphoma.
C. This disease is almost always driven by Epstein-Barr virus (EBV).
Rationale: EBV-associated staining is consistently negative in this disease.
D. IgH (immunoglobulin heavy locus) is almost always rearranged in this disease.
Rationale: The T-cell receptor is rearranged in 90% of cases (see Major Points of Discussion).
E. The cells in this disease typically express epithelial membrane antigen (EMA).
Rationale: This is important diagnostically because anaplastic large cell lymphoma must be distinguished from an epithelial neoplasm (see Major Points of Discussion).

Major points of discussion

- Anaplastic large cell lymphomas (ALCL) are divided by the World Health Organization into ALK-positive and ALK-negative types.
- ALK expression is usually secondary to t(2;5) and is prognostically favorable.
- ALCL represents approximately 50% of childhood high-grade lymphomas. Diffuse lymphadenopathy and B symptoms are common.
- The neoplastic cells are CD30$^+$ and approximately 90% have T-cell receptor (TCR) rearrangement. T-cell antigens are typically expressed, and when absent, the neoplasm is referred to as the null cell–type ALCL. This neoplasm is *not* driven by Epstein-Barr virus.
- If B-cell antigens are expressed on a morphologically similar neoplasm, the diagnosis of DLBCL is given, even in the presence of CD30 expression.
- EMA is often expressed. Because the cells can attain a cohesive pattern of growth, this neoplasm can mimic a carcinoma; a cytokeratin (CK) stain can be helpful in distinguishing the two.

12. A. The patient will likely have an elevated calcium level when serum chemistries are evaluated.

Rationale: Lytic lesions are not uncommon in adult T-cell leukemia/lymphoma (ATLL), and hypercalcemia is a common complication. In addition, the neoplastic cells can produce ectopic osteoclast-activating factor, which causes generalized bone resorption and calcium release.
B. With aggressive treatment and bone marrow transplantation, the patient's prognosis is good.
Rationale: The prognosis of ATLL (particularly the leukemic subtype) is poor (see Major Points of Discussion).
C. The patient's disease is related to a chronic parasitic infection that is endemic in the Caribbean islands.
Rationale: The causative agent of ATLL is human T-lymphotropic virus-1 (HTLV-1), a virus that is a member of the Retroviridae family.
D. The atypical cells will most likely be CD16 and CD56 positive.
Rationale: CD16 and CD56 are markers of NK cells and are not associated with ATLL.
E. The patient is immunocompromised because her bone marrow is likely replaced by neoplastic cells.
Rationale: The cells seen in the figure are the "flower cells" of ATLL. The neoplastic cells are CD4$^+$ cells that typically express CD25 and variably express Forkhead box P3 (FoxP3). These markers are those of regulatory T cells and are thought to contribute to the immunocompromised status in patients with ATLL. Opportunistic infections such as *Pneumocystis* pneumonia (PCP) are more closely related to defects in T-cell immunity, as opposed to decreased myelopoiesis as would occur in bone marrow replacement.

Major points of discussion

- ATLL is an aggressive neoplasm that is typified by the flower cells shown in Figure 11-10. The clinical presentation involves leukocytosis with atypical lymphocytes, lymphadenopathy, splenomegaly, skin involvement (erythema, papules, and nodules), T-cell–mediated immunosuppression, lytic bone lesions, and hypercalcemia.
- The causative agent of ATLL is HTLV-1, a retrovirus that is endemic in southern Japan, Brazil, South Africa, and the Caribbean. It can be contracted by sexual contact, exposure to contaminated blood, or breastfeeding.
- HTLV-1 is the causative agent of ATLL as well as tropical spastic paraparesis.
  - ATLL develops in approximately 1 in 40 infected people, with a latent period up to decades.
  - Tropical spastic paraparesis is characterized by myelopathy/neuropathy, which progresses over a discrete period for several years, leaving the patient with a fixed set of irreversible neurologic impairments (in this case, the patient's mother is presented as a case of HTLV-I-associated myelopathy/tropical spastic paraparesis).
- There are four clinical subtypes of ATLL: acute (leukemic), lymphomatous, chronic, and smoldering. Acute and lymphomatous types have poor prognoses, with overall survival of 2 and 11 months, respectively.
- The classic phenotype for ATLL is CD2$^+$, CD3$^+$, CD5$^+$, CD7$^-$, CD4$^+$, CD25$^+$, ±FoxP3$^+$. Because the neoplastic cells have a T-regulatory phenotype, these patients are immunocompromised.[2]

13. A. This disease is almost always associated with EBV in the Western world.

Rationale: Sporadic Burkitt lymphoma is EBV driven only in approximately 30% of cases.

B. Phenotypic analysis will likely show that these cells are CD10 negative.

Rationale: Burkitt lymphoma is a malignancy of germinal center origin; hence, the neoplastic cells are characteristically CD10 positive.

C. A histologic hallmark of this disease is the absence of tingible body macrophages.

Rationale: These neoplastic cells have an extremely high proliferation and turnover rate, and many tingible body macrophages are usually identified (starry-sky appearance).

D. Despite aggressive treatment with chemotherapy, the long-term prognosis is low.

Rationale: Sixty percent to 90% of patients with this disease are expected to be cured.

E. This disease usually involves the fusion of one of several genes to chromosome 8.

Rationale: The *c-Myc* gene on chromosome 8 is involved in the characteristic translocations of Burkitt lymphoma/leukemia.

Major points of discussion

- Burkitt lymphoma/leukemia is a mature B-cell malignancy of germinal center origin (CD10 positive). The leukemic form is equivalent to the FAB L3 B-ALL characterized by expression of CD20 and surface immunoglobulin (sIg) and absence of TdT.
- There are three clinicopathologic types of Burkitt lymphoma:
  - Endemic BL is a childhood disease mainly affecting those in equatorial Africa and is almost always EBV positive.
  - Sporadic BL is seen throughout the world, affecting children and young adults (median age, 30 years) and is EBV driven in approximately 30% of cases.
  - Immunodeficiency-associated BL, often in association with HIV, is not uncommonly the initial manifestation of the disease.
- Cytologically, the cells are characteristically medium sized with a deep-blue rim of cytoplasm and lipid-filled cytoplasmic vacuoles. Many mitotic figures are usually identified.
- In tissue, there is a characteristic starry-sky appearance due to the monotonous cell population and scattered tingible body macrophages. Ki-67 staining is typically positive in more than 95% of the cells.
- The cytogenetic hallmark of this malignancy is rearrangement of the *c-Myc* locus on chromosome 8 with a number of fusion partners (IgH-chromosome 14, Igλ-chromosome 2, Igκ-chromosome 22).
- Because the neoplastic cells have such a high turnover rate, aggressive chemotherapy can cure most patients with BL. Tumor lysis can occur after chemotherapy induction (hyperkalemia, hyperphosphatemia, hyperuricemia and hyperuricosuria, hypocalcemia, and consequent acute uric acid nephropathy and acute renal failure).

14. A. Cytomegalovirus (CMV).

Rationale: CMV can cause an infectious mononucleosis–like lymphadenitis with paracortical expansion and florid follicular hyperplasia; however, the presence of atrophic

follicles with onion-skin mantle zones is not a feature of this disease.

B. EBV.

Rationale: EBV can cause a variety of patterns within the lymph node, most classically infectious mononucleosis lymphadenitis with paracortical expansion and florid follicular hyperplasia. However, the presence of atrophic follicles with onion-skin mantle zones is not a feature of this disease.

C. Hepatitis C virus (HCV).

Rationale: HCV does not infect lymphoid tissues, although it is associated with cryoglobulinemia.

D. Human herpesvirus 8 (HHV-8).

Rationale: The lymph node in the figure shows plasma cell Castleman disease, which is associated with HHV-8 infection. This typically involves multiple lymph nodes and is frequently associated with HHV-8 and HIV infection.

E. Human T-lymphotropic virus 1 (HTLV-1).

Rationale: HTLV-1 is associated with development of ATLL and not Castleman disease.

Major points of discussion

- Lymph nodes affected by Castleman disease frequently show atretic follicles surrounded by concentric mantle cell lymphocytes, creating an onion-skin appearance.
- The atretic follicles in Castleman disease are often perforated by a single prominent venule, which enters at a 90-degree angle and creates a lollipop appearance.
- Castleman disease can be of the hyaline vascular, plasma cell, or plasmablastic variants.
- Plasma cell and plasmablastic Castleman disease are associated with HHV-8 and HIV infection and show expansion of plasmacytoid cells in the interfollicular areas.
- HHV-8–associated multicentric Castleman disease has a propensity to progress to large B-cell lymphoma.

15a. A. B-cell prolymphocytic leukemia (B-PLL).

Rationale: B-PLL is associated with high levels of prolymphocytes in the peripheral blood and a very high WBC count (generally $>100 \times 10^9$/L).

B. Chronic lymphocytic leukemia (CLL).

Rationale: The immunophenotype of the atypical lymphocytes is compatible with CLL; however, an absolute lymphocyte count of at least 5×10^9/L is required to render this diagnosis, and this patient has an absolute lymphocyte count of 4.55×10^9/L.

C. Hairy cell leukemia (HCL).

Rationale: The immunophenotype of the atypical lymphocytes shown in the figure is not compatible with HCL. HCL cells should be strongly positive for CD20 and tend to also be positive for CD25 and annexin A1.

D. Monoclonal B-cell lymphocytosis (MBL).

Rationale: MBL is diagnosed when a patient has a clonal population of B cells with a CLL-like phenotype but lacks a sufficiently high level of circulating lymphocytes to render this diagnosis.

E. Reactive lymphocytosis (RL).

Rationale: The presence of a monoclonal population of atypical lymphocytes with aberrant expression of CD5 is not compatible with RL.

15b. A. B-PLL.
Rationale: B-PLL is associated with high levels of prolymphocytes in the peripheral blood and a very high WBC count (generally $>100 \times 10^9$/L).
B. CLL.
Rationale: The immunophenotype and morphology are both consistent with CLL, and now the patient has a sustained (>3 months) absolute lymphocyte count greater than 5×10^9/L.
C. HCL.
Rationale: The immunophenotype and morphology of the atypical lymphocytes shown in the figure are not compatible with HCL. HCL cells should be strongly positive for CD20 and tend to also be positive for CD25 and annexin A1.
D. Large granular lymphocytic leukemia (LGL leukemia).
Rationale: LGL leukemia is a T-cell leukemia, and the neoplastic cells in this case are B cells.
E. MBL.
Rationale: The patient initially presented with MBL; however, because her lymphocyte count rose to a level of 44.72×10^9/L for more than 3 months, her disease progressed from MBL to CLL.

15c. A. CD38 expression.
Rationale: This is associated with an adverse prognosis in CLL.
B. Deletion 13q.
Rationale: Isolated deletion 13q is associated with a more favorable clinical course in CLL.
C. Deletion 17p.
Rationale: This is associated with an adverse prognosis in CLL.
D. Germline *IGHV* (immunoglobulin heavy variable cluster) gene.
Rationale: This is associated with an adverse prognosis in CLL. Mutated *IGHV* is associated with a better prognosis.
E. ZAP-70 (ζ-chain [T-cell receptor]-associated kinase 70) expression.
Rationale: This is associated with an adverse prognosis in CLL.

15d. A. ALL.
Rationale: CLL is a mature B-cell neoplasm and does not transform to a lymphoblastic leukemia.
B. Classic Hodgkin lymphoma (CHL).
Rationale: Although some CLL cases progress to CHL, it is more frequent that this disease transforms to a different entity.
C. Diffuse large B-cell lymphoma (DLBCL).
Rationale: CLL most commonly transforms to DLBCL when it progresses. The CLL to DLBCL transformation is referred to as *Richter transformation*.
D. LGL leukemia.
Rationale: LGL leukemia is a T-cell process, and CLL is a B-cell process and does not transform to a T-cell process.
E. Small lymphocytic lymphoma (SLL).
Rationale: SLL and CLL share the same phenotype and are differentiated by formation of tumor masses in SLL and peripheral blood involvement in CLL. Both are relative indolent B-cell neoplasms; however, the transformation described in the above vignette is highly aggressive.

Major points of discussion
■ MBL is characterized by a clonal proliferation of atypical B cells with a similar phenotype to CLL/SLL but with a lower absolute lymphocyte count ($<5 \times 10^9$/L).
■ CLL/SLL is a low-grade B-cell neoplasm.
■ CLL/SLL is characterized by CD5$^+$, CD23$^+$, CD20 dim, mature B cells.
■ The diagnosis of CLL requires an absolute lymphocyte count of at least 5×10^9/L for 3 months.
■ The diagnosis of SLL requires infiltration of organs or lymph nodes with a neoplastic infiltrate.
■ CLL/SLL can progress to CHL or DLBCL but more classically undergoes Richter transformation to DLBCL.
■ Several factors are associated with poor prognosis in CLL/SLL. These include CD38 and ZAP-70 expression, germline (unmutated) *IGHV* gene, del11q22-23, del17p, and del7q.
■ Isolated del13q14.3 and mutated *IGHV* gene are associated with a good prognosis in CLL/SLL.

16a. A. JAK2 V617F.
Rationale: The JAK2 V617F mutation is associated with other myeloproliferative neoplasms (polycythemia vera, primary myelofibrosis, and essential thrombocytosis) but not with CML.
B. Translocation t(9;22)(q34;q11.2).
Rationale: The diagnosis of CML requires the presence of the *BCR-ABL1* fusion protein resulting from the translocation of chromosomes 9 and 22. This translocation can be identified in 90% to 95% of cases by routine karyotype, whereas the remaining cases have variant or cryptic translocations resulting in this fusion protein.
C. Trisomy 8.
Rationale: Trisomy 8 can be found in other myeloproliferative/myelodysplastic neoplasms, MDSs, or AML but are not specific for or diagnostic of CML.
D. Translocation t(9;14)(p13;q32).
Rationale: Translocation t(9;14)(p13;q32) is associated with lymphoplasmacytic lymphoma but not with CML.
E. Deletion 5q.
Rationale: Deletion 5q is associated with various myeloid disorders. In patients with MDS, the presence of an isolated deletion 5q confers a good prognosis.

16b. A. AML with recurrent genetic abnormalities.
Rationale: The diagnosis of AML requires a blast count of at least 20% in either the peripheral blood or bone marrow.
B. t-AML.
Rationale: The diagnosis of AML requires a blast count of at least 20% in either the peripheral blood or bone marrow.
C. CML, AP.
Rationale: In the natural course of CML progression, patients may enter an AP when their course worsens and is unresponsive to therapy. When the blast count in the periphery reaches 20%, a diagnosis of BP or AML diagnosis can be made.
D. MDS/RAEB-II.
Rationale: Patients with RAEB-II do have peripheral blast counts of 6% to 19% or bone marrow blast counts of 10% to 19%; however, CML does not progress to MDS/RAEB-II.
E. BPDC.

Rationale: BPDC is a rare hematopoietic neoplasm arising characterized by skin lesions and frequent adenopathy; however, it is unrelated to CML.

16c. A. Bone marrow blast count.
B. Degree of bone marrow fibrosis.
C. Presence of cytogenetic abnormalities.
D. Response to targeted therapy.
Rationale: In the modern era, response to targeted (protein tyrosine kinase inhibitor) therapy is the most important prognostic factor.
E. Transfusion dependence.
Rationale for A, B, C, and E: In the modern era, these are not the most important prognostic factors. These are important prognostic factors in other myeloid neoplasms, including MDS and AML.

Major points of discussion

- CML is a myeloproliferative neoplasm characterized by proliferation of all myeloid elements with preserved maturation.
- Smears from patients with CML show full-spectrum maturation of all myeloid elements. The presence of basophils is often helpful in making the diagnosis on a peripheral blood or bone marrow aspirate smear.
- The presence of the BCR-ABL fusion protein caused by a t(9;22)(q34;q11.2) translocation is required for the diagnosis of CML.
- The JAK2 V617F mutation is seen in many myeloproliferative neoplasms, particular polycythemia vera; however, it is not specific or diagnostic for CML.
- In the modern era, CML is treated with imatinib (Gleevec), which is a tyrosine kinase inhibitor with activity against the BCR-ABL fusion protein. This has significantly improved survival.
- Failure of therapy in patients with CML is characteristic of progression to AP or BP of disease.
- Response to therapy with tyrosine kinase inhibitors is the most important prognostic factor in CML.[8]

17. A. A biopsy of this patient's rash will show epidermal involvement by the lesional cells.
Rationale: This patient has the characteristic presentation of Sézary syndrome (SS) and epidermotropism may be absent.
B. The lesional cells will have an NK phenotype.
Rationale: The cells of SS are characteristically CD4+ T cells. Loss of CD7 is typically seen.
C. Peripheral blood involvement of cutaneous lesions of this type is a strong indication that the bone marrow will also be involved.
Rationale: Bone marrow involvement is present in only a minority of patients with SS, even in late-stage disease.
D. Prognosis is affected by the degree of lymph node and/or peripheral blood involvement by the lesional cells.
Rationale: Although overall prognosis is poor, outcomes do depend on the extent of disease at diagnosis.
E. With aggressive treatment, this patient has an excellent prognosis.
Rationale: The overall prognosis of patients with SS is poor, with a 5-year survival rate of 10% to 20%.

Major points of discussion

- Mycosis fungoides (MF) and SS are both primary cutaneous T-cell lymphomas that have overlapping features but are distinct clinicopathologic entities.
- MF is an indolent disease with slow progression from patches to plaques to potential tumors of the skin with variable degrees of epidermal infiltration (lichenoid infiltrates to frank epidermotropism with Pautrier microabcesses). Stage is determined by the degree of skin, lymph node, and peripheral blood involvement and is predictive of prognosis.
- SS is a more aggressive disease with generalized erythroderma, lymphadenopathy, and the presence of characteristic Sézary cells. Epidermotropism is often absent. Prognosis is poor, with an overall 5-year survival rate of 10% to 20%.
- Sézary cells are clonally related T cells that have cerebriform nuclei on peripheral blood smear.
- The phenotype of the malignant cells is similar in MF and SS: CD2+, CD5+, CD3+, CD4+, and often loss of CD7.[12]

18. **A. Chloroacetate esterase (CAE) positivity is specific for the cells that are found in gate A.**
Rationale: CAE is specific for granulocytes.
B. The cells in gate B will be negative when stained with naphthyl acetate esterase staining.
Rationale: Naphthyl esterase (a *nonspecific esterase*) stains monocytes much stronger than cells of other hematopoietic lineages.
C. The cells in gate C will stain positive with Sudan Black B.
Rationale: Sudan Black B stains myeloblasts/myelocytes but not lymphoblasts/lymphocytes.
D. Myeloperoxidase staining is nearly 100% specific for the cells that are found in gate A.
Rationale: Myeloperoxidase is positive in both immature and mature neutrophils and mature monocytes.
E. The cells in gate C will be reactive when treated with nitroblue-tetrazolium (NBT).
Rationale: The NBT test is used to detect effective phagocytosis, which lymphocytes do not engage in.

Major points of discussion

- All hematopoietic cells except erythrocytes express CD45, so initially all CD45-positive cells are gated on. Forward scatter is roughly proportional to size, and side scatter is a reflection of the cytologic complexity of the cells (granules, vacuoles, nuclear complexity).
- Mature cells express CD45 brightly, and immature hematopoietic cells express CD45 dimly. The "blast gate" is characterized by low side scatter and dim CD45 expression and is, therefore, an area that is important to evaluate closely depending on the clinical context.
- After the "lymphocyte gate" (gate C on Figure 11-16) and the blast gate (gate D on the figure) are delineated, marker analysis can be analyzed by gating on either population.
- Many cytochemical stains for hematopoietic cells are nonspecific, but some are more specific for a particular lineage. Knowing these stains is most helpful in delineating blasts, that is, when morphologic determination is not possible (Table 11-5).[6]

Table 11-5

Myeloperoxidase (MPO)	+ Myeloblasts/mature granulocytes/ mature monocytes
	− Lymphoblasts/erythroblasts/ monoblasts/megakaryoblasts*
Sudan Black B	+ Myeloblasts/myelocytes, −lymphoblasts/lymphocytes
	+ Lipid vacuoles in Burkitt lymphoma
Periodic acid–Schiff	Acute lymphocytic lymphoma: rosary bead distribution
	AML: diffuse granular hue
Chloroacetate esterase	Specific for granulocytes
Nitroblue tetrazolium	Phagocytic cells with normal oxidative function (negative in chronic granulomatous disease)
Nonspecific esterases (i.e., naphthyl acetate esterase)	++++Monocytes, less so cells of the megakaryocytic, lymphocytic, granulocytic, erythrocytic lineages

*In blasts, absence of MPO does not necessarily imply lymphoid lineage.

19. A. Necrosis is an uncommon feature in lymph node biopsy of a patient with this disease.
Rationale: DLBCL is a rapidly growing neoplasm, and therefore, frank necrosis can be present in samples, obscuring the morphology in some cases.
B. CD10- or bcl6-positivity is prognostically unfavorable.
Rationale: CD10 and bcl6 (B-cell lymphoma 6) are germinal center markers that, when expressed, suggest germinal center origin and confer favorable prognosis compared with those with an activated B-cell (ABC) phenotype (see Major Points of Discussion).
C. The bone marrow is almost always involved when this disease is diagnosed.
Rationale: DLBCL is an aggressive lymphoma. As a rule of thumb, aggressive lymphomas are likely to present as a localized, rapidly growing mass.
D. A gene normally expressed in germinal centers is the most common cytogenetic abnormality.
Rationale: The most common translocation in DLBCL involves the 3q27 locus (approximately 30%), the site where the *bcl6* gene can be found. The *bcl6* gene is expressed in normal germinal centers.
E. The proliferation index (assessed by Ki-67 positivity) is almost universally greater than 90%.
Rationale: Although Ki-67 staining is usually high, it rarely exceeds 90% (approximately 10% of cases). This is important when differentiating a DLBCL from Burkitt lymphoma. Burkitt lymphoma universally has Ki-67 staining of more than 95%.

Major points of discussion
- DLBCL is an aggressive lymphoma. As such, compared with indolent lymphomas, which are characteristically widespread at diagnosis, these lesions are rapidly expanding and localized.
- Cytologically, the cells are large and have vesicular nuclear characteristics and several nucleoli. In tissue sections, the neoplastic cells diffusely efface the tissue architecture, have varying degrees of admixed small lymphocytes, and in many cases are associated with frank necrosis.
- The cells express pan-B-cell markers and variably express CD10, bcl6, bcl2, and MUM-1. Cases of DLBCL are characterized as germinal center (CD10- or bcl6-positive,

MUM-1 negative) or ABC (CD10 negative, MUM-1 positive). Germinal center DLBCL is prognostically favorable compared with the ABC counterpart.
- Translocations involving the bcl6 locus (3q27) and t(14;18) are recurrent and occur in about 30% and 10% of cases, respectively. No overt prognostic significance is associated with either.
- The proliferative index of DLBCL is high. However, Ki-67 positivity is typically found in less than 90% of cells. This feature is useful when discriminating this tumor from Burkitt lymphoma.[9]

20. A. These inclusions are rarely seen in conjunction with toxic granulation.
Rationale: These neutrophils contain Döhle bodies and are associated with pregnancy, infective and inflammatory states, and burns. They can often be associated with toxic granulation and, in severe states, vacuolation.
B. These inclusions demonstrate piled-up fragments of mitochondrial remnants on electron microscopy.
Rationale: Döhle bodies are composed of stacks of endoplasmic reticulum, not mitochondria.
C. These inclusions will be destroyed by treatment with ribonuclease.
Rationale: Döhle bodies are composed of piled-up rough endoplasmic reticulum. Because of the high RNA content, they will be destroyed when they are treated with ribonuclease.
D. These inclusions are a sign of a relatively slow turnover of neutrophils compared with systemic demands.
Rationale: Döhle bodies are associated with high turnover rates in neutrophils and appear more commonly in the progranulocyte stage of development.
E. These inclusions are more likely to be identified evenly distributed through the cell as opposed to on the periphery.
Rationale: True Döhle bodies typically appear around the periphery of the cells (as opposed to, for instance, Döhle-like bodies of the May-Hegglin anomaly that appear to be evenly distributed in the cytoplasm).

Major points of discussion
- Döhle bodies are seen in infective and inflammatory states (particularly burns), normal pregnancy, and congenital abnormalities such as the May-Hegglin anomaly. Other features on the peripheral smear (i.e., neutrophil leukocytosis and toxic granulation in the case of infection) or additional clinical information provided may help to identify the etiology of such inclusions.
- Toxic granulation can be seen in normal pregnancy, which can make the distinction between infection/ inflammation and pregnancy difficult in the setting of Döhle bodies in a peripheral smear evaluation, particularly in the absence of clinical information.
- Cytoplasmic vacuolation of neutrophils is more specific for systemic infection and acute alcohol poisoning.
- Granulocyte colony-stimulating factor therapy can cause left-shifted leukocytosis, toxic granulation, vacuolation, and Döhle bodies.

21. A. If the patient has a sibling, there is a 50% chance that he or she will also have the same disease.
Rationale: The inheritance of Fanconi anemia is autosomal recessive. Therefore, both parents must be carriers, and the chance of an affected sibling would be 25%.

B. Patients with this disease will have positive chromosome breakage studies.

Rationale: The patient described has classic clinical and laboratory features of Fanconi anemia. This is characterized by defects in DNA repair, and results of chromosome breakage studies will be positive.

C. Most patients with this condition never experience aplastic anemia.

Rationale: In most people with Fanconi anemia, aplastic anemia will develop before the age of 10 years.

D. Patients with this disorder are no more likely to develop a hematopoietic malignancy.

Rationale: A defect in DNA repair, Fanconi anemia causes accumulation of genetic defects over time that is focused on the hematopoietic system but affects epithelial cells as well.

E. A single gene is implicated in this disease.

Rationale: Fanconi anemia is an autosomal recessive disorder in 1 of 15 identified genes that are responsible for DNA repair.

Major points of discussion

- Fanconi anemia should be considered when a child presents with bone marrow failure, particularly in the presence of other clinical features suggesting the disease, such as abnormal skin pigmentation, skeletal abnormalities, mental retardation, short stature, and renal anomalies. This condition is more prevalent in Ashkenazi Jews and people of South African descent.
- Fanconi anemia is a disorder in 1 of 15 identified genes that are responsible for DNA repair, which causes the accumulation of genetic alterations in both hematopoietic as well as epithelial cells.
- Lymphocytes and fibroblasts from patients with Fanconi anemia are hypersensitive to drugs that cause DNA cross-linking, such as mitomycin C, and will have positive chromosome breakage studies.
- In most patients with Fanconi anemia aplastic anemia, will develop before the age of 10 years, and those who survive into adulthood have an increased risk of developing MDS, AML, or some type of epithelial cancer.
- Fanconi anemia is typically characterized by an autosomal recessive pattern of inheritance (a small percentage of genetic lesions that lead to Fanconi anemia are X-linked recessive).
- You should be familiar with other constitutional hematopoietic deficiencies:
  - Severe congenital neutropenia (SCN)
    - *ELA2* (neutrophil elastase) mutations (SCN2, cyclic neutropenia)
    - *HAX1* (hematopoietic cell–specific Lyn substrate–associated protein X-1) mutations (Kostmann syndrome)
  - Shwachman-Diamond syndrome
    - *SBDS* (Shwachman-Bodian-Diamond) gene
    - Exocrine pancreatic insufficiency, bone marrow dysfunction, skeletal abnormalities, and short stature
  - Diamond-Blackfan syndrome
    - Erythrocytic lineage only
  - Dyskeratosis congenita
    - Defect in telomerase maintenance (multiple genes)
    - Pleiotropic effects mimicking premature aging in many organ systems

  - One or more hematopoietic lineages affected
- Chédiak-Higashi syndrome
  - Microtubule polymerization defect (*LYST* gene [lysosomal trafficking regulator])
  - Anemia and neutropenia, recurrent infection (defect in phagocytosis), platelet dysfunction (first-wave aggregation only), oculocutaneous albinism, and neurologic defects
  - Abnormally giant granules in granulocytes that range in color from gray to red
- Glycogen storage disease type I
- WHIM syndrome
  - *W*arts, *h*ypogammaglobulinemia, *i*nfections, *m*yelokathexis (retention of neutrophils in bone marrow stroma)
  - Neutrophils only
- Wiskott-Aldrich syndrome
  - Eczema, thrombocytopenia, immune deficiency

22. A. The patient's flow cytometry will likely show a T-cell phenotype for the abnormal cells seen.

Rationale: It is important to be able to recognize buttock cells and to know that they represent cleaved centrocytic cells of follicular lymphoma. The phenotype of these abnormal cells will be that of a light-chain–restricted B-cell population.

B. Lymph node versus bone marrow grade discordance (high versus low) suggests a slightly better prognosis than high-grade concordance.

Rationale: Discrepancies within grade between the lymph node and bone marrow are not uncommonly seen and are prognostically relevant.

C. The patient's disease is associated with a translocation involving a cell cycle regulator gene.

Rationale: Follicular lymphoma, in most cases, is associated with t(14;18). This translocation creates a fusion of the immunoglobulin heavy locus (IgH) regulatory apparatus with the *bcl-2* (B-cell lymphoma 2) gene. This gene is an antiapoptotic gene, not a cell cycle regulator.

D. Bone marrow involvement is commonly found in this patient's disease and is typically characterized by a diffuse pattern of infiltration.

Rationale: The incidence of bone marrow involvement is high in follicular lymphoma. The pattern of bone marrow infiltration of follicular lymphoma, however, is characterized as paratrabecular. This pattern of bone marrow infiltration is also characteristic of T-cell-rich B-cell lymphoma.

E. The expression of CD10 is stronger in higher grade lesions of this type.

Rationale: CD10 expression tends to be bright or even negative as grade increases.

Major points of discussion

- FL accounts for approximately 20% of lymphomas diagnosed, with the highest incidence in the United States and Western Europe. FL is a disease primarily of the elderly; however, pediatric cases are reported and have distinct clinicopathologic characteristics. This is an indolent disease with a median survival of 8 to 10 years.
- Morphologically, FL will typically have back-to-back follicles with attenuated mantle zones, a low mitotic index, and paucity of tingible body macrophages. These

lesions are of germinal center origin, so they are usually CD10 positive and bcl6 positive, but not always.

- The cytogenetic hallmark of FL is the t(14;18), which juxtaposes the regulatory apparatus on the IgH (immunoglobulin heavy locus) locus and the antiapoptotic protein, bcl-2 (B-cell lymphoma 2). bcl-2 positivity within germinal centers helps to distinguish FL from reactive hyperplasia; however, FL can be bcl-2 negative. Note: bcl-2 positivity is *not* specific for FL.
- Grade is based on the number of centroblasts per high-power field: grade I, 0 to 5; grade II, 6 to 15; grade IIIA, greater than 15; grade IIIB, all centroblastic cells. As the grade of FL increases, so does the likelihood that the follicles will be negative for bcl-6, bcl-2, and CD10.
- Forty percent to 70% of patients present with bone marrow involvement, typically characterized by a focal paratrabecular distribution. A full characterization of the lymphoma cells in the bone marrow is essential because grade disconcordance has prognostic implications.
- Pediatric FL has a greater propensity to be localized, bcl-2 negative, t(14;18) negative, and higher grade, but are indolent. These lesions must be distinguished from clonal but reactive follicular hyperplasia, an entity that poses a pitfall in diagnosis. Additionally, such cases must be distinguished from a light-chain–restricted marginal zone hyperplasia, particularly in the tonsil or appendix.
- Transformation to a high-grade lymphoma is expected to occur in approximately 30% of cases of FL, and the resulting malignancy is typically highly resistant to chemotherapy.[13]

23. A. Cytogenetic studies play no role in prognosis in this disease.
Rationale: There are no known cytogenetic abnormalities that are specific for HCL, much less any that provide prognostic significance.
B. The villi that are seen on the lesional cells are characteristically polar.
Rationale: Cytologically, splenic marginal zone lymphoma cells can be distinguished from HCL cells in that former have polarized regions on the periphery that contain villi, whereas the cells in HCL typically have circumferential villi.
C. Marrow fibrosis is not a common feature in this disease.
Rationale: Marrow fibrosis is a common feature in HCL. Bone marrow aspirates often result in a dry tap.
D. Monocytosis is a common feature in this disease.
Rationale: Monocytopenia is the rule in HCL.
E. Diffuse adenopathy is usually present in patients with this disease.
Rationale: Adenopathy is uncommon in HCL. The most common sites of involvement are the spleen, peripheral blood, bone marrow, and the liver.

Major points of discussion
- HCL is a disease that affects predominantly older men. The classic presentation involves splenomegaly and features of pancytopenia.
- The cytologic features of HCL differ from the villous lymphocytes in splenic marginal zone lymphoma in that the villi are typically circumferential and nucleoli are not uniformly present or as distinct. In practical

hematopathology, flow cytometry is required to distinguish between the two.
- The bone marrow characteristically shows reticulin fibrosis (dry tap for aspirate). When aggregates of cells are present, a fried-egg appearance is described owing to large spaces between nuclei. Interstitial marrow involvement can be less obvious, which would be highlighted by immunohistochemical studies.
- The spleen will have red pulp involvement and "blood lakes."
- The phenotype of HCL is CD20$^+$, CD25$^+$, CD103$^+$, and tartrate-resistant acid phosphatase (TRAP)+.
- Monocytopenia is the rule. *Pitfall:* In automated cell counters, hairy cells can be counted as monocytes, potentially obscuring the monocytopenia that one would expect when evaluating HCL as a component of the differential diagnosis.
- Cytogenetic features are not characteristic and do not confer prognostically relevant information.
- Treatment with α-interferon or purine analogues results in an overall 10-year survival rate higher than 90%.

24. A. The main immunologic defect in this disease involves CD4$^+$ lymphocytes.
Rationale: Hemophagocytic lymphohistiocytosis is a disease of NK cells and CD8$^+$ dysregulation.
B. Hypoferritinemia is characteristic in this disease.
Rationale: High levels of ferritin are expected in hemophagocytic lymphohistiocytosis, partially owing to the overwhelming destruction of erythrocytes as well as the overwhelming inflammatory state of the patient.
C. Hemophagocytosis is necessary and sufficient to make this diagnosis.
Rationale: Hemophagocytosis is *neither* necessary *nor* sufficient to make the diagnosis of hemophagocytic lymphohistiocytosis (see Major Points of Discussion).
D. High levels of sCD25 are highly specific for this disease.
Rationale: Very high levels of CD25 (interleukin-2 receptor-α) are rarely seen in the absence of hemophagocytic lymphohistiocytosis.
E. The quantity of CD16$^+$/CD56$^+$ cells is characteristically reduced in this disease.
Rationale: NK cells are normal in quantity but have functional deficits in hemophagocytic lymphohistiocytosis.

Major points of discussion
- Hemophagocytic lymphohistiocytosis (HLH) is a heterogeneous disease that can be thought of as being primary (familial) or secondary (acquired); however, as more is being learned about the genetic etiologies between the two, it is becoming clear that there is significant overlap.
- In classic familial HLH, there is a disruption in the natural contraction of the immune response that seems to involve NK cells (and to a lesser extent T cells) and defects in granule-mediated cytotoxicity. There is usually not a quantitative defect in NK cells.
- The diagnosis of systemic HLH is based on:
  - Family history or molecular evidence of HLH *and/or*
  - The presence of at least five of the following:
    - Fever
    - Splenomegaly
    - Bicytopenia

○ Hypertriglyceridemia or hypofibrinogenemia
○ Hemophagocytosis
○ Hyperferritinemia
○ High sCD25
● Note: Rare hemophagocytic cells can be seen in a variety of clinical scenarios and should not be considered evidence of HLH unless prominent.

■ Forty percent of patients with familial HLH have defects in the perforin gene.
■ Secondary HLH is usually associated with an infectious etiology (EBV infection), autoimmune disease, or a neoplastic process.
■ Other genetic disorders can predispose a patient to developing HLH:
   1. Chédiak-Higashi syndrome
   2. Hermansky-Pudlak syndrome
   3. X-linked lymphoproliferative disease
■ Hematopoietic cell transplantation and treatment of inciting stimuli (infection/autoimmune disease/ neoplasm) are current strategies being used to treat HLH.[5]

25. **A. CD15$^+$ CD20$^-$ CD30$^+$ CD45$^-$ PAX5$^+$ LMP1$^+$.**
Rationale: The infiltrate shown in the image may represent CHL, DLBCL, T-cell histiocyte-rich B-cell lymphoma (TCRBCL), or another large cell lymphoma. Of these entities, CHL has the best prognosis and classically has this immunophenotype.
B. CD15$^-$ CD20$^+$ CD30$^+$ CD45$^+$ PAX5$^+$ LMP1$^+$.
Rationale: This immunoprofile is diagnostic of DLBCL. Although the infiltrate shown in the image may represent DLBCL, typically CHL has a better prognosis than DLBCL.
C. CD15$^-$ CD20$^+$ CD30$^-$ CD45$^+$ PAX5$^+$ LMP1$^-$.
Rationale: This immunoprofile is diagnostic of TCRBCL or nodular lymphocyte predominant Hodgkin lymphoma (NLPHL). The infiltrate shown in the image is not consistent with NLPHL but may represent TCRBCL. However, TCRBCL has a worse prognosis than classic Hodgkin lymphoma.
D. CD15$^-$ CD20$^-$ CD30$^+$ CD45$^+$ PAX5$^+$ LMP1$^+$.
Rationale: This immunoprofile is nonspecific.
E. CD15$^-$ CD20$^+$ CD30$^-$ CD45$^-$ PAX5$^-$ LMP1$^-$.
Rationale: This immunoprofile is nonspecific.

Major points of discussion
■ There is a wide differential diagnosis for large cell lymphomas, and these have widely varying prognoses based on subtype.
■ CHL has the immunophenotype of CD15$^+$ CD20$^-$ CD30$^+$ CD45$^-$ PAX5$^+$ and may be positive for LMP1.
■ CHL has a good prognosis.
■ CHL has a bimodal distribution and presents either in the young age group (15 to 35 years) or later in life.
■ DLBCL is characteristically positive for CD20, CD45, and PAX5 and may show CD30 and LMP1 expression.
■ TCRBCL is notable for large cells in a sea of histiocytes and T cells. The large cells are characteristically CD20$^+$, CD45$^+$, PAX5$^+$, but CD15$^-$, CD30$^-$, and LMP1$^-$.

26. A. An abundance of plasma cells is expected to be identified in this biopsy.
Rationale: The presence of many plasma cells is supportive of other reactive lymphadenopathies, such as lupus-related disease, not Kikuchi disease (see Major Points of Discussion).
B. The absence of neutrophils is characteristic of this disease.

Rationale: Despite regional necrosis, neutrophils are absent. Macrophages with crescent-shaped nuclei are seen.
C. This patient's clinical course will likely be characterized by lifelong intermittent disease.
Rationale: Spontaneous resolution with very little chance of recurrence is the rule in Kikuchi disease.
D. Human herpesvirus-6 (HHV-6) is the causative agent in this disease.
Rationale: No viral etiology has been ascribed to Kikuchi disease. The cause is not known.
E. CD4$^+$ cells are the predominant cells in affected lymph nodes.
Rationale: CD8$^+$ cells predominate and are the cells that are undergoing apoptosis in the areas with abundant karyorrhectic material.

Major points of discussion
■ Although Kikuchi disease is rare, it should be considered in the differential diagnosis of any necrotic lymphadenopathy, particularly in patients of Asian background who present with unilateral enlargement of lymph nodes (Table 11-6).
■ The histologic pattern is characterized by geographic necrosis with fibrinoid material/karyorrhectic debris and the *absence of neutrophils*. There are accumulations of histiocytes surrounding the necrotic regions, sometimes with crescentic nuclei or signet ring–like morphology.
■ The morphologic features in a lymph node taken from a patient with lupus can be similar. In lupus, hematoxylin bodies, neutrophils, abundant plasma cells, and occasionally vasculitis-like changes are seen. A rheumatologic workup to rule out lupus is suggested in these cases.
■ Key morphologic findings are seen in different causes of necrosis in lymph nodes. The exact etiology of Kikuchi disease is not known; however, it appears to be characterized by early apoptosis of CD8$^+$ cells, which predominate in the biopsy. No viral etiology is proposed at this time.
■ The prognosis for Kikuchi disease is excellent. Spontaneous resolution and only very rare recurrences are the rule.

Table 11-6

Infarction	Ischemic necrosis, no nuclear debris, usually entire lymph node
Tuberculosis/ leprosy/cat scratch	Epithelioid cells, giant cells, granulomas, organisms with special stains
Syphilis	Perivascular plasma cell infiltrates, thickened capsule (chronicity)
Bacterial infection	Neutrophils
Allergic reaction	Eosinophils
Herpes simplex	Viral inclusions

27. A. These findings are not associated with hematopoietic disease.
Rationale: Systemic mastocytosis (SM) can be found before, consequent with, or after the diagnosis of a hematopoietic malignancy, particularly that of myeloid lineage.
B. CD117 positivity in the cells seen in the patient's bone marrow biopsy is evidence of neoplasia.

Rationale: CD117 is positive on non-neoplastic (as well as neoplastic) mast cells.

C. Elevated histamine levels are highly specific for the patient's condition.

Rationale: Elevated histamine levels are not specific for systemic mastocytosis. This can occur in any hypereosinophilic condition.

D. Fibrosis is an uncommon feature in the bone marrow when this disease is identified.

Rationale: When the bone marrow is involved in mastocytosis, fibrosis is a common finding.

E. The patient's serum tryptase level will likely be elevated.

Rationale: Elevated tryptase is a consistent feature of systemic mastocytosis.

Major points of discussion

- Mastocytosis is a heterogeneous group of disorders that range in clinical presentation from self-limited disorders involving cutaneous lesions to more aggressive and lethal mast cell leukemia.
- Neoplastic mast cells express CD2 and CD25. Activating *KIT* mutations are evidence that mast cells are neoplastic. In the bone marrow, think of spindle cells or round cells in aggregates with lymphocytes and eosinophils and fibrosis.
- The diagnosis of SM involves:
  - Biopsy-proven multifocal aggregates of mast cells, a significant number demonstrating atypical morphology (e.g., spindle shape).
  - Activating mutations of *KIT*.
  - CD2 or CD25 expression by mast cells.
  - Elevated serum tryptase levels.
- Clinical features of SM include:
  - Constitutional symptoms.
  - Skin manifestations (pruritus, urticaria, dermatographia).
  - Mediator-related symptoms (flushing, hypotension, tachycardia).
  - Musculoskeletal complaints (bone pain, osteosclerosis/osteopenia/osteoporosis, myalgia).
- SM has a wide range of prognoses, depending on the categorization of the disease. Prognoses range from indolent to aggressive and lethal.
- Cutaneous mastocytosis (CM) can present as an urticarial/maculopapular rash, a diffuse peau d'orange–appearing rash, or a mastocytoma. CM may or may not be associated with systemic mastocytosis; therefore, organomegaly or elevated tryptase levels may not be present.
- CM in children has an excellent prognosis, and most patients will experience spontaneous regression at or around puberty. In adults, however, CM is associated with features of SM. In most patients, the disease will persist as an indolent disease.
- SM can be associated with non–mast cell hematopoietic malignancies.

28. A. Both of the patient's biologic parents are at least carriers of the genetic defect causing the patient's disorder.

Rationale: The patient described likely has the May-Hegglin anomaly, which has an autosomal dominant pattern of inheritance. Therefore, only one parent is required to have the mutation.

B. The patient has a defect in microtubule polymerization.

Rationale: The Chédiak-Higashi anomaly is characterized by a defect in microtubule polymerization. The morphologic features are markedly enlarged granules found in neutrophils, eosinophils, and lymphoid cells. In addition, the clinical features of this patient are not compatible with Chédiak-Higashi anomaly (see Major Points of Discussion).

C. When electron microscopy is performed, the inclusions seen within the cytoplasm of the neutrophils are enriched in degenerated organelles.

Rationale: The inclusions are composed of amorphous aggregations of myosin heavy chains type II.

D. The gene implicated in this patient's condition is implicated in numerous similar diseases.

Rationale: The gene affected in the May-Hegglin anomaly is *MYH-9* on chromosome 22q12-13; defects in this gene are responsible for other closely related large-platelet disorders such as Fechtner, Sebastian, and Epstein syndromes (see Major Points of Discussion).

E. This patient has a lysosomal storage disease.

Rationale: The Alder-Reilly anomaly is caused by Tay-Sachs or a mucopolysaccharidosis (see Major Points of Discussion). The clinical information given is not consistent with either.

Major points of discussion

- The May-Hegglin anomaly is characterized clinically by macrothrombocytopenia and varying degrees of sensorineural hearing loss, cataracts, nephritis, and polymorphonuclear Döhle-like bodies.
- It is a defect in the *MYH9* gene on chromosome 22, which encodes the non–muscle heavy chain myosin IIa protein and demonstrates an autosomal dominant pattern of inheritance.
- Other closely related diseases (Fechtner, Sebastian, and Epstein syndromes) are a result of defects in the same gene and cover the spectrum of clinical manifestations that is observed in patients with the May-Hegglin anomaly, albeit to varying degrees.
- Döhle-like inclusions in neutrophils are made of non–muscle myosin heavy chain IIa protein and are devoid of organelles. They differ from bona fide Döhle bodies in that they are characteristically found throughout the cytoplasm of the cell, and they are resistant to treatment with ribonuclease (Döhle bodies are composed of rough endoplasmic reticulum, therefore, having high RNA content).
- Chédiak-Higashi syndrome is a defect in microtubule polymerization (the *LYST* gene). Clinical features are anemia and neutropenia, recurrent infection (defect in phagocytosis), platelet dysfunction (first-wave aggregation only), oculocutaneous albinism, and neurologic defects. Large granules ranging in color from gray to red can be found in granulocytes, lymphocytes, and monocytes because of defective lysosomes.
- The Alder-Reilly anomaly results from Tay-Sachs disease or mucopolysaccharidosis. These inclusions are dark red to purple and involve all leukocytes, although only rarely monocytes. These can be difficult to distinguish from toxic granulation.

29a. A. Age, bone marrow blast percentage, cytopenias, FLT3 status.

Rationale: FLT3 status is not used to determine prognosis in MDS, and karyotype is important.

B. Age, bone marrow blast percentage, cytopenias, karyotype.
Rationale: The International Prognostic Scoring System (IPSS) stratifies patients into prognostic groups based on bone marrow blast percentage, cytopenias, and karyotype. When combined with age, this algorithm is a good predictor of survival.
C. Age, bone marrow blast percentage, FLT3 status, karyotype.
Rationale: FLT3 status is not used to determine prognosis in MDS, and the number of cytopenias is important.
D. Age, cytopenias, FLT3 status, karyotype.
Rationale: FLT3 status is not used to determine prognosis in MDS, and bone marrow blast percentage is important.
E. Bone marrow blast percentage, cytopenias, FLT3 status, karyotype.
Rationale: FLT3 status is not used to determine prognosis in MDS. The other three factors are those used in the IPSS staging classification; however, age can be combined with this score to predict survival.

29b. A. t(3;21).
Rationale: Translocation t(3;21) is associated with intermediate prognosis in MDS.
B. del(5q).
Rationale: Deletion del(5q) is associated with a good prognosis in MDS.
C. del(7q).
Rationale: Deletion del(7q) is associated with a poor prognosis in MDS.
D. +8.
Rationale: Trisomy 8 is associated with intermediate prognosis in MDS.
E. i(17q).
Rationale: Isochromosome i(17q) is associated with intermediate prognosis in MDS.

29c. **A. Refractory anemia with excess blasts II (RAEB-2).**
Rationale: The patient now has elevated myeloblasts accounting for 10% to 19% of bone marrow–nucleated elements.
B. Refractory anemia with ringed sideroblasts (RARS).
Rationale: RARS requires ringed sideroblasts to be seen on an iron stain, which is not provided. In addition, a diagnosis of RARS would not explain the increased number of blasts.
C. Refractory cytopenia with multilineage dysplasia (RCMD).
Rationale: This patient does have multilineage dysplasia; however, the presence of more than 5% bone marrow blasts brings the patient out of the RCMD category and into the RAEB category.
D. Refractory cytopenia with unilineage dysplasia.
Rationale: The patient has multilineage dysplasia (erythroid and myeloid) as well as increased bone marrow blasts.
E. Refractory neutropenia (RN).
Rationale: The patient has multilineage dysplasia and excess blasts. RN does not encompass these findings.

Major points of discussion
- MDS is a clonal hematopoietic stem cell disorder.
- MDS is characterized by cytopenias and dysplasia in one or more bone marrow lineages.

- Prognosis in MDS is determined by the IPSS score, which incorporates bone marrow blast percentage, karyotype, and number of cytopenias. Age can be added to the IPSS score to predict survival, with age over 60 years being a poor prognostic factor.
- Good prognostic karyotypes in MDS are normal karyotype, −Y, del(5q), and del(20q).
- Poor prognostic karyotypes in MDS are chromosome 7 anomalies and complex karyotypes (≥ 3 abnormalities).
- Intermediate prognostic karyotypes in MDS are any other abnormalities not classified as good or poor risk.
- Patients with MDS have a high risk for progression to AML with rising blast counts.

30a. A. Expression of CD56 by the lesional cells in the bone marrow biopsy favors a reactive condition.
Rationale: CD56 expression by plasma cells is indicative of neoplasia.
B. A perivascular distribution of suspicious cells is the histologic hallmark of neoplasia in this setting.
Rationale: Small collections of plasma cells surrounding vessels are not an uncommon finding in bone marrow biopsies.
C. Fibrosis is an uncommon feature in bone marrow biopsies in patients with this disease.
Rationale: Fibrosis is commonly seen in the marrow of a myeloma patient. Consider any fibrotic process when the aspirate is described as a dry tap.
D. Sampling error in bone marrow biopsies can be problematic in this disease because the infiltrate is often patchy.
Rationale: The pattern of bone marrow infiltration can indeed be patchy. An adequate core biopsy is necessary to rule out myeloma.
E. Cytoplasmic staining for immunoglobulin M (IgM) will likely be positive.
Rationale: It is rare that IgM will be produced by neoplastic plasma cells.

30b. A. Primary amyloidosis occurs in a minority of cases and is usually associated with κ light chains.
Rationale: Amyloidosis is not a prominent feature of multiple myeloma; however, the λ light chain is more amyloidogenic than the κ light chain.
B. In the United States, this disease is most commonly seen in African American men.
Rationale: This disease is more common in African Americans and is slightly more common in men that women.
C. The presence of clonal plasma cells comprising less than 10% of nucleated marrow elements rules out this diagnosis.
Rationale: It is essential to understand that the diagnosis of multiple myeloma is based on the integration of pathologic, clinical, and laboratory information (see Major Points of Discussion).
D. Decreased β₂-microglobulin is prognostically unfavorable.
Rationale: Elevated β₂-microglobulin is prognostically unfavorable.
E. The absence of a paraprotein on serum protein electrophoresis indicates the patient likely has a nonsecretory form of the disease.

Rationale: Nonsecretory myeloma is rare (2% of cases). In this situation, the patient likely has light-chain–only myeloma, and urine protein electrophoresis should be evaluated to look for Bence Jones paraproteinuria.

30c. A. Karyotypic analysis is usually sufficient to characterize the cytogenetic abnormalities in this disease.
Rationale: As plasma cells are difficult to culture, conventional cytogenetics identifies abnormalities in only approximately 30% of cases. FISH is able to detect chromosomal abnormalities in more than 90% of cases.
B. Cases with a hyperdiploid genotype characteristically contain gains in even-numbered chromosomes.
Rationale: Hyperdiploid myelomas typically have gains in odd-numbered chromosomes.
C. The t(11;14) induces constitutive tyrosine kinase activity and unregulated cell proliferation.
Rationale: The t(11;14) drives the *cyclin D1* locus, a cell cycle regulator gene.
D. Cytogenetics is of limited use in providing clinically prognostic information.
Rationale: There are many clear associations between cytogenetics and the prognosis of patients with plasma cell myeloma.
E. 17p13 deletion is prognostically unfavorable, with a median survival of about 1 year.
Rationale: This is equivalent to loss of *TP53*, conferring resistance to chemotherapy and overall poor prognosis.

Major points of discussion

- Although histologic examination of biopsies is required to establish the existence of a population of neoplastic cells, multiple myeloma is a diagnosis that incorporates clinical, laboratory, radiologic, and morphologic data.
- Multiple myeloma is diagnosed based on the following criteria:
  - Major criteria:
    - Marrow plasmacytosis (>30%).
    - Plasmacytoma on biopsy.
    - Presence of a monoclonal component (M-component) or secretion of a single clonal immunoglobulin.
    - Serum IgG > 3.5 g/dL, IgA > 2g/dL.
    - Urine > 1 g/24 hr of Bence Jones protein.
  - Minor criteria:
    - Marrow plasmacytosis (10% to 30%).
    - M-component present but less than as defined in the major criteria.
    - Presence of lytic bone lesions.
    - Normal immunoglobulins reduced to <50% of normal.
    - IgG < 600 mg/dL, IgA < 100 mg/dL, IgM < 50 mg/dL.
- A minimum of one major and one minor criterion or three minor criteria are necessary to make the diagnosis of multiple myeloma. The patient must be symptomatic with progressive disease.
- Monoclonal gammopathy of undetermined significance (MGUS) is characterized by the presence of an M-protein with no evidence of a plasma cell neoplasm, amyloidosis, or any other resultant disease. Patients with asymptomatic or smoldering myeloma produce a monoclonal protein (M-protein) at the levels seen in multiple myeloma and meet the diagnostic

criteria for multiple myeloma but are asymptomatic and do not have lytic bone lesions, anemia, renal insufficiency, hypercalcemia, or any end-organ damage. CRAB (hypercalcemia, renal insufficiency, anemia, bone lesions) indicates the presence of end-organ damage (Table 11-7).
- Basic histologic characteristics that favor reactive versus neoplastic plasma cells (Table 11-8).

Table 11-7

MGUS	Asymptomatic (Smoldering) Myeloma	Symptomatic Myeloma
Serum M-protein <30 g/L *and*	Serum M-protein >30 g/L *and/or*	Serum M-protein >30 g/L *and/or*
Clonal plasma cells <10% of BM nucleated elements *and*	Clonal plasma cells >10% of BM nucleated elements *and*	Clonal plasma cells >10% of BM nucleated elements/ plasmacytoma *and*
No end organ damage	*No* end organ damage	*With* end organ damage

BM, Bone marrow.

Table 11-8

Reactive	Neoplastic
Perivascular plasmacytosis	Interstitial plasmacytosis
Scattered plasma cells	Aggregates/sheets of plasma cells
Can be atypical (e.g., multinucleated, immature-appearing)	Frank atypia/blastic morphology *and/or*
	Cytoplasmic/nuclear inclusions such as Russell-Dutcher bodies
Polytypic	Monotypic (light-chain restricted)

- If myeloma is suspected, the degree of fibrosis should be quantified, and vascular structures should be carefully examined for the presence of amyloid. In addition, trabecular osteosclerosis can be a prominent finding.
- Monoclonal proteins produced by myeloma cells:
  - Heavy chains are most commonly immunoglobulin G (IgG) and IgA, followed by IgM.
  - Plasma cell leukemia is more associated with light-chain–only disease, IgD, and, IgE.
  - The λ light chain is more amyloidogenic than the κ light chain.
  - Flame cells are associated with IgA. These cells can be seen in non-neoplastic states.
- Outcome correlates with stage of disease. There are several staging strategies described.
  - The international staging system incorporates the albumin and β_2-microglobulin levels.
  - The staging system modified by Durie and Salmon incorporates the level of M-protein, the presence/ extent of or absence of lytic bony lesions, hemoglobin levels, and the presence or absence of renal dysfunction.
- Cytogenetics plays an important role in prognosis.
  - Common features are translocations involving the IgH locus and gains in *odd*-numbered chromosomes.

- Poor prognosis is associated with t(4;14), t(14;16), or 17p13.1 deletion (*TP53* locus).
- Patients with t(11;14) involving the *cyclin D1* locus or no cytogenetic abnormalities have the highest survival.
- Patients with 13q14 deletions alone show an intermediate prognosis.

31a. A. Age, bone marrow cell counts, bone marrow fibrosis, clinical presentation.
Rationale: Age and degree of bone marrow fibrosis may support a diagnosis of a myeloproliferative neoplasm but are not specific for a particular neoplasm.
B. Bone marrow cell counts, bone marrow fibrosis, duration of illness, mutation testing.
C. Bone marrow fibrosis, duration of illness, mutation testing, peripheral blood counts.
Rationale: Degree of bone marrow fibrosis may support a diagnosis of a myeloproliferative neoplasm, but is not specific for a particular neoplasm.
D. Bone marrow cell counts, duration of illness, mutation testing, peripheral blood counts.
Rationale: This patient has a myeloproliferative neoplasm. The bone marrow and peripheral counts along with duration and specific mutation testing can be used to classify the neoplasm.
E. Age, bone marrow cell counts, mutation testing, peripheral blood counts.
Rationale: Age may support a diagnosis of a myeloproliferative neoplasm but is not specific for a particular neoplasm.

31b. A. *BCR-ABL* translocation.
Rationale: The patient's symptoms, bone marrow aspirate, and peripheral blood counts are most consistent with polycythemia vera (PV). Among myeloproliferative neoplasms, *BCR-ABL* translocations are seen in CML.
B. *FGFR1* translocation.
Rationale: Among myeloproliferative neoplasms, fibroblast growth factor receptor-1 (*FGFR1*) translocations are seen in myeloid neoplasms with eosinophilia.
C. *JAK2* mutation.
Rationale: Greater than 95% of PV patients have Janus kinase 2 (JAK2) mutations (most commonly *JAK2* V617F followed by exon 12 mutation). However, these mutations are also present in other myeloproliferative neoplasms.
D. *MPL* mutation.
Rationale: Among myeloproliferative neoplasms, myeloproliferative leukemia virus (*MPL*) mutations are seen in essential thrombocytosis and primary myelofibrosis.
E. *PDGFRA* translocation.
Rationale: Among myeloproliferative neoplasms, *PDGFRA* translocations are seen in myeloid neoplasms with eosinophilia.

31c. A. Development of pure red cell aplasia.
Rationale: PV does not typically progress to red cell aplasia. In addition, this would fail to account for the resolution of thrombocytosis.
B. Leukemic transformation.
Rationale: Although PV may transform to acute leukemia, this is a rare event and would be associated with increased blast count (>20%) on peripheral blood or bone marrow aspirate smears.

C. Progression to spent phase.
Rationale: Approximately 20% of cases of PV progress to a "spent" or post-polycythemic phase in which blood counts resolve or cytopenias develop, and a leukoerythroblastic peripheral smear and marrow fibrosis may be seen.
D. Therapy-induced remission.
Rationale: PV is a chronic illness, and although phlebotomy or chemotherapy may be useful in reducing counts, it would be unlikely to induce a leukoerythroblastic peripheral smear or cause persistent changes with cessation of treatment as above.
E. Transformation to MDS.
Rationale: PV rarely transforms to MDS, and if it did, it would most likely be associated with marked dysplasia in one or more cell lines with single or multilineage cytopenias and variable degrees of blastemia.

Major points of discussion

- Myeloproliferative neoplasms (MPNs) are a group of clonal bone marrow disorders characterized by proliferation in the bone marrow with or without elevated peripheral blood counts.
- MPNs are frequently associated with atypical megakaryocytes and varying degrees of fibrosis on bone marrow biopsy.
- MPNs are characterized by bone marrow and peripheral cell counts and specific molecular alterations.
- CML is associated with *BCR-ABL* translocations.
- Myeloid neoplasms with eosinophilia are associated with platelet-derived growth factor receptor-α (*PDGFRA*), platelet-derived growth factor receptor-β (*PDGFRB*), and fibroblast growth factor receptor-1 (*FGFR1*) translocations.
- PV is associated with *JAK2* V617F and exon 12 mutations.
- PMF is associated with *JAK2* V617F and myeloproliferative leukemia virus W151L/K *(MPL W151L/K)* mutations.
- Essential thrombocytosis is associated with *JAK2* V617F and *MPL* W151L/K mutations.
- Mastocytosis is associated with *KIT* D816V mutations.
- PV often progresses to a spent or post-polycythemic phase with resolution of polycythemia; however, it may progress to a MDS or acute leukemia in rare cases.

32. A. CMV.
Rationale: CMV typically presents with a mononucleosis-like picture and does not cause specific red cell aplasia.
B. EBV.
Rationale: EBV typically presents with a mononucleosis-like picture and does not cause specific red cell aplasia. It is, however, associated with several lymphoproliferative disorders.
C. HHV-6.
Rationale: Human herpesvirus-6 can cause a viral illness with rash in children, but does not cause anemia or red cell aplasia.
D. HHV-8.
Rationale: HHV-8 is generally asymptomatic in immunocompetent individuals and is not associated with red cell aplasia. It is associated with Castleman disease, Kaposi sarcoma, and primary effusion lymphoma.

E. Parvovirus B19.
Rationale: Parvovirus B19 is a viral illness that typically affects school-aged children and initially presents with a viral prodrome followed by a "slapped-cheek" rash. It is also associated with pure red cell aplasia and characteristically shows giant normoblasts with viral inclusions on bone marrow aspirate smear.

Major points of discussion
- Fifth disease or erythema infectiosum is caused by parvovirus B19 and tends to occur in school-aged children.
- Parvovirus B19 infection is associated with a viral prodrome, anemia, and slapped-cheek malar rash.
- Parvovirus B19 is spread through respiratory secretions, placental transmission between a mother and fetus, and blood transfusions.
- The clinical course is usually mild in immunocompetent individuals, and treatment is usually not necessary.
- Parvovirus B19 can cause pure red cell aplasia.
- Parvovirus B19 infection leads to characteristic giant normoblasts with viral inclusions on a bone marrow aspirate smear.
- HHV-6 can cause a viral illness with rash in children but does not cause anemia or red cell aplasia.
- EBV typically presents with a mononucleosis-like picture and does not cause specific red cell aplasia. It is, however, associated with several lymphoproliferative disorders.
- HHV-8 is generally asymptomatic in immunocompetent individuals and is not associated with red cell aplasia. It is associated with Castleman disease, Kaposi sarcoma, and primary effusion lymphoma.
- CMV typically presents with a mononucleosis-like picture and does not cause specific red cell aplasia.

33. **A. Alder-Reilly anomaly.**
Rationale: Patients with Alder-Reilly anomaly have large numbers of coarse azurophilic granules in the cytoplasm of granulocytes. These resemble toxic granulations.
B. May-Hegglin anomaly.
Rationale: Patients with May-Hegglin anomaly have thrombocytopenia, giant platelets, and inclusion bodies in leukocytes, which resemble Döhle bodies.
C. MDS.
Rationale: Although patients with MDS may have neutrophils with similar morphologic features (bilobed or pince-nez morphology), this usually does not affect all neutrophils and is typically a disease of the elderly. Also, MDSs are not associated with developmental delay and epilepsy.
D. Myelokathexis.
Rationale: Patients with myelokathexis have markedly abnormal granulocytic nuclei rather than simple bilobation. This is also associated clinically with severe bacterial or fungal infections rather than developmental delay.
E. Pelger-Huët anomaly.
Rationale: Patients with Pelger-Huët anomaly have neutrophils with bilobed nuclei often connected by a thin strand of chromatin creating a pince-nez appearance. The chromatin shows a dark mature chromatin pattern, and this condition can be associated with developmental delay, epilepsy, and skeletal abnormalities.

Major points of discussion
- Pelger-Huët anomaly is an autosomal dominant abnormality of neutrophil morphology leading to bilobed nuclei separated by a thin strand of chromatin creating a pince-nez appearance.
- Pelger-Huët anomaly is clinically benign and does not lead to dysfunctional granulocytes.
- Pelger-Huët anomaly may be associated with developmental delay, epilepsy, and skeletal abnormalities in homozygotes.
- Alder-Reilly anomaly is characterized by neutrophils with numerous coarse azurophilic granules in the cytoplasm.
- May-Hegglin anomaly is characterized by thrombocytopenia, giant platelets, and Döhle-like inclusion bodies in the cytoplasm of leukocytes.
- MDS is a clonal hematopoietic stem cell disorder characterized by dysplasia in one or more myeloid lineages. Dysplasia in the granulocytic lineage may be associated with pseudo–Pelger-Huët neutrophils.
- Myelokathexis is characterized by markedly abnormal granulocytes and severe infections at an early age.

34. **A. An acid-fast bacillus causes this disease.**
Rationale: Rosai-Dorfman disease is not known to be related to an infectious etiology.
B. Central nervous system involvement has not been reported for this disease.
Rationale: There are numerous reports of central nervous system involvement by Rosai-Dorfman disease.
C. Plasmacytosis is infrequent in this disease.
Rationale: Plasma cell hyperplasia and associated polyclonal hypergammaglobulinemia are common features in Rosai-Dorfman disease. Occasionally Russell bodies are identified.
D. Expression of CD1a is concerning for malignancy.
Rationale: Expression of CD1a is seen in Langerhans cell histiocytosis, a malignant proliferation of histiocytes. It is necessary to rule out this disease in this setting.
E. Hemophagocytosis is characteristic of the disease.
Rationale: Although some degree of hemophagocytosis is possible, emperipolesis is more characteristic of Rosai-Dorfman disease.

Major points of discussion
- Sinus histiocytosis with massive lymphadenopathy (SHML; Rosai-Dorfman disease) affects patients of all age groups and is distributed worldwide.
- There is a profound accumulation of histiocytes that can cause the rapid enlargement of involved lymphoid tissue; however, this disease can also develop in the form of pseudo-tumors in almost any site, including the central nervous system. The etiology of SHML is not known.
- Patients usually feel well and seek medical attention with the sole concern of a swollen lymph node; however, SHML may also present with a short period of pharyngitis, night sweats, and/or fever.
- There is marked dilation of the sinuses with S100-positive/CD1a-negative histiocytes. The capsule will often be thickened and matted, and emperipolesis is common (more characteristic compared with hemophagocytosis).

- Lymph node plasmacytosis and polyclonal hypergammaglobulinemia are commonly seen.
- CD31, a cell-adhesion molecule usually found on endothelial cells, platelets, and granulocytes, is aberrantly expressed on histiocytes in SHML.
- SHML often undergoes spontaneous regression, and the prognosis is generally good. However, infiltration of vital organs and immune dysregulation are potential causes of death.

35. A. The patient has a histiocytic neoplasm.
Rationale: The clinical features coupled to the morphology of the cells seen in the aspirate should make you think of Gaucher disease, a lysosomal storage disease.
B. The histiocyte in the figure has accumulated heavy metal.
Rationale: The accumulated material in histiocytes in Gaucher disease is composed of glycolipids.
C. Histiocytes with this morphology are diagnostic of this patient's disease.
Rationale: Cells with a similar appearance can be seen in patients with clinical scenarios associated with increased cell turnover (i.e., myeloproliferative disorders), as well as with hyperlipidemia and hyperalimentation (i.e., parenteral nutrition).
D. This patient likely has a de novo mutation.
Rationale: Gaucher disease is an autosomal recessive disorder that is due to mutations in the glucocerebrosidase (GBA) gene located on chromosome 1q21.
E. Enzyme replacement therapy is available for this disease.
Rationale: Enzyme therapy is available and can prevent irreversible complications of this disease, underscoring the important of recognizing and evaluating Gaucher cells in hematopoietic specimens.

Major points of discussion
- Gaucher cells, Neimann-Pick cells, and sea-blue histiocytes are the most common storage disease–type histiocytes. These cells are not diagnostic of a particular lysosomal storage disease.
- Lysosomal storage diseases are diagnosed through genetic or biochemical analysis.
- Gaucher cells:
  - Voluminous, crinkly, eosinophilic cytoplasm.
  - Gaucher disease, myeloproliferative neoplasms, constitutional anemias.
- Niemann-Pick cells:
  - Foamy voluminous histiocytes with uniform vacuoles.
  - Niemann-Pick disease and other storage diseases, fat necrosis, hyperlipidemia, hypercholesterolemia, lipogranulomas.
- Sea-blue histiocytosis
  - Niemann-Pick and other lysosomal storage diseases, CML/myelodysplasia, leukemias/lymphomas, total parenteral nutrition.

36. A. t(3;14)(q27;q32).
Rationale: This translocation would be expected in BCL6-IGH (B-cell lymphoma 6–immunoglobulin heavy locus) rearrangement and may be found in diffuse large B-cell lymphoma.
B. t(8;14)(q24;q32).

Rationale: This translocation would be expected in MYC-IGH rearrangement and may be found in diffuse Burkitt lymphoma.
C. t(9;22)(q34;q11.2).
Rationale: This translocation would be expected in BCR-ABL rearrangement and may be found in CML.
D. t(11;14)(q13;q32).
Rationale: This translocation would be expected in CCND1-IGH (cyclin D1–immunoglobulin heavy locus) GH rearrangement and leads to overexpression of cyclin D1, which is the hallmark of mantle cell lymphoma.
E. t(14;18)(q32;q21).
Rationale: This translocation would be expected in BCL2-IGH (B-cell lymphoma 2–immunoglobulin heavy locus) rearrangement and may be found in follicular lymphoma.

Major points of discussion
- MCL is a B-cell lymphoma, which shows sheets of small to medium-sized B cells and often has scattered epithelioid histiocytes creating a starry-sky appearance.
- MCL typically presents late with lymphadenopathy, hepatosplenomegaly, bone marrow, and peripheral blood involvement.
- MCL shows a marked male predominance (2:1 or greater).
- The neoplastic cells of MCL are characteristically IgM$^+$, IgD$^+$, CD5$^+$, CD19$^+$, CD20$^+$, CD43$^+$, and cyclin D1$^+$, but CD10$^-$ and Bcl6$^-$.
- The pathogenic molecular alteration driving nearly all cases of MCL is the CCND1-IGH (cyclin D1–immunoglobulin heavy locus) rearrangement caused by the t(11;14)(q13;q32) translocation, which leads to constitutive cyclin D1 activity.
- DLBCL may show a BCL6 rearrangement but is characterized by a diffuse proliferation of large B cells and rarely shows strong immunoglobulin M (IgM) and IgD expression.
- BL is often associated with MYC rearrangement but is often found in extranodal sites and consists of monomorphic sheets of intermediate-sized cells, which have a cohesive appearance and squared-off borders.
- CML is a myeloproliferative neoplasm characterized by the BCR-ABL translocation.
- FL is usually associated with a BCL2 rearrangement but should show back-to-back follicles and should be positive for CD10 by flow cytometry.[1]

37. A. FL.
Rationale: The lymph node does not show a back-to-back follicular architecture, and the neoplastic cells are negative for CD10 by flow cytometry. Both of these features are inconsistent with FL.
B. MCL.
Rationale: The neoplastic cells are negative for CD5, which is atypical for MCL.
C. Marginal zone lymphoma.
Rationale: Morphologically, nodal marginal zone lymphoma shows reactive follicles surrounded by and sometimes infiltrated with neoplastic cells. The neoplastic cells are light-chain restricted and show the following immunophenotype: CD19$^+$, CD20$^+$, CD79a$^+$, CD5$^-$, CD10$^-$, CD23$^-$, and cyclin D1$^-$.

D. Reactive lymph node.
Rationale: The cells show light-chain restriction by flow cytometry, which should not occur in a nonneoplastic condition.
E. SLL.
Rationale: SLL shows sheets of neoplastic cells with effacement of lymph node architecture and proliferation centers. The neoplastic cells are positive for CD5. Neither of these is seen in this case.

Major points of discussion
- Most patients with nodal marginal zone lymphoma present with asymptomatic localized or generalized adenopathy.
- Morphologically, nodal marginal zone lymphoma shows reactive follicles surrounded by and sometimes infiltrated with neoplastic cells. These neoplastic cells are composed of marginal zone B cells, plasma cells, and transformed cells.
- The immunophenotype of marginal zone lymphoma cells is generally CD19$^+$, CD20$^+$, CD79a$^+$, CD5$^-$, CD10$^-$, CD23$^-$, and cyclin D1$^-$.
- Sixty percent to 80% of patients with nodal marginal zone lymphoma survive 5 years or longer.
- FL is characterized by a follicular pattern of growth with back-to-back follicles that efface the lymph node architecture. These follicles have attenuated or lost mantle cuffs and lack tingible body macrophages. The neoplastic cells are CD5$^-$, CD10$^+$, CD19$^+$, CD20$^+$, CD43$^-$, Bcl2$^+$, Bcl6$^+$, and cyclin D1$^-$.
- MCL characteristically shows a vaguely nodular or diffuse pattern of growth, and the neoplastic cells are CD5$^+$, CD10$^-$, CD19$^+$, CD20$^+$, CD43$^+$, and cyclin D1$^+$.
- SLL involving lymph nodes is characterized by effaced architecture with sheets of neoplastic small cells with admixed proliferation centers. The neoplastic cells are generally CD5$^+$, CD19$^+$, CD20$^+$, CD23$^+$, CD43$^+$ CD79a$^+$, and CD10$^-$.

38. A. Lymphocyte-depleted Hodgkin lymphoma.
Rationale: This is a subtype of classic Hodgkin lymphoma, and therefore, the large cells should be CD15$^+$, CD30$^+$, and CD45$^-$. This subtype almost always shows a diffuse growth pattern rather than the nodular pattern seen in this lymph node.
B. Lymphocyte-rich Hodgkin lymphoma (LRCHL).
Rationale: Although the pattern of growth for LRCHL is nodular as seen in this case, LRCHL is a subtype of classic Hodgkin lymphoma. Therefore, the large cells should be CD15$^+$, CD30$^+$, and CD45$^-$.
C. Mixed-cellularity Hodgkin lymphoma.
Rationale: Although the pattern of growth for MCCHL is nodular as seen in this case, MCCHL is a subtype of classic Hodgkin lymphoma. Therefore, the large cells should be CD15$^+$, CD30$^+$, and CD45$^-$.
D. Nodular lymphocyte-predominant Hodgkin lymphoma (NLPHL).
Rationale: The nodular growth pattern with numerous lymphocytes and admixed large cells is consistent with NLPHL. The large cells show a phenotype as described in the question. Expanded follicular dendritic cell meshworks are seen with CD21 or CD23 stains.
E. Nodular sclerosis Hodgkin lymphoma (NSCHL).

Rationale: Although the pattern of growth for NSCHL is nodular as seen in this case, NSCHL is a subtype of classical Hodgkin lymphoma. Therefore, the large cells should be CD15$^+$, CD30$^+$, and CD45$^-$.

Major points of discussion
- Hodgkin lymphomas are a group of lymphomas characterized by scattered large cells amid a background of mixed other cell types. The mixture of other cell types and pattern of growth as well as phenotype of the large cells determine the subtype of Hodgkin lymphoma.
- The classic Hodgkin lymphomas (CHLs) are lymphocyte depleted, lymphocyte rich, mixed cellularity, and nodular sclerosis.
- The phenotype of the large cells in CHLs is CD15$^+$, CD30$^+$, CD45$^-$, and CD20 dim/$-$. CHLs often show evidence of EBV infection.
- The non-CHL is nodular lymphocyte-predominant Hodgkin lymphoma. The large cells have the phenotype of large B cells (CD15$^-$, CD30$^-$, CD20$^+$, and CD45$^+$) and are generally negative for EBV infection.
- NSHL is the most easily distinguished morphologically by its nodular growth pattern with collagen bands separating the nodules and collections of mixed inflammatory cells in the nodules.
- NLPHL shows a nodular or nodular and diffuse infiltrate of mostly lymphocytes and histiocytes with admixed large cells that often have convoluted and/or multilobated nuclei, which have been called popcorn cells. Expanded follicular dendritic cell meshworks are seen with CD21 or CD23 stains.

39. A. Anemia.
Rationale: The presence of anemia is a minor criterion in making the diagnosis of PMF. The major criteria to make this diagnosis are (1) megakaryocytic proliferation and atypia, (2) not meeting World Health Organization (WHO) criteria for other myeloid neoplasms, and (3) clonal molecular change or, in the absence of a marker of clonality, exclusion of other causes of fibrosis.
B. Bone marrow fibrosis.
Rationale: The presence of bone marrow fibrosis is a nonspecific finding and by itself is not a major criterion in making the diagnosis of PMF. The major criteria to make this diagnosis are (1) megakaryocytic proliferation and atypia, (2) not meeting WHO criteria for other myeloid neoplasms, and (3) clonal molecular change or in the absence of a marker of clonality, exclusion of other causes of fibrosis.
C. Increased blast count.
Rationale: The presence of increased blast count is not related to the diagnosis of PMF. It is useful in stratifying MDS and making a diagnosis of acute leukemia. The major criteria to make this diagnosis are (1) megakaryocytic proliferation and atypia, (2) not meeting WHO criteria for other myeloid neoplasms, and (3) clonal molecular change or in the absence of a marker of clonality, exclusion of other causes of fibrosis.
D. JAK2 V617F mutation.
Rationale: The presence of a clonal molecular alteration is a major criterion to make the diagnosis of PMF. The other major criteria are (1) megakaryocytic proliferation and atypia, and (2) not meeting WHO criteria for other myeloid neoplasms.
E. Splenomegaly.

Rationale: The presence of splenomegaly is a minor criterion in making the diagnosis of PMF. The major criteria to make this diagnosis are (1) megakaryocytic proliferation and atypia, (2) not meeting WHO criteria for other myeloid neoplasms, and (3) clonal molecular change or, in the absence of a marker of clonality, exclusion of other causes of fibrosis.

Major points of discussion

- PMF is a myeloproliferative neoplasm and tends to affect patients in their sixth to seventh decade of life.
- Many patients with PMF are asymptomatic and present with splenomegaly or anemia, leukocytosis, and/or thrombocytosis.
- Early PMF may present with only thrombocytosis and must be distinguished from essential thrombocytosis (ET), another myeloproliferative neoplasm.
- To diagnosis PMF, all three major and two minor WHO criteria must be met. The major criteria are (1) megakaryocytic proliferation and atypia, (2) not meeting WHO criteria for other myeloid neoplasms, and (3) clonal molecular change or in the absence of a marker of clonality, exclusion of other causes of fibrosis. The minor criteria are (1) leukoerythroblastosis, (2) increase in serum lactate dehydrogenase, (3) anemia, and (4) splenomegaly.
- The most common clonal molecular alterations in PMF are JAK2 V617F and MPL W151L/K.

40a. A. Bruton tyrosine kinase *(BTK).*
Rationale: Mutations in *BTK* are associated with X-linked agammaglobulinemia, but the presence of only modestly decreased immunoglobulins and lack of infectious history argue against this entity.
B. CD40 ligand *(CD40L).*
Rationale: Mutations in *CD40L* are associated with X-linked hyper-IgM syndrome, but the presence of modestly decreased IgM and lack of infectious history argue against this entity.
C. Inducible T-cell costimulator *(ICOS).*
Rationale: Mutations in ICOS are associated with common variable immunodeficiency (CVID); however, *ICOS* is located on chromosome 2 and should therefore affect both sexes equally. In addition, most cases of CVID are due to sporadic mutations, and therefore, there should be no family history. These argue against a diagnosis of CVID in this patient.
D. Myosin 5A *(MYO5A).*
Rationale: Mutations in *MYO5A* are associated with Griscelli syndrome; however, Griscelli syndrome is autosomal recessive and is often associated with disorders of hair and skin. This patient suffers from an X-linked immunodeficiency, which is not associated with any dermal manifestations.
E. Signaling lymphocyte activation molecule *(SLAM).*
Rationale: Mutations in SLAM are associated with Duncan disease, also known as, X-linked lymphoproliferative syndrome. The patient presents with many of the features of this illness, including pancytopenia with lymphocytosis, mild decrease in immunoglobulins, and family history of X-linked illness.

40b. A. CMV.
Rationale: CMV is not associated with Duncan disease.

B. EBV.
Rationale: Duncan disease is thought to be related to an uncontrolled response to EBV infection.
C. HHV-8.
Rationale: HHV-8 is associated with Castleman disease, plasmablastic lymphoma, and Kaposi sarcoma but not with Duncan disease.
D. HIV-1.
Rationale: HIV-1 is not associated with Duncan disease.
E. HTVL-1.
Rationale: HTLV-1 is associated with ATLL but not with Duncan disease.

Major points of discussion

- Duncan disease is an X-linked immunodeficiency related to mutations in SLAM and XIAP proteins.
- Patients with Duncan disease have an exaggerated immune response to EBV infection, which causes fever, pharyngitis, lymphadenopathy, hepatosplenomegaly, and atypical lymphocytosis. Serum immunoglobulins may be reduced or absent, or there may be a polyclonal hypergammaglobulinemia.
- The average age of onset for Duncan's disease is 2.5 years, and there is 100% mortality by age 40 years. Most patients die from bone marrow failure or hepatic necrosis.
- The only curative therapy for Duncan disease is allogeneic stem cell transplantation.
- Duncan syndrome is also called X-linked lymphoproliferative syndrome because it is associated with variable lymphocytic proliferations, which range from circulating lymphocytosis to lymphoid infiltrates of various organs including the bone marrow, spleen, and central nervous system.
- X-linked agammaglobulinemia is a rare X-linked recessive immunodeficiency characterized by recurrent bacterial infections, which initially present as maternal immunoglobulins are lost (age 4 to 12 months). It is due to a mutation in the *BTK* gene.
- Hyper–immunoglobulin M (IgM) syndrome is a heterogeneous group of immunodeficiencies associated with elevated defective IgM in the presence of decreased IgA and IgG levels. Most cases are X-linked; however, approximately 30% are autosomal recessive.
- CVID consists of a heterogeneous group of immunodeficiencies characterized by defective antibody formation. These patients suffer from hypogammaglobulinemia, usually of all classes, although occasionally only affecting IgG. There are several genes associated with this group of disorders, and it can be inherited in an autosomal dominant, autosomal recessive, or X-linked fashion.
- Griscelli syndrome is an autosomal recessive disease characterized by hypopigmentation of hair and skin, fever, neutropenia, thrombocytopenia, and recurrent infections.[4]

41. A. This patient has acute leukemia and should be treated immediately with chemotherapy.
Rationale: Transient abnormal myelopoiesis (TAM) occurs in approximately 10% of newborns with trisomy 21 and most commonly regresses spontaneously within several months. In the absence of progressive organomegaly or evidence of liver dysfunction, chemotherapy is usually not necessary.

B. The prognosis of AML in young children with this cytogenetic abnormality is worse than in patients in the same age group with normal cytogenetics.
Rationale: Children with trisomy 21 in whom AML develops typically have *GATA-1* mutations and have a better prognosis than children with normal cytogenetics.
C. This condition will likely regress, and the patient will have no greater chance of developing acute leukemia than children with normal cytogenetics in his age group.
Rationale: As the name implies, TAM usually regresses spontaneously; however, in 20% to 30% of these patients, acute, nontransient leukemia will develop within 3 years.
D. Aside from leukocytosis, thrombocytopenia is the most prominent cytopenia is this clinical situation.
Rationale: A low platelet count is common in patients with transient abnormal myelopoiesis.
E. The cells in the figure are expected to be of lymphoid lineage.
Rationale: As the name implies, myeloid lineage is expected in TAM in newborns with trisomy 21. The expected phenotype is that of megakaryoblasts.

Major points of discussion
- TAM occurs in approximately 10% of newborns with trisomy 21.
- There is an abnormal proliferation of myeloid precursors, typically megakaryocytes. CD61 immunohistochemistry can be useful is assigning the megakaryocytic lineage to such cells in tissue sections.
- TAM will typically resolve spontaneously within the first few months of life. Organomegaly and liver disease occur in a significant proportion of these patients and can be fatal. Only in such a circumstance would aggressive chemotherapy be warranted. Other patients can be completely asymptomatic.
- There is a substantial risk (20% to 30%) for the development of nontransient acute leukemia within the first 3 years of life in patients with TAM. The preleukemic phase can be associated with dysplasia and features of refractory cytopenia of childhood.
- The prognosis of AML in this setting (typically associated with *GATA-1* mutation) is better than in cytogenetically normal children.
- Other clinical features include thrombocytopenia, vesicular skin disease, marrow fibrosis (teardrop cells), and if in utero, hydrops fetalis.
- Patients with trisomy 21 have an increased incidence of all types of leukemia in all age groups.[3]

References

1. Baron BW, Nucifora G, McCabe N, et al. Identification of the gene associated with the recurring chromosomal translocations t(3;14)(q27;q32) and t(3;22)(q27;q11) in B-cell lymphomas. Proc Natl Acad Sci U S A 1993;90:5262–5266.
2. Beltran B, Quiñones P, Morales D, et al. Different prognostic factors for survival in acute and lymphomatous adult T-cell leukemia/lymphoma. Leuk Res 2011;35:334–339.
3. Brink DS. Transient leukemia (transient myeloproliferative disorder, transient abnormal myelopoiesis) of Down syndrome. Adv Anat Pathol 2006;13:256–262.
4. Chadha SN, Amrol D. *X*-linked lymphoproliferative disease presenting as pancytopenia in a 10-month-old boy. Case Report Med 2010;2010:517178.
5. Filipovich AH. Hemophagocytic lymphohistiocytosis (HLH) and related disorders. Hematology Am Soc Hematol Educ Program 2009;127–131.
6. Freeman R, King B. Technique for the performance of the nitro-blue tetrazolium (NBT) test. J Clin Pathol 1972;25:912–914.
7. Goryczyca W, Sun ZY, Cronin W, et al. Immunophenotypic pattern of myeloid populations by flow cytometry analysis. Methods Cell Biol 2011;103:221–266.
8. Iida S, Rao PH, Nallasivam P, et al. The t(9;14)(p13;q32) chromosomal translocation associated with lymphoplasmacytoid lymphoma involves the PAX-5 gene. Blood 1996;88:4110–4117.
9. Miller TP, et al. Prognostic significance of the Ki-67-associated proliferative antigen in aggressive non-Hodgkin's lymphomas: a prospective Southwest Oncology Group trial. Blood 1994; 83:1460–1466.
10. Seegmiller AC, Kroft SH, Karandikar NJ, et al. Characterization of immunophenotypic aberrancies in 200 cases of B acute lymphoblastic leukemia. Am J Clin Pathol 2009; 132:940–949.
11. Sevilla DW, Colovai AI, Emmons FN, et al. Hematogones: a review and update. Lymphoma 2010;51:10–19.
12. Sibaud V, Beylot-Barry M, Thiébaut R, et al. Bone marrow histopathologic and molecular staging in epidermotropic T-cell lymphomas. Am J Clin Pathol 2003; 119:414–423.
13. Swerdlow SH. Pediatric follicular lymphomas, marginal zone lymphomas, and marginal zone hyperplasia. Am J Clin Pathol 2004;122(Suppl):S98–109.

CHAPTER 12

HEMATOLOGY: Platelets (Qualitative and Quantitative)

Jeffrey S. Jhang, Richard O. Francis

QUESTIONS

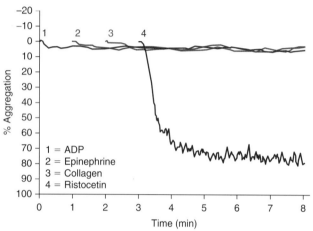

Figure 12-1 Platelet aggregation study. Curves represent aggregation in platelet-rich plasma with the addition of agonists.

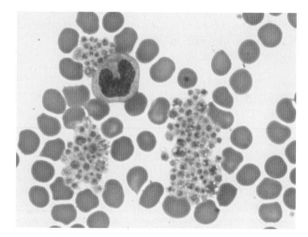

Figure 12-2 Wright-Giemsa–stained peripheral blood smear.

1. A 2-year-old boy is brought by his mother to his pediatrician with a history of easy bruising and nosebleeds. Results of a complete blood cell count (CBC) and iron studies show a hypochromic microcytic anemia. Platelet aggregation studies for this patient are shown in Figure 12-1. Which platelet receptor is defective in this disorder?
   - A. GPIb/V/IX.
   - B. GPIIb/IIIa.
   - C. P2Y$_{12}$.
   - D. GPIa.
   - E. GPVI.

2. A 45-year-old woman with no prior past medical history presents to the employee health office for routine preemployment screening. Her CBC results are shown in Table 12-1. You review the peripheral blood smear (Figure 12-2) and recommend repeating the CBC. Which is the best tube type for collecting the next sample?
   - A. Potassium ethylenediaminetetraacetic acid (EDTA) tube at 4°C.
   - B. Foil-wrapped potassium EDTA tube.
   - C. 3.2% sodium citrate tube.
   - D. Glass tube with no additives.
   - E. Serum separator tube.

Table 12-1

Test	Patient	Reference Range	Units
WBC	5.8	3.5-9.1	10^3/μL
RBC	4.73	4.3-5.6	10^{12}/L
Hemoglobin	14.5	13.3-16.2	g/dL
Hematocrit	43.0	38.8-46.4	%
MCV	90.9	79.0-93.3	fL
MCH	30.6	26.7-31.9	pg
MCHC	33.7	32.3-35.9	g/dL
RDW	12.0	<14	%
PLT	3	165-415	10^3/μL

Table 12-2

Test	Preoperative	Postoperative Day 5	Reference Range	Units
Hematology				
WBC	7.0	6.8	3.5-9.1	$10^3/\mu L$
RBC	4.3	4.4	4.3-5.6	$10^{12}/L$
Hemoglobin	14.0	14.1	13.3-16.2	g/dL
Hematocrit	42.3	42.0	38.8-46.4	%
PLT	380	165	165-415	$10^3/\mu L$
MPV	8.2	8.6	6.4-11	fL
Coagulation				
APTT	33.5	36.4	26.3-39.4	s
PT	13.2	13.1	12.7-15.4	s
Fibrinogen	305	310	233-496	mg/dL
D-dimer	225	300	220-740	ng/mL FEU
Chemistry				
BUN	40	45	7-20	mg/dL
Creatinine	2.1	2.2	0.6-1.2	mg/dL
AST	20	22	12-38	U/L
ALT	27	24	7-41	U/L
LDH	145	151	115-221	U/L

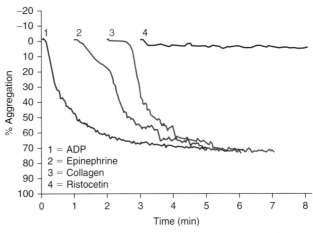

Figure 12-3 Light transmission platelet aggregation with agonists.

3a. A 58-year-old woman with a history of renal insufficiency underwent surgery for a total knee replacement. She is placed on low-molecular-weight heparin following her surgery for deep vein thrombosis (DVT) prophylaxis. On postoperative day 5 the patient complains of left calf pain and swelling is noted on physical exam. Duplex ultrasonography demonstrates venous thrombosis in the left leg. Laboratory results from the day before surgery and postoperative day 5 are shown in Table 12-2. A peripheral blood smear from postoperative day 5 is notable only for mild thrombocytopenia. What is the most likely diagnosis?

A. Immune thrombocytopenic purpura (ITP).
B. Heparin-induced thrombocytopenia (HIT).
C. Thrombotic thrombocytopenic purpura (TTP).
D. Disseminated intravascular coagulation (DIC).
E. Hemodilution.

3b. Based on the clinical suspicion and available laboratory results, which therapeutic intervention should be made for this patient?

A. Perform daily plasmapheresis.
B. Discontinue heparin.
C. Transfuse platelets.
D. Discontinue heparin and begin treating with a direct thrombin inhibitor.
E. Discontinue heparin and begin warfarin.

4. A 6-year-old Iranian boy is brought to his pediatrician by his mother for frequent nosebleeds and gingival bleeding, which are occasionally severe. There is no history of bleeding disorders in the mother, father, or two older brothers. The CBC shows hemoglobin 11.8 g/dL and platelets $160 \times 10^9/L$. Light transmission aggregometry on platelet-rich plasma is shown in Figure 12-3. If this patient is transfused platelets, which isoantibody is most likely going to render the platelet transfusion ineffective?

A. Anti-GPIa/IIa.
B. Anti-GPIbα.
C. Anti-GPIIb/IIIa.
D. Anti-GPVI.
E. Anti–HPA-1a.

5. Which of the following is found in platelet α-granules?

A. Adenosine diphosphate (ADP).
B. Magnesium.
C. Platelet-derived growth factor (PDGF).
D. Pyrophosphate.
E. Serotonin.

6. Which inherited platelet disorder is associated with a defect in a platelet membrane surface glycoprotein?

A. Quebec platelet syndrome.
B. Chediak-Higashi syndrome.
C. Wiskott-Aldrich syndrome.
D. Bernard-Soulier (BS) syndrome.
E. Gray platelet syndrome.

7. Which platelet function test is considered to be an in vivo assay?

A. Turbidometric aggregometry.
B. Bleeding time (BT).
C. PFA-100.
D. Vasodilator-stimulated phosphoprotein (VASP) phosphorylation assay.
E. Cone and plate analyzer.

8. Which of the following prolongs the BT?

A. Cool skin.
B. Hematocrit of 25%.
C. Platelet count of $200 \times 10^9/L$.
D. Pregnancy.
E. Repeating the BT within 4 hours.

9. Which inherited platelet disorder has the classical finding of "large peroxidase-positive granules" in neutrophils?
   A. May-Hegglin anomaly.
   B. Chediak-Higashi syndrome.
   C. BS syndrome.
   D. Hermansky-Pudlak syndrome.
   E. Gray platelet syndrome.

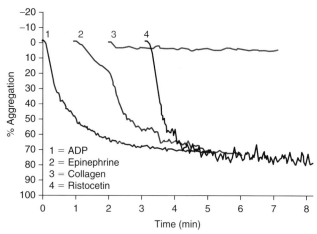

Figure 12-4 Light transmission aggregometry on platelet-rich plasma with adenosine diphosphate (ADP) (5 μmol/L), epinephrine (5 μmol/L), collagen (2 μg/mL), and ristocetin (1.0 mg/mL).

10. A 32-year-old Japanese woman with systemic lupus erythematosus presents with frequent epistaxis. The platelet count is normal. The BT is 15 minutes (reference range, <7 minutes). Light transmission aggregometry is performed as shown in Figure 12-4. The platelet function studies suggest the presence of an autoantibody against which platelet receptor?
    A. GPIbα.
    B. GPIIb/IIIa.
    C. GPVI.
    D. P2Y$_1$.
    E. P2Y$_{12}$.

11. Which assay assesses platelet function under shear conditions?
    A. Cone and plate analyzer.
    B. VerifyNow.
    C. Impedance aggregometry.
    D. Assays that measure thromboxane (Tx) A$_2$ metabolites.
    E. Turbidometric aggregometry.

12. Which inherited platelet disorder is associated with a mutation in the gene for the thrombopoietin (TPO) receptor (*MPL*)?
    A. May-Hegglin anomaly.
    B. Amegakaryocytic thrombocytopenia with radioulnar synostosis.
    C. Scott syndrome.
    D. Wiskott-Aldrich syndrome.
    E. Congenital amegakaryocytic thrombocytopenia.

13. Which of the following is found in platelet-dense bodies?
    A. β-Thromboglobulin.
    B. Calcium.
    C. Fibrinogen.
    D. P-selectin.
    E. von Willebrand factor (vWF).

14. Which type of sample is used for flow cytometry–based detection of activated GPIIb/IIIa?
    A. Fresh nonanticoagulated blood.
    B. Whole blood.
    C. Serum.
    D. Platelet-rich plasma (PRP).
    E. Platelet-poor plasma (PPP).

15. The decreased presence of which marker, detected by flow cytometry, is used for a definitive diagnosis of Glanzmann thrombasthenia?
    A. CD63.
    B. CD41.
    C. CD154.
    D. CD49b.
    E. CD29.

16. Which component of platelet α-granules can be reliably detected in platelets from patients with gray platelet syndrome?
    A. Factor V.
    B. β-Thromboglobulin.
    C. Fibrinogen.
    D. P-selectin.
    E. Platelet factor 4.

17. Which inherited platelet disorder is associated with oculocutaneous albinism?
    A. Sebastian syndrome.
    B. Wiskott-Aldrich syndrome.
    C. Hermansky-Pudlak syndrome.
    D. Paris-Trousseau/Jacobsen syndrome.
    E. BS syndrome.

Table 12-3

Test	Patient	Reference Range	Units
WBC	8.0	3.5-9.1	10^3/μL
RBC	4.8	4.3-5.6	10^{12}/L
Hemoglobin	14.2	13.3-16.2	g/dL
Hematocrit	42.8	38.8-46.4	%
MCV	90.0	79.0-93.3	fL
PLT	20	165-415	10^3/μL
MPV	20	9-13	fL

18. A 19-year-old woman with a history of bruising and thrombocytopenia her entire life presents to a hematologist. Her review of systems is otherwise negative. Results of her CBC are shown in Table 12-3, and examination of the peripheral smear demonstrates platelets the size of the surrounding red blood cells (RBCs) and Döhle-like bodies in neutrophils. This presentation is most consistent with which platelet disorder?
    A. BS syndrome.
    B. May-Hegglin anomaly.
    C. Epstein syndrome.
    D. Fechtner syndrome.
    E. Glanzmann thrombasthenia.

19. Which inherited platelet disorder is due to a defect in α-granules?
   A. Paris-Trousseau/Jacobsen syndrome.
   B. Chediak-Higashi syndrome.
   C. BS syndrome.
   D. Hermansky-Pudlak syndrome.
   E. Glanzmann thrombasthenia.

20. Which platelet function test uses conditions of high shear blood flow to test platelet function?
   A. Plateletworks.
   B. Thromboelastography.
   C. VerifyNow.
   D. Light transmission aggregometry.
   E. PFA-100.

Table 12-4

Test	Patient	Reference Range	Units
WBC	6.1	3.04-9.06	$\times 10^9$/L
RBC	3.57	4.3-5.6	$\times 10^{12}$/L
Hemoglobin	11.2	13.3-16.2	g/dL
Hematocrit	32.9	38.8-46.4	%
MCV	92.0	79.0-93.3	fL
MCH	31.4	26.7-31.9	pg
MCHC	34.2	32.3-35.9	g/dL
RDW	14.8	<4	%
PLT	161	165-415	$\times 10^9$/L

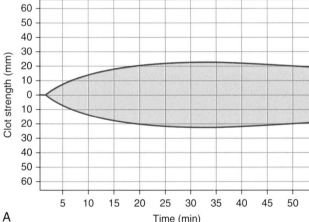

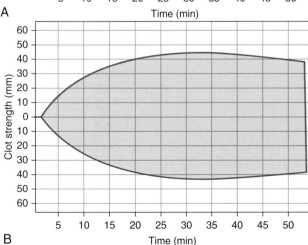

Figure 12-5 A, Patient thromboelastogram. **B.** Normal donor thromboelastogram.

21. A surgeon has completed coronary artery bypass surgery on a 72-year-old man and would like to close the chest, but there is still significant oozing. The CBC is shown in Table 12-4. The surgeon orders thromboelastography and the results with the addition of heparinase are shown in Figure 12-5. Given the results of the thromboelastogram, what is the most appropriate blood product/derivative to administer?
   A. Recombinant factor VIIa.
   B. Fresh frozen plasma.
   C. Platelets.
   D. Prothrombin complex concentrates.
   E. RBCs.

22. Which platelet function test uses detection of platelet aggregation as its end point?
   A. Plateletworks.
   B. PFA-100.
   C. Cone and plate analyzer.
   D. VASP.
   E. Thromboelastography.

Table 12-5

Test	Patient	Reference Range	Units
Hematology			
WBC	7.8	3.5-9.1	10^3/μL
RBC	4.5	4.3-5.6	10^{12}/L
Hemoglobin	13.5	13.3-16.2	g/dL
Hematocrit	40.7	38.8-46.4	%
PLT	5	165-415	10^3/μL
MPV	9.2	6.4-11	fL
Coagulation			
APTT	33.5	26.3-39.4	sec
PT	13.2	12.7-15.4	sec
Fibrinogen	505	233-496	mg/dL
D-dimer	222	220-740	ng/mL FEU
Chemistry			
BUN	10	7-20	mg/dL
Creatinine	0.6	0.6-1.2	mg/dL
AST	16	12-38	U/L
ALT	25	7-41	U/L
LDH	150	115-221	U/L

23. A 27-year-old pregnant woman in her tenth week of pregnancy presents to her physician with a complaint of new-onset bruising, epistaxis, and gum bleeding. Pertinent laboratory values are listed in Table 12-5. Examination of the smear demonstrated thrombocytopenia and normal RBC morphology. What is the most likely cause of this patient's presentation?
   A. TTP.
   B. ITP.
   C. DIC.
   D. Syndrome of hemolysis, elevated liver enzymes, and low platelet count (HELLP).
   E. Hemolytic uremic syndrome (HUS).

24. Which platelet receptor is blocked by the antiplatelet agent abciximab?
   A. α2β1.
   B. GPIbα.

    C. GPIIb/IIIa.
    D. P2X$_1$.
    E. P2Y$_{12}$.

25. Which receptor is blocked by the pharmaceutical agent clopidogrel?
    A. GPIbα.
    B. GPIIb/IIIa.
    C. GPVI.
    D. P2X$_1$.
    E. P2Y$_{12}$.

26. Which platelet disorder is associated with inadequate exposure of negatively charged phospholipids on the platelet surface?
    A. Sebastian syndrome.
    B. Fechter syndrome.
    C. Scott syndrome.
    D. Epstein syndrome.
    E. Chediak-Higashi syndrome.

27. What is the basis for using thromboelastography as a platelet function test?
    A. Activation-dependent changes in platelet surface marker expression.
    B. In vivo cessation of blood flow by a newly formed platelet plug.
    C. Shear-induced platelet adhesion.
    D. Rate and quality/strength of clot formation.
    E. Platelet-to-platelet aggregation.

28. Which platelet function test is immunoassay based?
    A. VerifyNow.
    B. PFA-100.
    C. Measurement of serum TxB$_2$.
    D. Measurement of activated GPIIb/IIIa.
    E. Plateletworks.

29. Which inherited platelet disorder is associated with a defect in platelet signal transduction?
    A. Arthrogryposis–renal dysfunction–cholestasis.
    B. Paris-Trousseau/Jacobsen syndrome.
    C. Chediak-Higashi syndrome.
    D. Tx synthase deficiency.
    E. Hermansky-Pudlak syndrome.

30. Which assay is considered the historical gold standard for platelet function testing?
    A. PFA-100.
    B. Impedance aggregometry.
    C. Turbidometric aggregometry.
    D. Measurement of TxA2 metabolites.
    E. Measurement of activated GPIIb/IIIa by flow cytometry.

31. Which test is considered the gold standard for assessing the P2Y$_{12}$ antagonist effect?
    A. Turbidometric aggregometry.
    B. Thromboelastography.
    C. Plateletworks.
    D. VASP phosphorylation.
    E. VerifyNow.

32. Which inherited platelet disorder is associated with immunodeficiency?
    A. BS syndrome.
    B. Scott syndrome.
    C. Glanzmann thrombasthenia.
    D. Quebec platelet syndrome.
    E. Wiskott-Aldrich syndrome.

33. Which analyte measured in urine best reflects systemic TxA$_2$ formation?
    A. 2,3-dinor TxB$_2$.
    B. 11-dehydro-TxB$_2$.
    C. Prostaglandin G$_2$.
    D. TxA$_2$.
    E. TxB$_2$.

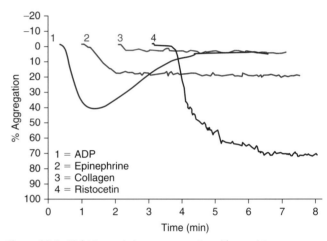

Figure 12-6   Light transmission aggregometry with agonists.

34. Which disorder most likely explains the findings on the platelet aggregation studies shown in Figure 12-6?
    A. Aspirin therapy.
    B. BS syndrome.
    C. Clopidogrel therapy.
    D. Glanzmann thrombasthenia.
    E. von Willebrand disease, type III.

35. Which medication can lead to thrombocytosis?
    A. Amphotericin.
    B. Furosemide.
    C. Piperacillin/tazobactam.
    D. Romiplostim.
    E. Tacrolimus.

36. Which mutation is most commonly present in essential thrombocythemia?
    A. *BCR-ABL* fusion gene.
    B. *EPO* mutation.
    C. *JAK2* V617F.
    D. *MPL* mutation.
    E. *PML-RAR* fusion gene.

37. Which of the following could best explain a falsely elevated platelet count enumerated on an impedance-based automated hematology analyzer?
    A. Macrothrombocytes.
    B. Microclots.
    C. Platelet satellitism.
    D. Pseudothrombocytopenia (PTCP).
    E. Schistocytes.

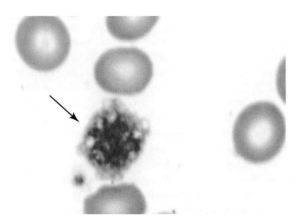

Figure 12-7 Wright-Giemsa–stained peripheral blood smear.

38. Which condition is most associated with the object indicated by the arrow in Figure 12-7?
    A. Babesiosis.
    B. Gray platelet syndrome.
    C. Myelodysplastic syndrome.
    D. Pseudothrombocytopenia.
    E. Wiskott-Aldrich syndrome.

39. Which source of platelets would be the best choice for transfusion in a neonate born with an intracranial hemorrhage to a woman with a history of a pregnancy loss due to neonatal alloimmune thrombocytopenia (NAIT)?
    A. Maternal platelets.
    B. Whole blood–derived random donor platelets.
    C. Paternal platelets.
    D. Single-donor platelets.
    E. Washed single-donor platelets.

40. Which of the following is an acceptable sample for performing platelet function studies by light transmission aggregometry on PRP?
    A. 3.2% sodium citrate, light-blue top tube.
    B. K_2-ethylenediaminetetraacetic acid (K_2EDTA), purple top tube.
    C. Lithium heparin, green top tube.
    D. No additive, red top tube.
    E. Serum separator, gold top tube.

41. An 8-year-old boy is admitted with bacterial meningitis. His CBC shows a platelet count of 721×10^9/L. Which of the following represents the best advice for the primary physician regarding this patient's platelet count?
    A. Perform apheresis immediately.

B. Perform apheresis followed by hydroxyurea treatment.
C. Treat with hydroxyurea.
D. No additional therapy is necessary.
E. Perform a splenectomy.

Table 12-6

Test	Patient	Reference Range	Units
WBC	7.7	3.04-9.06	$\times 10^9$/L
Hemoglobin	11.3	13.3-16.2	g/dL
Hematocrit	34.3	38.8-46.4	%
PLT	5	165-415	$\times 10^9$/L
Reticulocytes	14.6	<1	%
PT	12.4	12.7-15.4	sec
aPTT	30.3	26.3-39.4	sec
Fibrinogen	467	233-496	mg/dL
Haptoglobin	<7	30-200	mg/dL
LDH	392	115-221	U/L
Total bilirubin	2.9	0.3-1.3	mg/dL
Direct bilirubin	0.9	0.0-0.4	mg/dL

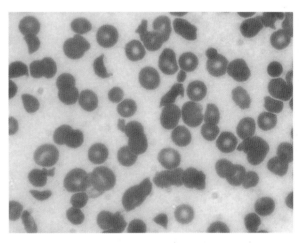

Figure 12-8 Wright-Giemsa–stained peripheral blood smear (high power).

42. A 42-year-old man with end-stage renal disease underwent a deceased donor renal transplant 6 months ago. He was discharged home on tacrolimus and prednisone. Several weeks later he is seen in his physician's office complaining of fatigue, shortness of breath, and bruising on the soles of his feet. His CBC and relevant laboratory studies are shown in Table 12-6. His peripheral blood smear is shown in Figure 12-8. Which of the following best accounts for the laboratory and peripheral blood smear findings?
    A. DIC.
    B. Drug-induced thrombocytopenia.
    C. ITP.
    D. TTP.
    E. Warm autoimmune hemolytic anemia (WAIHA).

43. A 63-year-old man with diabetes, hypertension, and hyperlipidemia is discharged from the hospital on clopidogrel after being treated for an acute myocardial infarction. Several

weeks later he is admitted with a second acute myocardial infarction. Which gene is associated with insufficient clopidogrel-induced platelet dysfunction?
* A. *CYP2C19*2*.
* B. *CYP1A1*.
* C. *CYP2C9*1*.
* D. *UGT1A6* T181A A > G.
* E. *VKORC*1 GG.

44. Your laboratory would like to perform "spot" checks of platelet counts reported from a new hematology analyzer using the Fonio method. The laboratory uses a 10 × ocular lens and a 100 × objective lens. The analyzer reports a platelet count of 200×10^9/L. Which of the following represents the approximate number of platelets per high-power field (HPF) that the technologist should count to correlate well with the analyzer?
    * A. 1.
    * B. 2.
    * C. 5.
    * D. 10.
    * E. 20.

45. A 79-year-old man with diabetes, hypertension, and hyperlipidemia underwent a single-vessel coronary artery bypass graft 4 years ago. His hospitalization was complicated by HIT without thrombotic complications, and his platelet count returned to normal after discontinuation of heparin. He is now admitted for a reoperation to perform a three-vessel coronary artery bypass. The anti-heparin/platelet factor-4 immunoglobulin G (IgG) enzyme-linked immunosorbent assay (ELISA) result is negative and the serotonin release assay result is negative. What is the most appropriate intraoperative management for anticoagulation of the bypass circuit?
    * A. Anticoagulation with unfractionated heparin.
    * B. Anticoagulation with bivalirudin.
    * C. Anticoagulation with argatroban.
    * D. Cancel surgery indefinitely.
    * E. Delay surgery until anti-heparin/platelet factor-4 IgG, IgA, and IgM ELISA is performed.

Table 12-7

Test	Patient	Reference Range	Units
WBC	5.8	3.5-9.1	10^3/μL
Hemoglobin	14.5	13.3-16.2	g/dL
PLT	22	165-415	10^3/μL
Blood type	O positive		
RBC antibody screen	Negative	Negative	

46. A 22-year-old woman has a history of ITP as a child. She was successfully treated, but she does not know what the treatment consisted of and she has not had any recurrences. She now presents to her obstetrician at 12 weeks of pregnancy for her first prenatal visit. She denies bleeding, including epistaxis, vaginal bleeding, petechiae, and bruising. Laboratory studies are shown in Table 12-7. What is the best choice for treating this patient?

* A. Azathioprine.
* B. Cyclophosphamide.
* C. Corticosteroids.
* D. Rituximab.
* E. Splenectomy.

Table 12-8

Test	Patient	Reference Range	Units
WBC	5.8	3.5-9.1	10^3/μL
Hemoglobin	14.5	13.3-16.2	g/dL
PLT	22	165-415	10^3/μL
Blood type	O positive		
RBC antibody screen	Negative	Negative	

47. A 51-year-old man undergoes presurgical testing prior to a right hernia repair. A CBC, blood type, and red cell antibody screen are performed as shown in Table 12-8. There is no active bleeding. A review of the peripheral blood smear does not show pseudothrombocytopenia. A diagnosis of ITP is made. What would be a first-line treatment for this patient?
    * A. Apheresis.
    * B. Dapsone.
    * C. Corticosteroids.
    * D. Rituximab.
    * E. Splenectomy.

48. A platelet count is performed on a normal adult volunteer using an impedance-based analyzer. Which of the following best describes the platelet histogram (*y*-axis: frequency; *x*-axis size 2 to 20 fL) reported by the analyzer?
    * A. Fonio distribution.
    * B. Fourier transform of *t*-distribution.
    * C. Gaussian (normal) distribution.
    * D. Negatively (left) skewed distribution.
    * E. Positively (right) skewed distribution.

49. Which platelet antigen is most commonly implicated in NAIT?
    * A. HPA-1a.
    * B. HPA-1b.
    * C. HPA-2a.
    * D. HPA-3b.
    * E. HPA-4a.

50. Which platelet receptor is activated by thrombin?
    * A. GPIIb/IIIa.
    * B. GPVI.
    * C. P2X1.
    * D. P2Y$_{12}$.
    * E. Protease-activated receptor 1 (PAR-1).

Table 12-9

Cartridge	Result	Reference Range
Collagen/epinephrine (Col/Epi)	89 sec	<120 sec
Collagen/adenosine diphosphate (Col/ADP)	113 sec	<180 sec

51. Which of the following is most consistent with the results shown in Table 12-9 for the PFA-100 platelet function analyzer?
    A. Aspirin, 325 mg per day.
    B. BS syndrome.
    C. Glanzmann thrombasthenia.
    D. Gray platelet syndrome.
    E. Scott syndrome.

52. How many platelets are produced in 1 day by the average adult under normal physiologic circumstances?
    A. 10^6
    B. 10^9
    C. 10^{11}
    D. 10^{12}
    E. 10^{15}

53. Which clinical manifestation is most characteristic of patients with abnormal platelet function?
    A. Minimal bleeding from superficial cuts.
    B. Deep muscle hematomas.
    C. Delayed bleeding.
    D. Hemarthrosis.
    E. Petechiae.

54. Which of the following is the ligand for CD110 (the *c-mpl* gene product)?
    A. Erythropoietin (EPO).
    B. Granulocyte colony-stimulating factor (G-CSF).
    C. PDGF.
    D. Signal transducer and activator of transcription 1 (STAT1).
    E. TPO.

55. A 17-year-old woman with chronic ITP receives a TPO mimetic after her platelet count fails to increase after trials of corticosteroids, Rh immune globulin, and splenectomy. Which of the following is a long-term complication of TPO mimetics that her physician should advise her about?
    A. Bone marrow reticulin deposition.
    B. Berry aneurysms with intracranial hemorrhage.
    C. Pancreatitis.
    D. Portal vein aneurysms.
    E. Retinal detachment.

56. Which of the following is stored in the Weibel-Palade bodies of endothelial cells?
    A. ADAMTS13.
    B. Factor VIII.
    C. Fibronectin.
    D. Tx A2.
    E. vWF.

ANSWERS

1. A. GPIb/V/IX.
   Rationale: Quantitative or qualitative defects in the platelet glycoprotein complex GPIb/V/IX lead to BS syndrome. GPIbα binds to vWF under conditions of high shear stress.
   B. GPIIb/IIIa.
   Rationale: Patients with Glanzmann thrombasthenia have a defect in platelet aggregation. GPIIb/IIIa is the central receptor mediating platelet adhesion through binding to fibrinogen and/or vWF.
   C. P2Y$_{12}$.
   Rationale: This receptor for ADP is targeted by antiplatelet agents such as clopidogrel and ticagrelor.
   D. GPIa.
   E. GPVI.
   Rationale: These receptors bind to collagen.

   Major points of discussion
   ■ Glanzmann thrombasthenia is a rare autosomal recessive disorder characterized by mucocutaneous bleeding (gingival bleeding, epistaxis, petechiae, ecchymosis, menorrhagia, and excess bleeding with dental extraction).
   ■ Glanzmann thrombasthenia is caused by decreased production or dysfunctional platelet glycoprotein GPIIb/IIIa complex. Absence of binding to fibrinogen and/or vWF leads to this bleeding disorder.

   ■ Platelet aggregation studies show an absence of aggregation with ADP, epinephrine, and collagen. Aggregation with ristocetin is normal because GPIIb/IIIa is not involved with the GPIbα–vWF interaction.
   ■ Platelet receptors mediate adhesion, activation, and aggregation of platelets. Defects in these receptors can be due to mutations or exogenous substances that inhibit their function.
   ■ Defects in platelet function can be characterized based on the type of the dysfunction (e.g., adhesion, activation, aggregation). For example, BS syndrome is characterized by a defect in platelet adhesion.
   ■ Inherited defects in collagen-binding receptors (e.g., glycoprotein VI) are rare.[15]

2. A. Potassium ethylenediaminetetraacetic acid (EDTA) tube at 4°C.
   Rationale: PTCP is almost exclusively caused by the presence of EDTA and is thought to be enhanced at colder temperatures.
   B. Foil-wrapped potassium EDTA tube.
   Rationale: Foil wrapping would not prevent pseudothrombocytopenia. Foil is used for light-sensitive analytes, such as bilirubin, erythrocyte protoporphyrin, and carotene.
   C. 3.2% sodium citrate tube.

Rationale: In the absence of EDTA, platelet clumps are less likely to form and an accurate automated platelet count can be determined.

D. Glass tube with no additives.

Rationale: A glass tube with no additives would clot the sample and remove coagulation factors and platelets. However, if analyzed when the sample is very fresh, an accurate platelet count may be obtained with this approach.

E. Serum separator tube.

Rationale: A serum separator tube would clot the sample and remove coagulation factors and platelets.

Major points of discussion

- PTCP is characterized by a falsely low platelet count on automated cell counters due to platelet clumping.
- PTCP is most commonly caused by autoantibodies that recognize platelet antigens (neoantigens) when combined with EDTA. It probably involves the GPIIb/IIIa complex.
- A way to avoid PTCP is to use a different anticoagulant (e.g., sodium citrate, sodium oxalate, and heparin) when collecting samples. In a subset of patients, it still may not be possible to obtain an accurate platelet count using an alternative anticoagulant.
- The peripheral blood smear should always be manually reviewed when the automated platelet count is low. This precaution prevents the inappropriate treatment of a falsely low platelet count with steroids, cyclophosphamide, splenectomy, and/or rituximab, which can have devastating consequences.
- Platelet satellitosis is also associated with EDTA autoantibodies that cause falsely low platelet counts on automated cell counters. Platelets adhere to the surface of neutrophils or monocytes and are not counted by the instrument.[3]

3a. A. Immune thrombocytopenic purpura (ITP).

Rationale: The platelet count would be expected to be lower in ITP. Clinical presentation is better for HIT.

B. Heparin-induced thrombocytopenia (HIT).

Rationale: The treatment of the patient with heparin, the timing and degree of thrombocytopenia, and the presence of thrombosis are all consistent with HIT.

C. Thrombotic thrombocytopenic purpura (TTP).

Rationale: No schistocytes are found upon examination of the peripheral smear, the LDH is not elevated, and the hemoglobin is stable, making TTP unlikely.

D. DIC.

Rationale: The coagulation parameters, including the activated partial thromboplastin time (aPTT), prothrombin time (PT), fibrinogen, and D-dimer are all within the reference range, and these would be abnormal in DIC.

E. Hemodilution.

Rationale: The decreased platelet count is most likely not due to hemodilution, because the other parameters in the CBC are stable.

3b. A. Perform daily plasmapheresis.

Rationale: Plasmapheresis is not a first-line therapy for HIT.

B. Discontinue heparin.

Rationale: Heparin should be discontinued; however, HIT is suspected, which puts the patient at an increased risk of thrombosis. Therefore an alternate anticoagulant should be given.

C. Transfuse platelets.

Rationale: There is no evidence of bleeding, and the platelet count is at the lower limit of normal with no evidence of decreased platelet function. Therefore, platelet transfusion would not be appropriate.

D. Discontinue heparin and begin treating with a direct thrombin inhibitor.

Rationale: Heparin should be discontinued and the patient should start an alternate anticoagulant.

E. Discontinue heparin and begin warfarin.

Rationale: Heparin should be discontinued; however, warfarin is inappropriate in the acute setting.

Major points of discussion

- HIT is an immune-mediated response to treatment with heparins.
- HIT antibodies are directed toward platelet factor 4 (PF4) in complex with heparin.
- HIT antibodies can develop in response to both unfractionated heparin (UFH) and low-molecular-weight heparin (LMWH). Due to its smaller molecular size, LMWH has a decreased capacity to bind to PF4 tetramers and generate HIT antibodies. Patients treated with LMWH are 2 to 3 times less likely to develop HIT antibodies than are patients treated with UFH.
- HIT antibodies are necessary, but not sufficient, to cause clinical symptoms of HIT (thrombocytopenia and thrombosis).
- The hallmark of HIT is an otherwise unexplained thrombocytopenia beginning 4 to 14 days after heparin administration. Thrombocytopenia can present with a platelet count less than 100 to $150 \times 10^3/\mu L$ or can present as a 30% to 50% decrease in platelet count from the preheparin baseline.
- Patients with HIT have an increased risk of thrombotic complications, such as venous or arterial thrombosis and skin lesions (necrosis or erythematous lesions). Thrombosis is estimated to occur in 30% of HIT patients with thrombocytopenia.
- Patients who initially present without thrombosis have up to a 50% risk of a thrombotic complication within the following 30 days if not treated with a non-heparin anticoagulant.
- Laboratory assays for HIT include immunological and functional assays. Immunological assays include ELISA to detect the presence of HIT antibodies. Functional assays, such as the serotonin release assay (SRA) and heparin-induced platelet aggregation (HIPA) assay, detect the presence of HIT antibodies that cause platelet aggregation. The SRA is considered the gold standard assay for HIT antibodies.
- When HIT is suspected, heparin should be discontinued and an alternate, rapidly acting anticoagulant should be started immediately.[21]

4. A. Anti-GPIa/IIa.

Rationale: Light transmission aggregometry is not consistent with a defect in GPIa/IIa, which is a collagen receptor.

B. Anti-GPIbα.

Rationale: The platelets from patients with BS syndrome aggregate with physiologic agonists, but do not aggregate when induced with ristocetin. In the absence of GPIb/IX/V, isoantibodies against GPIb can form, leading to ineffective responses to platelet transfusions.

C. Anti-GPIIb/IIIa.

Rationale: Patients with Glanzmann thrombasthenia have absent or nonfunctioning platelet glycoprotein GPIIb/IIIa. Thus, platelet binding to fibrinogen and vWF is impaired and platelets do not aggregate with physiologic agonists. The absence of only ristocetin-induced platelet aggregation suggests a defect in the GPIb/V/IX complex.

D. Anti-GPVI.

Rationale: The light transmission aggregometry results in this case are not consistent with a defect in GPVI, which is a collagen receptor.

E. Anti–IIPA-1a.

Rationale: HPA-1 is an antigen that is commonly implicated in posttransfusion purpura. The light transmission aggregometry results in the case presented would not be seen in this disorder.

Major points of discussion

- BS syndrome is an autosomal recessive disorder caused by genetic lesions in GPIb/IX/V complex such that platelets do not adhere to vWF.
- BS syndrome shows thrombocytopenia with giant platelets, a lack of ristocetin-induced platelet aggregation, and a decreased response to thrombin-induced aggregation,
- GPIbα contains vWF and thrombin binding sites.
- Bleeding in BS syndrome can be mild to severe, with vascular factors contributing to the severity. Almost all patients with BS syndrome require platelet transfusion at some time in their life. The level of residual glycoprotein remaining on the platelets does not correlate with bleeding tendency. Isoantibodies against missing antigens can block the function of transfused platelets.
- Thrombocytopenia with normal bone marrow megakaryocytes can lead to a misdiagnosis of ITP, rather than BS syndrome, with resulting incorrect treatment.
- Giant platelets may be counted as red cells on automated cell counters, which can lead to artifactually lower platelet counts.[12]

5. A. Adenosine disphosphate (ADP).

Rationale: ADP is found in platelet-dense bodies.

B. Magnesium.

Rationale: Magnesium is found in platelet-dense bodies.

C. Platelet-derived growth factor (PDGF).

Rationale: PDGF is found in platelet α-granules.

D. Pyrophosphate.

Rationale: Pyrophosphate is found in platelet-dense bodies.

E. Serotonin.

Rationale: Serotonin is found in platelet-dense bodies.

Major points of discussion

- α-Granules are platelet organelles that are round to oval. They are more numerous and less electron dense than dense bodies.
- α-Granules contain PDGF, β-thromboglobulin, PF4, vWF, fibrinogen, factor V, and other proteins.

- Dense bodies contain adenosine triphosphate (ATP), ADP, serotonin, pyrophosphate, magnesium, and calcium.
- Abnormal or deficient α-granules can lead to platelet dysfunction, such as in gray platelet syndrome.
- In gray platelet syndrome, α-granules are normally formed, but their contents leak from the organelle. Therefore, the α-granules are empty and the platelet does not have its usual granular appearance.

6. A. Quebec platelet syndrome.

Rationale: Quebec platelet syndrome is associated with a defect of the α-granules.

B. Chediak-Higashi syndrome.

Rationale: Chediak-Higashi syndrome is associated with a defect of the β-granules.

C. Wiskott-Aldrich syndrome.

Rationale: Wiskott-Aldrich syndrome is associated with defects in platelet signal transduction and maintenance of the cytoskeleton.

D. Bernard-Soulier (BS) syndrome.

Rationale: BS syndrome is associated with a defect of the membrane GPIb-IX-V complex.

E. Gray platelet syndrome.

Rationale: Gray platelet syndrome is associated with a defect of the α-granules.

Major points of discussion

- Inherited platelet disorders characterized by severe disorders of platelet function include the following:
  - Wiskott-Aldrich syndrome
  - Glanzmann thrombasthenia
  - BS syndrome
- BS syndrome is characterized by deficiency of the GPIb/V/IX complex and manifests with bleeding, thrombocytopenia, and large platelets.
- There are fewer than 1000 estimated cases of BS syndrome worldwide. It is inherited as an autosomal recessive disorder. The genetic defects are in the *GPIBA*, *GPIBB*, and *GP9* genes (genes encoding GPIb and GPIX, respectively; no defects in the gene encoding GPV have been described)
- Bleeding often starts in childhood with frequent nosebleeds, gum bleeding, and easy bruising.
- Diagnosis: Platelets fail to aggregate with ristocetin and the diagnosis can be confirmed using flow cytometry to analyze GPIb-α surface density.[4,9]

7. A. Turbidometric aggregometry.

Rationale: Turbidometric aggregometry is considered the gold standard for platelet function testing; however, it is not an in vivo test.

B. Bleeding time (BT).

Rationale: The BT is considered an in vivo platelet function test.

C. PFA-100.

Rationale: The PFA-100 measures the time required for the cessation of blood flow in an in vitro assay.

D. Vasodilator-stimulated phosphoprotein (VASP) phosphorylation assay.

Rationale: The VASP phosphorylation assay is a flow cytometry–based in vitro assay.

E. Cone and plate analyzer.

Rationale: The cone and plate analyzer is an in vitro assay that measures shear-induced platelet adhesion.

Major points of discussion

- The basis of the BT is the in vivo cessation of blood flow by a newly formed platelet plug.
- Procedure: A blood pressure cuff is applied at a standardized pressure (40 mm Hg) over the upper arm. A standardized cut is made on the volar surface of the forearm. A piece of filter paper is used to absorb the blood every 30 seconds (care must be taken not to dislodge the clot). The time when blood is no longer absorbed is the BT and has a reference range of less than 7 minutes.
- Major disadvantages of the BT are that it is invasive, can lead to scarring, and has low reproducibility.
- Qualitative platelet disorders and von Willebrand disease can prolong the BT.
- Nonetheless, there are many causes of a prolonged or shortened BT. The BT is inversely proportional to the hematocrit and the platelet count. Therefore, the test should not be performed in the presence of anemia or thrombocytopenia.[10,18,22]

8. A. Cool skin.
B. Hematocrit of 25%.
Rationale: This prolongs the bleeding time (BT).
C. Platelet count of 200×10^9/L.
Rationale: A normal platelet count should not affect the BT.
D. Pregnancy.
E. Repeating the BT within 4 hours.
Rationale for A, D, and E: This shortens the BT.

Major points of discussion

- The BT has traditionally been used to screen for abnormal platelet function and von Willebrand disease.
- It has high variability due to physiologic variation, operator dependence, and technical variation.
- The BT is performed by applying a blood pressure cuff at a standard pressure (e.g., 40 mm Hg), making a cut(s) on the volar surface of the forearm using a spring-loaded device, absorbing the blood away from the site of injury every 30 seconds using absorbent paper, and then determining the time it takes from the making the cut to cessation of bleeding (no blood on the paper).
- The BT is highly operator dependent due to variability in how the cuts are made (e.g., pressure applied, direction of the cut), how the blood is blotted away because the clot can be inadvertently dislodged with the filter paper, location of cuts made on the arm, and so on.
- Lower hematocrit and platelet count are independently associated with an increased BT. Therefore, the clinician should be cautious when the test is performed for anemic or thrombocytopenic patients. In addition, high cuff pressure, deep or long cuts, location, and residual alcohol from cleaning the site can all prolong the BT.
- Physiologic and other variables can also decrease the BT. Repeating the BT within 4 hours, cool skin, age, gender, ethnicity (e.g., Eskimo), pregnancy, and acute-phase reactions can shorten the BT.
- Although traditionally used, the BT is not thought to predict bleeding. A prolonged or normal BT does not mean that the patient will or will not bleed during surgery, respectively.

9. A. May-Hegglin anomaly.
Rationale: Döhle-like bodies in neutrophils on May-Grünwald-Giemsa–stained peripheral blood are suggestive of MYH-9–related syndromes (of which May-Hegglin anomaly is one).
B. Chediak-Higashi syndrome.
Rationale: Large peroxidase-positive granules in both hematopoietic (neutrophils) and nonhematopoietic cells are found.
C. BS syndrome.
Rationale: Absent ristocetin-induced platelet aggregation is a key finding in BS syndrome. Large platelets are also seen.
D. Hermansky-Pudlak syndrome.
Rationale: Large peroxidase-positive granules are not found in the Hermansky-Pudlak syndrome, which, like Chediak-Higashi syndrome, is associated with oculocutaneous albinism.
E. Gray platelet syndrome.
Rationale: A classical finding in gray platelet syndrome is a lack of α-granules when platelets are examined by electron microscopy.

Major points of discussion

- Inherited platelet disorders characterized by disorders of platelet granules include idiopathic dense-granule disorder (δ-storage pool disease); Hermansky-Pudlak syndrome; Chediak-Higashi syndrome; gray platelet syndrome; Paris-Trousseau/Jacobsen syndrome; and idiopathic α- and dense-granule storage pool disease.
- The dense-granule disorders include Hermansky Pudlak syndrome; Chediak-Higashi syndrome; and idiopathic dense-granule deficiency.
- Dense granules are lysosome-related organelles in platelets and megakaryocytes and are members of a family of cell-type-specific organelles that also includes melanosomes, and lytic granules of cytotoxic T lymphocytes and natural killer cells. As such, dense granule disorders are usually part of a more complex congenital disorder with defects in several other lysosome-related organelles.
- Dense-granule disorders typically present with mild to moderate bleeding, with easy bruising, epistaxis, menorrhagia, and the potential for significant bleeding in the setting of trauma or surgery.
- Dense-granule disorders may result in defects in platelet aggregation ranging from abnormal responses to all agonists to more subtle changes, such as abnormal responses to low concentrations of agonists.
- Characteristic aggregometry features include an absence of the secondary wave of aggregation in response to epinephrine; a delayed and reduced response to collagen; impaired aggregation to low concentrations of agonists, such as arachidonic acid and thrombin receptor agonist peptide (TRAP); and high concentrations of ADP eliciting full, irreversible aggregation.
- A reduction in both the content and ratio of ADP to ATP, or absence of release of ATP, is diagnostic of a platelet dense-granule disorder.
- A reduction in the number, or absence, of dense granules can be confirmed by electron microscopy.
- Some characteristics of Chediak-Higashi syndrome include the following: estimated number of cases worldwide: less than 1000; autosomal recessive; genetic

defect: *LYST* gene; oculocutaneous albinism, infections, and a lymphoproliferative accelerated phase; death usually occurs before age 10.

- Diagnosis: The presence of very large peroxidase-positive cytoplasmic granules in hematopoietic (e.g., neutrophils) and nonhematopoietic cells is a classical finding in Chediak-Higashi syndrome and helps distinguish it from the Hermansky-Pudlak syndrome.[4,9]

10. A. GPIbα.
Rationale: In this case, the platelet function study would show an absence of ristocetin-induced platelet aggregation, but normal aggregation with the other agonists.
B. GPIIb/IIIa.
Rationale: In this case, the platelet function study would show an absence of aggregation with ADP, epinephrine, and collagen, but the ristocetin results would be normal.
C. GPVI.
Rationale: GPVI is a collagen binding and signaling receptor. In this case, abnormal aggregation with collagen would be expected.
D. P2Y$_1$.
E. P2Y$_{12}$.
Rationale for D and E: P2Y$_{12}$ is an ADP receptor. In this case, the aggregation assay would be expected to show an abnormal ADP response.

Major points of discussion
- GPVI and integrin α2β1 (GPIa-IIa) are the major collagen receptors on platelets. GPVI is thought to be the major signaling collagen receptor.
- Autoantibodies against the collagen receptor have been described.
- Blockade of collagen receptor(s) by autoantibodies would decrease collagen-induced platelet aggregation.
- GPVI-deficient platelets have also been described; this is more commonly found among the Japanese.
- Under high shear stress, collagen receptors are unlikely to result in platelet adhesion. The platelet GPIbα-vWF interaction is most important for platelet adhesion under high shear stress.[23]

11. A. Cone and plate analyzer.
Rationale: The cone and plate analyzer evaluates high shear platelet adhesion onto a surface.
B. VerifyNow.
Rationale: The VerifyNow assay does not use shear conditions.
C. Impedance aggregometry.
Rationale: Impedance aggregometry does not use shear conditions.
D. Assays that measure thromboxane (Tx) A$_2$ metabolites.
Rationale: Assays that measure TxA$_2$ metabolites are immunoassays that measure stable Tx metabolites in the serum or urine.
E. Turbidometric aggregometry.
Rationale: Turbidometric aggregometry does not use shear conditions.

Major points of discussion
- The basis of the cone and plate analyzer (CPA) is shear-induced platelet adhesion. A whole blood sample is placed into a sample well. The platelets then aggregate

against the wall of the sample well under high shear stress. The nonadherent cells are washed away and the platelet aggregates are then stained.
- The number of aggregates, the average size of the aggregates, and the percentage of the total area covered by aggregates are measured by an image analyzer.
- The aggregation of platelets in this system is dependent on vWF, fibrinogen, platelet GPIbα and GPIIb/IIIa, and the platelet release reaction.
- CPA instruments are commercially available and can be used with a small sample volume, do not require any manual sample preparation, and produce rapid results. They have a small footprint and can be used at the point of care for near patient testing. Small sample volumes are required; therefore, it is an ideal platelet analyzer for pediatric samples.
- The disadvantage of the CPA instrument is that it is not widely used and clinical experience is limited. Similar to the BT and PFA-100, the CPA is dependent on the hematocrit and platelet count.[10,18,22]

12. A. May-Hegglin anomaly.
Rationale: May-Hegglin anomaly is associated with mutation of *MYH9* gene.
B. Amegakaryocytic thrombocytopenia with radioulnar synostosis.
Rationale: Amegakaryocytic thrombocytopenia with radioulnar synostosis is associated with a mutation of the *HOXA11* gene.
C. Scott syndrome.
Rationale: Scott syndrome is associated with mutation of the *ABCA1* gene.
D. Wiskott-Aldrich syndrome.
Rationale: Wiskott-Aldrich syndrome is associated with mutation of the *WAS* gene.
E. Congenital amegakaryocytic thrombocytopenia.
Rationale: Congenital amegakaryocytic thrombocytopenia is associated with mutation of the *MPL* gene.

Major points of discussion
- Inherited platelet disorders are rare causes of bleeding.
- Inherited platelet disorders characterized by abnormalities of platelet number include:
  - MYH9 disorders (May-Hegglin anomaly, Sebastian syndrome, Fechter syndrome, Epstein syndrome)
  - Congenital amegakaryocytic thrombocytopenia
  - Amegakaryocytic thrombocytopenia with radioulnar synostosis
  - Thrombocytopenia absent radius syndrome
  - X-linked thrombocytopenia with dyserythropoiesis
- Congenital amegakaryocytic thrombocytopenia is characterized by thrombocytopenia with virtually complete absence of megakaryocytes from the bone marrow.
- There are fewer than 100 cases estimated worldwide.
- It is inherited in an autosomal recessive inheritance pattern.
- The genetic defect is in the *MPL* gene (thrombopoietin receptor gene)
- Congenital amegakaryocytic thrombocytopenia usually presents during the neonatal period, or soon after, with bleeding and severe thrombocytopenia.
- Definitive confirmation requires molecular analysis of the *MPL* gene.[4,9]

13. A. β-Thromboglobulin.
Rationale: α-Granules contain β-thromboglobulin.
B. Calcium.
Rationale: Dense bodies contain calcium, magnesium, and pyrophosphate.
C. Fibrinogen.
Rationale: α-Granules contain fibrinogen.
D. P-selectin.
Rationale: α-Granules contain P-selectin.
E. von Willebrand factor (vWF).
Rationale: α-Granules contain vWF.

Major points of discussion
- Dense bodies are round, electron-opaque (dark) platelet organelles when visualized by electron microscopy.
- They have a distinct appearance on electron microscopy referred to as a bull's-eye.
- Dense bodies contain ADP, ATP, serotonin, calcium, magnesium, and pyrophosphate.
- The other type of organelles found in platelets are the α-granules, which are less dense and more numerous by electron microscopy.
- α-Granules contain PDGF, β-thromboglobulin, factor V, P-selectin, fibrinogen, vWF, PF4, and other proteins.
- Absent or abnormal α- and dense granules can lead to abnormal platelet function, such as in gray platelet syndrome and Hermansky-Pudlak syndrome, respectively.
- It should be noted that connections between α-and dense granules may occur in the Golgi apparatus, in which case they may have shared contents.

14. A. Fresh nonanticoagulated blood.
Rationale: Fresh nonanticoagulated blood is required for the Görög thrombosis test, an assay that assesses high shear–dependent platelet function and thrombolysis.
B. Whole blood.
Rationale: Whole blood samples are used for flow cytometry–based platelet function tests.
C. Serum.
Rationale: Serum is used for measuring TxA2 metabolites in the blood.
D. Platelet-rich plasma (PRP).
Rationale: Preparation of PRP is a step in the sample preparation for turbidometric aggregometry.
E. Platelet-poor plasma (PPP).
Rationale: Preparation of PPP is a step in the sample preparation for turbidometric aggregometry.

Major points of discussion
- Platelet function studies have historically been used to investigate the cause of unexplained bleeding. The majority of platelet-related bleeding can be attributed to defects of primary hemostasis, such as von Willebrand disease, inherited platelet disorders, and drug-induced platelet dysfunction.
- Platelet function tests are also increasingly used to monitor the therapeutic efficacy of antiplatelet agents used to treat patients at high risk for atherothrombosis.
- Platelet function studies may be classified based on the testing principle:
  - In vivo cessation of blood flow by the platelet plug
  - In vitro cessation of high shear blood flow by the platelet plug
  - Shear-induced platelet adhesion

- Platelet aggregation
- Changes in expression of surface markers following activation
- Intracellular signaling following activation
- Release of substances from platelets following activation
- Evaluation of platelet contribution to clot strength
- Flow cytometry–based assays can measure activation-dependent changes in the expression of platelet surface markers.
- Platelet surface markers that are measured in these assays include P-selectin, activated GPIIb/IIIa, and leukocyte-platelet aggregates.
- Characteristics of assays involving activation-dependent changes in platelet surface marker expression:
  - Sample: whole blood
  - Advantage: small sample volume
  - Disadvantage: requires complex sample preparation, a flow cytometer, and a high level of technical experience[10,18,22]

15. A. CD63.
Rationale: CD63 is decreased/absent in Hermansky-Pudlak syndrome.
B. CD41.
Rationale: CD41 (GPIIb) is decreased/absent in Glanzmann thrombasthenia.
C. CD154.
Rationale: CD154 is the CD40 ligand.
D. CD49b.
Rationale: CD49b (GPIa) is a component of the collagen receptor (GPIa/IIa).
E. CD29.
Rationale: CD29 (GPIIa) is a component of the collagen receptor (GPIa/IIa).

Major points of discussion
- Glanzmann thrombasthenia is characterized by a deficiency or functional defect in glycoprotein IIb/IIIa.
- Glanzmann thrombasthenia is characterized by a normal platelet count, normal platelet morphology, a prolonged BT, and defective platelet aggregation.
- Glanzmann thrombasthenia characteristics:
  - Estimated number of cases worldwide: less than 1000
  - Autosomal recessive
  - Genetic defects: *ITGA2B*, *ITGB3* (genes encoding GPIIb and GPIIIa, respectively)
  - Presentation: Most initial presentations are during the first 5 years of life with purpura or petechiae in the neonatal period or excessive bruising during early childhood.
- A definitive diagnosis is made by flow cytometry using antibodies against GPIIb (CD41) and GPIIIa (CD61).[4,9]

16. A. Factor V.
Rationale: Platelet factor V is absent in gray platelet syndrome.
B. β-Thromboglobulin.
Rationale: β-Thromboglobulin is absent in gray platelet syndrome.
C. Fibrinogen.
Rationale: Platelet fibrinogen is absent in gray platelet syndrome.
D. P-selectin.

Rationale: P-selectin is retained in Gray platelet syndrome.
E. Platelet factor 4.
Rationale: Platelet factor 4 is absent in gray platelet syndrome.

Major points of discussion

- Inherited platelet disorders characterized by disorders of the platelet granules include idiopathic dense-granule disorder (δ-storage pool disease); Hermansky-Pudlak syndrome; Chediak-Higashi syndrome; gray platelet syndrome; Paris-Trousseau/Jacobsen syndrome; and idiopathic α- and dense-granule storage pool disease.
- α-Granule disorders include gray platelet syndrome; Paris-Trousseau or Jacobsen syndrome; Quebec platelet syndrome; and arthrogryposis–renal dysfunction–cholestasis.
- Gray platelet syndrome is characterized by a lack of α-granules when the platelets are analyzed by electron microscopy. The contents of α granules that are both synthesized by the megakaryocyte (PF4, β-thromboglobulin, and PDGF) and taken up from the blood (factor V and fibrinogen) are lacking. P-selectin, an α-granule marker, is retained.
- There are fewer than 100 cases worldwide. Gray platelet syndrome has both autosomal recessive and autosomal dominant patterns of inheritance. The genetic defects may involve several genes.
- Platelets appear "gray" (due to lack of α-granules), misshapen, and slightly large (macrothrombocytopenia) on peripheral blood smear.
- Electron microscopy of platelets shows decreased numbers or absence of α-granules.
- Clinically, patients have a variable bleeding disorder (mild to severe) associated with both abnormal platelet function and thrombocytopenia.[4,9,19]

17. A. Sebastian syndrome.
Rationale: Sebastian syndrome is not associated with oculocutaneous albinism.
B. Wiskott-Aldrich syndrome.
Rationale: Wiskott-Aldrich syndrome is not associated with oculocutaneous albinism.
C. Hermansky-Pudlak syndrome.
Rationale: Hermansky-Pudlak syndrome is associated with oculocutaneous albinism.
D. Paris-Trousseau/Jacobsen syndrome.
Rationale: Paris-Trousseau/Jacobsen syndrome is not associated with oculocutaneous albinism.
E. BS syndrome.
Rationale: BS syndrome is not associated with oculocutaneous albinism.

Major points of discussion

- Dense granules are lysosome-related organelles in platelets and megakaryocytes and are members of a family of cell type–specific organelles that also includes melanosomes, lytic granules of cytotoxic T lymphocytes, and natural killer cells. As such, dense granule disorders are usually part of a more complex congenital disorder with defects in several other lysosome-related organelles.
- Dense-granule disorders typically present with mild to moderate bleeding with easy bruising, epistaxis,

menorrhagia, and the potential for significant bleeding in the setting of trauma or surgery.
- Dense-granule disorders may result in defects in platelet aggregation, ranging from abnormal responses to all agonists to more subtle changes, such as abnormal responses to low concentrations of agonists.
- Hermansky-Pudlak syndrome characteristics:
  - Estimated number of cases worldwide: more than 1000
  - Genetically, clinically, and biologically diverse
  - Most common genetic disorder in Puerto Rico
  - Autosomal recessive
  - Genetic defects: *HPS1, AP3B1/HPS2, HPS3, HPS4, HPS5, HPS6, DTNBP1, HPS8* genes (protein products may affect trafficking of proteins to new organelles)
  - Affects platelet dense granules and melanosomes
  - Other important features: oculocutaneous albinism (common to all forms); pulmonary fibrosis, granulomatous colitis, neutropenia, and mild immunodeficiency (characteristic of certain forms)[4,9]

18. A. BS syndrome.
Rationale: Neutrophil inclusions would not be present.
B. May-Hegglin anomaly.
Rationale: Presents with thrombocytopenia, giant platelets, and Döhle-like inclusions in neutrophils without hearing loss, nephritis, or cataracts.
C. Epstein syndrome.
Rationale: Characterized by thrombocytopenia, giant platelets, hearing loss, and nephritis. Döhle-like bodies are not present.
D. Fechtner syndrome.
Rationale: Characterized by thrombocytopenia, giant platelets, Döhle-like inclusions in neutrophils, hearing loss, nephritis, and cataracts.
E. Glanzmann thrombasthenia.
Rationale: Does not present with thrombocytopenia.

Major points of discussion

- Congenital macrothrombocytopenia syndromes include May-Hegglin anomaly, Sebastian syndrome, Fechtner syndrome, Epstein syndrome, BS syndrome, gray platelet syndrome, and X-linked macrothrombocytopenia with dyserythropoiesis.
- May-Hegglin anomaly, Sebastian syndrome, Fechtner syndrome, and Epstein syndrome are MYH9-related diseases that are characterized by mutations in the myosin heavy chain 9 (*MYH9*) gene.
- MYH9-related disorders all have giant platelets (i.e., platelets at least the size of RBCs) and are distinguished by the presence or absence of Döhle-like inclusions, hearing loss, nephritis, and cataracts.
- The majority of the *MYH9* mutations show autosomal dominant inheritance.
- Most patients with MYH9-related disorders do not have clinically significant bleeding problems.[4]

19. A. Paris-Trousseau/Jacobsen syndrome.
Rationale: Paris-Trousseau/Jacobsen syndrome is characterized by the presence of giant α-granules.
B. Chediak-Higashi syndrome.
Rationale: Chediak-Higashi syndrome is associated with a defect of the dense granules.
C. BS syndrome.

Rationale: BS syndrome is associated with a defect in the GPIb/V/IX complex.
D. Hermansky-Pudlak syndrome.
Rationale: Hermansky-Pudlak syndrome is associated with a defect of the dense granules.
E. Glanzmann thrombasthenia.
Rationale: Glanzmann thrombasthenia is associated with a defect of GPIIb/IIIa.

Major points of discussion

- α-Granule disorders include the following:
  - Gray platelet syndrome
  - Paris-Trousseau or Jacobsen syndrome
  - Quebec platelet syndrome
  - Arthrogryposis–renal dysfunction–cholestasis
- Paris-Trousseau/Jacobsen syndrome is characterized by the presence of giant α-granules in a low percentage of platelets.
- Associated congenital abnormalities include mental retardation, cardiac abnormalities, and craniofacial abnormalities.
- Paris-Trousseau/Jacobsen syndrome characteristics:
  - Estimated number of cases worldwide: less than 100
  - Autosomal recessive
  - Genetic defect: 11q23 deletion (includes the *FLI1* gene, which is important for megakaryopoiesis)
  - Presentation: mild bleeding diathesis[4,9]

20. A. Plateletworks.
Rationale: The Plateletworks assay does not use high shear blood flow conditions to test platelet function.
B. Thromboelastography.
Rationale: Thromboelastography does not use high shear blood flow conditions to test platelet function.
C. VerifyNow.
Rationale: The VerifyNow assay does not use high shear blood flow conditions to test platelet function.
D. Light transmission aggregometry.
Rationale: Light transmission aggregometry does not use high shear blood flow conditions to test platelet function.
E. PFA-100.
Rationale: The PFA-100 uses high shear blood flow conditions to test platelet function.

Major points of discussion

- The basis of the platelet function analyzer-100 (i.e., PFA-100) is the cessation of high shear blood flow in vitro by a newly formed platelet plug. It was created as a more physiologically relevant and standardized method to screen for disorders of primary hemostasis (i.e., to replace the BT).
- The PFA-100 is a whole blood assay where blood flows at physiologic shear stress through an aperture that is coated with a choice of physiological agonists (collagen/ADP, collagen/epinephrine). The interval from the start of the test until the aperture becomes occluded is the closure time.
- Characteristics of the PFA-100 assay:
  - Sample: whole blood
  - Advantages: small sample volume; no sample preparation
  - Disadvantages: dependent on vWF, hematocrit, and platelet count.

- Interpretation:
  - ADP normal and EPI normal = normal
  - ADP normal and EPI abnormal = aspirin, nonsteroidal antiinflammatory drugs (NSAIDs)
  - ADP abnormal and EPI abnormal = BS syndrome, Glanzmann thrombasthenia, von Willebrand disease, and so on.
- If the PFA-100 test result is normal, then further testing is usually not performed because of its excellent negative predictive value.
- However, if the test result is positive, confirmatory testing with light transmission or whole blood aggregometry is necessary.[10,18,22]

21. A. Recombinant factor VIIa.
B. Fresh frozen plasma.
C. Platelets.
Rationale: The decreased maximum amplitude with a sufficiently hemostatic platelet count (>50 mg/dL) suggests that there is platelet dysfunction. A platelet transfusion may be useful.
D. Prothrombin complex concentrates.
Rationale for A, B, and D: The thromboelastogram does not suggest a coagulation factor deficiency.
E. RBCs.
Rationale: A hemoglobin level higher than 10 g/dL is adequate for a patient with cardiac disease.

Major points of discussion

- Thromboelastography is performed by adding whole blood to a cuvette. A pin attached to a torsion wire is inserted into the sample and either the cup or the pin is oscillated. As the clot forms, the amount of torque required to move the pin or cup is plotted on the *y*-axis (clot strength) and time is plotted on the *x*-axis.
- The pattern can be interpreted to provide information on the hemostatic status of the patient, which can guide component therapy, especially during cardiothoracic surgery.
- The *R* value is the time from the initiation of the test to the initial formation of the clot. It is reflective of coagulation factor activation. A prolonged *R* value would suggest the presence of a coagulation factor deficiency and fresh frozen plasma would be indicated.
- Maximal aggregation (MA) is a measure of the clot strength and is the amplitude of the curve. It is reflective of platelet number or function. A decreased MA would suggest that platelets are indicated.
- If the MA decreases at an interval shorter than normal, then clot lysis is accelerated, as seen in excessive fibrinolysis. A antifibrinolytic agent may be indicated in this circumstance.

22. **A. Plateletworks.**
Rationale: The Plateletworks assay uses detection of platelet aggregation as its end point.
B. PFA-100.
Rationale: The PFA-100 is based on high shear blood flow.
C. Cone and plate analyzer.
Rationale: The cone and plate analyzer uses shear-induced platelet adhesion as its end point.

D. VASP.
Rationale: The VASP phosphorylation assay does not use detection of platelet aggregation as its end point. It is a flow cytometry–based assay.
E. Thromboelastography.
Rationale: Thromboelastography uses global clot formation as its end point.

Major points of discussion

- Platelet function studies have historically been used to investigate the cause of unexplained bleeding. Platelet function tests are now increasingly used to monitor the therapeutic efficacy of antiplatelet agents that treat patients at high risk for atherothrombosis.
- The basis of the Plateletworks assay is platelet aggregation and is performed by counting platelets from a sample before and after activation using agonists.
- The main use of this assay is the measurement of residual platelet reactivity after the administration of an antiplatelet agent following an acute cardiovascular or neurovascular event. If the residual reactivity remains high, the patient may be at risk of a secondary myocardial infarction or stroke, respectively.
- Steps in performing the assay:
  1. Measure baseline platelet count from a whole blood sample anticoagulated with EDTA (first sample).
  2. Measure platelet count from a second sample that is collected in the presence of a platelet agonist (e.g., collagen, ADP, or arachidonic acid).
  3. Uninhibited platelets in the presence of the agonists will become activated, aggregate, and will not be counted as individual platelets in this second sample.
  4. The difference in platelet counts between the two samples provides a measure of aggregation and a ratio of the two counts yields a percentage inhibition.
- The advantage of this test is that it requires minimal sample preparation. The disadvantage is that it is an indirect test. It assumes that the decrease in platelet count is proportional to amount of platelet aggregation.[10,18,22]

23. A. TTP.
Rationale: An elevated lactate dehydrogenase (LDH) in serum and schistocytes on the peripheral smear would be expected.
B. ITP.
Rationale: The only abnormality that would be expected in ITP is a low platelet count.
C. DIC.
Rationale: DIC often presents with a prolonged PT and APTT, increased LDH, and schistocytes on the peripheral smear.
D. Syndrome of hemolysis, elevated liver enzymes, and low platelet count (HELLP).
Rationale: HELLP presents with elevated aspartate aminotransferase (AST), alanine aminotransferase (ALT), LDH, and schistocytes on the peripheral smear.
E. Hemolytic uremic syndrome (HUS).
Rationale: HUS presents with elevated LDH, blood urea nitrogen (BUN), and creatinine, as well as changes in RBC morphology, including schistocytes.

Major points of discussion

- ITP is the most common autoimmune disorder noted during pregnancy.
- It is important to understand the normal physiologic changes that occur during pregnancy. For example, the platelet count is expected to decrease by approximately 10% during a normal pregnancy and the greatest decrease is during the third trimester.
- The differential diagnosis of thrombocytopenia during pregnancy includes ITP, gestational thrombocytopenia (GTP), TTP, HUS, DIC, and the HELLP syndrome.
- Antiplatelet antibodies in ITP are usually directed against the GPIIb/IIIa or GPIb-IX-V platelet proteins.
- The majority of antibodies are IgG, are able to cross the placenta and can cause fetal or neonatal ITP.[5,11]

24. A. $\alpha 2\beta 1$.
Rationale: $\alpha 2\beta 1$ is a platelet collagen receptor and is not blocked by abciximab.
B. GPIbα.
Rationale: GPIbα is a platelet vWF receptor involved in platelet adhesion and is not blocked by abciximab.
C. GPIIb/IIIa.
Rationale: Abciximab contains antibody Fab fragments that block GPIIb/IIIa (αIIbβ3). It is used to treat acute coronary syndromes and for percutaneous coronary intervention (i.e., cardiac catheterization).
D. P2X$_1$.
Rationale: P2X$_1$ is the platelet ATP receptor and is not blocked by abciximab.
E. P2Y$_{12}$.
Rationale: P2Y$_{12}$ is the platelet ADP receptor and is not blocked by abciximab.

Major points of discussion

- Abciximab is an antiplatelet agent containing Fab fragments that bind to and specifically block the GPIIb/IIIa platelet receptor.
- GPIIb/IIIa is required for platelet aggregation. Platelets aggregate by GPIIb/IIIa to fibrinogen or vWF. These interactions bridge platelets via fibrinogen and vWF.
- Other GPIIb/IIIa inhibitors include tirofiban (a nonpeptide agent) and eptifibatide (a heptapeptide agent). All three GPIIb/IIIa inhibitors have different platelet GPIIb/IIIa binding sites.
- Abciximab is used in percutaneous coronary interventions and for acute coronary syndromes.
- Glanzmann thrombasthenia is an inherited bleeding disorder caused by a GPIIb/IIIa deficiency.

25. A. GPIbα.
Rationale: There are no Food and Drug Administration (FDA)-approved pharmaceuticals that inhibit GPIbα.
B. GPIIb/IIIa.
Rationale: GPIIb/IIIa can be pharmaceutically blocked by abciximab, tirofiban, and eptifibatide.
C. GPVI.
Rationale: Currently, there are no FDA-approved pharmaceuticals that inhibit GPVI.
D. P2X$_1$.
Rationale: P2X$_1$ is an ATP receptor and is not specifically blocked by clopidogrel.

E. P2Y$_{12}$.
Rationale: Clopidogrel is a strong antiplatelet agent that blocks P2Y$_{12}$, the platelet ADP receptor.

Major points of discussion

- P2Y$_{12}$ and P2Y$_1$ are both platelet ADP receptors. However, P2Y$_{12}$ is more important for platelet activation. P2X$_1$ is an ATP receptor.
- Clopidogrel is a pharmaceutical agent that specifically blocks the P2Y$_{12}$ receptor and is a strong antiplatelet medication.
- Other medications that block the P2Y$_{12}$ receptor and are used as antiplatelet agents include ticlopidine, prasugrel, and cangrelor.
- Clopidogrel and other P2Y$_{12}$ receptor blockers are used for prophylaxis against secondary acute coronary and neurovascular thrombosis and in patients who cannot tolerate aspirin.
- Clopidogrel "resistance"—that is, the lack of platelet inhibition with standard doses of clopidogrel—can be caused by variable hepatic transformation of clopidogrel into its active form by polymorphisms of the *CYP2C19* gene. Genetic testing may be useful to determine the appropriate dose or if a change in medication is indicated.

26. A. Sebastian syndrome.
Rationale: Sebastian syndrome is associated with macrothrombocytopenia.
B. Fechter syndrome.
Rationale: Fechter syndrome is associated with macrothrombocytopenia.
C. Scott syndrome.
Rationale: Scott syndrome is associated with inadequate exposure of negatively charged phospholipids.
D. Epstein syndrome.
Rationale: Epstein syndrome is associated with macrothrombocytopenia.
E. Chediak-Higashi syndrome.
Rationale: Chediak-Higashi syndrome is associated with a dense-granule defect.

Major points of discussion

- Scott syndrome is characterized by a disorder of phospholipid exposure (reduced exposure of negatively charged phospholipids upon platelet activation).
- This lack of phospholipid exposure leads to a significantly reduced ability to promote tenase and prothrombinase activity on platelet surfaces.
- There are fewer than 10 cases of this syndrome reported worldwide. It has an autosomal recessive inheritance pattern. The exact gene defect for this disorder has not been definitively identified. At least one case is due to a mutation in transmembrane protein 16 F (TMEM16F).
- Patients present with bleeding following invasive procedures. There are also reports of postpartum bleeding.
- The diagnosis can be made using flow cytometry (by annexin V labeling) to assess whether phosphatidyl serine becomes exposed following platelet activation.
- The only known treatment is transfusion of normal donor platelets.[4,9]

27. A. Activation-dependent changes in platelet surface marker expression.
Rationale: Flow cytometry to detect various proteins, such as P-selectin and platelet surface activated GPIIb/IIIa, or to identify leukocyte-platelet aggregates, is used to evaluate activation-dependent changes in platelet surface marker expression.
B. in vivo cessation of blood flow by a newly formed platelet plug.
Rationale: The BT measures the time required for in vivo cessation of blood flow by a newly formed platelet plug.
C. Shear-induced platelet adhesion.
Rationale: The cone and plate analyzer evaluates shear-induced platelet adhesion.
D. Rate and quality/strength of clot formation.
Rationale: Thromboelastography evaluates the rate and quality/strength of clot formation.
E. Platelet-to-platelet aggregation.
Rationale: Aggregometry evaluates platelet-to-platelet aggregation.

Major points of discussion

- Platelet function studies have historically been used to investigate the cause of unexplained bleeding. The majority of platelet-related bleeding can be attributed to defects of primary hemostasis, such as von Willebrand disease, inherited platelet disorders, and drug-induced platelet dysfunction.
- Platelet function tests are also increasingly used to monitor the therapeutic efficacy of antiplatelet agents used to treat patients at high risk for atherothrombosis.
- The basis of using thromboelastography to evaluate platelet function is to evaluate the contribution of platelets to clot strength in a whole blood sample.
- Advantages of thromboelastography: It measures global coagulation (i.e., clotting factors, platelets, fibrinolysis) and can potentially be used at the point of care (e.g., in the operating room).
- Disadvantages of thromboelastography: To test the platelet-specific contribution to clot formation and strength, additional platelet activators (arachidonic acid or ADP) must be used, thereby increasing the complexity of the test.[10,18,22]

28. A. VerifyNow.
Rationale: The VerifyNow assay is based on platelet aggregation.
B. PFA-100.
Rationale: The PFA-100 is based on high shear blood flow.
C. Measurement of serum TxB$_2$.
Rationale: Measurement of serum thromboxane B$_2$, a metabolite of TxA2, uses an immunoassay.
D. Measurement of activated GPIIb/IIIa.
Rationale: Measurement of activated GPIIb/IIIa is based on flow cytometry.
E. Plateletworks.
Rationale: The Plateletworks assay is based on platelet aggregation.

Major points of discussion

- Platelet function tests are also increasingly used to monitor the therapeutic efficacy of antiplatelet agents used to treat patients at high risk for atherothrombosis.

- The substances measured in assays based on platelet secretion following activation include platelet-derived microparticles (by flow cytometry), serum TxB_2, urinary 11-dehydrothromboxane B_2, plasma sCD40L, plasma GPV, and α-granule constituents in plasma (e.g., PF4, β-thromboglobulin, and soluble P-selectin).
- Serum TxB_2, urinary 11-dehydrothromboxane B_2, plasma sCD40L, plasma GPV, and α-granule constituents are measured using immunoassays.
- Serum TxB_2 and urinary 11-dehydrothromboxane B_2 are indirect measures and are not platelet specific.
- Serum TxB_2 measures the capacity of platelets to synthesize TxA2 and is a measure of the antiplatelet effect of aspirin.[10,18,22]

29. A. Arthrogryposis–renal dysfunction–cholestasis.
Rationale: Arthrogryposis–renal dysfunction–cholestasis is associated with a defect in the α-granules.
B. Paris-Trousseau/Jacobsen syndrome.
Rationale: Paris-Trousseau/Jacobsen syndrome is associated with a defect in the α-granules.
C. Chediak-Higashi syndrome.
Rationale: Chediak-Higashi syndrome is associated with a defect in the δ-granules.
D. Tx synthase deficiency.
Rationale: Tx synthase deficiency is associated with a defect in platelet signal transduction.
E. Hermansky-Pudlak syndrome.
Rationale: Hermansky-Pudlak syndrome is associated with a defect in the dense granules.

Major points of discussion
- Inherited platelet disorders characterized by disorders of receptors and signal transduction include the following:
  - Platelet cyclooxygenase deficiency
  - Tx synthase deficiency
  - Tx A2 receptor defect
  - ADP receptor defect $(P2Y_{12})$
- In general, patients with this class of defects present with abnormal primary hemostasis manifested by mild bleeding. Platelet number and morphology are usually normal.
- Tx synthase deficiency or a defect in the TxA2 receptor presents with an aspirin-like defect, but a thorough medication history will not show any ingestion of aspirin or aspirin-containing medications.
- There is marked impairment of platelet aggregation in response to arachidonic acid; aggregation with ADP and collagen are also reduced. Aggregation with Tx analogs and ristocetin are normal.
- These cases are diagnosed when there is an abnormal secondary wave of aggregation, but there are normal dense granules on electron microscopy and an absence of aspirin ingestion.[4,9]

30. A. PFA-100.
Rationale: The PFA-100 assay is not considered the historical gold standard for platelet function testing.
B. Impedance aggregometry.
Rationale: Impedance aggregometry is not considered the historical gold standard for platelet function testing.
C. Turbidometric aggregometry.

Rationale: Turbidometric aggregometry is considered the historical gold standard for platelet function testing.
D. Measurement of TxA2 metabolites.
Rationale: Measurement of TxA2 metabolites is not considered the historical gold standard for platelet function testing. These metabolites are not specific for platelets.
E. Measurement of activated GPIIb/IIIa by flow cytometry.
Rationale: Measurement of activated GPIIb/IIIa by flow cytometry is not considered the historical gold standard for platelet function testing.

Major points of discussion
- Platelet function studies have historically been used to investigate the cause of unexplained bleeding. The majority of platelet-related bleeding can be attributed to defects of primary hemostasis, such as von Willebrand disease, inherited platelet disorders, and drug-induced platelet dysfunction. Platelet function tests are also increasingly used to monitor the therapeutic efficacy of antiplatelet agents used to treat patients at high risk for atherothrombosis.
- The basis of platelet aggregometry is platelet-to-platelet aggregation in response to various platelet agonists.
- Turbidometric (light transmittance) aggregometry measures platelet-to-platelet aggregation in PRP in response to classic agonists. The assay is time consuming because PPP and PRP must be prepared from whole blood. In addition, most of the steps in this assay are manual and are of high complexity. Nonetheless, this test is considered the gold standard for platelet function testing.
- Impedance aggregometry measures changes in impedance in response to classic agonists. It is a whole blood assay.
- Classic agonists include collagen, ADP, epinephrine, arachidonic acid, thrombin, TRAP, phorbol 12-myristate 13-acetate (PMA), ristocetin, and U44619 (a TxA2 analog).
- Both impedance and turbidometric aggregometry are used to diagnose a variety of inherited and acquired platelet defects.[10,18,22]

31. A. Turbidometric aggregometry.
Rationale: Turbidometric aggregometry is considered the gold standard overall for platelet function testing, but not specifically for assessing the $P2Y_{12}$ antagonist effect.
B. Thromboelastography.
Rationale: Thromboelastography is not considered the gold standard for assessing the $P2Y_{12}$ antagonist effect.
C. Plateletworks.
Rationale: The Plateletworks assay is not considered the gold standard for assessing the $P2Y_{12}$ antagonist effect.
D. VASP phosphorylation.
Rationale: VASP phosphorylation is considered the gold standard for assessing the $P2Y_{12}$ antagonist effect.
E. VerifyNow.
Rationale: The VerifyNow assay is not considered the gold standard for assessing the $P2Y_{12}$ antagonist effect.

Major points of discussion
- Platelet function studies have historically been used to investigate the cause of unexplained bleeding. Platelet function tests are also increasingly used to monitor the

therapeutic efficacy of antiplatelet agents used to treat patients at high risk for atherothrombosis.
- The basis of the VASP phosphorylation assay is measurement of activation-dependent signaling by flow cytometry.
- It is a whole blood assay considered the gold standard for assessing the P2Y$_{12}$ antagonist effect.
- Its major disadvantage is that it requires complex sample preparation, a flow cytometer (i.e., high capital investment), and a high level of technical experience.
- P2Y$_{12}$ inhibitors used as antiplatelet agents include clopidogrel, prasugrel, cangrelor, and ticagrelor.[10,18,22]

32. A. BS syndrome.
Rationale: BS syndrome is not associated with immunodeficiency.
B. Scott syndrome.
Rationale: Scott syndrome is not associated with immunodeficiency.
C. Glanzmann thrombasthenia.
Rationale: Glanzmann thrombasthenia is not associated with immunodeficiency.
D. Quebec platelet syndrome.
Rationale: Quebec platelet syndrome is not associated with immunodeficiency.
E. Wiskott-Aldrich syndrome.
Rationale: Wiskott-Aldrich syndrome is associated with immunodeficiency.

Major points of discussion
- Wiskott-Aldrich syndrome presents with thrombocytopenia, small platelets, eczema, and immunodeficiency.
- Estimated number of cases worldwide: less than 1000.
- X-linked inheritance; genetic defect: *WAS* gene.[4,9]
- Bleeding manifestations: bruising and purpura in the neonatal period with an increased risk of intracranial hemorrhage and bleeding after circumcision.
- Eczema develops during first year of life.
- Immunodeficiency is manifested by infections (most commonly bacterial) that occur in the first 6 months of life.
- Confirmatory molecular diagnosis is obtained by analyzing the *WAS* gene.

33. A. 2,3-dinor TxB$_2$.
Rationale: 2,3-dinor TxB$_2$ is formed by β-oxidation of TxA$_2$. Compared with 11-dehydro-TxB$_2$, it has a shorter half-life and is present in smaller amounts in urine.
B. 11-dehydro-TxB$_2$.
Rationale: 11-dehydro-TxB$_2$ is formed by dehydrogenation of TxB$_2$. Compared with 2,3-dinor TxB2, it is more abundant in urine and has a longer half-life.
C. Prostaglandin G$_2$.
Rationale: Prostaglandin G$_2$ is rapidly converted to PGH$_2$ by prostaglandin G/H synthase.
D. TxA$_2$.
Rationale: TxA$_2$ is rapidly hydrolyzed to TxB$_2$.
E. TxB$_2$.
Rationale: TxB$_2$ is rapidly metabolized and only a small fraction is excreted into urine. It is also produced during storage of blood samples.

Major points of discussion
- Platelet activation (e.g., by GPIbα:vWF binding) is thought to produce arachidonic acid from membrane phospholipids through the action of phospholipase A2.
- Cyclooxygenase is required to convert arachidonic acid to prostaglandin G$_2$, which is then quickly converted to PGH$_2$. PGH$_2$ is then converted to TxA$_2$ by Tx synthase.
- TxA$_2$ is rapidly hydrolyzed to form TxB$_2$, which is also rapidly metabolized and cleared from the circulation.
- Clinically, measuring TxA$_2$ metabolites has been used to assess the effectiveness of aspirin therapy. If aspirin therapy is effective in inhibiting cyclooxygenase, then TxA$_2$ levels should be significantly reduced.
- TxB$_2$ is mainly metabolized into 11-dehydro-TxB$_2$ and 2,3-dinor-TxB$_2$. Small amounts of both are excreted in the urine unchanged.
- TxB$_2$ is also formed during blood storage, so it is not a useful marker for TxA$_2$ formation.
- 11-dehydro- TxB$_2$ and 2,3-dinor-TxB$_2$ are found in urine and can be measured as markers of TxA$_2$ formation. 11-dehydro-TxB$_2$ is considered the better marker because of its longer half-life, greater abundance in urine, and less variability.[7]

34. A. Aspirin therapy.
Rationale: Aspirin irreversibly inhibits cyclooxygenase, which leads to impaired TxA2 production, and platelet aggregation is inhibited. The secondary wave of aggregation is usually missing after ADP or epinephrine agonists. Collagen aggregation is impaired. Ristocetin aggregation is unaffected.
B. BS syndrome.
Rationale: BS syndrome is the absence of the GPIb/V/IX complex, which leads to defective binding of vWF. Ristocetin aggregation is absent, but ADP, epinephrine, and collagen all induce aggregation.
C. Clopidogrel therapy.
Rationale: Clopidogrel inhibits the P2Y$_{12}$ receptor, which is the main receptor for ADP. Aggregation with ADP should not be present.
D. Glanzmann thrombasthenia.
Rationale: Glanzmann thrombasthenia is a disorder of GPIIb/IIIa. Aggregation with ADP, epinephrine, and collagen are absent, and ristocetin-induced aggregation is normal.
E. von Willebrand disease, type III.
Rationale: von Willebrand disease, type III shows the absence of vWF multimers. Ristocetin would not induce aggregation.

Major points of discussion
- Platelet activation (e.g., GPIbα:vWF binding) is thought to produce arachidonic acid from membrane phospholipids through the action of phospholipase A2.
- Cyclooxygenase is required for converting arachidonic acid to prostaglandin G2, which is then quickly converted to PGH2. PGH2 is then converted to Tx (TxA2) by Tx synthase.
- TxA2 binds to the thromboxane receptor by an autocrine or paracrine mechanism. TxA2 is essential for recruiting additional platelets into the nascent clot.

- Aspirin irreversibly inhibits cyclooxygenase by acetylation of a serine residue and strongly inhibits platelet function. NSAIDs reversibly inhibit cyclooxygenase and may transiently inhibit platelet function.
- Aspirin is effective for primary and secondary prophylaxis against myocardial infarction and cerebrovascular ischemic events.

35. A. Amphotericin.
Rationale: Amphotericin is a common cause of drug-induced thrombocytopenia.
B. Furosemide.
Rationale: Furosemide has been implicated as a cause of drug-induced thrombocytopenia.
C. Piperacillin/tazobactam.
Rationale: Piperacillin/tazobactam is a common cause of drug-induced thrombocytopenia.
D. Romiplostim.
Rationale: Romiplostim is a TPO analog that stimulates platelet production.
E. Tacrolimus.
Rationale: Tacrolimus is a cause of drug-induced thrombocytopenia, including TTP.

Major points of discussion

- Thrombocytosis can be reactive or due to a myeloproliferative disorder. Platelet counts can reach up to and exceed 1 million/μL.
- Reactive causes of thrombocytosis include infection, inflammation, splenectomy, hyposplenism, surgery, and iron deficiency anemia.
- Thrombocytosis can also be caused by myeloproliferative disorders such as essential thrombocytosis, polycythemia vera, and chronic myelogenous leukemia.
- TPO agonists such as eltrombopag and romiplostim, which are used to treat chronic refractory ITP, can lead to thrombocytosis.
- Reactive thrombocytosis is generally not treated because it does not increase the risk of thrombosis.
- Thrombocytosis due to a myeloproliferative disorder increases the risk of thrombosis at very high platelet counts (e.g., >1 million/μL). It is treated with aspirin, hydroxyurea, or anagrelide or with plateletpheresis as single or combination therapy.

36. A. *BCR-ABL* fusion gene.
Rationale: The Philadelphia chromosome results in the *BCR-ABL* fusion gene; it is associated with chronic myelogenous leukemia.
B. *EPO* mutation.
Rationale: Mutation of the EPO gene is not involved in the pathogenesis of essential thrombocythemia (ET).
C. *JAK2* V617F.
Rationale: *JAK2* V617F is found in 50% of patients with ET.
D. *MPL* mutation.
Rationale: *MPL* mutations are found in 4% of patients with ET.
E. *PML-RAR* fusion gene.
Rationale: The *PML-RAR* fusion gene is found in acute promyelocytic leukemia.

Major points of discussion

- Myeloproliferative disorders overproduce mature blood cells; in the case of ET, platelets are predominantly

overproduced; in polycythemia vera, red cells are overproduced.
- There is a high rate of thrombosis seen in patients with ET.
- According to the 2008 World Health Organization (WHO) guidelines, the diagnosis of ET requires the following:
  1. A platelet count greater than 450×10^9/L
  2. Megakaryocyte proliferation on bone marrow biopsy and/or aspirate; megakaryocytes must be enlarged and mature; an absence of granulopoiesis or erythropoiesis
  3. Not meeting WHO criteria for polycythemia vera, primary myelofibrosis, chronic myelogenous leukemia, myelodysplastic syndrome, or other myeloid disorder
  4. Demonstration of the *JAK2* V617F mutation or no evidence of reactive thrombocytosis in the absence of a clonal marker
- Patients with ET can be asymptomatic or they can present with vasomotor symptoms (e.g., headache, light-headedness, syncope). More serious complications result from thrombosis or hemorrhage. Although the platelet count is increased, the platelets that are produced do not function normally, which increases the risk for bleeding.
- The normal function of the JH2 (Janus homology 2) domain is to negatively regulate the JH1 (Janus homology 1) catalytic domain. The *JAK2* V617F mutation is located in the JH2 autoinhibitory domain, which leads to autonomous JAK2 function.
- The *JAK2* V617F mutation is present in 50% of patients with ET; 4% of patients have *MPL* mutations (i.e., in the TPO receptor).[25]

37. A. Macrothrombocytes.
Rationale: Large platelets can be counted as red cells, causing a falsely low platelet count.
B. Microclots.
Rationale: Platelets can become part of microclots, causing a falsely low platelet count.
C. Platelet satellitism.
Rationale: Platelets can adhere to the periphery of white cells, causing a falsely low platelet count.
D. Pseudothrombocytopenia (PTCP).
Rationale: PTCP, caused by anti-EDTA/platelet antibodies, results in the formation of platelet clumps. This causes a falsely low platelet count.
E. Schistocytes.
Rationale: Schistocytes, which are red cell fragments created by mechanical shear stress, can be small enough to be counted as platelets by impedance-based analyzers. This causes a falsely elevated platelet count.

Major points of discussion

- Impedance-based automated hematology analyzers enumerate platelets by passing blood through an electrical field. As cells pass through the electrical field, they act as a dielectric and deflect the field. The area of the deflection is proportional to the size of the cell, and the number of cells per volume is determined by the total number of such deflections.
- The cell count is determined by creating a histogram of cell frequency (*y*-axis) versus the cell size (*x*-axis). In

general, platelets range from 2 to 20 fL in size (this is instrument dependent); therefore, the area under the curve from 2 to 20 fL is the platelet count. Red cells can be enumerated by performing the same calculations between roughly 50 and 250 fL in size.

- The mean platelet volume is the average of the distribution from 2 to 20 fL.
- Microorganisms, extracellular parasites (e.g., Babesia), cytoplasmic cell fragments (e.g., in acute myeloid leukemia), schistocytes (e.g., in burns, TTP), and severely microcytic red cells can be counted as platelets. These could cause falsely elevated platelet counts.
- Optical measurement of platelets is an alternative to impedance counting. Optical counting may include a fluorescent dye to help distinguish platelets from other cell types and particles. For example, schistocytes would be the size of a platelet but would not fluorescently stain like a platelet. Therefore, these two populations can be separated.[16,26]

38. A. Babesiosis.
Rationale: Extracellular *Babesia* can be mistaken for normal platelets. These organisms usually measure 1 to 2 μm, whereas giant platelets are larger than 10 μm.
B. Gray platelet syndrome.
Rationale: Platelets in gray platelet syndrome are usually normal in size but can be enlarged. However, the platelets lack the basophilic granules, which gives them a hypogranular, gray, amorphous appearance.
C. Myelodysplastic syndrome.
Rationale: Giant platelets are associated with various conditions, including myelodysplastic syndrome and leukemias.
D. Pseudothrombocytopenia.
Rationale: In pseudothrombocytopenia, many agglutinated platelets are seen; these agglutinates should not be mistaken for giant platelets.
E. Wiskott-Aldrich syndrome.
Rationale: Wiskott-Aldrich syndrome is associated with thrombocytopenia and small platelets.

Major points of discussion
- Giant platelets are 10 to 20 μm in diameter. They are larger than a normal red cell or a normal lymphocyte nucleus.
- The cytoplasm can be blue-gray with bluish granules on Wright-Giemsa stain. The periphery may be scalloped or ruffled.
- Giant platelets can be mistaken for reticulocytes (polychromatophilic red cells), non–megakaryocyte cell fragments (e.g., cytoplasmic fragments of blast cells), neutrophils, megakaryocytes, and agglutinated platelets.
- Giant platelets are associated with various acquired and inherited diseases. Most of them are premalignant or malignant (e.g., myelodysplastic syndrome, acute leukemia, multiple myeloma). They can also be formed as a physiologic response to splenectomy, hemorrhage, and ITP.
- Inherited disorders associated with giant platelets include BS syndrome, the May-Hegglin anomaly, and familial macrothrombocytopenia.
- Small platelets are seen in Wiskott-Aldrich syndrome, an X-linked immune deficiency associated with eczema and thrombocytopenia.

39. A. Maternal platelets.
Rationale: Maternal platelets will lack the antigen to which the maternal antibody is directed against. However, the plasma will contain maternal antibodies that would be transfused along with the platelets. Some transfusion medicine physicians recommend volume reducing or washing the maternal platelets before transfusion.
B. Whole blood–derived random donor platelets.
Rationale: Random donor platelets would most likely carry the antigen implicated in NAIT.
C. Paternal platelets.
Rationale: Paternal platelets will express the antigen that immunized the mother of the newborn. Therefore, they are a poor choice for transfusion.
D. Single-donor platelets.
E. Washed single-donor platelets.
Rationale: Single-donor platelets will most likely carry the antigen implicated in NAIT. The plasma from such a donor is unlikely to contain the antiplatelet antibodies implicated in NAIT; therefore, washing would not be useful. There is also some concern that washing platelets decreases their number and functionality.

Major points of discussion
- NAIT can occur when the mother does not express a high-frequency platelet antigen (e.g., HPA-1a) and the fetus expresses the antigen inherited from the father. Maternal alloimmunization can occur from a previous pregnancy or the current pregnancy. The maternal antiplatelet antibodies can be transferred across the placenta and cause severe thrombocytopenia in the fetus/neonate.
- NAIT is a cause of severe fetal/neonatal thrombocytopenia that can lead to severe bleeding, including intracranial hemorrhage and death. The greatest risk in neonates is during the first 96 hours after birth and generally resolves after 2 weeks. However, most cases of intracranial hemorrhage occur in utero.
- If the antibody specificity is known, then platelets can be obtained from rare platelet donors who do not express the corresponding antigen. Approximately 95% of cases are caused by maternal alloimmunization to the HPA-1, -2, -3, -5, or -15 antigens. Anti-HPA-1a is the most commonly detected antibody.
- Laboratory testing that shows maternal serum reacting with paternal platelets in the presence of a negative HLA class I antibody screen supports the presence of an anti-HPA antibody. If the reaction of maternal serum is against a large number of random donor platelets, then an antibody against a high-frequency platelet antigen should be considered.
- Another cause of severe fetal/neonatal thrombocytopenia that should be considered is the transplacental transfer of maternal antiplatelet autoantibodies in a mother with idiopathic thrombocytopenic purpura. In this case, the maternal platelet count would also be low.
- Although maternal antigen-negative platelets are an optimal source for transfusing the affected neonate, if they are not available, then random donor platelets (apheresis- or whole blood–derived) would be the next best choice for emergently providing platelets to treat bleeding. Nonetheless, attempts to provide antigen-negative donor platelets should be made.[1]

40. **A. 3.2% sodium citrate, light-blue top tube.**
Rationale: Sodium citrate is a weak calcium chelator and is the anticoagulant of choice for platelet function studies.
B. K$_2$-ethylenediaminetetraacetic acid (K$_2$EDTA), purple top tube.
Rationale: K$_2$EDTA is a strong calcium chelator and is not used in platelet function studies.
C. Lithium heparin, green top tube.
Rationale: Heparin affects platelets by decreasing the response to epinephrine and collagen agonists. In addition, spontaneous aggregation can occur due to the presence of physiological concentrations of calcium in the anticoagulant.
D. No additive, red top tube.
E. Serum separator, gold top tube.
Rationale: Clotting in these tubes will consume platelets.

Major points of discussion

- Platelet function studies by light transmission aggregometry require an anticoagulated sample to prepare PRP and platelet-poor plasma.
- Samples are drawn into 3.2% sodium citrate anticoagulant in a ratio of 9 parts whole blood to 1 part sodium citrate. Sodium citrate is a weak chelator of calcium and inhibits clotting. However, some unbound calcium remains available for platelet aggregation.
- EDTA cannot be used for this purpose because it binds 10 times more calcium than sodium citrate, making calcium less available, which will blunt platelet aggregation responses. Heparin has physiological levels of calcium and spontaneous platelet aggregation can occur. Acid-citrate-dextrose (ACD) has a low pH, which decreases platelet aggregation. Therefore, these anticoagulants should not be used.
- Anticoagulant levels should be adjusted if the hematocrit (HCT) is elevated because the decreased plasma volume leads to over-anticoagulation of the sample. Some unbound calcium is required for platelet aggregation to occur.
- Anticoagulant volume $= (1.85 \times 10^{-3})(100 - \text{HCT}_{percent})(V_{blood})$.
- Samples should be prepared and analyzed within 4 hours of sample collection, preferably in less than 2 hours, because platelets undergo activation during prolonged storage.[8,14]

41. A. Perform apheresis immediately.
B. Perform apheresis followed by hydroxyurea treatment.
C. Treat with hydroxyurea.
Rationale: Apheresis and hydroxyurea do not a have a role in treating reactive thrombocytosis.
D. No additional therapy is necessary.
Rationale: Reactive thrombocytosis is not associated with an increased risk of thrombosis. Thrombocytosis caused by myeloproliferative disorders does require treatment when platelet counts are in the range of 1 million/μL or higher.
E. Perform a splenectomy.
Rationale: Splenectomy does not a have a role in reactive thrombocytosis.

Major points of discussion

- Thrombocytosis is associated with myeloproliferative disorders such as chronic myelogenous leukemia, polycythemia vera, and essential thrombocytosis.
- Secondary thrombocytosis is a reactive response to bacterial and viral infection, surgery, trauma, iron deficiency, and inflammatory states.
- Other causes of secondary thrombocytosis include rebound after chemotherapy or splenectomy.
- Secondary thrombocytosis rarely requires intervention because it is not associated with an increased risk of thrombosis.
- Because they are associated with an increased risk of thrombosis, high platelet counts in patients with primary thrombocytosis are treated with cytoreductive therapy (e.g., hydroxyurea), aspirin, and/or plateletpheresis.[6,26]

42. **A. DIC.**
Rationale: The absence of coagulation abnormalities is less consistent with DIC than with TTP. Although the PT, aPTT, and fibrinogen can be normal in DIC, more often the consumption of coagulation factors leads to a prolonged PT and aPTT, as well as to low fibrinogen levels.
B. Drug-induced thrombocytopenia.
Rationale: Medications are a common cause of thrombocytopenia and should always be considered as an explanation. However, in this case, medications alone do not explain the microangiopathic hemolytic anemia along with the thrombocytopenia.
C. ITP.
Rationale: ITP presents with thrombocytopenia in the absence of other hematologic abnormalities (e.g., anemia, leukopenia). Therefore, the presence of microangiopathic hemolytic anemia in this case is not consistent with ITP.
D. TTP.
Rationale: TTP is a microangiopathic hemolytic anemia that presents with hemolytic anemia with schistocytes on the peripheral blood smear and thrombocytopenia. Classically, TTP is accompanied by mental status changes, fever, and renal failure, but these three findings may not always be present. In this case, the TTP is drug induced (i.e., by tacrolimus).
E. Warm autoimmune hemolytic anemia (WAIHA).
Rationale: WAIHA alone does not present with low platelets or schistocytes.

Major points of discussion

- The laboratory studies show a microangiopathic hemolytic anemia (i.e., low hemoglobin, elevated reticulocytes, low haptoglobin, elevated bilirubin and LDH, and schistocytes) and thrombocytopenia. In the absence of DIC, the most likely diagnosis is TTP.
- TTP is classically associated with a pentad of signs/symptoms: fever, mental status changes, microangiopathic hemolytic anemia, thrombocytopenia, and renal failure. However, all five findings may not be present in all cases.
- Congenital TTP is caused by an inherited deficiency of the ADAMTS13 enzyme. ADAMTS13 cleaves ultralarge multimers of vWF. A deficiency in ADAMTS13 leads to an excess of ultralarge VWF multimers, platelet thrombi, and shear stress of red cells that leads to hemolysis. Simple plasma infusion can replace the enzyme in congenital TTP.
- Idiopathic TTP is caused by an autoantibody against ADAMTS13 that leads to its deficiency. Subsequently, ultralarge VWF multimers and platelet thrombi form,

which causes hemolysis by the shearing of red cells. The treatment of choice in antibody-mediated TTP is plasmapheresis using fresh frozen plasma as the replacement fluid. This procedure removes the autoantibody from the circulation and provides ADAMTS13 in the plasma replacement fluid. Immunosuppressants, usually steroids, are administered to inhibit antibody production.

■ Drug-induced TTP is caused by multiple medications; cyclosporine, tacrolimus, clopidogrel, mitomycin C, and gemcitabine are the ones most commonly reported. Treatment requires the cessation of the medication inducing the TTP. Although plasmapheresis is often used, it may not be beneficial in drug-induced TTP.[13]

43. A. *CYP2C19*2.*
Rationale: Clopidogrel metabolism to its active metabolite is slower with the *2 or *3 polymorphisms of the p450 enzyme gene *CYP2C19*.
B. *CYP1A1.*
Rationale: This gene encodes the enzyme that metabolizes the R isomer of warfarin into its inactive metabolites.
C. *CYP2C9*1.*
Rationale: CYP2C9 metabolizes *S*-warfarin to its inactive metabolites.
D. *UGT1A6* T181A A>G.
Rationale: UGT1A6 encodes for UDP-glucuronosyl-transferase 1A6, which metabolizes aspirin.
E. *VKORC1* GG.
Rationale: The *VKORC1* gene encodes the vitamin K epoxide reductase complex involved in vitamin K recycling and warfarin anticoagulation.

Major points of discussion
■ ADP released from activated platelets can bind to the $P2Y_1$ or the $P2Y_{12}$ receptors to activate other platelets. The $P2Y_{12}$ receptor, when bound to ADP, is the more potent activator of platelets.
■ Clopidogrel is a $P2Y_{12}$ antagonist that is commonly used as an antiplatelet agent for secondary prophylaxis after an acute ischemic cardiovascular or cerebrovascular event.
■ Clopidogrel is metabolized to an active metabolite that has the antiplatelet activity. It is metabolized to its active form by the P450 enzyme CYP2C19.
■ Polymorphisms in the *CYP2C19* gene are associated with "normal" or "slow" metabolism of clopidogrel to its active form. *CYP2C19*1* encodes the protein with normal clopidogrel metabolism, whereas *CYP2C19*2* or *3* is associated with slower metabolism.
■ Patients receiving clopidogrel for secondary prophylaxis against stroke or myocardial infarction may still have an event. Some of these cases may be due to inadequate clopidogrel-induced platelet inhibition (clopidogrel resistance) due to reduced clopidogrel metabolism.

44. A. 1.
Rationale: This is equivalent to approximately 20×10^9/L.
B. 2.
Rationale: This is equivalent to approximately 40×10^9/L.
C. 5.
Rationale: This is equivalent to approximately 100×10^9/L.
D. 10.
Rationale: This is equivalent to approximately 200×10^9/L.

E. 20.
Rationale: This is equivalent to approximately 400×10^9/L.

Major points of discussion
■ The gold standard method for counting platelets is the Neubauer chamber manual counting method. However, it is an imprecise method with high intra- and interoperator variability.
■ The Fonio method for estimating platelets is based on review of a peripheral blood smear using a light microscope. Using a ×10 ocular and ×100 objective lens, the average number of platelets per HPF can be determined. The platelet estimate is [(20) × (average number of platelets per HPF)].
■ If there are 10 platelets per HPF, then the platelet estimate using the Fonio method would be 200×10^9/L.
■ Modern hematology analyzers measure the platelet count using impedance-, optical-, fluorescence-, or antibody-based methods.
■ Automated analyzers are more accurate, reproducible, and less labor intensive than manual methods.

45. A. Anticoagulation with unfractionated heparin.
Rationale: Anticoagulation with unfractionated heparin for a remote history of HIT with negative immunologic and functional assays for HIT is recommended for patients undergoing cardiovascular surgery.
B. Anticoagulation with bivalirudin.
Rationale: In patients with acute HIT and positive immunologic and functional assay results for HIT, delay of cardiovascular surgery until assay results are negative is recommended. However, bivalirudin can be administered if surgery cannot be delayed.
C. Anticoagulation with argatroban.
Rationale: In patients with remote HIT undergoing percutaneous coronary intervention and who have negative immunologic and functional assay results for HIT, a nonheparin alternate anticoagulant can be used (e.g., bivalirudin, argatroban, danaparoid).
D. Cancel surgery indefinitely.
Rationale: Cardiovascular surgery can be performed with remote HIT and negative immunologic and functional assay results for HIT. Alternatively, bivalirudin can be used if surgery cannot be delayed.
E. Delay surgery until anti-heparin/platelet factor-4 IgG, IgA, and IgM ELISA is performed.
Rationale: Delaying surgery until anti-heparin/platelet factor-4 IgG, IgA, IgM ELISA is negative when the IgG assay result is already negative will not change anticoagulation management for this patient.

Major points of discussion
■ HIT is an immune complication of heparin therapy that can lead to life-threatening arterial and venous thrombosis.
■ HIT is characterized by a drop in the platelet count by approximately 50% within 5 to 10 days of the initiation of heparin therapy and can be associated with the development of thrombosis.
■ The anti-heparin/PF4 ELISA assay result is often used to screen for the antibodies implicated in causing HIT. Although this assay is highly sensitive, it has poor specificity. The serotonin release assay is a functional assay that assesses the presence of anti-heparin/PF4

antibodies that can activate platelets. This assay has high sensitivity and specificity (98% and 95%, respectively).

- If a patient has a remote history of HIT with negative immunologic and functional assay results for HIT, unfractionated heparin can be used for cardiovascular surgery.
- If a patient has acute HIT with positive immunologic and functional assays for HIT, unfractionated heparin should not be used for cardiovascular surgery. Surgery can be delayed until the assay results are negative and then unfractionated heparin can be used. If surgery cannot be delayed, then an agent such as bivalirudin can be used as an alternate anticoagulant.[17]

46. A. Azathioprine.
Rationale: Azathioprine is not recommended as a first-line treatment in a pregnant patient with ITP.
B. Cyclophosphamide.
Rationale: Cyclophosphamide is cytotoxic and teratogenic and should not be used in pregnancy.
C. Corticosteroids.
Rationale: Corticosteroids or intravenous immunoglobulin are the first-line treatments of ITP in pregnancy.
D. Rituximab.
Rationale: Rituximab is a second-line treatment for ITP.
E. Splenectomy.
Rationale: Splenectomy is a second-line treatment and surgery can be difficult because the gravid uterus presents a large obstacle.

Major points of discussion

- ITP is a clinical diagnosis of exclusion. Patients present with isolated low platelet counts without abnormalities in the red cell and white cell lineages. Other causes of thrombocytopenia should be excluded. For example, PTCP should be excluded by examining the peripheral blood smear. In ITP, the bone marrow biopsy shows normal erythropoiesis and myelopoiesis and increased megakaryocytes.
- ITP is caused by autoantibodies against platelet antigens. The antibody-coated platelets are cleared by the reticuloendothelial system. Recent evidence suggests that there is a concomitant platelet production defect.
- First-line treatment of ITP in adults includes corticosteroids, intravenous immunoglobulin (IVIG), and intravenous Rh immune globulin in Rh-positive patients. A longer course of corticosteroids is preferred over a shorter course of corticosteroids or IVIG. IVIG and Rh immunoglobulin are preferred, if steroids are contraindicated (e.g., uncontrolled diabetes mellitus).
- Pregnant patients should be treated in the same manner as adult patients, so corticosteroids and IVIG are suggested as first-line treatments. However, randomized controlled trials in pregnant patients have not been performed.
- When pregnant patients with ITP are delivering, the method of delivery is based on the current recommendations for the obstetric indication.
- Neonates born to women with ITP are at increased risk of thrombocytopenia.[20]

47. A. Apheresis.
Rationale: Plasmapheresis is not used in the treatment of ITP.
B. Dapsone.

Rationale: Dapsone is a second-line treatment for ITP.
C. Corticosteroids.
Rationale: A long course of corticosteroids is the first choice for the treatment of ITP in adults with platelet count less than 30/μL.
D. Rituximab.
Rationale: Rituximab is a second-line treatment for ITP.
E. Splenectomy.
Rationale: Splenectomy is used for patients with ITP in whom corticosteroid therapy has failed. Aside from the morbidity and mortality from the surgical procedure, there is also the long-term risk of infection and sepsis from encapsulated bacteria such as *Meningococcus, Pneumococcus,* and *Haemophilus.*

Major points of discussion

- ITP is a clinical diagnosis of exclusion. Patients present with isolated low platelet counts without abnormalities in the red cell and white cell lineages. Other causes of thrombocytopenia should be excluded. For example, PTCP should be excluded by examining the peripheral blood smear.
- Bone marrow biopsy shows normal erythropoiesis and myelopoiesis and increased megakaryocytes.
- ITP is caused by autoantibodies against platelet antigens. The antibody-coated platelets are cleared by the reticuloendothelial system. Recent evidence suggests there is a concomitant platelet production defect.
- First-line treatment of ITP includes corticosteroids, IVIG, and intravenous Rh immune globulin in Rh-positive patients. A longer course of corticosteroids is preferred over a shorter course of corticosteroids or IVIG. IVIG and Rh immunoglobulin are preferred if steroids are contraindicated.
- Second-line treatments for patients unresponsive to first-line therapy include rituximab, dapsone, and splenectomy. Splenectomy is avoided in pediatric patients because of the long-term risk of sepsis from encapsulated bacteria such as *Meningococcus, Pneumococcus,* and *Haemophilus.*
- Platelet transfusion is generally not useful because the transfused platelets are cleared at the same rate as the patient's own platelets. However, if there is significant bleeding or bleeding risk, then platelet transfusion may be indicated.[20]

48. A. Fonio distribution.
Rationale: Fonio is a method for counting platelets, not a distribution of platelets.
B. Fourier transform of *t*-distribution.
Rationale: This is irrelevant for platelet counting.
C. Gaussian (normal) distribution.
Rationale: Red cells have a normal distribution when presented as a histogram.
D. Negatively (left) skewed distribution.
Rationale: Platelets do not have a left skewed distribution; it is right skewed.
E. Positively (right) skewed distribution.
Rationale: The platelet histogram is right skewed.

Major points of discussion

- Many hematology analyzers still use impedance-based methods to measure the platelet size and number. However, optical-, fluorescence-, and antibody-based methods are also used.

- The platelet distribution (histogram) provides information beyond just the platelet count. It provides the platelet distribution width (PDW; platelet anisocytosis), mean platelet volume (MPV; average size), and the total platelet count (area under the curve).
- The platelet distribution is positively (right) skewed. Taller on the left side (small particles) than the right side (larger particles) of the distribution.
- The mean platelet volume (MPV) can be calculated as: MPV (fL) = Platelet crit (%)/Platelet count (10^9/L).
- An increase in larger platelets would increase the right side of the platelet distribution and also increase the MPV. An increase in larger platelets suggests new platelet production after platelet destruction (e.g., immune thrombocytopenia, TTP) or marrow recovery (e.g., after bone marrow transplant).

49. A. HPA-1a.
Rationale: HPA-1a (or, equivalently, PLA1) is a common platelet antigen that is most often implicated in NAIT. Antibodies recognizing it account for up to 80% of serologically confirmed cases of NAIT.
B. HPA-1b.
Rationale: HPA-1b (or, equivalently, PLA2) is rarely implicated in NAIT.
C. HPA-2a.
Rationale: HPA-2a is implicated in fewer than 1% of NAIT cases.
D. HPA-3b.
Rationale: HPA-3b is rarely implicated in NAIT.
E. HPA-4a.
Rationale: HPA-4a is commonly implicated in NAIT in Asian populations, but is not the most common among all ethnic groups.

Major points of discussion
- NAIT is a disorder caused by maternal alloantibodies formed against platelet antigens of the fetus/neonate that were inherited from the father.
- Antiplatelet antibodies cross the placenta and lead to platelet clearance and fetal/neonatal thrombocytopenia.
- NAIT increases the risk of intracerebral hemorrhage in utero, perinatally, and postnatally.
- The platelet antigen HPA-1a (or, equivalently, PLA1) is most commonly implicated in NAIT.
- Diagnostic workup includes antigen phenotyping and/or genotyping of maternal, paternal, and fetal platelet antigens.
- Treatment may include fetal monitoring and intrauterine or postdelivery platelet transfusion with antigen-negative platelets (often collected from the mother).[1]

50. A. GPIIb/IIIa.
Rationale: GPIIb/IIIa on platelets binds to vWF and fibrinogen to mediate platelet aggregation.
B. GPVI.
Rationale: GPVI on platelets binds to collagen and mediates platelet adhesion under low shear stress.
C. P2X1.
Rationale: ATP binds to the P2X1 receptor and increases intracellular calcium.
D. P2Y$_{12}$.
Rationale: ADP binds to the platelet P2Y$_{12}$ and the P2Y$_1$ receptors to mediate platelet activation.

E. Protease-activated receptor 1 (PAR-1).
Rationale: The most potent activator of platelets is mediated by the thrombin–PAR-1 interaction.

Major points of discussion
- Platelets interact with their environment using numerous receptors for vWF, fibrinogen, thrombin, ADP, ATP, Tx, serotonin, and others to mediate platelet plug formation.
- Adhesion is mediated by platelet GPIbα binding to subendothelial vWF and platelet GPVI binding to subendothelial collagen.
- Aggregation is mediated by platelet GPIIb/IIIa binding to fibrinogen and vWF.
- Platelets are also activated when specific receptors are bound to their ligands—for example: ADP-P2Y$_{12}$ or P2Y1; ATP-P2X1; serotonin-serotonin receptor; thromboxane-thromboxane receptor; epinephrine–α-adrenergic receptor, and so on.
- Thrombin is the most potent activator of platelets via the PAR-1 and PAR-4 receptors. Thrombin activates the platelet by irreversibly cleaving the first extracellular loop of the PAR, leading to a tethered ligand.
- Antiplatelet pharmaceuticals have been used for primary and secondary prophylaxis of acute myocardial infarction and cerebrovascular accidents (e.g., clopidogrel-P2Y12).

51. A. Aspirin, 325 mg per day.
Rationale: Therapeutic aspirin effect would show a prolonged closure time with collagen (Col) and epinephrine (Epi; Col/Epi) and a normal closure time with Col/ADP.
B. BS syndrome.
Rationale: Both Col/Epi and Col/ADP would be prolonged in BS syndrome.
C. Glanzmann thrombasthenia.
Rationale: Both Col/Epi and Col/ADP would be prolonged in Glanzmann thrombasthenia.
D. Gray platelet syndrome.
Rationale: Both Col/Epi and Col/ADP would be prolonged in gray platelet syndrome
E. Scott syndrome.
Rationale: Scott syndrome is a disorder of platelet procoagulant activity caused by defective exposure of platelet membrane phosphatidyl serine upon platelet activation.

Major points of discussion
- The PFA-100 platelet function analyzer is a whole blood–based test that measures platelet function under conditions similar to in vivo conditions of high shear stress flow. It is a commonly used test for screening for von Willebrand disease and platelet function disorders.
- In this test, whole blood flows through an orifice coated with collagen and a platelet agonist (Epi or ADP) under high shear stress. As platelets adhere to the orifice and become activated, a platelet plug is formed and closes the orifice.
- The time it takes for a sample to close the orifice is called the closure time. A normal closure time with Col/Epi and Col/ADP suggests normal platelet function.

- However, the PFA-100 test may not be sensitive enough to detect mild von Willebrand disease and mild platelet function disorders.
- Scott syndrome is a disorder of platelet procoagulant activity caused by defective exposure of platelet membrane phosphatidyl serine upon platelet activation. In this disorder, the PFA-100 closure time would be expected to be normal for both the Col/Epi and Col/ADP cartridges.

52. A. 10^6
B. 10^9
C. 10^{11}
D. 10^{12}
E. 10^{15}
Rationale: Approximately 10^{11} platelets are produced by an adult on a daily basis under normal, physiologic conditions.

Major points of discussion

- The lifespan of a platelet is approximately 7 to 10 days.
- Production of platelets can increase approximately 10-fold under physiologic stress.
- TPO is a factor that stimulates megakaryocytes to produce additional platelets.
- TPO analogs, such as eltrombopag and romiplostim, can be used to stimulate platelet production.

53. A. Minimal bleeding from superficial cuts.
Rationale: Persistent bleeding from superficial cuts is characteristic of platelet disorders.
B. Deep muscle hematomas.
Rationale: Deep hematomas are characteristic of coagulation factor deficiencies.
C. Delayed bleeding.
Rationale: Delayed postoperative bleeding is characteristic of coagulation factor deficiencies.
D. Hemarthrosis.
Rationale: Joint bleeding is characteristic of coagulation factor deficiencies.
E. Petechiae.
Rationale: Petechiae are seen in platelet-type bleeding.

Major points of discussion

- Platelet-type bleeding is characterized by petechiae, persistent bleeding from superficial cuts, menorrhagia, and mucosal bleeding, such as gum bleeding and epistaxis.
- Coagulation disorders are characterized by deep hematomas, minimal bleeding from superficial cuts, hemarthroses, and delayed postoperative bleeding.
- Platelet disorders are more commonly seen in women than men. Coagulation disorders are more commonly seen in men because of the sex-linked inheritance.
- von Willebrand disease is a quantitative or qualitative disorder of vWF. Platelet function is normal, but bleeding characteristic of a platelet disorder is seen (e.g., mucosal bleeding, epistaxis, petechiae, menorrhagia). This is due to the impaired ability of platelets to adhere to the subendothelium in the absence of vWF.
- In severe von Willebrand disease, factor VIII levels can be decreased and bleeding characteristic of a coagulation factor deficiency can be seen. This is due to the decreased stability of factor VIII in the absence of vWF.

54. A. Erythropoietin (EPO).
Rationale: EPO is an essential factor for red cell production and initiates its action by binding to EpoR (the EPO receptor).
B. Granulocyte colony-stimulating factor (G-CSF).
Rationale: G-CSF stimulates the proliferation and maturation of cells of the neutrophil lineage. It binds to the G-CSF receptor.
C. PDGF.
Rationale: PDGF stimulates mesenchymal cell proliferation and signals through the PDGF receptor α and β subunits.
D. Signal transducer and activator of transcription-1 (STAT-1).
Rationale: STAT-1 is a downstream target involved in intracellular signaling. It is not an extracellular ligand.
E. TPO.
Rationale: TPO is the ligand for the *c-mpl* gene product, the TPO receptor. It stimulates platelet production by acting on megakaryocytes and platelets.

Major points of discussion

- TPO stimulates megakaryocyte proliferation and differentiation, as well as platelet production.
- TPO is the ligand for CD110, the TPO receptor. The *c-mpl* gene encodes the CD110 protein.
- After binding TPO, CD110 forms dimers, leading to phosphorylation and activation of CD110, Janus kinases (JAKs), signal transducers and activators of transcription (STATs), and other downstream pathways, including mitogen-activated protein (MAP) kinases.
- Liver parenchymal and endothelial cells, as well as bone marrow stromal cells, are the main sites of TPO production.
- A recombinant form of TPO was used as a pharmaceutical, but trials were stopped when study volunteers developed anti-TPO autoantibodies and subsequent thrombocytopenia.
- Current TPO mimetics stimulate the TPO receptor but are not structurally related to TPO. Therefore, autoantibodies recognizing TPO are not a long-term complication.
- However, the TPO mimetics have long-term side effects of thromboembolism, hepatic toxicity, and bone marrow reticulin deposition.
- TPO mimetics are used as a second-line treatment for chronic immune thrombocytopenia when there is a risk of bleeding.

55. **A. Bone marrow reticulin deposition.**
Rationale: TPO mimetics may increase the risk or progression of bone marrow reticulin deposition.
B. Berry aneurysms with intracranial hemorrhage.
Rationale: TPO mimetics are not associated with aneurysms or bleeding. However, they can be associated with thromboembolic complications.
C. Pancreatitis.
Rationale: TPO mimetics can cause hepatotoxicity but are not known to be a risk for pancreatitis.
D. Portal vein aneurysms.
Rationale: Portal vein thrombosis, but not aneurysms, can be seen with TPO mimetics.
E. Retinal detachment.
Rationale: Cataracts may increase with TPO mimetics, but retinal detachment is not a complication.

Major points of discussion

- TPO mimetics, such as eltrombopag and romiplostim, stimulate megakaryocytes to produce platelets.
- These agents are used as a second-line treatment of chronic ITP when patients do not respond to treatment with corticosteroids, intravenous globulins, or splenectomy and when there is a risk of bleeding. They should not be used solely to normalize platelet counts.
- TPO mimetics can also be used to increase the platelet count in patients with hepatitis C so they qualify to receive α-interferon.
- Long-term complications of therapy include hepatotoxicity, thromboembolism, increased blast counts, and cataracts.
- TPO mimetics can either initiate or worsen bone marrow deposition of reticulin-type collagen. They should not be used in patients with myelodysplastic syndrome.[2]

56. A. ADAMTS13.
   B. Factor VIII.
   C. Fibronectin.
   D. Tx A2.
   Rationale: ADAMTS13, factor VIII, fibronectin, and TxA$_2$ are not stored in endothelial Weibel-Palade bodies.

E. vWF.
Rationale: vWF and P-selectin are stored in Weibel-Palade bodies.[24]

Major points of discussion

- Weibel-Palade bodies are secretory organelles found in endothelial cells.
- They appear as oval or elongated organelles with a whorled or fingerprint-like appearance on electron microscopy.
- Weibel-Palade bodies store vWF and P-selectin. vWF participates in primary hemostasis by binding platelets to the subendothelium and also stabilizes factor VIII in the plasma. P-Selectin participates in leukocyte adhesion.
- Qualitative or qualitative disorders of vWF can lead to a mild to severe bleeding disorder known as von Willebrand disease.
- Other proteins contained in Weibel-Palade bodies include interleukin 8, endothelin, and tissue plasminogen activator.
- Desmopressin-induced increase in VWF is most likely due to the direct release of multimeric vWF from Weibel Palade bodies.

References

1. Arnold DM, Smith JW, Kelton JG. Diagnosis and management of neonatal alloimmune thrombocytopenia. Transf Med Rev 2008;22:255–267.
2. Basciano PA, Bussell JB. Thrombopoietin-receptor agonists. Curr Opin Hematol 2012;19:392–398.
3. Bizzaro N, Brandalise M. EDTA-dependent pseudothrombocytopenia. Association with antiplatelet and antiphospholipid antibodies. Am J Clin Pathol 1995;103–107.
4. Bolton-Maggs PH, Chalmers EA, Collins PW, et al. A review of inherited platelet disorders with guidelines for their management on behalf of the UKHCDO. Br J Haematol 2006;135:603–633.
5. Bremme KA. Haemostatic changes in pregnancy. Best Pract Res Clin Haematol 2003;16:153–168.
6. British Committee for Standards in Haematology. Guideline for investigation and management of adults and children presenting with a thrombocytosis. Br J Haematol 2010;149:352–375.
7. Catella F, Lawson JA, Fitzgerald DJ, et al. Analysis of multiple thromboxane metabolites in plasma and urine. Adv Prostaglandin Thromboxane Leukot Res 1987;17B:611–613.
8. Clinical Laboratory Standards Institute (CLSI). Platelet function testing by aggregometry; approved guideline. CLSI document H58-A.Wayne, PA: Clinical Laboratory Standards Institute, 2008.
9. D'Andrea G, Chetta M, Margaglione M. Inherited platelet disorders: thrombocytopenias and thrombocytopathies. Blood Transf 2009;7:278–292.
10. Favaloro EJ, Lippi G, Franchini M. Contemporary platelet function testing. Clin Chem Lab Med 2010;48:579–598.
11. Franchini M. Hemostasis and pregnancy Thromb Haemost 2006;95:401–413.
12. Geddis AE, Kaushansky K. Inherited thrombocytopenias: toward a molecular understanding of disorders of platelet production. Curr Opin Pediatr 2004;16:15–24.
13. George JN. How I, treat patients with thrombotic thrombocytopenic purpura-hemoytic uremic syndrome. Blood 2000;96:1223–1229.
14. Hayward CPM, Moffat KA, Raby A, et al. Development of North American consensus guidelines for medical laboratories that perform and interpret platelet function testing using light transmission aggregometry. Am J Clin Pathol 2010;134:955–963.
15. Jennings LK. Mechanisms of platelet activation: Need for new strategies to protect against platelet-mediated atherothrombosis. Thromb Haemost 2009;102:248–257.
16. Kickler TS. Clinical analyzers. Advances in automated cell counting. Analyt Chem 1999;71:363R–365R.
17. Linkins LA, Dans AL, Moores LK, et al. Treatment and prevention of heparin-induced thrombocytopenia:antithrombotic therapy and prevention of thrombosis, 9th ed. American College of Chest Physicians Evidence-based clinical practice guidelines Chest 2012;141(suppl):e495S–e530S.
18. Michelson AD. Platelet function testing in cardiovascular diseases. Circulation 2004;110:e489–e493.
19. Monteferrario D, Bolar NA, Marneth AE, et al. A dominant-negative GFI1B mutation in the gray platelet syndrome. N Engl J Med 2014;370:245–253.
20. Neunert C, Lim W, Crowther M, et al. The American Society of Hematology 2011 evidence-based practice guidelines for immune thrombocytopenia. Blood 2011;117:4190–4207.
21. Prechel M, Walenga JM. The laboratory diagnosis and clinical management of patients with heparin-induced thrombocytopenia: an update. Semin Thromb Hemost 2008;34:86–96.
22. Rechner AR. Platelet function testing in clinical diagnostics. Hamostaseologie 2011;31:79–87.
23. Sugiyama T, Okuma M, Ushikubi F, et al. A novel platelet aggregating factor found in a patient with defective collagen induced platelet aggregation and autoimmune thrombocytopenia. Blood 1987;69:1712–1720.
24. Valentijn KM, Sadler JE, Valentijn JA, et al. Functional architecture of Weibel-Palade bodies. Blood 2011;117:5033–5043.
25. Vannucchi AM, Guglielmelli P. JAK2 mutation-related disease and thrombosis. Semin Thromb Hemost 2013;39:496–506.
26. Vora AJ, Lilleyman JS. Secondary thrombocytosis. Arch Dis Child 1993;68:88–90.

CHAPTER **13**

BODY FLUIDS AND CLINICAL MICROSCOPY

Anjali Saqi

QUESTIONS

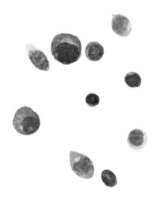

Figure 13-1 Diff-Quick stain of cerebrospinal fluid.

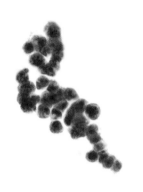

Figure 13-2 Papanicolaou stain of cerebrospinal fluid.

1. A patient underwent a lumbar puncture and cerebrospinal fluid (CSF) was obtained. No additional clinical history was provided. Based on the image in Figure 13-1, the patient would most likely have which one of the following?
   A. Normal findings.
   B. Bacterial meningitis.
   C. Aseptic meningitis.
   D. Parasitic infection.
   E. Lymphoma.

2. A 79-year-old woman with a history of breast carcinoma and smoking presented with multiple brain masses. Figure 13-2 shows the cells in the CSF obtained by lumbar puncture. These findings are most consistent with which one of the following diagnoses?
   A. Metastatic breast carcinoma.
   B. Metastatic lung small cell carcinoma.
   C. Metastatic melanoma.
   D. Metastatic lymphoma.
   E. Metastatic lung adenocarcinoma.

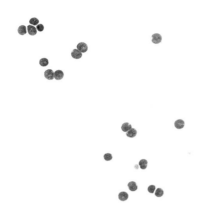

Figure 13-3   Diff-Quick stain of cerebrospinal fluid.

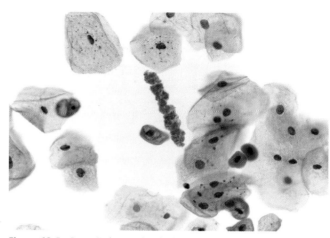

Figure 13-5   Papanicolaou stain of urine.

3. The CSF specimen in Figure 13-3, obtained by lumbar puncture from a 5-year-old boy, most likely represents which one of the following entities?
   A. Aseptic meningitis.
   B. Chronic lymphocytic leukemia/small lymphocytic lymphoma (CLL/SLL).
   C. Acute lymphoblastic leukemia (ALL).
   D. Medulloblastoma.
   E. Bacterial meningitis.

5. A 50-year-old man with no significant past medical history presented with microhematuria. The image in Figure 13-5 is from his voided urine cytology specimen. Which one of the following is the best diagnosis in this case?
   A. Granular cast.
   B. Hyaline inclusion body.
   C. Corpora amylacea.
   D. Trichomoniasis.
   E. Calcium oxalate crystal.

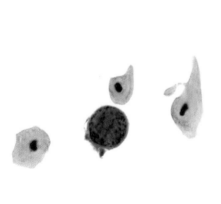

Figure 13-4   Papanicolaou stain of urine.

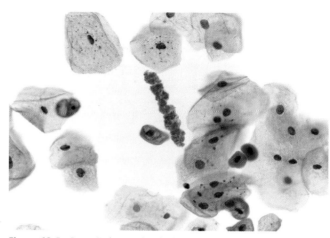

Figure 13-6   Papanicolaou stain of urine.

4. A 45-year-old man with a history of renal transplantation presented to his urologist for routine follow-up. The image in Figure 13-4 is from his voided urine cytology specimen. Which one of the following is the best diagnosis in this case?
   A. Positive for malignant cells; urothelial carcinoma.
   B. Positive for malignant cells; renal clear cell (conventional) carcinoma.
   C. Negative for malignant cells; polyomavirus infection.
   D. Negative for malignant cells; hyaline inclusion bodies.
   E. Negative for malignant cells; renal tubular cells.

6. A 39-year-old woman presented with symptoms of a urinary tract infection. A voided urine specimen was sent to the laboratory for further analysis. Several large cells were noted in the specimen, similar to the one seen in the center of Figure 13-6. Which one of the following is the best diagnosis for this type of cell?
   A. Endometrial cell.
   B. Squamous cell.
   C. Renal tubular cell.
   D. Basal cell.
   E. Umbrella cell.

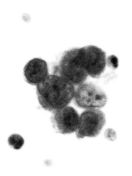

Figure 13-7 Papanicolaou stain of urine.

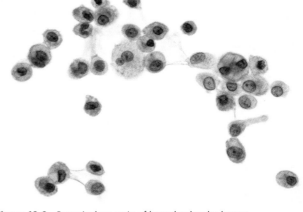

Figure 13-9 Papanicolaou stain of bronchoalveolar lavage.

7. A 92-year-old woman presented with gross hematuria. A voided urine specimen was sent for evaluation, and cells seen in Figure 13-7 were identified. Which one of the following is the best diagnosis for this specimen?
   A. Negative for malignant cells; umbrella cells.
   B. Positive for malignant cells; urothelial carcinoma.
   C. Negative for malignant cells; instrumentation effect.
   D. Positive for malignant cells; lymphoma.
   E. Negative for malignant cells; vaginal contamination.

9. As part of routine follow-up, a 45-year-old man with a history of lung transplantation underwent bronchoscopy and a bronchoalveolar lavage (BAL) was obtained. The BAL had the cells seen in Figure 13-9. Which one of the following is the best diagnosis based on this case?
   A. Positive for malignant cells; adenocarcinoma.
   B. Positive for malignant cells; lymphoma.
   C. Negative for malignant cells; benign bronchial cells.
   D. Negative for malignant cells; pulmonary alveolar macrophages.
   E. Negative for malignant cells; benign squamous cells.

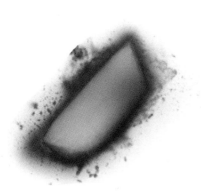

Figure 13-8 Diff-Quick stain of urine.

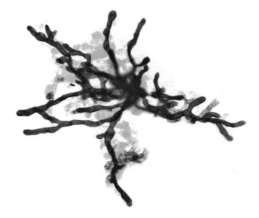

Figure 13-10 Gomori methenamine silver stain of bronchoalveolar lavage.

8. A 69-year-old man with microhematuria had a voided urine specimen submitted for evaluation. Numerous crystals were seen as in Figure 13-8. Which one of the following is the best diagnosis for these crystals?
   A. Calcium oxalate crystals; pathologic.
   B. Triple phosphate crystals; nonpathologic.
   C. Uric acid crystals; pathologic.
   D. Cystine crystals; nonpathologic.
   E. Tyrosine crystals; nonpathologic.

10. As a routine follow-up, a 45-year-old man with a history of lung transplantation had a BAL. Which one of the following is the best diagnosis based on the findings in Figure 13-10?
   A. Herpes simplex virus.
   B. *Candida* sp.
   C. *Aspergillus* sp.
   D. Cytomegalovirus.
   E. *Pneumocystis carinii.*

11. A patient presented with a pleural effusion with numerous mesothelial cells and eosinophils. Which one of the following is the most common cause of an eosinophilic effusion?
   A. Pneumothorax.
   B. Drug reaction.
   C. Parasitic infection.
   D. Rheumatoid arthritis.
   E. Systemic lupus erythematosus.

   A. Aspergillosis.
   B. Mucormycosis.
   C. Histoplasmosis.
   D. *Pneumocystis* infection.
   E. Cryptococcosis.

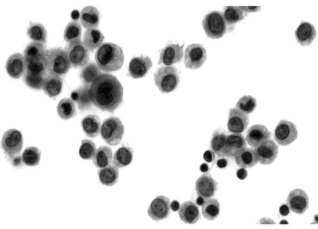

Figure 13-13 Papanicolaou stain of pleural effusion.

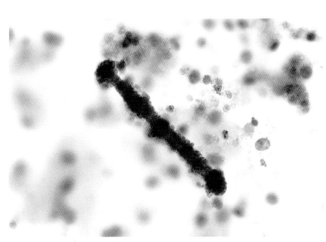

Figure 13-11 Papanicolaou stain of bronchoalveolar lavage.

12. A 42-year-old man presented with pneumonia. Imaging studies showed a pulmonary infiltrate and a minute, ill-defined, pleural-based thickening. The patient underwent a BAL. Based on Figure 13-11, the patient likely has which one of the following?
   A. Carcinoma.
   B. Mesothelioma.
   C. Pulmonary hemorrhage.
   D. Aspiration pneumonia.
   E. Asbestos exposure.

14. An 89-year-old man with shortness of breath and symptoms of pneumonia had a chest x-ray that demonstrated a small pleural effusion. The types of cells seen in the aspiration are shown in Figure 13-13. Which one of the following is the best diagnosis?
   A. Negative; tuberculosis.
   B. Malignant; adenocarcinoma.
   C. Negative; mostly histiocytes.
   D. Malignant; lymphoma.
   E. Negative; mostly mesothelial cells.

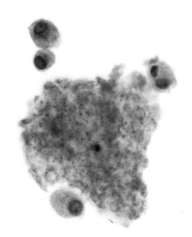

Figure 13-12 Papanicolaou stain of bronchoalveolar lavage.

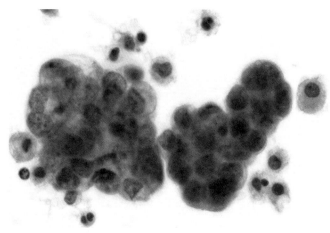

Figure 13-14 Papanicolaou stain of pleural effusion.

13. A 39-year-old woman with human immunodeficiency virus–acquired immunodeficiency syndrome (HIV-AIDS) presented with fever, cough, and pulmonary infiltrates. She underwent a BAL. Based on Figure 13-12, which one of the following is the best diagnosis?

15. Figure 13-14 shows the cells in a pleural effusion from a 70-year-old man. Which one of the following is the best diagnosis?
   A. Malignant; lymphoma.
   B. Benign; histiocytes.
   C. Malignant; mesothelioma.
   D. Benign; mesothelial cells.
   E. Malignant; adenocarcinoma.

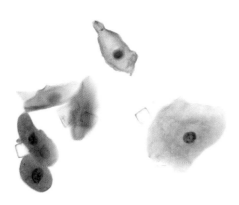

Figure 13-15 Papanicolaou stain of urine.

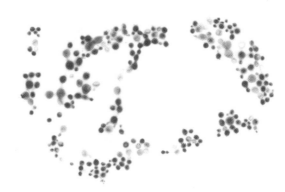

Figure 13-17 Diff-Quik stain of cerebrospinal fluid.

16. A voided urine specimen was submitted for evaluation. No additional clinical history was provided. Which one of the following is seen in Figure 13-15?
    A. Uric acid crystals.
    B. Cystine crystals.
    C. Tyrosine crystals.
    D. Calcium oxalate crystals.
    E. Sulfadiazine crystals.

18. A 50-year-old woman who is HIV positive presented with headaches and fevers. The findings shown in Figure 13-17 of the CSF obtained by lumbar puncture are most consistent with which one of the following diagnoses?
    A. Toxoplasmosis.
    B. Cryptococcus.
    C. Chondrocytes.
    D. Contamination (starch).
    E. Parasitic infection.

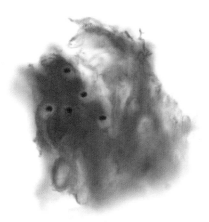

Figure 13-16 Papanicolaou stain of cerebrospinal fluid.

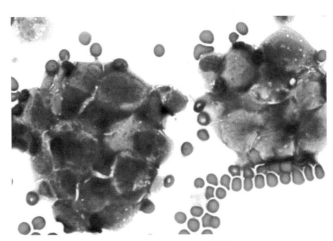

Figure 13-18 Diff-Quik stain of cerebrospinal fluid.

17. A patient underwent a lumbar puncture and CSF was obtained. No additional clinical history was provided. Based on the image in Figure 13-16, the patient would most likely be considered to have which one of the following entities?
    A. Chondrocytes.
    B. Traumatic tap.
    C. Glioblastoma multiforme (GBM).
    D. Signet ring adenocarcinoma.
    E. Old hemorrhage.

19. The CSF specimen in Figure 13-18 was obtained by lumbar puncture from a 5-year-old boy. The findings are most consistent with which one of the following diagnoses?
    A. Normal findings.
    B. Bacterial meningitis.
    C. Aseptic meningitis.
    D. Medulloblastoma.
    E. Small cell carcinoma.

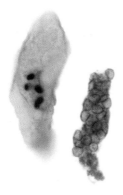

Figure 13-19 Papanicolaou stain of urine.

Figure 13-21 Papanicolaou stain of urine.

20. A voided urine specimen was submitted for evaluation. No additional clinical history was provided. Based on the image in Figure 13-19, which one of the following is the best interpretation?
   A. White blood cell cast; no clinical significance.
   B. White blood cell cast; clinically significant.
   C. Red blood cell cast; no clinical significance.
   D. Red blood cell cast; clinically significant.
   E. Renal tubular epithelial cell casts; clinically significant.

22. A voided urine specimen was submitted for evaluation. No additional clinical history was provided. Which one of the following is seen in Figure 13-21?
   A. Uric acid crystals.
   B. Cystine crystals.
   C. Tyrosine crystals.
   D. Calcium oxalate crystals.
   E. Sulfadiazine crystals.

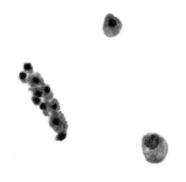

Figure 13-20 Papanicolaou stain of urine.

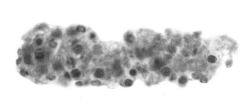

Figure 13-22 Papanicolaou stain of urine.

21. A voided urine specimen was submitted for evaluation. No additional clinical history was provided. Based on the image in Figure 13-20, which one of the following is the best interpretation?
   A. White blood cell cast; no clinical significance.
   B. White blood cell cast; clinically significant.
   C. Red blood cell cast; no clinical significance.
   D. Red blood cell cast; clinically significant.
   E. Renal tubular epithelial cell cast; clinically significant.

23. A voided urine specimen was submitted for evaluation. No additional clinical history was provided. Based on Figure 13-22, which one of the following is the best interpretation?
   A. White blood cell cast; no clinical significance.
   B. White blood cell cast; clinically significant.
   C. Red blood cell cast; no clinical significance.
   D. Red blood cell cast; clinically significant.
   E. Renal tubular epithelial cell casts; clinically significant.

ANSWERS

1. A. Normal findings.
Rationale: A normal CSF is sparsely cellular and contains only a few small, mature-appearing lymphocytes and monocytoid cells, which have moderate cytoplasm and folded or kidney bean–shaped nuclei.
B. Bacterial meningitis.
Rationale: CSF from a patient with bacterial meningitis is likely to be rich in neutrophils. However, neutrophils accompanied by numerous red blood cells are suggestive of peripheral blood contamination. Toxoplasmosis meningoencephalitis and early stages of viral meningitis are also in the differential diagnosis for a CSF sample with increased neutrophils.
C. Aseptic meningitis.
Rationale: CSF, as seen in Figure 13-1, from a patient with aseptic meningitis is likely to have increased numbers of lymphocytes. Plasma cells and monocytoid cells may also be present. An infectious organism, usually a virus, often causes aseptic meningitis. However, bacteria, fungi, systemic diseases, and medications can also lead to aseptic meningitis.
D. Parasitic infection.
Rationale: The presence of numerous eosinophils, which is a rare finding in CSF, is suggestive of a parasitic infection, such as one caused by *Taenia solium* or *Angiostrongylus cantonensis*.
E. Lymphoma.
Rationale: Numerous lymphoid cells are present in the CSF from a patient with lymphoma. However, the cells are more monotonous than the polymorphous population illustrated in the image.

Major points of discussion
- Microscopic description: A polymorphous population of small, intermediate, and large lymphocytes that are present singly.
- Normal CSF is sparsely cellular with only rare lymphocytes and monocytoid cells.
- Neutrophils in a CSF may be a "red herring" if numerous red blood cells from peripheral blood are present as a result of a traumatic tap.
- The differential diagnosis for a CSF with numerous lymphocytes includes a reactive process and lymphoma.
- A reactive process generally has a polymorphous population of lymphoid cells, including smaller and larger cells, as well as plasma cells. Lymphoma tends to have a more monomorphic population of lymphocytes.
- Flow cytometry may be necessary to confirm the diagnosis of lymphoma, especially when a low-grade lymphoma composed of smaller lymphocytes is suspected.[1]

2. A. Metastatic breast carcinoma.
Rationale: Metastatic breast carcinoma is among the most commonly encountered malignancies in adult women. Other common malignancies seen in CSF samples from adults include lung carcinoma, melanoma, lymphoma, and leukemia. Breast carcinoma cells occur singly or in clusters and lack nuclear molding.

B. Metastatic lung small cell carcinoma.
Rationale: Small cell carcinoma, as seen in Figure 13-2, has cells with scant cytoplasm, nuclear molding, and no nucleoli. The lung is often a source of occult primary tumors presenting as brain metastases, as in this case. There is morphological overlap between small cell carcinoma and medulloblastoma, but the latter predominantly affects children.
C. Metastatic melanoma.
Rationale: Metastatic melanoma is also among the common tumors presenting in the CSF. Melanoma can take on many morphological forms, including pigmented or nonpigmented, epithelioid or spindled, single cells or clusters, and monotonous or pleomorphic. However, melanoma cells lack the nuclear molding seen in this figure.
D. Metastatic lymphoma.
Rationale: Malignant lymphoid cells tend to occur singly and not in clusters. Nuclear molding is not a feature of lymphomas. In addition, diffuse large B-cell lymphoma, a subtype of lymphoma, likely involves the CSF and has coarse chromatin, prominent nucleoli, and irregular nuclear contours.
E. Metastatic lung adenocarcinoma.
Rationale: Lung adenocarcinoma, like breast carcinoma, consists of atypical epithelial cells present singly and in clusters. Sometimes the clusters form rounded structures resembling glands, and the cells have intracytoplasmic mucin, suggestive of an adenocarcinoma.

Major points of discussion
- Microscopic description: These cells are tightly cohesive, with nuclei that lack prominent nucleoli but have speckled chromatin that demonstrate molding, that is, nuclei conforming to the contours of adjacent cells.
- Lymphoid cells occur singly and do not form tight cohesive clusters. Numerous lymphoid cells are often accompanied by lymphoglandular bodies, which are pale-blue cytoplasmic fragments of different shapes and approximately the size of the red blood cells present in the background.
- Nuclear molding is evident in clusters and is defined as cohesive cell nuclei conforming to the contour of adjacent cells.
- Nuclear molding is seen in small cell carcinomas and medulloblastomas.
- Small cell carcinoma affects adults, whereas medulloblastoma affects children.
- Carcinomas present as single cells and cell clusters.
- Conspicuous nucleoli are not a feature of small cell carcinoma but may be seen in adenocarcinoma.
- Small cell carcinomas can arise in various organs. Clinical history, not morphology, is useful in determining the primary site.[1]

3. A. Aseptic meningitis.
Rationale: The CSF from a patient with aseptic meningitis typically has a polymorphous lymphoid population consisting of small, intermediate, and few large lymphocytes, some of which may appear atypical. Plasma cells and monocytoid cells can also be seen in the background.

B. Chronic lymphocytic leukemia/small lymphocytic lymphoma (CLL/SLL).
Rationale: CLL/SLL is composed of small lymphocytes, which are round to slightly irregular. CLL/SLL is a neoplasm of adulthood. Lymphomas, although they can have a morphologic appearance similar to that seen in Figure 13-3, tend to affect adults. Therefore, the clinical history, especially the age of the patient, is critical in formulating a differential diagnosis and arriving at the correct diagnosis.
C. Acute lymphoblastic leukemia (ALL).
Rationale: ALL arises in the bone marrow and most commonly affects children between the ages of 2 and 7 years. Lymphoblasts vary in size from small blasts with scant cytoplasm to larger cells with moderate cytoplasm. The age and clinical history are useful in interpreting the CSF in this setting. A diagnosis of ALL is usually established first, and then a lumbar puncture is performed to evaluate involvement of the central nervous system.
D. Medulloblastoma.
Rationale: Medulloblastoma, a small, round blue cell tumor of childhood, is also in the differential diagnosis in this case. Nuclear molding in medulloblastoma can aid in distinguishing it from ALL and other lymphoid entities, which occur as single, noncohesive cells. Nucleoli in medulloblastoma may be inconspicuous or prominent.
E. Bacterial meningitis.
Rationale: The CSF from a patient with bacterial meningitis will predominantly have neutrophils, rather than lymphoid cells, as seen in this case.

Major points of discussion
- Microscopic description: Increased numbers of single lymphoid cells with scant cytoplasm. All the cells are enlarged and of similar size. (In the lower third of the image, there is a single red blood cell that is useful in evaluating the size of the lymphoid cells.)
- Lymphoid cells occur singly.
- Cell type (epithelial, lymphoid, or other), distribution (single or clusters), and age (child or adult) aid in narrowing the differential diagnosis.
- The differential diagnosis for a cellular CSF with lymphoid cells also includes a reactive process and lymphoma.
- A polymorphous population of lymphocytes is suggestive of a reactive process.
- A monotonous population of lymphocytes is likely to represent lymphoma. Confirmation with ancillary studies, such as flow cytometry, may be necessary for low-grade lymphomas composed of smaller lymphoid cells that lack prominent nucleoli.
- Medulloblastoma affects the pediatric population. ALL affects young children between the ages of 2 and 7 years and has a second peak later in adulthood.[1]

4. A. Positive for malignant cells; urothelial carcinoma.
Rationale: Urothelial carcinoma in a voided urine specimen presents as atypical urothelial cells present singly and/or in clusters. Atypical features include a high nuclear/cytoplasmic ratio, hyperchromasia, coarse chromatin, and irregular nuclear borders. At times, large nucleoli may be present.
B. Positive for malignant cells; renal clear cell (conventional) carcinoma.

Rationale: Renal clear cell (conventional) carcinoma is the most common renal cell carcinoma, but is infrequently seen in voided urine specimens. Tumor cells have abundant cytoplasm that is vacuolated and round to slightly irregular nuclei. Nucleoli may be inconspicuous or prominent, depending on the grade of the tumor.
C. Negative for malignant cells; polyomavirus infection.
Rationale: Urothelial cells infected by polyomavirus (BK virus), as in this case, can mimic carcinoma because of the increased nuclear size and hyperchromasia; therefore, they are sometimes referred to as "decoy cells." The cells occur singly and the nuclei are round, homogeneous, and smudgy. Although human polyomavirus can affect immunocompromised patients, it can also be found in urine specimens of patients with no predisposing conditions.
D. Negative for malignant cells; hyaline inclusion bodies.
Rationale: Hyaline inclusion bodies are eosinophilic cytoplasmic inclusions of varying sizes frequently seen in degenerating urothelial cells.
E. Negative for malignant cells; renal tubular cells.
Rationale: Renal tubular cells are small cells, approximately the size of lymphocytes, with granular cytoplasm and dark nuclei.

Major points of discussion
- Microscopic description: A cell with nuclear hyperchromasia is surrounded by three benign urothelial cells. Relative to the adjacent urothelial cells, the abnormal cell has a high nuclear/cytoplasmic ratio, an atypical feature.
- Decoy cells are infected by human polyomavirus, also known as BK virus.
- Decoy cells are seen in both immunosuppressed and immunocompetent patients.
- The chromatin pattern is helpful in distinguishing between urothelial carcinoma and human polyomavirus–infected cells.
- The chromatin in urothelial carcinoma tends to be coarse.
- The nucleus is smudgy or glassy in a decoy cell.[1]

5. A. Granular cast.
Rationale: All casts appear as long tubular structures. Granular casts, as represented in Figure 13-5, are physiologic and may be present in normal urine specimens. Increased numbers of granular casts may be seen following physical stress. Other types of casts, including red blood cell casts, white blood cell casts, fatty casts, and degenerated renal tubular casts, are associated with underlying renal disease.
B. Hyaline inclusion body.
Rationale: Hyaline inclusion bodies, also known as globular inclusions or Melamed-Wolinska bodies, are round, red, eosinophilic, cytoplasmic structures of varying sizes thought to represent lysosomes. They are often present in degenerated urothelial cells. Most importantly, they do not represent viral inclusions.
C. Corpora amylacea.
Rationale: Corpora amylacea are round structures with concentric laminations derived from prostatic secretions.
D. Trichomoniasis.
Rationale: In urine specimens, trichomoniasis usually represents contamination from the female genital tract, but it may also be a source of prostatitis. The *Trichomonas* organism is pear shaped, with flagella that are sometimes visible.

E. Calcium oxalate crystal.
Rationale: Crystals are commonly seen in urine specimens and most are clinically insignificant. They can be of various shapes and sizes. Calcium oxalate crystals typically resemble an envelope, although they can take on other morphologic forms.

Major points of discussion

- Microscopic description: A long tubular structure with a granular consistency is present amongst benign squamous cells (the larger cells) and benign urothelial cells (the smaller cells).
- Casts in the urine occur as long tubular structures and corpora amylacea are round.
- Granular casts are relatively common in urine specimens and usually have no clinical significance.
- It is important to distinguish casts from parasites. Casts have a homogeneous granular appearance, whereas some internal structures may be seen in parasitic worms.
- Not to be mistaken for viral inclusions, hyaline inclusion bodies are red structures of varying sizes present in the cytoplasm of urothelial cells.
- *Trichomonas* may be difficult to identify due to its small size and relatively pale staining nucleus. On low magnification, the organisms resemble amorphous debris, but the nucleus and characteristic pear shape are better appreciated on higher magnification. Inflammation and a "dirty"-appearing background provide clues to the diagnosis.[1]

6. A. Endometrial cell.
Rationale: Endometrial cells are sometimes found incidentally in urine specimens obtained from women. Endometrial cells form tight three-dimensional clusters, and each cell is approximately the size of a lymphocyte and has a slightly irregular nucleus.
B. Squamous cell.
Rationale: Squamous cells can be similar in size to umbrella cells. Unlike umbrella cells, normal squamous cells have more homogenous and less grainy cytoplasm. When present in large numbers in voided urine specimens obtained from women, squamous cells likely represent vaginal contamination.
C. Renal tubular cell.
Rationale: Renal tubular cells are small cells, approximately the size of lymphocytes. Unlike umbrella cells, they have scant cytoplasm and a dark-staining nucleus.
D. Basal cell.
Rationale: Basal (i.e., transitional) cells also have slightly granular cytoplasm, like umbrella cells. However, they are intermediate in size; they are smaller than umbrella cells, but larger than renal tubular cells.
E. Umbrella cell.
Rationale: An umbrella cell, as seen in Figure 13-6, is a normal finding in urine specimens. They are larger than all other urothelial cells and can have one or multiple nuclei. The low nuclear/cytoplasmic ratio distinguishes them from malignant cells. Histologically, umbrella cells cap the basal (i.e., transitional) cells.

Major points of discussion

- Microscopic description: A large cell, characterized by its binucleation and low nuclear/cytoplasmic ratio, is present in the center of the image among normal squamous cells.
- Umbrella cells and squamous cells can be similar in size and represent the largest cells in urine specimens.
- Renal tubular cells are the smallest epithelial cells in urine specimens.
- The two types of cells that are multinucleated in urine specimens include umbrella cells and multinucleated giant cells.
- Multinucleated giant cells are typically present in patients with a history of urothelial carcinoma treated with bacillus Calmette–Guérin. The cytoplasm of these cells is less granular than that of umbrella cells.
- Umbrella cells can have a single nucleus or multiple nuclei.[1]

7. A. Negative for malignant cells; umbrella cells.
Rationale: In a normal voided urine specimen, urothelial cells occur singly. Although umbrella cells are large and can have multiple nuclei, they have low nuclear/cytoplasmic ratios and lack hyperchromasia, compatible with a benign process.
B. Positive for malignant cells; urothelial carcinoma.
Rationale: Cells from urothelial carcinomas can present singly and/or in clusters. High nuclear/cytoplasmic ratios, hyperchromasia, coarse chromatin, and nuclear irregularities, as seen in Figure 13-7, distinguish malignant cells from benign urothelial cells.
C. Negative for malignant cells; instrumentation effect.
Rationale: Benign transitional cells may occur as clusters if they are obtained during/following instrumentation or catheterization. In these scenarios, the "clusters" often consist of two-dimensional sheets and the cells lack atypical features, such as high nuclear/cytoplasmic ratios, hyperchromasia, coarse chromatin, and nuclear irregularities.
D. Positive for malignant cells; lymphoma.
Rationale: In a cytology preparation, lymphoid cells, whether in urine or body fluid from another site, occur singly. Cell clusters are suggestive of an epithelioid origin.
E. Negative for malignant cells; vaginal contamination.
Rationale: Urine specimens from women frequently have an abundance of benign squamous cells that likely originated in the vagina. However, squamous cells do not always represent vaginal contamination in women and are also present in urine specimens obtained from men. In these scenarios, the squamous cells likely originate from metaplasia in the trigone of the bladder or urethra. Benign squamous cells occur singly and have low nuclear/cytoplasmic ratios.

Major points of discussion

- Microscopic description: The image shows a cluster of hyperchromatic urothelial cells with coarse chromatin, irregularly shaped nuclei, and high nuclear/cytoplasmic ratios. (Note the size of these cells relative to the neutrophil and red blood cells in the background.)
- Malignant urothelial cells occur singly and/or in clusters.
- Umbrella cells and squamous cells are the largest cells in urine specimens, but their low nuclear/cytoplasmic ratios differentiate them from malignant cells.
- Coarse chromatin is useful in discerning urothelial carcinoma from decoy cells, which have smudgy chromatin.

- Clusters of urothelial cells may be seen in patients who have undergone catheterization or instrumentation (e.g., cystoscopy). Calculi in the urinary tract can also lead to shedding of urothelial clusters in urine specimens.
- In addition to the cytological features, a clinical history of calculi or cystoscopy is useful in determining the origin of cell clusters.[1]

8. A. Calcium oxalate crystals; pathologic.
Rationale: Most crystals have no clinical relevance. Crystals are commonly found in urine specimens and their presence in urine is related to pH, concentration, and temperature. Calcium oxalate crystals are not pathologic. Typically, they are square to rectangular in shape with a cross resembling the backside of an envelope, but they may also take other forms and be ovoid or dumbbell-shaped.
B. Triple phosphate crystals; nonpathologic.
Rationale: Triple phosphate crystals are rectangular in shape and bear resemblance to coffin lids; they are not clinically significant.
C. Uric acid crystals; pathologic.
Rationale: Uric acid crystals are not pathologic. They can have different shapes, including flat plates and pointed ovals.
D. Cystine crystals; nonpathologic.
Rationale: The presence of cystine crystals may signify cystinuria or cystine calculi. Cystine crystals are hexagonal and laminated.
E. Tyrosine crystals; nonpathologic.
Rationale: Tyrosine crystals may be seen in patients with liver disease. They look like thin needles in clusters.

Major points of discussion
- Most crystals have no clinical significance.
- Cystine and tyrosine crystals are suggestive of underlying disease.
- Crystals of the same compound can take on different shapes and sizes.
- The presence of crystals in a urine specimen is often related to pH and temperature.
- A specimen may have rare or numerous crystals.[1,2]

9. A. Positive for malignant cells; adenocarcinoma.
Rationale: Adenocarcinoma in the lung presents as cell clusters and usually with single cells. The cytoplasm of the cells can be vacuolated like macrophages, but the atypia, consisting of high nuclear/cytoplasmic ratios, hyperchromasia, and nuclear irregularities, distinguishes adenocarcinoma from benign cells. Poorly differentiated carcinomas may have all of the above listed atypical features, whereas the atypia in well-differentiated adenocarcinomas may be focal and subtle.
B. Positive for malignant cells;lymphoma.
Rationale: Following transplantation, patients are at risk for developing lymphoma. Lymphoid cells occur singly but are smaller and have scant cytoplasm compared with macrophages.
C. Negative for malignant cells; benign bronchial cells.
Rationale: Occasional bronchial cells are present in BAL specimens. Depending on their orientation, bronchial cells may appear as columnar cells with terminal bars and cilia, or as two-dimensional honeycombed sheets. Monotony and blandness of the cells are useful in recognizing that they are benign.

D. Negative for malignant cells; pulmonary alveolar macrophages.
Rationale: Numerous pulmonary alveolar macrophages are normally seen in BAL specimens. They occur singly, have low nuclear/cytoplasmic ratios, vacuolated cytoplasm, round to ovoid nuclei, and no hyperchromasia.
E. Negative for malignant cells; benign squamous cells.
Rationale: Benign squamous cells, often representing oral/upper airway contamination, are occasionally encountered in BALs. Unlike pulmonary alveolar macrophages, which are vacuolated, squamous cells have a dense, homogeneous cytoplasm.

Major points of discussion
- Microscopic description: Numerous singly dispersed cells with vacuolated cytoplasm and low nuclear/cytoplasmic ratios are present. Some of the cells are binucleated.
- A few types of cells, including bronchial cells and squamous cells, can be present in a BAL, but pulmonary alveolar macrophages are the most common cell type.
- Macrophages typically do not form clusters and occur as single cells.
- The low nuclear/cytoplasmic ratio, rather than the large size of macrophages (relative to adjacent inflammatory or red blood cells), is helpful in establishing that they are benign cells.
- The presence of cilia on a cell generally excludes a malignant diagnosis.
- At times, bronchial cells can be large and have multiple nuclei, but the presence of cilia suggests that they are benign cells with reactive changes.[1]

10. A. Herpes simplex virus.
Rationale: Cells infected with herpes tend to be multinucleated and have nuclear molding and smudgy chromatin.
B. *Candida* sp.
Rationale: *Candida* may appear as budding yeast or pseudohyphae.
C. *Aspergillus* sp.
Rationale: *Aspergillus* is a fungus with hyphae that show septation and acute 45-degree branching.
D. Cytomegalovirus.
Rationale: Cells infected with cytomegalovirus have intranuclear inclusions surrounded by a halo.
E. *Pneumocystis carinii*.
Rationale: In a BAL, *P. carinii* can be identified by the presence of foamy alveolar casts. A silver stain can be performed to confirm the diagnosis.

Major points of discussion
- After lung transplantation, patients are at risk for developing infections and lymphoma.
- Immunosuppressed patients, such as those with HIV-AIDS, are also at risk for opportunistic infections.
- An alveolar cast of *P. carinii* appears as a sheet of amorphous material.
- The Gomori methenamine silver stain highlights pneumocystis and other fungal organisms, such as *Aspergillus*, *Candida*, and *Mucor*.
- *Candida* organisms, associated with benign squamous cells in a BAL specimen, suggest that the specimen may represent oral contamination.[1,3–5]

11. A. Pneumothorax.

Rationale: Eosinophilic effusions are most commonly caused by prior sampling (e.g., placement of a chest tube for iatrogenic pneumothorax caused by a transthoracic lung biopsy) and the introduction of air or blood into the pleural space.

B. Drug reaction.

Rationale: A drug reaction can lead to eosinophils in an effusion, but it is a less common cause of an eosinophilic effusion.

C. Parasitic infection.

Rationale: A parasitic infection can lead to eosinophilia in an effusion, but it is a less common cause of an eosinophilic effusion.

D. Rheumatoid arthritis.

Rationale: A pleural effusion from a patient with rheumatoid arthritis is typically rich in macrophages and has abundant granular debris. Occasional lymphocytes and neutrophils may be seen. Eosinophils are not typically associated with rheumatoid pleuritis.

E. Systemic lupus erythematosus.

Rationale: An effusion from a patient with lupus pleuritis may have characteristic lupus erythematosus (LE) cells, which consist of neutrophils or macrophages with eccentrically-located nuclei and ingested degenerated material. This material, called a hematoxylin body, has a glassy, homogeneous appearance. Eosinophils are not associated with systemic lupus erythematous.

Major points of discussion

- Effusions can have lymphocytes, neutrophils, and/or eosinophils.
- Eosinophils are frequently associated with parasitic infections, but their presence in a pleural effusion is most commonly linked to introduction of air into the pleural space.
- The differential diagnosis for eosinophils in a pleural effusion includes infection and drug reaction.
- Abundant granular debris in an effusion is associated with rheumatoid arthritis.
- A hematoxylin body or LE cell may be seen in patients with lupus.[1,3-5]

12. A. Carcinoma.

Rationale: Figure 13-11 shows predominantly pulmonary macrophages, which is a normal finding in BAL specimens. Pulmonary macrophages have low nuclear/cytoplasmic ratios, nuclei with fine chromatin, and abundant vacuolated cytoplasm. Most carcinomas will form at least some clusters, have cells with high nuclear/cytoplasmic ratios, and contain nuclei with irregular contours and coarse chromatin.

B. Mesothelioma.

Rationale: Mesothelioma usually presents in a pleural effusion (and not in a BAL specimen) as cell clusters and single cells. In contrast, macrophages tend to occur singly. Also, the presence of an asbestos body signifies asbestos exposure, but it is not a sine qua non of mesothelioma.

C. Pulmonary hemorrhage.

Rationale: A patient with pulmonary hemorrhage will have hemosiderin-laden macrophages, characterized by golden-brown, intracytoplasmic particles of varying sizes. No hemosiderin is seen in the macrophages in this figure.

D. Aspiration pneumonia.

Rationale: The presence of food particles and inflammation in a BAL specimen is highly suggestive of aspiration.

E. Asbestos exposure.

Rationale: The figure demonstrates an elongated, dumbbell-shaped structure with a clear core coated by iron; this is consistent with an asbestos body. Patients with asbestos exposure may have asbestos bodies in the lung parenchyma and pleural plaques (thickening), as described in this patient. An asbestos body is a form of a ferruginous body. Non-asbestos ferruginous bodies have black or brown cores, in contrast to the clear cores seen in asbestos bodies.

Major points of discussion

- Microscopic description: A structure with an elongated, iron-coated, dumbbell shape and clear core.
- An asbestos body is a subtype of a ferruginous body.
- A clear core is suggestive of an asbestos body.
- A non-asbestos ferruginous body has a black or brown core.
- Identification of an asbestos body in a BAL specimen indicates that the person has had asbestos exposure.
- The presence of an asbestos body does not signify that the patient has mesothelioma.[1,3-5]

13. A. Aspergillosis.

Rationale: *Aspergillus* sp. pneumonia tends to affect immunosuppressed individuals. *Aspergillus* is a fungal organism that is characterized by septated hyphae with acute, 45-degree angle branching.

B. Mucormycosis.

Rationale: Mucormycosis is typically seen in patients with underlying hematopoietic malignancies or diabetes mellitus. Relative to *Aspergillus*, *Mucor* organisms have broader hyphae that are nonseptated and have irregular branching.

C. Histoplasmosis.

Rationale: Histoplasmosis may be asymptomatic or symptomatic, especially in immunosuppressed patients. The organisms are often intracellular, within macrophages, and consist of narrow-based, round to ovoid-shaped, budding yeast.

D. *Pneumocystis* infection.

Rationale: Immunosuppressed patients, such as those with HIV-AIDS, are susceptible to *P. carinii* infection. Vacuolated foamy casts are diagnostic of the organisms. A silver stain highlights the cysts.

E. Cryptococcosis.

Rationale: Immunocompetent and immunosuppressed patients are at risk for developing infections with *Cryptococcus neoformans*. Microscopically, *C. neoformans* consists of narrow-budding yeast surrounded by a mucinous capsule.

Major points of discussion

- Microscopic description: Amorphous foamy material with the configuration of a pulmonary alveolus is present in the center of this image. Pulmonary alveolar macrophages are seen in the background.
- The differential for budding yeast includes *Candida* sp., *Histoplasma capsulatum*, and *C. neoformans*.
- *Histoplasma* organisms are typically intracellular, within macrophages.

- The thickness of hyphae, septation, and angle of hyphal branching are useful in differentiating among *Candida*, *Aspergillus*, and *Mucor*.
- A mucicarmine stain is helpful in confirming a diagnosis of *Cryptococcus*.
- Occasionally strands of mucus and elastic fibers can mimic fungi. A silver stain is helpful in differentiating between these mimics and fungi.[1,3-5]

14. A. Negative; tuberculosis.
Rationale: An effusion from a patient with tuberculosis is composed predominantly of lymphocytes and rare mesothelial cells. A similar pattern may be observed in effusions from patients with lymphoma/leukemia, recent cardiac surgery, or sarcoidosis. Clinical history and ancillary tests are helpful is determining the etiology of the lymphocytes.
B. Malignant; adenocarcinoma.
Rationale: Carcinomas in fluids will occur as clusters and single cells. A second cell population that does not resemble mesothelial cells or histiocytes can be helpful in identifying adenocarcinoma. Features helpful in making a diagnosis of malignancy include cells with high nuclear/cytoplasmic ratios, prominent nucleoli, enlarged cells, and irregular nuclear contours. Poorly differentiated carcinomas may have all of these features, whereas well-differentiated carcinomas may lack some of these characteristics.
C. Negative; mostly histiocytes.
Rationale: Most benign effusions are composed of mesothelial cells and histiocytes, which tend to occur as single cells. In contrast to mesothelial cells, histiocytes have more vacuolated cytoplasm, folded or bean-shaped nuclei, and no "windows."
D. Malignant; lymphoma.
Rationale: Lymphomas present as single cells, and the type of lymphoma dictates other cytologic features. For example, an effusion caused by a diffuse large B-cell lymphoma has large lymphoid cells with prominent nucleoli. In contrast, one caused by follicular lymphoma is composed of relatively smaller cells with cleaved nuclei.
E. Negative; mostly mesothelial cells.
Rationale: Mesothelial cells tend to have dense cytoplasm. When they do aggregate, mesothelial cells have a small space or window between them resulting from intervening long microvilli.

Major points of discussion
- Microscopic description: Cells with foamy vacuolated cytoplasm and ovoid to kidney-shaped nuclei. There is also a single cell of a different type with dense cytoplasm (mid left).
- Pleural effusions and ascites fluid typically have a combination of mesothelial cells and histiocytes.
- Both mesothelial cells and histiocytes are normal constituents of the pleural and peritoneal cavities.
- Benign mesothelial cells and histiocytes are present as single cells. In pelvic washing specimens, mesothelial cells shed as two-dimensional sheets.
- Identification of clusters of epithelioid cells and two-celled populations suggest malignancy. Immunostains may be necessary to confirm the morphologic impression and determine the identity of the primary tumor.

- Lymphocytes, whether benign or neoplastic, occur as single cells. Lymphocytes are smaller than mesothelial cells and histiocytes.[1]

15. A. Malignant; lymphoma.
Rationale: Lymphomas present predominantly as single cells. The morphology varies with the type of lymphoma, ranging from small cells to large cells with prominent nucleoli.
B. Benign; histiocytes.
Rationale: Histiocytes are present singly, have foamy cytoplasm, and low nuclear/cytoplasmic ratios.
C. Malignant; mesothelioma.
Rationale: Because the cells in both mesotheliomas and adenocarcinomas form cell clusters, distinguishing between them can be challenging and immunostains are often required for definitive diagnosis. Morphologic features in favor of mesothelioma include the presence of windows and dense cytoplasm. Cytoplasmic vacuolization and signet ring cells support a diagnosis of adenocarcinoma.
D. Benign; mesothelial cells.
Rationale: In effusions, benign mesothelial cells tend to occur singly. If they aggregate, mesothelial cells have a space or window between them. In addition, they have round nuclei and dense cytoplasm.
E. Malignant; adenocarcinoma.
Rationale: Figure 13-14 shows two populations of cells. There are smaller cells that are singly dispersed and represent an admixture of benign mesothelial cells and histiocytes. The second population is composed of larger atypical cells present mostly as cohesive clusters, consistent with adenocarcinoma. The presence of vacuolated cytoplasm aids in rendering a diagnosis of adenocarcinoma and in distinguishing these cell clusters from those of mesothelioma.

Major points of discussion
- Microscopic description: Hyperchromatic cell clusters, with focal vacuolization and high nuclear/cytoplasmic ratios, are noted. In the background are a rare mesothelial cell, a few histiocytes, and inflammatory cells.
- A signet ring cell has an intracytoplasmic vacuole that compresses the nucleus to one side. These cells are characteristic of adenocarcinomas.
- In a malignant effusion, the presence of vacuolated cytoplasm is typical of adenocarcinoma.
- The presence of psammoma bodies (spherical concentrically laminated collections of calcium) in a malignant effusion is characteristic of an adenocarcinoma.
- Abundant extracellular mucin in a malignant effusion is consistent with adenocarcinoma.
- Dense cytoplasm and windows between malignant cells are suggestive of mesothelioma. However, immunostains are typically performed to confirm the morphological impression.[1]

16. A. Uric acid crystals.
Rationale: Uric acid crystals can have various shapes. Some uric acid crystals are hexagonal. In contrast to cystine crystals, uric acid crystals are birefringent under polarized light. Increased numbers of uric acid crystals may be

associated with increased urates in patients undergoing therapy for leukemia/lymphoma.

B. Cystine crystals.

Rationale: Cystine crystals, like some uric acid crystals, are hexagonal with equal or unequal sides. Unlike uric acid crystals, thin forms of cystine crystals do not polarize. Cystinuria, an autosomal recessive disease, may lead to the development of calculi in the urinary tract.

C. Tyrosine crystals.

Rationale: Tyrosine crystals occur as groups of fine needles and may coexist with leucine crystals, which are spherical. Tyrosine crystals are present in patients with underlying liver disease who are unable to metabolize the amino acid.

D. Calcium oxalate crystals.

Rationale: The image shows urothelial cells, the two cells in the lower left with more opaque cytoplasm; and squamous cells, which have more transparent cytoplasm. Interspersed are square crystals. (Diagonal lines are not illustrated here.) Calcium oxalate crystals are colorless squares with intersecting diagonal lines resembling an envelope. Dumbbell-shaped and ovoid forms also occur. Large numbers of calcium oxalate crystals may suggest the presence of chronic renal disease or toxicity from ethylene glycol or methoxyflurane.

E. Sulfadiazine crystals.

Rationale: Drugs excreted in the urine may form crystals. The configuration of the sulfadiazine crystals depends on the specific drug. One form appears as wheat sheaves.

Major points of discussion

- Crystals formed from the same substance can have various shapes.
- Abnormal crystals include cystine, tyrosine, leucine, and sulfadiazine.
- Uric acid crystals and cystine crystals can be hexagonal.
- Uric acid crystals, unlike some cystine crystals, are birefringent under polarized light.
- Crystal formation in urine is dependent on pH, temperature, and concentration of the substance.

17. A. Chondrocytes.

Rationale: Cartilage-containing chondrocytes, as seen in Figure 13-16, are sometimes present in CSF specimens. The cells can be present singly or in clusters. The combination of chondrocyte lacunae, which create paranuclear clearing, and large size can sometimes be mistaken for neoplastic epithelial cells. The slide shows chondrocytes with surrounding clear lacunae in cartilage.

B. Traumatic tap.

Rationale: A traumatic tap is composed of numerous red blood cells from peripheral blood contamination. Presence of cartilage is not an indication of a traumatic tap.

C. Glioblastoma multiforme (GBM).

Rationale: Cells from a GBM are large and have highly pleomorphic nuclei with coarse chromatin.

D. Signet ring adenocarcinoma.

Rationale: Cells from a signet ring cell carcinoma can be present singly or as clusters. In contrast to chondrocytes, adenocarcinoma has hyperchromatic and angulated nuclei, but sometimes the cells can appear bland. Signet ring cells contain mucin, which usually displaces the nucleus to the periphery. The nuclei of chondrocytes tend to be centrally located.

E. Old hemorrhage.

Rationale: A CSF with old hemorrhage will have hemosiderin-laden macrophages, which consist of macrophages with intracellular refractile, golden-brown pigment.

Major points of discussion

- Chondrocytes have no pathologic significance.
- Chondrocytes can be present as single cells or clusters.
- Chondrocytes are obtained from inadvertent sampling of cartilage.
- Numerous red blood cells, not chondrocytes, are suggestive of a traumatic tap.
- Chondrocytes can be mistaken for adenocarcinoma, including one with signet ring cell features.

18. A. Toxoplasmosis.

Rationale: Toxoplasma gondii causes meningoencephalitis in immunocompromised hosts. The crescent-shaped organisms are present either intracellularly or extracellularly. The background shows a mixture of neutrophils and mononuclear cells.

B. Cryptococcus.

Rationale: C. neoformans, as seen in Figure 13-17, is a fungus that can be seen in the CSF of both healthy and immunocompromised hosts. The yeast vary in size, have narrow-based budding, and the capsule is mucin positive. The amount of inflammation in the background can be variable.

C. Chondrocytes.

Rationale: Rarely, contamination by chondrocytes may be seen in CSF specimens as a result of inadvertent sampling of the vertebral column. In contrast to *Cryptococci,* chondrocytes are much larger and are surrounded by a thick matrix. The large size of chondrocytes may also be mistaken for a malignant neoplasm.

D. Contamination (starch).

Rationale: Starch, typically a contaminant from glove powder, can be mistaken for *Cryptococcus.* Unlike *Cryptococcus,* starch displays a Maltese cross under polarized light in the center and has no capsule or budding forms.

E. Parasitic infection.

Rationale: Parasitic infections are accompanied by numerous eosinophils. The structures in this figure represent fungi, and no significant inflammatory component is present.

Major points of discussion

- Microscopic description: Numerous round to ovoid organisms of varying sizes. The paler-staining periphery represents the capsule. Rare cryptococci demonstrate budding at their bases.
- *Toxoplasma* tachyzoites are present both intracellularly and extracellularly.
- Toxoplasma organisms (3 to 6 μm) are smaller than cryptococci, which range from 5 to 15 μm in diameter.
- A capsule surrounds cryptococci.
- Cryptococci demonstrate narrow-based budding.
- The capsule of cryptococci stains with mucicarmine. There are also capsule-deficient forms of cryptococci.

19. A. Normal findings.

Rationale: Normal CSF is typically sparsely cellular with rare, mature-appearing lymphocytes and monocytoid cells. These usually occur as singly dispersed cells.

B. Bacterial meningitis.
Rationale: Bacterial meningitis in CSF contains mostly neutrophils. Similar to lymphocytes and monocytoid cells, neutrophils occur as singly dispersed cells.
C. Aseptic meningitis.
Rationale: In contrast to a CSF with normal findings, a specimen from a patient with aseptic meningitis is more cellular and has a mixture of lymphocytes, plasma cells, and monocytoid cells.
D. Medulloblastoma.
Rationale: Medulloblastoma, as seen in this figure, is a small, round blue cell tumor that occurs primarily in children. Identification of nuclear molding is useful in distinguishing medulloblastoma from lymphoma/leukemia, another small, round blue cell tumor. Metastatic small cell carcinoma also demonstrates nuclear molding, but it affects primarily adults.
E. Small cell carcinoma.
Rationale: Small cell carcinoma has cells with scant cytoplasm, nuclear molding, and no nucleoli. The lung is often a source of occult primary tumors presenting as brain metastases. There is morphological overlap between small cell carcinoma and medulloblastoma, but the latter predominantly affects children.

Major points of discussion
- Microscopic description: Two atypical clusters of cells in a background of red blood cells. The medulloblastoma cells are large relative to the red blood cells. In addition, they have irregular nuclear contours and demonstrate nuclear molding—a feature that distinguishes them from lymphoid cells.
- Normal CSF has rare cells.
- Small, round blue cell tumors include lymphoma/leukemia, small cell carcinoma, and medulloblastoma.
- Nuclear molding may be present in medulloblastoma and small cell carcinoma.
- Small cell carcinoma lacks nucleoli.
- Small cell carcinoma is more likely to be seen in adults, whereas medulloblastoma affects children.

20. A. White blood cell cast; no clinical significance.
Rationale: White blood cell casts are elongated structures with variable numbers of white blood cells.
B. White blood cell cast; clinically significant.
Rationale: These casts are clinically relevant and seen in patients who have tubulointerstitial disease and renal transplant rejection.
C. Red blood cell cast; no clinical significance.
Rationale: Red blood cell casts are associated with glomerulonephritis.
D. Red blood cell cast; clinically significant.
Rationale: Figure 13-9 demonstrates an epithelial cell adjacent to a tubular structure composed of numerous red blood cells, consistent with a red blood cell cast. Red blood cells casts are elongated structures containing outlines of red blood cells and are a sign of bleeding within nephrons.
E. Renal tubular epithelial cell casts; clinically significant.
Rationale: Renal tubular casts can resemble white blood cell casts. Identification of cells with relatively abundant granular cytoplasm is characteristic of renal tubular epithelial casts. Several disease states, including tubular

necrosis, viral disease, and drug toxicity, are associated with renal tubular casts.

Major points of discussion
- Urinary casts are cylindrical structures formed in the kidney.
- When dislodged, casts can be detected in urine specimens.
- Casts can be associated with pathologic and nonpathologic conditions.
- Casts can be composed of various cell types, including red blood cells, leukocytes, and renal tubular cells.
- The width of a cast can vary. Broader casts arise from dilated tubules/ducts, whereas thinner ones form in compressed tubules.

21. A. White blood cell cast; no clinical significance.
Rationale: White blood cell casts are elongated structures with variable numbers of white blood cells.
B. White blood cell cast; clinically significant.
Rationale: These casts are clinically relevant and seen in patients who have tubulointerstitial disease and renal transplant rejection.
C. Red blood cell cast; no clinical significance.
Rationale: Red blood cell casts are associated with renal disease.
D. Red blood cell cast; clinically significant.
Rationale: Red blood cells casts are elongated structures containing outlines of red blood cells and are a sign of bleeding within nephrons.
E. Renal tubular epithelial cell cast; clinically significant.
Rationale: The image shows two larger urothelial cells and a tubular structure composed of renal tubular cells, consistent with a renal tubular cast. Moderate and granular cytoplasm typical of renal tubular cells is helpful in distinguishing renal tubular cell casts from white blood cell casts. Renal tubular casts, as seen in Figure 13-20, can resemble white blood cell casts. Identification of cells with relatively abundant granular cytoplasm is characteristic of renal tubular epithelial casts. Several disease states, including tubular necrosis, viral disease, and drug toxicity, are associated with renal tubular casts.

Major points of discussion
- Urinary casts are cylindrical structures formed in the kidney.
- When dislodged, casts can be detected in urine specimens.
- Casts can be associated with pathologic and nonpathologic conditions.
- Casts can be composed of various cell types, including red blood cells, leukocytes, and renal tubular cells.
- The width of a cast can vary. Broader casts arise from dilated tubules/ducts, whereas thinner ones form in compressed tubules.

22. **A. Uric acid crystals.**
Rationale: The image shows two hexagonal crystals compatible with uric acid crystals. Uric acid crystals can have various shapes. Some uric acid crystals are hexagonal, as seen in Figure 13-21. In contrast to cystine crystals, uric acid crystals are birefringent under polarized light. Numerous

uric acid crystals may be associated with increased urates in patients undergoing therapy for leukemia/lymphoma.
B. Cystine crystals.
Rationale: Cystine crystals, like some uric acid crystals, are hexagonal with equal or unequal sides. Unlike uric acid crystals, thin forms of cystine crystals do not polarize. Cystinuria, an autosomal recessive disease, may lead to the development of calculi in the urinary tract.
C. Tyrosine crystals.
Rationale: Tyrosine crystals occur as groups of fine needles and may coexist with leucine crystals, which are spherical. Tyrosine crystals are present in patients with underlying liver disease who are unable to metabolize the amino acid.
D. Calcium oxalate crystals.
Rationale: Calcium oxalate crystals are colorless squares with intersecting diagonal lines resembling an envelope. Dumbbell-shaped and ovoid forms also occur. Large numbers of calcium oxalate crystals may suggest the presence of chronic renal disease or toxicity from ethylene glycol or methoxyflurane.
E. Sulfadiazine crystals.
Rationale: Drugs excreted in the urine may form crystals. The configuration of the sulfadiazine crystals depends on the specific drug. One form appears as wheat sheaves.

Major points of discussion

- Crystals formed from the same substance can have various shapes.
- Abnormal crystals include cystine, tyrosine, leucine, and sulfadizine.
- Uric acid crystals and cystine crystals can be hexagonal.
- Uric acid crystals, unlike some cystine crystals, are birefringent under polarized light.
- Crystal formation in urine is dependent on pH, temperature, and concentration of the substance.

23. A. White blood cell cast; no clinical significance.
Rationale: White blood cell casts are elongated structures with variable numbers of white blood cells.
B. White blood cell cast; clinically significant.
Rationale: The image demonstrates a tubular structure with interspersed lymphocytes, consistent with a white blood cell cast. White blood cell casts, as seen in Figure 13-22, are clinically relevant and seen in patients who have tubulointerstitial disease and renal transplant rejection.
C. Red blood cell cast; no clinical significance.
Rationale: Red blood cell casts are associated with renal disease.
D. Red blood cell cast; clinically significant.
Rationale: Red blood cells casts are elongated structures containing outlines of red blood cells and are a sign of bleeding within nephrons.
E. Renal tubular epithelial cell casts; clinically significant.
Rationale: Renal tubular casts can resemble white blood cell casts. Identification of cells with relatively abundant granular cytoplasm is characteristic of renal tubular epithelial casts. Several disease states, including tubular necrosis, viral disease, and drug toxicity, are associated with renal tubular casts.

Major points of discussion

- Urinary casts are cylindrical structures formed in the kidney.
- When dislodged, casts can be detected in urine specimens.
- Casts can be associated with pathologic and nonpathologic conditions.
- Casts can be composed of various cell types, including red blood cells, leukocytes, and renal tubular cells.
- The width of a cast can vary. Broader casts arise from dilated tubules/ducts, whereas thinner ones form in compressed tubules.

References

1. Cibas ES, Ducatman BS. Cytology. Diagnostic Principles and Clinical Correlates. 3rd ed. Philadelphia: Saunders Elsevier, 2009.
2. Henry JB. Clinical Diagnosis and Management by Laboratory Methods. 20th ed. Philadelphia: WB Saunders, 2001.
3. Katzenstein AA. *Katzenstein and Askin's Surgical Pathology of Non-Neoplastic Lung Disease.* Philadelphia: Saunders Elsevier, 2006.
4. Leslie KO, Wick MR. *Practical Pulmonary Pathology.* Philadelphia: Elsevier, 2005.
5. Travis WD, Colby TV, Koss MN, et al. *Non-Neoplastic Disorders of the Lower Respiratory Tract.* Washington, DC: American Registry of Pathology and the Armed Forces Institute of Pathology, 2002.

CHAPTER 14

COAGULATION:
Hemostasis and Thrombosis (Anticoagulation, Thrombophilias, Fibrinolysis)

Richard O. Francis, Jeffrey S. Jhang

QUESTIONS

1. An 18-year-old man with a history of von Willebrand disease (vWD) is scheduled to undergo wisdom-tooth extraction. In preparation for his procedure, his hematologist is planning to perform a trial of desmopressin (DDAVP) to see whether he responds. In which one of the following types of von Willebrand disease has DDAVP been known to cause thrombocytopenia?
   A. Type 1.
   B. Type 3.
   C. Type 2B.
   D. Type 2A.
   E. Type 2M.

Table 14-1

Test	Patient	Reference Range	Units
aPTT	50.2	26.3-39.4	sec
PT	13.6	12.7-15.4	sec

2. A 2-month-old boy with a history of gut malrotation is scheduled to undergo corrective surgery. Preoperative laboratory tests include coagulation screening tests as shown in Table 14-1. The surgery is performed without any bleeding complications. Which one of the following clotting factors has similar or higher activity levels in younger children than in adults?
   A. Fibrinogen.
   B. Factor II.
   C. Factor X.
   D. Factor XI.
   E. Prekallikrein.

Table 14-2

Test	Patient	Reference Range	Units
Platelets	210	165-415	10^9/L
Bleeding time	>12	<7	min
FVIII:C	70	56-191	%
vWF:Ag	25	52-214	%
vWF:RCo	<5	51-215	%
Blood group	O+		

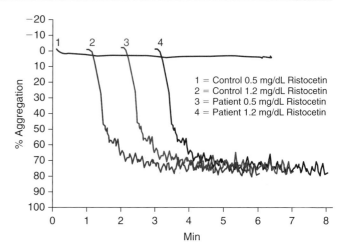

Figure 14-1 Ristocetin-induced platelet aggregation using platelet-rich plasma from the patient and normal control. Light transmission aggregations with low-dose ristocetin (0.5 mg/mL) and high-dose ristocetin agonists are shown for the patient and normal control.

3. A 4-year-old girl with epistaxis and significant bleeding with loss of her baby teeth is brought to her pediatrician by her mother. The patient had a laboratory evaluation, including an evaluation for vWD. The relevant laboratory findings are shown in Table 14-2. A ristocetin-induced platelet aggregation study was performed (Figure 14-1). Which one of the following steps would be most useful in distinguishing the disorders that could account for these findings?
   A. Desmopressin (DDAVP) challenge.
   B. Cryoprecipitate challenge.
   C. Platelet function analyzer (PFA)-100.
   D. Partial thromboplastin time (PTT) mixing study.
   E. von Willebrand factor (vWF) multimer analysis.

Table 14-3

Test	Patient	Reference Range	Units
vWF Antigen	40	50-150	% mean of normal
Ristocetin cofactor activity	42	50-150	% mean of normal
Factor VIII	35	50-150	%
Ristocetin-induced platelet aggregation	70	>65% aggregation	
vWF multimers	Normal distribution	Normal distribution	

4a. A 20-year-old woman with a history of menorrhagia was recently diagnosed with vWD. Her laboratory results are shown in Table 14-3. Which one of the following types of vWD is most consistent with the laboratory values?
   A. Type 3.
   B. Type 2N.
   C. Type 2A.
   D. Type 2M.
   E. Type 1.

4b. The initial diagnosis of the patient was delayed because vWF antigen and activity results were within the reference range when she was initially evaluated 2 years earlier. In the interim, however, she continued to have menorrhagia, prompting reevaluation and the subsequent diagnosis of type of vWD in Question 4a. Which one of the following is the most likely reason that vWD was not diagnosed on her initial visit?
   A. The patient is blood type O, and these individuals tend to have higher baseline vWF antigen levels than those with other blood groups.
   B. At the time of initial evaluation the patient was taking oral contraceptives, which are known to increase vWF levels.
   C. The blood sample for testing was transported to the laboratory at room temperature instead of the preferred temperature of 4°C.
   D. At the time of the initial evaluation, the patient had not recently exercised, and a lack of physical activity is known to increase vWF levels.
   E. vWF levels are known to decrease with increasing age.

5. Which one of the following is an acquired cause of factor VII deficiency?
   A. Left ventricular assist device.
   B. Inflammatory bowel disease.
   C. Phytonadione therapy.
   D. Heparin therapy.
   E. Ganciclovir therapy.

6. Which one of the following clotting factors has the longest plasma half-life?
   A. Factor VII.
   B. Factor X.
   C. Factor II.
   D. Factor XIII.
   E. Factor VIII.

7. Which one of the following is a rare complication of congenital factor VII deficiency?
   A. Epistaxis.
   B. Thrombosis.
   C. Menorrhagia.

   D. Central nervous system bleeding.
   E. Postoperative bleeding.

8. A 3-day-old infant, born by normal spontaneous delivery without complications, is brought to the emergency department with vomiting, lethargy, and pallor. On physical examination, the anterior fontanelle is bulging, and a cephalohematoma is diagnosed. A complete blood cell count shows a hemoglobin of 7.2 g/dL (11.0 to 13.0 g/dL), platelet count of 254 (165 to 415 × 10^9/L), prothrombin time (PT) of 62.4 seconds (12.3 to 14.6 seconds), and activated partial thromboplastin time (aPTT) of 32.1 seconds (24.0 to 34.6 seconds). The PT corrects into the reference range when mixed 1:1 with pooled normal plasma. Which one of the following factors is most likely to be decreased in this patient?
   A. Factor V.
   B. Factor VII.
   C. Factor VIII.
   D. Factor IX.
   E. Factor XI.

9. Which one of the following reasons makes it difficult to treat actively bleeding patients with congenital factor VII deficiency using recombinant factor VIIa?
   A. Formation of anti–factor VII antibodies.
   B. Short half-life of recombinant factor VIIa.
   C. Requirement for high doses (120 µg/kg).
   D. Contamination with activated factors II, IX, and X.
   E. Need to overlap with heparin therapy.

Table 14-4

Mixing study*	Control	Patient	Mix
Immediate mix	32.4	112.1	39.4
37°C separate (control)	31.7	104.4	39.3
37°C together	31.7	104.4	48.5

*Activated partial thromboplastin time in seconds.

10a. A 28-year-old man with known hemophilia A is seen in the emergency department at 3 AM with hemarthrosis after getting into a fight at a local bar. He occasionally develops hemarthrosis and has received factor replacement therapy. The patient's factor VIII activity is reported as less than 1%. The patient weighs 100 kg, and 2500 IU of factor VIII concentrates was administered. The following morning, a right forearm muscle hematoma was expanding and the affected joint was not improving. A factor VIII level 12 hours after administration was 4%. A 1:1 mixing study and a 2-hour incubated mixing study were performed. Which one of the following is the best explanation for the clinical and laboratory findings shown in Table 14-4?
   A. Consistent with factor VIII half-life.
   B. Consistent with inadequate dosing of factor VIII.
   C. Inadequate reconstitution of lyophilized product.
   D. Presence of a lupus anticoagulant (LAC).
   E. Factor VIII inhibitor.

10b. The desired target for factor VIII activity was 50% in this patient. Which one of the following is the correct initial dose of factor VIII concentrate that should be administered?
   A. 750 IU.
   B. 1000 IU.
   C. 2500 IU.
   D. 3500 IU.
   E. 5000 IU.

Table 14-5

Test	Patient	Reference Range	Units
PT	13.4	12.7-15.4	sec
aPTT	112.1	26.3-39.4	sec
Fibrinogen	278	233-496	mg/dL

11a. An 8-year-old boy presents to the emergency department with a left knee hemarthrosis and persistent bleeding from a cut after falling while playing tennis. The parents were told that their child has hemophilia but they do not know what type. He has never had any bleeding and has not received any clotting factors. His coagulation studies are shown in Table 14-5, and a 1:1 mixing study with pooled normal plasma shows correction of the aPTT into the reference range. Which one of the following is the most likely factor that is deficient in this patient?
   A. Factor II.
   B. Factor VII.
   C. Factor VIII.
   D. Factor X.
   E. Factor V.

11b. The patient has never been transfused and has not received factor replacement therapy. A factor IX activity is reported as less than 1% and factor VIII as 82%. The patient weighs 30 kg, and a target of 50% factor IX activity is desired. Which one of the following is the appropriate dose of recombinant factor IX replacement?
   A. 75 IU.
   B. 210 IU.
   C. 750 IU.
   D. 1500 IU.
   E. 5000 IU.

12. What is the biologic half-life of factor IX?
   A. 5 hours.
   B. 12 hours.
   C. 24 hours.
   D. 48 hours.
   E. 96 hours.

13. Which one of the following clinical manifestations is characteristic of patients with a coagulation factor deficiency?
   A. Petechiae.
   B. Superficial hematomas.
   C. Epistaxis.
   D. Delayed bleeding.
   E. Gum bleeding.

14. Which one of the following coagulation factor proteins is vitamin K dependent?
   A. Factor XII.
   B. Factor II.
   C. Factor VIII.
   D. Factor V.
   E. Factor XIII.

15. Polymorphisms in which one of the following genes is associated with variable response to warfarin therapy?
   A. *VKORC1*.
   B. *CYP2D9*.
   C. *ABCB1*.
   D. *CYP3A4*.
   E. *CYP2J2*.

16. A 32-year-old Ashkenazi Jewish woman, 38 weeks pregnant (G2P1001), is in active labor and is failing to progress. A cesarean delivery is planned. During the delivery of her first child, she bled profusely and required transfusion of 2 U of packed red cells. At her obstetrician's office, records show that she has a complete blood cell count with a hemoglobin of 10.2 g/dL (11.0 to 13.0 g/dL), platelets 254 (165 to 415 × 109/L), PT 13.4 seconds (12.3 to 14.6 seconds), and aPTT 54.1 seconds (24.0 to 34.6 seconds). The patient's aPTT corrected into the reference range when mixed 1:1 with pooled normal plasma. Factor levels are factor VIII 180% (50% to 150%), factor IX 107% (50% to 150%), and factor XI 12% (50% to 150%). Which one of the following is the best choice to treat active bleeding in this patient?
   A. Recombinant activated factor VII, 90 μg/kg.
   B. Fresh frozen plasma (FFP), 15 mL/kg.
   C. Recombinant factor VIII.
   D. Fibrin glue.
   E. Recombinant factor XI.

17. Which one of the following coagulation protein deficiencies is not associated with a bleeding disorder?
   A. Factor II (prothrombin).
   B. Factor VII.
   C. Factor XI.
   D. Factor XII.
   E. Factor XIII.

Table 14-6

Test	Patient	Reference Range	Units
PT	14.7	12.7-15.4	sec
aPTT	>180	26.3-39.4	sec

18. A 73-year-old man's coagulation studies are shown in Table 14-6. A 1:1 mixing study corrected the patient's plasma aPTT into the reference range. When the incubation time of the patient plasma with the aPTT reagent was increased to 10 minutes, the aPTT decreased to 30.6 seconds. Which one of the following disorders is consistent with these findings?
   A. LAC.
   B. Protein C deficiency.
   C. Factor XIII deficiency.
   D. Prekallikrein deficiency.
   E. High-molecular-weight kininogen deficiency.

19. Your laboratory performs a factor X activity assay using a minimum of three dilutions of patient plasma. The three plasma dilutions exceed the allowable within-run coefficient of variation. Which one of the following disclaimers should be reported with the result?
   A. Factor deficiency.
   B. Inhibitor pattern.
   C. Noncalibrated curve.
   D. Linear range.
   E. Between-subject variability.

20. Which one of the following acquired coagulation factor deficiencies is associated with primary systemic amyloidosis?
   A. Factor II.
   B. Factor VII.
   C. Factor VIII.
   D. Factor X.
   E. Factor XII.

Table 14-7

Test	Patient	Reference Range	Units
PT	13.6	12.7-15.4	sec
aPTT	33.4	26.3-39.4	sec
Fibrinogen	386	233-496	mg/dL
Thrombin time	17.7	15.3-18.5	sec
D-Dimer	550	220-740	ng/mL FEU
White blood cell count	7.2	6.2-13.0	$\times 10^9$/L
Hemoglobin	12.0	12.8-16.9	g/dL
Hematocrit	36.2	34.4-50.8	%
Platelets	289	128-309	$\times 10^9$/L

FEU, fibrinogen-equivalent unit.

21. A 5-day-old infant has delayed bleeding from the umbilical cord stump. Laboratory studies are shown in Table 14-7. A 5 M urea test is performed on the patient's sample and shows rapid dissolution of the clot (decreased clot stability). Which one of the following disorders is the most likely to be the cause of bleeding?
    A. α_2-Antiplasmin deficiency.
    B. Dysfibrinogenemia.
    C. Factor XIII deficiency.
    D. Fibrinolysis.
    E. High-molecular-weight kininogen deficiency.

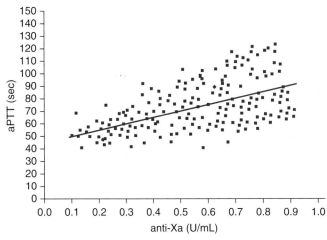

Figure 14-2 Linear regression line for aPTT vs. anti-Xa.

22. Your laboratory is validating a new aPTT reagent. To determine the heparin therapeutic range, samples from heparinized patients are tested with the aPTT reagent and then an anti-Xa assay is performed. The linear regression line is shown in Figure 14-2. Which one of the following is the best therapeutic range according to this Brill-Edwards experiment?
    A. 40 to 120 seconds.
    B. 40 to 60 seconds.
    C. 60 to 80 seconds.
    D. 60 to 120 seconds.
    E. 80 to 120 seconds.

23. For which one of the following clinical situations would thrombophilia testing be most indicated?
    A. 45-year-old man with a second cousin who had a venous thrombosis.
    B. 49-year-old man with hypertension, hyperlipidemia, and diabetes with first stroke.
    C. 55-year-old man with first mesenteric vein thrombosis.
    D. 35-year-old woman with first spontaneous abortion in first trimester.
    E. 45-year-old woman taking oral contraceptives.

24. Which of the following can lead to falsely low protein S activity on a PTT-based protein S activity assay?
    A. Decreased factor VIII activity.
    B. Decreased factor V activity.
    C. Direct thrombin inhibitor.
    D. Factor V Leiden mutation.
    E. Pregnancy.

Table 14-8

Test	Patient	Reference Range	Units
PT	14.1	12.7-15.4	sec
aPTT	70.2	26.3-39.4	sec
aPTT (1:1 mix with pooled normal plasma)	49.8	26.3-39.4	sec

25a. A 29-year-old woman who has had three consecutive spontaneous abortions over the past 2 years presents to her physician complaining of pain, swelling, and redness in her left leg. Ultrasound of her lower extremities reveals a deep venous thrombosis (DVT) in her left leg. She has no history of prior DVT. Her complete blood cell count is normal. Coagulation study results are shown in Table 14-8. Which one of the following is the most likely cause of the prolongation of the aPTT?
    A. Factor VIII deficiency.
    B. Severe factor VII deficiency.
    C. LAC.
    D. Disseminated intravascular coagulation (DIC).
    E. Factor IX inhibitor.

25b. Which one of the following must be demonstrated during laboratory testing to identify an LAC?
    A. Phospholipid independence of the inhibitor.
    B. Phospholipid dependence of the inhibitor.
    C. Mixing study in which the aPTT corrects into the reference range.
    D. Prolongation of a phospholipid-independent clotting test.
    E. Mixing study where the aPTT prolongation is time dependent.

25c. Which one of the following is an antiphospholipid antibody that is evaluated for the diagnosis of antiphospholipid antibody syndrome?
    A. Anti–glomerular basement membrane (anti-GBM) antibody.
    B. Antinuclear antibody.
    C. Anti-Jo-1 antibody.
    D. Anti–ADAMTS-13 antibodies.
    E. Anti-β_2-glycoprotein 1 antibodies.

Table 14-9

Test	Patient	Reference Range	Units
PT	14.1	12.7-15.4	sec
aPTT	70.2	26.3-39.4	sec
aPTT (1:1 mix with pooled normal plasma)	49.8	26.3-39.4	sec

25d. The patient is tested for the presence of an anticardiolipin (aCL) antibody following baseline coagulation studies (Table 14-9). A high-titer aCL antibody is detected. Which one of the following best describes whether the patient meets the criteria for the diagnosis of antiphospholipid antibody syndrome (APS) at this time?

   A. A history of three consecutive spontaneous abortions and the presence of aCL antibody are diagnostic for APS.

   B. A DVT and positive mixing study showing the presence of an inhibitor are diagnostic for APS.

   C. An arterial thrombosis is necessary to diagnose APS.

   D. An antiphospholipid antibody must be demonstrated on more than one occasion to meet the diagnostic criteria for APS.

   E. Detection of any antiphospholipid antibody is itself diagnostic of APS.

26. Which one of the following is the best therapy to treat the findings shown in Figure 14-3, B?

   A. Tranexamic acid.

   B. Aspirin.

   C. Packed red blood cell transfusion.

   D. Plasma transfusion.

   E. Platelet transfusion.

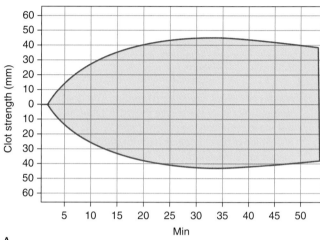

A

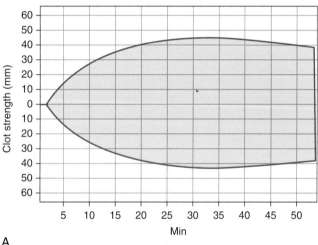

A

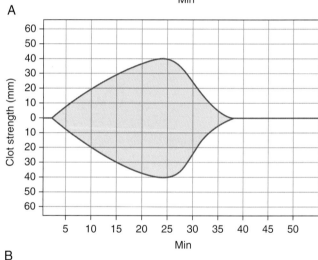

B

Figure 14-4 **A,** Normal thromboelastogram. **B,** The patient's thromboelastogram.

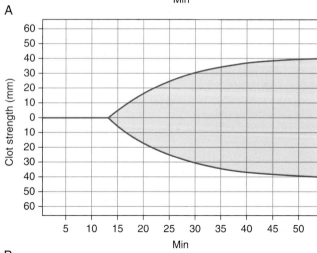

B

Figure 14-3 **A,** Normal thromboelastogram. **B,** The patient's thromboelastogram.

27. Which one of the following is the best therapy to treat the findings shown in Figure 14-4, *B*?

   A. Tranexamic acid.

   B. Heparin.

   C. Packed red blood cell transfusion.

   D. Plasma transfusion.

   E. Platelet transfusion.

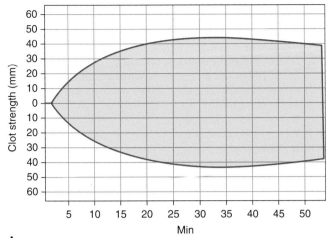

A

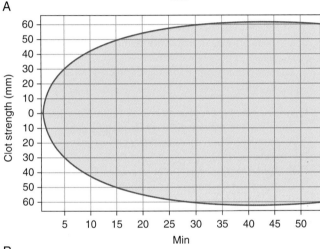

B

Figure 14-5 **A**, Normal thromboelastogram. **B**, The patient's thromboelastogram.

28. Which one of the following is the best therapy to treat the findings shown in Figure 14-5, *B*?
    A. Tranexamic acid.
    B. Heparin.
    C. Packed red blood cell transfusion.
    D. Plasma transfusion.
    E. Platelet transfusion.

29. Which one of the following assays is the best method for measuring antithrombin (AT) activity?
    A. Chromogenic amidolytic.
    B. Enzyme-linked immunoassay (ELISA).
    C. Latex particle immunoturbidometric.
    D. DNA analysis.
    E. Heparin-binding site inhibition.

30. Which one of the following tests is the most sensitive in detecting dysfibrinogenemia?
    A. Antigenic-based fibrinogen.
    B. Fibrometer-based fibrinogen.
    C. Nephelometry.
    D. Reptilase time.
    E. Thrombin time.

31. Which one of the following is the closest approximation of the prevalence of the factor V Leiden mutation in Caucasian Americans?

A. 0.5%.
B. 1%.
C. 5%.
D. 15%.
E. 25%.

32. Which one of the following is an acquired cause of low AT activity?
    A. Increased heparin cofactor II.
    B. L-Asparaginase therapy.
    C. Hematuria.
    D. Menopause.
    E. Warfarin therapy.

33. Your laboratory performs a second-generation modified functional activated protein C (APC) resistance screen by determining the activated protein C resistance (APCR) ratio of an aPTT. Which one of the following situations will most likely cause a false-positive result?
    A. Protein S level of 20%.
    B. Warfarin therapy.
    C. Heparin 0.7 U/mL.
    D. LAC.
    E. Liver dysfunction.

34. Which one of the following can increase protein C activity in an aPTT-based assay?
    A. Elevated factor VIII activity.
    B. Factor V Leiden.
    C. LAC.
    D. Warfarin therapy.
    E. Thrombosis.

35. Which one of the following disorders can present with purpura fulminans and DIC in newborns?
    A. Double heterozygous protein S and AT deficiency.
    B. Dysfibrinogenemia.
    C. Homozygous factor V Leiden.
    D. Homozygous protein C deficiency.
    E. Homozygous prothrombin 20210G>A mutation.

36. Which one of the following is an effect associated with heparin therapy?
    A. Activation of osteoclasts.
    B. Development of anti–heparin polyvinyl sulfate antibodies.
    C. Development of Hollenhorst plaques.
    D. Hypokalemia.
    E. Hirsutism.

37. The international sensitivity index (ISI) of the thromboplastin used in your laboratory is 1.26 according to the package insert. You perform the PT with this reagent in 120 normal donors and find the arithmetic mean to be 13.5 seconds, the geometric mean 13.7 seconds, and the standard error 3.5%. A patient's PT is 19.8 seconds using this reagent. Which one of the following is the closest value for the international normalized ratio (INR) for this patient? (Note: A calculator to determine the value is allowed.)
    A. 1.45
    B. 1.47
    C. 1.59
    D. 1.62
    E. 5.67

38. A 64-year-old man develops a DVT after a right total hip replacement. Before initiating heparin therapy, laboratory studies show a PT of 14.8 seconds (12.7 to 15.4) and an aPTT of 29.3 seconds (26.3 to 39.4). The heparin therapeutic range is an aPTT of 60 to 80 seconds. Heparin therapy is initiated with a bolus of 5000 IU and then 1000 IU/hr. Six hours later, the aPTT is 35 seconds. Another bolus of 5000 IU of heparin is administered, and the infusion is increased to 1500 IU/hr. The aPTT 6 hours later is 44 seconds. An antI-Xa level is performed and found to be 1.1 IU/mL. Which one of the following is the most likely explanation for these findings?

  A. LAC.
  B. AT deficiency.
  C. Acquired factor VIII deficiency.
  D. APCR.
  E. Increased heparin cofactor II activity.

39. A 55-year-old man requires heparin reversal after cardiopulmonary bypass for aortic valve repair. Which one of the following is the best method for reversal of the anticoagulant effect of unfractionated heparin (UFH) in this patient?

  A. FFP.
  B. Vitamin K.
  C. Cryoprecipitate.
  D. Prothrombin complex concentrates.
  E. Protamine sulfate.

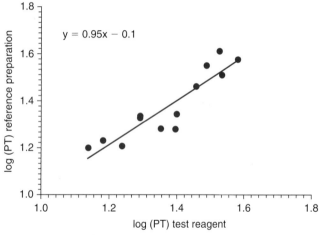

Figure 14-6 A double logarithmic plot of the prothrombin time (PT) of the international reference preparation versus a test thromboplastin reagent.

40. The PT for 13 normal donors and patients receiving stable warfarin therapy is tested with a reference thromboplastin and your new thromboplastin preparation (test reagent). A double logarithmic plot of the PT (seconds) of the reference preparation versus the test thromboplastin reagent is shown along with the regression equation (Figure 14-6). If the ISI of the reference preparation is 1.0, which one of the following is the best estimation of the ISI of the test reagent?

  A. 0.1
  B. 0.90
  C. 0.95
  D. 1.0
  E. 1.1

41. Which one of the following is an adverse effect of warfarin therapy?

  A. Avascular necrosis.
  B. Transmissible spongiform encephalopathy.

  C. Purple toe syndrome.
  D. Immune thrombocytopenia.
  E. Hollenhorst plaque.

42. Several hemostatic changes occur during the different stages of the liver transplant procedure. Which one of the following stages of liver transplantation is associated with hypercoagulability?

  A. Pre-anhepatic.
  B. Anhepatic to reperfusion.
  C. Postreperfusion.
  D. Postoperative.
  E. During surgical dissection and mobilization of the diseased liver.

43. Which one of the following is the mechanism of thrombosis associated with AT III deficiency?

  A. Endothelial cell cytotoxicity and disturbance of vascular hemostatic mechanisms.
  B. Failure to generate APC.
  C. Failure of APC to inactivate factors Va and VIIIa.
  D. Failure to generate plasmin.
  E. Failure to inhibit factors IIa (thrombin), Xa, and other activated factors.

44. Which one of the following is a recognized mechanism for thrombosis in patients with dysfibrinogenemia?

  A. Abnormal fibrinogen neutralizes tissue plasminogen activator (tPA).
  B. Abnormal fibrinogen inhibits protein C activity.
  C. Abnormal fibrinogen resists fibrinolysis.
  D. Abnormal fibrinogen induces cytotoxicity and disrupts vascular hemostatic mechanisms.
  E. Abnormal fibrinogen disrupts the activation of plasminogen.

45. Which one of the following is the mechanism of thrombosis in the setting of factor V Leiden?

  A. Failure to generate APC.
  B. Neutralization of tissue plasminogen activator (tPA).
  C. Endothelial cell toxicity and disruption of vascular hemostatic mechanisms.
  D. Activated protein C is unable to inactivate factor Va.
  E. Failure to inhibit thrombin.

46. Which one of the following is the mechanism for thrombosis in the setting of heparin cofactor II deficiency?

  A. Failure to inhibit thrombin.
  B. Failure to activate plasminogen.
  C. Failure to inhibit factor IIa (i.e., thrombin), factor Xa, and other activated factors.
  D. Failure to generate APC.
  E. Neutralization of tPA.

47. Which one of the following anticoagulant factors is solely produced by the liver?

  A. Protein C.
  B. AT.
  C. Protein S.
  D. Plasminogen.
  E. Tissue factor pathway inhibitor.

48. Which one of the following procoagulant hemostatic factors is produced solely by the liver?

  A. Factor VIII.
  B. Fibrinogen.

C. Factor V.

D. Plasminogen activator inhibitor.

E. Plasminogen.

49. Which one of the following is the mechanism of thrombosis associated with hyperhomocysteinemia?
   A. Failure to generate APC.
   B. Failure to inhibit factor IIa (i.e. thrombin), factor Xa, and other activated factors.
   C. Failure to activate plasminogen.
   D. Endothelial cell toxicity and disruption of vascular hemostatic mechanisms.
   E. Failure of APC to inactivate factors Va and VIIIa.

50. Which one of the following statements most accurately reflects the utility of routine coagulation tests to predict bleeding or thrombotic risk in liver disease?
   A. There is good evidence to support the use of routine coagulation tests for predicting bleeding or thrombotic risk in liver disease.
   B. There is good evidence that the PT, not the PTT, is useful in predicting bleeding or thrombotic risk in liver disease.
   C. There is no good evidence to support the use of routine coagulation tests for predicting bleeding or thrombotic risk in liver disease.
   D. There is good evidence to support the use of the PTT for predicting bleeding or thrombotic risk in liver disease.
   E. There is good evidence to support the use of the thrombin time for predicting bleeding or thrombotic risk in liver disease.

51. Which one of the following disorders is associated with neutralization of tPA?
   A. Protein C deficiency.
   B. AT deficiency.
   C. Factor V Leiden.
   D. Heparin cofactor II deficiency.
   E. Excess plasminogen activator inhibitor 1 activity.

52. Which one of the following mechanisms for thrombosis is associated with plasminogen deficiency?
   A. Failure of APC to inactivate factors Va and VIIIa.
   B. Failure to inhibit thrombin.
   C. Failure to generate plasmin.
   D. Failure to generate APC.
   E. Failure of activated protein C to inactivate factor Va.

53. Which one of the following is the mechanism of thrombosis in protein C deficiency?
   A. Failure to inhibit factor IIa, factor Xa, and other activated factors.
   B. Failure to generate APC.
   C. Failure to generate plasmin.
   D. Endothelial cell toxicity and disturbance of vascular hemostatic mechanisms.
   E. Failure of APC to inactivate factors Va and VIIIa.

54. Which one of the following is the mechanism of thrombosis in protein S deficiency?
   A. Failure to inhibit thrombin.
   B. Failure of APC to inactivate factors Va and VIIIa.
   C. APC fails to inactivate factor Va because of a highly conserved point mutation.
   D. Failure to activate plasminogen.
   E. An acquired abnormality in fibrin results in decreased fibrinolysis.

55. Which one of the following is the mechanism of thrombosis associated with tPA deficiency?
   A. Endothelial cell toxicity and disruption of vascular hemostatic mechanisms.
   B. Failure of APC to inactivate factors Va and VIIIa.
   C. Failure to generate APC.
   D. Failure to activate plasminogen.
   E. Failure to inhibit factor IIa, factor Xa, and other activated factors.

ANSWERS

1. A. Type 1.
   Rationale: A trial of DDAVP is usually a first-line treatment to increase release of normal vWF and should not cause thrombocytopenia.
   B. Type 3.
   Rationale: DDVAP most likely will be ineffective in increasing vWF levels but should not cause thrombocytopenia.
   C. Type 2B.
   Rationale: The vWF gain-of-function mutation increases platelet aggregation and thrombocytopenia.
   D. Type 2A.
   Rationale: DDVAP will lead to release of the smaller vWF multimers that may be adequate for hemostasis and should not cause thrombocytopenia.
   E. Type 2M.
   Rationale: Although there is decreased binding of vWF to GPIb/V/IX, increased amounts can mediate hemostasis and should not cause thrombocytopenia.

Major points of discussion
- Desmopressin (DDAVP) is a synthetic form of vasopressin that causes release of vWF from Weibel-Palade bodies in endothelial cells.
- Types 1 and 3 vWD are characterized by quantitative deficiencies of normal vWF.
- Type 2A vWD is caused by a mutation in the vWF protease cleavage site, leading to increased enzymatic cleavage and a lack of high- and intermediate-molecular-weight multimers.
- Type 2B vWD is caused by a gain-of-function-mutation in the platelet GPIb/V/IX binding site of vWF, leading to a "stickier" vWF.
- Type 2M vWD is caused by a loss-of-function-mutation in the platelet GPIb/V/IX binding site of vWF, leading to decreased binding of vWF to platelets.
- Type 2N vWD is caused by a mutation in the factor VIII binding site of vWF.

- Thrombocytopenia following DDAVP administration in type 2B vWD is usually transient and often is not associated with bleeding or thrombosis.
- DDAVP may be cautiously considered for patients with type 2 vWD.[18]

2. A. Fibrinogen.
Rationale: Similar levels in young children and adults.
B. Factor II.
C. Factor X.
D. Factor XI.
E. Prekallikrein.
Rationale: Lower levels in young children than adults.

Major points of discussion
- The hemostatic system of the neonate is physiologically immature and may manifest as prolongation of coagulation screening tests (PT and PTT).
- Interpretation of screening tests, as well as clotting factor activities, should be based on age-specific reference intervals.
- Clotting factors with lower levels in young children than in adults include the vitamin K–dependent factors (II, VII, IX, and X), as well as factors V, XI, and XII, prekallikrein, and high-molecular-weight kininogen.
- Clotting factors with similar or higher levels in young children than in adults include fibrinogen, factor VIII, and vWF.
- Because of the age-related changes in clotting factor levels that occur early in life, repeat testing at a later age may be necessary to exclude or confirm a diagnosis of bleeding related to a factor deficiency in a neonate.[1]

3. A. Desmopressin (DDAVP) challenge.
Rationale: The DDAVP challenge is a clinical test to measure increased vWF:Ag and vWF:RCo activity after the administration of DDAVP. DDAVP is contraindicated in platelet-type vWD.
B. Cryoprecipitate challenge.
Rationale: Platelet-type vWD (PT-vWD) and type 2B vWD can present with similar clinical and laboratory findings. PT-vWD is caused by gain-of-function mutation in the platelet glycoprotein GPIbα that leads to increased binding to vWF. Type 2B vWD is caused by gain-of-function mutation in the platelet-binding domain of vWD. Although presentation can be variable, both disorders can have thrombocytopenia, increased bleeding time, decreased FVIII activity, and increased vWF:Ag/RCo ratio. Both also aggregate with low concentrations of ristocetin, whereas normal controls do not. However, the addition of cryoprecipitate containing normal vWF leads to spontaneous aggregation of PT-vWD platelets, whereas type 2B vWD will not.
C. Platelet function analyzer (PFA)-100.
Rationale: This is a screening test that can detect vWD, but it cannot distinguish between type 2B vWD and PT-vWD.
D. Partial thromboplastin time (PTT) mixing study.
Rationale: If the PTT is elevated because of decreased FVIII activity, then the mixing study will correct. Both type 2B and PT-vWD can present with decreased FVIII activity.
E. von Willebrand factor (vWF) multimer analysis.
Rationale: Type 2B vWD and PT-vWD have loss of high-molecular-weight vWF multimers.

Major points of discussion
- Type 2B vWD is caused by a gain-of-function mutation in vWF that leads to increased binding to platelets.
- PT-vWD is caused by a gain-of-function mutation in GPIbα that leads to increased binding to vWF.
- Type 2B vWD and PT-vWD have similar clinical and laboratory findings. Although variable, patients classically present with thrombocytopenia, decreased vWF:Ag and vWF:ristocetin cofactor activity (RCo), increased vWF:Ag/vWF:RCo ratio, lack of high-molecular-weight vWF multimers, decreased FVIII:C, and abnormal ristocetin-induced platelet aggregation.
- It is important to distinguish these two disorders because the treatment will differ. Administration of vWF/FVIII concentrates in vWF type 2B would be effective, whereas in PT-vWD, it would not. Desmopressin (DDAVP) is contraindicated in PT-vWD.
- The cryoprecipitate challenge is a laboratory test that tests spontaneous platelet aggregation after the addition of cryoprecipitate containing normal vWF. The challenge will lead to spontaneous aggregation in PT-vWD, but not in type 2B vWD.[9]

4a. A. Type 3.
Rationale: Results consistent with type 3 vWD are markedly decreased vWF antigen level; markedly decreased vWF activity; markedly decreased factor VIII activity; multimer analysis demonstrating an absence of high, intermediate, and small bands; and absent ristocetin-induced platelet aggregation.
B. Type 2N.
Rationale: Results consistent with type 2N vWD are normal vWF antigen level; normal vWF activity; markedly decreased factor VIII activity; multimer analysis demonstrating high, intermediate, and small bands; and normal ristocetin-induced platelet aggregation.
C. Type 2A.
Rationale: Results consistent with type 2A vWD are normal to mildly decreased vWF antigen level, vWF activity lower than the antigen level, normal factor VIII level, multimer analysis demonstrating absent high and intermediate bands, and decreased ristocetin-induced platelet aggregation.
D. Type 2M.
Rationale: Results consistent with type 2M vWD are normal to mildly decreased vWF antigen level; vWF activity lower than the antigen level; normal factor VIII level; multimer analysis demonstrating high, intermediate, and small bands; and decreased ristocetin-induced platelet aggregation.
E. Type 1.
Rationale: Results consistent with type 1 vWD are mildly decreased vWF antigen level; mildly decreased vWF activity; mildly decreased factor VIII activity; multimer analysis demonstrating high, intermediate, and small bands; and normal or decreased ristocetin-induced platelet aggregation.

4b. A. The patient is blood type O, and these individuals tend to have higher baseline vWF antigen levels than those with other blood groups.

Rationale: Incorrect because blood group O individuals tend to have lower baseline vWF antigen levels than those with other blood groups.

B. At the time of initial evaluation the patient was taking oral contraceptives, which are known to increase vWF levels.

Rationale: vWF is an acute-phase reactant that increases during pregnancy and when taking oral contraceptives.

C. The blood sample for testing was transported to the laboratory at room temperature instead of the preferred temperature of 4°C.

Rationale: Transporting the sample at 4°C would have caused the vWF levels to have been artifactually low because of cryoprecipitation of the vWF. Samples should be transported to the laboratory at room temperature.

D. At the time of the initial evaluation, the patient had not recently exercised, and a lack of physical activity is known to increase vWF levels.

Rationale: Exercise and physical stress are known to increase vWF levels.

E. vWF levels are known to decrease with increasing age.

Rationale: The age-related decrease in vWF levels occurs from birth until approximately 180 days of life. After this time, the levels are the same as in adults.

Major points of discussion

- Several factors affect vWF levels and can confound the diagnosis of vWD.
- vWF is an acute-phase reactant and therefore is increased by stress, inflammation, pregnancy, and oral contraceptives. Repeated testing is necessary in some cases to identify low vWF levels.
- Medical conditions that can decrease vWF levels or activity include autoimmune/antibody-induced inhibition or clearance and destruction of vWF by increased shear stress (e.g., left ventricular assist devices).
- ABO blood type has an effect on plasma vWF levels. Individuals with group O blood type have approximately 25% lower vWF levels than individuals with other blood types.
- vWF levels tend to be higher in neonates than adults.
- Approximately 30% of variation in vWF levels is heritable.[18]

5. A. Left ventricular assist device.

Rationale: Left ventricular assist devices can cause acquired vWD.

B. Inflammatory bowel disease.

Rationale: Lack of absorption of vitamin K leads to vitamin K deficiency with decreased activity of factors II, VII, IX, and X and proteins C and S; these are the vitamin K–dependent coagulation factors.

C. Phytonadione therapy.

Rationale: Phytonadione is vitamin K, and its administration should increase levels of vitamin K–dependent coagulation factors (factors II, VII, IX, and X and proteins C and S).

D. Heparin therapy.

Rationale: Heparin therapy does not affect levels of factor VII. Heparin therapy can decrease levels of AT.

E. Ganciclovir therapy.

Rationale: Antibiotics decrease gut flora and lead to vitamin K deficiency with decreased levels of factor II, VII, IX, and X; these are the vitamin K–dependent coagulation factors. Ganciclovir is an antiviral and should not lead to factor VII deficiency.

Major points of discussion

- Normal vitamin K levels require an appropriate diet, normal gastrointestinal absorption, and a normal gut bacterial flora.
- Acquired factor VII deficiency can be due to acquired vitamin K deficiency (e.g., diet, antibiotic therapy, total parenteral nutrition, and gastrointestinal malabsorption), liver disease, and warfarin therapy.
- Vitamin K is required for the γ-carboxylation of the vitamin K–dependent coagulation factors (factors II, VII, IX, and X and proteins C and S). In the absence of vitamin K and γ-carboxylation, these factors are not active.
- Recycling vitamin K requires enzymes that are inhibited by warfarin, which leads to inactive vitamin K–dependent coagulation and anticoagulation factors. Exogenous administration of vitamin K (phytonadione) is used as an antidote for the warfarin effect.
- Antibiotics can alter gut flora, which leads to vitamin K deficiency. Hospitalized patients are often taking antibiotics and may be NPO or receiving total parenteral nutrition, which can make them vitamin K deficient.
- Hemorrhagic disease of the newborn can be seen in neonates who do not get adequate vitamin K across the placenta before delivery.
- The vitamin K–dependent factors II, VII, IX, and X and proteins C and S are produced in the liver. Decreased synthetic ability of the liver leads to decreased coagulation factor levels.

6. A. Factor VII.

Rationale: Factor VII has a half-life of approximately 5 hours.

B. Factor X.

Rationale: Factor X has a half-life of approximately 40 hours.

C. Factor II.

Rationale: Factor II has a half-life of approximately 65 hours.

D. Factor XIII.

Rationale: Factor XIII has a half-life of approximately 200 hours.

E. Factor VIII.

Rationale: Factor VIII has a half-life of approximately 10 hours.

Major points of discussion

- The half-lives of the coagulation factors vary and this is important when considering factor replacement therapy (dosing schedule) as well as anticoagulant therapy.
- For example, recombinant factor VIIa is dosed every 2 hours, factor VIII every 12 hours, and factor IX every 24 hours.
- Factor VII has the shortest half-life.
- Factor XIII has the longest half-life.
- The approximate plasma half-lives of the clotting factors are as follows:
  - Factor I: 90 hours
  - Factor II: 65 hours
  - Factor V: 15 to 36 hours
  - Factor VII: 5 hours
  - Factor VIII: 10 hours
  - Factor IX: 25 hours
  - Factor X: 40 hours
  - Factor XI: 45 to 80 hours
  - Factor XII: 50 to 70 hours
  - Factor XIII: 200 hours

7. A. Epistaxis.
Rationale: This is a common complication.
B. Thrombosis.
Rationale: This is a rare complication of congenital factor VII deficiency and is associated with surgery and sometimes recombinant factor VIIa therapy.
C. Menorrhagia.
Rationale: Up to 60% of women with congenital factor VII deficiency have menorrhagia.
D. Central nervous system bleeding.
Rationale: Occurs most commonly in the first 6 months of life.
E. Postoperative bleeding.
Rationale: Up to 30% of patient will bleed after surgery.

Major points of discussion
- Congenital factor VII deficiency is caused by homozygosity or double heterozygosity for mutations in the factor VII gene that cause decreased production or function of factor VII.
- It is an autosomal recessive disorder and has an incidence of 1 in 500,000.
- The genotype and factor activity level in congenital factor VII deficiency do not correlate well with clinical bleeding.
- Clinical manifestations include epistaxis, mucosal bleeding, soft tissue hematomas, hemarthrosis, menorrhagia, and postoperative bleeding.
- Thrombosis is a rare complication of congenital factor VII deficiency and is more commonly seen during surgical interventions or replacement therapy.[16]

8. A. Factor V.
Rationale: PT and aPTT are generally prolonged in this setting.
B. Factor VII.
Rationale: A normal aPTT and a prolonged PT that corrects with mixing with pooled normal plasma are characteristic of congenital factor VII deficiency.
C. Factor VIII.
D. Factor IX.
E. Factor XI.
Rationale: Hemophilia A, B, and C are characterized by a prolonged aPTT and a normal PT

Major points of discussion
- An isolated elevation of the PT (with a normal aPTT), along with a clinical history of bleeding, suggests congenital factor VII deficiency or acquired causes, such as liver disease, vitamin K deficiency, and warfarin therapy.
- A mixing study with pooled normal plasma should correct the prolonged PT when a factor deficiency is present.
- Clinical manifestations of congenital factor VII deficiency include epistaxis, mucosal bleeding, soft tissue hematomas, hemarthrosis, menorrhagia, postoperative bleeding, and uncommonly, thrombosis.
- Recombinant factor VIIa at a low dose of 20 to 30 µg/kg is used to treat congenital factor VII deficiency.
- Although plasma infusions can be used for treatment in this setting, there is a risk for volume overload, other transfusion reactions, and transfusion transmitted infection.

9. A. Formation of anti–factor VII antibodies.
Rationale: Formation is possible but extremely rare in patients with congenital factor VII deficiency.
B. Short half-life of recombinant factor VIIa.
Rationale: Recombinant factor VIIa must be administered every 2 hours because of the short half-life.
C. Requirement for high doses (120 µg/kg).
Rationale: Low doses (20 to 30 µg/kg) are usually given; this is a much lower dose than for patients with factor VIII inhibitors.
D. Contamination with activated factors II, IX, and X.
Rationale: Activated prothrombin concentrates can have activated factors II, VII, IX, and X. However, recombinant factor VIIa does not contain the activated factors II, IX, and X.
E. Need to overlap with heparin therapy.
Rationale: Initiation of warfarin requires heparin overlap, but recombinant factor VIIa is not used for anticoagulation and does not require heparin overlap.

Major points of discussion
- Recombinant factor VIIa (rVIIa) at a low dose of 20 to 30 µg/kg is used in the treatment of congenital factor VII deficiency.
- Although plasma infusions have been used, there is risk for volume overload and other transfusion reactions, as well as transfusion-transmitted infection.
- The biological half-life of rFVIIa is 2 hours, so it may have to be administered frequently until bleeding ceases.
- rFVIIa in vivo action is inhibited by tissue factor pathway inhibitor (TFPI).
- rFVIIa is also used to treat bleeding in patients with hemophilia A or B with inhibitors or patients with acquired factor VIII or IX inhibitors.

10a. A. Consistent with factor VIII half-life.
Rationale: The half-life of factor VIII is 12 hours, so approximately 25% of factor VIII activity should remain after 12 hours (the administered dose should result in 50% peak factor VIII levels). The mixing study in this case is consistent with an inhibitor.
B. Consistent with inadequate dosing of factor VIII.
Rationale: The dose is calculated correctly for factor VIII replacement: body weight (kg) × desired % increase × 0.5 IU/kg.
C. Inadequate reconstitution of lyophilized product.
Rationale: The mixing study is not consistent with a factor deficiency.
D. Presence of a lupus anticoagulant (LAC).
Rationale: An LAC could produce an isolated elevated PTT without correction on a mixing study. However, the time dependence of the antibody and bleeding, rather than thrombosis, suggests that this is less likely an LAC.
E. Factor VIII inhibitor.
Rationale: The percentage recovery of factor activity is too low after 12 hours, and the mixing study shows a time-dependent inhibitor. These findings are most consistent with a factor inhibitor.

Major points of discussion
- An alloantibody against factor VIII should be considered when an appropriate dose of factor VIII is administered but the desired increase in factor activity is not reached.

- Anti–factor VIII antibodies can be detected on coagulation studies by performing a mixing study. A mixing study is performed by mixing one volume of patient plasma with one volume of pooled normal plasma. If a factor deficiency is present, the pooled normal plasma will correct the prolonged aPTT. However, the presence of an alloantibody will inhibit the factor VIII in both the patient plasma and the pooled normal plasma.
- LACs can also inhibit coagulation by interfering with the phospholipid surfaces that coagulation factors require for their activity. However, the inhibitor activity is usually seen upon immediate mixing and with incubation. In addition, LACs are more likely to cause thrombosis, not bleeding.
- Anti–factor VIII alloantibodies are generally weaker antibodies than LACs, and with incubation, their inhibition will strengthen. Therefore, the immediate mix may correct, and then with incubation for 1 to 2 hours, the aPTT will prolong as the antibody's binding is enhanced.
- The strength of an antibody should be determined using a Bethesda assay, which measures the titer of the antibody. The higher the Bethesda units (BUs), the greater the strength of the antibody. A BU reflects the amount of inhibitor that will inactivate half of the factor activity.
- If there are fewer than 5 BUs, then overwhelming the inhibitor with increasing factor replacement can be attempted (i.e., give a very large dose of factor VIII). However, if there are more than 5 BUs, then alternate concentrates (e.g., porcine factor VIII) or bypassing agents (e.g., factor VIII inhibitor bypassing activity, prothrombin complex concentrates, recombinant factor VIIa) should be used to treat active bleeding.

10b. A. 750 IU.
B. 1000 IU.
Rationale: These doses are too low for weight and target goal.
C. 2500 IU.
Rationale: This dose may be appropriate for factor VIII replacement.
D. 3500 IU.
E. 5000 IU.
Rationale: These doses are too high. The target should be 50%.

Major points of discussion
- Factor VIII is dosed based on the current factor activity, the desired factor activity, and the weight.
- Calculated dose in units = [% Change in factor activity desired] × [Body weight (kg)] × 0.5 IU/kg.
- For this patient, assuming factor VIII activity of 0%, a target of 50%, and body weight of 100 kg: Calculated dose = 50% × 100 kg × 0.5 IU/kg = 2500 IU.
- The target goal for hemarthrosis, gastrointestinal bleeding, and dental extraction is 50%; major surgery and intracranial hemorrhage should have a target goal of 100%.
- The half-life of factor VIII is 12 hours, so the maintenance dose (50% of loading dose) should be administered approximately every 12 hours.

11a. A. Factor II.
Rationale: Factor II deficiency should affect both the PT and the aPTT.
B. Factor VII.
Rationale: Factor VII deficiency is usually associated with an elevated PT and a normal aPTT.
C. Factor VIII.
Rationale: An isolated aPTT in the setting of clinical bleeding can be caused by factor VIII, factor IX, and factor XI deficiencies.
D. Factor X.
Rationale: The PT and aPTT are usually affected in factor X deficiency.
E. Factor V.
Rationale: The PT and aPTT are usually affected in factor V deficiency.

Major points of discussion
- Hemophilia A is caused by a deficiency in factor VIII.
- Hemophilia A is inherited in an X-linked recessive manner so that males are affected more than females. Females can develop hemophilia A by inheriting two affected alleles, having Turner syndrome (XO), or having skewed lyonization.
- Factor deficiencies associated with an elevated aPTT but a normal PT include factors VIII, IX, XI, and XII; prekallikrein; and high-molecular-weight kininogen deficiencies. Deficiencies in prekallikrein, factor XII, and high-molecular-weight kininogen are not associated with an increased risk for bleeding.
- An elevated PTT caused by a factor deficiency can be corrected in vitro by mixing patient plasma with pooled normal plasma (mixing study) if an inhibitor is not present.
- Hemophilia A is classified into severe (<1% activity), moderate (1% to 5%), and mild (>5% to 30%).
  - Severe hemophilia is associated with spontaneous bleeding.
  - Moderate hemophilia is associated with bleeding with minor trauma or surgery.
  - Mild hemophilia usually requires a greater degree of trauma or invasive procedures to cause bleeding.
- Clinical manifestations include hemarthrosis, deep soft tissue hematomas, hematuria, intracranial hemorrhage, and gastrointestinal bleeding.

11b. A. 75 IU.
B. 210 IU.
C. 750 IU.
Rationale: These doses are too low for weight and target goal.
D. 1500 IU.
Rationale: This dose may be appropriate.
E. 5000 IU.
Rationale: This dose is too high.

Major points of discussion
- Factor IX is dosed based on the current factor activity, the desired factor activity, and the weight.
- Calculated dose in units = % Change in factor activity desired × Body weight (kg) × 1.0 IU/kg.
- For this patient, assuming factor IX activity of 0%, weight of 30 kg, and desired factor level of 50%: Calculated dose = 50% × 30 kg × 1.0 IU/kg = 1500 IU.

- Target goal for hemarthrosis is 50%; major surgery has a target of 100%.
- The half-life of factor IX is 18 to 24 hours, so the maintenance dose (50% of loading dose) should be administered approximately every 24 hours.
- In addition, factor IX distributes into the extravascular space, so recovery of factor activity after infusion may not reliably be 100%. Therefore, a correction factor to increase the dose to account for the loss of intravascular recovery may be required based on empirical studies for a specific patient.

12. A. 5 hours.
Rationale: The half-life of factor VII is approximately 5 hours.
B. 12 hours.
Rationale: The half-life of factor VIII is 12 hours.
C. 24 hours.
Rationale: The half-life of factor IX is 18 to 24 hours.
D. 48 hours.
Rationale: The half-life of factor XI is approximately 50 hours.
E. 96 hours.
Rationale: The half-life of fibrinogen is approximately 4 days.

Major points of discussion
- Replacement therapy with factor IX is used in patients with hemophilia B.
- Targets of 50% are desirable for joint bleeding, dental procedures, hematuria, and gastrointestinal bleeding.
- Higher targets of 100% are desirable for soft tissue hematomas, intracranial hemorrhage, and surgery.
- The half-life of factor IX is 18 to 24 hours, which means a loading dose should be provided and then a maintenance dose (usually one half the loading dose) administered every 24 hours.
- Administration of recombinant factor IX can have 60% to 80% recovery because of the rapid extravascular distribution of the factor after administration.

13. A. Petechiae.
B. Superficial hematomas.
Rationale: Deep hematomas are characteristic of coagulation deficiencies.
C. Epistaxis.
D. Delayed bleeding.
Rationale: Delayed postoperative bleeding is characteristic of coagulation deficiencies.
E. Gum bleeding.
Rationale for A, C, and E: Seen in platelet-type bleeding.

Major points of discussion
- Coagulation factor deficiencies are characterized by deep hematomas, hemarthroses, and delayed postoperative bleeding.
- Coagulation factor deficiencies are inherited in an X-linked recessive (factor VIII or factor IX deficiency), autosomal recessive (factor VII or XI deficiency), or autosomal dominant (vWD) manner.
- Petechiae, persistent bleeding from superficial cuts, and mucosal bleeding such as gum bleeding characterize platelet-type bleeding.
- Coagulation factor deficiencies are more commonly seen in men because of sex-linked inheritance.
- It is important to keep in mind that abnormalities of the blood vessels may also lead to bleeding disorders.

14. A. Factor XII.
B. Factor II.
Rationale: Factors II, VII, IX, and X and proteins C and S are vitamin K–dependent factors.
C. Factor VIII.
D. Factor V.
E. Factor XIII.
Rationale for A, C, D, and E: These factors are not vitamin K dependent.

Major points of discussion
- The vitamin K–dependent coagulation proteins include factors II, VII, IX, and X and proteins C, S, and Z.
- Vitamin K is a cofactor for γ-carboxylation of glutamic acid residues of the vitamin K–dependent coagulation proteins.
- The carboxylation of glutamic acid residues results in the chelation of calcium ions and allows the proteins to bind to the phospholipids on the platelet cell membranes to promote the assembly of coagulation factor complexes on the platelet surface.
- Without sufficient vitamin K, γ-carboxylation does not take place, the proteins are unable to bind to phospholipids, and coagulation proteins cannot interact, making them functionally inactive.
- Warfarin exerts its effect by inhibiting vitamin K 2,3-epoxide reductase, thereby blocking regeneration of the active form of vitamin K, leading to a lack of γ-carboxylation.

15. A. *VKORC1.*
Rationale: VKORC1 single-nucleotide polymorphisms are associated with variable metabolism of warfarin.
B. *CYP2D9.*
Rationale: CYP2C9, not *CYP2D9,* is a hepatic P450 enzyme associated with variable metabolism of warfarin.
C. *ABCB1.*
Rationale: Encodes P-glycoprotein, a drug efflux pump, that may be involved in dabigatran availability.
D. *CYP3A4.*
E. *CYP2J2.*
Rationale: Involved in the metabolism of rivaroxaban.

Major points of discussion
- Warfarin is metabolized by oxidation in the liver by CYP2C9. The mechanism of action of warfarin is the inhibition of the vitamin K epoxide reductase complex, subunit 1.
- *VKORC1* and *CYP2C9* are two genes with single-nucleotide polymorphisms that predict variable response to warfarin metabolism.
- CYP2C9 is a P450 enzyme involved in warfarin metabolism. The variant alleles *CYP2C9*2* and *CYP2C9*3* metabolize warfarin more slowly and may require a lower initial dose.
- *VKORC1* encodes the vitamin K epoxide reductase gene. Variable alleles are associated with variable metabolism of warfarin. Individuals with the group A haplotype produce less VKORC1, and lower warfarin doses are needed in these patients.
- The *CYP2C9* and *VKORC1* alleles are found in different frequencies based on ethnic background. For example, the *VKORC1* group A haplotype associated with lower warfarin requirements is present in 89% of Asians, but

the group B haplotype is seen more in whites and African Americans.[22]

16. A. Recombinant activated factor VII, 90 µg/kg.
Rationale: This may be considered for life-threatening bleeding, but it is not the standard therapy for factor XI deficiency,
B. Fresh frozen plasma (FFP), 15 mL/kg.
Rationale: This is the correct loading dose of plasma for factor XI deficiency.
C. Recombinant factor VIII.
Rationale: The patient most likely has factor XI deficiency.
D. Fibrin glue.
Rationale: Fibrin glue can be used for dental extraction, but not for uterine bleeding.
E. Recombinant factor XI.
Rationale: This is not available as a U.S. Food and Drug Administration (FDA)-approved drug.

Major points of discussion
- Factor XI deficiency (hemophilia C) is an autosomal recessive disorder and therefore is seen equally in males and females.
- It is more commonly seen in patients with an Ashkenazi Jewish background.
- Patients may have a range of clinical manifestations from no bleeding tendency to severe bleeding. Factor XI levels do not correlate well with the bleeding risk.
- The aPTT is prolonged, and the PT is normal. The prolonged aPTT can be corrected by a 1:1 mix with pooled normal plasma. Homozygotes and compound heterozygotes have factor XI levels of less than 15%.
- Mild bleeding episodes may not have to be treated. However, factor levels above 30% are generally desired before surgery.
- If treatment is required, a loading dose of 15 to 20 mL/kg of FFP is administered, followed by a 3 to 6 mL/kg dose every 12 hours. Factor XI has a half-life of approximately 50 hours.
- For severe bleeding, recombinant factor VIIa has been used, including in patients with factor XI inhibitors. These indications are not approved by the FDA for use with recombinant factor VIIa.

17. A. Factor II (prothrombin).
Rationale: Factor II deficiency is associated with hematomas and hemarthroses.
B. Factor VII.
Rationale: Congenital and acquired factor VII deficiencies are associated with bleeding.
C. Factor XI.
Rationale: Factor XI deficiency is associated with variable degrees of bleeding from asymptomatic to severe. Factor levels do not predict bleeding manifestations.
D. Factor XII.
Rationale: Factor XII deficiency is *not* associated with bleeding.
E. Factor XIII.
Rationale: Factor XIII deficiency is associated with bleeding.

Major points of discussion
- Factor XII (Hageman factor) is a coagulation protein that autoactivates when exposed to negatively charged

surfaces. It is a component of the intrinsic pathway. Factor XIIa acts as a serine protease that activates factor XI, prekallikrein, and C1 esterases.
- Factor XII deficiency results in an elevated aPTT with a normal PT. However, factor XII deficiency is not associated with bleeding. Rather, factor XII deficiency is thought to have delayed arterial thrombosis.
- Factor VII deficiency is associated with bleeding that is treated with recombinant factor VIIa or plasma.
- Factor XIII cross-links fibrin and stabilizes a clot. Deficiency of factor XIII is associated with bleeding. Screening for factor XIII deficiency is performed by measuring clot stability in 5M urea.[20,26]

18. A. LAC.
Rationale: In the presence of an LAC, the mixing study would not correct and autoactivation would not be seen.
B. Protein C deficiency.
Rationale: Protein C deficiency is not associated with an elevated aPTT, correction of a mixing study, or autoactivation.
C. Factor XIII deficiency.
Rationale: Factor XIII deficiency does not show an elevated aPTT, correction of a mixing study, or autoactivation.
D. Prekallikrein deficiency.
Rationale: Prekallikrein deficiency is associated with increased aPTT (intrinsic pathway), correction with a mixing study (deficiency), and autoactivation.
E. High-molecular-weight kininogen deficiency.
Rationale: High-molecular-weight kininogen deficiency is associated with increased aPTT (intrinsic pathway) and correction with a mixing study (deficiency), but autoactivation is not a characteristic.

Major points of discussion
- The contact system consists of factor XII, factor XI, and prekallikrein (serine protease zymogens) and the nonenzymatic cofactor high-molecular-weight kininogen.
- Deficiencies in the contact system proteins can result in an elevated aPTT with a normal PT. A mixing study with pooled normal plasma would correct the aPTT (i.e., deficiency, not an inhibitor).
- Factor XII, prekallikrein, and high-molecular-weight kininogen deficiencies are not associated with bleeding.
- Complete normalization of prolonged aPTT following prolonged incubation is characteristic of prekallikrein deficiency and is caused by autoactivation of factor XII (activation of factor XII by factor XIIa).
- Although autoactivation of factor XII has been described with LACs, normalization of the aPTT into the reference range does not occur. In addition, LACs are not associated with correction after mixing with pooled normal plasma.[2]

19. A. Factor deficiency.
Rationale: Agreement among dilutions of the patient sample does not indicate a factor deficiency.
B. Inhibitor pattern.
Rationale: An inhibitor pattern shows nonparallelism. In nonparallelism, dilutions of patient plasma do not provide the same factor activity within allowable error.
C. Noncalibrated curve.
D. Linear range.

Rationale: A calibration curve is determined using dilutions of calibrator, not a patient sample. The linear range is determined after the best-fit curve is fit to the calibration points and the widest linear range.
E. Between-subject variability.
Rationale: The variability in this experiment is within subjects at three patient plasma dilutions. Between-subject variability would be determined between two subjects.

Major points of discussion

- Factor activity for intrinsic factors is determined using PTT-based assays. A reference curve for a factor is constructed by determining the factor activity after diluting a calibrator (that has a known factor activity traceable to a World Health Organization standard) using plasma deficient for the factor being assayed. The percentage factor activity is plotted against the PTT, usually using a log-linear or log-log transformation. The factor activity in a patient sample is determined by measuring the PTT using two or more dilutions of patient sample and then reading the activity from the reference curve.
- The one-stage coagulation factor assay is an example of a parallel line bioassay. In this type of assay, the results are reliable when the curves of reference and patient plasma are parallel. If there is nonparallelism, the factor activity results should be considered incorrect.
- A common reason for nonparallelism is the presence of LACs or other nonspecific inhibitors.
- If three or more patient dilutions are used and they do not agree within a set tolerance limit, the assay is demonstrating an inhibitor pattern. A nonspecific inhibitor should be suspected.
- The presence of anticoagulants will interfere with clotting times and may underestimate factor activities.
- The presence of LACs will interfere with coagulation factor activity and can underestimate coagulation factor activity.
- Elevated factor VIII levels (acute-phase reactant) can shorten the PTT and thus overestimate factor activity.
- If nonparallelism is encountered using a factor assay with multiple dilutions, a chromogenic factor assay should be performed.[25]

20. A. Factor II.
B. Factor VII.
C. Factor VIII.
D. Factor X.
Rationale: This deficiency is associated with systemic amyloidosis.
E. Factor XII.
Rationale for A, B, C, and E: These deficiencies are not associated with systemic amyloidosis.

Major points of discussion

- Systemic amyloidosis is associated with acquired factor X deficiency.
- Amyloid fibers are thought to bind directly to factor X.
- Treatment consists of FFP or prothrombin complex concentrate infusions.
- Acquired factor X deficiency can result from vitamin K deficiency or liver disease, although the deficiency is usually not isolated; it is usually associated with decreased factors II, VII, and IX.
- Respiratory infections, thymoma, and malignancies (e.g., renal carcinoma, adrenal adenocarcinoma, acute myeloid

leukemia) have also been reported to be associated with acquired factor X deficiency.
- Congenital factor X deficiency is rare (1 per 500,000). Acquired inhibitors to factor X are uncommon.

21. A. α_2-Antiplasmin deficiency.
Rationale: α_2-Antiplasmin deficiency would show normal clot dissolution in the 5M urea test.
B. Dysfibrinogenemia.
Rationale: Dysfibrinogenemia would show a prolonged thrombin time.
C. Factor XIII deficiency.
Rationale: The rapid clot dissolution in 5M urea is characteristic of factor XIII deficiency.
D. Fibrinolysis.
Rationale: An elevated D-dimer would be expected if bleeding were caused by fibrinolysis.
E. High-molecular-weight kininogen deficiency.
Rationale: High-molecular-weight kininogen deficiency would cause a prolongation of the aPTT and is not a cause of bleeding.

Major points of discussion

- The differential diagnosis of a bleeding disorder with a normal PT and aPTT includes factor XIII deficiency, disorders of fibrinolysis, and disorders of platelets.
- Factor XIII deficiency is a rare, autosomal recessive disorder. Factor XIII cross-links fibrin through peptide bonds. The clots from these patients dissolve rapidly in 5M urea or in 1% monochloracetic acid.
- Factor XIII deficiency is associated with delayed umbilical stump bleeding, bleeding after circumcision, hematomas, soft tissue bleeding, and recurrent spontaneous abortions.
- Factor XIII deficiency is treated with cryoprecipitate or factor XIII concentrates (Europe).
- Patients with α_2-antiplasmin deficiency have a bleeding tendency because of decreased inactivation of plasmin, which leads to excess fibrinolysis.
- The PT and aPTT are normal in α_2-antiplasmin deficiency. Solubility in 5M urea is normal. However, the euglobulin lysis time is shortened. Euglobulin is formed when plasma is acidified, and it contains important fibrinolytic factors such as plasminogen, tPA, and α_2-antiplasmin. Deficiency will result in a markedly accelerated lysis time.
- Fibrinolytic disorders are treated with antifibrinolytics, such as ϵ-aminocaproic acid.[12]

22. A. 40 to 120 seconds.
Rationale: This corresponds to 0.1 to 0.9 U/mL anti-Xa.
B. 40 to 60 seconds.
Rationale: This corresponds to 0.1 to 0.3 U/mL anti-Xa.
C. 60 to 80 seconds.
Rationale: This corresponds to 0.3 to 0.7 U/mL anti-Xa.
D. 60 to 120 seconds.
Rationale: This corresponds to 0.3 to 0.9 U/mL anti-Xa.
E. 80 to 120 seconds.
Rationale: This corresponds to 0.7 to 0.9 U/mL anti-Xa.

Major points of discussion

- UFH is a glycosaminoglycan consisting of repeating sulfated disaccharides with chains from 3 to 30 kDa in size.

- Heparin binds to AT and accelerates its activity 1000-fold, leading to the inactivation of coagulation factors IIa, Xa, IXa, and XIa.
- UFH is the most common injectable anticoagulant and is used for the treatment of acute coronary syndromes, venous thromboembolism (VTE), and atrial fibrillation. It is also used as the anticoagulant in cardiac bypass and extracorporeal membrane oxygenation circuits.
- UFH is monitored by following the aPTT. The sensitivity of the aPTT to heparin concentration varies from lot to lot of aPTT reagent. Therefore, the therapeutic range should be established with each new lot of aPTT reagent.
- The Brill-Edwards method of establishing the UFH therapeutic range requires samples from patients currently on UFH therapy, but not on warfarin (the PT should be in the reference range). UFH anti-Xa activity and the aPTT are measured on each sample. A linear regression is performed; the aPTT corresponding to 0.3 to 0.7 U/mL anti-Xa activity is read from the regression line. The aPTT range is set as the therapeutic range. If heparin-protamine titration is used, then 0.2 to 0.4 U/mL heparin would be used to determine the therapeutic range.
- UFH is usually administered as a bolus dose and then a constant infusion. The half-life of heparin is 1 to 2 hours. Therefore, heparin therapy is usually monitored by measuring the aPTT every 6 hours while it is adjusted.
- Adverse reactions to heparin include heparin-induced thrombocytopenia, osteopenia, and hyperkalemia.
- Heparin is reversed by administered protamine; FFP is not used to reverse heparin.[11]

23. A. 45-year-old man with a second cousin who had a venous thrombosis.
Rationale: Testing should be performed when there are first-degree relatives with VTE.
B. 49-year-old man with hypertension, hyperlipidemia, and diabetes with first stroke.
Rationale: Testing should be performed when there is spontaneous thrombosis, in the *absence* of such risk factors as mentioned previously, in a patient younger than 50 years.
C. 55-year-old man with first mesenteric vein thrombosis.
Rationale: Thrombosis at unusual sites, such as mesenteric vein, portal vein, splenic vein, renal vein, and cerebral sinus, without other risk factors is an indication for thrombophilia testing.
D. 35-year-old woman with first spontaneous abortion in first trimester.
Rationale: Testing should be performed for recurrent spontaneous abortions and abortions in the second and third trimesters of pregnancy.
E. 45-year-old woman taking oral contraceptives.
Rationale: Testing should be performed for women intending to conceive or to start oral contraceptives when there is a first-degree relative with a thrombophilia.

Major points of discussion

- Venous thromboembolic disease occurs in 1 to 2 per 1000 adults. Approximately 60% of patients with an unprovoked stroke have an underlying inherited thrombophilia.

- Acquired risk factors for thrombophilia include malignancy, older age, estrogen replacement, immobilization (e.g., orthopedic surgery), chronic inflammation, and antiphospholipid antibodies.
- Laboratory testing is recommended only for a select population of patients.
- Indications for testing for patients with VTE:
  - Spontaneous thrombosis in a young patient (<50 years old)
  - Recurrent VTE
  - First-degree relatives with VTE
  - Thrombosis at unusual sites, such as mesenteric vein, portal vein, splenic vein, renal vein, and cerebral sinus, without other risk factors
- Laboratory testing for thrombophilia can include APCR/factor V Leiden, proteins C and S deficiency, prothrombin G20210A mutation, AT deficiency, homocysteine levels, elevated factor VIII activity, antiphospholipid antibodies (e.g., LAC, aCL antibodies, anti-β_2-glycoprotein I antibodies).[3]

24. A. Decreased factor VIII activity.
Rationale: Elevated factor VIII levels can falsely decrease protein S activity in PTT-based assays.
B. Decreased factor V activity.
Rationale: Factor V is normalized in the assay with protein S–deficient plasma, and factor Va is also added.
C. Direct thrombin inhibitor.
Rationale: Direct thrombin inhibitors overestimate the protein S level.
D. Factor V Leiden mutation.
Rationale: Factor V Leiden mutation and other causes of APCR can lead to a falsely low protein S activity on a PTT-based protein S activity assay.
E. Pregnancy.
Rationale: Protein S levels decrease with pregnancy, which is a normal physiologic response. It is a true decrease in the protein S activity.

Major points of discussion

- Protein S deficiency can be an inherited or acquired cause of thrombophilia. Protein S is a cofactor for APC, which inactivates factors Va and VIIIa.
- Acquired causes of protein S deficiency include vitamin K deficiency, warfarin therapy, liver disease, thrombosis, oral contraceptives, and estrogen replacement therapy.
- PTT-based protein S assays are performed by diluting patient plasma with protein S–deficient plasma. Fixed amounts of APC and factor Va are added. Prolongation of the PTT is proportional to the amount of protein S in the sample (low protein S → less factor Va inactivated → shorter PTT).
- PTT-based assays can be affected by LACs, APCR/factor V Leiden, elevated factor VIII activity, direct thrombin inhibitors, and heparin therapy.
- Protein S circulates as free protein S and as C4 binding protein (C4bp)-bound protein S. C4bp-bound protein S is not active.
- Total protein S = C4bp – protein S + free protein S.[27]

25a. A. Factor VIII deficiency.
Rationale: aPTT for the 1:1 mix should have corrected into the reference range.

B. Severe factor VII deficiency.
Rationale: There should be a prolongation of the PT.
C. LAC.
Rationale: The prolonged aPTT, failure of the aPTT to correct in the mixing study, and the DVT are consistent with the presence of an LAC.
D. Disseminated intravascular coagulation (DIC).
Rationale: Both the PT and aPTT would be prolonged and thrombocytopenia would be expected in DIC.
E. Factor IX inhibitor.
Rationale: An inhibitor to factor IX would be expected to present with bleeding, not clotting.

25b. A. Phospholipid independence of the inhibitor.
Rationale: LACs are phospholipid dependent.
B. Phospholipid dependence of the inhibitor.
Rationale: LACs prolong clotting times by binding to phospholipids and interfering with their ability to provide a surface for the clotting cascade.
C. Mixing study in which the aPTT corrects into the reference range.
Rationale: Because an LAC is an inhibitor, the aPTT should not correct into the reference range.
D. Prolongation of a phospholipid-independent clotting test.
Rationale: A phospholipid-dependent clotting test should be prolonged because LACs interfere with phospholipids.
E. Mixing study where the aPTT prolongation is time dependent.
Rationale: Time-dependent prolongation of the aPTT upon incubation is suggestive of the presence of an inhibitor to a specific coagulation factor, not an LAC.

25c. A. Anti–glomerular basement membrane (anti-GBM) antibody.
Rationale: Antibody against type IV collagen found in the GBM and alveolar basement membrane.
B. Antinuclear antibody.
Rationale: Antibody associated with systemic lupus erythematosus (SLE).
C. Anti–Jo-1 antibody.
Rationale: Antibody associated with polymyositis.
D. Anti–ADAMTS-13 antibodies.
Rationale: Antibody associated with idiopathic thrombotic thrombocytopenic purpura.
E. Anti–β_2-glycoprotein 1 antibodies.
Rationale: One of three major types of antiphospholipid antibodies.

25d. A. A history of three consecutive spontaneous abortions and the presence of aCL antibody are diagnostic for APS.
B. A DVT and positive mixing study showing the presence of an inhibitor are diagnostic for APS.
C. An arterial thrombosis is necessary to diagnose APS.
Rationale: Arterial, venous, and small vessel thromboses are all a part of the clinical criteria for diagnosing APS.
D. An antiphospholipid antibody must be demonstrated on more than one occasion to meet the diagnostic criteria for APS.
Rationale for A, B, and D: As part of the criteria, antiphospholipid antibodies should be detected on two or more occasions, at least 12 weeks apart.
E. Detection of any antiphospholipid antibody is itself diagnostic of APS.

Rationale: Diagnosis of APS requires at least one clinical criterion and one laboratory criterion to be met.

Major points of discussion

- Antiphospholipid antibody syndrome (APS; APLAS) is an acquired autoimmune condition characterized by clinical features of thrombosis and/or pregnancy loss, along with persistent antiphospholipid antibodies (APLA).
- Thrombosis can be venous, arterial, or microvascular. Microvascular thrombosis may manifest as "catastrophic antiphospholipid syndrome" that typically involves multiorgan failure (lungs, brain, kidneys).
- According to criteria defining APS, APS is present if at least one of the following clinical and one of the following laboratory criteria are met:
- Clinical criteria:
  - Vascular thrombosis: one or more clinical episodes of arterial, venous, or small vessel thrombosis.
  - Pregnancy morbidity: (a) one or more unexplained deaths of a morphologically normal fetus at or beyond the tenth week of gestation; (b) one or more preterm births of a morphologically normal neonate before the thirty-fourth week of gestation because of eclampsia or severe pre-eclampsia, or recognized features of placental insufficiency; (c) three or more unexplained consecutive spontaneous miscarriages before the tenth week of gestation, with maternal anatomic or hormonal abnormalities and paternal and maternal chromosomal causes excluded.
- Laboratory criteria:
  - LAC present in plasma, on two or more occasions at least 12 weeks apart
  - ACL antibody of immunoglobulin G (IgG) and/or IgM isotype in serum or plasma, present in medium or high titer, on two or more occasions, at least 12 weeks apart
  - Anti–β_2-glycoprotein 1 antibody of IgG and/or IgM isotype in serum or plasma, present on two or more occasions at least 12 weeks apart
- LAC activity is an in vitro phenomenon defined by prolongation of a phospholipid-dependent coagulation test that is not caused by an inhibitor to a specific coagulation factor. Criteria for the laboratory diagnosis of an LAC include the following:
  - Prolongation of a phospholipid-dependent clotting test
  - Demonstration of presence of an inhibitor by mixing tests
  - Demonstration of the phospholipid dependence of the inhibitor

  Present on two or more occasions 12 weeks apart
- Two or more phospholipid-based screening tests should be used to detect LACs. Options for these tests include a low phospholipid concentration PTT, dilute Russell viper venom time, kaolin clotting time, and dilute PT. A confirmatory step using high phospholipid concentration, platelet neutralizing agent, or LAC-insensitive reagent should be performed to demonstrate phospholipid dependence.
- ELISAs are used to detect aCL and anti–β_2-glycoprotein 1 antibodies.[3,13]

26. A. Tranexamic acid.
Rationale: Tranexamic acid is an antifibrinolytic agent. The thromboelastogram shows a coagulation deficiency.
B. Aspirin.
Rationale: Aspirin is an antiplatelet agent. The thromboelastogram shows a coagulation deficiency.
C. Packed red blood cell transfusion.
Rationale: Packed red blood cells are used to treat anemia, not hemostatic defects. The thromboelastogram shows a coagulation deficiency.
D. Plasma transfusion.
Rationale: Plasma is used to replace coagulation factors and natural anticoagulants. The thromboclastogram shows a coagulation deficiency, so this would be the appropriate therapy. The R value is prolonged in this case.
E. Platelet transfusion.
Rationale: Platelet transfusions are used to treat quantitative or qualitative platelet disorders. The thromboelastogram shows a coagulation deficiency.

Major points of discussion

- Thromboelastography is an assay that uses whole blood and measures the overall ability of blood to form a clot.
- A small wire is rotated in a well filled with whole blood (or the well is rotated), and an activator is added. In addition, heparin neutralizers can be added so that testing can be performed during cardiac bypass. As the clot forms, the resistance on the wire or cup increases. This resistance (measured in arbitrary millimeter units) is graphed over time to produce the thromboelastogram.
- Thromboelastography can show specific defects of platelets, coagulation, and/or fibrinolysis.
- The time from initiation of the test to the beginning of clot resistance is called the R time and indicates the function of coagulation factors. The rate of clot formation is indicated by the time it takes to reach 20 mm of clot strength.
- The α angle gives information about fibrin production and clot strength.
- The maximal amplitude achieved reflects platelet function.
- Excess fibrinolysis is reflected in the formation of a clot that dissolves faster than normal.
- The R time is increased in this thromboelastogram, which suggests a coagulation factor deficiency. Therefore, plasma transfusions would be the appropriate therapy.[7,15]

27. **A. Tranexamic acid.**
Rationale: Tranexamic acid is an antifibrinolytic agent. This thromboelastogram shows fibrinolysis.
B. Heparin.
Rationale: Heparin would be the most appropriate therapy for a hypercoagulable state. This thromboelastogram shows fibrinolysis.
C. Packed red blood cell transfusion.
Rationale: Packed red cells are used to treat anemia, not hemostatic defects. This thromboelastogram shows fibrinolysis.
D. Plasma transfusion.
Rationale: Plasma is used to replace coagulation factors and natural anticoagulants. This thromboelastogram shows fibrinolysis.
E. Platelet transfusion.

Rationale: Platelets are used to treat quantitative or qualitative platelet disorders. This thromboelastogram shows fibrinolysis.

Major points of discussion

- Thromboelastography is an assay that uses whole blood and measures the overall ability of blood to form a clot. See Question 29 for additional details on the methodology.
- The LY30 measures the percentage decrease in amplitude 30 minutes after maximal amplitude. The LY60 measures the percentage decrease in amplitude 60 minutes after maximal amplitude.
- The reference range for the LY30 is about 7.5% but is activator dependent (e.g., celite activated or whole blood).
- The LY30 is a measure of clot lysis (i.e., fibrinolysis).
- Excess fibrinolysis is reflected in the formation of a clot that dissolves faster than normal.
- Antifibrinolytic medications include aminocaproic acid, aprotinin, and tranexamic acid.

28. A. Tranexamic acid.
Rationale: Tranexamic acid is an antifibrinolytic agent. This thromboelastogram shows a hypercoagulable state.
B. Heparin.
Rationale: Heparin would be the most appropriate therapy for a hypercoagulable state.
C. Packed red blood cell transfusion.
Rationale: Packed red cells are used to treat anemia, not hemostatic defects. This thromboelastogram shows a hypercoagulable state.
D. Plasma transfusion.
Rationale: Plasma is used to replace a balance of normal levels of coagulation factors and natural anticoagulants. This thromboelastogram shows a hypercoagulable state, and the levels of natural anticoagulants in plasma would not be therapeutically sufficient.
E. Platelet transfusion.
Rationale: Platelet transfusions are used to treat quantitative or qualitative platelet disorders. This thromboelastogram shows a hypercoagulable state.

Major points of discussion

- Thromboelastography (TEG) is an assay that uses whole blood and measures the overall ability of blood to form a clot. See question 29 for additional details on the methodology.
- A hypercoagulable state can be measured using TEG by detecting a decreased R time and increased maximal amplitude (MA).
- Causes of hypercoagulability include the postoperative state, oral contraceptives, pregnancy, deficiencies of natural anticoagulants, and cancer.
- Thrombocytosis can increase coagulability on TEG by increasing the MA.
- Hypercoagulability on TEG may suggest a role for antiplatelet agents (e.g., aspirin) or anticoagulants (e.g., heparin, warfarin).[7,15]

29. **A. Chromogenic amidolytic.**
Rationale: This is a functional assay.
B. Enzyme-linked immunoassay (ELISA).
C. Latex particle immunoturbidometric.

Rationale: These are measures of antigen, not function.
D. DNA analysis.
Rationale: This is a molecular method that may allow prediction of the phenotype based on the genotype, but does not directly measure activity.
E. Heparin-binding site inhibition.
Rationale: There is no such assay that is routinely available clinically. If there were an existing assay to measure this, it would miss the other types of mutations, such as those of the reactive site.

Major points of discussion

- Chromogenic amidolytic assays measure the functional activity of AT. Excess thrombin is added to patient plasma with heparin. AT will then inactivate thrombin, leaving a residual amount of thrombin. A thrombin substrate is added, and the cleavage product is measured. AT activity is inversely proportional to the residual thrombin. The assay can also be factor Xa based because AT also inhibits factor Xa.
- There are several assays that measure AT antigen levels. ELISA-based assays, immunodiffusion, and latex particle immunoturbidometric methods are the most common.
- Type I AT deficiency is a decreased level of functionally normal AT. Antigen assays would be low, and functional assay would be low (i.e., quantitative defect).
- Type II AT deficiency is a functionally abnormal AT present in normal quantities. Antigen assays would be normal, and functional assay would be low (i.e., qualitative defect).
- Argatroban, a direct thrombin inhibitor (DTI), will affect thrombin-based functional assays, but not factor Xa–based functional assays.[28]

30. A. Antigenic-based fibrinogen.
Rationale: Measures all fibrinogen regardless of functional activity.
B. Fibrometer-based fibrinogen.
Rationale: Can be falsely low in mechanical-based clotting assay for fibrinogen.
C. Nephelometry.
Rationale: A method for antigenic measurement of fibrinogen, which measures all fibrinogen regardless of functional activity.
D. Reptilase time.
Rationale: Not as sensitive as the thrombin time.
E. Thrombin time.
Rationale: Prolonged in all congenital forms of dysfibrinogenemia except fibrinogens Oslo I and Valhalla.

Major points of discussion

- Dysfibrinogenemias are disorders of fibrinogen structure, which may or may not lead to abnormal function.
- Dysfibrinogenemias can be congenital or acquired. The most common causes of acquired dysfibrinogenemia are associated with liver disease.
- Among dysfibrinogenemias, 55% are asymptomatic, 25% are associated with bleeding only, and 20% are associated with thrombosis with or without bleeding.
- The thrombin time is performed by adding a low concentration of thrombin to platelet-poor plasma and measuring the time to clot formation. It is sensitive but is not a very specific test for dysfibrinogenemias. It can

be prolonged in the presence of heparin, fibrin degradation products, hypofibrinogenemia, antibovine thrombin antibodies (secondary to fibrin glue), and others.
- The reptilase time is performed by adding *Bothrops atrox* snake venom to platelet-poor plasma and measuring the time to clot formation. Reptilase time is prolonged in similar situations such as thrombin time, but it is not sensitive to heparin inhibition. Therefore, a prolonged thrombin time with normal reptilase time suggests the presence of heparin.
- Antigenic measurement of fibrinogen can be performed with immunoassays. Decreased functional fibrinogen with normal antigenic fibrinogen suggests the presence of a functional abnormality of fibrinogen.[10]

31. A. 0.5%.
Rationale: 0.45% of Asian Americans have the factor V Leiden mutation.
B. 1%.
Rationale: 1.2% of African Americans and 1.25% of Native Americans have the factor V Leiden mutation.
C. 5%.
Rationale: 5.2% of Caucasian Americans have the factor V Leiden mutation.
D. 15%.
Rationale: In some areas of Europe, the prevalence of the factor V Leiden mutation can be as high as 10% to 15% (e.g., Greece).
E. 25%.
Rationale: This is a very high prevalence; it has not been described in general populations of the United States or Europe.

Major points of discussion

- Factor V Leiden (FVL) is an inherited thrombophilia that increases the risk for VTE.
- The FVL mutation is a mutation of factor V at the APC cleavage site (1691G>A). APC is 10 times slower in inactivating FVL than wild-type factor V.
- FVL is the most common mutation (>90%) causing APCR. APCR is caused by other factor V mutations (i.e., FV Cambridge, FV Liverpool, R485K mutation, R2 haplotype, A/G allele).
- FVL is the most common genetic risk factor for VTE. It is found in 20% to 25% of patients with VTE and 50% of cases of familial VTE.
- The FVL mutation is seen in 3% to 8% of the general American and European populations. However, the prevalence of the FVL mutation is much lower in African Americans, Native Americans, and Asian Americans.[14]

32. A. Increased heparin cofactor II.
Rationale: Increases AT activity.
B. L-Asparaginase therapy.
Rationale: Decreases AT activity.
C. Hematuria.
Rationale: Proteinuria, not hematuria, decreases AT levels.
D. Menopause.
Rationale: Postmenopausal levels of AT activity increase.
E. Warfarin therapy.
Rationale: Anticoagulation increases AT activity.

Major points of discussion

- AT is a natural anticoagulant that inactivates thrombin and factors Xa, IXa, XIa, and XIIa.

- Administration of UFH can accelerate AT activity 1000-fold.
- Congenital AT deficiency is seen in 0.02% to 0.17% of the general population and 0.5% to 4.9% of patients with VTE (i.e., very rare).
- AT levels are decreased in liver disease, active thrombosis, surgery, DIC, sepsis, inflammatory bowel disease, L-asparaginase therapy, nephrotic syndrome, oral contraceptive therapy, and pregnancy.
- AT levels can be increased by warfarin and argatroban anticoagulation as an artifact of function-based assays.[28]

33. **A. Protein S level of 20%.**
   Rationale: Protein S level of less than 20% could cause false-positive results in the first-generation assay, but usually not in the second-generation assay. The second-generation assays normalize vitamin K–dependent factors by the addition of factor V–deficient plasma. However, protein S activity may be low in factor V–deficient plasmas, and this could influence the result.
   B. Warfarin therapy.
   C. Heparin 0.7 U/mL.
   Rationale: Second-generation APCR assays include the addition of polybrene to neutralize unfractionated and low-molecular-weight heparin.
   D. LAC.
   Rationale: This is the most likely cause of a false-positive result in the second-generation APCR assay.
   E. Liver dysfunction.
   Rationale for B and E: Second-generation APCR assays normalize vitamin K–dependent factors by the addition of factor V–deficient plasma.

Major points of discussion
- The first-generation functional assay for APCR was an aPTT performed with and without the addition of APC. The APCR ratio was calculated as aPTT/aPTT with APC. An APCR ratio of less than 2.0 indicates an individual screening positive for APCR.
- First-generation assays were subject to false-negative and false-positive results because of factor deficiencies, the presence of heparin, warfarin therapy, and LACs.
- Second-generation, modified functional APCR assays are performed after diluting the sample with factor V–deficient plasma to replace any factor deficiencies, thus removing the effect of warfarin therapy or protein C deficiency. The assay also adds polybrene to neutralize unfractionated and low-molecular-weight heparin.
- Factor V–deficient plasma could have low protein S activity because of the manufacturing process. Therefore, protein S deficiency can still produce false-positive results.
- LACs are still problematic in second-generation assays, although dilution with factor V–deficient plasma dilutes the antibody and its effect.
- APCR assays are 100% sensitive for detecting factor V Leiden.[29]

34. A. Elevated factor VIII activity.
   Rationale: Increased factor VIII activity will underestimate the protein C activity.
   B. Factor V Leiden.
   Rationale: APCR, caused by FVL, will underestimate the protein C activity. It would not affect a dilute Russell viper venom–based assay.

C. LAC.
Rationale: Artifactual elevation of protein C activity can be seen in aPTT-based assays in the presence of LACs.
D. Warfarin therapy.
Rationale: Warfarin inhibits the carboxylation of vitamin K–dependent factors such as protein C so that its activity is reduced.
E. Thrombosis.
Rationale: Thrombosis can incorporate protein C into natural anticoagulant complexes, decreasing the detected protein C activity levels. Testing should not be performed immediately after an acute thrombotic event.

Major points of discussion
- Protein C activity can be measured using a Russell viper venom–based or aPTT-based assay. An activator of protein C is added to plasma, such as the snake venom Protac, to convert the protein C to APC. Increased APC will then inactivate factors Va and VIIIa, prolonging the Russell viper venom time (RVVT) or aPTT in these assays. Therefore, the more protein C, the more factors Va and VIIIa are inactivated, and the more prolonged the aPTT or RVVT will be.
- Protein C deficiency can be inherited, acquired, or an artifact of the testing system.
- Inherited causes of protein C deficiency are seen in 0.14% to 0.5% of the general population and in 3% of patients with a first VTE; it increases the risk for VTE by sevenfold.
- Acquired causes of protein C deficiency include vitamin K deficiency, warfarin therapy, liver disease, thrombosis, surgery, DIC, and L-asparaginase therapy.
- In aPTT-based assays, protein C levels may be overestimated when there is an LAC or DTI. aPTT-based assays may also underestimate protein C activity in the presence of increased factor VIII activity and FVL.
- Chromogenic assays are not subject to the same artifacts as clot-based assays.[28]

35. A. Double heterozygous protein S and AT deficiency.
   B. Dysfibrinogenemia.
   C. Homozygous factor V Leiden.
   D. Homozygous protein C deficiency.
   Rationale: Severe protein C deficiency as seen in homozygous protein C mutations can present in the newborn period with purpura fulminans and DIC.
   E. Homozygous prothrombin 20210G>A mutation.
   Rationale for A, B, C, and E: These increase the risk for thrombosis but are not characteristic causes of this presentation.

Major points of discussion
- Severe protein C deficiency (homozygous protein C deficiency) can present as life-threatening purpura fulminans and DIC.
- Purpura fulminans is characterized by ecchymotic skin lesions that spontaneously become necrotic. Purpura fulminans is often associated with DIC.
- Protein C is a vitamin K–dependent natural anticoagulant. Activated protein C, with its cofactor protein S, inactivates factors VIIIa and Va.
- Heterozygous hereditary protein C deficiency is seen in 3% of patients with their first VTE and in only 0.14% to 0.5% of the general population.

- Protein C deficiency increases the risk for VTE by sevenfold.[5]

36. A. Activation of osteoclasts.
Rationale: Osteoporosis due to suppression of osteoblasts and activation of osteoclasts develops with unfractionated and, more often, low-molecular-weight heparin.
B. Development of anti–heparin polyvinyl sulfate antibodies.
Rationale: Heparin-induced thrombocytopenia can be a serious complication of heparin therapy. Antibodies against heparin–platelet factor 4 can lead to immune thrombocytopenia. Polyvinyl sulfate complexes with heparin are used in ELISA-based anti–heparin platelet factor 4 assays.
C. Development of Hollenhorst plaques.
Rationale: Cholesterol emboli in the eyes (Hollenhorst plaques) are not a complication of heparin therapy.
D. Hypokalemia.
Rationale: Hyperkalemia is an uncommon side effect of heparin therapy.
E. Hirsutism.
Rationale: Alopecia, not hirsutism, can be seen with heparin therapy.

Major points of discussion
- Bleeding is the major, serious consequence of heparin therapy, especially in patients with uncontrolled blood pressure, liver disease, and stroke.
- Osteoporosis caused by osteoclast activation and osteoblast suppression can develop, especially with long-term therapy with low-molecular-weight heparin.
- Less common complications include increased liver enzymes, alopecia, and hyperkalemia.
- Administering protamine sulfate reverses heparin anticoagulation.[8]

37. A. 1.45
Rationale: This is the ratio of PT to arithmetic mean. It is not the INR.
B. 1.47
Rationale: This is the ratio of the PT to geometric mean. It is not the INR.
C. 1.59
Rationale: INR = (PT/geometric mean)^{ISI}.
D. 1.62
Rationale: This is (PT/arithmetic mean)^{ISI}. It is not the INR.
E. 5.67
Rationale: This is the PT/standard error. It is not the INR.

Major points of discussion
- The PT is determined by adding a thromboplastin and calcium to platelet-poor plasma and measuring the time to clot formation.
- The PT measures extrinsic coagulation factors and is used to monitor warfarin therapy. Warfarin anticoagulation prevents the carboxylation of vitamin K–dependent coagulation factors (factor II, VII, IX, and X and proteins C and S).
- The sensitivity of each thromboplastin reagent to vitamin K–dependent coagulation factors can differ significantly from manufacturer to manufacturer and lot to lot. The INR was developed so that patients taking warfarin could have their warfarin therapy monitored by different laboratories.

- Each thromboplastin should have an ISI determined by testing it against an international or working reference preparation, which are thromboplastins available in several different preparations (e.g., rabbit, human, recombinant) from the World Health Organization.
- To determine the INR of a patient's PT, the geometric mean of the normal donor population for an individual laboratory must be determined by testing 120 normal donors. The arithmetic mean is not acceptable.
- INR = (PT/PT$_{GeoMean}$)^{ISI}.
- Log (INR) = ISI × PT/PT$_{GeoMean}$.
- PT/PT$_{GeoMean}$ is often referred to as the PT ratio.
- The target INR depends on the patient's condition; in most cases, the treatment goal is an INR between 2 and 3.

38. A. LAC.
Rationale: Although an LAC increases the risk for DVT, it does not explain the heparin resistance. LACs usually prolong the PT and/or aPTT.
B. AT deficiency.
Rationale: Inherited or acquired AT deficiency affects heparin therapy because heparin is not able to accelerate AT effectively if AT is present in low amounts.
C. Acquired factor VIII deficiency.
Rationale: The aPTT should be prolonged before initiation of therapy. Heparin resistance is seen with elevated factor VIII activity.
D. APCR.
Rationale: APCR, most commonly caused by the FVL mutation, is a risk factor for DVT. However, it should not lead to heparin resistance.
E. Increased heparin cofactor II activity.
Rationale: Heparin cofactor II binds heparin, which leads to inactivation of factor IIa. This would not lead to heparin resistance.

Major points of discussion
- Heparin acts as a cofactor for AT and accelerates the ability for AT to inactivate factors such as factors IIa (thrombin), IXa, Xa, and XIa.
- The aPTT is usually used to monitor UFH therapy. After a bolus dose and infusion, the aPTT is checked after 6 hours to determine whether the aPTT is in the therapeutic range. Depending on the aPTT, heparin can be adjusted to achieve the target based on being over, under, or at target.
- However, if heparin is administered and the aPTT does not increase, heparin resistance should be considered. Usually, if more than 25,000 to 35,000 IU of heparin is administered in a 24-hour period without achieving the therapeutic target (as measured by aPTT or activated clotting time) constitutes heparin resistance. Anti-Xa activity of the heparin can be determined. If the anti-Xa is elevated out of proportion to the measured aPTT, then heparin resistance should be considered.
- Common causes for heparin resistance are elevated factor VIII activity (acute-phase reactant), congenital or acquired AT deficiency, increased heparin clearance, and increased heparin-binding proteins.
- Treatment can consist of switching to an alternate anticoagulant such as argatroban. In addition, administering AT through infusion of plasma or AT concentrates may be useful. Monitoring with anti-Xa activity instead of aPTT may be useful.

39. A. FFP.
Rationale: FFP may accentuate the anticoagulant effect by providing additional AT.
B. Vitamin K.
Rationale: Vitamin K is used for the reversal of warfarin.
C. Cryoprecipitate.
Rationale: Cryoprecipitate has no role in the reversal of heparin therapy.
D. Prothrombin complex concentrates.
Rationale: Prothrombin complex concentrates can be used for warfarin therapy but are not useful for heparin reversal.
E. Protamine sulfate.
Rationale: Protamine sulfate is the treatment of choice for reversal of heparin.

Major points of discussion
- UFH accelerates the anticoagulant activity of AT, which inactivates factors Xa, IIa (thrombin), IXa, and XIa.
- UFH has a half-life of 1 hour, so it takes 5 to 6 hours to be cleared.
- UFH can be reversed by administering protamine, which is an arginine-rich (positively charged) protein that binds to the negatively charged heparin.
- Dosing of protamine for heparin reversal: Administer 100 mg of protamine for each 100 IU/mL of heparin activity.
- The main side effect of protamine is allergic reactions that can be severe (anaphylaxis). It can also cause hypotension, bradycardia, and hypertension/pulmonary hypertension.
- Protamine is also used to reverse the anticoagulant effect of low-molecular-weight heparin, but it only partially reverses the effect of low-molecular-weight heparin.

40. A. 0.1
Rationale: The y-intercept is not used in the calculation of the ISI of a test reagent.
B. 0.90
Rationale: This is equal to the ISI + y-intercept, which is not the correct equation.
C. 0.95
Rationale: The ISI of the test reagent = ISI reference preparation × Slope of regression line.
D. 1.0
Rationale: The ISI of the test reagent would be 1.0 if the slope of the regression line were 1.0.
E. 1.1
Rationale: This is equal to the ISI of the reference preparation – the y-intercept, which is not the correct equation.

Major points of discussion
- The PT is determined by adding a thromboplastin and calcium to platelet-poor plasma and measuring the time to clot formation. The PT measures extrinsic coagulation factors and is used to monitor warfarin therapy. Warfarin prevents the carboxylation of vitamin K–dependent coagulation factors (factors II, VII, IX, and X and proteins C and S).
- The sensitivity of each thromboplastin reagent to vitamin K–dependent coagulation factors can differ significantly from manufacturer to manufacturer and lot to lot. The INR was developed so that patients taking warfarin could have their warfarin therapy monitored by different laboratories.
- Each thromboplastin should have an ISI determined by testing it against an international or working reference preparation, which are thromboplastins available in several different preparations (e.g., rabbit, human, recombinant) from the World Health Organization.
- To determine the ISI of a reagent, the PT is performed using both the international reference preparation or working reference preparation on a group of normal donors and patients on stable warfarin therapy. A double logarithmic plot of a donor/patient's PT using the reference and test reagent is plotted, and a linear regression is calculated. The ISI is determined in terms of this slope.
- ISI of test reagent − ISI of the reference preparation × Slope.
- In this example, ISI = $1.0 \times 0.95 = 0.95$.
- The ISI is used to determine the international normalized ratio:
  - $INR = (PT/PT_{GeoMean})^{ISI}$.
  - $Log\,(INR) = ISI \times PT/\,PT_{GeoMean}$.
  - $PT/\,PT_{GeoMean}$ is often referred to as the PT ratio.[23]

41. A. Avascular necrosis.
Rationale: Osteoporosis is a side effect of warfarin, but bone necrosis is not.
B. Transmissible spongiform encephalopathy.
Rationale: Warfarin is chemically synthesized; it is not derived from animals or human tissue.
C. Purple toe syndrome.
Rationale: Purple toe syndrome is a side effect of warfarin occurring approximately 8 weeks after warfarin initiation.
D. Immune thrombocytopenia.
Rationale: Heparin-induced thrombocytopenia is seen with heparin therapy.
E. Hollenhorst plaque.
Rationale: Hollenhorst plaque is composed of cholesterol emboli that most likely dislodge from an atheromatous plaque in the internal carotid and become lodged within the retinal artery; it is not an adverse consequence of warfarin therapy.

Major points of discussion
- Warfarin decreases the vitamin K coagulation factors II, VII, IX, and X and proteins C and S. The half-life of protein C (8 hours) and protein S is shorter than factors II, IX, X (2 to 5 days, 1 day, 2 days, respectively). Therefore, until the anticoagulant effect of warfarin initiation is reached, heparin must be administered to prevent the prothrombotic effect of decreased protein C and protein S.
- Warfarin skin necrosis typically appears 3 to 10 days after warfarin initiation if heparin is not overlapped. Lack of the overlap results in clot formation and necrosis of skin, which is more common on the penis, thighs, buttocks, and breasts. It is more common in obese, middle-aged women.
- Purple toe syndrome is a rare complication appearing 3 to 8 weeks after initiation of therapy. Cholesterol emboli deposit in the skin of the feet, causing pain and the purple color.
- Most adverse events associated with warfarin are related to hemorrhage, which is seen in 1% to 3% of patients treated with warfarin. There are many drug-drug

interactions that may increase the risk for bleeding. Bleeding can be mild with bruising and epistaxis, or it can be severe with intracranial hemorrhage and stroke, gastrointestinal bleeding, intraabdominal bleeding, and compartment syndrome.
■ Osteoporosis and allergic reactions can also occur.

42. A. Pre-anhepatic.
Rationale: The pre-anhepatic stage is characterized by a mild deterioration in baseline coagulopathy.
B. Anhepatic to reperfusion.
Rationale: During this stage, there is a loss of coagulation factor synthesis and clearance as well as hyperfibrinolysis, which can lead to severe bleeding.
C. Postreperfusion.
Rationale: During the postreperfusion stage, there is resolution of fibrinolysis, restoration of coagulation factor synthesis and clearance, and a heparin-like effect from the donor liver.
D. Postoperative.
Rationale: Hypercoagulability during the postoperative stage is related to the early recovery of procoagulants, elevated factor VIII, and delayed recovery of AT, protein C, and protein S.
E. During surgical dissection and mobilization of the diseased liver.
Rationale: This refers to the pre-anhepatic stage. The pre-anhepatic stage is characterized by a mild deterioration in baseline coagulopathy.

Major points of discussion
■ Because of the essential role of the liver in the production and clearance of hemostatic factors, orthotopic liver transplantation is a formidable hemostatic challenge.
■ The stages of liver transplantation are:
  ● Pre-anhepatic (surgical dissection and mobilization)
  ● Anhepatic to reperfusion (from occlusion of hepatic vasculature to reperfusion)
  ● Postreperfusion
  ● Postoperative
■ The hemostatic changes associated with each stage of transplantation have been described.
■ A mild deterioration in baseline coagulopathy is noted in the pre-anhepatic stage and is mostly related to the preexisting coagulopathy.
■ The anhepatic to reperfusion stage is associated with a loss of coagulation factor synthesis and clearance and hyperfibrinolysis that can lead to severe bleeding. There is also an increase in tPA that may be caused by reduced clearance and increased release from the ischemic endothelium of the donor liver.
■ During the postreperfusion stage, there is restoration of coagulation factor synthesis and clearance by the transplanted liver, resolution of hyperfibrinolysis, thrombocytopenia, and a heparin-like effect from the donor liver. The resolution of hyperfibrinolysis may be attributed to increased clearance of tPA and increased production of plasminogen activator inhibitor 1. Thrombocytopenia may be caused by sequestration of platelets in the sinusoids of the donor liver. And the heparin-like effect from the donor liver is associated with heparinization of the donor before harvest and the release of heparinoids from the ischemic donor liver endothelium.

■ The postoperative stage is characterized by thrombocytopenia and hypercoagulability. Thrombocytopenia may be caused by platelet activation/consumption in the graft and sequestration owing to hypersplenism. Hypercoagulability is attributed to the early recovery of procoagulants and elevated factor VIII with concomitant delayed recovery of AT, protein C, and protein S. In addition, the hypercoagulability may be exacerbated by the use of antifibrinolytics.[24]

43. A. Endothelial cell cytotoxicity and disturbance of vascular hemostatic mechanisms.
Rationale: This is the mechanism for thrombosis associated with homocysteinemia.
B. Failure to generate APC.
Rationale: This is the mechanism of thrombosis associated with protein C deficiency.
C. Failure of APC to inactivate factors Va and VIIIa.
Rationale: This is the mechanism of thrombosis associated with protein S deficiency.
D. Failure to generate plasmin.
Rationale: This is the mechanism of thrombosis associated with plasminogen deficiency.
E. Failure to inhibit factors IIa (thrombin), Xa, and other activated factors.
Rationale: Through its interaction with heparin and heparin-like glycosaminoglycans, AT III inhibits factors IIa (thrombin), Xa, and other activated factors.

Major points of discussion
■ AT is a natural anticoagulant that inactivates factor IIa (thrombin), factor Xa, and several other coagulation factors.
■ Heparin is a cofactor that accelerates the binding of AT to thrombin and factor Xa.
■ AT deficiency is associated with an increased risk for VTE.
■ AT deficiency can be inherited or acquired (e.g., liver disease, sepsis, nephrotic syndrome, cardiothoracic surgery/bypass).
■ AT deficiency is associated with heparin resistance. In these cases, therapeutic targets of the activated clotting time or aPTT can be achieved after administering plasma or AT concentrates.[6,19]

44. A. Abnormal fibrinogen neutralizes tissue plasminogen activator (tPA).
Rationale: Neutralization of tPA is the mechanism of thrombosis associated with excess plasminogen activator inhibitor 1 activity.
B. Abnormal fibrinogen inhibits protein C activity.
Rationale: This is not a recognized mechanism of thrombosis caused by dysfibrinogenemia.
C. Abnormal fibrinogen resists fibrinolysis.
Rationale: This is one of two recognized mechanisms for thrombosis caused by dysfibrinogenemia.
D. Abnormal fibrinogen induces cytotoxicity and disrupts vascular hemostatic mechanisms.
Rationale: This is the mechanism of thrombosis associated with homocysteinemia.
E. Abnormal fibrinogen disrupts the activation of plasminogen.
Rationale: This is the mechanism of thrombosis associated with tPA deficiency.

Major points of discussion

- Dysfibrinogenemias are qualitative disorders of fibrinogen. Antigenic levels of fibrinogen would be normal, but the functional activity is decreased.
- The pattern of inheritance is autosomal dominant.
- Dysfibrinogenemias classically show an elevated thrombin time and an elevated reptilase time. An elevated thrombin time and normal reptilase time would suggest the presence of heparin.
- Clinically, approximately half of the patients with dysfibrinogenemias are asymptomatic, and the other half present with bleeding or thrombosis, or both.
- Two mechanisms used to explain most cases of thrombosis associated with dysfibrinogenemia are (1) abnormal thrombin binding sites on fibrin results in elevated thrombin levels and increased clot formation; and (2) abnormal fibrinogen forms a fibrin clot that is resistant to plasmin degradation.[4,6]

45. A. Failure to generate APC.
Rationale: This is the mechanism for thrombosis associated with protein C deficiency.
B. Neutralization of tissue plasminogen activator (tPA).
Rationale: This is the mechanism for thrombosis associated with excess plasminogen activator inhibitor 1 activity.
C. Endothelial cell toxicity and disruption of vascular hemostatic mechanisms.
Rationale: This is the mechanism for thrombosis associated with homocysteinemia.
D. Activated protein C is unable to inactivate factor Va.
Rationale: Because of a highly conserved point mutation in factor V, APC is unable to cleave factor Va.
E. Failure to inhibit thrombin.
Rationale: This is the mechanism for thrombosis associated with heparin cofactor II deficiency.

Major points of discussion

- Protein C is a natural anticoagulant that, when activated to APC, combines with its cofactor, protein S, to inactivate factors Va and VIIIa.
- APCR is an inherited thrombophilia caused by an abnormal factor V that is resistant to inactivation by APC.
- The factor V Leiden *(FVL)* gene mutation is the most common cause of APCR. Approximately 5% of North American Caucasians carry the *FVL* gene.
- In patients with an *FVL* mutation, APC fails to inactivate factor Va because of a highly conserved point mutation (G1628A), leading to an amino acid substitution (R485K) in factor V, leading to APCR and an increased risk for thrombosis.
- The factor V Liverpool variant is caused by a point mutation (T1250C), resulting in an amino acid substitution (I359T) that also leads to APCR and an increased risk for thrombosis.
- The factor V Cambridge variant is caused by a point mutation (G1091C), resulting in an amino acid substitution (R306T) that leads to APCR; however, it is *not* associated with an increased risk for thrombosis.[6]

46. A. **Failure to inhibit thrombin.**
Rationale: This is the mechanism for thrombosis in the setting of heparin cofactor II deficiency.
B. Failure to activate plasminogen.

Rationale: This is the mechanism for thrombosis associated with tPA deficiency.
C. Failure to inhibit factor IIa (i.e., thrombin), factor Xa, and other activated factors.
Rationale: This is the mechanism for thrombosis associated with AT deficiency.
D. Failure to generate APC.
Rationale: This is the mechanism for thrombosis associated with protein C deficiency.
E. Neutralization of tPA.
Rationale: This is the mechanism for thrombosis associated with excess plasminogen activator inhibitor 1 activity.

Major points of discussion

- Heparin cofactor II (HCII) is a serine protease inhibitor (serpin) that inactivates thrombin (factor IIa), but it does not have activity against other coagulation factors.
- HCII requires heparin, heparan sulfate, or dermatan sulfate as a cofactor.
- HCII appears to act as an adjunct to AT, and evidence suggests that its deficiency alone does not lead to an increased risk for thrombosis; however, it may increase the risk for thrombosis when there is a concomitant AT deficiency.
- HCII activity can be measured in vitro by measuring its anti–factor IIa activity in the presence of dermatan sulfate. Alternatively, HCII can be measured antigenically using an ELISA-based method.
- Testing for HCII deficiency is not recommended as part of a thrombophilia evaluation.[6,21]

47. A. Protein C.
B. AT.
C. Protein S.
D. Plasminogen.
Rationale: Plasminogen is only choice produced in the liver.
E. Tissue factor pathway inhibitor.
Rationale for A, B, C, and E: TFPI is produced both in the liver and in extrahepatic sites.

Major points of discussion

- The liver is the major site of synthesis of both procoagulant and anticoagulant proteins.
- The procoagulant factors produced by the liver include factors II (prothrombin), VII, IX, X, XI, XII, V, and VIII, plasminogen activator inhibitor 1 (PAI-I), α_2-antiplasmin, and thrombin activatable fibrinolysis inhibitor (TAFI).
- The anticoagulant factors produced by the liver include AT, protein C, protein S, TFPI, and plasminogen.
- Factor V, factor VIII, PAI-1, AT, protein C, protein S, and TFPI are also synthesized by extrahepatic sites.
- Hemostatic changes found in liver disease lead to rebalancing of the coagulation system; reduction of procoagulant and fibrinolytic factors is offset by a concomitant decrease of anticoagulant and antifibrinolytic proteins.
- Patients with liver disease therefore may be at risk for both bleeding and thrombotic complications.[24]

48. A. Factor VIII.
B. Fibrinogen.
Rationale: Fibrinogen is synthesized only in the liver.
C. Factor V.
D. Plasminogen activator inhibitor.

Rationale for A, C, and D: Plasminogen activator inhibitor is produced both in the liver and in extrahepatic sites.
E. Plasminogen.
Rationale: Plasminogen is a fibrinolytic factor that is produced solely by the liver and is not a procoagulant factor.

Major points of discussion

- The liver is the major site of synthesis of both procoagulant and anticoagulant proteins.
- The procoagulant factors produced by the liver include factors II, VII, IX, X, XI, XII, V, and VIII, PAI-I, α_2-antiplasmin, and TAFI.
- The anticoagulant factors produced by the liver include AT, protein C, protein S, TFPI, and plasminogen.
- Factor V, factor VIII, PAI-1, AT, protein C, protein S, and TFPI are also synthesized by extrahepatic sites.
- Hemostatic changes found in liver disease lead to rebalancing of the coagulation system; reduction of procoagulant and fibrinolytic factors is offset by a concomitant decrease of anticoagulant and antifibrinolytic proteins.
- Patients with liver disease therefore may be at risk for both bleeding and thrombotic complications.

49. A. Failure to generate APC.
Rationale: This is the mechanism of activation associated with protein C deficiency.
B. Failure to inhibit factor IIa (i.e., thrombin), factor Xa, and other activated factors.
Rationale: This is the mechanism of thrombosis associated with AT deficiency.
C. Failure to activate plasminogen.
Rationale: This is the mechanism of thrombosis associated with tPA deficiency.
D. Endothelial cell toxicity and disruption of vascular hemostatic mechanisms.
Rationale: This is the mechanism of thrombosis associated with hyperhomocysteinemia.
E. Failure of APC to inactivate factors Va and VIIIa.
Rationale: This is the mechanism of thrombosis associated with protein S deficiency.

Major points of discussion

- Hyperhomocysteinemia is an inherited thrombotic disorder caused by a metabolic defect.
- Homocysteine is an intermediate amino acid formed during the conversion of methionine to cysteine; the enzyme cystathionine-β-synthase is required.
- Moderate elevations of homocysteine may be a risk factor for atherothrombotic disease and VTE.
- Elevation of homocysteine can be caused by inherited defects of metabolism, nutritional deficiencies of vitamin cofactors, acquired diseases, and medications.
- Vitamin supplementation with folate, vitamin B_6, and vitamin B_{12} can decrease homocysteine levels, but their clinical usefulness as prophylaxis against arterial and venous thrombotic events is questionable.[6]

50. A. There is good evidence to support the use of routine coagulation tests for predicting bleeding or thrombotic risk in liver disease.

B. There is good evidence that the PT, not the PTT, is useful in predicting bleeding or thrombotic risk in liver disease.
Rationale: The PT is not a good predictor of bleeding or thrombotic risk in patients with liver disease; in addition, the INR should not be used.
C. There is no good evidence to support the use of routine coagulation tests for predicting bleeding or thrombotic risk in liver disease.
Rationale for A and C: Routine coagulation tests are poor predictors of bleeding and thrombotic risk in patients with liver disease.
D. There is good evidence to support the use of the PTT for predicting bleeding or thrombotic risk in liver disease.
Rationale: There is no evidence that the PTT is a good predictor of bleeding or thrombotic risk in patients with liver disease.
E. There is good evidence to support the use of the thrombin time for predicting bleeding or thrombotic risk in liver disease.
Rationale: There is no evidence that the thrombin time is a good predictor of bleeding or thrombotic risk in patients with liver disease.

Major points of discussion

- The liver is the major site of synthesis of both procoagulant and anticoagulant proteins.
- The procoagulant factors produced by the liver include factors II, VII, IX, X, XI, XII, V, and VIII, PAI-I, α_2-antiplasmin, and TAFI.
- The anticoagulant factors produced by the liver include AT, protein C, protein S, TFPI, and plasminogen.
- Factor V, factor VIII, PAI-1, AT, protein C, protein S, and TFPI are also synthesized by extrahepatic sites.
- Hemostatic changes found in liver disease lead to rebalancing of the coagulation system; reduction of procoagulant and fibrinolytic factors is offset by a concomitant decrease of anticoagulant and antifibrinolytic proteins.
- Patients with liver disease therefore may be at risk for both bleeding and thrombotic complications.
- Although there is currently no evidence that routine coagulation tests are useful for predicting bleeding or thrombotic risk in liver disease, investigators are exploring the value of global coagulation assays such as thrombin generation and thromboelastography in this clinical scenario.[24]

51. A. Protein C deficiency.
Rationale: This deficiency results in failure to generate APC.
B. AT deficiency.
Rationale: This deficiency results in failure to inhibit factor IIa (i.e., thrombin), factor Xa, and other activated factors.
C. Factor V Leiden.
Rationale: This variant factor V protein results in the failure of APC to inactivate factor Va.
D. Heparin cofactor II deficiency.
Rationale: This deficiency results in failure to inhibit factor IIa.
E. Excess plasminogen activator inhibitor 1 activity.
Rationale: Excess plasminogen activator inhibitor 1 activity will inhibit tPA inhibitor activity, leading to increased clot stability.

Major points of discussion

- PAI-1 is a serine protease inhibitor (serpin) that regulates fibrinolysis by inhibiting tPA and urokinase.
- tPA activates plasminogen to plasmin. Plasmin degrades fibrinogen and fibrin to its degradation products.
- Excess PAI-1 activity decreases tPA levels and decreases plasminogen activation, leading to decreased plasmin and decreased fibrinolysis.
- Excess PAI-1 activity can lead to arterial and venous thrombotic disorders, such as VTE and myocardial infarction.
- Congenital deficiencies of PAI-1 lead to a bleeding disorder because tPA is inadequately inactivated and leads to excess fibrinolysis.[6]

52. A. Failure of APC to inactivate factors Va and VIIIa.
    Rationale: This is the mechanism for thrombosis associated with protein S deficiency.
    B. Failure to inhibit thrombin.
    Rationale: This is the mechanism for thrombosis associated with heparin cofactor II deficiency.
    C. Failure to generate plasmin.
    Rationale: Failure to generate plasmin results in increased clot stability.
    D. Failure to generate APC.
    Rationale: This is the mechanism for thrombosis associated with protein C deficiency.
    E. Failure of activated protein C to inactivate factor Va.
    Rationale: This is the mechanism for thrombosis associated with FVL.

Major points of discussion

- Plasminogen is a zymogen that is activated to plasmin by the serine proteases tPA and urokinase.
- Plasmin degrades fibrinogen and fibrin with the primary role of dissolving thrombi.
- Both homozygous and heterozygous forms of plasminogen deficiency have been described; they can be qualitative defects (active site mutations; type II) or quantitative defects (type I). It is a very rare disorder.
- Patients can be asymptomatic or present with a history of thrombosis. They can also have ligneous conjunctivitis with pseudomembranes covering the eyes (other organs can also be affected). The pseudomembranes are caused by the accumulation of fibrin and are more commonly found in patients with type I deficiencies.
- It has not been clearly established if plasminogen deficiency alone is sufficient to cause a hypercoagulable state.[6,17]

53. A. Failure to inhibit factor IIa, factor Xa, and other activated factors.
    Rationale: This is the mechanism for thrombosis associated with AT III deficiency.
    B. Failure to generate APC.
    Rationale: Protein C deficiency results in a lack of APC and an inability to inactivate factors Va and VIIIa.
    C. Failure to generate plasmin.
    Rationale: This is the mechanism for thrombosis in plasminogen deficiency.
    D. Endothelial cell toxicity and disturbance of vascular hemostatic mechanisms

Rationale: This is the mechanism for thrombosis associated with homocysteinemia.
E. Failure of APC to inactivate factors Va and VIIIa.
Rationale: This is the mechanism for thrombosis associated with protein S deficiency.

Major points of discussion

- Protein C is a vitamin K–dependent natural anticoagulant. It is a zymogen that is converted to APC by thrombin.
- Thrombomodulin on endothelial surfaces accelerates the activation of protein C to APC.
- APC, along with its cofactor protein S, inactivates factors Va and VIIIa.
- Protein C deficiency is a rare inherited disorder that is associated with an increased risk for VTE. Type I defects are quantitative defects of normal protein C and type II defects are qualitative defects.
- Protein C deficiency should not be confused with APCR, which is caused by a mutation in factor V that makes it resistant to inactivation by APC. The most common mutation causing APCR is FVL, which may be present in up to 50% of North American Caucasians.[6]

54. A. Failure to inhibit thrombin.
    Rationale: This is the mechanism for thrombosis associated with heparin cofactor II deficiency.
    B. Failure of APC to inactivate factors Va and VIIIa.
    Rationale: Activated protein C requires the activity of its cofactor, protein S, to inactivate factors Va and VIIIa.
    C. APC fails to inactivate factor Va because of a highly conserved point mutation.
    Rationale: This is the mechanism for thrombosis associated with FVL.
    D. Failure to activate plasminogen.
    Rationale: This is the mechanism for thrombosis associated with tPA deficiency.
    E. An acquired abnormality in fibrin results in decreased fibrinolysis.
    Rationale: This is the mechanism for thrombosis associated with dysfibrinogenemia.

Major points of discussion

- Protein S is a vitamin K–dependent protein that is a cofactor for APC. Activated protein C inactivates factors Va and VIIIa. This pathway is an important part of the natural anticoagulant system.
- Protein S circulates bound to C4 binding protein (C4bp) or as free protein S (Total protein S = Free protein S + Protein S:C4bp).
- Approximately 65% of protein S is bound to C4bp, and the remainder is free protein S. Only the free form has cofactor activity.
- Protein S deficiency is an inherited, autosomal dominant disorder that is a risk factor for VTE. However, inherited protein S deficiency is not common.
- Assays for protein S include total protein S antigen, free protein S antigen, and total protein S activity. Antigenic assays are immunologically based, whereas activity is measured by clot-based assays using platelet poor plasma.
- Type I protein S deficiency is a quantitative disorder of normal protein S. Type II is a qualitative disorder of quantitatively normal protein S. Type III is a disorder of normal total protein S, but decreased free protein S and increased bound protein S.

■ It is important to note that there is a physiologic decrease in protein S during pregnancy. Therefore, a physiologic decrease in protein S should not be misinterpreted as protein S deficiency. Other possible causes of decreased protein S activity include warfarin therapy, vitamin K deficiency, and liver disease.[6,27]

55. A. Endothelial cell toxicity and disruption of vascular hemostatic mechanisms.
Rationale: This is the mechanism of thrombosis associated with hyperhomocysteinemia.
B. Failure of APC to inactivate factors Va and VIIIa
Rationale: This is the mechanism of thrombosis associated with protein S deficiency.
C. Failure to generate APC.
Rationale: This is the mechanism of thrombosis associated with protein C deficiency.
D. Failure to activate plasminogen.
Rationale: Failure to activate plasminogen to plasmin results in increased clot stability.

E. Failure to inhibit factor IIa, factor Xa, and other activated factors.
Rationale: This is the mechanism for thrombosis associated with AT deficiency.

Major points of discussion
■ tPA is a serine protease (serpin) expressed by endothelial cells and acts as an activator of fibrinolysis.
■ tPA converts plasminogen to plasmin. Plasmin functions to degrade fibrinogen and fibrin.
■ Recombinant tPA is a pharmaceutical agent that is used therapeutically for acute ischemic cerebrovascular events, pulmonary embolism, and other thrombotic disorders.
■ Increased endogenous tPA activity can lead to excessive fibrinolysis and bleeding.
■ tPA deficiency can lead to hypofibrinolysis and a risk for thrombosis.

References

1. Andrew M, Paes B, Johnston M. Development of the hemostatic system in the neonate and young infant. Am J Pediatr Hematol Oncol 1990;12:95–104.
2. Asmis LM, Sulzer I, Furlan M, et al: Prekallikrein deficiency: the characteristic normalization of the severely prolonged aPTT following increased preincubation time is due to autoactivation of factor XII. Thromb Res 2002;105:463–470.
3. Ballard RB, Marques MB. Pathology consultation on the laboratory evaluation of thrombophilia. Am J Clin Pathol 2012;137:553–560.
4. de Moerloose P, Boehlen F, Neerman-Arbez M. Fibrinogen and the risk of thrombosis. Semin Thromb Hemost 2010;36:7–17.
5. Dreyfus M, Magny JF, Bridey F, et al: Treatment of homozygous protein C deficiency and neonatal purpura fulminans with a purified protein C concentrate. N Engl J Med 1991;325:1565–1568.
6. Florell SR, Rogers GM. Inherited thrombotic disorders: an update. Am J Hematol 1997;54:53–60.
7. Ganter MT, Hofer CK. Coagulation monitoring: current techniques and clinical use of viscoelastic point-of-care coagulation devices. Anesth Analg 2008;106:1366–1375.
8. Gray E, Mulloy B, Barrowcliffe TW. Heparin and low-molecular-weight heparin. Thromb Haemost 2008;99:807–818.
9. Hamilton A, Ozelo M, Leggo J, et al: Frequency of platelet type versus type 2B VWD: an international registry based study. Thromb Haemost 2011;105(3):501–508.
10. Hayes T. Dysfibrinogenemia and thrombosis. Arch Pathol Lab Med 2002;126:1387–1390.
11. Hoffman M. Heparins: clinical use and laboratory monitoring. Lab Med 2010;41:621–626.
12. Hsieh L, Nugent D. Factor XIII deficiency. Haemophilia 2008;14:1190–1200.
13. Keeling D, Mackie I, Moore GW, et al: Guidelines on the investigation and management of antiphospholipid syndrome. Br J Haematol 2012;157:47–58.
14. Kujovich JL, Factor V Leiden thrombophilia. Genet Med 2011;13(1):1–16.
15. Luddington RJ. Thromboelastography/thromboelastometry. Clin Lab Haematol 2005;27:81–90.
16. Mariani G, Herrmann FH, Schulman S, et al: Thrombosis in inherited factor VII deficiency. J Thromb Haemost 2003;1(10):2153–2158.
17. Mehta R, Shapiro AD. Plasminogen deficiency. Hemophilia 2008;14:1261–1268.
18. Nichols WL, Hultin MB, James AH, et al: von Willebrand disease (VWD): evidence-based diagnosis and management guidelines, the National Heart, Lung, and Blood Institute (NHLBI) Expert Panel report (USA). Haemophilia 2008;14:171–232.
19. Patnaik MM, Moll S. Inherited antithrombin deficiency: a review. Hemophilia 2008;14:1229–1239.
20. Ratnoff OD, Busse RJ, Sheon RP. The demise of John Hageman. N Engl J Med 1968;279:760–761.
21. Rau JC, Mitchell JW, Fortenberry YM, et al: Heparin cofactor II: discovery, properties, and role in controlling vascular homeostasis. Semin Thromb Hemost 2011;37:339–348.
22. Reider MJ, Reiner AP, Gage BF, et al: Effect of VKORC1 haplotypes on transcriptional regulation and warfarin dose. N Engl J Med 2005;352:2285–2293.
23. Riley RS, Rowe D, Fisher LM. Clinical utilization of the international normalized ratio (INR). J Clin Lab Anal 2000;14:101–114.
24. Roberts LN, Patel RK, Arya R. Haemostasis and thrombosis in liver disease. Br J Haematol 2009;148:507–521.
25. Ruinemans-Koerts J, Peterse-Stienissen I, Verbruggen B. Non-parallelism in the one-stage coagulation factor assay is a phenomenon of lupus anticoagulants and not of individual factor inhibitors. Thromb Haemost 2010;104:1080–1082.
26. Stavrou E, Schmaier AH. Factor XII: what does it contribute to our understanding of the physiology and pathophysiology of hemostasis & thrombosis. Thromb Res 2010;125:210–215.
27. Ten Kate MK, Van Der Meer J. Protein S deficiency: a clinical perspective. Haemophilia 2008;14:1222–1228.
28. Van Cott EM, Khor B. Laboratory tests for antithrombin deficiency. Am J Hematol 2010;85:947–950.
29. Van Cott EM, Soderberg BL, Laposata M. Activated protein C resistance, the factor V Leiden mutation, and a laboratory testing algorithm. Arch Pathol Lab Med 2002;126:577–582.

CHAPTER 15

IMMUNOLOGY, IMMUNOGENETICS

George Vlad, Raphael Clynes, Adriana I. Colovai,
Elena-Rodica Vasilescu

QUESTIONS

1. Which one of the following assays provides the most complete picture of a transplant candidate's antibody status?
   A. Complement-dependent cytotoxicity (CDC) against a reference panel of T and B cells.
   B. Flow cytometry (FC) crossmatch with donor peripheral blood mononuclear cells and panel reactive antibody (PRA) testing.
   C. Solid-phase assays (SPAs).
   D. CDC against a reference panel of T cells and B cells and SPAs.

Table 15-1

	CDC Crossmatch		FC Crossmatch	
	T cell	**B cell**	**T cells**	**B cells**
Scenario A	Neg	Pos	Pos	Pos
Scenario B	Pos	Neg	Pos	Neg
Scenario C	Neg	Pos	Neg	Pos
Scenario D	Pos	Pos	Neg	Neg

2a. Consider the following CDC and FC crossmatch results shown in Table 15-1. Which crossmatch result presents the highest risk of rejection?
   A. Scenario A.
   B. Scenario B.
   C. Scenario C.
   D. Scenario D.

2b. Referring to the same alloantibody testing methods and results described above, which set of crossmatch results requires additional testing?
   A. Scenario A.
   B. Scenario B.
   C. Scenario C.
   D. Scenario D.

2c. Referring to the same alloantibody testing methods and results described above, which positive crossmatch is due to an IgM antibody?
   A. Scenario A.
   B. Scenario B.
   C. Scenario C.
   D. Scenario D.

3. A kidney transplant patient is treated with pulse corticosteroids and rituximab after acute mediated rejection is detected as outlined by the Banff criteria (graft dysfunction, C4d deposition detected in the biopsy, and circulating alloantibodies). The patient eventually undergoes nephrectomy. Although the level of circulating anti–human leukocyte antigen (HLA) antibodies was low during the rejection episode (mean fluorescence intensity [MFI] ~2000, by SPAs), the level continues to rise steadily. After nephrectomy, the MFI values reach 10,000 at day 7 and 12,000 at day 21. Which one of the following accounts for this phenomenon?
   A. Nephrectomy was incomplete; residual tissues left behind continue to be rejected and generate a humoral response.
   B. Anti-donor HLA antibodies continue to be produced after nephrectomy; however, the graft no longer adsorbs them.
   C. The readings are an artifact of the rituximab treatment, which can persist in circulation many months after the treatment.
   D. The histocompatibility lab switched reagent lots, and the new reagents are much better than the old ones at detecting the antibodies against the specific allele of the donor in this case.

Table 15-2

Father	A1 A2	B44 B60	DR4 DR13
Mother	A3 A24	B7 B56	DR15 DR16
Child 1	A2 A3	B44 B7	DR4 DR15
Child 2	A2 A24	B44 B56	DR4 DR16
Child 3	A1 A3	B60 B7	DR13 DR15
Child 4	A1 A24	B60 B56	DR4 DR16

From 2011 Annual Report of the U.S. Organ Procurement and Transplantation Network and the Scientific Registry of Transplant Recipients: Transplant Data 2004–2010. Department of Health and Human Services, Health Resources and Services Administration, Healthcare Systems Bureau, Division of Transplantation, Rockville, MD; United Network for Organ Sharing, Richmond, VA; University Renal Research and Education Association, Ann Arbor, MI.

4. A family typing at the *HLA-A/-B/-DR* loci is shown in Table 15-2. Which one of the following children has HLA gene recombination?
   A. Child 1.
   B. Child 2.
   C. Child 3.
   D. Child 4.

5. A patient who underwent successful kidney transplantation 20 years ago loses his allograft to chronic rejection. He is listed for retransplantation. His HLA typing performed at a different institution shows the following results:

   HLA-A1/A26
   HLA-B42/B16
   HLA-DR3/DR4

   As a standard procedure, a recipient blood sample is retyped at his current institution with the following results:

   HLA-A1/A26
   HLA-B42/B38
   HLA-DR17/DR4

   Which one of the following would account for this discrepancy?
   A. Splits of HLAs, indistinguishable by old serologic typing methods.
   B. Egregious errors of the previous histocompatibility lab.
   C. Egregious errors of the current histocompatibility lab.
   D. The donor's HLAs are detected in the patient's blood.

6. A patient with end-stage renal disease who is highly sensitized is considered for an antibody reduction protocol with plasmapheresis and intravenous immunoglobulin (IVIg). Which one of the following parameters should determine the number of plasmapheresis courses to be administered?
   A. Number of mismatched antigens.
   B. Number of previous transplants.
   C. The PRA percentage.
   D. Titer of donor-specific antibodies.

7. A transplantation patient who is not presensitized to any HLAs receives a 5/6 matched allograft. The typing results are as follows:

   Patient: HLA-A2, -A3, -B7, -BX, -DR7, -DR11
   Donor: HLA-A2, -A3, -B7, -B27, -DR7, -DR11

   The patient develops de novo alloantibodies detected on routine serum monitoring on 50% of a panel of cells (PRA ~50%). SPAs using individual HLA-coated beads show antibodies reacting with over 20 HLA-B specificities, including HLA-B27. The serum also shows positive reactions against HLA-A23, -24, -25, and -32. The patient's medical history records no other sensitizing events other than the transplant. Which one of the following is the best explanation?
   A. The patient produced donor-specific antibodies to a likely mismatched allele of HLA-A2 (which is present in about 40% of the population) not represented on the SPA beads but cross-reacts with multiple HLA-A and -B alleles.
   B. The patient produced multiple anti-HLA antibodies against mismatched, nontyped loci (HLA-C, -DQ, -DP), which cross-react with multiple HLA-A and -B alleles.
   C. The patient produced antibodies against the β-2 microglobulin chain of HLA class I expressed by half of the cell panel and used by all the HLA alleles identified by SPAs.
   D. The patient produced a single antibody against the epitope Bw4 present in HLA-B27 and many HLA-A and -B alleles.

8. In kidney transplantation, living related donors represent an important source of donated organs and tend to have significantly better outcomes. A distinct advantage of donation from a relative is the possibility of good donor-recipient antigen matching; first-degree related donors (i.e., parents, children) might share one haplotype with the recipient. However, not all donor-recipient pairings are created equal. Which one of the following is the worst pairing among first-degree relatives?
   A. Mother donates to child.
   B. Father donates to child.
   C. Child donates to mother.
   D. Child donates to father.

9. Which one of the following is a prediction of compatibility based on the patient's alloantibody status compared with specific donors' antigens?
   A. Auto-crossmatch.
   B. Direct crossmatch.
   C. Virtual crossmatch.
   D. Flow crossmatch.

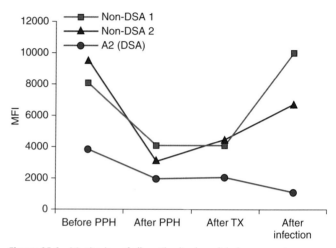

Figure 15-1 Monitoring of alloantibodies by solid phase assay in a sensitized allograft recipient. The evolution of three alloantibodies through desensitization protocol, transplantation, and an infection event. DSA, Donor specific antibodies; MFI, mean fluorescence intensity; PPH, plasmapheresis; TX, transplant.

10. A heart transplant candidate is broadly presensitized, displaying antibodies against more than 80% of the cell panel (PRA >80%). The antibody specificities established by SPAs include the common HLA-A2, present with a frequency of more than 40% in many human populations; however, this is not listed as an unacceptable antigen due to the apparently low amounts of this antibody (MFI = 3800). He is desensitized using plasmapheresis and IGIg and receives an HLA-A2+ heart on the basis of a negative crossmatch. A few months after transplantation, he experiences a severe infection with *Streptococcus pneumoniae*. Immunosuppression is lowered and the infection clears with antibiotics. However, after this episode the patient describes heart failure symptoms and the ejection fraction seems to have significantly decreased compared with the preinfection measurements. Antibody monitoring shows that multiple anti-HLA non–donor-specific antibodies are sharply upregulated, although the only donor-specific antibody (anti–HLA-A2) is disappearing (MFI = 1100) (Figure 15-1). Which one of the following is the best explanation for these observations?
    A. Graft dysfunction is caused by a thrombus.
    B. Graft dysfunction caused by a humoral response against the pathogen, which cross-reacts with non-HLA heart antigens.
    C. Antibody-mediated rejection caused by complement-fixing non–donor-specific antibodies that cross-react with donor HLA alleles.
    D. Antibody-mediated rejection caused by the anti–HLA-A2 antibody, which increased along with other anti-HLA antibodies as a consequence of the infection.

11. In which one of the following situations would HLA allele-level typing be most useful for the identification of an HLA-identical sibling?
    A. Mother: *DR1 DR15*; father: *DR3, DR7*.
    B. Mother: *DR1 DR3*; father: *DR4, DR7*.
    C. Mother: *DR1 DRX*; father: *DR1, DR4*.
    D. Mother: *DR11 DR4*; father: *DR3, DR7*.

Table 15-3

Serum	T-Cell Crossmatch Result	B-Cell Crossmatch Result
Negative control serum	Neg	Neg
Positive control serum	Pos	Pos
Patient serum, untreated	Neg	Neg
Patient serum, dithiothreitol treated	Pos	Pos

12. The results of a CDC crossmatch are indicated in Table 15-3. Which one of the following conclusions can be drawn?
    A. The results are invalid.
    B. The serum contains a donor-specific IgG antibody and a blocking IgM antibody.
    C. The serum contains a donor-specific IgM antibody and a blocking IgG antibody.
    D. The serum contains a donor-specific IgA antibody.

13. Which one of the following features is shared by HLA class I and II molecules?
    A. Types of T cells they stimulate.
    B. Types of cells that express them.
    C. The chromosome on which they are located.
    D. Types of antigens they present.
    E. Types of cells that contain a β-2 microglobulin subunit.

14. Which one of the following describes the reaction of an antibody with antigens that are similar, but not identical, to the antigen that stimulated antibody production?
    A. Co-dominance.
    B. Cross-reactivity.
    C. Memory response.
    D. Mixed lymphocyte reaction.
    E. PRA.

15. Which one of the following types of serum antibodies is detected by standard FC crossmatch performed with donor lymphocytes?
    A. Anti-donor HLA class I IgG.
    B. Anti-donor HLA class I and class II IgG.
    C. Anti-donor non-HLA IgG.
    D. Anti-donor lymphocyte IgG.
    E. Cytotoxic anti-donor HLA IgG and IgM.

16. In which one of the following situations is high-resolution HLA class I and class II typing most important?
    A. Living related kidney transplantation in patients with high PRA.
    B. Liver transplantation.
    C. Stem cell transplantation: unrelated donor.
    D. Stem cell transplantation: two haplotype–matched related donor.
    E. ABO-incompatible renal transplantation.

17. Which one of the following laboratory tests involves direct recognition of alloantigens by T lymphocytes?
    A. FC crossmatch.
    B. CDC crossmatch.
    C. HLA typing using sequence-specific oligonucleotides (SSOs).
    D. Mixed lymphocyte culture.
    E. Mitogen T-cell stimulation.

18. As part of the immunologic evaluation of a renal transplant candidate, anti-HLA antibody screening was performed by CDC and SPA. Using an HLA-typed cell panel, CDC screening indicated that no PRAs (PRA=0%) were present in the patient's serum. However, SPA using single HLA-coated beads revealed the presence of serum IgG antibodies reactive to *HLA-A2, -A28, -A9,* and *-B17*. These results indicate which one of the following?
    A. There is a high probability that the CDC crossmatch with an *HLA-A2* donor will be positive.
    B. There is an increased risk of acute antibody-mediated rejection if the patient received an *HLA-A2* transplant.
    C. There is a high risk of hyperacute rejection if the patient received an *HLA-A2* transplant.
    D. Transplantation with an *HLA-A2* graft is contraindicated even if the CDC crossmatch is negative.
    E. The results of the CDC and solid-phase immunoassays are discordant and, therefore, they are invalid.

19. Which one of the following statements about lymph nodes is correct?
    A. Dendritic cells enter the germinal centers through high endothelial venules.
    B. Long-lived plasma cells reside primarily in the germinal center and paracortical areas.
    C. Antigen-independent proliferation of B cells occurs in lymph nodes.
    D. Activated T cells are absent from germinal centers.
    E. Affinity maturation of B cells occurs in the germinal center.

20. A kidney transplant patient receiving chronic immunosuppressive medication presents with lymphadenopathy. He was Epstein-Barr virus (EBV) negative before transplantation and received an allograft from an EBV-positive donor. FC of a biopsy shows both Ig κ and λ staining of the B-cell gate. Which one of the following is true?
    A. The patient is not at risk for EBV lymphoma.
    B. EBV reactivation in immunocompromised patients is due to humoral insufficiency and can be overcome with IVIg treatment.
    C. B-cell proliferation in EBV lymphoproliferative disorders is due to B-cell receptor–mediated B-cell recognition of EBV antigens.
    D. The receptor for EBV viral entry on B cell is the complement receptor CD21.
    E. EBV lymphoma is less commonly seen in pediatric transplants since posttransplant lymphoproliferative disorder is due to EBV reactivation from prior infection.

21. A patient with systemic lupus erythematosus (SLE) is awaiting a kidney transplant. The FC crossmatch with a potential donor is positive both on T cells and B cells, but so is the auto-crossmatch. Which one of the following is the best course of action in this case?

A. Proceed with the transplant because the auto-crossmatch establishes the threshold of a negative reaction.

B. Rule out this donor because the crossmatch is positive regardless of the auto-crossmatch results.

C. Do not transplant. These are autoantibodies (auto-crossmatch–positive) that recognize the same antigen on donor cells and, therefore, will destroy the transplanted kidney as well.

D. Perform SPA testing to determine whether the antibodies are anti-HLA antibodies, and if yes, whether they are donor specific.

Table 15-4

Patient	A*02:01, A*03:01
Donor 1	A*02:01, A*03:04
Donor 2	A*02:01, A*01:01

22a. The *HLA-A* locus typing of a patient who is a bone marrow transplant candidate and two potential donors are shown in Table 15-4. Which donor is "the best" match?

A. Donor 1 due to the allele mismatch with the patient, *A*03:01* vs. *A*03:04.*

B. Donor 2 due to the antigen mismatch with the patient, *A*03:01* vs. *A*01:01.*

C. No difference between donors 1 and 2 regarding the impact of mismatch on graft survival.

D. Depends on where the mismatched amino acid(s) lie in the HLA structure.

22b. Would a third donor (donor 3) typing as *A*02:01, A*02:305 N* be a better choice than donors 1 and 2?

A. Yes. Donor 3 is better than donor 2, but equivalent to donor 1.

B. No. Donor 3 has an exotic allele, which is highly likely to elicit allorecognition and trigger graft-versus-host disease (GVHD).

C. Yes. Donor 3 has a perfectly matched allele *A*02:01* and a null allele *A*02:305 N*, which does not contribute to the allorecognition.

D. No. Homozygosity or single-allele expression at one locus in the donor may trigger GVHD.

23. The likelihood of a mother and her daughter being HLA identical (assuming no consanguinity in the family) is closest to which one of the following percentages?

A. 75%.

B. 50%.

C. 25%.

D. 16.7%.

E. 0%.

24. Which one of the following is *true* about antigen presentation by HLA molecules?

A. There are an unlimited amount of peptides that can be presented from a single protein.

B. HLA haplotypes can contribute to immune responsiveness to a specific virus or vaccine.

C. Only extracellular antigens can be presented on HLA class II molecules.

D. Only intracellular antigens can be presented on HLA class I molecules.

E. Only the amino acid sequence determines the immunogenicity of peptides loaded onto HLA molecules.

25. A transplant recipient with swollen glands, high fever, and fatigue presents to the emergency department. A peripheral smear of the blood shows high numbers of "atypical" lymphocytes and a second sample is sent for FC. Which one of the following statements is true?

A. In infectious mononucleosis, the atypical lymphocytes are likely a large number of CD20+ B-cell blasts.

B. In infectious mononucleosis, the atypical lymphocytes are likely a large number of activated CD8+ T cells.

C. B-cell leukemia can be excluded if the atypical cells are surface B-cell receptor negative.

D. EBV-positive serology is seen in around 50% of adults.

E. Stable integration of the EBV genome into chromosomal DNA of infected B cells is required for latency.

26. Which one of the following statements is true regarding the alloreactive cellular infiltrates?

A. Cytokine receptors for interleukins (ILs)-2, -4, -7, -9, -15, and -21 signal through a common gamma chain–associated receptor activating JAK3 kinase.

B. T-cell production of interferon (IFN)-γ, IL-12, and IL-17 augments the cellular immune response.

C. Cyclosporine blocks T-cell receptor signaling via inhibition of the tyrosine kinase nuclear factor of activated T cells (NFAT).

D. Toll-like receptors recognize only microbial constituents and activate innate immune cells through necrosis factor (NF)- κB.

E. Regulatory T cells have the capacity to induce tolerance by killing self-reactive effector T cells.

27. Which one of the following explains why an individual does not normally make an immune response to a self-protein?

A. Self-proteins cannot be processed into peptides.

B. Peptides from self-proteins cannot bind to HLA class I molecules.

C. Peptides from self-proteins cannot bind to HLA class II molecules.

D. Lymphocytes reactive to self-proteins are inactivated by deletion, anergy, or receptor editing.

E. Developing lymphocytes cannot rearrange V genes required to produce a receptor for self-proteins.

28. A patient with active rheumatoid arthritis feels ill with low-grade fever, malaise, morning stiffness, and fatigue. Which one of the following proteins or cytokines is most likely responsible for these symptoms?

A. Complement components.

B. Rheumatoid factor.

C. Tumor necrosis factor (TNF) and IL-1.

D. IL-4 and IL-10.

Table 15-5

| | CDC Crossmatch | | FC Crossmatch | | Luminex | |
	T cells	B cells	T cells	B cells	Class I	Class II
Patient cells	Neg	Neg	Neg	Neg		
Donor cells	Neg	Neg	Neg	Weak pos	Weak pos	Neg

29a. A patient with end-stage renal disease (ESRD) is evaluated for a living unrelated kidney transplant. The results of histocompatibility testing by SPAs (Luminex with mixed antigen beads) and CDC and FC crossmatches between patient sera and patient lymphocytes and between patient sera and donor lymphocytes are shown in Table 15-5. Which one of the following best explains these results?

   A. A non-HLA antibody.
   B. An HLA class I antibody.
   C. An HLA class II antibody.
   D. An autoantibody.
   E. Major histocompatibility complex (MHC) class I polypeptide-related sequence A (MICA) antigen antibody.

Table 15-6

	CDC Crossmatch		FC Crossmatch		Luminex	
	T cells	B cells	T cells	B cells	Class I	Class II
Crossmatch with donor	Neg	Neg	Neg	Neg	Neg	Neg

29b. The results of the pretransplant crossmatch are shown in Table 15-6. The transplant proceeds and the patient undergoes induction therapy with rituximab. If the testing were repeated 1 week after transplant, what would the results most likely show?

A.

	CDC Crossmatch		FC Crossmatch		Luminex	
	T cells	B cells	T cells	B cells	Class I	Class II
Crossmatch with donor	Neg	Neg	Neg	Neg	Neg	Neg

B.

Crossmatch with donor	Neg	Pos	Neg	Pos	Weak pos	Neg

C.

Crossmatch with donor	Pos	Pos	Pos	Pos	Weak pos	Neg

D.

Crossmatch with donor	Neg	Neg	Neg	Pos	Neg	Pos

29c. Which one of the following tests offers additional information about the anti-HLA class I antibody present in this serum, complementing the testing results described in the previous question?

   A. PRAs.
   B. Luminex/SPA with single antigen beads.
   C. T- and B-cell CDC crossmatch with anti-human globulin.
   D. High-resolution typing of the recipient and donor.

30. Which one of the following diseases is associated with *HLA-DQB1*06:02*?

   A. Narcolepsy.
   B. Celiac disease.
   C. Ankylosing spondylitis.
   D. Behçet's disease.

31. In transplantation, the T-cell contribution to allograft rejection is caused primarily by direct recognition of the donor's MHC molecules by clonal T-cell receptors (TCRs). This strong recognition is based on which one of the following?

   A. Recipient peptides presented on donor MHC class II molecules to recipient T cells.
   B. Complementarity-determining regions (CDRs) of recipient TCR stably binding the polymorphic domains of the donor MHC.
   C. Stable binding of CD4 co-receptor molecules to nonself MHC class II alleles.
   D. Stable binding of CD8 co-receptor molecules to nonself MHC class I alleles.
   E. Stable binding of both CD4 co-receptor molecules to nonself MHC class II alleles and stable binding of CD8 co-receptor molecules to nonself MHC class I alleles.

32. Which one of the following treatments used in transplantation can cause a false-positive FC crossmatch?

   A. Cyclosporin A.
   B. Rituximab.
   C. Prednisone.
   D. Mycophenolate mofetil.

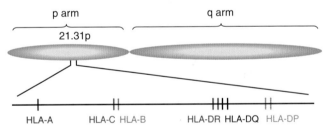

Figure 15-2 Schematic representation of the HLA locus genomic organization. This figure demonstrates the organization of the different HLA class I and class II genes on chromosome 6p21.31.

33. Assuming there are no recombination hot spots in the HLA chromosome region, which HLA gene pair displays the highest recombination frequency (Figure 15-2)?

   A. *HLA-A* and *HLA-DP*.
   B. *HLA-B* and *HLA-DR*.
   C. *HLA-DR* and *HLA-DQ*.
   D. *HLA-A* and *HLA-DR*.

34. An allograft transplant recipient who received a kidney from an older HLA-identical brother (*HLA-A/B/C/DR* typed, 8/8 identity) is experiencing graft dysfunction 4 months after transplantation. A biopsy reveals cellular infiltrates with the majority being T cells. Which one of the following is the most likely basis of T-cell reactivity in this case?

   A. Drug toxicity.
   B. Crossover event at the *HLA-DQ* locus.
   C. Age of the donated organ.
   D. The direct recognition pathway.
   E. The indirect recognition pathway.

35. According to current (2011) national transplant statistics published by the United Network for Organ Sharing (UNOS), heart, kidney, and liver primary allograft survival rates are roughly 70% at 5 years. Which one of the following is true regarding lung allograft survival?
    A. It is much better than other solid organs because the lung is an immune-privileged site.
    B. It is much worse than other solid organs due to the inflammation elicited by airborne antigens.
    C. It is about in line with other solid organs because rejection is histocompatibility driven and other organ-specific factors play only minor roles.
    D. All lung allografts are lost within 5 years due to bronchiolitis obliterans syndrome (BOS).

36. Which one of the following molecular HLA designations shows the correct use of nomenclature to identify a particular allele?
    A. DR*03:01:01.
    B. DRB1*030101.
    C. DRB1*03:01:01.
    D. DRB103:01:01.

37. Hyperacute rejection distinguishes itself from other types of acute and chronic rejection through the extreme alacrity of its onset. Immunologically, the speed of this reaction is explained by its reliance on which one of the following?
    A. Preformed donor-specific antibodies and complement deposition.
    B. Preformed donor-specific antibodies and alloreactive T cells.
    C. Preformed donor-specific antibodies, de novo antibody production against the graft, and complement deposition.
    D. De novo antibody production against the graft and complement deposition.

38a. SPAs are the newest methods used in histocompatibility testing for alloantibody detection. SPA tests for alloantibodies rely on which one of the following?
    A. Beads coated with antigen(s).
    B. Magnetic beads.
    C. FC.
    D. Anti-human globulin (AHG)–augmented CDC crossmatch.

38b. Which one of the following can cause interference in the identification of anti-HLA antibody specificity by SPA (Luminex)?
    A. Cells with poor viability binding antibodies nonspecifically.
    B. Absence of the target allele on testing beads.
    C. Instrument sensitivity.
    D. Assay interference by medications.

39. Which one of the following is an advantage of SPAs with single antigen beads in histocompatibility testing?
    A. Identification of complement fixing antibodies.
    B. Prediction of a negative effect on graft survival.
    C. Identification of HLA specificities of antibodies.
    D. Prediction of acute cellular rejection (ACR) risk.

40. A kidney transplant candidate underwent a thorough pre-transplant antibody study. Serum testing on a panel of cells from 70 individuals (PRA) shows that her serum lyses five (7%) of the cells, all of which are *HLA-B27+*. SPAs

Table 15-7 Testing Methodology in Brief

Method	Reaction			Readout
PRA	Patient serum	+ Cells from 70 individuals (selected as a good representation of the HLA makeup of the population)	+ Complement	Cell lysis detected by microscopy
CDC crossmatch	Patient serum (±DTT)	+ Donor cells	+ Complement	Cell lysis detected by microscopy
SPA	Patient serum	+ HLA-coated beads	+ Anti-human IgG antibody, phycoerythrin (PE conjugated)	Serum antibody deposition on HLA-coated beads detected by phycoerythrin (PE) fluorescence

CDC, Complement-dependent cytotoxicity; PE, phycoerythrin; PRA, peripheral blood mononuclear cells and panel reactive antibody testing; SPA, solid-phase assay.

performed on the same serum indicate that the patient has two antibodies against *HLA-B27* and *HLA-B35*, and they both present roughly similar MFI values (6000-7000). A child of the patient (who is *HLA-B27+*) and a sibling (who is *HLA-B35+*) volunteer for donation. The CDC crossmatch reactions with the child's cells (*HLA-B27+*) are positive in the presence or absence of dithiothreitol (DTT), but the CDC crossmatch with the *HLA-B35+* sibling's cells is negative. Which one of the following is the best explanation for this observation and the best recommendation for transplantation (Table 15-7)?
    A. The anti–*HLA-B27* is an IgM antibody, and transplantation with the child's kidney is an acceptable option.
    B. The anti–*HLA-B35* is an IgG1 or IgG3 antibody, and transplantation with the sibling's kidney is *not* acceptable.
    C. The anti–*HLA-B27* is an IgG antibody and transplantation with the child's kidney is an acceptable option.
    D. The anti–*HLA-B35* is an IgG2 or IgG4 antibody, and transplantation with the sibling's kidney is an acceptable option.

41. A female leukemia patient received a bone marrow allograft. She is blood type O+ and shows high titers of anti-A and anti-B antibodies. Her donor is a male of blood type AB+. At 3 months posttransplant, the patient has the following data entered into her medical record: 100% white blood cells (WBCs) of donor origin by karyotyping Y chromosome–carrying cells. The recipient ABO testing yields O+ results. Which one of the following is the likely explanation for these results?
    A. The WBC karyotyping is wrong due to interference by anti-donor (ABO) antibodies.
    B. The ABO typing was performed on a different patient's sample.
    C. The ABO results were obtained by back typing and front typing should be performed.
    D. Both results are correct; donor bone marrow produces WBCs while recipient bone marrow produces red blood cells.

42. Posttransplant de novo anti-HLA antibodies develop in an allograft recipient with no history of sensitization (pretransplant). Which one of the following can be caused by these de novo antibodies?
    A. A positive crossmatch.
    B. Recurrence of the original disease.
    C. Hyperacute rejection episodes.
    D. Chronic rejection.

43. Which one of the following statements is true?
    A. Anti-CD20 humanized monoclonal antibody eliminates plasma cells more effectively than circulating B cells.
    B. Anti-CD25 monoclonal antibody therapy can reduce alloreactive B-cell responses.

C. Administration of IVIg can increase the titer of alloreactive antibodies.
D. Bortezomib is a proteosome inhibitor that induces apoptosis by accumulation of large amounts of protein.

44. Which one of the following includes all of the generally accepted signs of antibody-mediated rejection of a solid organ allograft?
    A. Anti-HLA antibodies alone.
    B. Circulating donor-specific antibodies, Cd4 deposition in the graft, and graft dysfunction.
    C. Donor-specific antibodies, C4d deposition in the graft, and ejection fraction less than 40%.
    D. Biopsy IgG immunofluorescence, C4b deposition in the graft, and graft dysfunction.

ANSWERS

1. A. Complement-dependent cytotoxicity (CDC) against a reference panel of T and B cells.
B. Flow cytometry (FC) crossmatch with donor peripheral blood mononuclear cells and panel reactive antibody (PRA) testing.
Rationale: PRA testing is less sensitive than other methods and cannot distinguish anti-human leukocyte antigen (HLA) antibodies from non-HLA antibodies. In highly sensitized patients (PRA >80%), the HLA specificities cannot be defined. FC cannot determine complement fixation or HLA specificity.
C. Solid-phase assays (SPAs).
Rationale: SPAs have high sensitivity and can be used to determine anti-HLA antibody specificities but cannot determine whether the antibodies are complement fixing.
D. CDC against a reference panel of T cells and B cells and SPAs.
Rationale: These two methods (PRA and SPA) provide the most comprehensive picture of allosensitization. PRA can be used to determine the ability of the antibodies to fix complement, whereas SPAs can detect low titers of alloantibodies and define their HLA specificities.

Major points of discussion
■ Each antibody detection method currently in use has advantages and disadvantages. A combination of methodologies, which cover each other's "blind spots," is necessary to gain the most information about the sensitization status of a patient.
■ PRA testing performed by CDC detects IgG and IgM complement fixing antibodies. The pattern of reaction against T cells and/or B cells can hint to the nature of the anti-HLA antibodies. T-cell–positive and B-cell–positive reactions signal the presence of anti-HLA class I antibodies, whereas T-cell–negative and B-cell–positive reactions reveal anti-HLA class II antibodies. PRAs can detect antibodies against other (non-HLA) antigens if they are expressed on the cells used for testing.
■ PRA cannot detect the presence of antibodies that do not fix complement. Although the HLA typing of the cells forming a panel is known, it is sometimes impossible to ascertain the specificities of the antibodies in the serum of a highly sensitized patient (i.e., PRA >90%).

■ SPAs use collections of beads coated with mixtures or individual HLAs. This allows resolution of the antibodies' HLA specificities. SPAs have a limit of detection that surpasses that of any other test currently used. SPAs also allow a relative quantification of the antibodies by the mean fluorescence intensity (MFI) readouts.
■ SPAs also have several limitations. Generally, only HLAs are coated onto SPA beads; therefore, non-HLA antibodies cannot be detected. SPAs are not designed to detect IgM antibodies. It cannot distinguish between complement fixing and nonfixing antibodies.
■ PRA and SPA technologies complement each other nicely, as each method provides information not available from the other.[4,21,22]

2a. A. Scenario A.
Rationale: This appears to be a case of HLA class I and class II sensitization with an anti-HLA class II donor-specific antibody, which also fixes complement (CDC crossmatch B cells +). An IgG anti-HLA class I antibody is also detected but is either of insufficient titer, affinity, or wrong isotype subtype to fix complement.
B. Scenario B.
Rationale: This appears to be a non-HLA antibody to an antigen present on T cells and not B cells. An iatrogenic effect of monoclonal antibody therapy such as muromonab-CD3 (trade name Orthoclone OKT3) or anti-thymocyte globulin (ATG) should be suspected.
C. Scenario C.
Rationale: The results suggest a complement fixing (CDC+) anti-HLA class II antibody (B cells+), without any anti-HLA class I antibodies.
D. Scenario D.
Rationale: This result is due to one or more IgM isotype antibody(ies), which is(are) not detectable by FC crossmatch but can fix complement. Despite their ability to fix complement, IgM antibodies do not present a grave danger to allografts.

2b. A. Scenario A.
Rationale: Unambiguous result: HLA class I and class II sensitization, with a class II donor-specific antibody that also fixes complement (CDC crossmatch B cell +).

B. Scenario B.
Rationale: Ambiguous result: It could be a non-HLA antibody present on T cells and not B cells or an iatrogenic effect of anti–T-cell monoclonal antibody therapy such as muromonab-CD3 or ATG. Further testing by SPAs with single antigen beads or enzyme-linked immunosorbent assay (ELISA) may elucidate this.
C. Scenario C.
Rationale: Unambiguous result: A complement fixing (CDC+) anti-HLA class II antibody (B cells+), with no anti-HLA class I antibodies detected.
D. Scenario D.
Rationale: Unambiguous result: This result is due to an IgM isotype antibody(ies), which is(are) not detectable by FC crossmatch but can fix complement.

2c. A. Scenario A.
B. Scenario B.
C. Scenario C.
Rationale: A positive FC crossmatch implies an IgG antibody.
D. Scenario D.
Rationale: This result is due to one or more IgM isotype antibody(ies), which is(are) not detectable by FC crossmatch but can fix complement. Standard FC crossmatch methodology is designed to detect only IgG antibodies.

Major points of discussion
- CDC crossmatch can detect complement fixing IgG and IgM antibodies against donor cells.
- FC crossmatch is designed to detect the binding of IgG to donor cells but not their complement fixing ability.
- Anti-HLA class I antibodies in serum will give T-cell– and B-cell–positive crossmatch reactions due to the expression of HLA class I (i.e., HLA-A, -B, -C) on all cells.
- Anti-HLA class II antibodies in serum will give only B-cell–positive crossmatch reactions since only antigen-presenting cells (APCs) such as B cells express HLA class II antigens (i.e., HLA-DR, -DQ, -DP).
- No HLA distribution explains a T+B– crossmatch reaction. Certain anti–T-cell antibody treatments often used in transplantation (such as Orthoclone OKT3, ATG) may, however, result in a T+B– crossmatch.

3. A. Nephrectomy was incomplete; residual tissues left behind continue to be rejected and generate a humoral response.
Rationale: Following immune reactions, it is thought that some antigen is always retained by follicular dendritic cells in the lymph nodes maintaining long-term memory responses. Antigen storage and increases in circulating antibodies can occur regardless of the "thoroughness" of the nephrectomy.
B. Anti-donor HLA antibodies continue to be produced after nephrectomy; however, the graft no longer adsorbs them.
Rationale: Anti-donor HLA antibodies are secreted by plasma cells. These plasma cells can be long lived and are not vulnerable to rituximab treatment due to downregulation of surface CD20 antigen. After nephrectomy, plasma cells continue to produce antibodies, but the graft no longer acts as a sink for the circulating antibodies.

C. The readings are an artifact of the rituximab treatment, which can persist in circulation many months after the treatment.
Rationale: Whereas rituximab can interfere with a B-cell crossmatch, SPAs use beads coated only with HLAs. Therefore, antibodies against antigens other than HLA cannot be detected in SPAs.
D. The histocompatibility lab switched reagent lots, and the new reagents are much better than the old ones at detecting the antibodies against the specific allele of the donor in this case.
Rationale: Clinical labs must test reagents for efficacy and consistency from lot to lot. Although not inconceivable, this is an extremely remote possibility.

Major points of discussion
- Solid organ allografts can adsorb a large amount of donor-specific alloantibodies. Circulating levels of antibodies can be misleadingly low because of adsorption by the graft.
- Rituximab can persist in the circulation of patients for months and can interfere with some antibody testing methodologies. As an anti–B-cell antibody, rituximab causes false-positive results in CDC assays using B cells.
- SPAs, which use beads coated with specific antigens (usually HLAs), have several advantages, including the following:
  - Excellent sensitivity
  - Ability to resolve antibody specificity (if an anti-HLA antibody)
  - Immunity to interference from most monoclonal antibody therapies currently used since those target antigens are not coated onto the beads
- SPAs also suffer from a few shortcomings:
  - Inability to distinguish harmful complement fixing antibodies from non–complement fixing ones,
  - Inability (using the standard SPA procedures) to identify antibody isotypes other than IgG
  - Inability to detect antibodies to non-HLAs[1,19,22]

4. A. Child 1.
B. Child 2.
C. Child 3.
D. Child 4.
Rationale: If the parental haplotypes are designated as:
a: *A2 B44 DR4*
b: *A1 B60 DR13*
c: *A3 B7 DR15*
d: *A24 B56 DR16*
The family haplotype makeup is:
Father a/b
Mother c/d
Child 1 a/c
Child 2 a/d
Child 3 b/c
Child 4: a+b/d

Major points of discussion
- Chromosomal crossover (or crossing over) is an exchange of genetic material between homologous chromosomes.

- The frequency of crossover between two loci is directly proportional to the distance between the two genes on the chromosomes.
- The genetic identity between a parent and a child is exactly 50%.
- There is a 25% chance that siblings will be 100% HLA matched or 100% mismatched by inheriting the same or the other parental HLA haplotypes. There is a 50% chance that siblings will be 50% HLA matched.
- Chromosomal crossover events can yield unexpected HLA matching between siblings, such as 8/10 HLA matching (when 0/10, 5/10, or 10/10 identity is expected). Allele-level matching is extremely important in bone marrow transplantation, and crossover events bear great importance in donor selection.
- Family studies aim to establish the parental haplotypes by tracking which HLA alleles "travel" together.

5. **A. Splits of HLAs, indistinguishable by old serologic typing methods.**
Rationale: HLA nomenclature was initially assigned according to common alloantibodies that recognized them. It was later recognized that some antibodies detected multiple antigens and the nomenclature was redefined by renaming the old antigen into the two or more newly discovered "splits." For example, *HLA-B16* split into B38 and B39 and *HLA-DR3* became DR17 and DR18.
B. Egregious errors of the previous histocompatibility lab.
C. Egregious errors of the current histocompatibility lab.
Rationale: The first and second typings are actually concordant.
D. The donor's HLAs are detected in the patient's blood.
Rationale: A kidney does not shed sufficient amounts of antigens or cells into the circulation of a recipient to interfere with HLA typing.

Major points of discussion
- HLA nomenclature began by assigning each locus consecutive numbers corresponding to new anti-HLA antibodies discovered (*HLA-A1, -A2,* etc).
- It was realized early on that some anti-HLA antibodies recognized multiple HLAs, hence the need to "split" what was formerly thought to be a single antigen into newly discovered subtypes, that is, *B16→B38, B39; B17→B57, B58.*
- With the advent of genetics, HLA loci were discovered to be much more polymorphic than could ever be classified by serology. For example, at the genetic level, *HLA-B57* appeared to be a collection of alleles *B*57:01, B*57:02,* etc.
- In this nomenclature convention (i.e., *B*57:01*), the first two numbers represent the serologically defined antigen and the second two represent the allelic subtype.
- Finally, in 2011 a new nomenclature was introduced to address the problem that arises at loci that have more than 99 genetically defined alleles—that is, *HLA-B*5799* would be the last allele in which the genetic resolution can be described by two digits. The newest nomenclature looks like *HLA-B*57:01:02*, and the last two digits define alleles of *B*57:01* with silent mutations.
- Patients with long allograft survival times may have typing results in their charts and medical records conforming to outdated nomenclatures.[9,20]

6. A. Number of mismatched antigens.
Rationale: The number of mismatches does not determine the amount of donor-specific antibodies in circulation.
B. Number of previous transplants.
Rationale: The number of previous transplants does not determine the amount of donor-specific antibodies in circulation.
C. The PRA percentage.
Rationale: Even in a patient with high PRA (i.e., >80%), the antibodies may not be donor specific.
D. Titer of donor-specific antibodies.
Rationale: High titers of donor-specific antibodies can result in hyperacute rejection. Lowering these titers to levels at which the patient no longer has a positive crossmatch with the donor is paramount before proceeding with the transplant.

Major points of discussion
- Presensitization with donor-specific antibodies may result in hyperacute rejection and immediate loss of the graft.
- A cytotoxicity crossmatch is a useful tool in screening against such reactions.
- However, there are such highly sensitized patients for whom a donor is nearly impossible to find; that is, the patient will have at least one antibody against any combination of HLAs. Without desensitization protocols, these patients' access to lifesaving organ transplantation would be blocked or severely limited.
- Desensitization protocols, usually relying on plasmapheresis and IVIg, can be used to reduce the titers of antibodies present in the patient's circulation and inhibit the production of more antibodies from plasma cells.
- If the titers of antibodies against a donor can be lowered sufficiently so as not to yield a positive CDC crossmatch, the patient may be safely transplanted.

7. A. The patient produced donor-specific antibodies to a likely mismatched allele of *HLA-A2* (which is present in about 40% of the population) not represented on the SPA beads but cross-reacts with multiple *HLA-A* and *-B* alleles.
Rationale: Whereas the A2 serotype is indeed present in 40% of many human populations, individual HLA alleles (i.e., *A*02:04*) are present in smaller fractions and, hence, would not justify a 50% PRA. Cross-reactivity of antibodies between closely related HLAs is common, but they usually involve a few antigens, not dozens.
B. The patient produced multiple anti-HLA antibodies against mismatched, nontyped loci (*HLA-C, -DQ, -DP*), which cross-react with multiple *HLA-A* and *-B* alleles.
Rationale: Two facts make this scenario implausible: (1) If anti-*HLA-C/DQ/DP* reactions occurred, the SPA failed to detect them, and (2) the cross-reactivity of antibodies across loci is simply not as extensive as it would need to be for this explanation to be true.
C. The patient produced antibodies against the β-2 microglobulin chain of HLA class I expressed by half of the cell panel and used by all the HLA alleles identified by SPAs.
Rationale: The β-2 microglobulin is a nonpolymorphic chain in all HLA class I molecules. It is a self-antigen for the recipient, so the patient should not be able to make antibodies against it. If such an autoantibody should arise, it would test positive on 100% of the panel.

D. The patient produced a single antibody against the epitope Bw4 present in *HLA-B27* and many *HLA-A* and *-B* alleles.
Rationale: Bw4 is a "public epitope" composed of four residues. It appears on many *HLA-B* and some *HLA-A* alleles.

Major points of discussion
■ There are several epitopes common to many HLA alleles. These are often referred to as "public epitopes."
■ The Bw4 antigen consists of four amino acids at positions 80-83 in HLA class I molecules. It is present on alleles *HLA-B5 (51, 52, 5102, 5103), 0802, 0803, 13, 17 (57, 58), 1809, 27, 37, 38 (16), 44 (12), 47, 49 (21), 53, 5607, 59, 63, 67, 77,* and *HLA-A23, 24, 25, 32.*
■ The Bw6 epitope consists of 4 amino acids: NLRG 80-83 at positions 80-83 in HLA class I molecules. It is present on alleles *HLA-B7, 703, 8, 1309, 18, 2708, 2712, 2718, 35, 39 (16), 3901, 3902, 4005, 4406, 4409, 45 (12), 46*, 4702, 48, 50 (21), 54 (22), 55 (22), 56 (22), 60 (40), 61 (40), 62 (15), 64 (14), 65 (14), 67, 71 (70), 72 (70), 73, 75 (15), 76 (15), 78, 81.*
■ Only a handful of HLA-B alleles have neither Bw4 nor Bw6 (*HLA-B1806, -B4601, -B5503,* and *-B7301*).
■ A transplant recipient who has only one Bw epitope can form antibodies against the other Bw epitope.
■ Bw4/6 antibodies can have a major impact on the donor pool available to the presensitized patient.

8. A. Mother donates to child.
Rationale: This may be the best pairing. Some evidence suggests that antigens make it across the placental barrier, and children establish central tolerance to maternal antigens providing the basis for better transplant outcomes than other parent-child pairings.
B. Father donates to child.
C. Child donates to mother.
Rationale: Fetal antigens (of paternal genetic origin) can be transferred to the mother during the pregnancy, and the mother's immune system can form antibodies against them. This can represent a presensitization event for a child-to-mother organ transplant, and the rejection risk is higher than in the other donor-recipient pairings shown here.
D. Child donates to father.
Rationale for B and D: The donor and recipient share one half of their genetic material, including one half of all the HLAs (all loci). This scenario does not have any additional benefits or detractions like the mother-child scenarios.

Major points of discussion
■ Central tolerance is established very early in the life of an individual, and it ensures that adaptive immunity components do not react to "self" antigens.
■ A main component of central tolerance is the negative selection of self-reactive T cells and B cells in the thymus and bone marrow. Positive selection of self-cognate T cells also occurs, ensuring that T and B cells possess functional T-cell receptors and B-cell receptors, respectively, and giving rise to T regulatory cells.
■ Maternal antigens crossing the placental barrier can participate in the central tolerance being established in the fetus, thus accounting for better mother-to-child allograft survival.
■ Fetal antigens crossing the placental barrier cannot participate in the central tolerance establishment in the

mother, which by the time of the pregnancy is largely shut down. Thus, the mother's adult immune system recognizes these antigens as exogenous and can create antibodies to them.
■ Pregnancy constitutes a well-documented allosensitizing event.

9. A. Auto-crossmatch.
Rationale: Auto-crossmatch is defined as the patient's serum reactivity with his or her own cells.
B. Direct crossmatch.
Rationale: Direct crossmatch is defined as the patient's serum reactivity with his or her donor's cells.
C. Virtual crossmatch.
Rationale: Crossmatch results can be accurately predicted when the patient's antibody specificities have been identified using recombinant single HLA bead technologies and the potential donor HLA type is known.
D. Flow crossmatch.
Rationale: Flow crossmatch analyzes the reactivity of patient's serum alloantibodies with a donor's cells by FC.

Major points of discussion
■ The advent of SPAs has allowed the characterization of circulating alloantibodies with unprecedented sensitivity and specificity.
■ The technology consists of an ELISA reaction where the antigen(s) are fixed on a solid phase (microbeads). A laser-based detection system allows quantification of the amount of antibody detected based on MFI readings.
■ An important caveat of the technology is that, although it provides accurate information on the antibodies' specificities and quantity, it does not provide any qualitative information. Most importantly, it does not detect the complement-fixing ability of the antibodies detected.
■ A virtual crossmatch relies on SPA measurements of the circulating antibodies in a transplant patient, then refusing donor offers from individuals who express HLAs to which antibodies were detected.
■ This method carries the risk of denying access to transplantation of terminally ill patients who, although having high titers of alloantibodies in circulation, do not have complement-fixing antibodies and, therefore, may fare well with a negative CDC crossmatch transplant.

10. A. Graft dysfunction is caused by a thrombus.
Rationale: Sepsis can in fact cause thrombus formation; however, no mention is made of the patient being septic.
B. Graft dysfunction caused by a humoral response against the pathogen, which cross-reacts with non-HLA heart antigens.
Rationale: β-Hemolytic streptococci, but not *S. pneumoniae,* can induce anti-myosin antibodies by molecular mimicry.
C. Antibody-mediated rejection caused by complement-fixing non–donor-specific antibodies that cross-react with donor HLA alleles.
Rationale: Cross-reactivity of anti-HLA antibodies with closely related HLA alleles has been long documented. Antibodies classified as non–donor-specific remained in circulation at high levels throughout this patient's history.

However, they caused neither a positive crossmatch nor hyperacute/acute rejection, so they are not the likely cause of humoral rejection.

D. Antibody-mediated rejection caused by the anti–HLA-A2 antibody, which increased along with other anti-HLA antibodies as a consequence of the infection.
Rationale: Humoral immunity including anti–HLA-A2 antibody production increased as a consequence of the infection. Solid organs can absorb a large amount of antibodies and the levels of circulating anti-A2 antibody misleadingly appear to decrease during rejection.

Major points of discussion

- Antibody testing methods test the levels/titers of *circulating* antibodies.
- Organs can adsorb a large amount of donor-specific antibodies.
- Infections and lapses in immunosuppression can increase humoral immunity nonspecifically.
- Increases in circulating antibodies accompanied by decreases in donor-specific antibodies could be indicative of deposition of donor-specific antibodies into the graft.
- Decreases of circulating donor-specific antibodies can support an antibody-mediated rejection diagnosis, rather than rule it out.

11. A. Mother: *DR1 DR15*; father: *DR3, DR7*.
B. Mother: *DR1 DR3*; father: *DR4, DR7*.
C. Mother: *DR1 DRX*; father: *DR1, DR4*.
Rationale: This family will benefit most from allele-level typing for the identification of an HLA-identical sibling. Allele-level typing of the parents' HLA genes will identify the subtypes of the *DR1* gene carried by the mother and father. Allele-level typing of the children will facilitate the identification of parental HLA haplotypes and recognition of HLA-identical siblings.
D. Mother: *DR11 DR4*; father: *DR3, DR7*.
Rationale for A, B, and D: HLA-identical siblings can be identified with low-resolution (antigen-level) HLA typing in this family.

Major points of discussion

- HLA matching of stem cell recipients and donors is essential for the success of stem cell transplantation.
- Molecular methods using genomic DNA analysis are used to identify the HLA type of stem cell transplant recipients and donors. These methods include polymerase chain reaction (PCR) and DNA sequencing based methods.
- Low-resolution HLA typing methods provide generic, antigen-level HLA typing data. Such methods use PCR-based techniques.
- High-resolution HLA typing methods provide allele-level HLA typing data. Such methods use PCR- and DNA sequencing–based techniques.
- The types of tissues most often used for HLA typing of stem cell recipients and donors are peripheral blood, umbilical cord, bone marrow, and buccal swabs.
- HLA laboratories performing HLA typing for stem cell transplantation follow the guidelines of the National Bone Marrow Donor Registry.[2,16]

12. A. The results are invalid.
Rationale: This pattern of reactivity can occur in donor-recipient crossmatching.
B. The serum contains a donor-specific IgG antibody and a blocking IgM antibody.
Rationale: A blocking IgM antibody may interfere with donor-specific IgG antibody, resulting in a negative crossmatch. This effect is abolished on treatment of the serum with a reducing agent, such as DTT.
C. The serum contains a donor-specific IgM antibody and a blocking IgG antibody.
Rationale: A donor-specific IgM antibody typically causes a positive crossmatch with the untreated serum and a negative crossmatch with the DTT-treated serum.
D. The serum contains a donor-specific IgA antibody.
Rationale: Cytotoxic anti-lymphocyte IgA antibodies are extremely rare. In addition, the pattern of serum reactivity is consistent with the presence of a blocking IgM antibody.

Major points of discussion

- Serum anti-HLA antibodies may occur as a result of sensitization to HLAs through the following:
  - Pregnancy
  - Transfusion
  - Transplantation
- Anti-HLA antibodies can be detected by the following:
  - CDC using a panel of HLA-typed cells
  - FC using HLA-coated beads
  - CDC or FC crossmatch using donor cells to detect anti-donor HLA antibodies.
- Serum anti-HLA IgG antibodies are considered the most deleterious to the graft. The clinical significance of anti-lymphocytic IgM antibodies is not clearly understood.
- To assess the cytotoxic activity of anti-lymphocytic antibodies, sera are tested in the presence and absence of DTT. DTT is a reduction agent, which destroys IgM structures.
- A serum containing anti-donor IgG antibodies will cause a positive crossmatch when tested with or without prior treatment with DTT.
- A serum containing anti-donor IgM antibodies, but not IgG antibodies, will cause a positive crossmatch when tested without DTT treatment and a negative crossmatch when tested after DTT treatment.

13. A. Types of T cells they stimulate.
Rationale: HLA class I and class II molecules stimulate CD8$^+$ and CD4$^+$ T lymphocytes, respectively.
B. Types of cells that express them.
Rationale: Most cells express HLA class I antigens. However, expression of HLA class II is restricted to antigen presenting cells, such as dendritic cells, monocytes, macrophages and B lymphocytes.
C. The chromosome on which they are located.
Rationale: Both HLA class I and class II genes are located on human chromosome 6.
D. Types of antigens they present.
Rationale: HLA class I predominantly presents peptides derived from intracellular proteins, whereas HLA class II presents mostly peptides derived from extracellular and membrane proteins.

E. Types of cells that contain a β-2 microglobulin subunit.
Rationale: Only HLA class I proteins contain a β-2 microglobulin subunit.

Major points of discussion
- HLAs are the most polymorphic genes in the human genome.
- HLA genes are co-dominantly expressed in each individual.
- HLA proteins bind peptides derived from self and foreign protein antigens. HLA-peptide complexes are exposed on the cell surface of APCs and interact with the T-cell receptor of cytotoxic or helper T cells.
- HLA class I proteins bind 9– to 12–amino acid long peptides from mostly intracellular proteins and interact with the T-cell receptor of CD8$^+$ cytotoxic T cells.
- HLA class II proteins bind 12– to 16–amino acid long peptides from mostly extracellular and membrane proteins and interact with the T-cell receptor of CD4$^+$ helper T cells.
- Recognition of foreign peptides presented in the context of self-HLA results in activation of T cells.

14. A. Co-dominance.
Rationale: Co-dominance is the relationship between two alleles from a single locus, which contribute equally to the phenotype.
B. Cross-reactivity.
Rationale: See Major Points of Discussion.
C. Memory response.
Rationale: Memory response is the enhanced immune response that occurs on reexposure to antigen.
D. Mixed lymphocyte reaction.
Rationale: Mixed lymphocyte reaction is an in vitro assay that measures T-cell proliferation triggered by HLA-mismatched cells.
E. PRA.
Rationale: PRA is a measure of anti-human antibodies present in the patient serum. PRA estimates the percentage of individuals in a population who will be excluded as transplant donors for that patient because of a positive crossmatch.

Major points of discussion
- An adaptive immune response is specific to the antigen (immunogen) that stimulated it. However, many naturally occurring immunogens display multiple epitopes that stimulate a variety of immune responses.
- Cross-reactivity is the reaction between an antibody and an antigen in which the antigen differs from the immunogen.
- In a broader sense, cross-reactivity applies to other immune responses as well. For example, despite the high specificity of T-cell responses, some T-cell clones may react against more than a single antigen.
- Cross-reactivity of immune cells has been documented in humans. For example, influenza virus–specific CD8$^+$ T cells were shown to react against hepatitis virus antigen.
- Cross-reactivity contributes to the vigorous response of T cells to allogeneic major MHC. T cells, which have been exposed to antigens, may cross-react with allogeneic cells.

15. A. Anti-donor HLA class I IgG.
B. Anti-donor HLA class I and class II IgG.
C. Anti-donor non-HLA IgG.
Rationale: These types of antibodies may cause a positive FC crossmatch. However, a positive FC crossmatch is most frequently caused by anti-donor HLA class I and/or class II antibodies.
D. Anti-donor lymphocyte IgG.
Rationale for A, B, and D: FC crossmatch performed with donor lymphocytes detects anti-donor HLA class I and class II antibodies as well as non-HLA antibodies, which bind to donor cells. In addition, FC crossmatch also detects anti-donor non-HLA antibodies.
E. Cytotoxic anti-donor HLA IgG and IgM.
Rationale: This test does not assess cytotoxicity.

Major points of discussion
- Sensitization to HLA and production of anti-HLA antibodies occurs through blood transfusions, pregnancy, or previous transplantation.
- Anti-donor HLA antibodies are associated with increased risk of allograft rejection and graft loss.
- To detect donor-specific antibodies in the serum of a transplant candidate, the patient's serum is crossmatched with donor lymphocytes. A positive crossmatch is primarily due to anti-donor HLA antibodies.
- CDC crossmatch is performed prior to transplantation to detect donor-specific cytotoxic antibodies.
- FC crossmatch is performed prior to transplantation to assess the level of serum antibodies that bind to donor cells. This type of crossmatch is more sensitive than CDC crossmatch.
- To reduce the titer of anti-HLA antibodies prior to transplantation, several desensitization protocols, such as plasmapheresis and treatment with IVIg or rituximab, are used.

16. A. Living related kidney transplantation in patients with high PRA.
B. Liver transplantation.
Rationale: High-resolution HLA class I and class II typing is not required in solid organ transplantation. Many liver transplant programs do not require HLA class I and class II typing at any level of resolution. Anti-HLA allele-specific antibodies are rare.
C. Stem cell transplantation: unrelated donor.
D. Stem cell transplantation: two haplotype–matched related donor.
Rationale: High-resolution HLA class I and class II typing is required in stem cell transplantation. In the setting of unrelated donor transplantation, high-resolution typing is particularly important because of the higher probability of an allele-level mismatch between the donor and recipient. A single mismatch detected with either low-resolution or high-resolution DNA testing is associated with higher mortality. The risk is compounded with two or more mismatches.
E. ABO-incompatible renal transplantation.
Rationale: High-resolution HLA class I and class II typing will not add useful information to that provided by low-resolution typing in the setting of ABO-incompatible transplantation.

Major points of discussion

- HLA typing is an important component of the immunologic evaluation of transplant candidates.
- Low-resolution (antigen-level) HLA typing of recipient and donor is required for most solid organ transplants.
- High-resolution (allele-level) HLA typing of recipient and donor is required for stem cell transplantation.
- HLA matching is crucial for the success of stem cell transplantation. Lack of HLA matching may lead to graft failure and graft-versus-host disease, two major complications of stem cell transplantation.
- PCR- and DNA sequencing–based methods are most often used for HLA typing.

17. A. FC crossmatch.
Rationale: This test detects the recipient's antibodies that bind to donor lymphocytes.
B. CDC crossmatch.
Rationale: This test detects recipient's antibodies that are able to kill donor lymphocytes.
C. HLA typing using sequence-specific oligonucleotides (SSOs).
Rationale: HLA typing using SSOs involves DNA isolation and SSO hybridization. It does not involve T-lymphocyte recognition of alloantigens.
D. Mixed lymphocyte culture.
Rationale: This test measures proliferation of T lymphocytes in response to direct recognition of cell surface alloantigens, in particular allogeneic HLA.
E. Mitogen T-cell stimulation.
Rationale: This test measures proliferation of T lymphocytes in response to a mitogen and does not involve recognition of alloantigens.

Major points of discussion

- Direct recognition of allogeneic HLA occurs through the interaction of T-cell receptors on the surface of host (responding) cells and allogeneic HLA proteins displayed on the surface of donor (stimulating) APCs.
- Direct recognition of alloantigens results in a vigorous immune response, which leads to graft rejection. The ability of responding T cells to react against allogeneic cells can be assessed in vitro by measuring T-cell proliferation in a mixed lymphocyte culture.
- Indirect recognition of allogeneic HLAs occurs through the interaction of T-cell receptors on the surface of host (responding) cells and peptides derived from allogeneic HLA proteins, presented in the context of self-HLA.
- Indirect recognition of allogeneic HLAs results in activation of discrete subsets of T cells. However, as a result of continuous shedding of proteins from the graft, T-cell activation by the indirect recognition pathway is an ongoing process, which contributes to graft rejection.
- Host CD4$^+$ T helper cells activated by direct and/or indirect alloantigen recognition pathways promote activation and differentiation of antibody producing B cells. Production of anti-donor HLA antibodies may lead to irreversible rejection of the allograft by the mechanism known as complement-mediated cytotoxicity.

18. A. There is a high probability that the CDC crossmatch with an *HLA-A2* donor will be positive.
Rationale: It is unlikely that the CDC crossmatch will be positive because the patient's serum does not contain detectable cytotoxic antibodies.
B. There is an increased risk of acute antibody-mediated rejection if the patient received an *HLA-A2* transplant.
Rationale: Patients with preformed donor-specific antibodies are at increased risk of acute antibody-mediated rejection compared with patients without donor-specific antibodies.
C. There is a high risk of hyperacute rejection if the patient received an *HLA-A2* transplant.
Rationale: There is no evidence that anti-donor HLA antibodies detected exclusively by solid-phase immunoassay cause hyperacute rejection.
D. Transplantation with an *HLA-A2* graft is contraindicated even if the CDC crossmatch is negative.
Rationale: The presence of a donor-specific antibody that is undetectable by CDC is not considered a contraindication for transplantation.
E. The results of the CDC and solid-phase immunoassays are discordant and, therefore, they are invalid.
Rationale: CDC and solid-phase immunoassays have different sensitivity levels in detecting anti-HLA antibodies. Solid-phase immunoassays are more sensitive than CDC-based assays and may detect low-titer/low-strength antibodies.

Major points of discussion

- Anti-donor HLA antibodies are associated with increased risk of allograft rejection and graft loss.
- Cytotoxic donor-specific antibodies may cause hyperacute or acute antibody-mediated rejection.
- Sensitization to HLAs can occur through the following:
  - Pregnancy
  - Blood transfusion
  - Transplantation
- The techniques frequently used for the detection and identification of serum anti-HLA antibodies are:
  - CDC assay using a panel of HLA-typed cells.
  - FC assays using HLA-coated beads. They may be performed on a multiplex platform.
  - CDC or FC crossmatch with donor lymphocytes.
- Virtual crossmatch determines whether a transplant candidate has anti-donor HLA antibodies and is at increased risk of rejection. Virtual crossmatch is positive if the HLA antibodies detected in the patient's serum are specific for the donor HLA. This assessment facilitates the selection of the most suitable donor for an HLA-sensitized patient.

19. A. Dendritic cells enter the germinal centers through high endothelial venules.
Rationale: Lymphocytes enter lymph nodes from the blood through high endothelial venules, whereas most dendritic cells enter the lymph node from the tissue through the lymphatics into the cortical sinus.
B. Long-lived plasma cells reside primarily in the germinal center and paracortical areas.
Rationale: Long-lived plasma cells reside primarily in the bone marrow.
C. Antigen-independent proliferation of B cells occurs in lymph nodes.

Rationale: Antigen-independent stages of B cell development occur in the bone marrow. Antigen-dependent proliferation occurs in the secondary lymphoid organs (lymph nodes and spleen).

D. Activated T cells are absent from germinal centers.
Rationale: Activated T cells and B cells are the mutually dependent driving force of the germinal center response. B-cell presentation of antigen to T cells activates responding T cells, which in turn drive B-cell activation.

E. Affinity maturation of B cells occurs in the germinal center.
Rationale: B-cell somatic hypermutation and class switching require CD40 engagement by CD40L-expressing helper T cells in the germinal center. Defective CD40 signaling is responsible for the hyper IgM syndrome.

Major points of discussion
- A lymph node is a small secondary lymphoid organ of the immune system that is distributed widely throughout the body.
- The lymph node acts a major communication hub between APCs and T cells.
- Tissue-resident macrophages and dendritic cells enter the local draining lymph node through afferent lymphatics and present phagocytosed antigen to cognate T cells.
- B cells, which encountered cognate antigen, form germinal centers in the lymph node where they proliferate, differentiate, class switch, and affinity mature their B-cell receptors (through somatic hypermutation).
- The B-cell evolution through the germinal center is highly dependent on follicular dendritic cells (which sustain their activation with antigen) and T-cell help in the form of costimulation (CD40-CD40L, CD86-CD28 molecular cross-talk) and cytokines.

20. A. The patient is not at risk for EBV lymphoma.
Rationale: Although there is evidence of B-cell polyclonality with mixed κ/λ light chain expression, clonal expansion is not excluded and the CD43 dim subset should be assessed for evidence of clonality.
B. EBV reactivation in immunocompromised patients is due to humoral insufficiency and can be overcome with IVIg treatment.
Rationale: Defective cell-mediated immunity, in particular reduced activity of EBV-specific effector memory CD8 T-cell activity, is likely to be responsible for this failure of immune surveillance.
C. B-cell proliferation in EBV lymphoproliferative disorders is due to B-cell receptor–mediated B-cell recognition of EBV antigens.
Rationale: EBV-related posttransplant lymphoproliferative disorder is due to the activation of EBV-infected B cells by EBV-encoded oncoproteins.
D. The receptor for EBV viral entry on B cell is the complement receptor CD21.
Rationale: See Major Points of Discussion.
E. EBV lymphoma is less commonly seen in pediatric transplants since posttransplant lymphoproliferative disorder is due to EBV reactivation from prior infection.
Rationale: Primary EBV infection in the posttransplant period is a major cause of EBV posttransplant lymphoproliferative disorder in the pediatric population in

which 50% or more of recipients may not have been previously exposed to EBV.

Major points of discussion
- Donor/recipient viral serology matching plays in important role in transplantation, having a major impact on mortality and morbidity.
- Allografts can transfer infection to a previously unexposed individual.
- In the United States, over 90% of the adult population is EBV seropositive and 50% to 80% is cytomegalovirus (CMV) positive. Seroprevalence is age dependent.
- Upon chronic immunosuppression, viral infections, which are kept under immunologic control in healthy individuals, can reactivate and become life threatening.
- Posttransplant lymphoproliferative diseases (PTLDs) are dependent on the transplanted organ and level of immunosuppression. The highest incidence of PTLDs is observed in small bowel and multiple organ transplants (5% to 20%), followed by thoracic allografts (2% to 10%), and then by renal and liver transplants (1% to 5%).[6,15]

21. A. Proceed with the transplant because the auto-crossmatch establishes the threshold of a negative reaction.
Rationale: A negative control (serum from a nonsensitized donor) is included in the flow crossmatch test, and it serves to establish the negative threshold for the crossmatch reaction.
B. Rule out this donor because the crossmatch is positive regardless of the auto-crossmatch results.
C. Do not transplant. These are autoantibodies (auto-crossmatch positive) that recognize the same antigen on donor cells and, therefore, will destroy the transplanted kidney as well.
D. Perform SPA testing to determine whether the antibodies are anti-HLA antibodies, and if yes, whether they are donor specific.
Rationale: The SLE diagnosis and the positive auto-crossmatch suggest that an autoantibody might be present. Patients with autoantibodies are clinically manageable and fare quite well after transplantation, so this is not an absolute contraindication to transplantation. However, it is certain that the patient has antibodies in circulation and the presence of a donor-specific anti-HLA antibodies must be ruled out.

Major points of discussion
- Autoantibodies can be a major contributing factor to organ failure in autoimmune diseases. For instance, anti-neutrophil cytoplasmic antibody (ANCA) leads to vasculitis and rapidly progressive glomerulonephritis, resulting in end-stage renal disease (ESRD).
- The relapse of the original autoimmune disease can happen after transplantation and contribute to the attrition of allografts.
- However, patient and graft survival rates in transplanted autoimmune patients can approach those of nonautoimmune patients. For example, in kidney allograft recipients who displayed ANCAs before transplantation, the vasculitis relapse rate was 0.02 per patient-year and graft survival rates were 100% at 1 year,

93.4% at 5 years, and 67.4% at 10 years, in a Johns Hopkins study.
- Kidney transplant is a safe and effective option for treating ESRD secondary to ANCA-associated vasculitis.
- Autoimmune disease relapses are rare with current immunosuppression.[7]

22a. A. Donor 1 due to the allele mismatch with the patient, *A*03:01* vs. *A*03:04*.
Rationale: Allele mismatches are dangerous in bone marrow transplantation, reducing the 1-year survival by about 10% for every mismatch.
B. Donor 2 due to the antigen mismatch with the patient, *A*03:01* vs. *A*01:01*.
Rationale: Antigen mismatches are dangerous in bone marrow transplantation and can result in graft versus host disease or poor engraftment, reducing the 1-year survival by about 10% for every mismatch.
C. No difference between donors 1 and 2 regarding the impact of mismatch on graft survival.
Rationale: Allele- and antigen-level mismatches appear equally deleterious in terms of the impact on graft survival.
D. Depends on where the mismatched amino acid(s) lie in the HLA structure.
Rationale: Most polymorphic sites in HLA molecules lie in the α helices flanking the peptide groove and interact with the T-cell receptor's complementarity-determining regions (CDRs).

22b. A. Yes. Donor 3 is better than donor 2, but worse than donor 1.
Rationale: All three donors would be considered to have one mismatch at the *HLA-A* locus to the recipient.
B. No. Donor 3 has an exotic allele, which is highly likely to elicit allorecognition and trigger graft-versus-host disease (GVHD).
Rationale: All allele groups designated by identical first numbers (i.e., all *A*02* alleles) are similar enough that they are hardly distinguishable by serology methods. In this case, *A*02:305 N* differs by a single nucleotide deletion from *A*02:01:01*; however, this causes it to be a null allele, which yields no protein.
C. Yes. Donor 3 has a perfectly matched allele *A*02:01* and a null allele *A*02:305 N*, which does not contribute to the allorecognition.
D. No. Homozygosity or single-allele expression at one locus in the donor may trigger GVHD.
Rationale: The donor cells would recognize the host A*03:01 as allogeneic/nonself, and this recognition could be the basis of a GVHD reaction. Donor homozygosity at a locus counts as a mismatch in stem cell transplantation. Therefore, donor 3 is not a better choice than either donor 1 or 2.

Major points of discussion
- GVHD is one of the additional challenges that stem cell transplantation presents compared with solid organ transplantation.
- Allele-level HLA mismatches are sufficient to trigger the allorecognition of the entire host body by the transplanted immune system.
- A study by Lee et al.[22] has shown that high-resolution DNA (allele) matching for *HLA-A, -B, -C,* and *-DRB1* (8/8 match) was the minimum level of matching associated with the highest survival.

- A single mismatch detected by low- or high-resolution DNA testing at *HLA-A, -B, -C,* or *-DRB1* (7/8 match) was associated with higher mortality (relative risk, 1.25; 95% CI, 1.13-1.38; *P*<.001) and 1-year survival of 43% compared with 52% for 8/8 matched pairs.
- Single mismatches at *HLA-B* or *HLA-C* appear better tolerated than mismatches at *HLA-A* or *HLA-DRB1*. Mismatching at two or more loci compounded the risk.
- Mismatching at *HLA-DP* or *-DQ* loci and donor factors other than HLA type were not associated with survival. In multivariate modeling, patient age, race, disease stage, and CMV status were as predictive of survival as donor HLA matching.
- In a heterozygous recipient, an immune system generated from homozygous bone marrow donor (or a donor expressing only one allele) can recognize the mismatched allele as nonself and trigger GVHD.[12]

23. A. 75%.
B. 50%.
C. 25%.
D. 16.7%.
E. 0%.
Rationale: Since a child inherits one HLA haplotype from each parent, a child will typically be 50% matched to each parent. Exceptions in which children are 100% HLA matched to a parent can occur when the parents share HLA haplotypes—that is, closely related parents, isolated communities with a strong founder effect, and so on.

Major points of discussion
- The HLA inheritance follows classic Mendelian inheritance principles for diploid organisms.
- The HLA genes are located on chromosome 6p21 and are inherited together as a haplotype (except for rare crossover events within the locus).
- Therefore, children are exactly haplo-identical to their parents, inheriting one HLA haplotypes (50% of their HLA makeup) from each parent.
- The only exception is when one haplotype (or both) are represented in both parents.
- Due to the highly polymorphic nature of the HLA genes, when parents share identical haplotypes, some level of shared ancestry can be inferred.

24. A. There are an unlimited amount of peptides that can be presented from a single protein.
Rationale: Peptides bind to HLA molecules through anchor residues to specific HLA molecules. Each HLA molecule has specific anchor residue requirements for binding that limit the potential peptides that can be presented from even large proteins. Although each HLA molecule can present only a limited number of peptides, HLA diversity within the human population is likely to be important evolutionarily to enable a broad capacity of antigen-presenting structures to broaden responsiveness to microbes across the population.
B. HLA haplotypes can contribute to immune responsiveness to a specific virus or vaccine.
Rationale: Since HLA molecules vary according to their ability to bind specific amino acid sequences, some HLA molecules are better than others in presenting specific viral peptides to T cells. For example, specific HLA alleles correlate

with hepatitis B vaccine responsiveness as a result of their differing ability to present hepatitis B virus surface antigen peptides to helper T cells.

C. Only extracellular antigens can be presented on HLA class II molecules.

Rationale: While the exogenous pathway is the dominant pathway for HLA class II loading by peptides in the endosomal system, intracellular antigens can be presented as well, including by means of autophagy.

D. Only intracellular antigens can be presented on HLA class I molecules.

Rationale: Although the endogenous pathway is the dominant pathway for HLA class I loading, the cross-presentation pathway also allows extracellular antigens to be presented.

E. Only the amino acid sequence determines the immunogenicity of peptides loaded onto HLA molecules.

Rationale: Classic HLA molecules can present modified peptides. Although binding to the HLA molecule strictly requires anchor amino acid interactions with the HLA groove, the polypeptide can have linked glycosylations or other modifications that protrude from the cleft and interact with T-cell receptor contacts, thus contributing to the immunologic "epitope." Moreover, nonclassic HLA molecules can present glycolipids as, for instance, cell wall constituents of tuberculosis.

Major points of discussion

- Antigen presentation is a process by which specialized cells (APCs; i.e., macrophages, dendritic cells, and others) capture antigens and then enable their recognition by T cells.
- Unlike B cells, T cells recognize antigens only in the context of an MHC molecule. The recognition of a foreign antigen by T cells and its subsequent activation is predicated on the stable biochemical interaction between the TCR and the peptide-MHC complex on APCs.
- Not all peptides can be loaded in all MHC molecules. Protein fragments must conform to a certain biochemical topology compatible with the MHC molecule.
- MHC class I molecules (HLA-A, -B, -C) are ubiquitously and highly expressed on most tissues. They present intracellular proteins, which are derived from the organism's own genome or from intracellular pathogens such as viruses. Only CD8$^+$ T cells can be primed by presentation from MHC class I molecules.
- MHC class II molecules (HLA-DR, -DP, -DQ) are expressed mostly by APCs and are loaded with proteins of extracellular origin following endocytosis. Only CD4$^+$ T cells can be primed by presentation from MHC class II molecules.
- The compartmentalization of intracellular-protein/class I/CD8 versus extracellular-protein/class II/CD4 is not absolute. Cross-presentation is the process by which some APCs allow extracellular antigen to be leaked out of the endosomes, loaded, and presented by MHC class I molecules. Thus, dendritic cells can prime both CD4$^+$ and CD8$^+$ T cells to phagocytose antigens.[5,8]

25. A. In infectious mononucleosis, the atypical lymphocytes are likely a large number of CD20$^+$ B-cell blasts.

Rationale: Primary EBV infection is associated with a reactive lymphocytosis that includes circulating EBV-specific CD8$^+$ T cells.

B. In infectious mononucleosis, the atypical lymphocytes are likely a large number of activated CD8$^+$ T cells.

Rationale: See Major Points of Discussion.

C. B-cell leukemia can be excluded if the atypical cells are surface B-cell receptor negative.

Rationale: Pre–B-cell leukemia staining will identify cytoplasmic μ chains, which are identified only by staining of permeabilized cells.

D. EBV-positive serology is seen in around 50% of adults.

Rationale: In the adult population, EBV-positive serology is more than 90%.

E. Stable integration of the EBV genome into chromosomal DNA of infected B cells is required for latency.

Rationale: The EBV genome can exist in infected B cells either episomally or integrated into the chromosome.

Major points of discussion

- The transplant patient population is at increased risk for EBV infection as a result of the immunosuppressive regimens used to prevent allograft rejection.
- Immunosuppression is nonspecific. It inhibits the immune response against the allograft, but it also reduces the immune surveillance against viral infections and tumors.
- The majority (50% to 80%) of posttransplant lymphoproliferative disorder biopsy samples test positive for EBV.[15]

26. **A. Cytokine receptors for interleukins (ILs)-2, -4, -7, -9, -15, and -21 signal through a common gamma chain–associated receptor activating JAK3 kinase.**

Rationale: Genetic deficiency in the common gamma chain results in X-linked severe combined immunodeficiency, including loss of B, T, and natural killer (NK) cells caused by the loss of IL-2, -7, and -15. Anti-inflammatory agents targeting the JAK3 tyrosine kinase are in clinical development to treat autoimmunity and to prevent/treat solid organ transplant rejection.

B. T-cell production of interferon (IFN)-γ, IL-12, and IL-17 augments the cellular immune response.

Rationale: These cytokines are potent proinflammatory agents that boost cellular immunity, but APCs are the primary sources of IL-12. IFN-γ is made by T helper (Th)1 cells and NK cells, and IL-17 is made by Th17 cells.

C. Cyclosporine blocks T-cell receptor signaling via inhibition of the tyrosine kinase nuclear factor of activated T cells (NFAT).

Rationale: NFAT is a transcription factor (not a kinase) activated on T-cell receptor activation of T cells and drives the transcription of T-cell–derived cytokines, including IL-2. Cyclosporine prevents the dephosphorylation of NFAT by binding to cyclophilin.

D. Toll-like receptors recognize only microbial constituents and activate innate immune cells through necrosis factor (NF)-κB.

Rationale: Toll-like receptors (TLRs) certainly recognize microbial constituents and signal through the NF-κB transcription factor. However, it has become clear that TLRs can recognize self/endogenous ligands. For instance, endosomal TLRs TLR7 and TLR9 are activated by CpG motifs in chromatin and ribonuclear proteins, respectively, and HMGB-1 is a ligand for TLR4. Thus, innate activation by self- and graft-derived ligands could contribute to autoimmunity and graft rejection.

E. Regulatory T cells have the capacity to induce tolerance by killing self-reactive effector T cells.
Rationale: Regulatory T cells are not thought to have cytolytic capacity. Regulatory T cells inhibit APCs and responding T cells through the production of anti-inflammatory cytokines IL-10 and transforming growth factor (TGF)-β and through contact-dependent mechanisms.

Major points of discussion
- T-cell activation on recognition of presented antigen results in proliferation and cytokine production.
- The effector function of CD4$^+$ Th cells is largely dependent on the cytokine repertoire secreted on activation.
- Th1 cells produce IFN-γ and enhance the killing activity of CD8$^+$ cytotoxic T lymphocytes.
- Th2 cells produce IL-4, -5, -6, -10, and -13 and enhance humoral responses from B cells.
- Th17 effector cytokines are IL-17, -21, and -22, and they play an important role in antimicrobial immunity at epithelial/mucosal barriers.
- T regulatory cells (some of which have been shown to act through IL-10 and TGF-β) inhibit the reactivity of other T cells to antigens.

27. A. Self-proteins cannot be processed into peptides.
B. Peptides from self-proteins cannot bind to HLA class I molecules.
Rationale: HLA class I molecules primarily present intracellular self-peptides.
C. Peptides from self-proteins cannot bind to HLA class II molecules.
Rationale: Phagocytes can take up and present necrotic or apoptotic cells and material, which include self-antigens.
D. Lymphocytes reactive to self-proteins are inactivated by deletion, anergy, or receptor editing.
Rationale: Negative selection generally ensures that a lymphocyte expressing a receptor reactive to a self-protein is eliminated by deletion, anergy induction, or receptor editing in the case of an autoreactive B cell.
E. Developing lymphocytes cannot rearrange V genes required to produce a receptor for self-proteins.
Rationale: Such rearrangements can happen, but self-reactive cells are negatively selected out.

Major points of discussion
- Central tolerance is the mechanism by which T-cell and B-cell populations are culled to only non–self-reactive clones.
- T- and B-cell clones that recognize self-peptides/epitopes do arise, but they are eliminated in the thymus or bone marrow, respectively, before they can enter the periphery.
- Positive selection of nonreactive cells with functional T-cell receptors or B-cell receptors also takes place. Positive

selection of self-cognate cells with regulatory function gives rise to "natural" T regulatory cell populations.
- According to some estimates, over 90% of the T cells generated in the thymus are never released into the periphery.
- Tissue-specific antigens are expressed in the thymus due to autoimmune regulator (AIRE) activation.
- A key concept of alloreactivity is that adaptive immune cells are educated to be tolerant to self-HLAs during their development; however, their reactivity to foreign HLAs expressed by an allograft was never screened out.

28. A. Complement components.
B. Rheumatoid factor.
C. Tumor necrosis factor (TNF) and IL-1.
D. IL-4 and IL-10.
Rationale: Patients with rheumatoid arthritis have elevated levels of proinflammatory cytokines TNF and IL-1 in their joints, which play a role in the pain, swelling, stiffness, and other symptoms associated with this disease.

Major points of discussion
- Rheumatoid arthritis is a chronic, systemic inflammatory process, which principally affects synovial joints.
- The disease association with HLA-DR4 suggests the activation of T cells to synovial antigens; however, depletion of B cells appears to be more effective in halting the disease.
- A remarkable deceleration of disease progression is observed in many cases by blockade of the cytokine TNF-α.
- Blockade of IL-1, IL-15, and IL-6 also has beneficial effects.
- These manifestations suggest that both the B- and T-cell compartments are involved, with presentation of antigens by B cells to T cells by HLA-DR eliciting T-cell help and consequent production of rheumatoid factors and antibodies to citrullinated peptides.

29a. A. A non-HLA antibody.
Rationale: Luminex SPAs can detect only anti-HLA antibodies.
B. An HLA class I antibody.
Rationale: In order of sensitivity, the methods listed are CDC < FC crossmatch < SPA/Luminex. A low-titer anti-HLA class I antibody would explain the Luminex/SPA reaction and the partial flow crossmatch–positive reaction on B cells (B cells express HLA class I and class II).
C. An HLA class II antibody.
Rationale: An anti-HLA class II antibody is inconsistent with the SPA results, which show only an anti-HLA class I antibody.
D. An autoantibody.
Rationale: Autoantibodies are not directed against HLAs, which are the only antigens coated on Luminex beads (the one exception is MHC class I polypeptide related sequence A [MICA] antigens).
E. Major histocompatibility complex (MHC) class I polypeptide related sequence A (MICA) antigen antibody.
Rationale: MICA antigens are distinguishable from HLA class I and class II on Luminex beads. They do not give positive reactions on B cells, as they are mostly expressed on stressed endothelial cells.

29b. A.

Rationale: Rituximab treatment affects some of the testing methodology.

B.

Rationale: Rituximab would give positive crossmatches by FC and CDC. It would not affect SPA results.

C.

Rationale: If the anti-HLA class I antibody detected pretransplantation is a donor-specific antibody and is induced by the allograft despite induction therapy, it would likely be first observed by the most sensitive method, which is the SPA/Luminex. It would likely also take longer than 1 week to generate positive crossmatches.

D.

Rationale: Rituximab treatment would not be detected by SPA/Luminex because the rituximab target, CD20, is not represented on the Luminex beads. CDC crossmatch, however, should have been positive on B cells.

29c. A. PRAs.

Rationale: PRA is a CDC-based method and the CDC crossmatch does not appear to detect this antibody. The PRA would not offer additional information.

B. Luminex/SPA with single antigen beads.

Rationale: Luminex/SPA with single antigen beads uses beads coated with individual antigens and can determine the HLA specificity of the anti–class I antibody present in this serum.

C. T- and B-cell CDC crossmatch with anti-human globulin.

Rationale: Anti-human globulin is used to enhance the sensitivity of the CDC crossmatch against T-cell targets. All B cells express B-cell receptors, which are essentially cell surface antibodies. The use of anti-human globulin on B cells would give a certain false-positive reaction.

D. High-resolution typing of the recipient and donor.

Rationale: Unlike in stem cell transplantation, solid organ recipients and donors are not HLA matched at the allele level. Such typing would give no additional information about the antibody present in this serum.

Major points of discussion

- In order of sensitivity, the antibody testing methodology can be arranged in the following order: CDC < FC < SPAs.
- A negative CDC crossmatch reaction allows a transplant to proceed with minimal risk of hyperacute rejection. The presensitization status of an allograft recipient may necessitate desensitization, induction therapies, and increased immunologic monitoring protocols by biopsy and serum antibody screening.
- Antibody therapies designed to eliminate immune cell lineages (i.e., rituximab) interfere with cell-based assays (CDC and FC).
- Humanized antibodies used for therapies can persist in circulation for months.
- SPAs detect only antibodies against antigens coated on the solid phase (i.e., HLA-antigen–coated beads for the Luminex method). As a result, SPA testing is not susceptible to the iatrogenic effects of antibody therapies.

30. **A. Narcolepsy.**

Rationale: Narcolepsy has one of the tightest known associations to an HLA allele. *DQB1*06:02* constitutes the major HLA susceptibility allele across all ethnic groups.

B. Celiac disease.

Rationale: Celiac disease is associated with *HLA-DQ2/DQ8*.

C. Ankylosing spondylitis.

Rationale: Ankylosing spondylitis is associated with *HLA-B27*.

D. Behçet's disease.

Rationale: Behçet's disease is associated with *HLA-B51*.

Major points of discussion

- Multiple human diseases are associated with HLA alleles.
- It is important to understand the difference between association and causation; HLA alleles associated with diseases may not always be pathogenic themselves. The culprit may be other (non-HLA) alleles specific to a human population, which also happens to be characterized by a high frequency of certain HLA alleles.
- In the case of *DQB1*06:02*, it is one of the strongest disease associations of an HLA allele described. Some 90% to 100% of patients with definite cataplexy carry this allele.
- The pathogenic role of *HLA-DQB1*06:02* has not been fully elucidated, but as in all HLA-disease associations, an autoimmune mechanism is strongly suspected.
- Recent studies describe a deficiency in hypocretin-secreting neurons in the hypothalamus of narcoleptic patients. *HLA-DQB1*06:02* was shown to bind hypocretin with high affinity, and presumably present it to T cells, triggering an autoimmune response.[3,17]

31. A. Recipient peptides presented on donor MHC class II molecules to recipient T cells.

Rationale: This process cannot be the basis of strong recognition between recipient T and donor cells because of the following:

- Recipient (self) peptides should not improve recipient TCR reaction to the donor MHC.
- Most allograft parenchyma and stroma do not express MHC class II antigens and are unable to present exogenous (recipient) antigens.
- Professional APCs of donor origin expressing MHC class II are not transferred in significant amounts to the recipient.
- Recipient antigen endocytosed by donor endothelium (which can express MHC class II in inflammatory conditions) can be presented after the onset of inflammation.

B. Complementarity-determining regions (CDRs) of recipient TCR stably binding the polymorphic domains of the donor MHC.

Rationale: The hypervariable CDRs of recipient TCR, which stably bind the polymorphic grooves of self MHC, have been negatively selected against in the recipient thymus. However, no such selection happened for the recipient CDRs/donor MHC pairing. This interaction can be very strong by itself and can only be made worse by presentation of donor (exogenous) peptides in the MHC groove.

C. Stable binding of CD4 co-receptor molecules to nonself MHC class II alleles.

D. Stable binding of CD8 co-receptor molecules to nonself MHC class I alleles.

E. Stable binding of both CD4 co-receptor molecules to nonself MHC class II alleles and stable binding of CD8 co-receptor molecules to nonself MHC class I alleles.
Rationale: CD8 and CD4 molecules bind to nonpolymorphic domains of MHC class I/II and, therefore, the strength of these interactions is not dependent on the MHC allele. If this were the case, all T cells would be alloreactive in MHC-mismatched transplantation. The alloresponse in transplantation is oligoclonal.

Major points of discussion
- There are two modalities of allorecognition by T cells: the direct and indirect pathways.
- The direct allorecognition pathway is driven by the stable binding of some of the TCRs of the recipient's T-cell clones to the donor MHC. This interaction with self-MHC is screened out in the thymus, and no strongly self-reactive TCRs are allowed to exit into the periphery. The interaction with donor MHC was never screened for in the same manner.
- The indirect allorecognition pathway is the transplantation equivalent of T cells' immunity to any foreign antigen. Exogenous (donor) antigens are phagocytosed by (recipient) APCs and presented to (recipient) T cells in the context of self-MHC.
- The direct allorecognition is the dominant process in HLA-mismatched transplantation.
- The indirect recognition is evidenced by rejection in transplantation between HLA-matched siblings (not identical twins). In this scenario, the HLA molecules are identical and cannot generate direct allorecognition, but they can present polymorphic molecules by means of the indirect pathway.
- Siblings can inherit the same maternal and paternal chromosome 6 (or HLA region only) but be genetically different at any other locus due to the stochastic nature of chromosome segregation during gametogenesis.[13,14]

32. A. Cyclosporin A.
Rationale: Cyclosporin A binds to the cytosolic protein cyclophilin in lymphocytes. This complex inhibits calcineurin, which is responsible for activating the transcription of IL-2. It is not an antibody, and it does not interfere with antibody binding to cells. Therefore, it does affect FC crossmatch results.
B. Rituximab.
Rationale: Rituximab is an anti-CD20 antibody, which is a marker of mature B cells. Its immunosuppressive effect is mediated by the depletion of the B-cell lineage. Rituximab is a humanized antibody and can remain in circulation for months after therapy. Therefore, if present in the patient's serum, it can bind B cells in an FC crossmatch reaction and give false-positive results.
C. Prednisone.
Rationale: Prednisone is not an antibody and does not interfere with antibodies binding to cells. Therefore, it does affect FC crossmatch results.
D. Mycophenolate mofetil.
Rationale: Mycophenolate mofetil (MMF) is an inhibitor of inosine monophosphate dehydrogenase (IMPDH), which is needed for guanine synthesis during T-cell and B-cell proliferative reactions. It is not an antibody and does not

interfere with antibody binding to cells. Therefore, it does affect FC crossmatch results.

Major points of discussion
- CDC crossmatch detects cytolytic activity in mixtures of a transplant candidate's sera with a potential donor's T cells and B cells in the presence of complement.
- If the patient is presensitized and has antibodies against the donor's alloantigens (most commonly, HLAs) in circulation, the serum will opsonize and fix complement on the donor cells, killing them.
- A positive CDC crossmatch is a strong contraindication for transplantation. Presensitized transplant recipients who have a positive CDC crossmatch with their donors may hyperacutely reject their allograft.
- A T- and B-cell–positive crossmatch indicates the presence of anti-HLA class I antibodies (since HLA class I is ubiquitously expressed on human tissues and cells).
- A B-cell–positive crossmatch with a negative T-cell crossmatch indicates the presence of anti-HLA class II antibodies since HLA class II is expressed only on APCs such as B cells.
- Anti-thymocyte globulin and basiliximab are antibodies against T-cell antigens. Rituximab is a humanized anti-CD20 antibody (a B-cell lineage–specific marker). All of these antibodies can give false-positive T- or B-cell CDC crossmatch results.

33. A. *HLA-A* and *HLA-DP.*
B. *HLA-B* and *HLA-DR.*
C. *HLA-DR* and *HLA-DQ.*
D. *HLA-A* and *HLA-DR.*
Rationale: The recombination frequency between two genes is directly proportional to the genomic distance between them. HLA-A and -DP are the farthest apart in the HLA region, exhibiting the highest recombination frequency. The HLA-DR and HLA-DQ genes display the tightest linkage.

Major points of discussion
- The frequency of crossover between two loci is directly proportional to the distance between the two genes on the chromosomes.
- Recombination between HLA genes is relatively rare since all HLA genes are contained together on chromosome 6p21.31.
- The *HLA-DR* and *-DQ* genes are in linkage disequilibrium, such that the DQ typing could be predicted fairly reliably from the DR typing.

34. A. Drug toxicity.
Rationale: Although some drugs are nephrotoxic, they do not elicit specific T-cell responses. Recipients of organs from HLA-identical siblings are likely to require less immunosuppression.
B. Crossover event at the *HLA-DQ* locus.
Rationale: This is conceivable but very unlikely. Crossover events are rare, especially between *HLA-DR* and *HLA-DQ* loci, which are very tightly linked.
C. Age of the donated organ.
Rationale: Age disparity, which can affect the quality of a donated organ, should not be a significant factor in sibling

donation. Age of the allograft itself is not a factor in eliciting T-cell responses.

D. The direct recognition pathway.

Rationale: The siblings are HLA identical; there is no direct recognition of nonself HLA in this case.

E. The indirect recognition pathway.

Rationale: Although the recipient and donor are 8/8 HLA matched, they are not genetically identical. Polymorphic gene products, previously unencountered by recipient T cells, can be processed by recipient APCs and presented to autologous T cells, thus eliciting an immune reaction.

Major points of discussion

- The direct allorecognition is the dominant process in HLA-mismatched transplantation by which recipient T cells recognize the allograft.
- In cases of organ transplantation from HLA-identical siblings, direct allorecognition cannot occur, since the MHC molecules of the donor and recipient are identical.
- Nevertheless, rejection of allografts from HLA-identical siblings does occur due to indirect allorecognition.
- Indirect allorecognition is the process by which an allopeptide is presented in the context of self-MHC molecules and elicits the activation of cognate T-cell clones.
- Siblings can inherit the same maternal and paternal chromosome 6 (or HLA region only) haplotypes but still be genetically different at any other polymorphic locus due to the stochastic nature of chromosome segregation during gametogenesis.
- Importantly, indirect allorecognition can occur in HLA-identical siblings but not in monozygotic twins (who are 100% genetically identical).
- In HLA-mismatched transplantation, direct and indirect allorecognition can occur in parallel, and the peptides providing the basis of indirect allorecognition can be derived from the mismatched donor MHC molecules.[13,14]

35. A. It is much better than other solid organs because the lung is an immune-privileged site.

Rationale: The lung does exhibit some immune privilege and is to tolerate various inhaled harmless airborne antigens; however, this does not extend to tolerance of allografts.

B. It is much worse than other solid organs due to the inflammation elicited by airborne antigens.

Rationale: Lung allografts fare significantly worse in the long term than other solid organ transplants partly due to exposure to exogenous airborne antigens and pathogens, which can initiate inflammation and allograft rejection in a previously tolerant patient (Table 15-8).

C. It is about in line with other solid organs because rejection is histocompatibility driven, and other organ-specific factors play only minor roles.

Rationale: Although HLAs and other histocompatibility factors may provide the basis of rejection, other factors can initiate rejection and have a serious impact on long-term survival.

D. All lung allografts are lost within 5 years due to bronchiolitis obliterans syndrome (BOS).

Table 15-8 Graft Survival (%)

Time	Heart	Kidney	Liver	Lung	Intestine
1 Year	87.1	91.9	83.3	83.1	76.9
3 Years	78.5	82.4	73.6	62.2	52.2
5 Years	71.5	72.0	67.3	46.2	38.2

From Organ Procurement and Transplantation Network. U.S. Department of Health and Human Services. Available at http://optn.transplant.hrsa.gov/latestData/step2.asp/.

Rationale: BOS has a significant impact on lung allograft survival, although not all lung allografts are lost within 5 years due to BOS.

Major points of discussion

- Lung and small bowel allograft survival is significantly worse than that for other solid organs.
- Lung allograft survival is affected by the complexity of the surgical procedure, area of exposure to the external environment, and size-matching requirements.
- Infections represent a major morbidity factor in transplantation. Some, such as bacterial pneumonia, are particular to lung transplantation, whereas others are the result of chronic immunosuppression and are common to many types of transplantation (i.e., CMV infections). Cystic fibrosis, one of the major pathologies addressed by lung transplantation, is notorious for its association with persistent airway infections.
- BOS is a lung-specific fibroproliferative reaction in the small airway lumens, leading to allograft dysfunction. BOS is caused by alloimmune, autoimmune, and nonimmunologic factors and has a major impact on lung allograft survival.

36. A. *DR*03:01:01.*

Rationale: The HLA-DR antigen is made up of a *DR* α and a *DR* β chain. The *HLA-DR* β chain could be encoded by several genetic loci: *HLA-DRB1, -DRB3, -DRB4,* and *-DRB5*. It impossible to know which gene/locus is being described by *DR*03:01:01.*

B. *DRB1*030101.*

Rationale: This represents an older, discontinued naming system: The first two numbers show the allele family, the third and fourth are used to show the specific allele, and the fifth and sixth show silent variations where the DNA sequence is unique but the coded protein remains the same. This system broke down when the number of alleles per family exceeded 99. Names written this way will be found in older literature.

C. *DRB1*03:01:01.*

Rationale: This name shows the new nomenclature instituted in 2010. The first two numbers show the allele family, the third and fourth are used to show the specific allele, and the fifth and sixth show silent variations where the DNA sequence is unique but the coded protein remains the same. Colons are used as delineators to allow for naming alleles in families with more than 99 members.

D. *DRB103:01:01.*

Rationale: Since there are multiple *HLA-DR* β loci (and they all make use of numbers, i.e., *DRB1, DRB3, DRB4, DRB5*), an asterisk is now placed between the locus designation and the allele number to avoid confusion.

Major points of discussion

- The HLA genes have a complex nomenclature system due to their significant polymorphism.
- An example is *HLA-B*44:02:01:02S*.
- HLAs are a group of genetic loci on chromosome 6. The function of the proteins encoded by these genes is peptide presentation to T cells.
- *HLA-B*; the letter after HLA- indicates the specific locus. It could be *A, B, C, DRB1, DRB3, DRB5, DQA1, DQB1*, and so on.
- *HLA-B*44*, the first numbers after the locus and asterisk, indicate an allele group. This was historically serologically defined (i.e., an HLA allele group recognized by a certain anti-serum).
- *HLA-B*44:02*; the second set of numbers represents a unique protein in the allele group *HLA-B*44*.
- *HLA-B*44:02:01*; the third number represents silent genomic variants that encode the same protein *HLA-B*44:02* (e.g., *HLA-B*44:02:01* and *HLA-B*44:02:02* transcribe identical protein but are encoded by slightly different genes).
- *HLA-B*44:02:01:02S*; the last set of numbers indicates different gene variants with differences in the noncoding regions.
- The letter at the end of the allele name could indicate a secreted form of the molecule (S), a null or nonexpressed allele (N), or a low-expressed allele (L).

37. A. Preformed donor-specific antibodies and complement deposition.

Rationale: To destroy a transplanted organ within hours, preformed antibodies must be present at the time of transplantation. Mechanistically, they destroy the organ by fixation of complement. Cellular or humoral adaptive immune responses may take several days to develop and cannot destroy the allograft as quickly.
B. Preformed donor-specific antibodies and alloreactive T cells.
Rationale: Priming alloreactive T cells is too slow to account for the fast destruction of the graft seen in hyperacute rejection.
C. Preformed donor-specific antibodies, de novo antibody production against the graft, and complement deposition.
D. De novo antibody production against the graft and complement deposition.
Rationale: Although de novo antibodies can kill graft cells in a complement-dependant manner, this process simply does not happen fast enough to account for hyperacute rejection. De novo antibody production requires the recognition of the graft by B cells, subsequent activation and proliferation of B cells, somatic hypermutation of the B-cell receptor (BCR), receiving T-cell help, class switching recombination, formation of plasma cells, and, finally, the buildup of sufficient amounts of specific antibodies to harm the graft. This process may take days or weeks, not hours.

Major points of discussion

- Allograft rejection is driven by humoral and/or cellular immune responses of the recipient. Both humoral (B lymphocyte/antibody) and cellular (T lymphocyte) immune responses are adaptive and, therefore, take weeks to fully develop.

- Hyperacute rejection manifests within minutes after transplant due to preexisting humoral immunity.
- In contrast, acute rejection is caused by the immune recognition of the graft after transplantation and development of alloreactive T cells or de novo antibody production. Acute rejection can take weeks to months to develop and is to some extent clinically manageable, if detected early.
- Chronic rejection describes the loss of allograft function in the long term due to processes such as fibrosis and vasculopathy of the allograft.
- Preexisting antibodies to donor antigens can be easily screened for using PRAs, SPAs, and other methods.
- Most solid organs are allocated on the basis of a negative crossmatch, which ensures that hyperacute rejection will not occur.

38a. A. Beads coated with antigen(s).

Rationale: SPAs detect alloantibodies reactive with an individual or mixtures of HLA antigens fixed on a solid surface (beads).
B. Magnetic beads.
Rationale: Magnetic beads are sometimes used in biomedical applications for cell separations, not antibody detection.
C. FC.
Rationale: FC is similar to SPAs in many respects (i.e.; using fluoresceinated antibodies to detect antigens through a combination of fluidics and laser detection); however, unlike older methods, SPA techniques do not measure cells (technically not "cytometry").
D. Antihuman globulin (AHG)-augmented CDC crossmatch.
Rationale: This is not a SPA. To detect cytotoxicity, CDC crossmatching requires antigen-bearing live target cells, not antigen coated on a solid phase.

38b. A. Cells with poor viability binding antibodies nonspecifically.

Rationale: SPAs do not test cells.
B. Absence of the target allele on testing beads.
Rationale: It is virtually impossible and impractical to represent all HLA alleles on individual beads for SPA testing. Therefore, an antibody that does not cross-react with the antigens coated on beads may be missed (i.e., an anti-HLA-B*0711 not reacting with the other HLA-B7 antigens coated on SPA beads, say HLA-B*0701, -B*0702, or -B*0703).
C. Instrument sensitivity.
Rationale: SPA instruments are exquisitely sensitive. Sensitivity would likely affect the limit of detection, not specificity detection.
D. Assay interference by medications.
Rationale: SPA specificity detection is not affected by medications. This includes the newer class of drugs consisting of humanized anti-human cell surface markers, such as rituximab (anti-CD20) and other medications that can interfere with cellular assays.

Major points of discussion

- Prediction of humoral alloimmune responses in transplant recipients is the objective of histocompatibility testing and depends on accurate donor typing and sensitive and specific detection of alloantibodies. The overwhelming majority of alloantibodies are directed against highly polymorphic HLAs.

- Antibody-mediated damage has been documented in the absence of detectable antibodies in circulation by cytotoxic screening methods, suggesting the need for more sensitive assays.
- In SPAs, purified molecules (usually HLA proteins) are coated on solid-phase media. On incubation with patient sera, the solid phase will adsorb any antibodies specific for the antigens coated, which can be subsequently detected with secondary fluorochrome-labeled reagents.
- SPA methods are extremely sensitive, detecting much smaller antibody titers than previously possible by cytotoxicity methods. However, the drawbacks of SPAs include the inability to detect antigens not represented on the solid phase and to distinguish between complement fixing and nonfixing antibodies.
- CDC methods test recipient sera against live target cells. This method is a much more physiologically relevant measurement of the harmful potential of a patient's serum upon contact with allogeneic cells. However, it requires the presence of certain quantities and quality of antibodies for a positive determination.

39. A. Identification of complement fixing antibodies.
Rationale: Standard SPA technologies do not test complement fixation.
B. Prediction of a negative effect on graft survival.
Rationale: SPA identifies any IgG-isotype anti-HLA antibodies, some of which may not be harmful to the graft.
C. Identification of HLA specificities of antibodies.
Rationale: Single antigen beads are coated with individual HLA molecules. The specificities of the alloantibodies present in the serum can be determined by its reactivity with specific beads.
D. Prediction of acute cellular rejection (ACR) risk.
Rationale: SPA is a technique for the detection of antibodies and, therefore, useful for determining antibody-mediated rejection (AMR) risk.

Major points of discussion

- Traditionally, the method used for antibody detection was the CDC assay.
- In recent years, SPAs have been introduced as methods for HLA antibody screening. Luminex is an SPA that consists of a series of polystyrene microspheres (beads) that are fluorochrome labeled and coated with mixtures of or individual HLAs. On incubation with a patient serum, alloantibodies directed against the coated antigens are deposited on the beads and are detected with a secondary (laser-excitable) fluorochrome-conjugated reagent.
- The detection of antibody deposition on specific beads (coated with known HLAs) indicates the specificity of the antibodies present.
- The intensity of the emission spectrum (read as MFI) gives information about the quantity of antibody present in the serum tested.
- The MFI quantification can reveal antibodies that are present in very low amounts and that would not be able

to cause donor cell lysis in a CDC crossmatch or yield a positive reaction in FC crossmatching.
- SPA does not yield any qualitative information about the antibodies detected (most importantly, the complement fixing ability).

40. A. The anti–*HLA-B27* is an IgM antibody, and transplantation with the child's kidney is an acceptable option.
Rationale: The anti–*HLA-B27* cannot be an IgM because the crossmatch reaction is positive even in the presence of DTT, which denatures IgM antibodies.
B. The anti–*HLA-B35* is an IgG1 or IgG3 antibody, and transplantation with the sibling's kidney is *not* acceptable.
Rationale: Both IgG1 and IgG3 are IgG isotypes that avidly fix complement; therefore, *HLA-B35* specificity would have been picked up by the PRA assay or CDC crossmatch (CDC crossmatch) tests (but was not).
C. The anti–*HLA-B27* is an IgG antibody and transplantation with the child's kidney is an acceptable option.
Rationale: The anti–*HLA-B27* is indeed an IgG antibody and it gives a positive CDC crossmatch; therefore, transplantation is *not* recommended.
D. The anti–*HLA-B35* is an IgG2 or IgG4 antibody, and transplantation with the sibling's kidney is an acceptable option.
Rationale: The anti–*HLA-B35* must be an IgG isotype (SPA detected) with low complement fixing ability (CDC crossmatch and PRA negative). The ability of human IgG subtypes to fix complement can be summarized by IgG3 > IgG1 > IgG2 > IgG4 = 0. Transplantation with the sibling's kidney is acceptable on the basis of a negative crossmatch.

Major points of discussion

- Alloantibodies are often, but not always, problematic in transplantation.
- Antibody testing methodologies have various advantages and disadvantages and should be used in combination to obtain the most complete picture of a patient's sensitization status.
- Advantages of CDC methods include the following:
  - Detection of the most harmful type of antibodies—namely, the ones that fix complement.
  - Detection of IgM and IgG isotypes' positive reactions in the absence or presence of DTT, respectively.
  - Differentiation between anti-HLA class I and class II antibodies (positive reactions with T and B cells or B cells only).
  - Ability to detect antibodies against non-HLAs.
  - The HLA specificity of antibodies can be resolved in patients who are not broadly presensitized.
- Disadvantages on CDC methods include the following:
  - Low sensitivity.
  - Possibility of yielding false-positive reactions in patients treated with monoclonal antibody therapies.
- Advantages of SPA testing methods include the following:
  - Excellent sensitivity.
  - Ability to identify the specificity of anti-HLA antibodies.
  - The HLA specificity of antibodies can be resolved by use of single antigen beads.

- Disadvantages of SPA testing methods include the following:
  - High sensitivity (i.e., low titer antibodies often do not yield a positive crossmatch and represent little danger to an allograft).
  - Inability to detect antibodies against any antigen not represented on the solid phase.
  - Inability to differentiate between complement fixing and nonfixing antibodies.
  - In most implementations of SPA testing, only IgG is detected.
  - Antibody detection may be flawed because the HLA alleles represented on the beads may be different than the one(s) expressed by the donor.
- When gauging the acceptability of alloantibodies in transplantation, the complement fixing ability should be considered; The ability of human IgG subtypes to fix complement can be summarized by IgG3 > IgG1 > IgG2 > IgG4 = 0.
- Antibodies that do not fix complement can act as blocking antibodies, masking the target antigens from recognition by T cells, B cells, and other complement fixing antibodies.

41. A. The WBC karyotyping is wrong due to interference by anti-donor (ABO) antibodies.
Rationale: ABO antigens are not present on WBCs and would be unlikely to affect the detection of the Y chromosome.
B. The ABO typing was performed on a different patient's sample.
Rationale: This is unlikely.
C. The ABO results were obtained by back typing and front typing should be performed.
Rationale: In back typing, the patient serum is mixed with type A and type B red cells. If the patient serum continues to contain anti-A and -B antibodies, the patient would appear to be blood type O. In reality, her red blood cells are probably of donor origin (AB), although the results of the forward typing are not listed.
D. Both results are correct; donor bone marrow produces WBCs, whereas recipient bone marrow produces red blood cells.
Rationale: Such segregation of lineages by bone marrow origin is unlikely.

Major points of discussion

- ABO incompatibility is of paramount importance in solid organ transplantation, possibly leading to hyperacute/acute graft loss. In stem cell transplantation, ABO incompatibility leads to poorer engraftment, but it is not immediately life threatening.
- The H antigen (which gives the ABO type) is a carbohydrate entity on the surface of red blood cells.
- ABO typing can be performed by front typing in which the patient's red blood cells are tested for reactivity with anti-sera of known (anti-A or anti-B) specificity.
- Alternatively, ABO typing is done by back typing in which patient serum is incubated with cells of known typing (group A or group B cells). A patient should have detectable antibodies to the antigens he or she does *not* possess.
- The difference between the two typing methodologies is that one actually tests the patient's cells, whereas the

other infers it from the antibody content of the patient's serum. Both tests are done in conjunction to ensure correct blood typing.

- After a successful ABO-incompatible stem cell transplant, circulating red cells are expected to be of donor origin, but the patient's anti-A/B antibodies may be detectable for months. The presence of such anti-A/B antibodies can adversely affect engraftment.

42. A. A positive crossmatch.
Rationale: By definition, de novo antibodies occur after transplantation; therefore, they cannot affect the crossmatch, which occurs before or concurrent with the transplant.
B. Recurrence of the original disease.
Rationale: The recurrence of the original disease (autoimmunity, viral hepatitis, and so on), which led to the failure of an organ, can adversely impact an allograft; however, formation of de novo anti-HLA antibodies is a largely independent process.
C. Hyperacute rejection episodes.
Rationale: Hyperacute rejection occurs shortly after transplantation due to preformed (not de novo) anti-donor antibodies.
D. Chronic rejection.
Rationale: Alloantibodies are a major contributing factor to chronic rejection. Some data suggest that anti-HLA class I antibodies trigger survival and proliferation signaling in endothelial cells, which leads over time to the occlusion of the blood vessels.

Major points of discussion

- De novo alloantibody development can lead to acute and chronic rejection and is a major cause of allograft attrition.
- Alloantibodies can attack the allograft directly by activating the complement cascade.
- In addition, alloantibodies can also trigger coagulation, production of fibrinogenic factors, and cell proliferation.
- Recent studies have shown that anti-HLA antibodies can activate the PI3K/Akt pathway and promote cell survival by means of Bcl-2 and Bcl-xL induction in endothelial cells. Thus, anti-HLA class I antibodies may contribute to the process of chronic allograft rejection by promoting endothelial cell survival and proliferation.
- Although HLA class I molecules themselves cannot signal this activation, it is hypothesized to be relayed through an HLA-associated chain.[10]

43. A. Anti-CD20 humanized monoclonal antibody eliminates plasma cells more effectively than circulating B cells.
Rationale: Nearly all B cells express CD20. Plasma cells do not express CD20 and are not depleted by anti-CD20 antibodies. Treatment with anti-CD20 depleting antibodies depletes B cells, which is more effective than elimination of existing plasma cells at preempting a humoral rejection.
B. Anti-CD25 monoclonal antibody therapy can reduce alloreactive B-cell responses.
Rationale: CD25 is a marker highly expressed by activated T cells (and regulatory cells) and to a much lesser extent on some B cells.
C. Administration of IVIg can increase the titer of alloreactive antibodies.

Rationale: IVIg administration can enhance clearance of IgG antibodies by overloading the receptor responsible for the long serologic half-life of IgG immunoglobulins—namely, the FcRn receptor expressed by endothelial cells.
D. Bortezomib is a proteosome inhibitor that induces apoptosis by accumulation of large amounts of protein.
Rationale: Bortezomib's main mechanism of action is thought to be as an inducer of plasma cell death by accumulation of misfolded immunoglobulins.

Major points of discussion

■ AMR presents some unique challenges in transplantation. Whereas in ACR episodes the main effectors are immune cells, which can be targeted for deletion with antibodies (e.g., antithymocyte globulin, basiliximab), antibodies are much more difficult to eliminate.

■ Anti-B cell humanized antibodies (e.g., rituximab) are somewhat effective at preventing a humoral response (by deleting the potentially alloreactive B cells). However, it is ineffective against an already formed humoral response because plasma cells downregulate their expression of CD20.

■ Plasmapheresis removes some of the alloantibodies in the circulation; however, it alone cannot block the continued secretion of alloantibodies from existing plasma cells. It is therefore usually administered together with IVIG.

■ The precise mechanism of action of IVIG is not fully understood, but it is postulated that it may affect the antibody homeostatic balance by acting on inhibitory Fc receptors downregulating antibody production. The formation of immune complexes and the introduction of anti-idiotypic antibodies may also be involved.

■ Bortezomib represents a new approach to inhibition of the humoral response by inhibiting the proteosome. It relies on the fact that cells, which produce large amounts of proteins, operate close to their apoptotic threshold due to the accumulation of large amounts of misfolded proteins. Proteosome inhibitors can push plasma cells beyond the apoptosis threshold by increasing the accumulation of misfolded proteins.

44. A. Anti-HLA antibodies alone.
Rationale: The presence of anti-HLA antibodies is not sufficient to diagnose antibody-mediated rejection. Many patients are presensitized and receive transplants despite anti-HLA antibodies that are either non–donor-specific or donor-specific but of insufficient titer or quality to harm the graft.
B. Circulating donor-specific antibodies, Cd4 deposition in the graft, and graft dysfunction.
Rationale: A combination of all three of these findings is the most conclusive indication of antibody-mediated rejection. They document the presence of antibodies (circulating donor-specific antibodies), their action in the graft (complement fixation by C4d), and their deleterious effect (impaired function).
C. Donor-specific antibodies, C4d deposition in the graft, and ejection fraction less than 40%.
Rationale: Ejection fraction is a common means of measuring heart allograft function but does not apply to solid organs in general.
D. Biopsy IgG immunofluorescence, C4b deposition in the graft, and graft dysfunction.
Rationale: IgG immunofluorescence is an older method of detecting Ig deposition in the graft. C4d deposition, not C4b, is a newer, commonly practiced methodology that is a sensitive marker for the presence of humoral rejection.

Major points of discussion

■ There is no universally accepted definition of AMR.
■ However, most clinicians and investigators currently accept that three components are crucial in the diagnosis of AMR.
■ First, graft dysfunction is indicative of rejection of an allograft. It can be a measurement of the ejection fraction for a heart allograft or creatinine levels compared with an established baseline for a renal allograft.
■ Second, deposition of C4d or Ig on the graft tissues and graft damage (by biopsy) is indicative of AMR.
■ Finally, the presence of donor-specific antibodies in the circulation can be indicative of AMR.
■ Importantly, not all three criteria are always observed together. AMR can be often asymptomatic, C4d deposition can be missed due to "sampling error," and donor-specific antibodies can disappear from circulation by being absorbed onto the graft.[11,18]

References

1. Book BK, Agarwal A, Milgrom AB, et al: New crossmatch technique eliminates interference by humanized and chimeric monoclonal antibodies. Transplant Proc 2005;37:640–642.
2. Bray RA, Hurley CK, Kamani NR, et al: National marrow donor program HLA matching guidelines for unrelated adult donor hematopoietic cell transplants. Biol Blood Marrow Transplant 2008;14(9 Suppl):45–53.
3. Caillat-Zucman S. Molecular mechanisms of HLA association with autoimmune diseases. Tissue Antigens 2009;73:1–8.
4. Cecka JM. Current methodologies for detecting sensitization to HLA antigens. Curr Opin Organ Transplant 2011;16:398–403.
5. Desombere I, Willems A, Leroux-Roels G. Response to hepatitis B vaccine: multiple HLA genes are involved. Tissue Antigens 1998;51:593–604.
6. Dharnidharka VR, Tejani AH, Ho PL, et al: Post-transplant lymphoproliferative disorder in the United States: young Caucasian males are at highest risk. Am J Transplant 2002;2:993–998.
7. Geetha D, Eirin A, True K, et al: Renal transplantation in antineutrophil cytoplasmic antibody-associated vasculitis: a multicenter experience. Transplantation 2011;91:1370–1375.
8. Heath WR, Carbone FR. Cross-presentation in viral immunity and self-tolerance. Nat Rev Immunol 2001;1:126–134.
9. Holdsworth R, Hurley CK, Marsh SGE, et al: The HLA dictionary 2008: a summary of HLA-A, -B, -C, -DRB1/3/4/5, and -DQB1 alleles and their association with serologically defined HLA-A, -B, -C, -DR, and -DQ antigens. Tissue Antigens 2009;72:95–170.
10. Jin YP, Jindra PT, Gong KW, et al: Anti-HLA class I antibodies activate endothelial cells and promote chronic rejection. Transplantation 2005;79:S19–S21.

11. Kobashigawa J, Crespo-Leiro MG, Ensminger SM, et al: Consensus Conference Participants. Report from a consensus conference on antibody-mediated rejection in heart transplantation. J Heart Lung Transplant 2011;30:252–269.

12. Liu Z, Colovai AI, Tugulea S, et al: Indirect recognition of donor HLA-DR peptides in organ allograft rejection. J Clin Invest 1996;98:1150–1157.

13. Liu Z, Sun YK, Xi YP, et al: Contribution of direct and indirect recognition pathways to T cell alloreactivity. J Exp Med 1993;177:1643–1650.

14. Nourse JP, Jones K, Gandhi MK. Epstein-Barr virus-related post-transplant lymphoproliferative disorders: pathogenetic insights for targeted therapy. Am J Transplant 2011;11: 888–895.

15. Nunes E, Heslop H, Fernandez-Vina M, et al: Definitions of histocompatibility typing terms. Blood 2011;118:180–183.

16. Peyron C, Faraco J, Rogers W, et al: A mutation in a case of early onset narcolepsy and a generalized absence of hypocretin peptides in human narcoleptic brains. Nat Med 2000;6:991–997.

17. Racusen LC, Solez K, Colvin RB, et al: The Banff 97 working classification of renal allograft pathology. Kidney Int 1999;55:713–723.

18. Solez K, Axelsen RA, Benediktsson H, et al: International standardization of criteria for the histologic diagnosis of renal allograft rejection: The Banff working classification of kidney transplant pathology. Kidney Int 1993;44:411–422.

19. Tait BD. The ever-expanding list of HLA alleles: changing HLA nomenclature and its relevance to clinical transplantation. Transplant Rev (Orlando) 2011;25:1–8.

20. Tait BD. Solid phase assays for HLA antibody detection in clinical transplantation. Curr Opin Immunol 2009;21:573–577.

21. Vlad G, Ho EK, Vasilescu ER, et al: Relevance of different antibody detection methods for the prediction of antibody-mediated rejection and deceased-donor kidney allograft survival. Hum Immunol 2009;70:589–594.

22. Lee SJ, Klein J, Haagenson M, et al: High-resolution donor-recipient HLA matching contributes to the success of unrelated donor marrow transplantation. Blood 2007;110:4576–4583.

CHAPTER 16

MICROBIOLOGY: Bacteriology, Mycobacteriology, Mycology

Phyllis Della-Latta, Richard C. Huard, Susan Whittier, Fann Wu

QUESTIONS

Bacteriology

1. Which one of the following statements best defines the minimum inhibitory concentration (MIC) of a bacterial pathogen to an antimicrobial agent?
   A. The MIC is the lowest drug level that can reach all sites of infection.
   B. The MIC is the amount of drug that can be administered in a single dose.
   C. The MIC is the lowest drug level that is bacteriostatic.
   D. The MIC is the lowest drug level that is nontoxic.
   E. The MIC is the lowest drug level that kills the bacterial pathogen.

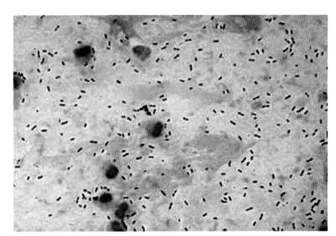

Figure 16-1 Photomicrograph showing gram-positive organisms along with neutrophils.

2. A 70-year-old man presents to his physician with a 2-day history of fever, malaise, chest pain, and a productive cough. No upper respiratory symptoms were noted. Laboratory testing shows an elevated peripheral blood leukocyte count and a chest radiograph shows lobar consolidation. The Gram stain of a sputum specimen sent for bacterial culture is shown in Figure 16-1. Which one of the following is the etiologic agent?
   A. *Moraxella catarrhalis.*
   B. *Legionella pneumophila.*
   C. *Mycoplasma pneumonia.*
   D. *Streptococcus pneumonia.*
   E. *Staphylococcus aureus.*

3. Gram-negative bacilli causing infections in health care settings often produce extended-spectrum β-lactamases (ESBLs). Which one type of the following antimicrobial agents is most appropriate for treating ESBL-producing pathogens?
   A. Carbapenems.
   B. Third-generation cephalosporins.
   C. First-generation cephalosporins.
   D. Second-generation cephalosporins.
   E. Aztreonam.

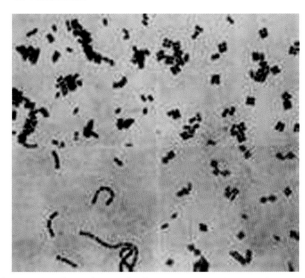

Figure 16-2 Photomicrographs showing gram-positive organisms.

4. A blood culture set was drawn from an adult patient with a fever of 101°F. The following day, the laboratory reported the presence of gram-positive cocci in the arrangement depicted in the Figure 16-2. What is the presumptive identification of this morphotype?
   A. *Staphylococcus aureus.*
   B. Coagulase-negative staphylococci.
   C. *Streptococcus pneumoniae.*
   D. Staphylococci.
   E. Enterococci.

5. A 70-year-old woman presents to her urologist with a urinary tract infection. Culture results indicate that the infecting pathogen is *Escherichia coli,* which has an MIC interpreted as

"intermediate" for the antimicrobial agent of choice. Which one of the following statements best describes this MIC interpretation for this antibiotic?

A. The patient is likely to not respond to treatment with this antibiotic.

B. This antibiotic may be efficacious either at higher doses or if concentrated in the urine.

C. Antibiotics with intermediate interpretations cannot be dosed at therapeutic levels.

D. An intermediate result indicates a technical error and must be repeated using the disk diffusion susceptibility method.

E. The intermediate category is interpreted as nonsusceptible.

6. The incidence and prevalence of etiologic agents causing sexually transmitted infections are underestimated due to diagnostic challenges and social stigma. Which one of the following statements regarding sexually transmitted infections is most accurate?

A. HIV acquisition is highest in the presence of sexually transmitted infections that cause discharge.

B. Nucleic acid amplification tests (NAATs) are the most sensitive and accurate method for detecting *Neisseria gonorrhea* and *Chlamydia trachomatis* infections.

C. Dark-field microscopic examination is used to diagnose herpes simplex ulcerative genital lesions.

D. *Haemophilus ducreyi* is the causative agent of lymphogranuloma venereum.

E. Syphilis is currently on the rise in the adolescent population in urban settings.

7. A 24-year-old immunocompetent farm worker who was 27 weeks pregnant presented with a fever of 102°F, headache, a 1-day history of diarrhea, and decreased fetal movements. Labor was induced and a stillborn infant was delivered vaginally. The Gram stain from a positive blood culture and colonial morphology on blood agar provided a presumptive identification (Figure 16-3). Which one of the following bacterial pathogens is the most likely cause of sepsis in this patient?

A. *Streptococcus agalactiae* (group B streptococci [GBS]).

B. *Chlamydia trachomatis.*

C. *Listeria monocytogenes.*

D. *Neisseria gonorrhoeae.*

E. *Campylobacter jejuni.*

8. A febrile 4-year-old child was admitted to the pediatric intensive care unit with a petechial rash and lethargy. A lumbar puncture revealed an elevated protein level of 200 mg/dL, a decreased glucose level of 30 mg/dL, and a predominance of neutrophils. A Gram stain of the cerebrospinal fluid revealed the pathogen shown in Figure 16-4. Which one of the following etiologic agents is the cause of the child's meningitis?

A. *Moraxella catarrhalis.*

B. *Haemophilus influenza.*

C. *Streptococcus pneumonia.*

D. *Neisseria meningitidis.*

E. *Listeria monocytogenes.*

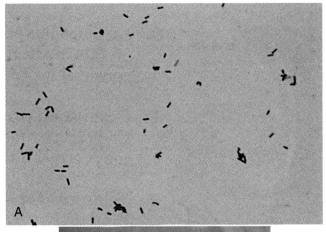

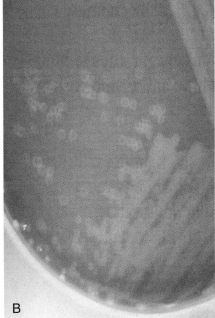

Figure 16-3 **A,** Photomicrograph of the Gram stain of the organism isolated from the blood of this patient. **B,** Colonial morphology and the type of hemolysis elicited by its growth.

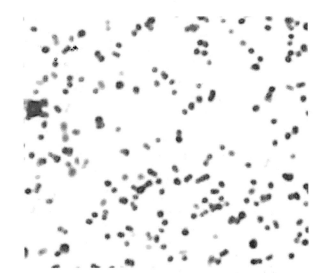

Figure 16-4 Photomicrograph illustrating Gram stain and the cellular morphology of a pathogen present in cerebrospinal fluid.

9. An 11-year-old patient presented to the emergency department with fever and axillary lymphadenopathy. Erythematous papules are noted on the right hand and forearm. A Gram stain and a Kinyoun acid-fast stain of a lymph node biopsy were both negative, as were cultures of the biopsy and blood cultures that were incubated for 5 days. The family has a 2-month-old kitten that they recently adopted from a shelter. The diagnosis was made using a serologic assay. Which one of the following is the most likely cause of the disease in this patient?
   A. *Streptobacillus moniliformis.*
   B. *Borrelia burgdorferi.*
   C. *Coxiella burnetii.*
   D. *Bartonella henselae.*
   E. *Mycobacterium haemophilum.*

10. A 5-year-old child presented to her pediatrician with bloody diarrhea of 2 days' duration accompanied by abdominal cramps and dehydration. She was afebrile. She had become symptomatic 4 days after consuming potato salad, a hamburger, and milk. Examination of growth of the stool specimen on sorbitol-MacConkey agar plates coupled with a positive enzyme immunoassay (EIA) stool test provided the diagnosis. Which one of the following is the most likely pathogen in this case?
   A. *Shigella sonnei.*
   B. Shiga toxin-producing *Escherichia coli.*
   C. *Salmonella enterica.*
   D. *Yersinia enterocolitica.*
   E. *Campylobacter jejuni.*

11. A 70-year-old woman presented to the emergency department with a fever of 102°C, a cough, and night sweats. She frequently visits Lebanon, where her family resides. Slow-growing, small coccobacillary rods were isolated from blood cultures after 48 hours on chocolate and sheep blood agar; no growth was observed on MacConkey plates. The pathogen was oxidase and urease positive and was identified by a rise in serologic titers. Which one of the following is the most likely etiologic agent?
   A. *Francisella tularensis.*
   B. *Mycobacterium tuberculosis.*
   C. *Brucella melitensis.*
   D. *Bordetella bronchiseptica.*
   E. *Haemophilus influenza.*

12. A 14-year-old male sustained a traumatic injury to his foot from a jagged seashell while at the beach. The next day he presented to the emergency department with a high fever and erythema, with diffuse swelling and purulent drainage from the foot and ankle. The Gram stain from drainage revealed the presence of curved gram-negative bacilli. Which one of the following is the most likely pathogen?
   A. *Pseudomonas aeruginosa.*
   B. *Haemophilus influenza.*
   C. *Vibrio vulnificus.*
   D. *Campylobacter jejuni.*
   E. *Pasteurella multocida.*

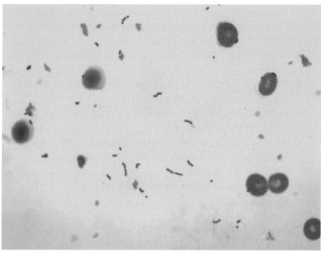

Figure 16-5 Photomicrographs showing gram-positive organisms. Several red blood cells from the blood culture bottle are also seen (×1000).

13. A full-term neonate developed a fever of 103°C at 3 days of age. The infant was irritable and not feeding well. Blood cultures were positive for the organism shown in Figure 16-5. Beta-hemolytic colonies were observed on sheep blood agar. A latex agglutination test confirmed the identity of the pathogen. Which one of the following is the mostly likely etiologic agent of this infant's bacteremia?
   A. *Enterococcus faecalis.*
   B. *Streptococcus pneumonia.*
   C. *Streptococcus agalactiae.*
   D. *Staphylococcus aureus.*
   E. *Staphylococcus epidermidis.*

14. Which one of the following Gram stain components acts as a counterstain?
   A. Safranin.
   B. Iodine.
   C. Crystal violet.
   D. Acetone alcohol.
   E. Methylene blue.

15. Which one of the following bacteriologic media is considered both differential and selective?
   A. 5% sheep blood agar.
   B. Chocolate agar.
   C. MacConkey agar.
   D. Brucella agar.
   E. Mueller Hinton agar.

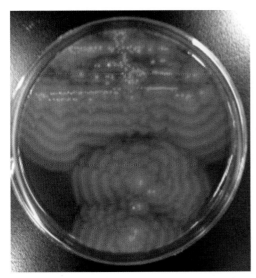

Figure 16-6 Colonial morphology of the pathogen. The results of this urine culture demonstrate waves of bacterial growth on a 5% sheep blood agar plate.

16. While in the medical intensive care unit, an 80-year-old man developed a catheter-related urinary tract infection. Urine was sent for culture and, after 24 hours of incubation, the organism shown in Figure 16-6 was observed. Rapid indole test results were negative. Which one of the following is the most likely etiologic agent of this patient's infection?
    A. *Escherichia coli.*
    B. *Proteus mirabilis.*
    C. *Pseudomonas aeruginosa.*
    D. *Proteus vulgaris.*
    E. *Serratia liquefaciens.*

17. An 80-year-old woman was admitted from a long-term care facility for worsening diarrhea. She had received antibiotics the previous week for a urinary tract infection. Endoscopy revealed the presence of pseudomembranous colitis. Which one of the following is the best treatment regimen to initiate?
    A. Dexamethasone.
    B. Clindamycin.
    C. Levofloxacin.
    D. Fluconazole.
    E. Vancomycin.

18. A 6-week-old infant presented to the pediatrician with a 7-day history of symptoms of a mild cold that progressed to paroxysms of coughing, gasping for breath, and vomiting. Upon admission to the hospital, a chest radiograph was taken and found to be normal. Nasopharyngeal swabs were diagnostic for the illness. Which one of the following is the most likely pathogen?
    A. *Staphylococcus aureus.*
    B. Group A streptococci (GAS).
    C. *Streptococcus pneumoniae.*
    D. *Bordetella pertussis.*
    E. *Moraxella catarrhalis.*

19. A 12-year-old child presented the emergency department with facial edema, a 3-day history of dark-colored urine, and a sore throat of 10 days' duration. Laboratory results showed hematuria and proteinuria. Urine and blood cultures were negative, and a throat culture grew β-hemolytic gram-positive cocci in chains. The presumptive diagnosis was acute glomerulonephritis. Which one of the following is the most likely etiologic agent of this disease?
    A. *Streptococcus pyogenes* (GAS).
    B. *Streptococcus agalactiae* (GBS).
    C. *Enterococcus faecium.*
    D. *Streptococcus pneumoniae.*
    E. *Streptococcus mutans.*

20. A patient presented to the emergency department with shortness of breath and fever. A chest radiograph revealed a left lower lobe infiltrate and right pleural effusion. His family indicated that he became symptomatic several days after visiting a petting zoo. Both blood cultures and pleural fluid grew oxidase-negative, small gram-negative coccobacilli on sheep blood agar, but there was no growth on MacConkey agar. Which one of the following is the most likely cause of the infection?
    A. *Pasteurella multocida.*
    B. *Capnocytophaga canimorsus.*
    C. *Burkholderia pseudomallei.*
    D. *Yersinia pestis.*
    E. *Francisella tularensis.*

21. A 7-month-old infant presented to the emergency department after 1 day of bloody diarrhea and fever. He was transferred to the pediatric intensive care unit in septic shock. Onset of symptoms occurred shortly after the family's purchase of an iguana. Stool and blood cultures yielded gram-negative bacilli that appeared as red colonies with a black center on xylose-lysine-deoxycholate and colorless colonies on MacConkey media. Which one of the following is the most likely etiologic agent causing this infection?
    A. *Shigella* spp.
    B. *Salmonella* spp.
    C. *Campylobacter jejuni.*
    D. *E. coli* O157:H7.
    E. *Yersinia enterocolitica.*

22. Gram-positive cocci in clusters were isolated from a breast abscess of a 30-year-old diabetic woman. The bacteria were slide-coagulase positive and tube coagulase negative. Both the pyrrolidonyl arylamidase (PYR) and ornithine decarboxylase tests were positive. Which one of the following is the most likely pathogen?
    A. *Staphylococcus aureus.*
    B. *Staphylococcus lugdunensis.*
    C. *Staphylococcus epidermidis.*
    D. *Staphylococcus schleiferi.*
    E. *Staphylococcus haemolyticus.*

23. Small, gram-negative coccobacilli grew from a blood culture collected from a patient with ventilator-associated pneumonia. The isolate was oxidase negative and nonmotile, produced colorless colonies on MacConkey agar, and was multi-drug resistant. Which one of the following is the most likely pathogen identified by this workup?
    A. *Escherichia coli.*
    B. *Klebsiella pneumoniae.*

C. *Acinetobacter baumannii.*
D. *Stenotrophomonas maltophilia.*
E. *Pseudomonas aeruginosa.*

24. Which one of the following methods is most commonly used in molecular epidemiology to generate strain-specific molecular fingerprints to determine microbial strain relatedness in a hospital setting?
   A. 16S rRNA gene sequencing.
   B. Staphylococcal cassette chromosome *mec* (SCC*mec*).
   C. Peptide nucleic acid fluorescent in situ hybridization.
   D. Pulsed-field gel electrophoresis (PFGE).
   E. Matrix-assisted laser desorption/ionization time of flight (MALDI-TOF) mass spectrometry.

25. A patient presented to the adolescent clinic with symptoms of dysuria and a purulent vaginal discharge. She gave a history of being sexually active with one partner over the past 2 months. A urine specimen tested positive for *Neisseria gonorrhoeae.* Which one of the following diagnostic tests is best for rapid detection of the etiologic agent?
   A. EIA.
   B. Gene sequencing.
   C. Cell culture.
   D. NAAT.
   E. Gram stain.

26. A 30-year-old woman with a prior history of recurrent episodes of cystitis presented to her private practitioner with urinary urgency and dysuria. A urinalysis and culture were ordered, and results were positive for leukocyte esterase, nitrite, and growth of more than 10^4 colony forming units (CFU)/mL of lactose-fermenting, oxidase-negative, indole-positive, gram-negative bacilli. Which one of the following is the most likely pathogen?
   A. *Klebsiella pneumoniae.*
   B. *Proteus mirabilis.*
   C. *Acinetobacter baumannii.*
   D. *Pseudomonas aeruginosa.*
   E. *Escherichia coli.*

27. A 23-year-old woman in her second trimester of pregnancy presented to her obstetrician with symptoms of malodorous vaginal discharge. Specimens were sent to the microbiology laboratory, where a Gram stain detected the cause of her bacterial infection. Which one of the following is the most likely cause of this infection?
   A. Bacterial vaginosis.
   B. *Chlamydia trachomatis.*
   C. *Trichomonas.*
   D. *Neisseria gonorrhoeae.*
   E. *Candida albicans.*

28. The foul-smelling purulent drainage from the surgical wound of a patient with a ruptured appendix was sent for culture. The Gram stain showed gram-negative bacilli, and the culture grew *Bacteroides fragilis, Citrobacter freundii, Klebsiella pneumoniae, Pseudomonas aeruginosa,* and *Escherichia coli.* Which one of the following anaerobic pathogens is the most likely cause of this infection?
   A. *Bacteroides fragilis.*
   B. *Enterobacter aerogenes.*

C. *Veillonella parvula.*
D. *Pseudomonas aeruginosa.*
E. *Escherichia coli.*

29. A 17-year-old patient with cystic fibrosis presented to her pulmonologist with increased respiratory secretions and difficulty breathing. A sputum specimen was sent for culture. Four days later a presumptive identification was obtained for a slow-growing, short, gram-negative nonlactose fermenter that was weakly oxidase positive. Which one of the following is the most likely etiologic agent?
   A. *Pseudomonas aeruginosa.*
   B. *Klebsiella pneumonia.*
   C. *Burkholderia cepacia* complex.
   D. *Acinetobacter lwoffii.*
   E. *Stenotrophomonas maltophilia.*

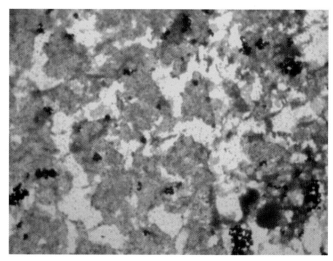

Figure 16-7 Photomicrograph showing gram-positive organisms isolated from the patient's blood.

30. As part of a rule-out sepsis workup, two sets of blood cultures were collected from a patient in the intensive care unit after a fever spike. Twelve hours later, another two sets were collected. All four blood culture sets were flagged as positive by the semiautomated blood culture system within 24 hours. The Gram stain was identical for all bottles and is shown in Figure 16-7. Which one of the following is the most likely etiologic agent of this patient's sepsis?
   A. *Bacillus* species.
   B. *Streptococcus pneumoniae.*
   C. *Clostridium* species.
   D. *Corynebacterium* species.
   E. *Enterococcus* species.

31. Rapid phenotypic tests are often used in the microbiology laboratory as an aid in the identification algorithm. Which one of the following phenotypic tests can differentiate enterococci from staphylococci?
   A. Indole production.
   B. The PYR reaction.
   C. The oxidase reaction.
   D. The catalase reaction.
   E. The hippurate reaction.

32. A positive blood culture obtained from a septic patient in the intensive care unit was reported as *Escherichia coli* resistant to piperacillin, ceftazidime, and aztreonam but susceptible to imipenem and cefoxitin. Which one of the following mechanisms of resistance does this pathogen exhibit?
A. CTX-M β-lactamase.
B. Metallo-β-lactamase.
C. Carbapenemase.
D. AmpC β-lactamase.
E. ESBL.

33. A 58-year-old man presented to the emergency department with fever and shortness of breath. A chest radiograph was consistent with pneumonia. A rapid urine antigen test revealed the likely causative agent, and he was discharged with a 2-week course of levofloxacin. Routine bacteriology cultures failed to recover the pathogen. Which one of the following is the most likely cause of his pneumonia?
A. *Legionella pneumophila.*
B. *Staphylococcus aureus.*
C. *Haemophilus influenza.*
D. *Mycobacterium tuberculosis.*
E. Influenza A.

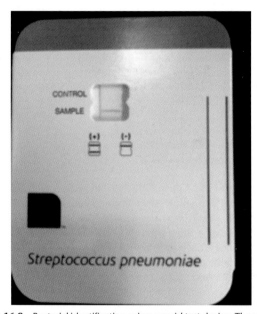

Figure 16-8 Bacterial identification using a rapid test device. The results of a urine specimen from a patient with community-acquired pneumonia are shown.

34. A rapid immunochromatographic assay was performed on a urine specimen collected from a patient suspected of having community-acquired pneumonia. Which one of the following statements best explains the results demonstrated in Figure 16-8?
A. The patient result is invalid because urine was tested instead of a respiratory secretion.
B. Patient results can be reported because this rapid device has a very high specificity.
C. Patient results can be reported because this rapid device has a very high sensitivity.
D. The result should be reported as negative because the control line is not present.

E. The patient result is invalid because the control line is not present.

35. An 88-year-old woman presented to the emergency department with signs and symptoms of pneumonia. She had shortness of breath, tachycardia, and a fever of 102°F. Sputum was obtained and sent for bacterial culture. Gram stain demonstrated many polymorphonuclear leukocytes and small, faintly staining gram-negative coccobacilli. After 24 hours, only the chocolate agar plate demonstrated growth. Which one of the following tests is most useful for identifying this pathogen?
A. Optochin susceptibility.
B. PYR reaction.
C. Bacitracin susceptibility.
D. X and V factor growth requirements.
E. Bile solubility.

36. An 18-year-old college student presented to her campus health clinic with complaints of sore throat, lymphadenopathy, and low-grade fever. A rapid "strep test" was negative. The student was not prescribed antibiotics based on a presumptive diagnosis of a virus infection. Due to persistent symptoms, a bacterial throat culture was obtained. Twenty-four hours later the pathogen was identified. Which one of the following is the most likely cause of her pharyngitis?
A. *Streptococcus* viridans group.
B. *Haemophilus influenza.*
C. *Streptococcus dysgalactiae* subspecies *equisimilis.*
D. *Streptococcus pneumonia.*
E. GBS.

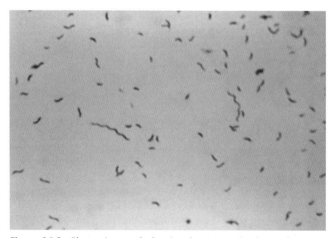

Figure 16-9 Photomicrograph showing the gram-stained organism isolated from the stool of a patient with diarrhea.

37. A family presented to a private practitioner with similar symptoms, including 1 week of diarrhea and abdominal pain. They had attended a picnic a few days prior to onset of their illness. Items consumed included chicken salad, watermelon, and bottled water. Stool specimens were sent for culture. The causative bacterial agent demonstrated in Figure 16-9 was isolated after 2 days of incubation in microaerophilic conditions. Which one of the following is the most likely etiologic agent?
A. *Helicobacter pylori.*
B. *Campylobacter jejuni.*
C. *Salmonella enteritidis.*
D. *Cryptosporidium parvum.*
E. *Clostridium difficile.*

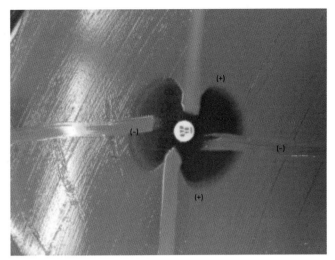

Figure 16-10   To perform the Hodge test for identifying KPC-carbapenemase producing organisms, an agar plate is streaked with a carbapenem-susceptible *Escherichia coli*, an ertapenem disk is placed in the center, and the test organisms are streaked out from the disk. This figure shows inactivation of ertapenem by a KPC-producing *Klebsiella pneumoniae* (+), distorting the zone of inhibition of *E. coli*. KPC-negative organisms are also demonstrated (−), which show no distortion of the zone of inhibition of *E. coli*.

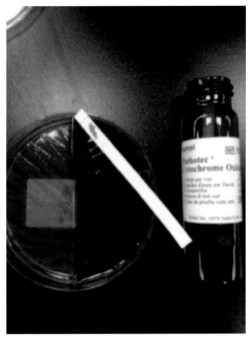

Figure 16-11   Colonial growth and oxidase test result of an organism cultured on a 5% sheep blood agar/MacConkey biplate.

38. An oxidase-negative, lactose-fermenting, gram-negative bacillus grew from a bronchoalveolar lavage specimen collected from a lung transplant recipient with pneumonia (Figure 16-10). The antimicrobial susceptibility test panel showed resistance to all antibiotics, including imipenem and ertapenem. It was only susceptible to tigecycline and polymyxin B. Which one of the following is the most likely pathogen?
    A. *Klebsiella pneumonia.*
    B. *Pseudomonas aeruginosa.*
    C. *Acinetobacter baumannii.*
    D. *Stenotrophomonas maltophilia.*
    E. *Serratia marcescens.*

39. Commercially available multiplex PCR assays are used to detect bloodstream infections caused by *Staphylococcus aureus* and methicillin-resistant *S. aureus* (MRSA). These methods are designed to detect pathogen-specific molecular targets directly from newly positive blood culture bottles showing gram-positive cocci in clusters. Which one of the following answers best describes the genetic regions targeted in these assays?
    A. Staphylococcal protein A (*spa*), SCC*mec*, and *mecA* gene.
    B. Staphylococcal Panton-Valentine leukocidin (PVL), *spa* gene, and *mecA* gene.
    C. Staphylococcal protein A (*spa*), SCC*mec-orfX* junction, and *vanA* gene.
    D. *nuc* gene, *mupA* gene, and *mecA* gene.
    E. SCC*mec-orfX* junction, *agr* gene, and *mecA* gene.

40. A 38-year-old male developed a wound infection while in the intensive care burn unit. A sample of the purulent exudate was sent for culture. The bacterial isolate and the oxidase test result, as demonstrated in Figure 16-11, best suggest the presumptive identification of which one of the following pathogens?
    A. *Acinetobacter baumannii.*
    B. *Klebsiella pneumoniae.*
    C. *Stenotrophomonas maltophilia.*
    D. *Pseudomonas aeruginosa.*
    E. *Escherichia coli.*

41. The microbiology laboratory evaluated a new agar media (agar B) developed to be both selective and differential for MRSA with claims of enhanced sensitivity. A total of 500 nares swabs were inoculated onto the laboratory's current MRSA agar (agar A, the gold standard) and onto agar B. Concordance was observed for 138 positive and 337 negative cultures. Fourteen specimens were positive on agar A and negative on agar B. Eleven specimens were positive on agar B and negative on agar A. Based on this data, which one of the following statements is correct?
    A. Agar B demonstrated a higher sensitivity of 96.8%.
    B. Agar B demonstrated a lower sensitivity of 90.8%.
    C. Agar B demonstrated a higher sensitivity of 96.0%.
    D. Agar B demonstrated a lower sensitivity of 95%.
    E. Agar B demonstrated a lower sensitivity of 92.6%.

42. Which one of the following set of parameters for performing antimicrobial susceptibility testing of aerobic, nonfastidious bacteria best follows established practice guidelines?
    A. 0.5 McFarland inoculum, Mueller Hinton agar, ambient air incubation.
    B. 1.0 McFarland inoculum, Mueller Hinton agar with 5% sheep blood agar, CO_2 incubation.
    C. 1.0 McFarland inoculum, Mueller Hinton agar with 5% sheep blood agar, ambient air incubation.
    D. 1.0 McFarland inoculum, Mueller Hinton agar, ambient air incubation.
    E. 0.5 McFarland inoculum, Mueller Hinton agar, CO_2 incubation.

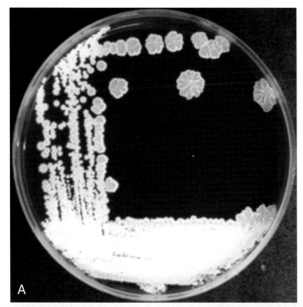

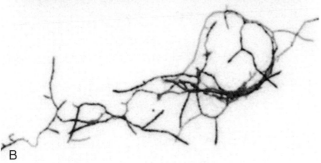

Figure 16-12 **A**, Colonial growth and cellular morphology of an organism cultured from sputum after 3 days on a blood agar plate. **B**, Cellular morphology using a modified acid-fast stain (×900).

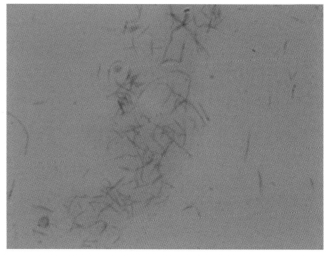

Figure 16-13 Photomicrograph showing cellular morphology by Gram stain (×1000) of the organism cultured from a brain abscess.

44. A 94-year-old woman presented to the emergency department with progressive, unilateral headaches of 3 weeks duration. Magnetic resonance imaging of her brain revealed the presence of an abscess. Purulent material was drained and sent for culture. The microscopic morphology on Gram stain is shown in Figure 16-13, and the anaerobic culture grew white colonies with a bread-crumb appearance. Which one of the following is the most likely etiologic agent of her brain abscess?
   A. *Prevotella intermedia.*
   B. *Porphyromonas asaccharolytica.*
   C. *Fusobacterium nucleatum.*
   D. *Bacteroides fragilis.*
   E. *Clostridium septicum.*

45. An elderly man was transferred from a nursing home to your hospital with low-grade fever, flank pain, hypothermia, dysuria, and nausea. His workup included blood cultures and a urine specimen. The urine specimen grew 10^4 non–β-hemolytic colonies of gram-positive cocci in pairs and chains on blood agar media. Which one of the following is the most likely agent causing this infection?
   A. GBS.
   B. *Enterococcus faecium.*
   C. *Staphylococcus saprophyticus.*
   D. GAS.
   E. *Staphylococcus aureus.*

43. A diabetic male patient status postheart transplant presented to the emergency department with a several-day history of fatigue, productive cough, and fever. Pulmonary imaging studies revealed bilateral nodular opacities, and direct exam of his sputum demonstrated gram-positive, beaded, partially acid-fast bacilli (Figure 16-12). Culture on day 3 produced chalky white colonies with aerial hyphae on solid media and filamentous, delicately branching bacilli in liquid culture. Which one of the following is the most likely pathogen?
   A. *Streptomyces griseus.*
   B. *Nocardia cyriacigeorgica.*
   C. *Rhodococcus equi.*
   D. *Gordonia sputa.*
   E. *Mycobacterium fortuitum.*

46. A 10-year-old girl presented to the emergency department with signs and symptoms of depression. Her mother reported disruptive behavior at school and suspects sexual abuse. Urine and vaginal discharge specimens were sent to the microbiology laboratory for analysis. Which one of the following statements best describes the tests that must be performed to optimize detection of sexually transmitted pathogens?
   A. NAATs and bacterial culture.
   B. Direct fluorescent antibody tests and serology.
   C. NAATs and serology.
   D. Viral culture and serology.
   E. Gram stain and NAATs.

47. A 48-year-old man presented to an outpatient clinic with a 1-week history of daily fevers to 102°F. On physical exam a new heart murmur was detected. He was referred to the emergency department for a transesophageal echocardiogram, which identified a vegetation on the aortic valve. Blood cultures were collected, and 24 hours later gram-positive cocci in pairs and tetrads were reported. The organism was α-hemolytic, PYR positive, leucine aminopeptidase (LAP) negative, and susceptible to vancomycin. Which one of the following is the most likely etiologic agent?

A. *Gemella haemolysans.*

B. *Aerococcus urinae.*

C. *Streptococcus pneumoniae.*

D. *Pediococcus acidilactici.*

E. *Aerococcus viridians.*

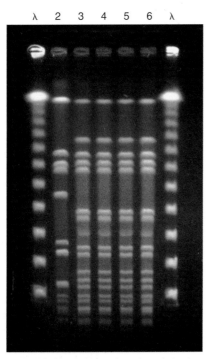

λ 2 3 4 5 6 λ

Figure 16-14   Pulsed-field gel electrophoresis analysis of methicillin-resistant *Staphylococcus aureus* isolates. Genetic profiles of these isolates were obtained by digesting chromosomal DNA with the *SmaI* restriction endonuclease. Lanes 1 and 7 are λ markers. Lane 2 is a control strain. Lanes 3 to 6 are isolates from individual patients.

48. The epidemiology team identified a cluster of MRSA infections in the surgical intensive care unit of an urban hospital. Two patients had MRSA bloodstream infections, and two had sternal wound infections within a 1-week timeframe. The microbiology laboratory analyzed these four isolates to determine strain relatedness using PFGE. The results are shown in Figure 16-14. Which one of the following statements best describes the relatedness of the patient isolates?

A. Indistinguishable.

B. Closely related.

C. Possibly related.

D. Different.

E. Inconclusive.

49. An 18-year-old patient was admitted to the hospital with fever, hypotension, altered mental status, and an erythematous abscess on her leg that was developing a blackened eschar. A diagnosis of necrotizing fasciitis was made. Blood cultures were collected, and the abscess was cultured. The Gram stain revealed gram-positive cocci in clusters. Which one of the following is the most likely etiologic agent?

A. *Vibrio vulnificus.*

B. *Bacillus anthracis.*

C. Beta-hemolytic *Streptococcus pyogenes* (GAS).

D. MRSA.

E. *Staphylococcus lugdunensis.*

Mycobacteriology

50. A 32-year-old HIV-positive patient presents to the emergency department with a chronic cough of 4 months' duration. The chest radiograph shows bilateral infiltrates. Respiratory specimens are submitted for detecting mycobacteria. Which one of the following statements best describes the rapid mycobacteriology tests that are used to detect these pathogens directly in clinical specimens?

A. Carbol fuchsin stain and the niacin test.

B. Fluorochrome stain and NAAT.

C. Giemsa stain and liquid culture.

D. Fluorochrome stain and nucleic acid sequencing.

E. DNA probe assay and high-pressure liquid chromatography.

51. A tissue biopsy obtained from a 5-year-old child with submandibular lymphadenitis was positive on direct examination for acid-fast bacilli. Nonchromogenic slow-growing colonies were observed only on chocolate agar at 30°C and not on standard mycobacterial media at 37°C. Which one of the following is the most likely etiologic agent?

A. *Mycobacterium bovis.*

B. *Mycobacterium haemophilum.*

C. *Mycobacterium avium.*

D. *Mycobacterium leprae.*

E. *Mycobacterium marinum.*

52. A thin, immunocompetent, 85-year-old woman presents with chronic obstructive pulmonary disease and a chronic cough. Sputum smears were acid-fast positive, and a nonchromogenic mycobacterial isolate grew from multiple specimens after 21 days of culture. Which one of the following is the most likely etiologic agent causing her infection?

A. *Mycobacterium abscessus.*

B. *Mycobacterium kansasii.*

C. *Mycobacterium avium* complex.

D. *Mycobacterium scrofulaceum.*

E. *Mycobacterium gordonae.*

53. A 43-year-old HIV-positive man presented to the emergency department with a 2-month history of fever, night sweats, cough with productive sputum, and a 20-pound weight loss. He was recently released from prison. Three sputum specimens were positive for acid-fast bacilli (AFB). Which one of the following statements best describes the conventional methods used for diagnosis and identification of this pathogen?
    A. A tuberculin purified protein derivative skin test is diagnostic for *Mycobacterium tuberculosis* when more than 10 mm of induration is seen.
    B. Culture on standard media used to isolate bacterial agents causing community-acquired pneumonia.
    C. Cavitary lesions on chest radiographs, which are diagnostic of tuberculosis.
    D. Culture on mycobacterial selective media, along with the use of DNA probes and biochemical tests.
    E. The use of NAATs identifying the *Mycobacterium avium* complex.

54. A 52-year-old man living in southern Louisiana presents with multiple, hyposensitive, irregularly shaped, annular macules on his arms and back and bilateral numbness of his hands. Kinyoun carbol fuchsin staining of a skin biopsy shows AFB, but culture of the biopsy tissue is negative. He reports no travel history outside the United States and frequently hunts deer and armadillos. Which one of the following is the most likely etiologic cause of his disease?
    A. *Trichophyton mentagrophytes.*
    B. *Borrelia burgdorferi.*
    C. *Treponema pallidum.*
    D. *Nocardia brasiliensis.*
    E. *Mycobacterium leprae.*

55. Which of the following statements best describes species of mycobacteria that are classified as nontuberculous mycobacteria?
    A. *Mycobacterium canetti, Mycobacterium africanum,* and *Mycobacterium fortuitum.*
    B. *Mycobacterium kansasii, Mycobacterium abscessus,* and *Mycobacterium avium-intracellulare* complex.
    C. *Mycobacterium avium-intracellulare* complex, *Mycobacterium microti,* and *Mycobacterium mucogenicum.*
    D. *Mycobacterium chelonae, Mycobacterium africanum,* and *Mycobacterium scrofulaceum.*
    E. *Mycobacterium gordonae, Mycobacterium bovis,* and *Mycobacterium kansasii.*

56. An asymptomatic health care worker from India had a positive tuberculin skin test. She had a history of Bacille Calmette-Guerin vaccination. Which one of the following tests should be performed to confirm the diagnosis of latent tuberculosis?
    A. Interferon-gamma release assay (IGRA).
    B. Purified protein derivative inoculation.
    C. Chest radiograph.
    D. Adenosine deaminase assay.
    E. Galactomannan assay.

57. A 29-year-old woman presented to her physician with a papular rash on her calf that developed 2 weeks after receiving a tattoo. A punch biopsy showed inflammatory cells but no microorganisms. Upon culture nonchromogenic, AFB grew within 7 days. The results of biochemical tests included negative iron uptake, positive citrate utilization, and NaCl intolerance. Which one of the following is the most likely etiologic agent?
    A. *Mycobacterium tuberculosis.*
    B. *Mycobacterium chelonae.*
    C. *Mycobacterium abscessus.*
    D. *Mycobacterium fortuitum.*
    E. *Mycobacterium szulgai.*

58. Which one of the following phenotypic methods can best be used to differentiate *Mycobacterium tuberculosis* from *Mycobacterium bovis*?
    A. Iron uptake.
    B. Urease.
    C. Growth on MacConkey agar.
    D. Niacin.
    E. Pigment production.

59. Subtyping of strains of *Mycobacterium tuberculosis* is important for epidemiologic purposes. Which one of the following methods is considered the current gold standard for molecular typing of *M. tuberculosis* isolates?
    A. Deletion typing.
    B. IS6110 restriction length polymorphism analysis.
    C. Spacer oligonucleotide typing (spoligotyping).
    D. Mycobacterial interspersed repetitive units/variable number tandem repeat (MIRU-VNTR) typing.
    E. Genome-wide single nucleotide polymorphism analysis.

60. A patient who immigrated to the United States from China presented to her clinician with a chronic productive cough and a 1-month history of treatment with isoniazid. A chest radiograph revealed a nodular infiltrate in the apex of the upper lobe. The patient had a positive tuberculin skin test. Which one of the following is the most effective initial treatment regimen?
    A. Isoniazid and rifampin, pending drug susceptibility results.
    B. Fluoroquinolone, pending drug susceptibility results.
    C. Second-line drugs (e.g., ethionamide, cycloserine, kanamycin), pending drug susceptibility results.
    D. Treatment with isoniazid, rifampin, pyrazinamide, and ethambutol, pending drug susceptibility results.
    E. Isoniazid plus ethambutol is adequate to avoid the hepatotoxicity of rifampin.

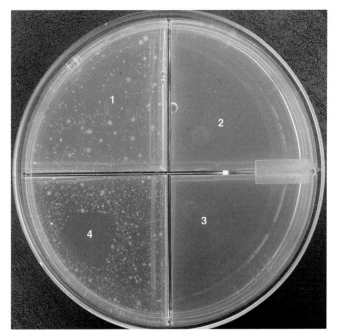

Figure 16-15 Agar proportion susceptibility test results for the organism isolated from a patient *with Mycobacterium tuberculosis. 1,* Isoniazid disk (1 μg); *2,* rifampin disk (5 μg); *3,* isoniazid disk (5 μg); *4,* drug-free control disk.

61. A patient with tuberculosis discontinued standard rifampin/ isoniazid/pyrazinamide/ethambutol (RIPE) therapy after 2 months and now presents with presumptive pulmonary tuberculosis and multiple sputum specimens that are acid-fast bacillus smear positive. Direct susceptibility by agar proportion was performed, with the results shown in Figure 16-15. Which one of the following statements provides the most accurate interpretation of these results?
    A. The isolate is isoniazid and rifampin susceptible.
    B. The isolate is a multi-drug-resistant tuberculosis strain.
    C. The isolate is rifampin monoresistant.
    D. The isolate is low-level isoniazid resistant and rifampin susceptible.
    E. The results cannot be interpreted due to culture contamination of the control quadrant.

62. A 2-year-old child presented to the emergency department with painless unilateral enlargement of a cervical lymph node. A fine-needle aspirate was performed, and the specimen was sent to the microbiology laboratory for culture. Which one of the following is the most likely pathogen?
    A. *Mycobacterium scrofulaceum.*
    B. *Mycobacterium gordonae.*
    C. *Mycobacterium mucogenicum.*
    D. *Mycobacterium kansasii.*
    E. *Mycobacterium abscessus.*

63. Which one of the following species of nontuberculous mycobacteria is not a photochromogen?
    A. *Mycobacterium avium.*
    B. *Mycobacterium kansasii.*
    C. *Mycobacterium marinum.*
    D. *Mycobacterium simiae.*
    E. *Mycobacterium asiaticum.*

64. Operational safety requirements are mandated to prevent transmission of *Mycobacterium tuberculosis* to personnel who process potentially infectious specimens and cultures. Which one of the following most accurately describes the correct safety practice(s) requirements to ensure personnel safety?
    A. A confined access room under negative pressure with an optional biologic safety cabinet (BSC).
    B. Air sterilization by ultraviolet light within a BSC and on the ceiling of the room to disinfect the ambient air.
    C. A room or suite that has a minimum of 20 air exchanges per hour to remove 99% of airborne particulates.
    D. A BSC in a controlled access area with the capacity to draw 75 to 100 linear feet of air per minute across the entire front opening for proper functioning of the HEPA filter.
    E. Respiratory protection using a HEPA-filtered respirator, such as the N95 or N100, and mandatory fit testing every 6 months.

65. AFB were detected in sputum specimens from a cluster of patients in your hospital. Cultures from respiratory specimens and water sources produced slow-growing, yellow pigmented AFB that grew optimally at 42°C, were arylsulfatase test positive, and were negative by commercial rRNA probe assays. Which one of the following is the most likely etiologic agent?
    A. *Mycobacterium avium* complex.
    B. *Mycobacterium xenopi.*
    C. *Mycobacterium abscessus.*
    D. *Mycobacterium kansasii.*
    E. *Mycobacterium mucogenicum.*

66. From the nontuberculous mycobacteria species listed below, which one is most often considered to be clinically relevant when isolated from the sputum of a patient with symptoms indicative of nontuberculous mycobacterial lung disease?
    A. *Mycobacterium mucogenicum.*
    B. *Mycobacterium lentiflavum.*
    C. *Mycobacterium terrae.*
    D. *Mycobacterium intracellulare.*
    E. *Mycobacterium gordonae.*

67. AFB were detected in a bronchoalveolar lavage specimen from a patient presenting with a chronic cough and a chest radiograph suspicious for tuberculosis. The nucleic acid hybridization probe test result was negative for *M. tuberculosis* complex and positive for another mycobacterial species. The isolate was yellow after exposure to light. Which one of the following is the most likely etiologic agent?
    A. *Mycobacterium xenopi.*
    B. *Mycobacterium scrofulaceum.*
    C. *Mycobacterium gordonae.*
    D. *Mycobacterium kansasii.*
    E. *Mycobacterium abscessus.*

68. Proper isolation practices in patients with suspected or confirmed pulmonary tuberculosis are the primary protective measures against the spread of tuberculosis to other patients and staff. Which one of the following statements most accurately reflects the infection control criteria for release from airborne isolation?
    A. Airborne isolation can be discontinued when another diagnosis is made that excludes tuberculosis and when three sputum specimens are AFB smear negative and NAAT negative.
    B. Airborne isolation can be discontinued when two sputum specimens are AFB smear negative and culture negative.
    C. Airborne isolation can be discontinued when the patient has received 48 hours of antituberculous therapy.
    D. Airborne precautions can be discontinued in young children when three expectorated sputum specimens are AFB smear negative and culture negative.
    E. Airborne isolation can be discontinued when two sputum specimens are AFB smear negative and nucleic acid probe test negative.

69. An 8-year-old child who recently traveled to rural Mexico presented to the pediatric emergency department with severe abdominal pain. She was taken to the operating room, where a nodular omental mass was noted near the colon. Peritoneal fluid and tissue specimens were sent to microbiology for analysis. A positive NAAT and molecular analysis identified the mycobacterial pathogen. Which one of the following species is the most likely etiologic agent?
    A. *Mycobacterium kansasii.*
    B. *Mycobacterium ulcerans.*
    C. *Mycobacterium bovis.*
    D. *Mycobacterium avium* complex.
    E. *Mycobacterium fortuitum.*

70. A 32-year-old HIV-positive patient presents to the emergency department with a chronic cough of 4 months' duration. The chest radiograph shows bilateral infiltrates. Respiratory specimens are submitted for analysis. Which one of the following statements best describes the rapid mycobacteriology tests that are used to detect these pathogens directly in clinical specimens?
    A. Carbol fuchsin stain and the niacin test.
    B. Fluorochrome stain and NAAT.
    C. Giemsa stain and liquid culture.
    D. Fluorochrome stain and nucleic acid sequencing.
    E. DNA probe assay and high-pressure liquid chromatography.

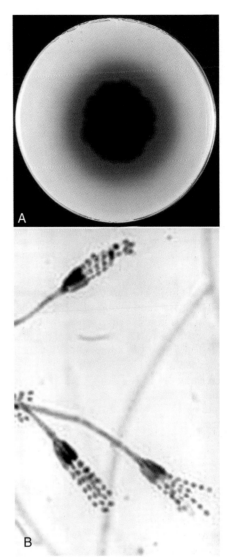

Figure 16-16 **A,** Reverse colony morphology on a Sabouraud agar plate after 3 days of culture at 30°C. **B,** Wet mount of the organism (×100).

Mycology

71. A 32-year-old, HIV-positive recent immigrant from Vietnam presented to the emergency department with fever, weight loss, and lymphadenopathy. Two sets of blood cultures were collected and became positive after 2 days of incubation. The organism demonstrated in Figure 16-16 was recovered after 72 hours of incubation at 30°C. Which one of the following is the most likely etiologic agent?
    A. *Penicillium marneffei.*
    B. *Aspergillus nidulans.*
    C. *Trichophyton rubrum.*
    D. *Fusarium solani.*
    E. *Cryptococcus neoformans.*

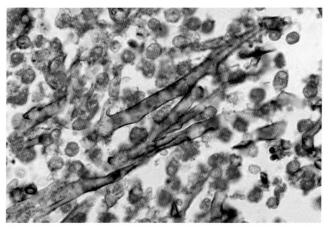

Figure 16-17 Methenemine silver stain of the fungal elements found in a needle aspirate of the maxillary sinus of a bone marrow transplant recipient.

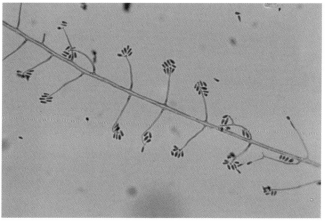

Figure 16-19 Photomicrograph showing a lactophenol cotton blue preparation of an organism obtained by 6 days of culture from a tissue biopsy (×500).

72. A 13-year-old female bone marrow transplant recipient presents with nasal congestion and a severe headache. A needle aspirate from the sinus reveals hyphae by light microscopy (Figure 16-17). Which one of the following organisms is the most likely cause of this infection?

- **A.** Mucormycosis.
- **B.** Aspergillosis.
- **C.** Candidiasis.
- **D.** Mycetoma.
- **E.** Rhinosporidiosis.

74. A 70-year-old gardener presented to the emergency department with a hyperkeratotic lesion on her left thumb and nodules tracking up her arm. A thermally dimorphic white mold grew from a tissue biopsy within 6 days. Microscopic morphology showed rosette-like clusters of conidia and conidia along the sides of the hyphae (Figure 16-19). Which one of the following is the most likely etiologic agent causing this infection?

- **A.** *Sporothrix schenckii* (sporotrichosis).
- **B.** *Fusarium solani* (fusariosis).
- **C.** *Penicillium marneffei* (penicilliosis).
- **D.** *Nocardia brasiliensis* (sporotrichoid nocardiosis).
- **E.** *Histoplasma capsulatum* (histoplasmosis).

75. Which one of the following media is differential for identifying *Cryptococcus neoformans*?

- **A.** Birdseed agar.
- **B.** Sabouraud dextrose agar.
- **C.** Mycosel agar.
- **D.** Potato dextrose agar.
- **E.** Brain heart infusion agar.

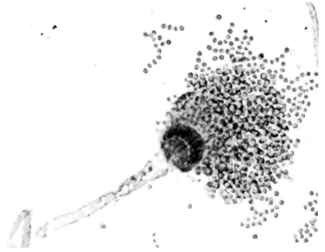

Figure 16-18 Photomicrograph showing cellular morphology of the organism isolated from the liver biopsy of a patient after 3 days of culture.

73. An 8-year-old boy presented with a 1-week history of fever and fatigue. Six months prior to this episode, he had a bone marrow transplant. Computed tomography scan revealed opacities in his liver, which were biopsied and sent for microbiologic and histologic examination. After 3 days of incubation, the microbiology laboratory reported the presence of the pathogen shown in Figure 16-18. Which one of the following is the most likely etiologic agent?

- **A.** *Aspergillus fumigates.*
- **B.** *Penicillium* spp.
- **C.** *Aspergillus niger.*
- **D.** *Fusarium solani.*
- **E.** *Aspergillus flavus.*

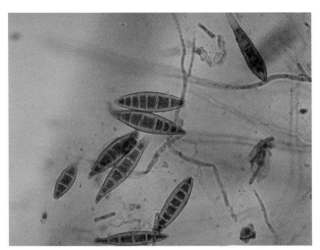

Figure 16-20 Photomicrograph showing a lactophenol cotton blue preparation of an organism obtained by 5 days of culture from a scalp lesion (×100).

76. A 5-year-old boy presented to his pediatrician with a 1-week history of a scalp lesion, described as scaly and noninflamed, with some hair loss at the site. The lesion was sampled and sent for bacterial and fungal cultures. After 5 days, growth was observed; smears of the colony were stained and examined microscopically. Which one of the following is the etiologic agent demonstrated in Figure 16-20?
    A. *Trichophyton tonsurans.*
    B. *Microsporum gypseum.*
    C. *Trichophyton schoenleinii.*
    D. *Epidermophyton floccosum.*
    E. *Microsporum canis.*

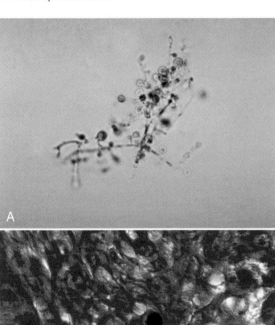

Figure 16-21 **A,** Photomicrograph showing a lactophenol cotton blue preparation of an organism obtained after culture at 25°C from a bronchoalveolar lavage specimen (×100). **B,** Gram stain results for this organism after culture at 37°C (×1000).

77. A 45-year-old man presented to the emergency department with a 1-week history of flulike symptoms, including fever, chills, cough, and myalgia. One month prior, he was camping in North Carolina but reported no tick bites. A bronchoalveolar lavage specimen was obtained. Two weeks later the etiologic agent was identified (Figure 16-21). Which one of the following is the most likely cause of his severe pneumonia?
    A. *Blastomyces dermatitidis.*
    B. *Histoplasma capsulatum.*
    C. *Sporothrix schenckii.*
    D. *Penicillium marneffei.*
    E. *Rhizomucor pusillus.*

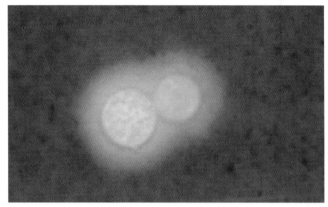

Figure 16-22 Photomicrograph showing an India ink preparation of cerebrospinal fluid obtained from an HIV-infected patient (×100).

78. A 68-year-old HIV-infected man presented to the emergency department with a 5-day history of headache, fever, and altered mental status. Cerebrospinal fluid was collected and sent for bacterial and fungal cultures. A direct examination demonstrated the organism shown in Figure 16-22. Which one of the following is the most likely etiologic agent?
    A. *Candida albicans.*
    B. *Cryptococcus neoformans.*
    C. *Streptococcus pneumoniae.*
    D. *Blastomyces dermatitidis.*
    E. *Neisseria meningitides.*

79. A 17-year-old male presented to his dermatologist complaining of a solitary lesion on his arm present for 1 week and now beginning to ulcerate. He works in an exotic bird pet store and recalls being bitten 2 weeks earlier. A biopsy was performed and a diagnosis was made based on growth of a brown-pigmented colony on birdseed agar. Which one of the following is the most likely etiologic agent?
    A. *Cryptococcus neoformans.*
    B. *Mycobacterium avium.*
    C. *Aspergillus niger.*
    D. *Exophiala dermatitidis.*
    E. *Trichophyton rubrum.*

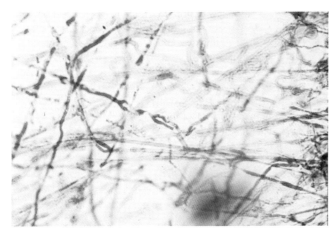

Figure 16-23 Photomicrograph showing a lactophenol cotton blue preparation of an organism obtained from a left ventricular assist device.

80. A 56-year-old man with refractory heart failure was placed on an emergent left ventricular assist device (LVAD) while awaiting a heart transplant. The LVAD malfunctioned due to a mechanical obstruction, necessitating surgery. Results from intraluminal material collected from the occluded LVAD were reported by pathology as fungal hyphae with 45-degree angle branching and by microbiology as a white mold with no phialides and few septae (Figure 16-23). Which one of the following fungi is the most likely etiologic agent?

    A. *Syncephalastrum racemosum.*
    B. *Penicillium* spp.
    C. *Aspergillus niger.*
    D. *Fusarium* spp.
    E. *Acremonium* spp.

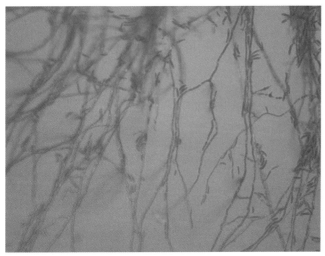

Figure 16-24 Photomicrograph showing a lactophenol cotton blue preparation of an organism obtained after culture for 48 hours of a corneal scraping (×100).

81. A 20-year-old college student presented to a student health facility complaining of blurred vision, excessive tearing, and sensitivity to light. She was referred to an ophthalmologist, who obtained a corneal scraping. This biopsy, as well as the student's contacts lenses and contact cleaning solution, were sent to the laboratory for culture. After 48 hours, the hyaline fungus shown in Figure 16-24 was recovered from all three specimens. Which one of the following is the most likely etiologic agent of her fungal keratitis?

    A. *Alternaria* spp.
    B. *Exophiala* spp.
    C. *Geotrichum* spp.
    D. *Torulopsis* spp.
    E. *Fusarium* spp.

82. Which one of the following statements most accurately describes the standard practice required to ensure a safe environment when processing specimens and/or cultures of potentially pathogenic fungi in the mycology laboratory?

    A. It is standard practice that all yeast and filamentous fungi (molds) are handled and processed under a BSC. Tape or shrink seals are required to seal all agar and broth media to protect against contamination or infection with dimorphic fungi (e.g., *Coccidioides immitis*).
    B. The use of a BSC is required for processing and handling molds, not yeast. Tape or shrink seals are required when using plated agar media; however, petri plates should not be used if *C. immitis* is suspected.
    C. The required location of the BSC used for handling fungal specimens and cultures is a confined access mycology facility. All agar slants and plates are required to be sealed by tape or shrink seals to prevent contamination.
    D. Slide cultures of suspect dimorphic fungi, in lieu of wet mount preparations, must be prepared in a BSC located within a confined access room.
    E. Mold species, such as *Aspergillus* and *Candida* species, are less infectious to laboratory workers; therefore, they can be handled and processed outside of a BSC.

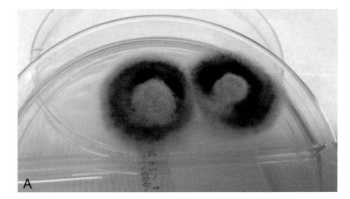

A

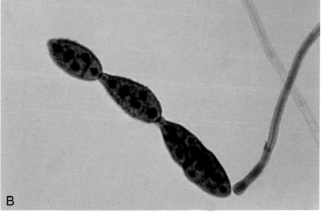

B

Figure 16-25 Growth of an organism on an inhibitory mold agarplate.

83. A 32-year-old male with a history of chronic sinusitis presented with nasal congestion, facial pain, and increased nasal secretions. A computed tomography scan demonstrated diffuse mucosal thickening involving both maxillary sinuses. Material was aspirated from his sinus cavities and sent for culture. In less than 1 week, the fungus shown in Figure 16-25 was isolated on inhibitory mold agar (reverse color is black). Which one of the following is the most likely etiologic agent of his sinusitis?
    A. *Aspergillus fumigates.*
    B. *Alternaria* spp.
    C. *Cryptococcus neoformans.*
    D. *Fusarium* spp.
    E. *Mucor* spp.

84. Which one of the following assays is most useful for the diagnosis of invasive aspergillosis?
    A. India ink examination.
    B. *Aspergillus* antibody EIA.
    C. Galactomannan antigen EIA.
    D. KOH examination.
    E. Calcofluor white examination.

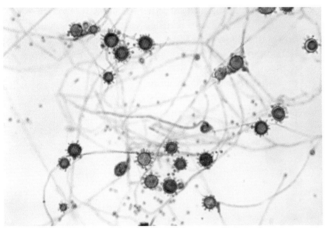

Figure 16-26 Photomicrograph showing a lactophenol cotton blue preparation of a pathogenic fungus obtained after 3 weeks of incubation at 25°C (×400).

85. The fungus shown in Figure 16-26 was isolated after 3 weeks of incubation at 25°C. Which one of the following is the most likely pathogen?
    A. *Paracoccidioides brasiliensis.*
    B. *Blastomyces dermatitidis.*
    C. *Sporothrix schenckii.*
    D. *Penicillium marneffei.*
    E. *Histoplasma capsulatum.*

86. Which one of the following differential tests is most useful for identifying *Candida albicans*?
    A. Urease test.
    B. Germ tube test.
    C. India ink examination.
    D. Phenol oxidase test.
    E. Rapid assimilation of trehalose.

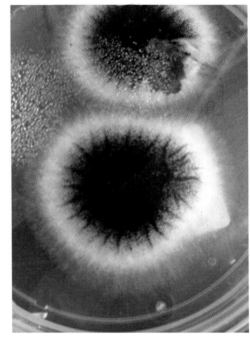

Figure 16-27 Colonial morphology of an organism isolated after 3 days of culture on Sabouraud dextrose agar.

87. A 57-year-old man was diagnosed with otomycosis at a travel medicine clinic. Cultures were positive after 3 days for the fungus demonstrated in Figure 16-27. Which one of the following is the most likely etiologic agent?
    A. *Aspergillus flavus.*
    B. *Exophiala dermatitidis.*
    C. *Aspergillus niger.*
    D. *Fonsecaea pedrosoi.*
    E. *Epidermophyton floccosum.*

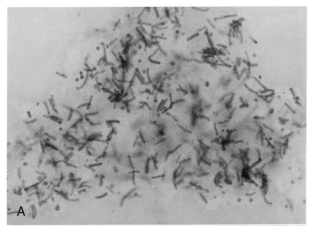

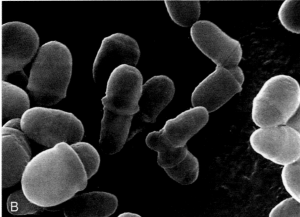

Figure 16-28 Gram stain (**A**) and scanning electron microscope image (**B**) showing cellular morphology of an organism growing in blood culture bottles inoculated with samples from a neonate.

88. A 17-day-old neonate became febrile and had an elevated white blood cell count. This premature infant was found to have congenital gastrointestinal abnormalities on delivery and was placed on parenteral nutrition. Blood cultures became positive after 48 hours of incubation, and Gram stain demonstrated yeast-like cells (Figure 16-28). Repeated subcultures of the positive bottle on routine bacteriologic media failed to recover the organism. Which one of the following is the most likely etiologic agent?

A. *Aspergillus fumigates.*
B. *Candida albicans.*
C. *Candida parapsilosis.*
D. *Malassezia turfur.*
E. *Cryptococcus neoformans.*

89. A patient presented to his private physician after noticing that several toenails on his right foot were thick and discolored. A culture was obtained and, after 10 days, a fungus was recovered. Microscopic examination revealed numerous teardrop microconidia along the sides of septate hyphae. Occasional long, narrow, thin-walled macroconidia were also observed. Which one of the following is the most likely etiologic agent?

A. *Trichophyton rubrum.*
B. *Microsporum canis.*
C. *Trichophyton tonsurans.*
D. *Epidermophyton floccosum.*
E. *Microsporum gypseum.*

90. A 73-year-old postsurgical patient became febrile and newly positive blood cultures revealed yeast on Gram stain. Which one of the following is the best rapid assay that can be used to obtain same-day identification of this pathogen?

A. Routine culture.
B. Chromagar *Candida* culture.
C. Peptide nucleic acid fluorescent in situ hybridization.
D. 16S rRNA gene sequencing.
E. Yeast identification panels.

ANSWERS

BACTERIOLOGY

1. A. The MIC is the lowest drug level that can reach all sites of infection.
Rationale: The MIC is based on achievable levels in serum.
B. The MIC is the amount of drug that can be administered in a single dose.
Rationale: The MIC value is independent of antimicrobial dosing regimens.
C. The MIC is the lowest drug level that is bacteriostatic.
Rationale: The MIC is the lowest concentration of antimicrobial agent that inhibits microbial growth.
D. The MIC is the lowest drug level that is nontoxic.
Rationale: The MIC value does not provide information regarding drug toxicity.
E. The MIC is the lowest drug level that kills the bacterial pathogen.
Rationale: The MIC is not a measure of bactericidal activity.

Major points of discussion
■ The Clinical Laboratory Standards Institute (CLSI) develops consensus guidelines for accurate antimicrobial susceptibility test methods and interpretation.
■ MICs are traditionally determined from serial two-fold dilutions of each antibiotic.
■ Isolated, pure bacterial colonies must be used for accurate susceptibility testing.
■ MIC results must be reported together with an interpretative category (i.e., susceptible, intermediate, or resistant) to guide clinician treatment strategies.
■ Although the agar dilution methodology is considered the gold standard, microbroth dilutions assays are commonly used in routine clinical laboratories.[22]

2. A. *Moraxella catarrhalis.*
Rationale: *M. catarrhalis* is a gram-negative diplococcus that can cause otitis media or sinusitis and bronchitis and pneumonia in patients with underlying chronic lung disease.
B. *Legionella pneumophila.*
Rationale: *L. pneumophila* is a poorly staining gram-negative bacillus. A rapid urine antigen assay is available for detecting this pathogen.
C. *Mycoplasma pneumonia.*

Rationale: Due to the absence of a cell wall, *M. pneumoniae* cannot be Gram stained. Laboratory diagnosis by NAAT is preferred over serologic tests or culture on specialized media.

D. *Streptococcus pneumonia.*
Rationale: S. pneumoniae are gram-positive, lancet-shaped diplococci. This pathogen is a common cause of community-acquired pneumonia. A rapid urine antigen assay is available for diagnosis.

E. *Staphylococcus aureus.*
Rationale: S. aureus stains as gram-positive cocci in clusters. Staphylococcal pneumonia is a known complication of influenza infection.

Major points of discussion

- The recommended therapy for pneumococcal pneumonia is high-dose penicillin G or a second- or third-generation cephalosporin. Antimicrobial susceptibility testing must be performed because penicillin resistance is common.
- Presentation with lobar consolidation on chest radiograph is suspicious for "typical" as opposed to "atypical" pneumonia in nonhospitalized patients. The most common etiologic agents in this category include *Streptococcus pneumoniae* and *Haemophilus influenzae*.
- The major virulence factor of *Streptococcus pneumoniae* is a polysaccharide capsule that consists of more than 90 antigenically distinct types. Type 3 is thought to be the most virulent.
- *Streptococcus pneumoniae* is differentiated from other streptococci by biochemical tests. It is bile soluble, α-hemolytic, and optochin (i.e., ethylhydrocupreine hydrochloride) susceptible.
- A single-dose 23-polyvalent vaccine (Pneumovax) is available to prevent infection by the most common serotypes of *Streptococcus pneumoniae*. It is recommended for individuals older than 65 and patients with chronic pulmonary, cardiac, liver, or renal disease, patients with asplenia and sickle cell disease, and diabetic and immunocompromised patients. In addition, a vaccine has been approved for children younger than 2 years.[44,68]

3. A. Carbapenems.
Rationale: This class of antibiotics, which includes imipenem, meropenem, and ertapenem, can be used to treat ESBL-producing bacteria.

B. Third-generation cephalosporins.
Rationale: This class of antibiotics, which includes ceftriaxone and ceftazidime, is inactivated by ESBL-producing bacteria.

C. First-generation cephalosporins.
Rationale: This class of antibiotics, which includes cefazolin and cephalothin, is inactivated by ESBL-producing bacteria.

D. Second-generation cephalosporins.
Rationale: This class of antibiotics, such as cefuroxime, is inactivated by ESBL-producing bacteria.

E. Aztreonam.
Rationale: This monobactam antibiotic is inactivated by ESBL-producing bacteria.

Major points of discussion

- *Klebsiella pneumoniae* and *Escherichia coli* are the two most common ESBL-producing bacteria.
- Cephamycins, such as cefoxitin and cefotetan, are not affected by ESBL-producing bacteria.

- ESBL enzymes are plasmid encoded and, therefore, are easily transferable among different bacteria.
- Hospitalized patients who are infected with ESBL-producing bacteria are placed on contact isolation to minimize the risk of transmission to other patients.
- Studies suggest that infections caused by ESBL isolates are associated with increased morbidity and mortality compared with infections caused by non–ESBL-producing organisms.[55]

4. A. *Staphylococcus aureus.*
Rationale: The figure depicts round, gram-positive cocci in clusters. A specific identification test is required to report *S. aureus* as the pathogen.

B. Coagulase-negative staphylococci.
Rationale: The figure depicts gram-positive cocci in clusters. A specific identification test is required to report coagulase-negative staphylococci as the organism.

C. *Streptococcus pneumoniae.*
Rationale: The morphotype of *S. pneumoniae* is lancet-shaped gram-positive cocci, predominately in pairs, but also in short chains. They do not appear in clusters.

D. Staphylococci.
Rationale: The figure depicts gram-positive cocci in clusters, which is consistent with staphylococci.

E. Enterococci.
Rationale: The morphotype of enterococci is gram-positive cocci in pairs and chains, not clusters.

Major points of discussion

- One blood culture set consists of two bottles (one aerobic and one anaerobic) obtained from one venipuncture site.
- Two to three blood culture sets, collected from separate venipuncture sites, must be drawn per septic episode.
- The bacterial morphotype consists of the shape, size, and arrangement of the microorganism (Table 16-1).
- All staphylococci, including *Staphylococcus aureus* and coagulase-negative staphylococci, appear as round gram-positive cocci on Gram stain.
- The accurate determination of the Gram stain morphotype can impact the choice of empiric therapy (see Table 16-1).

Table 16-1 Morphotypes of Gram-Positive Cocci

Microscopic Morphology	Suggestive of	Empiric Therapy
Gram-positive cocci clusters	Staphylococci	Vancomycin
Gram-positive cocci pairs and chains	Streptococci	β-Lactam antimicrobial agent
Gram-positive diplococci, lancet shaped	~~Staphylococcus~~ *Strep* *pneumoniae*	β-Lactam antimicrobial agent

5. A. The patient is likely to not respond to treatment with this antibiotic.
Rationale: The intermediate MIC interpretation does not necessarily predict treatment failure due to the ability of certain drugs to concentrate in the urine.

B. This antibiotic may be efficacious either at higher doses or if concentrated in the urine.

Rationale: Antimicrobial agents such as quinolones and β-lactams can concentrate in the urine, particularly with higher than normal dosing.

C. Antibiotics with intermediate interpretations cannot be dosed at therapeutic levels.

Rationale: The therapeutic dosage of antimicrobial agents depends on multiple factors, such as pharmacokinetic-pharmacodynamic data, host factors, and site of infection.

D. An intermediate result indicates a technical error and must be repeated using the disk diffusion susceptibility method.

Rationale: The intermediate category does not connote technical error, and whether repeat testing by MIC or disk diffusion should be undertaken is determined in consultation with the medical staff.

E. The intermediate category is interpreted as nonsusceptible.

Rationale: The nonsusceptible category is reserved for isolates for which only susceptible interpretive criteria have been designated by CLSI.

Major points of discussion

- MICs of antimicrobial agents are assigned as susceptible, intermediate, or resistant using interpretative criteria from CLSI based on usual dosage regimens, routes, and administration.
- Isolates that are initially susceptible can become intermediate or resistant after initiation of therapy; therefore, repeat testing of subsequent isolates from the same site may be warranted to detect the development of drug resistance.
- The category of "susceptible" implies that the isolate tested is inhibited by the usual achievable drug concentration, whereas the "resistant" category implies lack of inhibition or the presence of microbial resistance mechanisms.
- Antimicrobial agents that are used only for treating urinary tract infections should not be routinely reported against pathogens recovered from other sites of infection (e.g., nitrofurantoin).
- The most prevalent uropathogen causing uncomplicated cystitis and pyelonephritis is *Escherichia coli*. Hospital-specific antimicrobial susceptibility patterns of *Escherichia coli* should be considered when deciding on empiric therapy.[23,40]

6. A. HIV acquisition is highest in the presence of sexually transmitted infections that cause discharge.

Rationale: Genital ulceration has the highest risk of HIV acquisition due to the disruption of genital epithelium and recruitment of CD4 lymphocytes.

B. Nucleic acid amplification tests (NAATs) are the most sensitive and accurate methods for detecting *Neisseria gonorrhea* and *Chlamydia trachomatis* infections.

Rationale: NAATs improve the speed and sensitivity of *Neisseria gonorrhoeae* and *Chlamydia trachomatis* detection and allow for focused screening using urine specimens.

C. Dark-field microscopic examination is used to diagnose herpes simplex ulcerative genital lesions.

Rationale: Dark-field microscopy can be used to detect *Treponema pallidum* from the chancre of primary syphilis, with a sensitivity of approximately 80%.

D. *Haemophilus ducreyi* is the causative agent of lymphogranuloma venereum.

Rationale: Haemophilus ducreyi is the etiologic agent causing chancroid (soft chancre); in contrast, certain strains of *Chlamydia trachomatis* cause lymphogranuloma venereum.

E. Syphilis is currently on the rise in the adolescent population in urban settings.

Rationale: Syphilis rates have been increasing in the United States among HIV-positive men and men who have sex with men.

Major points of discussion

- *Chlamydia trachomatis* is the most prevalent etiologic agent causing sexually transmitted infections in the United States, followed by *Neisseria gonorrhoeae*.
- The most serious sequelae resulting from untreated *Chlamydia trachomatis* and *Neisseria gonorrhoeae* occur among women in the form of pelvic inflammatory disease, ectopic pregnancy, infertility, and chronic pelvic pain.
- Despite the decline of gonorrhea and syphilis in the United States, the prevalence of these sexually transmitted infections is increasing among men who have sex with men.
- Lymphogranuloma venereum is a systemic infection caused by invasive strains of *Chlamydia trachomatis* serovars L1, L2, and L3.
- Dual therapy of (ceftriaxone or cefixime) plus (azithromycin or doxycycline) for confirmed gonorrhea infection in adults and adolescents is recommended to also provide *Chlamydia trachomatis* coverage.[16]

7. A. *Streptococcus agalactiae* (group B streptococci [GBS]).

Rationale: Microscopically, GBS are gram-positive cocci in chains. These bacteria are also β-hemolytic on blood agar media.

B. *Chlamydia trachomatis*.

Rationale: C. trachomatis is an obligate intracellular bacteria that cannot be Gram stained and cannot be cultured on routine bacterial media.

C. *Listeria monocytogenes*.

Rationale: L. monocytogenes is a short gram-positive bacillus that is β-hemolytic on blood agar plates.

D. *Neisseria gonorrhoeae*.

Rationale: N. gonorrhoeae, a sexually transmitted pathogen, stains as gram-negative diplococci. It will not grow on blood agar plates and requires chocolate agar media for growth.

E. *Campylobacter jejuni*.

Rationale: C. jejuni presents as small, curved, faintly staining gram-negative bacilli with a characteristic "seagull" appearance. The bacteria are nonhemolytic on blood agar media.

Major points of discussion

- The natural reservoir of *L. monocytogenes* is the intestinal tract of humans and animals as well as soil and vegetable matter. The mode of transmission is via contaminated food, such as meat and dairy products. A unique characteristic is the pathogen's ability to replicate at refrigerated temperatures.
- *L. monocytogenes* exhibits transplacental transmission from mother to child, leading to stillbirth or premature delivery. To prevent infection, immunocompromised hosts and pregnant women should avoid eating soft cheeses, cold cuts, or undercooked hot dogs.
- *L. monocytogenes* has characteristic tumbling motility, exhibiting an umbrella-shaped pattern after overnight

incubation of a culture-stabbed tube of semisolid agar at room temperature. It is catalase positive and esculin positive.

- Therapeutic options for treating infections with *Listeria* include ampicillin or penicillin, with or without an aminoglycoside. Because antimicrobial resistance to the antimicrobial agents of choice has not occurred, routine susceptibility testing is not performed by the laboratory.
- The pathogenesis of *L. monocytogenes* is associated with virulence factors, such as actin to move within and between cells, hemolysins, and membrane proteins called internalins that mediate cell adherence and invasion.[52,61]

8. A. *Moraxella catarrhalis.*
Rationale: M. catarrhalis appear as gram-negative diplococci (i.e., in pairs), but rarely causes meningitis.
B. *Haemophilus influenza.*
Rationale: H. influenzae is a gram-negative coccobacillary pathogen that does not appear in pairs
C. *Streptococcus pneumoniae.*
Rationale: S. pneumoniae are gram-positive cocci, presenting on Gram stain as diplococci and short chains.
D. *Neisseria meningitides.*
Rationale: N. meningitides are gram-negative diplococci and can cause severe meningitis.
E. *Listeria monocytogenes.*
Rationale: L. monocytogenes is a gram-positive bacillus.

Major points of discussion

- Six capsular groups of *N. meningitidis* (A, B, C, W-135, X, and Y) are associated with invasive disease. Group A organisms, and less often those of group X, predominantly cause epidemics in Central Africa (the "meningitis belt"), whereas groups B, C, and W-135 commonly cause disease in industrialized nations.
- The human nasopharynx is the only known reservoir for *N. meningitidis* (meningococci). Transmission occurs via contaminated respiratory droplets in settings of close contact.
- A quadrivalent vaccine targeting the polysaccharide capsular antigens of *N. meningitidis* serogroups A, C, Y, and W135 is recommended in the United States for military recruits, asplenic patients, children older than 2 years, freshmen in college, incarcerated individuals, and laboratory workers. The current vaccine does not cover *N. meningitidis* group B due to the poor immunogenicity of its capsule.
- Chemoprophylaxis with rifampin, ciprofloxacin, or ceftriaxone is indicated for close contacts of patients with meningococcal meningitis.
- *N. meningitidis* can be identified using culture by sugar fermentation of glucose and maltose, and by serotyping for specific capsular antigen types.
- Treatment for meningococcal meningitis includes penicillin G, cephalosporins, chloramphenicol, and rifampin.[6]

9. A. *Streptobacillus moniliformis.*
Rationale: S. moniliformis is a fastidious gram-negative rod that requires extended incubation periods to culture. It is the etiologic agent of rat-bite fever and the symptoms do not

include lymphadenopathy. The diagnosis is made by culture.
B. *Borrelia burgdorferi.*
Rationale: B. burgdorferi is the etiologic agent of Lyme disease and is diagnosed using serology. It is transmitted by deer tick bites and causes an acute migrating erythematous rash but not lymphadenopathy.
C. *Coxiella burnetii.*
Rationale: C. burnetii (the Q fever agent) is a cause of culture-negative endocarditis. The diagnosis is based on serologic tests. It usually occurs in persons with exposure to cattle, such as farmers and veterinarians, and does not cause lymphadenopathy.
D. *Bartonella henselae.*
Rationale: B. henselae is the cause of cat-scratch disease and is usually transmitted from kittens to children younger than 18 years. It is difficult to culture in the laboratory, even with extended incubation periods. The diagnosis is based on elevated Bartonella titers by serology.
E. *Mycobacterium haemophilum.*
Rationale: M. haemophilum is a common cause of cervical lymphadenitis in children. However, this tissue usually shows the presence of AFB and the organism is easily cultured in the laboratory.

Major points of discussion

- *B. henselae* is a gram-negative bacillus that causes intraerythrocytic bacteremia in cats (the reservoir host) and is the most common *Bartonella* infection of humans worldwide. The spectrum of disease includes cat scratch disease, endocarditis, bacillary angiomatosis, and neuroretinitis. It is transmitted to humans by cat scratch or bite and, possibly, by cat flea bites.
- Classic cat scratch disease begins with an erythematous papule at the infected site and is characterized by fever and cervical or axillary lymphadenopathy that may suppurate.
- Uncomplicated cat scratch disease usually resolves in 1 month and is often treated with tetracyclines, macrolides, or aminoglycosides. Cat scratch disease may progress to infective endocarditis in patients who have a history of previous heart valve injury.
- Isolation of *B. henselae* is difficult because it is highly fastidious and often does not grow despite 2 to 6 weeks of culture. Diagnosis of infection is best confirmed by the serologic detection of antibodies in the patient's serum or by molecular detection of *B. henselae* DNA from the patient's tissues.
- A Warthin-Starry stain of infected tissue may demonstrate *Bartonella henselae* in chains, clumps, or filaments within areas of necrosis. Gram stains are usually negative.[5,26]

10. A. *Shigella sonnei.*
Rationale: S. sonnei causes severe inflammatory, often bloody, diarrhea accompanied by fever. It is most often contracted from contaminated water and vegetables, not beef. Growth characteristics on sorbitol-MacConkey agar plates are not diagnostic. Biochemical tests are required for identification.
B. *Shiga* toxin-producing *Escherichia coli.*
Rationale: Infection with *Shiga* toxin-producing *Escherichia coli* (STEC) manifests as bloody diarrhea and is commonly

contracted by ingestion of undercooked ground beef. Laboratory diagnosis includes failure to ferment sorbitol on sorbitol-MacConkey agar and a positive reaction with the EIA test for Shiga toxin.

C. *Salmonella enterica.*

Rationale: S. *enterica* causes bloody, watery diarrhea and is usually contacted from poultry, eggs, or peanut butter. The hallmark biochemical reactions that differentiate *Salmonella* from *Shigella* are hydrogen sulfide production and motility. Growth characteristics on sorbitol-MacConkey agar plates are not diagnostic, and *Shiga* toxin is not produced.

D. *Yersinia enterocolitica.*

Rationale: Y. *enterocolitica* causes watery, occasionally bloody, diarrhea, following consumption of contaminated water and undercooked meat, particularly pork. Cefsulodin-irgasan-novobiocin agar, but not sorbitol-MacConkey agar, is the selective media for growth. Shiga toxins are not produced.

E. *Campylobacter jejuni.*

Rationale: C. *jejuni* causes bloody diarrhea and is primarily transmitted by undercooked poultry or unpasteurized milk. MacConkey media will not support growth of this pathogen; campylobacter-selective agar, incubated at 42°C, under microaerophilic conditions is required. It is also *Shiga* toxin negative.

Major points of discussion

- STEC, previously called enterohemorrhagic *E. coli*, causes hemorrhagic colitis and hemolytic uremic syndrome (HUS). The incubation period for disease onset is 3 to 9 days.
- STEC is the main cause of infection-related renal failure in childhood and is associated with a mortality rate of 3% to 5%. In HUS, Shiga toxin is released in the gut, enters the bloodstream, and reaches the renal endothelium, where cellular damage occurs.
- The virulence factors produced by STEC strains include intimin adhesion and two Shiga toxins, Stx1 and Stx2 (also called "verotoxins"). The verotoxins are similar to the Shiga toxin expressed by *Shigella dysenteriae* serotype 1.
- Although the predominant serotype causing bloody diarrhea in the United States is O157, there are over 150 non–O157 STEC serotypes. The majority of non–O157 strains infecting humans belong to serotypes O26, O103, O111, O121, and O45.
- Unlike most O157:H7 STEC strains, the non–O157 *Escherichia coli* are able to ferment sorbitol on sorbitol-MacConkey agar. These non-O157:H7 samples that are Shiga toxin positive by EIA should be sent to the health department for serotyping.
- The appearance of stool specimens in acute diarrheal episodes is usually watery when pathogens with small bowel affinity are involved, such as *Cholera* spp., *Vibrio* spp., as well as parasites (e.g., *Giardia, Cryptosporidium* spp.) and viruses (e.g., Rotavirus, Adenovirus, Norovirus). Bloody diarrhea is characteristic of large bowel infections with STEC, *Shigella, Salmonella, Campylobacter,* and *Yersinia.*
- The key characteristics differentiating common pathogens causing foodborne diarrhea are found in Table 16-2.[30]

Table 16-2

Enteric Pathogen	Selective Growth Media	Key Reactions	Transmission
STEC O157	Sorbitol-MacConkey agar plate	Sorbitol fermentation with the O157:H7 strain	Undercooked beef, fresh spinach
Salmonella	MacConkey, Hektoen enteric agar	Motile, hydrogen sulfide production	Meat and poultry, undercooked eggs
Shigella	MacConkey, Hektoen enteric agar	Nonmotile	Contaminated water
Campylobacter	Charcoal-based media, Campy-CVA (antibiotics)	Gram stain: curved, gull-shaped; microaerophilic growth (high nitrogen)	Undercooked poultry, unpasteurized milk
Yersinia enterocolitica	MacConkey incubated 25-28°C, Cefsulodin-Irgasan-novobiocin agar	Growth at lower temperatures	Swine and cattle
Vibrio para-haemolyticus	TCBS agar	Salt-containing selective media (TCBS)	Seafood (oysters)

STEC, Shiga-toxin producing *E. coli*; TCBS, thiosulfate citrate bile salts sucrose.

11. A. *Francisella tularensis.*

Rationale: F. *tularensis* is a tiny coccobacillary pathogen that is designated as a select agent. This pathogen will only grow on chocolate agar or charcoal-yeast extract agar. All specimen handling and preliminary tests must be performed under a biologic safety cabinet. It is oxidase and urease negative.

B. *Mycobacterium tuberculosis.*

Rationale: M. *tuberculosis* cannot be recovered from routine blood cultures and will only grow on media designed to cultivate mycobacteria. M. *tuberculosis* requires an average of 3 to 6 weeks to grow on solid media selective for mycobacteria.

C. *Brucella melitensis.*

Rationale: B. *melitensis* is a slow-growing coccobacillary rod that is designated as a select agent. Serologic tests to detect antibodies specific for *Brucella* are diagnostic. The pathogen must be handled under a biologic safety cabinet, and automated identification systems must not be used for identification. It is oxidase and urease positive.

D. *Bordetella bronchiseptica.*

Rationale: B. *bronchiseptica* is a coccobacillary rod that grows on MacConkey agar plates within 24 hours. It is primarily a respiratory pathogen that is not identified by serologic monitors of serum levels. It is oxidase and urease positive. It is not designated as a select agent.

E. *Haemophilus influenza.*

Rationale: H. *influenzae* is a coccobacillary rod that grows in 24 hours on chocolate agar, not blood agar plates. Serologic and tests are not used to identify the pathogen.

Major points of discussion

- Brucellosis is a chronic granulomatous zoonotic infection transmitted to humans though infected animals, consumption of raw meat or unpasteurized dairy products, or by inhalation. *Brucella* species most frequently causing infections are *B. melitensis* (sheep and goats), *B. abortus* (cattle), *B. suis* (pigs), and, rarely, *B. canis* (dog). The disease occurs in shepherds, abattoir workers, veterinarians, and dairy industry professionals.
- Brucellosis is one of the most common infections that can be acquired in microbiology laboratories though routine workup of cultures outside of biologic safety cabinets. Procedures that place microbiologists at high risk of contracting the infection include aerosol-generating procedures, such as vortexing, centrifuging, mouth pipetting, catalase testing, or sniffing culture plates.
- *Brucella*-exposed individuals that are classified as high risk are advised to receive postexposure prophylaxis, which consists of a regimen of doxycycline and rifampin for 21 days. The 2012 postexposure recommendations for frequency of serologic testing at the Centers for Disease Control and Prevention (CDC) on all workers exposed to *Brucella* include at baseline and at 6, 12, 18, and 24 weeks postexposure.
- Symptom surveillance of postexposure events includes daily fever checks for febrile illness and symptom watch over a 24-week period after the last known exposure.
- Slow-growing coccobacillary gram-negative rods can be considered presumptive *Brucella* species when the patient history and symptoms, particularly when coupled with travel to an endemic area, are consistent with brucellosis. An isolate can be considered as presumptive *Brucella* when there is slow, scant growth on chocolate and blood agar and no growth on MacConkey agar.
- Suspicious *Brucella* isolates test positive for oxidase, urease, and catalase, and these procedures must be performed in a biologic safety cabinet. Timely notification of the clinician and public health officials is mandated when a *Brucella* isolate is suspected. Automated identification systems must not be used with when *Brucella* is suspected. PCR technology for identification at the species level is available at public health laboratories.[29,53]

12. A. *Pseudomonas aeruginosa.*
Rationale: P. aeruginosa is an elongated gram-negative bacillus.
B. *Haemophilus influenza.*
Rationale: H. influenzae is a small gram-negative coccobacillary organism that does not cause wound infections and cannot survive in saltwater.
C. *Vibrio vulnificus.*
Rationale: V. vulnificus is a curved gram-negative halophilic bacillus that infects wounds on exposure to contaminated seawater.
D. *Campylobacter jejuni.*
Rationale: C. jejuni is a curved, comma-shaped, gram-negative bacillus that causes gastroenteritis and cannot survive in salt water environments.
E. *Pasteurella multocida.*
Rationale: P. multocida are small gram-negative bacilli that cannot survive in salt water and are associated with infected animal bites or scratches.

Major points of discussion

- *Vibrio vulnificus* is a small, curved, gram-negative bacillus that is oxidase positive, motile, and ferments lactose. It requires 6% sodium chloride for growth and grows well on thiosulfate citrate bile salts sucrose (TCBS) agar.
- *V. vulnificus* causes severe wound infections after exposure to contaminated salt water. It is responsible for more than 90% of *Vibrio*-related deaths in the United States annually. This pathogen also causes infections related to ingestion of raw oysters.
- In immunocompromised persons, especially those with chronic liver disease, *V. vulnificus* often infects the bloodstream and rapidly progresses to septic shock
- The virulence factors present in *V. vulnificus* include the presence of a capsule, elastolytic protease, cytolysins, and collagenase.
- *V. vulnificus* is highly susceptible to most antibiotics. Tetracyclines or aminoglycosides are the treatments of choice. There is no vaccine available for preventing this disease.[46]

13. A. *Enterococcus faecalis.*
Rationale: Although enterococci can appear in short chains on Gram stain, they are not β-hemolytic and not a common cause of neonatal sepsis.
B. *Streptococcus pneumonia.*
Rationale: Streptococci appear as lancet-shaped diplococci on Gram stain and are not β-hemolytic.
C. *Streptococcus agalactiae.*
Rationale: S. agalactiae, also referred to as GBS, appear as cocci in chains on a Gram stain of a positive blood culture bottle. GBS is β-hemolytic and is a common cause of neonatal sepsis.
D. *Staphylococcus aureus.*
Rationale: Staphylococci, which can be β-hemolytic, appear as cocci in clusters on Gram stain.
E. *Staphylococcus epidermidis.*
Rationale: S. epidermidis appear as cocci in clusters on Gram stain and are not a common cause of neonatal sepsis.

Major points of discussion

- Invasive GBS disease is the leading cause of infectious disease in infants. Early onset GBS disease is most commonly associated with sepsis, pneumonia, and meningitis.
- Maternal GBS colonization is one of the most important risk factors for early onset GBS disease in newborns because of vertical transmission from GBS-colonized mothers to their babies.
- Maternal GBS screening is performed at 35 to 37 weeks of gestation. Because the gastrointestinal tract is the natural reservoir for GBS and the likely source of vaginal colonization, both the vagina and the rectum are sampled for GBS screening.
- Studies have demonstrated that maternal intrapartum prophylaxis with β-lactam antibiotics significantly reduces the rate of neonatal GBS colonization and the incidence of early onset GBS disease.
- Antimicrobial susceptibility testing of GBS isolates is necessary for penicillin-allergic women who are at high risk for anaphylaxis because resistance to clindamycin, a common agent used in this population, is increasing among GBS isolates.

- Molecular-based polymerase chain reaction assays for detecting GBS in selective enrichment broth are currently recommended by the CDC because they are more sensitive than culture-based methodologies.[13]

14. A. Safranin.
Rationale: Safranin is used in the final step of the Gram stain and enables visualization of gram-negative organisms.
B. Iodine.
Rationale: Iodine is the second step of the Gram stain and serves as a mordant for the crystal violet.
C. Crystal violet.
Rationale: Crystal violet is the primary stain and the first step of the process.
D. Acetone alcohol.
Rationale: Acetone alcohol is a decolorizing agent that removes the primary stain from gram-negative bacteria.
E. Methylene blue.
Rationale: Methylene blue is not a component of the Gram stain. It is sometimes used to show bacterial cell morphology and to analyze stool specimens for the presence of leukocytes.

Major points of discussion
- The Gram stain is a differential staining procedure used for microscopic examination of bacteria. It can be used for direct examination of clinical specimens as well as bacterial growth.
- Bacteria are classified based on the Gram stain reaction. Gram-positive organisms appear purple or deep blue, whereas gram-negative organisms appear red or pink.
- The cell wall components of bacteria impact the Gram stain reaction. Gram-negative organisms contain large amounts of lipopolysaccharide, which is degraded by the acetone alcohol decolorization step, thereby allowing the crystal violet to be washed out of the cell.
- Although mycobacteria may not always be visible by Gram stain, they can appear as beaded gram-positive bacilli.
- Organisms that lack a cell wall (e.g., *Mycoplasma*, *Chlamydia*) cannot be visualized by the Gram stain.

15. A. 5% sheep blood agar.
Rationale: 5% sheep blood agar is a nonselective medium that supports the growth of all bacteria other than fastidious organisms, such as *Haemophilus influenzae*.
B. Chocolate agar.
Rationale: Chocolate agar is a nonselective medium that supports the growth of all bacteria, including fastidious organisms, such as *Haemophilus influenzae*.
C. MacConkey agar.
Rationale: MacConkey agar is selective in that only gram-negative bacteria will be recovered, and it is differential because the ability to use lactose can be determined by visual inspection of the colony.
D. Brucella agar.
Rationale: Brucella agar is nonselective and often used for recovering anaerobic bacteria.
E. Mueller Hinton agar.
Rationale: Mueller Hinton agar is used for antimicrobial susceptibility testing and is neither selective nor differential.

Major points of discussion
- Sheep blood agar is useful for visualizing and classifying hemolysis. Beta hemolysis is characterized by complete lysis of the red blood cells, whereas alpha hemolysis is incomplete lysis and results in a greenish zone around the colony. Gamma hemolysis is used to describe the absence of hemolysis.
- Chocolate agar supports the growth of fastidious organisms because hemin and nicotinic adenine dinucleotide are present in the medium as a result of lysing red blood cells during preparation of the agar.
- MacConkey agar contains bile salts and crystal violet dye, both of which inhibit the growth of gram-positive bacteria. It also contains neutral red dye, which enables lactose-fermenting gram-negative bacteria to appear pink and nonlactose fermenting bacteria to appear colorless.
- Media selection is dependent on the source of the specimen. Urine specimens will be inoculated onto sheep blood agar and MacConkey plates, whereas respiratory specimens will also include chocolate agar for recovering *Haemophilus* and *Streptococcus pneumoniae*.
- For purposes of quality control, bacteriologic media are categorized as exempt or nonexempt. Nonexempt media must be tested with a panel of predefined American Type Culture Collection (ATCC) organisms prior to use with clinical samples. This is used to verify that the expected reactions are observed. Exempt media do not require this additional testing; however, media must be visually inspected prior to use for cracks, contamination, even filling, no bubbles, and so forth.[25]

16. A. E*scherichia coli.*
Rationale: E. coli is indole positive and does not swarm on blood agar.
B. *Proteus mirabilis.*
Rationale: P. mirabilis is indole negative and swarms on blood agar. The "waves" of swarming can be appreciated in the figure.
C. *Pseudomonas aeruginosa.*
Rationale: P. aeruginosa is an oxidase-positive lactose nonfermenter that does not swarm on blood agar.
D. *Proteus vulgaris.*
Rationale: P. vulgaris is indole positive and swarms on blood agar.
E. *Serratia liquefaciens.*
Rationale: S. liquefaciens is indole negative and does not swarm on blood agar.

Major points of discussion
- *Proteus* species are members of the family Enterobacteriaceae, which includes other gram-negative bacilli, such as *E. coli*, *Klebsiella*, and *Serratia*. Some *Proteus* species are covered with flagella that act in concert to produce swarming motility on solid media.
- Elderly patients are at higher risk for *Proteus* infections, particularly catheter-associated urinary tract infections. *P. mirabilis* is the most common species isolated.
- *P. mirabilis* and *P. vulgaris* are both urea positive. Only *P. vulgaris* is indole positive, and only *P. mirabilis* is ornithine decarboxylase (ODC) positive.
- Although *P. mirabilis* has no intrinsic resistance to β-lactam antibiotics, *P. vulgaris* is intrinsically resistant to ampicillin, as well as to first and second generation

cephalosporins, due to a chromosomal β-lactamase. For *P. vulgaris*, quinolones (i.e., ciprofloxacin, levofloxacin) or trimethoprim-sulfamethoxazole are usually first line agents for therapy.

- *Serratia* species are common health care–associated pathogens. Indwelling urinary catheters are a primary mode of transmission. This genus has inducible β-lactamases, which confer resistance to third-generation cephalosporins. Therefore, quinolones (e.g., ciprofloxacin, levofloxacin) or trimethoprim-sulfamethoxazole are usually first-line agents for therapy.

17. A. Dexamethasone.
Rationale: Dexamethasone is an antiinflammatory steroid that is often used to treat autoimmune diseases. It would not be used to treat *C. difficile* disease.
B. Clindamycin.
Rationale: Clindamycin is a risk factor for the development of *C. difficile* disease and, therefore, would not be used as therapy for this patient.
C. Levofloxacin.
Rationale: Levofloxacin is a quinolone antibiotic that has no activity against *C. difficile*.
D. Fluconazole.
Rationale: Fluconazole is an antifungal agent that has no activity against *C. difficile*.
E. Vancomycin.
Rationale: Vancomycin is an effective antibiotic for patients with *C. difficile* infection.

Major points of discussion
- *C. difficile* is a gram-positive, anaerobic, spore-forming bacillus. It is the most common cause of antibiotic-associated diarrhea.
- *C. difficile*'s ability to form spores enables it to last in the environment for extended periods of time, thereby facilitating patient-to-patient spread if rooms are not properly cleaned.
- Toxigenic strains of *C. difficile* are associated with disease. Toxins A and B both contribute to the pathogenesis and clinical symptoms of *C. difficile* infection. Pseudomembranous colitis is pathognomonic for *C. difficile*. Nontoxigenic strains do not cause disease.
- Molecular assays, such as the polymer chain reaction, that detect either toxin A or B are the most sensitive diagnostic tests. Culture is not clinically meaningful because both toxigenic and nontoxigenic strains will be recovered. EIAs should not be relied on due to lack of sensitivity for toxin detection.
- Depending on the severity of disease, patients with *C. difficile* infection are treated with either metronidazole (for mild to moderate disease) or vancomycin (for severe disease).

18. A. *Staphylococcus aureus*.
Rationale: *S. aureus* is an uncommon cause of upper respiratory infections; therefore, clinical presentation of infection does not include severe coughing.
B. Group A streptococci (GAS).
Rationale: Although group A streptococci can cause pharyngitis or tonsillitis, symptoms do not include paroxysms of coughing.
C. *Streptococcus pneumoniae*.

Rationale: *S. pneumoniae* causes sinusitis and lower respiratory tract infections. The pharynx is not affected; therefore, symptoms do not include repetitive coughing.
D. *Bordetella pertussis*.
Rationale: *B. pertussis* causes whooping cough, which is an upper respiratory infection characterized by a repetitive dry cough and gasping for breath. The site of infection is the nasopharynx.
E. *Moraxella catarrhalis*.
Rationale: *M. catarrhalis* causes otitis media or lower respiratory tract infections; severe coughing is not a symptom of infection.

Major points of discussion
- Pertussis is a highly contagious infection of the upper respiratory tract that is characterized by a paroxysmal stage with episodes of severe and violent coughing, described as "whooping," as air is rapidly inspired into the lungs past the swollen glottis.
- *Bordetella pertussis* is a minute, faintly staining, gram-negative coccobacillus. It produces several virulence factors, including adhesins and pertussis toxin.
- Real-time polymerase chain reaction assays are increasingly being used for detection and identification of *B. pertussis* due to their increased sensitivity compared with culture. Diagnosis is obtained by sampling the nasopharynx with rayon or Dacron swabs on plastic shafts because the pathogen binds to and multiples in the ciliated epithelial cells of the upper respiratory tract.
- *B. pertussis* can be isolated using the selective agar media Bordet-Gengou (potato infusion agar and sheep blood with cephalexin) or Regan-Lowe (charcoal agar with 10% horse blood and cephalexin). Growth is detected within 1 week of incubation at 35°C. A direct fluorescent antibody stain can be used to identify the pathogen.
- In the United States, children receive doses of the diphtheria, tetanus, and acellular pertussis vaccine (DTaP) at 2 months, 4 months, 6 months, 15 to 18 months, and 4 to 6 years of age. Erythromycin, clarithromycin, and azithromycin are preferred for treating pertussis in patients older than 1 month. For infants younger than 1 month, azithromycin is preferred for postexposure prophylaxis and treatment.[70]

19. A. ***Streptococcus pyogenes* (GAS).**
Rationale: *S. pyogenes* are β-hemolytic gram-positive cocci in chains that frequently cause pharyngitis. Acute glomerulonephritis can be a delayed sequela of infection.
B. *Streptococcus agalactiae* (GBS).
Rationale: GBS are β-hemolytic gram-positive cocci in chains that do not cause pharyngitis and are not nephritogenic.
C. *Enterococcus faecium*.
Rationale: *E. faecium* are α-hemolytic, gram-positive cocci in chains that do not infect the pharynx and do not cause glomerulonephritis.
D. *Streptococcus pneumoniae*.
Rationale: *S. pneumoniae* are α-hemolytic gram-positive diplococci that do not cause pharyngitis or result in glomerulonephritis.
E. *Streptococcus mutans*.
Rationale: *S. mutans* strains are α-hemolytic gram-positive cocci in chains that are found in the oral cavity and do not cause pharyngitis or glomerulonephritis.

Major points of discussion

■ The spectrum of disease due to GAS can be divided into superficial, invasive, toxin-mediated, and postinfectious diseases. GAS is the most common cause of bacterial pharyngitis and impetigo. Less common presentations include osteomyelitis, endocarditis, and severe neonatal infections.

■ Poststreptococcal glomerulonephritis (PSGN) is an acute inflammatory disorder of the renal glomerulus that is characterized by proliferative glomerular lesions. The disease is a delayed nonsuppurative sequela occurring 10 to 14 days after pharyngeal or cutaneous infection with certain nephritogenic strains of GAS. Rheumatic fever is another nonsuppurative complication of poststreptococcal infection.

■ Although the components of GAS involved in the pathogenesis of PSGN are not thoroughly understood, the type 12 M protein is thought to be important. In PSGN, antibodies against the bacterial components are deposited in the basement membrane of glomeruli. These immune complexes then activate an immune response leading to glomerulonephritis.

■ GAS are gram-positive cocci in chains, produce β hemolysis on blood agar, and are catalase negative and bacitracin susceptible. The pyrrolidonyl aminopepetidase (PYR) test is a rapid spot test that identifies both GAS and enterococci from culture. Rapid streptococcal antigen tests, which are performed directly from throat specimens, are often used in point-of-care settings. Due to the poor sensitivity of these assays, it is recommended that cultures be taken when results are negative. A DNA probe assay that uses nucleic acid hybridization for detection of GAS RNA directly from throat swabs is available, and Lancefield antigen grouping sera are used for type confirmation.

■ There is no specific treatment for PSGN. However, antibiotics, such as penicillin, should be used to treat active infections with nephritogenic strains and for prophylaxis of colonized family contacts.[10,47]

20. A. *Pasteurella multocida.*
Rationale: P. multocida, a causative agent of dog or cat bite infections, is a small, oxidase-positive, small, gram-negative coccobacillus.
B. *Capnocytophaga canimorsus.*
Rationale: C. canimorsus, often recovered from dog bite infections, is an oxidase-positive gram-negative, fusiform-shaped bacillus.
C. *Burkholderia pseudomallei.*
Rationale: B. pseudomallei, a small oxidase-positive, slightly curved, bipolar-staining, gram-negative bacillus, grows on MacConkey agar.
D. *Yersinia pestis.*
Rationale: Y. pestis is a plump gram-negative bacillus that can appear safety-pin shaped due to bipolar staining. It grows on MacConkey media.
E. ***Francisella tularensis.***
Rationale: F. tularensis is an oxidase-negative, small gram-negative coccobacillus that will not grow on MacConkey agar.

Major points of discussion

■ *F. tularensis,* the causative agent of tularemia, is highly infectious. Clinical manifestations of infection can be glandular, ulceroglandular, oculoglandular, systemic, or pneumonic. As few as 10 bacteria are sufficient to cause severe disease; therefore, any laboratory test must be performed within a certified biosafety cabinet and isolates sent to the state department of health or the CDC for definitive identification. Automated identification systems must not be used.

■ *F. tularensis* is a select agent considered to be a potential biologic threat that can pose a substantial risk to public health. It is therefore reportable to the state department of health and the CDC. The United States weaponized the pathogen between 1950 and 1960 during its offensive biowarfare program, and other countries are suspected to have weaponized it as well.

■ *F. tularensis* is a tiny, intracellular, faintly staining, gram-negative coccobacillus that is nonmotile and oxidase negative. It grows on cysteine-supplemented media, such as sheep blood agar, chocolate agar, and modified charcoal-yeast agar but will not grow on MacConkey plates. For definitive identification, a select-agent polymerase chain reaction platform, a direct fluorescent antigen test, and serologic assays are used.

■ Transmission of *F. tularensis* occurs through ticks, animal bites, cutaneous inoculation, ingestion, or handling infected animals. Human-to-human transmission does not occur. Tularemia remains widely enzootic to North America, Europe, and northern Asia. The incubation period is 2 to 10 days; mortality rates from untreated typhoidal and pneumonic forms of disease can be as high as 40%.

■ Treatment for tularemia includes administration of streptomycin, gentamicin, or doxycycline for 7 to 10 days. Penicillin and cephalosporins are not effective and should not be used to treat tularemia.[22,32]

21. A. *Shigella* spp.
Rationale: Species of *Shigella* cause gastroenteritis and invasive disease that are not transmitted by reptiles. They are H_2S negative and do not ferment lactose; therefore, colorless colonies grow on xylose-lysine-deoxycholate (XLD) and MacConkey media.
B. ***Salmonella* spp.**
Rationale: Several species of *Salmonella* can be transmitted via colonized reptiles, causing gastroenteritis and invasive disease. Colonies of *Salmonella* are black pigmented on XLD media due to H_2S production and colorless on MacConkey media, indicating nonlactose fermentation.
C. *Campylobacter jejuni.*
Rationale: Gastroenteritis and sepsis due to *C. jejuni* can be transmitted by farm animals or dogs, but not by reptiles. The pathogen cannot grow on either XLD or MacConkey media.
D. *E. coli* O157:H7.
Rationale: MacConkey media with sorbitol is needed for selection and differentiation of *E. coli* O157:H7 and not XLD. Gastroenteritis caused by pathogen transmission via cattle has been reported, but not via reptiles.
E. *Yersinia enterocolitica.*
Rationale: Although gastroenteritis due to *Y. enterocolitica* can be acquired from various animals, reptile transmission has not yet been reported. The pathogen is nonlactose fermenting and does not produce H_2S.

Major points of discussion

- Salmonellosis causes enteric fever by bacterial invasion of the bloodstream and acute gastroenteritis, resulting from foodborne infection or contact with colonized animals. Children younger than 5 years and immunocompromised individuals are at increased risk for invasive illness. Reptiles (e.g., lizards, snakes, and turtles) and amphibians (e.g., frogs, toads, newts, and salamanders) are commonly colonized with *Salmonella*, which are shed intermittently in their feces. Transmission occurs via unwashed hands after direct contact with the animals or their cages, or indirect contact from contaminated surfaces when animals roam freely throughout the home.
- Most *Salmonella* strains are motility positive, lactose negative, indole negative, urease negative, and H_2S positive. Commonly used selective media for *Salmonella* are Hektoen enteric, brilliant green agar, and XLD. Molecular platforms are being developed to detect *Salmonella* and other enteric pathogens through multiplex, real-time polymerase chain reaction assays.
- *Salmonella* strains may produce a thermolabile enterotoxin that bears a limited relatedness to cholera toxin. In addition, the pathogen produces a cytotoxin that inhibits protein synthesis and is immunologically distinct from Shiga toxin.
- *Salmonella* serotyping is based on the immunologic characterization of three surface structures: the O antigen, which is the outermost portion of the lipopolysaccharide surface of the cell; the H antigen, which is the filament protein of the bacterial flagella; and the Vi antigen, which is a capsular polysaccharide present in some serotypes. *Salmonella* serotypes *Enteritidis* and *Typhimurium* are the two most common in the United States.
- Recommendations are to treat most patients with uncomplicated *Salmonella* infections with supportive therapy and no antimicrobial agents. However, therapy such as quinolones (e.g., ciprofloxacin), third-generation cephalosporins (e.g., cefotaxime, ceftriaxone), or azithromycin are suggested if the infection has spread beyond the intestinal tract, if it is severe, or if the patient is immunocompromised.[15]

22. A. *Staphylococcus aureus.*
Rationale: *S. aureus* is slide and tube coagulase positive. Both the PYR and ODC tests are negative.
B. *Staphylococcus lugdunensis.*
Rationale: *S. lugdunensis* can be slide coagulase positive, but is tube coagulase negative. The PYR and ODC tests are positive.
C. *Staphylococcus epidermidis.*
Rationale: *S. epidermidis* is slide and tube coagulase negative, PYR negative, and ODC variable.
D. *Staphylococcus schleiferi.*
Rationale: *S. schleiferi* can be slide coagulase positive, but is tube coagulase negative. The PYR test is positive and ODC is negative.
E. *Staphylococcus haemolyticus.*
Rationale: *S. haemolyticus* is slide and tube coagulase negative, PYR positive, and ODC negative.

Major points of discussion

- *S. lugdunensis* can cause severe, aggressive infections, including endocarditis, sepsis, skin and soft tissue infections, and prosthetic joint infections. The overall mortality rate associated with *S. lugdunensis* endocarditis is high, with estimates from 50% to 73%. Its habitat is usually the lower extremities, particularly the perineum.
- *S. lugdunensis* expresses virulence factors similar to those of *S. aureus*, such as the ability to bind extracellular matrix proteins (e.g., vitronectin and fibrinogen). In addition, *S. lugdunensis* contains a virulence gene similar to the major regulatory determinant for virulence, the accessory gene regular (*agr*) of *S. aureus*. Biofilm formation plays a major role in the pathogenesis of *S. lugdunensis* infections, permitting attachment on implantable devices and providing protection from antibiotics and host immunity.
- Phenotypically, *S. lugdunensis* strains are catalase-positive, gram-positive cocci in clusters that can be either slide coagulase positive or negative but are usually tube coagulase negative. The PYR test is positive for *S. lugdunensis*, whereas *S. aureus* is PYR negative. The test for production of ODC is positive in *S. lugdunensis*, distinguishing it from the other coagulase-negative staphylococci.
- There are two tests to measure coagulase production: 1) the tube test, which detects extracellular free staphylococcal coagulase that converts fibrinogen to fibrin, and 2) the slide coagulase test, which detects the presence of cell wall bound "clumping factor." Due to the low sensitivity of the slide test for *S. aureus*, a negative result should be confirmed by the tube coagulase test. *S. lugdunensis* can be mistaken for *S. aureus* because it can test slide coagulase positive.
- Treatment of infections due to *S. lugdunensis* should be guided by susceptibility test results and severity of infection. They are more susceptible to antimicrobial agents than other coagulase negative staphylococci. The *mecA* gene is rarely present; therefore, methicillin resistance is rare. β-Lactam treatment is recommended over vancomycin whenever possible. Of interest, moxifloxacin is especially effective against the pathogen in biofilms.[37,57]

23. A. *Escherichia coli.*
Rationale: *E. coli* is an oxidase-negative, gram-negative bacillus that produces pink colonies on MacConkey agar, indicating lactose fermentation.
B. *Klebsiella pneumoniae.*
Rationale: *K. pneumoniae* is an oxidase-negative, gram-negative bacillus that produces pink colonies on MacConkey agar, indicating lactose fermentation.
C. *Acinetobacter baumannii.*
Rationale: *A. baumannii* is an oxidase-negative, nonmotile, small, gram-negative coccobacillus that produces colorless colonies on MacConkey agar, indicating that it is a nonlactose fermenter. These strains are multi-drug resistant.
D. *Stenotrophomonas maltophilia.*
Rationale: *S. maltophilia* is an oxidase-negative, motile gram-negative bacillus that that produces colorless colonies on MacConkey agar, indicating that it is a nonlactose fermenter.

E. *Pseudomonas aeruginosa.*
Rationale: P. aeruginosa is an oxidase-positive, motile, long gram-negative bacillus that produces colorless colonies on MacConkey agar, indicating that it is a nonlactose fermenter.

Major points of discussion

- *Acinetobacter baumannii* is an increasingly common nosocomial pathogen that causes ventilator-associated pneumonia, bacteremia, wound infections, urinary tract infections, and meningitis. The pathogen has been associated with outbreaks of bloodstream infections, osteomyelitis, and complicated skin and soft tissue infections in U.S. military and civilian personnel who were wounded while serving in Iraq and Afghanistan.

- *A. baumannii* is a nonfermentative, gram-negative, nonmotile, oxidase-negative coccobacillus. Its natural habitats are water and soil. Its ability to survive environmental desiccation for weeks contributes to its nosocomial transmission.

- The pathogenic determinants of *A. baumannii* include a novel pilus assembly system involved in biofilm formation and an outer membrane protein (Omp38) that causes apoptosis in human epithelial cells. Multiple pathogenicity islands have been found containing genes implicated in virulence, indicating that this organism devotes a considerable portion of its genes to pathogenesis.

- *A. baumannii* is highly resistant to antimicrobial agents and, at times, is pan-resistant due to its propensity to harbor diverse drug resistance mechanisms, including degradation enzymes against β-lactams, modification enzymes against aminoglycosides, altered binding sites for quinolones, efflux mechanisms, and changes in outer membrane proteins. Integrons containing resistance genes are common.

- *A. baumannii* infections are difficult to treat due to multidrug resistance. Carbapenems, due to their excellent bactericidal activity, are the most effective therapeutic option for treating susceptible strains. Among the β-lactamase inhibitors, sulbactam has the greatest intrinsic bactericidal activity. Amikacin and tobramycin appear to retain activity against many strains, but can only be used in combination therapy. Polymyxins are reserved for highly drug-resistant isolates and are used only in combination with rifampin or a carbapenem.[35,51]

24. A. 16S rRNA gene sequencing.
Rationale: 16S rRNA gene sequencing uses amplification of a targeted genetic region and specific primers to identify microorganisms but is not used to determine strain relatedness.
B. Staphylococcal cassette chromosome *mec* (SCC*mec*).
Rationale: SCC*mec*, which is the DNA cassette carrying the *mecA* gene determinant for methicillin resistance in staphylococci, has seven variants and various subtypes. SCC*mec* detection does not determine strain relatedness for epidemiologic purposes.
C. Peptide nucleic acid fluorescent in situ hybridization.
Rationale: Peptide nucleic acid fluorescent in situ hybridization uses specific probes to hybridize targeted

sequences for microbial identification, but this method cannot be used for strain subtyping.
D. Pulsed-field gel electrophoresis (PFGE).
Rationale: DNA fragments from isolates are placed in adjacent agarose gel lanes and are separated by electrophoresis into distinct band patterns that are compared to determine strain relatedness.
E. Matrix-assisted laser desorption/ionization time of flight (MALDI-TOF) mass spectrometry.
Rationale: In MALDI-TOF mass spectrometry, proteomics can be used for microbial identification and differentiation of microbial subtypes within a species but lack the discriminatory power to determine strain relatedness.

Major points of discussion

- Molecular strain typing methods in a hospital setting are most often applied to determine whether a cluster of infections in a particular medical unit is caused by a single clone or multiple strains. This technique directly impacts the successful control, prevention, and containment of hospital-acquired outbreaks through appropriate infection control interventions, such as patient cohorting.

- PFGE is the gold standard for genotypic microbial strain typing. In PFGE large DNA fragments (40 kb to 2000 kb) are generated by restriction endonuclease digestion of chromosomal DNA within agarose plugs. After plugs are added to an agarose gel, they are subjected to an apparatus with pulsed electric fields that separates the fragments into distinct patterns with resolution and number of bands amenable for accurate strain subtyping results.

- An essential feature of a successful molecular strain-typing test is high discriminatory power, which is the ability to generate distinct and discrete units of genetic information from different isolates at the subspecies level. Additional limiting factors are reproducibility, ease of use, and cost.

- Restriction endonucleases select unique nucleotide sequences and cut the microbial genome at specific recognition sites; therefore, they are highly pathogen specific (e.g., *SmaI* for *S. aureus*). They must produce DNA fragments in optimal numbers to generate assay results of high discrimination and resolution.

- Other molecular genotyping methods include random amplification of polymorphic DNA, multilocus sequence typing, restriction fragment length polymorphism, and amplified fragment length polymorphism.[38,71]

25. A. EIA.
Rationale: EIA testing is performed from genital samples and not urine specimens. It is less accurate for detecting *N. gonorrhoeae* than a NAAT.
B. Gene sequencing.
Rationale: Gene sequencing can identify bacteria from a pure culture. However, the assay sensitivity is too low to permit detection of *N. gonorrhoeae* from urine.
C. Cell culture.
Rationale: Tissue culture can be used to detect *Chlamydia trachomatis*, but not *N. gonorrhoeae*, from genital specimens only.

D. NAAT.

Rationale: Due to their high performance characteristics, NAATs are recommended for the rapid detection of *N. gonorrhoeae* from urine as well as genital specimens.

E. Gram stain.

Rationale: Gram stains of female vaginal specimens are not diagnostic for *N. gonorrhoeae,* even if gram-negative diplococci are observed, due to the presence of microscopically similar commensal flora. In addition, *N. gonorrhoeae* cannot be accurately observed from urine.

Major points of discussion

- Approximately 700,000 new cases of gonorrhea are diagnosed annually in the United States, second only to *Chlamydia trachomatis* infections as the most frequently reported sexually transmitted disease in the United States. Among women, gonococcal infections are often asymptomatic until complications, such as pelvic inflammatory disease, are recognized. Pelvic inflammatory disease can result in tubal scarring, infertility, and ectopic pregnancies.

- Commercial NAATs are available for detecting *N. gonorrhoeae* and *C. trachomatis* from urine, urethral, vaginal, and endocervical specimens. NAATs, which use polymerase chain reaction or transcription-mediated amplification technology, are recommended for detecting these pathogens due to their enhanced sensitivity and specificity, as compared with culture, and their ability to detect both pathogens in a single specimen.

- *N. gonorrhoeae* has several virulence factors involved in its pathogenesis: 1) pili, the adhesin that mediates attachment and stimulates phagocytosis, 2) outer membrane porin proteins that trigger phagocytosis, and 3) lipo-oligosaccharide surface proteins that contribute to the purulent response and to tissue damage.

- Except in pregnant women, test-of-cure, which is repeat testing 3 to 4 weeks after competing therapy, is not advised unless therapeutic compliance is in question, symptoms persist, or reinfection occurs.

- For treating uncomplicated urogenital, anorectal, and pharyngeal gonorrhea, public health laboratories recommend combination therapy with a single intramuscular dose of ceftriaxone (250 mg) plus a single oral dose of azithromycin (1 g). In 2007, emergence of fluoroquinolone-resistant *N. gonorrhoeae* in the United States prompted the CDC to no longer recommend fluoroquinolones for treatment. A recent trend toward increased cefixime MICs may result in a decline in efficacy.[16]

26. A. *Klebsiella pneumoniae.*

Rationale: *K. pneumoniae* is a lactose-fermenting gram-negative bacillus that is both oxidase and indole negative.

B. *Proteus mirabilis.*

Rationale: *P. mirabilis* is a nonlactose fermenting, gram-negative bacillus that is oxidase and indole negative.

C. *Acinetobacter baumannii.*

Rationale: *A. baumannii* is a nonlactose fermenting, gram-negative bacillus and is not a common community-acquired uropathogen.

D. *Pseudomonas aeruginosa.*

Rationale: *P. aeruginosa* is a nonlactose fermenting, gram-negative bacillus that is oxidase positive. It is not a common community-acquired uropathogen.

E. *Escherichia coli.*

Rationale: *E. coli* is a lactose-fermenting, gram-negative bacillus that is oxidase negative and indole positive. It is the predominant uropathogen causing uncomplicated cystitis.

Major points of discussion

- Urinary tract infections (UTIs) are the most common bacterial infection encountered in ambulatory care settings. An estimated 10% of women in the United States report at least one UTI per year, and the lifetime probability of infection is 60%. UTIs are also the most common hospital-acquired infection, primarily due to indwelling catheters.

- UTIs can be classified as asymptomatic bacteriuria, cystitis, and pyelonephritis, or simply as uncomplicated and complicated infections. The most frequent cause of uncomplicated community-acquired UTIs is *Escherichia coli* (75%-95%), but occasionally other uropathogens can cause infections (e.g., species of other Enterobacteriaceae, *Staphylococcus saprophyticus*, and enterococci). Complicated hospital-acquired UTIs are most often caused by *Pseudomonas, Klebsiella,* and *Proteus* species.

- Uropathogenic *E. coli* strains possess virulence factors encoded on pathogenicity islands that enhance their ability to colonize and infect the urinary tract. These virulence factors include fimbriae that bind to uroepithelial cells, siderophores that help gather iron from the host, hemolysins, and capsules.

- Enterobacteriaceae are a family of gram-negative bacteria that ferment lactose and are oxidase negative. They are routinely identified by semiautomated systems using miniaturized conventional biochemical tests. Rapid phenotypic methods, such as spot indole tests, can differentiate swarming *Proteus mirabilis* (indole negative) from *Proteus vulgaris* (indole positive). Differential agar media, such as MacConkey, can distinguish bacteria that are lactose fermenters (e.g., *E. coli, Klebsiella pneumoniae*) from non–lactose fermenters (e.g., *Proteus* spp., *Salmonella, Shigella*).

- First-line antimicrobial agents for treating uncomplicated cystitis due to uropathogenic *E. coli* strains include nitrofurantoin and trimethoprim-sulfamethoxazole. Rates of resistance to fluoroquinolones are on the rise.[40]

27. A. Bacterial vaginosis.

Rationale: Bacterial vaginosis (BV) is diagnosed by using the Nugent Gram stain criteria to determine a numerical score based on morphotypes and quantification of bacteria.

B. *Chlamydia trachomatis.*

Rationale: *C. trachomatis* is an intracellular organism that can be detected using cell culture or molecular amplification, but not Gram stain.

C. *Trichomonas.*

Rationale: *Trichomonas* is a parasite, not a bacterium; therefore, a Gram stain will not be diagnostic.

D. *Neisseria gonorrhoeae.*

Rationale: *N. gonorrhoeae* cannot be identified from vaginal discharge because commensal flora resembles that of gonococci.

E. *Candida albicans.*
Rationale: *Candida* spp. are fungi, not bacteria.

Major points of discussion

- BV is the most prevalent vaginal infection in women of reproductive age. It is associated with significant sequelae related to an increased incidence of pelvic inflammatory disease, mucopurulent cervicitis and endometritis, and increased risk of HIV acquisition. Acquisition is associated with sexual activity, either through transmission between partners or because sexual activity adversely impacts colonization with protective lactobacilli.

- The clinical diagnosis of BV is established when three of four Amsel's criteria are met: clue cells on vaginal microscopy, positive results on KOH amine testing, vaginal pH greater than 4.5, and a watery, "fishy" vaginal discharge. Clue cells are squamous epithelial cells densely coated with small coccobacilli.

- BV is a noninflammatory infection defined as an imbalance in normal vaginal flora as evidenced by a shift from predominately gram-positive lactobacilli to gram-negative anaerobic bacteria (e.g., *Prevotella* spp., *Mobiluncus* spp., *Gardnerella*, and *Bacteroides* spp.). It is hypothesized that vaginal lactobacilli play a critical protective role in the vagina by producing bactericidal and virucidal agents, including lactic acid and bacteriocins, which prevent overgrowth of pathogens and other opportunistic organisms.

- The gold standard for laboratory diagnosis of BV is the Nugent Gram stain classification. The Nugent score measures the numbers of lactobacilli, *Gardnerella* (gram-negative coccobacillary), and *Mobiluncus* (curved gram-variable bacilli) morphotypes in each oil-immersion field. A score of 0 to 3 is normal, 4 to 6 is intermediate, and 7 to 10 is consistent with BV.

- Treatment for BV includes metronidazole or clindamycin.[4,33]

28. A. *Bacteroides fragilis.*

Rationale: *B. fragilis* is an anaerobic, gram-negative bacterium that is the most frequent cause of intraabdominal infections.
B. *Enterobacter aerogenes.*
Rationale: *E. aerogenes* is not an anaerobe and is not a common cause of intraabdominal infections.
C. *Veillonella parvula.*
Rationale: Members of the genus *Veillonella* are predominant in the oropharynx, not the gastrointestinal tract. They are small, gram-negative, anaerobic cocci. They are not a common cause of intraabdominal infections.
D. *Pseudomonas aeruginosa.*
Rationale: *P. aeruginosa* is aerobic. It is not a common cause of intraabdominal infections.
E. *Escherichia coli.*
Rationale: *E. coli* is not an anaerobe and is not a common cause of intraabdominal infections.

Major points of discussion

- Anaerobic bacteria are a significant cause of life-threatening infections, including bacteremia, aspiration pneumonia, head and neck abscesses, pelvic inflammatory disease, sinusitis, intra-abdominal infections, and diabetic foot infections. A fetid odor, which is caused by the production of volatile short-chain fatty acids and amines, is a hallmark of anaerobic infections.

- Among the anaerobic gram-negative bacteria, the *Bacteroides* group are bile resistant; *Prevotella* are bile sensitive, pigmented and saccharolytic; and *Porphyromonas* are pigmented and asaccharolytic.

- Virulence factors produced by the anaerobes of the *Bacteroides* group include capsules, endotoxin, and succinic acid, which inhibit phagocytosis. Tissue destruction can be caused by various enzymes, such as collagenase, fibrinolysin, neuraminidase, heparinase, and hemolysins.

- Antimicrobial resistance of anaerobes is increasing; for example, approximately 97% of *Bacteroides* species produce β-lactamase, and resistance to clindamycin is on the rise. Anaerobes are naturally resistant to aminoglycosides and most quinolones. Resistance to tetracycline is prevalent.

- First-line therapy for anaerobic, gram-negative bacilli consists of β-lactam/β-lactamase inhibitor combination drugs (e.g., ampicillin-sulbactam, piperacillin-tazobactam), carbapenems (e.g., imipenem, meropenem), and metronidazole.

29. A. *Pseudomonas aeruginosa.*

Rationale: *P. aeruginosa* is a long, nonfermenting, gram-negative bacillus that produces a strong oxidase reaction within 30 seconds. This bacterium grows within 24 hours on routine media.
B. *Klebsiella pneumoniae.*
Rationale: *K. pneumoniae* is an oxidase-negative, lactose-fermenting, gram-negative bacillus that grows within 24 hours on routine media.
C. *Burkholderia cepacia* complex.
Rationale: The *B. cepacia* complex is a slow-growing, nonlactose fermenting, gram-negative bacillus that produces a weakly positive oxidase reaction.
D. *Acinetobacter lwoffii.*
Rationale: *A. lwoffii* is an oxidase-negative, nonlactose fermenting, gram-negative bacillus that grows within 24 hours on routine media.
E. *Stenotrophomonas maltophilia.*
Rationale: *S. maltophilia* is an oxidase-negative, nonlactose fermenting, gram-negative bacillus that grows within 24 hours on routine media.

Major points of discussion

- Cystic fibrosis (CF) is the most common life-shortening genetic disease among whites. The CF gene is located on chromosome 7 and codes for a chloride transmembrane regulator. CF is an autosomal recessive disease; therefore, the gene on both chromosomes must have a defect for the patient to be classified as having CF.

- Although *Pseudomonas aeruginosa* is the most commonly isolated organism in this patient population for all age groups, *Burkholderia cepacia* complex emerges as a pathogen in older teen and adult groups. The *B. cepacia* complex has a host of virulence factors; thus, acquisition of this organism by CF patients often leads to a rapid decline in health and sometimes death.

- The *B. cepacia* complex is composed of more than 17 genomovars that are phenotypically indistinguishable; therefore, all identifications are "presumptive" until molecular assays, such as 16S sequencing, confirm the identity. *B. multivorans* and *B. cenocepacia* account for more than 70% of strains recovered from CF patients.
- Members of the *B. cepacia* complex are slow-growing nonfermenters; therefore, they are difficult to isolate from the more rapidly growing organisms present in the respiratory specimen. Microbiology laboratories that process CF samples are required to use selective and differential media designed to inhibit growth of all bacteria other than the *B. cepacia* complex. Antimicrobials, such as vancomycin, polymyxin B, and gentamicin, are often used to suppress growth.
- The *B. cepacia* complex can be resistant to most antibiotics. There are no clinical trials to guide decision making; therefore, clinicians must assess each patient individually, taking into account in vitro antibiotic susceptibility data and previous clinical responses.

30. A. *Bacillus* species.
Rationale: Bacillus species stain as large gram-positive rods; the presence of spores can be observed. *Bacillus* species can also appear gram variable or sometimes gram negative.
B. *Streptococcus pneumoniae.*
Rationale: S. pneumoniae stain as gram-positive, lancet-shaped diplococci.
C. *Clostridium* species.
Rationale: Clostridium species stain as large gram-positive rods that can appear as "box cars." Certain species, such as *C. ramosum* and *C. innocuum*, appear to stain as gram negative.
D. *Corynebacterium* species.
Rationale: Corynebacterium species stain as small, gram-positive rods that group together in a palisade or "Chinese letter" pattern.
E. *Enterococcus* species.
Rationale: Enterococcus species stain as gram-positive cocci in pairs or short chains.

Major points of discussion

- There are more than 50 clinically relevant species of *Corynebacterium*. Because they are part of the normal microbiota of humans, the isolation of these bacteria from clinical specimens is not always medically significant. When evaluating positive cultures for determination of clinical relevance, factors to consider include demonstration of coryneform bacteria in the direct Gram stain, source of isolation (e.g., sterile body fluids), and, in the case of blood cultures, recovery from more than one set of bottles.
- *Corynebacterium* species will grow on routine blood-based agar media at 35 to 37°C within 24 hours. The characteristic Gram stain (e.g., with palisades) is very useful for preliminary identification.
- *Listeria monocytogenes* can also appear on Gram stain as short, positive rods (singly, pairs, or short chains). A catalase reaction can easily distinguish *Listeria* from *Corynebacterium*, the latter of which is catalase positive.
- There are several commercially available identification systems that can be used to identify coryneform bacteria (also referred to as diphtheroids) to the species level based

on fermentation and oxidation reactions and carbohydrate utilization.
- For treating systemic infections caused by corynebacteria, the physician must rely on antimicrobial susceptibility testing. Although many coryneform bacteria are susceptible to various agents (e.g., penicillins, macrolides, quinolones), certain species, such as *C. jeikeium* and *C. tuberculostearicum*, are more resistant. Oftentimes, removal of the indwelling device is also required.

31. A. Indole production.
Rationale: The indole test determines the ability of bacteria to split indole from tryptophan. It is useful for identifying many gram-negative bacilli, such as *Escherichia coli* and *Haemophilus influenzae.*
B. The PYR reaction.
Rationale: The PYR test detects pyrrolidonyl arylamidase activity in certain groups of bacteria, such as *Streptococcus pyogenes, Enterococcus* species, some coagulase-negative staphylococci, and some *Enterobacteriaceae.*
C. The oxidase reaction.
Rationale: The oxidase test for detecting cytochrome oxidase is used to identify *Neisseria* (oxidase positive) and to differentiate Enterobacteriaceae (mostly oxidase negative) from other bacilli, such as *Pseudomonas aeruginosa* and *Aeromonas* (oxidase positive).
D. The catalase reaction.
Rationale: The catalase test determines whether a bacterial species is able to convert hydrogen peroxide into water and oxygen. Staphylococci are catalase positive, whereas enterococci are catalase negative.
E. The hippurate reaction.
Rationale: The hippurate test, which determines the ability of bacteria to hydrolyze hippurate to glycine, aids in the presumptive identification of *Gardnerella vaginalis, Campylobacter jejuni, Listeria monocytogenes,* and GBS.

Major points of discussion

- Key biochemical reactions used to identify *Staphylococcus aureus* include the Gram stain (gram-positive cocci in clusters) and positive catalase and coagulase reactions. Colonial morphology, pigment production (light yellow), and β-hemolysis on sheep blood agar media also aid in the presumptive identification of *S. aureus*.
- Phenotypic reactions that aid in identifying staphylococci other than *S. aureus* include a negative coagulase test; a positive PYR test for *S. haemolyticus, S. lugdunensis, S. saprophyticus,* and *S. schleiferi*; and white, nonhemolytic colonies on agar.
- Key phenotypic reactions used to identify enterococci include the Gram stain (gram-positive cocci in pairs and short chains) and catalase negative, PYR positive, and α-hemolytic colonies on sheep blood agar media. Commercial systems are available to identify enterococcal species based on carbohydrate utilization. *Enterococcus faecalis* and *E. faecium* are the two most commonly encountered species.
- Selective and differential primary agar plates are available for the rapid identification of *S. aureus* and *Enterococcus* species. Mannitol salt agar incorporates mannitol and higher salt concentrations to enhance the growth of *S. aureus*, which will appear as yellow colonies on a light red agar. Bile esculin agar selects for the growth of

Enterococcus species, which appear as black colonies on a white agar.

■ Chromagar media, which are both selective and differential, are available for direct detection of *S. aureus* and MRSA from nares swabs and for direct detection of vancomycin-resistant *E. faecium* and *E. faecalis* from rectal swabs (Figure 16-29).

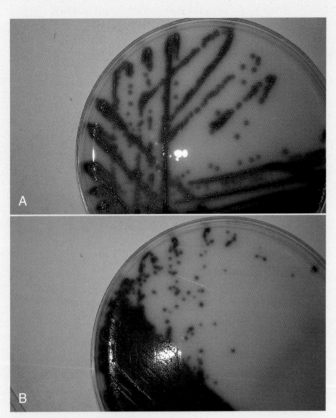

Figure 16-29 Plate morphology of colonies of vancomycin-resistant *Enteroccous faecalis* (**A**) and *E. faecium* (**B**).

32. A. CTX-M β-lactamase.
Rationale: The CTX-M β-lactamases belong to the ESBL group and, therefore, confer resistance to piperacillin, aztreonam and cefotaxime, but remain susceptible to ceftazidime. The treatment of choice is a carbapenem (e.g., meropenem, imipenem).
B. Metallo-β-lactamase.
Rationale: These enzymes hydrolyze all penicillins, all cephalosporins (including ceftazidime), and carbapenems (e.g., meropenem, imipenem), but are susceptible to aztreonam. They are often present in *Pseudomonas aeruginosa* and *Acinetobacter baumannii*.
C. Carbapenemase.
Rationale: Among the carbapenemases, the most common is *Klebsiella pneumoniae* carbapenemase. *Klebsiella pneumoniae* carbapenemase producers are resistant to all penicillins, all cephalosporins (including ceftazidime), aztreonam, and carbapenems (e.g., meropenem, imipenem).
D. AmpC β-lactamase.
Rationale: AmpC β-lactamases are cephalosporinases, hydrolyzing all β-lactam antibiotics except carbapenems (e.g., meropenem, imipenem) and cefepime. Strains are also resistant to cephamycins, such as cefoxitin. Gram-negative

bacteria that harbor these enzymes include *Serratia, Proteus, Acinetobacter, Citrobacter,* and *Enterobacter.*
E. ESBL.
Rationale: ESBL-producing bacteria are resistant to extended-spectrum penicillins (e.g., piperacillin), third-generation cephalosporins (e.g., ceftazidime), and aztreonam but remain susceptible to carbapenems (e.g., meropenem, imipenem) and cefoxitin.

Major points of discussion
■ ESBL-producing Enterobacteriaceae are a major problem worldwide. The most common ESBL-producing pathogens in the hospital environment include *Escherichia coli, Klebsiella pneumonia,* and *Proteus mirabilis.* Consequences of infections include increased length of hospital stay, increased hospital costs, improper antibiotic use, and increased mortality.
■ ESBLs are defined as β-lactamases that hydrolytically cleave the β-lactam ring, thus conferring resistance to the penicillins; first-, second-, and third-generation cephalosporins (e.g., ceftazidime); and aztreonam, but not the cephamycins (e.g., cefoxitin) or carbapenems (e.g., imipenem, meropenem). They are inhibited by β-lactamase inhibitors (e.g., clavulanic acid).
■ More than 300 types of ESBLs have been characterized, and they are often plasmid mediated. The first groups described were the TEM and SHV-types, and the cefotaxime-hydrolyzing CTX-M group, which are all present in *E. coli* and *K. pneumoniae*. These ESBLs groups were followed by the oxacillin hydrolyzing type present in *Pseudomonas aeruginosa*. The latest to be found is the Guiana extended spectrum group observed in *K. pneumoniae* and *P. aeruginosa*.
■ Detection of ESBL-producing bacteria is challenging. A confirmatory test is based on the principle that clavulanic acid restores the activity of either cefotaxime or ceftazidime, or both, for ESBL producers. If the MIC of ceftazidime and/or cefotaxime decreases by three or more twofold dilutions with clavulanic acid compared with the MIC for cefotaxime/ceftazidime alone, then ESBL production is confirmed.
■ Treatment with carbapenems, such as imipenem or meropenem, has demonstrated a high rate of clinical success among patients infected with ESBL-producing Enterobacteriaceae.

33. A. *Legionella pneumophila.*
Rationale: A rapid immunochromatographic assay is available for the detection of an *L. pneumophila* serogroup 1–specific urine soluble antigen. Special media are required for isolating Legionella in culture.
B. *Staphylococcus aureus.*
Rationale: There is no rapid urine-based assay for detecting *S. aureus*. In addition, routine bacteriologic cultures would have successfully recovered this organism.
C. *Haemophilus influenza.*
Rationale: There is no rapid urine-based assay for detecting *H. influenzae*. In addition, routine bacteriologic cultures would have successfully recovered this organism.
D. *Mycobacterium tuberculosis.*
Rationale: There is no rapid urine-based assay for detecting *M. tuberculosis*. Special media are required for isolating M. tuberculosis in culture.

E. Influenza A.
Rationale: There is no rapid urine-based assay for detecting influenza A. Rapid assays use nasopharyngeal aspirates or swabs to detect influenza A and B and respiratory syncytial virus. Influenza virus requires inoculating tissue culture cells and would not be detected in routine bacteriologic cultures.

Major points of discussion

- Legionellosis has two distinct clinical syndromes: Legionnaires disease, which manifests as severe pneumonia accompanied by multisystemic disease, and Pontiac fever, which is an acute, febrile, self-limited, viral-like illness. *L. pneumophila* serogroup 1 is responsible for 70% to 90% of cases of adult Legionnaires disease.
- Transmission occurs by means of aerosolization or aspiration of water contaminated with *Legionella* organisms. Wounds can become infected after contact with contaminated water. In adults, risk factors for legionellosis include cigarette smoking, alcoholism, and chronic lung disease.
- *Legionella* species are aerobic, motile, and nutritionally fastidious, pleomorphic gram-negative rods. Growth depends on using specialized media: buffered charcoal yeast extract agar, which contains L-cysteine and iron. Growth may take up to 7 days.
- A direct fluorescent antigen assay is commercially available detecting *Legionella* directly from respiratory specimens; however, cross-reactivity with other bacteria, such as *Pseudomonas aeruginosa*, limits the utility of this test.
- The choice of antibiotics used to treat *Legionella* infection includes those that can achieve high intracellular concentrations (e.g., macrolides, quinolones, ketolides, tetracyclines, rifampin) because the organism is often sequestered in macrophages. Quinolones, such as levofloxacin, are used most often. β-lactams and aminoglycosides are not clinically effective.

34. A. The patient result is invalid because urine was tested instead of a respiratory secretion.
Rationale: There are commercially available rapid devices to detect urine-soluble antigens for *Streptococcus pneumoniae* and *Legionella pneumophila* serogroup 1.
B. Patient results can be reported because this rapid device has a very high specificity.
C. Patient results can be reported because this rapid device has a very high sensitivity.
D. The result should be reported as negative because the control line is not present.
Rationale: Patient results cannot be released if the control line is absent.
E. The patient result is invalid because the control line is not present.
Rationale: For single-use devices, the control line serves as the positive internal control and the clear background serves as the negative internal control. Both controls must be acceptable for patient results to be valid.

Major points of discussion

- Regulatory agencies require that all new shipments and new lot numbers of reagents and kits must undergo quality control testing prior to use with clinical specimens.

If expected quality control results are not obtained, the reagents and/or kits are not approved for use.
- When performing quality control for kits and reagents, in addition to the controls provided by the manufacturer, previously characterized patient samples can be used to confirm acceptable performance.
- Expired reagents are not to be used to test clinical samples. It is important to be cognizant of the fact that individual kit components may have different expiration dates. The expiration date indicated by the manufacturer on the outside of the kit packaging must be adhered to.
- Kit components can never be interchanged. If an individual component is depleted, the entire kit needs to be discarded.
- Proper storage conditions must be maintained in order to ensure the integrity of reagents and kit components. The date that the reagent and/or kit is opened should be recorded on the container/box.

35. A. Optochin susceptibility.
Rationale: Inhibition of growth around an optochin disk (or P disk) is useful for presumptively identifying *Streptococcus pneumoniae*, which appears on Gram stain as gram-positive, lancet-shaped diplococci.
B. PYR reaction.
Rationale: The PYR test detects PYR activity in certain groups of bacteria, such as *Streptococcus pyogenes*, *Enterococcus* species, some coagulase-negative staphylococci, and some *Enterobacteriaceae*. The Gram stain for this patient is not consistent with any of these PYR positive bacteria.
C. Bacitracin susceptibility.
Rationale: Inhibition of growth around a bacitracin disk (A disk) is useful for identifying *Streptococcus pyogenes* (GAS), which appears on Gram stain as gram-positive cocci in chains.
D. X and V factor growth requirements.
Rationale: Growth of *Haemophilus influenzae* depends on the presence of X and V factors. Chocolate agar is an enriched medium and, therefore, supports growth.
E. Bile solubility.
Rationale: When colonies of *Streptococcus pneumoniae* are exposed to bile, the bacteria lyse and are no longer visible macroscopically or microscopically.

Major points of discussion

- Severe *Haemophilus influenzae* infections, such as meningitis, epiglottitis, and bacteremia have become rare since the introduction of childhood vaccination programs in developed countries. Less life-threatening infections that are common today include conjunctivitis, otitis media, sinusitis, and pneumonia.
- Rapid antigen detection assays directly from cerebrospinal fluid are available for *H. influenzae*, *Streptococcus pneumonia*, and *Neisseria meningitidis*; however, their sensitivity and specificity are lower than that of the Gram stain. Therefore, this test is discouraged and is not used by most microbiology laboratories in the United States.
- *H. influenzae* is a catalase-positive, gram-negative coccobacillary organism. Biochemical tests useful for differentiating the eight biotypes of *H. influenzae* include indole, ODC, and urease. A rapid porphyrin test can help distinguish *H. influenzae* from non–*H. influenzae* species.

- The requirement of X (protoporphyrin IX) and V (nicotinamide) factors for *H. influenzae* growth is commonly used for identification. The presumptive isolate is inoculated onto nonnutrient agar, X and V strips are applied, and the plate is incubated overnight. *Haemophilus* will only grow along the periphery of the strips containing both factors (also called satellite growth).
- For systemic infections, treatment with a third-generation cephalosporin is often warranted. For less severe infections, amoxicillin was previously commonly used; however, treatment failure due to the production of a plasmid-mediated β-lactamase became common. Therefore, the current treatment of choice is amoxicillin-clavulanate.

36. A. *Streptococcus* viridans group.
Rationale: Members of the *Streptococcus* viridans group are commensal oral flora and are not associated with bacterial pharyngitis.
B. *Haemophilus influenza.*
Rationale: Although the upper respiratory tract of some individuals may be colonized with *Haemophilus influenzae*, it is not a common cause of bacterial pharyngitis.
C. *Streptococcus dysgalactiae* **subspecies** *equisimilis.*
Rationale: Streptococcus dysgalactiae subspecies *equisimilis* is a common cause of pharyngitis in teens and young adults. The rapid strep tests are specific for GAS; therefore, culture is required for diagnosis of this organism.
D. *Streptococcus pneumonia.*
Rationale: Although the upper respiratory tract of some individuals may be colonized with *Streptococcus pneumonia*, it is not a common cause of bacterial pharyngitis.
E. GBS.
Rationale: Group B *Streptococcus* is not associated with bacterial pharyngitis.

Major points of discussion
- Beta-hemolytic streptococci have been classified as group A (*S. pyogenes*), group B (*S. agalactiae*), and groups C and G. Recently the large colony variants (>0.5 mm) of *Streptococcus* groups C and G were reclassified as *S. dysgalactiae* subsp. *equisimilis* (SDSE). These strains are pyogenic and often cause pharyngitis in adolescents. The small colony variants (≤0.5 mm) of groups C and G have been placed in the *S. anginosus* group, which are often harmless commensals that can occasionally cause abscesses.
- GAS remains the primary cause of bacterial pharyngitis, particularly in children. There are a multitude of rapid GAS antigen detection tests and they vary greatly in their performance characteristics. False-negative reactions may be related to poor sensitivity, inadequate specimen collection, or a low bacterial load at the site of infection. Therefore, it is recommended that negative rapid tests be backed up with culture. Culture also offers the advantage of detecting non-GAS causes of pharyngitis.
- SDSE is a common cause of upper respiratory tract infections and also infects skin and soft tissues, causing cellulitis, abscesses, and necrotizing fasciitis. SDSE shares many of the same virulence factors as GAS, including adhesions, pyogenic exotoxins, the M protein, and streptokinases.

- Other than colony size, SDSE strains can be differentiated from members of the *Streptococcus anginosus* group by a negative Voges-Proskauer reaction.
- SDSE isolates are uniformly susceptible to penicillin, which is the drug of choice. Severe infections may require the addition of an aminoglycoside; clindamycin is typically added for cases of toxic shock syndrome.

37. A. *Helicobacter pylori.*
Rationale: H. pylori is a curved gram-negative bacillus, but is difficult to culture and may take up to 1 week to grow. It is a major cause of gastritis and duodenal ulcers.
B. *Campylobacter jejuni.*
Rationale: C. jejuni, a causative agent of foodborne diarrheal disease, is a curved gram-negative bacillus and has been described as gull-wing shaped on microscopic exam. Growth requires microaerophilic conditions.
C. *Salmonella enteritidis.*
Rationale: S. enteritidis, a causative agent of foodborne diarrheal disease, is a gram-negative bacillus that can be recovered in 24 hours under routine incubation conditions.
D. *Cryptosporidium parvum.*
Rationale: Cryptosporidium is a parasite that has been associated with self-limited watery diarrhea. Use of a modified acid-fast stain is necessary to observe oocysts in stool specimens.
E. *Clostridium difficile.*
Rationale: C. difficile, a gram-positive anaerobic bacillus, is not associated with foodborne diarrheal disease. It is a primary cause of antibiotic-associated diarrhea.

Major points of discussion
- Globally, *Campylobacter jejuni* is the leading cause of foodborne bacterial diarrhea, putting it ahead of *Salmonella* and *Shigella*. Although many infected individuals remain asymptomatic, others develop watery or bloody diarrhea with ulcerations of the intestinal mucosa. Clinical features can last up to a week.
- *Campylobacter* species are part of the normal microbiota of birds. Up to 100% of poultry, including chickens, turkeys, and waterfowl, have asymptomatic infections in their intestinal tracts. The pathogen is primarily acquired from fecally contaminated water, unpasteurized milk, or undercooked poultry and meats. Transmission can also occur through cross-contamination of utensils and food preparation areas.
- *C. jejuni* is a slender, curved gram-negative bacillus with gull-wing morphology. It is microaerophilic, growing best on selective media, in 5% to 10% oxygen with increased carbon dioxide at 42°C for 72 hours. The pathogen displays characteristic darting motility and is oxidase, catalase, and hippurate positive.
- *C. jejuni* is thought to be a major cause of Guillain-Barré syndrome, a serious paralytic condition. Symptoms of Guillain-Barré syndrome usually occur 1 to 3 weeks after the onset of *Campylobacter* enteritis.
- Therapy for the diarrheal illness usually consists of fluid and electrolyte replacement. In cases of more severe disease, erythromycin and azithromycin are effective.

38. A. *Klebsiella pneumoniae.*
Rationale: K. pneumoniae is an oxidase-negative, lactose-fermenting, gram-negative bacillus that is the most

common KPC carbapenemase-producing pathogen. Emerging multi-drug-resistant strains exhibit resistance to all penicillins, all cephalosporins (including ceftazidime), aztreonam, and carbapenems (e.g., meropenem, imipenem).
B. *Pseudomonas aeruginosa.*
Rationale: P. aeruginosa is an oxidase-positive, nonlactose fermenting, gram-negative bacillus. It can be multidrug resistant due to metallo-β-lactamase production and porin mutations.
C. *Acinetobacter baumannii.*
Rationale: A. baumannii is an oxidase-negative, nonlactose fermenting, gram-negative bacillus that is frequently multidrug resistant. Among its resistance mechanisms are AmpC β-lactamases.
D. *Stenotrophomonas maltophilia.*
Rationale: S. maltophilia is an oxidase-negative, nonlactose fermenting, gram-negative bacillus that is inherently resistant to nearly all antibiotics. Susceptibility is limited to trimethoprim-sulfamethoxazole, Timentin, and fluoroquinolones.
E. *Serratia marcescens.*
Rationale: S. marcescens is an oxidase-negative, lactose-fermenting, gram-negative bacillus that produces AmpC β-lactamases that hydrolyze all β-lactam antibiotics except carbapenems and cefepime.

Major points of discussion

■ *Klebsiella pneumoniae* is a frequent cause of hospital-acquired infections. Pneumonia involves the necrotic destruction of alveolar spaces, formation of cavities, and production of blood-tinged sputum. This pathogen also causes sepsis, wound infections, and urinary tract infections.

■ Carbapenemases confer resistance to all β-lactamases, including carbapenems (e.g., imipenem, meropenem, doripenem, ertapenem), penicillins, monobactams, and cephalosporins. They are most commonly found in *K. pneumoniae*. Carbapenemases are grouped as molecular classes A, B, and D. Class A are predominantly KPC, which are found in *K. pneumoniae*, other Enterobacteriaceae, and *Serratia marcescens*. Class B comprise the metallo-β-lactamases, such as IMP, VIM, and SPM, which are produced by *Pseudomonas aeruginosa, Acinetobacter, Stenotrophomonas maltophilia*, and Enterobacteriaceae. The OXA carbapenemases are produced by *Acinetobacter baumannii*.

■ The production of KPC-mediated resistance can be illustrated using the Hodge (clover leaf) test. After an agar plate is streaked with a carbapenem-susceptible *E. coli*, an ertapenem disk is placed in the center and test organisms are streaked out from the disk. The figure shows inactivation of ertapenem by a KPC-producing *K. pneumoniae* (+), distorting the zone of inhibition of *E. coli*. KPC-negative organisms are also demonstrated (–), which show no distortion of the zone of inhibition of *E. coli*.

■ Hospital-acquired infections due to multi-drug-resistant strains are increasing with *A. baumannii, P. aeruginosa*, and KPC-producing *K. pneumoniae*. Therapeutic choices are severely limited with multi-drug-resistant pathogens, and they are often only susceptible to colistin/polymyxin B and tigecycline. In addition, infection control measures, such as contact precautions and, possibly, active surveillance testing, need to be implemented.

■ Polymyxin B and colistin (polymyxin E) are used to treat carbapenem-resistant bacteria, such as *K. pneumoniae, P. aeruginosa*, and *A. baumannii*. In vitro testing guidelines have not yet been set by the CLSI; however, the broth or E test methods are preferred over disk diffusion.

39. A. Staphylococcal protein A (*spa*), SCC*mec*, and *mecA* gene.
Rationale: The *spa* gene is specific for *S. aureus*. SCCmec is the genetic element carrying *mecA*, which is inserted by transposition into the *orfX* gene. The *mecA* gene encodes the protein conferring methicillin (oxacillin) resistance.
B. Staphylococcal Panton-Valentine leukocidin (PVL), *spa* gene, and *mecA* gene.
Rationale: PVL is a cytotoxin produced by the *lukS* and *lukF* genes associated with virulence in some strains of MRSA (e.g., the USA300 strain); it is not useful in detecting *S. aureus* species.
C. Staphylococcal protein A (*spa*), SCC*mec-orfX* junction, and *vanA* gene.
Rationale: Vancomycin resistance is carried by the *vanA* gene. It resides in enterococci and is not a marker for detecting methicillin resistance.
D. *nuc* gene, *mupA* gene, and *mecA* gene.
Rationale: The *nuc* gene has been used as a specific marker for *S. aureus*. However the plasmid-mediated *mupA* gene confers high-level resistance to mupirocin, not to methicillin (oxacillin).
E. SCC*mec-orfX* junction, *agr* gene, and *mecA* gene.
Rationale: The accessory gene regulator (*agr*) operon controls many virulence pathways in *S. aureus*. It has not been developed as a marker for identifying this species.

Major points of discussion

■ Methicillin resistance results from the acquisition of the *mecA* gene, which codes for the production of penicillin-binding protein 2a (PBP2a). PBP2a acts as a β-lactam resistant transpeptidase that causes resistance to the penicillins, cephalosporins, carbapenems, and monobactams. There is a latex agglutination test containing monoclonal antibodies for detecting PBP2a from pure colonies on agar media.

■ There are several SCC*mec* types and subtypes, each with a different genetic content. Larger elements, such as SCC*mec* types II and III, possess additional resistance genes that can confer resistance to erythromycin and/or the aminoglycosides and tetracycline.

■ In PCR-based assays, a *S. aureus* specific target (e.g., *spa* or *nuc*) that excludes other pathogens is essential. Other targets for assay incorporation include the SCC*mec* and the *mecA* gene. SCC*mec* is a mobile genetic element integrated into the *S. aureus* open reading frame (*orfX*) at the region that carries the methicillin resistance determinant *mecA*. Molecular assays for MRSA detection that target only the SCC*mec-orfX* junction without inclusion of the *mecA* gene can produce false-positive results due to SCC*mec* variants with missing or incomplete *mecA* genes.

■ Rapid, multiplex, PCR assays can detect MRSA infections within hours. Rapid identification of infected sites by direct testing from positive blood cultures, wounds/skin, and soft tissues can guide targeted antimicrobial therapy and can decrease lengths of hospital stay, health care costs, and morbidity, and mortality.

- The objective of nasal MRSA screening programs is to identify carriers to consider decolonization to decrease their individual risk of infection. For MRSA, carriers identified by screening should receive contact precautions or decontamination to decrease risk of infection and diminish the reservoir and risk of cross-transmission. Decolonization usually relies on intranasal mupirocin ointment, with or without chlorhexidine soap. However, widespread use of chlorhexidine and mupirocin could result in the emergence of resistance.[41,45]

40. A. *Acinetobacter baumannii.*
Rationale: A. baumannii, a lactose nonfermenter, produces pink colonies on MacConkey agar and is oxidase negative (colorless reaction on the strip). The commercially available strip for cytochrome oxidase production turns purple-blue when positive and is colorless when negative.
B. *Klebsiella pneumoniae.*
Rationale: K. pneumoniae, a lactose fermenter, appears pink and mucoid on MacConkey agar and is oxidase negative.
C. *Stenotrophomonas maltophilia.*
Rationale: S. maltophilia, a lactose nonfermenter, is oxidase negative.
D. *Pseudomonas aeruginosa.*
Rationale: P. aeruginosa, a lactose nonfermenter, grows colorless colonies on MacConkey agar and is oxidase positive as indicated by the purple-blue reaction.
E. *Escherichia coli.*
Rationale: E. coli, a lactose fermenter, appears pink on MacConkey agar and is oxidase negative.

Major points of discussion
- Burn patients are at risk for severe disease because their protective skin barrier has been compromised and their circulatory system is disrupted. In addition to *Pseudomonas aeruginosa,* other common pathogens recovered from burn patients include *Staphylococcus aureus, Enterococcus* species, *Acinetobacter,* and other members of the Enterobacteriaceae.
- *P. aeruginosa* are aerobic, motile, long, slender, gram-negative bacilli. Macroscopic features include flat colonies with a metallic sheen, β-hemolysis on sheep blood agar, and a characteristic sweet grape-like odor. *P. aeruginosa* can produce diffusible pigments resulting in colonies that appear green, red, yellow, or brown. Most *Pseudomonas* species are oxidase positive, with the exception of *P. luteola* and *P. oryzihabitans. P. aeruginosa* is unique among the more common species because of the ability to grow at 42°C.
- *P. aeruginosa* is an opportunistic pathogen that causes various infections, including ventilation-associated pneumonia, meningitis, malignant otitis externa, sepsis, endocarditis, osteomyelitis, osteochondritis, and folliculitis. Virulence factors produced by *P. aeruginosa* include exotoxin A (like diphtheria toxin) and cytotoxins.
- A mucoid phenotype of *P. aeruginosa* is prevalent in cystic fibrosis patients. This is due to overproduction of alginate. Other characteristics of mucoid *P. aeruginosa* include slow growth, loss of motility, and loss of pigment production.

- Treatment of burn wound infections includes debridement of necrotic tissue, early grafting, and pathogen-specific antimicrobial therapy. Effective antibiotics for *P. aeruginosa* include piperacillin/tazobactam, ceftazidime, and a combination of an aminoglycoside (e.g., tobramycin) with an anti-pseudomonal β-lactam, such as ticarcillin.

41. A. Agar B demonstrated a higher sensitivity of 96.8%.
Rationale: 96.8% represents the specificity, not the sensitivity, of agar B.
B. Agar B demonstrated a lower sensitivity of 90.8%.
Rationale: 90.8% represents the sensitivity of agar B; agar A, as the gold standard, detected more positives samples.
C. Agar B demonstrated a higher sensitivity of 96.0%.
Rationale: 96.0% represents the negative predictive value of agar B.
D. Agar B demonstrated a lower sensitivity of 95%.
Rationale: 95% represents the percentage of concordant results.
E. Agar B demonstrated a lower sensitivity of 92.6%.
Rationale: 92.6% represents the positive predictive value of agar B.

Major points of discussion
- Diagnostic tests vary in their sensitivity, specificity, and positive and negative predictive values. Therefore, validation of new assays by the microbiology laboratory is a critical component of the decision-making process. Factors to be considered, other than performance characteristics, include cost, turn-around time, space requirements, ease of use, and ease of interpretation.
- Sensitivity is defined as the proportion of individuals with a disease that are correctly identified by the test (i.e., the percentage of true positives [TP]). In this scenario, the total number of true positives using the gold standard assay (agar A) is $14 + 138 = 152$. To obtain the sensitivity, apply the following formula using the number of TP and false negatives (FN):

$$\text{Sensitivity (\%)} = [(TP)/(TP + FN)] \times 100$$

- Specificity is defined as the proportion of individuals without the disease that are correctly identified (true negatives [TN]). In this scenario the total number of true negatives using the gold standard assay (agar A) is $11 + 337 = 351$. To obtain the percent specificity, apply the following formula using the number of TN and FP:

$$\text{Specificity (\%)} = [(TN)/(TN + FP)] \times 100$$

- Positive predictive value (PPV) takes into consideration how many agar B positives were falsely positive. In this scenario: $138/138 + 11$. In a low prevalence population, the incidence of false positives is more likely. To obtain the positive predictive value, apply the following formula:

$$PPV = [TP/(TP + FP)] \times 100$$

- Negative predictive value (NPV) takes into consideration how many agar B negatives were falsely negative. In this scenario: $337/14 + 337$. High negative predictive values are essential for screening assays. To obtain the negative predictive value, apply the following formula:

$$[TN/(TN + FN0)] \times 100$$

42. **A. 0.5 McFarland inoculum, Mueller Hinton agar, ambient air incubation.**
Rationale: CLSI requires these conditions for susceptibility testing.
B. 1.0 McFarland inoculum, Mueller Hinton agar with 5% sheep blood agar, CO_2 incubation.
C. 1.0 McFarland inoculum, Mueller Hinton agar with 5% sheep blood agar, ambient air incubation.
D. 1.0 McFarland inoculum, Mueller Hinton agar, ambient air incubation.
Rationale: A 1.0 McFarland standard contains too many organisms. Mueller Hinton agar with 5% sheep blood agar is used for testing fastidious organisms.
E. 0.5 McFarland inoculum, Mueller Hinton agar, CO_2 incubation.
Rationale: Incubation must be under non-CO_2 conditions.

Major points of discussion
- Mueller Hinton is the agar medium of choice for antimicrobial susceptibility testing of nonfastidious bacteria. It demonstrates acceptable batch-to-batch reproducibility, contains minimal inhibitors that might affect test results (i.e., trimethoprim and tetracycline), and supports the growth of most pathogens. Other formulations of Mueller Hinton agar designed for fastidious bacteria include Mueller Hinton with sheep blood, *Haemophilus* test media, and a gonococci (GC) agar base with growth supplements.
- The standardized bacterial inoculum is 0.5 McFarland, which is equivalent to 1 to 2×10^8 CFU/mL. The use of overinoculated or underinoculated suspensions could adversely affect susceptibility results. False susceptible results are considered very major errors, whereas false resistant results are classified as major errors.
- All commercially available, semiautomated susceptibility platforms require that a set of defined quality control organisms be tested on a weekly basis. If expected results are not obtained, patient susceptibility results cannot be released.
- If a new antibiotic or antibiotic panel is implemented, susceptibility testing must be performed for 20 or 30 consecutive days. If no more than 1 out of 20, or 3 out of 30, MICs for each antibiotic/organism combination is outside of the acceptable range, quality control testing can be performed weekly.
- Some examples of why quality control may fail include use of quality control organisms not recommended by the manufacturer, improper storage, contamination, use of expired materials, incorrect inoculum, or clerical error. If the quality control failure cannot be resolved in a timely fashion, the decision may be made to withhold that antibiotic from clinical reporting and/or to find an alternative testing method.[22]

43. A. *Streptomyces griseus.*
Rationale: *Streptomyces* species produce chalky white colonies with aerial hyphae and appear as long-branching filaments but are gram positive and modified acid-fast stain negative.
B. *Nocardia cyriacigeorgica.*
Rationale: *N. cyriacigeorgica* is a gram-positive, partially acid-fast, filamentous branching rod that forms chalky white colonies with aerial hyphae and grows within 3 days.
C. *Rhodococcus equi.*
Rationale: *R. equi* are gram-positive, nonbranching coccobacilli that are modified acid-fast positive. They grow within 24 hours as salmon-pink colonies that do not produce aerial hyphae.
D. *Gordonia sputa.*
Rationale: *Gordonia* are gram-positive, partially acid-fast, short nonbranching bacilli that do not produce aerial hyphae.
E. *Mycobacterium fortuitum.*
Rationale: *M. fortuitum* is a weakly gram-positive, acid-fast positive bacillus that does not produce aerial hyphae.

Major points of discussion
- *Nocardia* are phylogenetically closely related to mycobacteria and ubiquitously found in soil and aquatic habitats. The majority of species (>30) are known to cause human disease, primarily pulmonary and disseminated infections of immunocompromised hosts and cutaneous disease in immunocompetent patients.
- Identification of *Nocardia* to the species level is important because of species-specific differences in pathogenicity and resistance to antimicrobial agents. Mortality rates may be as high as 50% in disseminated disease.
- *Nocardia* are best identified to the species level by molecular methods, such as sequencing of the *16S rRNA*, *hsp65*, *rpoB*, or *secA* genes.
- No controlled trials have been performed to determine the most effective therapy for nocardiosis; however, trimethoprim/sulfamethoxazole is considered the standard of therapy. For severe infections, amikacin is combined with this drug combination or with imipenem.
- The former *Nocardia asteroides* complex has been reclassified into the following clinically important species: *N. cyriacigeorgica*, *N. farcinica*, *N. abscessus*, *N. nova* complex, and *N. transvalensis* complex.[7,59]

44. A. *Prevotella intermedia.*
Rationale: Microscopically, *P. intermedia* are small, gram-negative, coccobacilli; colonies are black pigmented and fluoresce brick-red.
B. *Porphyromonas asaccharolytica.*
Rationale: Microscopically, *P. asaccharolytica* are tiny gram-negative, coccobacilli; colonies are black pigmented and fluoresce brick-red.
C. *Fusobacterium nucleatum.*
Rationale: Microscopically, *F. nucleatum* are long slender, gram-negative bacilli; colonies are white, rough, and bread-crumb like.
D. *Bacteroides fragilis.*
Rationale: Microscopically, *B. fragilis* are small, gram-negative bacilli; colonies are nonpigmented with concentric rings around the edge of the colony.
E. *Clostridium septicum.*
Rationale: Microscopically, *C. septicum* are pleomorphic, spore-forming, gram-positive bacilli that sometimes produce long, thin filaments. Colonies are β-hemolytic, are flat with irregular margins, and demonstrate swarming.

Major points of discussion

- In addition to *Fusobacterium*, other anaerobic bacteria associated with brain abscesses include *Peptostreptococcus*, *Prevotella*, and *Porphyromonas*. The major habitat of these anaerobic bacteria is the oral cavity, particularly around teeth and gingival surfaces, where there is lower oxygen tension and reduced oxidation-reduction potential. These organisms cause various infections, including pleuropulmonary infections, brain abscesses, chronic sinusitis, osteomyelitis, and septic arthritis.

- Proper specimen collection and transport are critical preanalytic factors to consider when anaerobic infections are on the differential diagnosis. Aspiration of the abscess fluid and immediate transfer to an anaerobic transport vial is required. Sampling the fluid or infected tissue with a swab compromises the recovery of anaerobes, which should be rejected as unacceptable specimens.

- Recovery of anaerobes requires special media and incubation conditions. Media types should include nonselective, selective, and enrichment (Table 16-3). Various methods are available for anaerobic incubation, including glove box chambers, jars, and pouches. The correct atmosphere for anaerobic incubation is 85% N_2, 10% H_2, and 5% CO_2.

- *Fusobacterium nucleatum*, the most common species found in clinical specimens, is relatively biochemically inactive. Most *Fusobacterium* species are indole positive, and *F. necrophorum* can be differentiated based on a positive lipase reaction. Molecular analysis may be necessary for identification to the species level.

- Penicillins are the treatment of choice for *Fusobacterium* infections. Alternatives include cephalosporins (such as cefoxitin and cefotetan), metronidazole, or clindamycin.

Table 16-3 Culture Media for Anaerobic Bacteria

Media	Type	Comments
CDC anaerobic blood agar	Nonselective	Supplemented with yeast extract, hemin, vitamin K_1, and L-cystine.
Anaerobic phenyethylalcohol blood agar	Selective	Phenyethylalcohol inhibits the growth of enteric bacteria that may be present in the specimen.
Anaerobic kanamycin-vancomycin blood agar	Selective	Kanamycin inhibits most facultative gram-negative rods and vancomycin inhibits gram-positive bacteria.
Anaerobic laked paromomycin-vancomycin blood agar	Selective	Paromomycin inhibits most facultative gram-negative rods and vancomycin inhibits gram-positive bacteria. Laked blood (i.e., freezing and thawing blood) allows early recognition of pigmented *Prevotella*.
Thioglycolate broth	Enriched	Supplemented with hemin and vitamin K_1.

45. A. GBS.
Rationale: GBS are β-hemolytic, gram-positive cocci in pairs and chains that infrequently cause urinary tract infections, particularly among men.
B. *Enterococcus faecium*.
Rationale: E. faecium is non–β-hemolytic and is a frequent cause of urinary tract infections in the elderly, particularly those that reside in long-term care facilities and hospitals.
C. *Staphylococcus saprophyticus*.
Rationale: S. saprophyticus is a uropathogen in adolescents and young adult women. The microscopic morphology is gram-positive cocci in clusters.
D. GAS.
Rationale: GAS is not a cause of urinary tract infections and is β-hemolytic on blood agar.
E. *Staphylococcus aureus*.
Rationale: S. aureus is a rare causative agent of urinary tract infections and microscopically presents as gram-positive cocci in clusters.

Major points of discussion

- Complicated urinary tract infections (UTIs) occur in patients with functional abnormalities (e.g., diseases of the urethra, bladder, or prostate) that impede urine flow or in those with indwelling urinary catheters. They also occur in hosts with altered defenses (e.g., the elderly, diabetics, renal transplant recipients) that predispose the patient to treatment failure or complications. Severe sequelae in patients with complicated UTIs include urosepsis, renal scarring, or end-stage disease. Most UTIs in younger women are uncomplicated, whereas those of older women are often complicated. Among men, uncomplicated UTIs are uncommon.

- The elderly are especially susceptible to acquiring complicated UTIs, particularly in nursing home or hospitalized settings. Geriatric patients with UTIs can be afebrile and can present with a wide range of symptoms, including hypothermia, nausea, vomiting, abdominal pain, or respiratory distress. The misdiagnosis of UTI in this population is high (20% to 40%).

- Detection of UTIs depends on urine culture. The current practice is to consider 10^4 to 10^5 CFU/mL of urine positive for a UTI. However, counts as low as 10^2 to 10^3 CFU/mL can be significant, particularly with pathogens such as *Staphylococcus saprophyticus* and enterococci.

- Enterococci are a frequent cause of UTIs among hospitalized patients and those residing in long-term care facilities. They are intrinsically resistant to antibiotics, including β-lactams, aminoglycosides, and vancomycin. Vancomycin-resistant enterococci are most common in *E. faecium*. Six types of vancomycin resistance genes (VanA through G and L) have been described; however, VanA is most prevalent. VanA-type vancomycin resistance is transferred via a transposon (i.e., Tn*1546*).

- Antibiotic therapy should be considered for any patient with symptoms of a UTI and a culture positive for a urinary tract pathogen, even as low as 10^3 CFU/mL. Removal of indwelling urinary catheters should be considered and antibiotic therapy should be guided by urine culture and susceptibility results. For uncomplicated UTI therapy, nitrofurantoin, fosfomycin, and fluoroquinolones are considered. For pyelonephritis and complicated UTIs, daptomycin, linezolid, and quinupristin-dalfopristin can be considered.[40,65]

46. A. NAATs and bacterial culture.
Rationale: Culture for *C. trachomatis* and *N. gonorrhoeae* from genital sites and urine are not indicated when NAATs are performed.
B. Direct fluorescent antibody tests and serology.
Rationale: DFA tests for *C. trachomatis* detection are not recommended due to low sensitivity compared with NAATs.
C. NAATs and serology.
Rationale: NAATs test for *C. trachomatis* and *N. gonorrhoeae* from both urine and vaginal specimens and serologic tests detect HIV.
D. Viral culture and serology.
Rationale: Culture for herpes simplex virus is not diagnostic for sexual abuse.
E. Gram stain and NAATs.
Rationale: The Gram stain from a vaginal discharge to detect *N. gonorrhoeae* is nonspecific in females. Although the Gram stain can be used to detect BV using the Nugent score, this infection is an inconclusive indicator for sexual abuse.

Major points of discussion
- The indications for testing children for sexually transmitted diseases (STDs) include physical signs or symptoms of an STD (e.g., vaginal discharge or pain, genital itching, odor, ulcers or lesions, and urinary symptoms); evidence of genital, oral, or anal penetration or an ejaculate; request by the patient or parent; a sibling or another child or adult in the household or the child's immediate environment who has an STD; or if a suspected assailant is known to have an STD or to be at high risk for STDs.
- CDC guidelines state that NAATs can be used as a more sensitive and accurate alternative to culture to detect *Chlamydia trachomatis* and *Neisseria gonorrhoeae* in vaginal specimens or urine from girls and urethral specimens or urine from boys. The NAATs must be FDA cleared and must test for two different molecular targets for each pathogen. Extragenital specimens (e.g., from the pharynx and anus), are not FDA cleared for testing for *C. trachomatis* and *N. gonorrhoeae* by commercially available NAATs. Therefore, cultures should be taken from these sites. All specimens should be retained for additional testing, if necessary.
- Pathogens diagnostic for sexual abuse include *Chlamydia trachomatis*, *N. gonorrhoeae*, HIV, and syphilis. *Trichomonas vaginalis* is highly suspicious for abuse, genital herpes is suspicious for abuse, and BV is inconclusive. Of note, only approximately 3% to 5% of prepubertal children evaluated for sexual abuse have an STD.
- With assault cases, *C. trachomatis* and *N. gonorrhoeae* must be tested for from any site of penetration or attempted penetration, using either an FDA-cleared NAAT or culture; *T. vaginalis* should be tested for by NAAT or culture.
- The culture sensitivity of *C. trachomatis* and *N. gonorrhoeae* in cases of child abuse is extremely low; 25% to 30% of *Chlamydia* and 5% to 10% of gonorrhea are missed by culture.[16]

47. A. *Gemella haemolysans.*
Rationale: Microscopically, *G. haemolysans* are gram-positive cocci in pairs and short chains. It is α-hemolytic on blood agar, PYR positive, LAP positive, and susceptible to vancomycin.
B. *Aerococcus urinae.*
Rationale: Microscopically, *A. urinae* are gram-positive cocci in pairs and tetrads. It is α-hemolytic on blood agar, PYR negative, LAP positive, and susceptible to vancomycin.
C. *Streptococcus pneumonia.*
Rationale: *S. pneumoniae* are gram-positive, lancet-shaped cocci in pairs. It is α-hemolytic on blood agar, PYR negative, LAP negative, and susceptible to vancomycin.
D. *Pediococcus acidilactici.*
Rationale: *P. acidilactici* are gram-positive cocci in pairs and tetrads. It is α-hemolytic, PYR negative, LAP positive, and resistant to vancomycin.
E. *Aerococcus viridians.*
Rationale: *A. viridans* are gram-positive cocci in pairs and tetrads. It is α-hemolytic, PYR positive, LAP negative, and susceptible to vancomycin.

Major points of discussion
- Infective endocarditis (IE) is an infection of the endocardial surface of the heart, which may include one or more heart valves. Fever is present in approximately 90% of patients with IE, and heart murmurs are heard in approximately 85% of patients. Other classic signs of IE include petechiae, subungual (splinter) hemorrhages in the nail beds, and Osler nodes (tender subcutaneous nodules on the finger tips).
- The bacteria most commonly associated with infective endocarditis include *S. aureus*, *Streptococcus viridans*, *Streptococcus-like organisms*, and enterococci. These pathogens have the ability to resist the bactericidal action of complement and possess fibronectin receptors for the surface of fibrin-platelet thrombi.
- To diagnose subacute IE, three to five sets of blood cultures should be collected over 24 hours. This will detect more than 90% of cases in patients who have not recently received antibiotics. For acute IE, three sets may be drawn over 30 minutes to document continuous bacteremia.
- The identification of *Streptococcus*-like bacteria to the genus level relies heavily on Gram stain arrangement, PYR, LAP, and vancomycin susceptibility. In addition to *Pediococcus*, other vancomycin-resistant bacteria in this group include *Leuconostoc* and *Globicatella*. It is often necessary to use 16S sequencing to identify these bacteria to the species level.
- Antimicrobial testing guidelines have not been established for many of the *Streptococcus*-like bacterial pathogens, such as *Aerococcus*. The empiric antimicrobial therapy of choice for infective endocarditis caused by these organisms is a combination of penicillin and gentamicin.

48. **A. Indistinguishable.**
Rationale: All four patient isolates showed identical restriction enzyme band patterns; therefore, they belong to the same clone.
B. Closely related.
Rationale: To be considered closely related, the band patterns would need to differ from each other by one to three bands.
C. Possibly related.
Rationale: To be considered possibly related, the patient isolates would need to differ by four to six bands.

D. Different.
Rationale: Isolates with more than six band differences are interpreted as distinctly different strains and, therefore, epidemiologically unrelated.
E. Inconclusive.
Rationale: When there are too many DNA fragments present on a gel, the patterns cannot be compared and no results can be reported.

Major points of discussion

- PFGE is the most common method used for microbial strain typing of nosocomial pathogens in a hospital setting. It is used in epidemiologic investigations to determine whether a cluster of infections in a particular medical unit is caused by a single clone or multiple strains. Detecting the outbreak source through strain typing can directly affect infection control practices, particularly patient cohorting and surveillance investigations, to prevent and contain hospital-acquired outbreaks and pathogen transmission.
- Isolates used for strain typing for epidemiologic investigations are obtained from patients or the environment defined by the infection control team. Strains that are indistinguishable (i.e., the same PFGE band pattern), closely related (i.e., differ by 1 to 3 bands), or possibly related (i.e., differ by 4 to 6 bands) are presumed to be derived from a common clone. The interpretation of the gel patterns must be made in concert with other clinical parameters considered in the epidemiologic investigation.
- In PFGE patterns, each lane represents an isolate recovered from a patient. Genetic profiles are obtained by digestion of chromosomal DNA with a restriction endonuclease that is highly pathogen specific. The PFGE patterns of isolates representing the outbreak strain will be indistinguishable from each other and distinctly different from those of epidemiologically unrelated strains.
- PFGE patterns can be altered by random genetic events, including point mutations and insertions and deletions of bacterial DNA. On the basis of fragment-for-fragment comparisons, each isolate's pattern is then classified for its relatedness to the outbreak pattern. Patterns that differ from the outbreak pattern by two to three fragment differences are considered to be closely related to the outbreak strain. Four to six band differences are considered to be possibly related to the outbreak strain.
- PFGE restriction fragment patterns can be analyzed by computer-assisted programs. These programs demonstrate enhanced capability of comparing DNA fragment patterns present on multiple gels. Investigators can create a searchable database of PFGE fragment patterns for interlaboratory comparison and to facilitate cluster analysis.[45,66]

49. A. *Vibrio vulnificus.*
Rationale: *V. vulnificus* is a gram-negative bacillus that can cause toxic cutaneous infections, which are not characterized by eschar formation.
B. *Bacillus anthracis.*
Rationale: *B. anthracis* is a gram-positive bacillus that is classified as a select agent. Cutaneous infections begin as a papule, resembling an insect bite, followed by vesicles that heal as eschars.

C. Beta-hemolytic *Streptococcus pyogenes* (GAS).
Rationale: GAS are gram-positive cocci in chains that commonly cause impetigo, alone or with *S. aureus*. Lesions present as multiple papules and pustules, not abscesses. They form crusts on healing, not eschars.
D. MRSA.
Rationale: Community-associated MRSA are gram-positive cocci in clusters causing subcutaneous infections that lead to necrotizing fasciitis with characteristic eschar formation.
E. *Staphylococcus lugdunensis.*
Rationale: *S. lugdunensis* are gram-positive cocci in clusters that can cause cutaneous infections that are not characterized by necrotizing fasciitis or eschar formation.

Major points of discussion

- Community-associated MRSA is the leading cause of skin and soft tissue infections in the United States. Community-associated MRSA differs from hospital-associated MRSA by the lack of traditional risk factors associated with hospital-associated MRSA, differences in bacterial virulence factors, and resistance to fewer antibiotics. Many community-associated MRSA isolates are resistant only to β-lactams and macrolides; however, resistance to other antimicrobial agents is increasing. These strains have caused outbreaks among prisoners, people engaging in athletic activities (football, wrestling), military recruits, and men who have sex with men.
- The predominant community-associated MRSA strains that cause serious infections in the United States belong to two major clones identified by PFGE; they are named USA300 and USA400 by the CDC. Some of the virulence factors expressed by these clones include Panton-Valentine leukocidin, variants of enterotoxins Q and K, and a high prevalence of α-toxin and enterotoxin B. Panton-Valentine leukocidin is an intracellular pore-forming toxin that induces polymorphonuclear cell death by necrosis or apoptosis. In addition, USA300 contains the arginine catabolic mobile element, which inhibits polymorphonuclear cell production.
- Suppurative skin infections can lead to necrotizing fasciitis, necrotizing pneumonia, severe sepsis, and Waterhouse-Friderichsen syndrome. Necrotizing fasciitis is a subcutaneous infection that tracks along fascial planes and extends well beyond the superficial signs of infection. Diagnosis is suggested by the following features: treatment failure, hard wooden feel of the subcutaneous tissue extending beyond the lesion itself, systemic toxicity with altered mental status, and skin necrosis.
- An eschar is sometimes called a "black wound" because the wound is covered with thick, dry, black, necrotic tissue. It can be observed in necrotizing fasciitis, cutaneous anthrax, and spider bites, particularly from the brown recluse spider.
- Primary treatment of simple skin and soft tissue infections due to community-associated MRSA includes incision and drainage, and possibly clindamycin or trimethoprim-sulfamethoxazole. Antimicrobial therapy, consisting of vancomycin, daptomycin, or linezolid, is indicated in cases of rapidly progressing cellulitis, abscesses in areas that are difficult to drain, septic phlebitis, and other severe infections requiring hospitalization.[50,58]

MYCOBACTERIOLOGY

50. A. Carbol fuchsin stain and the niacin test.
Rationale: Carbol fuchsin stains are recommended for detecting AFB in mycobacterial cultures. The niacin test is performed from growth on solid media.
B. Fluorochrome stain and NAAT.
Rationale: The fluorochrome stain is recommended for detecting AFB directly from specimens. NAATs can identify *Mycobacterium tuberculosis* complex from specimens.
C. Giemsa stain and liquid culture.
Rationale: Giemsa stains are not used for detecting AFB; liquid culture media does not provide a rapid assay.
D. Fluorochrome stain and nucleic acid sequencing.
Rationale: The fluorochrome stain is recommended for detecting AFB in clinical specimens. Nucleic acid sequencing cannot be performed directly on clinical specimens.
E. DNA probe assay and high-pressure liquid chromatography.
Rationale: DNA probe assays and high-pressure liquid chromatography are used to identify mycobacteria from culture and not directly from clinical specimens.

Major points of discussion

- Culture using both solid and liquid media is the gold standard for isolating mycobacteria. Biochemical tests, such as the niacin test, can be used to identify mycobacteria to the species level.
- NAATs for identifying *M. tuberculosis* complex must be performed in conjunction with culture and should be tested on acid-fast smear–positive respiratory specimens.
- DNA probe assays are commonly used to identify *M. tuberculosis* complex, *M. avium* complex, *M. kansasii*, and *M. gordonae* from acid-fast smear positive cultures.
- *M. bovis* and the vaccine strain, *M. bovis* bacillus Calmette Guerin (BCG), are members of the *M. tuberculosis* complex that should be differentiated from the other species in the complex, especially in initial isolates.
- Once growth is detected on culture media, mycobacteria can be rapidly identified to the species level by DNA probes, DNA sequencing, line probes, or high-pressure liquid chromatography.
- To screen for AFB in clinical specimens, fluorochrome-stained smears (examined under low power magnification) are recommended over carbol fuchsin stains, which require oil immersion. Increased sensitivity and rapid smear examination are the advantages of fluorescent stains.[27]

51. A. *Mycobacterium bovis*.
Rationale: M. bovis is a slow growing, nonchromogenic pathogen that grows on standard mycobacterial culture media at 37°C.
B. *Mycobacterium haemophilum*.
Rationale: M. haemophilum is a nonchromogenic, slow-growing pathogen that requires iron-supplemented media and incubation at 30°C for growth.
C. *Mycobacterium avium*.

Rationale: M. avium is a slow growing, nonchromogenic pathogen that grows on standard mycobacterial culture media at 37°C.
D. *Mycobacterium leprae*.
Rationale: M. leprae cannot be cultured in the laboratory by routine methods.
E. *Mycobacterium marinum*.
Rationale: M. marinum is a rapid growing, photochromogen that grows on all standard mycobacterial media at 30°C.

Major points of discussion

- In immunosuppressed patients, skin lesions are the most common presenting symptom of *M. haemophilum* infection.
- *M. haemophilum* is the second most common cause of lymphadenitis after *M. avium* in the pediatric population.
- Patients with *M. haemophilum* lymphadenitis are most often treated by excisional surgery of skin lesions followed by multiple antibiotics such as clarithromycin, fluoroquinolones, and rifamycin for 12 to 24 months.
- Pigment and growth characteristics are used to identify mycobacteria to the species level.
- Mycobacterial lymphadenitis in children can also be caused by *M. scrofulaceum*.[49]

52. A. *Mycobacterium abscessus*.
Rationale: M. abscessus is a rapid grower that usually causes skin and soft tissue infections or postoperative wound infections.
B. *Mycobacterium kansasii*.
Rationale: M. kansasii is a photochromogen causing pulmonary disease.
C. *Mycobacterium avium* complex.
Rationale: M. avium complex is a slow-growing nonchromogen, often causing chronic pulmonary obstructive disease with fibronodular bronchiectasis.
D. *Mycobacterium scrofulaceum*.
Rationale: M. scrofulaceum is a scotochromogen and is a rare cause of childhood cervical lymphadenitis and other clinical syndromes.
E. *Mycobacterium gordonae*.
Rationale: M. gordonae is a nonpathogenic scotochromogen.

Major points of discussion

- *M. avium* complex includes *M. avium* and *M. intracellulare* as well as several other less commonly isolated species.
- *M. avium* complex is the most common cause of nontuberculous mycobacterial disease, causing lymphadenitis (usually in children), soft tissue infections, and disseminated disease in immunocompromised patients, such as HIV patients with a CD4+ count of less than 50/μL.
- Patients exposed to *M. avium* complex present in recreational hot tubs may develop a hypersensitivity pneumonitis-like syndrome.
- The innate resistance to chlorination and ozonization compared to other nontuberculous mycobacteria may explain the high prevalence of *M. avium* complex lung disease.

- Fibronodular bronchiectasis of the right middle lobe and lingua is a frequently seen manifestation of *M. avium* complex disease in thin, elderly women. Cavitary lung disease involving the upper lobes, similar to pulmonary tuberculosis, can occur in older males with a history of tobacco or alcohol abuse.
- *M. avium* complex colonial morphology is distinguished from other nontuberculous mycobactcria as shown in the Table 16-4. It is a slow-growing, nonchromogen with detectable growth on solid media after 3 to 6 weeks and in liquid media after 1 to 2 weeks.[34]

Table 16-4 Runyoun Classification of Nontuberculous Mycobacteria

Runyoun Group	Classification	Growth Rate	Pigment Production
I	Photochromogen	Slow growing >7 days	Colony pigment production occurs after exposure to light
II	Scotochromogen	Slow growing >7days	Pigment production in colonies is independent of the presence of light
III	Non-photochromogen	Slow growing >7days	Nonpigmented colonies
IV	Rapid grower	Rapid grower <7 days	Mostly nonpigmented

53. A. A tuberculin purified protein derivative skin test is diagnostic for *Mycobacterium tuberculosis* when more than 10 mm of induration is seen.
Rationale: The purified protein derivative skin test is a screening test that is nonspecific and insensitive as a method of diagnosing tuberculosis. As such, it is not a diagnostic tool for identifying *M. tuberculosis*.
B. Culture on standard media used to isolate bacterial agents causing community-acquired pneumonia.
Rationale: This patient's specimens were AFB-positive and should be processed and identified by methods used in the mycobacteriology laboratory.
C. Cavitary lesions on chest radiographs, which are diagnostic of tuberculosis.
Rationale: The presentation of pulmonary tuberculosis as cavitary lesions on chest radiograph is most common among immunocompetent hosts; in contrast, pulmonary infiltrates predominate in the HIV/AIDS patient population.

D. **Culture on mycobacterial selective media, along with the use of DNA probes and biochemical tests.**
Rationale: Conventional methods for mycobacterial species identification from culture include the use of DNA probes and biochemical tests.
E. The use of NAATs identifying the *Mycobacterium avium* complex.
Rationale: NAATs for MAC detection directly from clinical specimens are not currently available for use in diagnosis.

Major points of discussion
- HIV-positive patients with CD4+ T cell counts of less than 200/μL usually present with pulmonary infiltrates and not with cavitary lesions on chest radiographs due to the inability of these patients to develop cell-mediated immune responses to mycobacterial infection.
- The tuberculin skin test, also known as the intradermal Mantoux or purified protein derivative test, is considered positive when an induration of 5 mm or more is seen in immunosuppressed individuals (e.g., HIV patients or organ transplant recipients).
- Key biochemical reactions that differentiate *M. tuberculosis* from *M. bovis* are niacin positivity, production of nitrate reductase, production of pyrazinamidase, and resistance to thiophene-2-carboxylic acid hydrazide. In industrialized nations, genotypic tests are replacing phenotypic methods for identification at the species level (Table 16-5).
- *M. avium* complex infection usually presents as disseminated disease in patients with HIV/AIDS with CD4+ T cell counts of less than 50/μL, whereas tuberculosis can occur in HIV-infected patients with higher CD4+ T cell counts.
- The primary drug regimen for treatment of tuberculosis is isoniazid, rifampin, pyrazinamide, and ethambutol. Whenever an isolate is resistant to rifampin or any two other primary drugs, then second-line drugs are used, including capreomycin, ethionamide, kanamycin, fluoroquinolones, amikacin, p-aminosalicylic acid, and streptomycin.
- Both broth and solid media are recommended for growth of mycobacteria. The most commonly used solid media include egg-based modified Lowenstein-Jensen tubes and agar-based 7H10 or 7H11 plates. Selective media containing antibiotics can also be used.[1,34]

Table 16-5 Conventional Methods for Identification of *Mycobacterium tuberculosis* complex

	L-J Colony Morphology	68°F Catalase	Niacin	Nitrate	Pyrazinamidase	TCH Susceptibility
M. tuberculosis	Rough	Negative	Positive	Positive	Positive	Resistant
M. bovis	Smooth	Negative	Negative	Negative	Negative	Susceptible
M. africanum	Rough	Negative	Variable	Negative	Positive	Variable
M. canettii	Smooth	Negative	Positive	Positive	Positive	Resistant

L-J, Lowenstein-Jensen; TCH, thiophene-2 carboxylic acid hydrazide.

54. A. *Trichophyton mentagrophytes.*
Rationale: *T. mentagrophytes* is a dermatophyte that causes ringworm (tinea corporis) on the dermis of the extremities and is contracted via contact with infected persons, pets, or farm animals. However, this pathogen is not acid fast and most commonly causes raised red rings with an area of central healing rather than numb macular lesions.
B. *Borrelia burgdorferi.*
Rationale: *B. burgdorferi* is the etiologic agent of Lyme disease; contact with deer and/or deer ticks is a known risk factor. Unlike the case described, this spirochete is not acid fast and causes an acute migrating erythematous rash.
C. *Treponema pallidum.*
Rationale: Secondary syphilis, caused by *T. pallidum* infection, presents as a maculopapular eruption rather than annular macules. *T. pallidum* is a spiral-shaped, non–acid-fast bacterium that is best visualized using dark field microscopy.
D. *Nocardia brasiliensis.*
Rationale: *N. brasiliensis* is a cause of sporotrichoid nocardiosis, a lymphocutaneous syndrome originating on the hands or arms. *N. brasiliensis* is a partially acid-fast, branching gram-positive bacillus and is readily cultured in the laboratory.
E. *Mycobacterium leprae.*
Rationale: Contact with *M. leprae*–infected nine-banded armadillos, commonly found in the southern United States, is a known risk factor for leprosy. *M. leprae* cannot currently be grown in the routine laboratory; tissue biopsies may demonstrate the presence of AFB.

Major points of discussion
- Leprosy (Hansen's disease) is a granulomatous disease affecting the upper respiratory tract and peripheral nerves. Untreated leprosy can result in significant morbidity and mortality. Disfigurement and permanent damage to the skin, nerves, limbs, and eyes are also possible outcomes.
- Skin lesions are the primary external sign of leprosy. It manifests as several forms, ranging from mild tuberculoid leprosy, to borderline forms (the most common), to severe lepromatous leprosy.
- The lepromin skin test is used to determine the type of leprosy. It involves the injection of a standardized extract of inactivated *M. leprae* under the skin. Patients with tuberculoid and borderline tuberculoid leprosy will have a positive skin reaction. It is not recommended as the primary mode of diagnosis.
- *M. leprae* can be present in high quantities in nasal secretions; human-to-human transmission most likely occurs via respiratory droplets. The average incubation period for leprosy is 2 to 5 years, but longer periods of up to 30 years from exposure have been reported.
- *M. leprae* is the main etiologic agent of leprosy, but a second, newly recognized species, *Mycobacterium lepromatosa*, is now recognized as a cause of diffuse lepromatous leprosy.

- *M. leprae* is an obligate intracellular pathogen that cannot be cultured in the laboratory. *M. leprae* can be propagated in nine-banded armadillos as a result of their lower resting body temperature (30 to 35°C).
- Treatment consists of a 12-month regimen of rifampin, dapsone, and clofazimine.[62]

55. A. *Mycobacterium canetti, Mycobacterium africanum,* and *Mycobacterium fortuitum.*
Rationale: *M. canetti* is not an nontuberculous mycobacteria (NTM); it is a member of the *M. tuberculosis* complex.
B. *Mycobacterium kansasii, Mycobacterium abscessus,* and *Mycobacterium avium-intracellulare* complex.
Rationale: *M. kansasii* is second to *M. avium-intracellulare* complex as a cause of NTM lung disease. *M. abscessus* is a rapid-growing NTM that causes more than 80% of pulmonary infections. *M. avium-intracellulare* complex are NTM that cause pulmonary disease, such as bronchiectasis.
C. *Mycobacterium avium-intracellulare* complex, *Mycobacterium microti,* and *Mycobacterium mucogenicum.*
Rationale: *M microti* is not an NTM but is a member of the *M. tuberculosis* complex.
D. *Mycobacterium chelonae, Mycobacterium africanum,* and *Mycobacterium scrofulaceum.*
Rationale: *M. africanum* is not an NTM but is a member of the *M. tuberculosis* complex.
E. *Mycobacterium gordonae, Mycobacterium bovis,* and *M. kansasii.*
Rationale: *M. bovis* is not an NTM but is a member of the *M. tuberculosis* complex.

Major points of discussion
- NTM, previously referred to as atypical mycobacteria, are often classified as either slow growing (>7 days) or rapidly growing (<7 days) in culture. Within these groups, NTM are differentiated by the presence or absence of pigment.
- The major reservoirs for NTM are water, soil, and animals. The majority are usually nonpathogenic in immunocompetent individuals. MAC is the most common environmental NTM that causes disease in HIV-infected individuals.
- NTM comprise over 130 mycobacterial species that are not within the *M. tuberculosis* complex. This complex includes *M. tuberculosis, M. bovis, M. bovis* BCG, *M. africanum, M. caprae, M. microti,* and *M. pinnipedii.*
- NTM can be identified to the species level by phenotypic characteristics, biochemical testing, DNA probes, nucleic acid amplification, or gene sequencing.
- CLSI recommends microbroth dilution for susceptibility testing. There are CLSI guidelines for testing *M. avium* complex, *M. kansasii, M. marinum,* and rapidly growing mycobacteria.[67]

56. A. **Interferon-gamma release assay (IGRA).**
Rationale: IGRAs are blood tests that detect interferon-gamma released from lymphocytes of individuals infected

with *M. tuberculosis*. False-positive reactions do not occur when testing BCG vaccinated individuals.

B. Purified protein derivative inoculation.

Rationale: The purified protein derivative test is a tuberculin skin test containing a sterile *M. tuberculosis* filtrate. The antigens present can result in false-positives with BCG-vaccinated individuals.

C. Chest radiograph.

Rationale: Chest radiographs are not used to diagnose latent tuberculosis. They are diagnostic tools used to evaluate the degree of active infection or disease in the lungs.

D. Adenosine deaminase assay.

Rationale: Elevated adenosine deaminase levels are found in pleural and pericardial effusions of patients with tuberculosis as well as other disorders. It cannot diagnose latent tuberculosis.

E. Galactomannan assay.

Rationale: The Galactomannan test is an EIA used to diagnose invasive aspergillosis, not latent tuberculosis.

Major points of discussion
- The IGRA is based on the principle that peripheral blood lymphocytes of individuals infected with *M. tuberculosis* will produce detectable levels of the interferon-gamma cytokine when exposed to *M. tuberculosis* antigens.
- The two currently available commercial IGRAs are an EIA (QuantiFERON TB) and an enzyme-linked immunospot test (T-SPOT). Both tests are unable to distinguish latent from active disease.
- The limitations of tuberculin skin tests include technical problems in administration and reading, the need for more than one visit, false-negatives due to anergy and reversion at old age, and false-positives due to BCG vaccination. The advantages of tuberculin skin tests include low cost, no need for special equipment, and a long history of clinical experience.
- Unlike tuberculin skin tests, IGRAs contain two or three *M. tuberculosis* antigens that do not cross react with BCG or *M. Avium* complex. However, these antigens can cross react, causing false-positives, with *M. kansasii*, *M. marinum*, and *M. szulgai*.
- Foreign-born individuals primarily develop tuberculosis through reactivation of latent infection, whereas most U.S.-born individuals develop disease through recent transmission.

57. A. *Mycobacterium tuberculosis*.

Rationale: *M. tuberculosis* is slow growing (>14 days) and rarely causes skin and soft tissue infections.

B. *Mycobacterium chelonae*.

Rationale: *M. chelonae* is a species of rapidly growing mycobacteria that can cause cutaneous infections. It is iron

uptake negative, uses citrate as substrate, and cannot grow in the presence of 5% NaCl.

C. *Mycobacterium abscessus*.

Rationale: *M. abscessus*, a rapidly growing mycobacteria species that can cause skin infections, is citrate test negative, and is tolerant of growth in 5% NaCl.

D. *Mycobacterium fortuitum*.

Rationale: *M. fortuitum* is iron uptake test positive. It is the only common rapidly growing mycobacteria species that is nitrate test positive.

E. *Mycobacterium szulgai*.

Rationale: *M. szulgai* is pigmented (i.e., scotochromogenic) and slow growing (>7 days).

Major points of discussion
- Rapidly growing mycobacteria are opportunistic pathogens that cause a wide spectrum of diseases, including pulmonary, disseminated, skin and soft tissue, bone and joint, ocular keratitis, otitis media, and catheter-related infections. Isolation from sterile sites, or multiple isolates from nonsterile sites, is an indicator of true infection.
- Rapidly growing mycobacteria are ubiquitous in the environment and may form biofilms. They are relatively resistant to standard disinfectants and are frequently found in tap water.
- Recognized tattoo-related sources of rapidly growing mycobacteria cutaneous infections include unsafe hygienic practices (e.g., the use of tap water to wash equipment or dilute ink) and ink contamination during the manufacturing process.
- Rapidly growing mycobacteria form mature colonies on solid agar within 7 days. Although they can be identified using phenotypic tests (Table 16-6), definitive identification is obtained by molecular methods (e.g., gene sequencing).
- Rapidly growing mycobacteria identification to the species level can affect therapeutic choice because of differences in intrinsic resistance. *M. chelonae* is generally susceptible to antibiotics to which *M. abscessus* is resistant (e.g., tobramycin, macrolides, and linezolid) while being resistant to antibiotics that are active against *M. abscessus* (e.g., cefoxitin and amikacin). *M. fortuitum* is susceptible to a range of antimicrobial agents with the exception of macrolides.[9,17]

58. A. Iron uptake.

Rationale: Iron uptake is a useful test to differentiate *M. chelonae* from *M. fortuitum*, but it cannot differentiate *M. tuberculosis* from *M. bovis*.

B. Urease.

Rationale: *M. tuberculosis* and *M. bovis* cannot be differentiated because they both hydrolyze urea due to the

Table 16-6 Culture-Based Identification of the Most Commonly Isolated Nonpigmented Rapidly Growing Mycobacteria

Species	Colony Morphology	Iron Uptake	NaCl Tolerance	Citrate	Nitrate	Mannitol
M. abscessus	Smooth/rough	−	+	−	−	−
M. chelonae	Rough	−	−	+	−	−
M. fortuitum	Rough	+ (rust)	+	−	+	−
M. mucogenicum	Smooth	+ (tan)	−	+	−	+

production of urease. The urease test is useful in identifying some scotochromogenic and nonchromogenic mycobacteria.

C. Growth on MacConkey agar.

Rationale: MacConkey agar can be used to distinguish rapid growing mycobacteria. It cannot differentiate among species within the *M. tuberculosis* complex.

D. Niacin.

Rationale: M. tuberculosis, in contrast to *M. bovis,* accumulates niacin due to the inability to metabolize nicotinic acid; hence, the biochemical test strip for niacin detection is positive with *M. tuberculosis* and negative with *M. bovis.*

E. Pigment production.

Rationale: Both *M. tuberculosis* and *M. bovis* are nonchromogenic. No species of *M. tuberculosis* complex produces the yellow to orange pigment that characterizes some NTM.

Major points of discussion

- The discriminatory phenotypic methods that can distinguish *Mycobacterium tuberculosis* from *M. bovis* are niacin, nitrate, thiophene-2-carboxylic acid hydrazide, susceptibility or resistance to pyrazinamide, and colonial morphology (Table 16-7).

- Molecular methods for identifying *M. tuberculosis* and *M. bovis* provide rapid results. These include DNA sequence analysis of direct repeat regions or single nucleotide polymorphisms. In addition, the presence of absence of particular deletions can be discriminatory. Intrinsic resistance to pyrazinamide can also be detected using DNA sequence analysis.

- *M. bovis* is the etiologic agent for tuberculosis in warm-blood animals, mainly cattle. It can be transmitted from animal-to-human and person-to-person through inhalation of infectious droplet nuclei. Patients most susceptible to *M. bovis* infection include those born outside the United States, of Hispanic ethnicity, younger than 15 years, and with HIV infection.

- Abdominal tuberculosis is more often caused by *M. bovis* than *M. tuberculosis* and is transmitted to humans through the ingestion of unpasteurized, contaminated dairy products, such as Mexican cheese. *M. bovis* is prevalent in dairy herds in some parts of Mexico, whereas it has been nearly eradicated in U.S. and Canadian cattle herds.

- Distinguishing between *M. tuberculosis* and *M. bovis* is important for determining epidemiologic profiles to track the incidence and transmission of *M. bovis.* In

addition, treatment of *M. bovis* infection is the same as that for *M. tuberculosis,* except for pyrazinamide in *M. bovis* due to intrinsic resistance.[43]

59. A. Deletion typing.

Rationale: This technique is used to identify the species within the *M. tuberculosis* complex and to differentiate lineages of *M. tuberculosis.*

B. IS*6110* restriction length polymorphism analysis.

Rationale: Restriction length polymorphism analysis (RFLP) using IS*6110* as a probe is currently the best genotypic method to determine strain relatedness.

C. Spacer oligonucleotide typing (spoligotyping).

Rationale: This is a first-line molecular epidemiologic method that lacks the discriminatory power of IS*6110*-RFLP.

D. Mycobacterial interspersed repetitive units variable number tandem repeat (MIRU-VNTR) typing.

Rationale: MIRU-VNTR is an increasingly used first-line fingerprinting method that may eventually replace IS*6110*-RFLP, once the method is better refined and standardized.

E. Genome-wide single nucleotide polymorphism analysis.

Rationale: Single nucleotide polymorphism analysis is used to characterize the position of isolates within the *M. tuberculosis* complex phylogenetic structure and is not useful for strain differentiation.

Major points of discussion

- Genotyping of *M. tuberculosis* complex is important for differentiating patient isolates, cluster analyses, and contact investigations. *M. tuberculosis* isolates with identical or highly similar DNA fingerprints are said to be clustered and the proportion of clustering in a population is thought to reflect the amount of recent transmission.

- IS*6110* is a mobile transposable genetic element that varies in copy number (0 to ≥ 25) and location throughout the *M. tuberculosis* complex genome. IS*6110*-RFLP has several limitations, such as being labor intensive, lacking automation, and having a limited degree of discriminatory power with strains containing 6 or fewer copies of IS*6110*.

- MIRU-VNTR typing requires PCR amplification followed by band size analysis of independent loci dispersed throughout the *M. tuberculosis* complex genome. Variability in MIRU-VNTR results from a modulation in the number of consensus repeats and, thus, band sizes, at each locus.

- Spoligotyping analyzes the presence or absence of 43 spacer sequences within the direct-repeat region of the *M. tuberculosis* complex genome by the reverse-hybridization of labeled PCR products to a membrane spotted with oligonucleotides corresponding to each spacer. Spoligotyping cannot delineate clusters as finely as IS*6110*-

Table 16-7 Phenotypic Differentiation of *Mycobacterium tuberculosis* from *M. bovis*

Species	Niacin	Nitrate Reduction	TCH	Pyrazinamide	Colonial Morphology
M. tuberculosis	Positive	Positive	Resistant	Susceptible	Rough
M. bovis	Negative	Negative	Susceptible	Resistant	Smooth

TCH, Thiophene-2-carboxylic acid hydrazide.

RFLP or MIRU-VNTR typing, but is useful for cluster analyses of strains with 6 or fewer copies of IS*6110*.

■ The combination of spoligotyping and MIRU-VNTR analysis may eventually provide better discrimination of clusters than IS*6110*-RFLP, and, therefore, is considered as an emerging epidemiologic tool.[3]

60. A. Isoniazid and rifampin, pending drug susceptibility results.
Rationale: Initial treatment with only two drugs is not recommended. Pyrazinamide and ethambutol must be added to isoniazid and rifampin, pending drug susceptibility test results.
B. Fluoroquinolone, pending drug susceptibility results.
Rationale: Monotherapy with any drug will not eradicate *Mycobacterium tuberculosis* and can lead to the emergence of resistant strains.
C. Second-line drugs (e.g., ethionamide, cycloserine, kanamycin), pending drug susceptibility results.
Rationale: Second-line agents (e.g., ethionamide, cycloserine, kanamycin, capreomycin, para-aminosalicyclin acid) are less efficacious and more toxic than first-line drugs. They are reserved for proven multi-drug-resistant cases.
D. Treatment with isoniazid, rifampin, pyrazinamide, and ethambutol, pending drug susceptibility results.
Rationale: These first-line drugs, particularly isoniazid and rifampin, are the cornerstones of effective treatment. This regimen is used unless susceptibility tests indicate that the isolate is multi-drug-resistant tuberculosis.
E. Isoniazid plus ethambutol is adequate to avoid the hepatotoxicity of rifampin.
Rationale: A four-drug regimen is the standard of care for tuberculosis.

Major points of discussion
■ The basic first-line treatment regimen for active tuberculosis includes 6 months of directly observed therapy with isoniazid, rifampin, pyrazinamide, and ethambutol. Treatment can be shortened to 4 months in patients with less severe disease.
■ Most tuberculosis cases in the United States occur among foreign-born persons from endemic areas. This population is more likely than U.S.-born individuals to harbor drug-resistant strains of *M. tuberculosis*.
■ Multi-drug-resistant tuberculosis is defined as tuberculosis with resistance to at least isoniazid and rifampin. Extensively drug-resistant tuberculosis is also resistant to the fluoroquinolones and at least one of the injectable second-line drugs (e.g., amikacin or capreomycin).
■ Resistance to anti-tuberculous agents is considered primary when it occurs before initiating therapy, or secondary when it occurs in the setting of inadequate therapy, such as monotherapy or noncompliance.
■ Drug susceptibility testing must be performed on all initial *M. tuberculosis* isolates. For multi-drug-resistant isolates, extensive susceptibility tests against the second-line drugs must performed. Phenotypic assays are the current gold standard. However, molecular tests for drug resistance markers are increasingly being used.[19]

61. A. The isolate is isoniazid and rifampin susceptible.
Rationale: There is no growth in the rifampin quadrant, indicating rifampin susceptibility, but there is growth in the quadrant with the 1 μg isoniazid disk, indicating isoniazid resistance.
B. The isolate is a multi-drug-resistant tuberculosis strain.
Rationale: Multi-drug-resistant tuberculosis is defined as resistance to both isoniazid and rifampin; the lack of growth in the rifampin quadrant indicates rifampin susceptibility.
C. The isolate is rifampin monoresistant.
Rationale: There is no growth in the quadrant with the rifampin disk, indicating rifampin susceptibility, but there is growth in the quadrant with the 1 μg isoniazid disk, indicating isoniazid resistance.
D. The isolate is low-level isoniazid resistant and rifampin susceptible.
Rationale: There is growth in the quadrant with the 1 μg isoniazid disk, but no growth in the quadrants with the 5 μg isoniazid and rifampin disks.
E. The results cannot be interpreted due to culture contamination of the control quadrant.
Rationale: There must be growth in the drug-free control quadrant to count colonies and compare with growth in quadrants containing antituberculosis drugs.

Major points of discussion
■ For the agar proportion method, the number of colony-forming units growing on drug-containing medium (supplemented 7H10 agar) is compared with the number growing on the drug-free quadrant. If the number of colony-forming units on the drug-containing media is greater than 1% of the colony forming units on drug-free medium, then the strain is considered resistant.
■ There are many mutations in several genes and gene promoter regions that are known to confer isoniazid resistance in *M. tuberculosis*. High-level isoniazid resistance is associated with a mutation of the catalase-peroxidase gene (*katG*) at codon 315. Low-level isoniazid resistance occurs most often as a result of mutation of the promoter of the *mabA-inhA* gene complex.
■ Molecular-based testing for rifampin resistance is increasingly used as a surrogate for multi-drug-resistant tuberculosis, because approximately 95% of rifampin-resistant tuberculosis strains are isoniazid resistant.
■ Select mutations that cause low-level isoniazid resistance also confer ethionamide cross-resistance.
■ It has been suggested that patients with low-level isoniazid resistant tuberculosis (i.e., isoniazid resistance at 0.2 mg/L [1 μg disk], but susceptibility at 1.0 mg/L [5 μg disk]) may be treated with high-dose isoniazid as part of their regimen. However, the clinical significance and effectiveness of the use of isoniazid in the setting of low-level isoniazid resistance is unclear.[19]

62. A. Mycobacterium scrofulaceum.
Rationale: M. scrofulaceum causes enlarged cervical lymph nodes (i.e., scrofula) in children.
B. *Mycobacterium gordonae*.
Rationale: M. gordonae, a nonpathogenic contaminant present in tap water and soil, rarely causes disease.
C. *Mycobacterium mucogenicum*.

Rationale: M. mucogenicum commonly causes posttraumatic wound infections and catheter-related sepsis.
D. *Mycobacterium kansasii*.
Rationale: M. kansasii commonly causes lower respiratory disease with clinical symptoms resembling *M. tuberculosis*.
E. *Mycobacterium abscessus*.
Rationale: M. abscessus is a skin and soft tissue pathogen that can also cause pulmonary infections and disseminated disease in immunocompromised individuals.

Major points of discussion

- *Mycobacterium scrofulaceum* is second to *M. avium* complex as the most common cause of cervical lymphadenitis in children. It can also present as cutaneous lesions.
- *M. scrofulaceum* is identified using routine biochemical assays, line probe assays, or gene sequencing. Although there are currently no commercially available probe tests for identification, this organism has a unique 16S rRNA sequence that is targeted for gene sequencing analysis.
- *M. scrofulaceum* is a slow-growing, yellow-pigmented, scotochromogen that tests negative for niacin and nitrate reduction and positive for the 68°C and semiquantitative catalase tests.
- With the exception of rapidly growing mycobacteria, susceptibility testing for NTM is not standardized by CLSI.
- Treatment for cervical lymphadenitis is surgical excision and/or treatment with clarithromycin combined with ethambutol or rifabutin.[39]

63. A. *Mycobacterium avium*.

Rationale: M. avium, the most frequent cause of nonmycobacterial pulmonary disease, is nonpigmented.
B. *Mycobacterium kansasii*.
Rationale: M. kansasii, a pulmonary pathogen that presents clinically similar to tuberculosis, is a photochromogen.
C. *Mycobacterium marinum*.
Rationale: M. marinum is a photochromogen and can cause skin and soft tissue infections.
D. *Mycobacterium simiae*.
Rationale: M. simiae is weakly photochromogenic and is rarely clinically relevant.
E. *Mycobacterium asiaticum*.
Rationale: M. asiaticum, a rare cause of pulmonary infection, is a photochromogen.

Major points of discussion

- Photochromogenic mycobacteria are nonpigmented when incubated in the dark but produce deep yellow to orange carotenoid pigments when exposed to light.
- Scotochromogens produce a yellow to orange pigment when grown either in the light or the dark. Nonphotochromogens remain nonpigmented either in the dark or after light exposure.
- To differentiate photochromogens from scotochromogens, three tubes of egg-based media are inoculated and incubated. Two tubes are wrapped in aluminum foil to block all light and one is left

uncovered to permit light exposure. When growth is detected, one tube is unwrapped and exposed to light for another 3 to 5 hours if it is nonpigmented. The tube is then rewrapped, reincubated, and examined for pigment production at 24, 48, and 72 hours.
- Photochromogens include *M. kansasii* and *M. marinum*, which are definitively pathogenic, and *M. asiaticum* and *M. simiae*, which are potentially pathogenic.
- Scotochromogens include both potential pathogens (e.g., *M. scrofulaceum* and *M. szulgai*) and common saprophytes (e.g., *M. gordonae* and *M. flavescens*).[31]

64. A. A confined access room under negative pressure with an optional biologic safety cabinet (BSC).

Rationale: All specimens and cultures must be processed and handled under a BSC located within a confined access facility. Handling these potentially infectious samples require procedures that generate aerosols.
B. Air sterilization by ultraviolet light within a BSC and on the ceiling of the room to disinfect the ambient air.
Rationale: The CDC states that ultraviolet light is not required for sterilization or decontamination. Ultraviolet lights are limited by a number of factors, including limited penetration power, relative humidity, temperatures below 77°F, air movement, cleanliness, and age.
C. A room or suite that has a minimum of 20 air exchanges per hour to remove 99% of airborne particulates.
Rationale: The appropriate number of air exchanges per hour is 6 to 12 to ensure removal of 99% of airborne particulates within 30 to 45 minutes.
D. A BSC in a controlled access area with the capacity to draw 75 to 100 linear feet of air per minute across the entire front opening for proper functioning of the HEPA filter.
Rationale: If the airflow is less than 75 linear feet per minute, as detected by the gauge on the front of the BSC, the HEPA filters may be clogged and need replacement by a qualified technician.
E. Respiratory protection using a HEPA-filtered respirator, such as the N95 or N100, and mandatory fit testing every 6 months.
Rationale: Annual fit testing is required if N95 or N100 respirators are used.

Major points of discussion

- The risk of *M. tuberculosis* infection is 3 to 5 times greater among workers in the mycobacteriology laboratory than other laboratory workers. The production of aerosols, particularly droplet nuclei less that 5 μm, can be hazardous to personnel not trained in safety practices.
- For all mycobacteriology procedures that require centrifugation, aerosol-free safety cups with O-ring sealed closures are recommended. Specimens must be centrifuged for at least 15 minutes at more than 3000 *g*. Safety carriers are opened inside a BSC in case of tube breakage.
- The personnel protective equipment worn within the mycobacteriology laboratory includes impermeable protective gowns that have back closures and fitted sleeve cuffs. These must be either disposed of in the laboratory or laundered by the institution.

■ A biosafety level 3 facility is recommended when working with cultures suspected or confirmed to contain *M. tuberculosis*, and at least biosafety level 2 practices with clinical specimens from suspect or known cases of tuberculosis. All rooms must have negative pressure of 6 to 12 air exchanges per hour and a means to monitor negative pressure.

■ Tuberculin skin testing or IGRAs are performed annually for employees working in the mycobacteriology laboratory (Occupational Health and Safety Administration requirement). All laboratory workers with newly recognized positive tuberculin skin testing or IGRA tests should be promptly evaluated for clinically active tuberculosis .[27,28]

65. A. *Mycobacterium avium* complex.
Rationale: M. avium complex isolates are nonpigmented and positive with commercial test probes.
B. *Mycobacterium xenopi.*
Rationale: M. xenopi are pigmented, grow best at 42 to 45°C, and are arylsulfatase test positive.
C. *Mycobacterium abscessus.*
Rationale: M. abscessus are nonpigmented and grow rapidly within 7 days.
D. *Mycobacterium kansasii.*
Rationale: M. kansasii strains are pigmented and positive with commercial test probes.
E. *Mycobacterium mucogenicum.*
Rationale: M. mucogenicum are nonpigmented and grow rapidly within 7 days.

Major points of discussion

■ *M. xenopi* is a cause of chronic respiratory, joint, and soft tissue infections, as well as disseminated disease in immunocompromised hosts, such as patients with acquired immune deficiency syndrome. Underlying lung disease and exposure to water systems that contain *M. xenopi* are risk factors for *M. xenopi* infection in immunocompromised patients.

■ In the United States, pulmonary infections due to *M. xenopi* occur less frequently than with *M. avium* complex and *M. kansasii*. Cavitary upper-lobe radiologic findings are common with *M. xenopi* and *M. kansasii* infections.

■ The recommended antimicrobial treatment for *M. xenopi* includes a combination of macrolide, rifampin, and ethambutol with moxifloxacin. In vitro susceptibility tests may need to be performed at 42 to 45°C and for extended periods of incubation.

■ Molecular methods, such as gene sequencing of *16S rRNA*, *hsp65*, or *rpoB* targets are rapidly replacing conventional biochemicals for the identification *M. xenopi* and other mycobacterial isolates.

■ Water supplies can become contaminated when biofilms form on pipes. Nosocomial outbreaks have been reported for multiple NTM species, including *M. xenopi*. Other sources of infection by NTM include bronchoscopes and hemodialysis equipment.[8,34]

66. A. *Mycobacterium mucogenicum.*
Rationale: M. mucogenicum is a rapidly growing mycobacteria that rarely causes lung disease.
B. *Mycobacterium lentiflavum.*

Rationale: M. lentiflavum has not been identified as a cause of lung infection.
C. *Mycobacterium terrae.*
Rationale: M. terrae is a nonpathogenic species of the *M. terrae* complex (which also includes *M. arupensis*, *M. nonchromogenicum*, and *M. hiberniae*).
D. *Mycobacterium intracellulare.*
Rationale: M. intracellulare is a species of the *M. avium* complex that frequently causes pulmonary infections.
E. *Mycobacterium gordonae.*
Rationale: M. gordonae is nonpathogenic and is considered a water contaminant when isolated from respiratory specimens.

Major points of discussion

■ NTM are ubiquitous in the environment (e.g., soil and water). Their clinical significance on isolation from a patient specimen depends on their known pathogenicity, site of isolation, as well as the patient's immune status and clinical presentation.

■ The isolation of an NTM species is more likely to be considered clinically relevant if it is recovered from a sterile body site or from multiple specimens.

■ *M. avium* complex is a slow-growing NTM that is most commonly identified in the United States using the AccuProbe system. This test uses targeted DNA probes that hybridize with complex-specific 16s rRNA.

■ *M. avium* complex is associated with pulmonary infections in patients with preexisting respiratory disease (e.g., chronic obstructive pulmonary disease, cervical lymphadenitis, and disseminated disease).

■ The pathogenesis of *M. avium* complex infections is not clearly understood, but it is known to be acquired by inhalation or ingestion and not by human-to-human transmission. MAC is known to thrive in hot water, resulting in pulmonary illness in healthy individuals who frequently use hot tubs. It is postulated that the forced air jets in these tubs aerosolize the organism, which is subsequently inhaled.[8,39]

67. A. *Mycobacterium xenopi.*
Rationale: M. xenopi can cause pulmonary or disseminated infections. They are scotochromogens, producing pigment in the absence of light. There are currently no commercial nucleic acid probe tests available for its identification.
B. *Mycobacterium scrofulaceum.*
Rationale: M. scrofulaceum is associated with cervical adenitis and bone infections. It is a scotochromogen, and there are currently no commercial nucleic acid probe tests available for its identification.
C. *Mycobacterium gordonae.*
Rationale: M. gordonae is a tap water scotochromogen that is considered nonpathogenic. Strains can be identified by nucleic acid hybridization probe testing.
D. *Mycobacterium kansasii.*
Rationale: M. kansasii are photochromogenic and present clinically as pulmonary disease resembling classical tuberculosis with cavitary lesions. Strains can be identified by nucleic acid hybridization probe testing.
E. *Mycobacterium abscessus.*
Rationale: M. abscessus is a nonpigmented, rapidly growing mycobacteria species for which there are currently no

commercial nucleic acid probe tests available for its identification.

Major points of discussion

- Although *M. kansasii* can cause pulmonary infection that is clinically indistinguishable from tuberculosis, person-to-person transmission has not been documented. The reservoir appears to be water, with infection likely by aerosolization. It is highly endemic in regions of the southern and central United States.
- *M. kansasii* is a slow growing, photochromogen that is the second most common cause of NTM pulmonary disease in the United States (after *M. avium* complex). Biochemically, the species is niacin negative, nitrate positive, and catalase positive.
- The recommended antimicrobial treatment for *M. kansasii* includes a combination of rifampin, ethambutol, and isoniazid (or clarithromycin). In vitro susceptibility tests need to be performed for rifampin only, as treatment failure is associated with resistance to this antibiotic. *M. kansasii* is innately resistant to pyrazinamide.
- Most *M. kansasii* infections in humans are caused by a single subtype that tests positive by the current commercial nucleic acid probe assay, although probe-negative subtypes of *M. kansasii* have been identified.
- *M. kansasii* can be identified and differentiated from other mycobacteria by gene sequencing using various targets, such as heat shock protein (*hsp65*) or the B subunit of the RNA polymerase (*rpoB*) gene.[8,34]

68. A. Airborne isolation can be discontinued when another diagnosis is made that excludes tuberculosis and when three sputum specimens are AFB smear negative NAAT negative.
Rationale: Patients with a suspicion high enough to start tuberculosis medication require a clinical response after at least 1 week of antituberculous treatment in addition to the required laboratory test criteria.
B. Airborne isolation can be discontinued when two sputum specimens are AFB smear negative and culture negative.
Rationale: The guidelines for discontinuing tuberculosis isolation are exclusive of *M. tuberculosis* culture results because the turnaround time for culture negatives require up to 6 to 8 weeks of isolation. At least 3 AFB-negative smears are needed before airborne isolation is discontinued.
C. Airborne isolation can be discontinued when the patient has received 48 hours of antituberculous therapy.
Rationale: NAATs and AFB smear data must be used when evaluating whether to discontinue airborne isolation. Patients must remain on airborne precautions until the patient has shown decreased clinical symptoms after 1 week of therapy.
D. Airborne precautions can be discontinued in young children when three expectorated sputum specimens are AFB smear negative and culture negative.
Rationale: Collecting spontaneously produced sputum specimens in young children is problematic; thus, gastric aspiration or sputum induction are feasible alternatives.

E. Airborne isolation can be discontinued when two sputum specimens are AFB smear negative and nucleic acid probe test negative.
Rationale: At least three AFB smears are needed to increase the sensitivity of the stain; probe assays are only used to identify *M. tuberculosis* from culture.

Major points of discussion

- All patients at high risk for tuberculosis must be on airborne isolation in a negative pressure room (≥ 12 air exchanges per hour), if they have pulmonary symptoms (e.g., cough) or an abnormal chest radiograph. Staff members and visitors entering the patient's room must wear a respirator (e.g., an N-95 mask) and gown.
- High-risk patients include 1) patients from endemic areas, 2) those with known contact with active infectious tuberculosis cases, 3) HIV-positive patients, 4) injecting drug users, 5) homeless persons, 6) prisoners, 7) those with a past history of tuberculosis, and 8) immunosuppressed patients receiving chemotherapy or steroids with an abnormal chest radiograph.
- Operating rooms are under positive pressure; therefore, patients with confirmed or suspected tuberculosis who require surgical procedures should be scheduled as the last case in the operating room at the end of the day.
- The NAAT, which detects *M. tuberculosis* complex, should be performed on at least one respiratory specimen from each patient for whom there is a reasonable index of suspicion for tuberculosis. NAATs do not replace the need for AFB smears and culture and are never used as the definitive test to exclude tuberculosis.
- Although young children with active tuberculosis are not generally considered infectious, they have been identified as a probable source of hospital-acquired transmission of *M. tuberculosis*. Infected children require frequent suctioning and/or mechanical ventilation; therefore, consideration should be given to using airborne transmission precautions during these procedures.[12,14]

69. A. *Mycobacterium kansasii.*
Rationale: *M. kansasii*, a pulmonary pathogen, would not be detected by NAAT, which is currently specific for members of the *M. tuberculosis* complex.
B. *Mycobacterium ulcerans.*
Rationale: *M. ulcerans* causes chronic skin ulcers and not abdominal infection. This species would not be detected by NAAT, which is currently specific for members of the *M. tuberculosis* complex.
C. *Mycobacterium bovis.*
Rationale: *M. bovis* can cause abdominal tuberculosis. The NAAT test is positive for *M. tuberculosis* complex, which includes *M. bovis*. *M. bovis* is specifically identified by gene deletion analysis and biochemical tests.
D. *Mycobacterium avium* complex.
Rationale: *M. avium* complex causes pulmonary or disseminated infections. This complex would not be detected by NAAT, which is currently specific for members of the *M. tuberculosis* complex.
E. *Mycobacterium fortuitum.*
Rationale: There is currently no NAAT available for rapidly growing mycobacteria.

Major points of discussion

- Outbreaks of abdominal tuberculosis have been observed in the United States in areas bordering Mexico due to the consumption of *queso fresco*, or homemade cheese that is made with unpasteurized milk. In India, abdominal infection with *M. tuberculosis* complex is the second most common extrapulmonary site of infection (~9%).
- Four modes of transmission can lead to tuberculosis enteritis: swallowing infected sputum, hematogenous spread from active pulmonary or miliary tuberculosis, ingestion of contaminated milk or food, or contiguous spread from adjacent organs.
- The affinity of *M. tuberculosis* complex for the ileocecal region of the intestine may be due to relative stasis and abundant lymphoid tissue in this area. *M. bovis*, a member of the *M. tuberculosis* complex, commonly causes this infection.
- *M. bovis* is an important causative agent of abdominal tuberculosis since it frequently infects cows and humans. In Mexico, 17% of cattle are colonized or infected with *M. bovis*.
- Laboratory testing for *M. bovis* identification includes gene deletion analysis and *pncA* gene sequencing to detect pyrazinamide resistance. The NAAT for *M. tuberculosis* complex detects *M. bovis* as well as *M. tuberculosis*.[43,69]

70. A. Carbol fuchsin stain and the niacin test.
Rationale: Carbol fuchsin stains are recommended for detection of AFB in mycobacterial cultures. The niacin test is performed from growth on solid media.
B. Fluorochrome stain and NAAT.
Rationale: The fluorochrome stain is recommended for detection of AFB directly from specimens; NAATs can identify *M. tuberculosis* complex from specimens.
C. Giemsa stain and liquid culture.
Rationale: Giemsa stains are not used for detection of AFB, and using liquid culture media does not provide a rapid assay.
D. Fluorochrome stain and nucleic acid sequencing.
Rationale: The fluorochrome stain is recommended for detecting AFB in clinical specimens. Nucleic acid sequencing cannot be performed directly on clinical specimens.
E. DNA probe assay and high-pressure liquid chromatography.
Rationale: DNA probe assays and high-pressure liquid chromatography are used to identify mycobacteria from culture and not directly from clinical specimens.

Major points of discussion

- Culture using both solid and liquid media is the gold standard for isolating mycobacteria. Biochemical tests, such as the niacin test, can be used to identify mycobacteria to the species level.
- NAATs for identifying the *Mycobacterium tuberculosis* complex must be performed in conjunction with culture and should be tested on acid-fast, smear-positive respiratory specimens.
- DNA probe assays are commonly used to identify *Mycobacterium tuberculosis* complex, *Mycobacterium*

avium complex, *Mycobacterium kansasii*, and *Mycobacterium gordonae* from acid-fast smear-positive cultures.
- *Mycobacterium bovis* and the vaccine strain, *Mycobacterium bovis* BCG, are members of the *Mycobacterium tuberculosis* complex that should be differentiated from the other species in the complex, especially in initial isolates.
- Once growth is detected on culture media, mycobacteria can be rapidly identified to the species level by DNA probes, DNA sequencing, line probes, or high-pressure liquid chromatography.
- Fluorochrome-stained smears (examined under low-power magnification) are recommended over carbol fuchsin stains, which require oil immersion, when screening for AFB in clinical specimens. Increased sensitivity and rapid smear examination are the advantages of fluorescent stains.[27]

MYCOLOGY

71. A. *Penicillium marneffei.*
Rationale: P. marneffei produces a red diffusible pigment and microscopic morphology demonstrates flask-shaped phialides and chains of round conidia.
B. *Aspergillus nidulans.*
Rationale: A. nidulans does not produce a diffusible pigment and microscopic morphology demonstrates biseriate phialides and round conidia.
C. *Trichophyton rubrum.*
Rationale: T. rubrum does not produce a diffusible pigment and microscopic morphology demonstrates tear-shaped microconidia.
D. *Fusarium solani.*
Rationale: F. solani does not produce a diffusible pigment and microscopic morphology demonstrates sickle-shaped septated macroconidia.
E. *Cryptococcus neoformans.*
Rationale: C. neoformans is an encapsulated yeast and does not produce a diffusible pigment.

Major points of discussion

- *P. marneffei*, endemic in Southeast Asia, is a common cause of infections in immunocompromised hosts but can also cause disease in immunocompetent individuals who have travelled to that area.
- *P. marneffei* demonstrates thermal dimorphism (mold at 30°C and yeast at 37°C); growth is inhibited by cyclohexamide.
- Transmission of *P. marneffei* is most likely airborne, via inhalation of conidia from an environmental reservoir (often associated with exposure to bamboo rats).
- Other *Penicillium* species are not dimorphic and demonstrate septate hyphae in tissue, whereas *P. marneffei* are present in a yeast-like form.
- *P. marneffei* is typically highly susceptible to miconazole, itraconazole, and ketoconazole but resistant to fluconazole.

72. A. Mucormycosis.
Rationale: Mucor species contain fungal elements that are largely nonseptate with irregular branching.
B. Aspergillosis.

Rationale: Aspergillus species have hyaline septate hyphae with branching at 45-degree angles.

C. Candidiasis.

Rationale: Candida species form pseudohyphae that show distinct constrictions at the septa and form budding yeast cells.

D. Mycetoma.

Rationale: Fungi and bacteria causing mycetoma appear as aggregates of intertwined filaments rather than individual hyphae.

E. Rhinosporidiosis.

Rationale: Rhinosporidium seeberi invades mucocutaneous tissue and appears as round mature sporangia containing endospores.

Major points of discussion

- Zygomycetes are a fungal class that are mostly nonseptate. Most fungi in this class that cause infection belong to the order Mucorales, which includes *Rhizopus, Mucor, Rhizomucor,* and *Absidia*.
- The hyphae of the Mucorales fungi are nonseptate and branching is nondichotomous, irregular, and sometimes at right angles.
- Mucormycosis can invade the lung, nasal, sinus, brain, and mucous membranes.
- Fungi causing mucormycosis can be differentiated from aspergillosis by the morphology of the hyphae and by the presence of chlamydospores in the hyphae.
- Differential characteristics of commonly encountered pathogens causing mucormycosis include rhizoid production and sporangiophore pigment (Table 16-8).

73. A. *Aspergillus fumigates.*

Rationale: A. fumigates have uniseriate, compact phialides on the top portion of the vesicle and round, smooth conidia.

B. *Penicillium* spp.

Rationale: Penicillium spp. demonstrates flask-shaped phialides and chains of round conidia.

C. *Aspergillus niger.*

Rationale: A. niger demonstrates biseriate phialides that radiate around the entire vesicle and rough, dark conidia.

D. *Fusarium solani.*

Rationale: F. solani demonstrates sickle-shaped septated macroconidia.

E. *Aspergillus flavus.*

Rationale: A. flavus demonstrates uniseriate and biseriate phialides over most of the vesicle and slightly rough conidia.

Major points of discussion

- *Aspergillus* infections occur in 2% to 26% of bone marrow transplant recipients and in 1% to 15% of solid-organ transplant recipients, with an associated mortality rate ranging from 74% to 92%.
- *Aspergillus fumigatus* grows rapidly, and by 3 days in culture demonstrates a green surface with a narrow white border.
- *Aspergillus niger* grows with a black surface and a white border, whereas *Aspergillus flavus* grows with a yellow-green to olive surface.
- A differentiating characteristic of *A. fumigatus* is its ability to grow at 45°C.
- Voriconazole is the current drug of choice for invasive aspergillosis. When compared with amphotericin, it is better tolerated by the patient and is associated with improved survival.[64]

74. A. *Sporothrix schenckii* (sporotrichosis).

Rationale: S. schenckii is a thermally dimorphic fungus causing a tracking nodular infection. The rate of growth (<7 days) and production of rosette-like conidial clusters differentiate this fungus from other thermally dimorphic fungi.

B. *Fusarium solani* (fusariosis).

Rationale: F. solani commonly produces erythematous nodules with central necrosis and is not thermally dimorphic. *Fusarium* species are readily identified by their banana-shaped macroconidia.

C. *Penicillium marneffei* (penicilliosis).

Rationale: P. marneffei is a thermally dimorphic, rapidly growing (≤3 days) mold that produces a red pigment on solid media. Skin infections are rare and present as generalized skin papules.

D. *Nocardia brasiliensis* (sporotrichoid nocardiosis).

Rationale: N. brasiliensis causes sporotrichoid nocardiosis, a similar tracking lymphocutaneous syndrome originating on the hands or arms following an inoculation injury. Microscopic examination demonstrates gram-positive, branching rods.

E. *Histoplasma capsulatum* (histoplasmosis).

Rationale: H. capsulatum is a thermally dimorphic mold that is extremely slow-growing and produces macroconidia covered with nodules. Pulmonary infection is the most common manifestation.

Major points of discussion

- Thermally dimorphic fungi convert from the mold form to the yeast form at a higher temperature (e.g., 25 to 30°C vs. 37°C; Table 16-9).
- Also known as rose gardener's disease, sporotrichosis is caused by percutaneous inoculation. Lymphocutaneous disease is the most common manifestation.

Table 16-8 Characteristics of Representatives of Mucorales

Fungus	Rhizoids	Sporangiophores	Optimal Growth Temp (°C)	Pathogenicity
Rhizopus	Present	Unbranched, brown	45-50, inhibited by cycloheximide	Most common pathogen
Mucor	Absent	Branched, hyaline	≤37	Opportunistic, occasional
Rhizomucor	Few	Branched, dark brown	38-58	Opportunistic, occasional
Absidia (Lichtheimia)	Present	Fine branches, hyaline	45-50	Uncommon pathogen

Table 16-9 Thermally Dimorphic Fungi

	Rate of Growth	Colony Features	Microscopic Morphology	
			Mold	Yeast
Penicillum marneffei	Rapid (3-4 days)	Tan, red on reverse	Septate hyphae with branched brush-like conidiophores	Oval arthroconidia that fragment at septa, no budding
Sporothrix schenckii	Moderately rapid (<7days)	White-orange, sometimes black	Branched septate hyphae with rosette-like conidia and conidia singly along hyphae	Round-oval to elongated budding cells
Blastomyces dermatitidis	Slow (≥14 days)	Cream-tan	Branched septate hyphae with single round conidia	Broad-based large round-oval budding cells
Histoplasma capsulatum	Slow (15-20 days)	White-brown	Branched septate hyphae with pear-shaped microconidia and knobby macroconidia	Narrow-based small round-oval budding cells
Paracoccidiodes braziliensis	Slow (~21 days)	Cream-tan	Nonbranching septate hyphae with intercalating and terminal chlamydosphores	Large, ship's wheel shape, multiple budding cells with narrow connections

- Sporotrichosis usually presents with nodular skin lesions, although the lungs, joints, bones, and brain may be affected. It may be misdiagnosed as pyoderma gangrenosum due to the large cutaneous ulcerations that often develop.
- Sporotrichosis can occur in domestic animals, especially cats, and is considered an occupational hazard for veterinarians.
- Itraconazole is the current antifungal of choice. In addition, 3 to 6 months of topical potassium iodide can cure cutaneous sporotrichosis.[48]

75. A. Birdseed agar.
Rationale: C. neoformans can be differentiated from other fungi by producing phenol oxidase, which permits the production of melanin, resulting in dark brown colonies.
B. Sabouraud dextrose agar.
Rationale: Sabouraud dextrose agar supports the growth of most fungi and is not differential for *C. neoformans.*
C. Mycosel agar.
Rationale: Mycosel agar contains chloramphenicol to inhibit bacterial growth and cyclohexamide to inhibit *A. fumigatus.*
D. Potato dextrose agar.
Rationale: Potato dextrose agar is used to stimulate the production of conidia and pigment, both of which can be helpful for identifying many fungi. It is not differential for *C. neoformans.*
E. Brain heart infusion agar.
Rationale: Brain heart infusion agar is enriched and suitable for isolating fastidious fungi, such as *Histoplasma capsulatum.* It is not differential for *C. neoformans.*

Major points of discussion
- Selective media allow certain types of organisms to grow and inhibits the growth of other organisms. For example, inhibitory mold agar is an enriched media that aids in the recovery of fungi but also contains antibiotics to inhibit bacteria.
- Differential media are used for differentiating closely related organisms. For example, only *C. neoformans* and *Cryptococcus gattii* produce brown colonies on birdseed agar, whereas all other yeasts are cream to beige colored.

- For most fungal cultures, a combination of media is used to optimize recovery of clinically significant fungi. Fungal media, with and without antifungal and antibacterial agents, are used.
- After inoculation, most fungal media are incubated at 30°C. If thermally dimorphic fungi are suspected (i.e., *Histoplasma, Blastomyces, Sporothrix*), additional media are incubated at 35 to 37°C.
- *C. gattii,* a recently recognized pathogen, is morphologically indistinguishable from *C. neoformans.* The use of selective/differential canavanine glycine bromothymol blue agar is recommended (*C. gattii* turns the agar blue, whereas *C. neoformans* does not grow).

76. A. *Trichophyton tonsurans.*
Rationale: T. tonsurans, a common cause of scalp infections in the United States, is characterized by numerous microconidia and rarely produces macroconidia.
B. *Microsporum gypseum.*
Rationale: The macroconidia of *M. gypseum,* an uncommon cause of scalp infections, are thin walled with rounded ends.
C. *Trichophyton schoenleinii.*
Rationale: T. schoenleinii causes favus, a severe, chronic scalp infection. Microconidia and macroconidia are both absent.
D. *Epidermophyton floccosum.*
Rationale: E. floccosum is not associated with scalp infections and produces short macroconidia containing two to six cells.
E. *Microsporum canis.*
Rationale: The macroconidia of *M. canis,* a common cause of scalp infections, are thick walled with tapered ends.

Major points of discussion
- *Microsporum canis* can cause scalp (i.e., tinea capitis) and skin (i.e., tinea corporis) infections, typically in children. Most infections are acquired by exposure to infected dogs or cats.
- On Sabouraud's dextrose agar, *M. canis* colonies are flat, spreading, and white to cream colored. Colonies usually have a bright golden yellow to brownish-yellow reverse pigment.

- The macroconidia of *M. canis* are typically spindle shaped with five to 15 cells, verrucose, thick walled, and often have a terminal knob. Club-shaped microconidia may be found along the septate hyphae.
- Ectothrix hair invasion is characterized by the development of arthroconidia on the exterior of the hair shaft, which destroys the hair cuticle. Under a Wood lamp, infected hairs fluoresce bright green-yellow. Etiologic agents include *Microsporum canis* and *M. gypseum*.
- Endothrix hair invasion is characterized by the development of arthroconidia within the hair shaft only. Infected hairs do not fluoresce under a Wood lamp. Etiologic agents include *Trichophyton tonsurans* and *T. violaceum*.
- Griseofulvin was the first effective oral therapy for tinea capitis. Newer antifungal medications, such as itraconazole and terbinafine, are commonly used as alternative therapeutic agents for tinea capitis.

77. A. *Blastomyces dermatitidis.*

Rationale: B. dermatitidis is a slow-growing, thermally dimorphic fungus, which means that it grows as a mold at 25°C and as a yeast at 37°C.
B. *Histoplasma capsulatum.*
Rationale: Although *H. capsulatum* is a thermally dimorphic fungus, conversion to the yeast phase is difficult. Yeast cells are small, round, or oval budding cells as opposed to the broad-based budding shown in the figure.
C. *Sporothrix schenckii.*
Rationale: S. schenckii is a thermally dimorphic fungus that takes approximately 7 days to mature. The yeast phase demonstrates fusiform budding cells, often referred to as cigar bodies.
D. *Penicillium marneffei.*
Rationale: P. marneffei is a rapidly growing (<3 days), thermally dimorphic fungus. The yeast-like phase demonstrates nonbudding round to oval arthroconidia.
E. *Rhizomucor pusillus.*
Rationale: R. pusillus is not a thermally dimorphic fungus. It is a zygomycete that does not have a yeast phase.

Major points of discussion

- Inhalation of airborne, microscopic fungal spores from the environment (predominantly moist soil) can lead to blastomycosis. In the United States, *B. dermatitidis* is endemic in the Southeast and Midwest.
- Although antigen assays are available for urine and serum, culture is highly recommended for diagnosis. Antibody can be detected using immunodiffusion or complement fixation methods for diagnosis; however, these are often negative during acute infection. In addition, false positives can occur with *Histoplasma* and *Coccidioides*.
- The mold phase is characterized by septate hyphae with short or long conidiophores and a round conidia at the apex (i.e., resembling a lollipop). The yeast phase demonstrates thick-walled cells with broad-based budding.
- Definitive identification is based on exoantigen and DNA probe results.
- Itraconazole is commonly used to treat blastomycosis. More severe infections may require amphotericin B.

78. A. Candida albicans.

Rationale: C. albicans is a yeast that does not demonstrate broad-base budding and cannot be visualized on an India ink preparation.
B. *Cryptococcus neoformans.*
Rationale: C. neoformans is a yeast that demonstrates broad-base budding and can be visualized on an India ink preparation due to the presence of a capsule.
C. *Streptococcus pneumoniae.*
Rationale: S. pneumoniae is a bacterium that appears as gram-positive diplococci and cannot be visualized on an India ink preparation.
D. *Blastomyces dermatitidis.*
Rationale: B. dermatitidis is a dimorphic fungus that has both a yeast and a mold form depending on the temperature of growth. It cannot be visualized on an India ink preparation.
E. *Neisseria meningitides.*
Rationale: N. meningitidis is a bacterium that appears as small gram-negative diplococci and cannot be visualized on an India ink preparation.

Major points of discussion

- *C. neoformans* is a ubiquitous yeast that is primarily associated with pneumonia and meningitis. Immunocompetent individuals can be exposed to this organism and remain asymptomatic. However, people with defective cell-mediated immunity, such as HIV or transplant patients, can develop life-threatening disease.
- The India ink preparation can be used to detect *Cryptococcus* directly from cerebrospinal fluid. Identification must be confirmed by culture and biochemical analysis.
- Cerebrospinal fluid glucose concentrations are usually lower than normal, whereas cerebrospinal fluid protein concentrations are usually elevated. Cerebrospinal fluid leukocyte counts are 20/μL or higher, with a lymphocyte predominance. In HIV-infected individuals, these markers may appear normal due to these patients' inability to mount an adequate inflammatory response.
- In fixed tissues, *C. neoformans* can be distinguished from other nondematiaceous fungi with the Fontana-Masson stain, which detects melanin precursors in the cell wall. The mucicarmine stain can also be used to visualize the capsule.
- Treatment of cryptococcal meningitis consists of amphotericin B, with or without flucytosine, for 2 weeks, followed by fluconazole for a minimum of 8 to 10 weeks.

79. A. *Cryptococcus neoformans.*

Rationale: Birdseed agar is differential for *C. neoformans* and *C. gattii.* These organisms produce phenol oxidase, which breaks down a substrate in the medium and produces melanin. Other yeasts will appear beige or cream colored.
B. *Mycobacterium avium.*
Rationale: M. avium, an NTM, does not grow on birdseed agar.
C. *Aspergillus niger.*
Rationale: A. niger, a mold commonly associated with otitis externa, cannot be identified by growth on birdseed agar.
D. *Exophiala dermatitidis.*

Rationale: E. dermatitidis, a dematiaceous mold associated with central nervous system infections, cannot be identified by growth on birdseed agar.
E. *Trichophyton rubrum.*
Rationale: T. rubrum, a dermatophyte that can infect the skin and nails, cannot be identified by growth on birdseed agar.

Major points of discussion

- *Cryptococcus* spp. can be recovered on various media, including Sabouraud dextrose agar, sheep blood agar, and inhibitory mold agar, which contains chloramphenicol. It will not grow on Mycosel agar due to the presence of cycloheximide.
- The two most common species of *Cryptococcus* are C. *neoformans* (serotypes A and D) and *C. gattii* (serotypes B and C). Strains of serotype D are more likely to be found in skin lesions. *C. neoformans* infections are more common in immunocompromised patients, whereas infections with *C. gattii* are more common in immunocompetent individuals.
- Primary cutaneous infections are typically characterized by a history of trauma or direct inoculation and the development of a single lesion at the site of inoculation, which eventually ulcerates. Birds can be colonized with *Cryptococcus* spp., and the fungus is often spread through aerosolization of dried feces.
- C. *neoformans* and *C. gattii* are difficult to differentiate from each other. A recently developed agar medium containing canavanine, glycine and bromothymol blue (CGB) is effective. *C. gattii* colonies appear dark blue, whereas *C. neoformans* colonies are colorless.
- Primary cutaneous cryptococcal disease can currently be treated with oral fluconazole or itraconazole.

80. A. *Syncephalastrum racemosum.*
Rationale: S. racemosum has white to gray colonies, and its hyphae branch at a 45-degree angle. There are no phialides and few septae.
B. *Penicillium* spp.
Rationale: Penicillium spp. usually produce green-colored colonies, with septate hyphae and phialides that produce chaining conidia.
C. *Aspergillus niger.*
Rationale: The colonies of *A. niger* quickly turn black, and the septate hyphae have 45-degree angle branching. Phialides radiate round the entire vesicle.
D. *Fusarium* spp.
Rationale: Fusarium spp. produce pink or violet colonies, and the hyphae are septate. Phialides produce large sickle-shaped macroconidia.
E. *Acremonium* spp.
Rationale: Colonies of *Acremonium* are often red, and the septate hyphae produce tubelike phialides.

Major points of discussion

- *Syncephalastrum racemosum* is a ubiquitous, saprophytic fungus found in soil and decaying plant debris. It belongs to the order Mucorales and has been reported as a rare cause of systemic and nail infections.
- *S. racemosum* may resemble *Aspergillus* or *Fusarium* spp. on microscopic examination because all three can show dichotomous branching, often at a 45-degree angle.

In contrast to the numerous septate hyphae of *Aspergillus* or *Fusarium* spp., *Syncephalastrum* is sparsely septate. Phialides, which are specialized cells that produce conidia (conidiogenous) without increasing length, are absent in *Syncephalastrum.*

- LVADs can be used to salvage a patient in cardiogenic shock and can be used as a bridge to transplantation. The devices are equipped with alarms if they malfunction. Should there be an obstruction, the parts should be cultured and the source of the contaminant investigated.
- The identification of filamentous fungi by phenotypic methods includes colonial and microscopic morphology, biochemical tests, and growth on differential media. Culture remains the gold standard for mold identification, but it is cumbersome, technically challenging, and has a prolonged turn around time for results. Molecular methods are increasingly used for fungal identification due to increased sensitivity, ease of use, and rapid results.
- There are only limited data regarding treatment of *Syncephalastrum* infections. Amphotericin B, ketoconazole, and itraconazole MICs are low, whereas those of voriconazole are relatively high.[48,60]

81. A. *Alternaria* spp.
Rationale: Alternaria spp. are dematiaceous or pigmented molds and have large brown conidia that have transverse and longitudinal septations.
B. *Exophiala* spp.
Rationale: Exophiala spp. are dematiaceous or pigmented molds and produce single-celled conidia that aggregate at the apex of the conidiophore.
C. *Geotrichum* spp.
Rationale: Geotrichum spp. are yeast that produce arthroconidia, which occurs when the hyphae break into segmented cells.
D. *Torulopsis* spp.
Rationale: Torulopsis spp. are yeast that produce small oval yeast cells with single terminal buds.
E. *Fusarium* spp.
Rationale: Fusarium spp. are hyaline or nonpigmented molds characterized by canoe-shaped macroconidia.

Major points of discussion

- Keratitis, an inflammation of the cornea, can be caused by bacteria, viruses, amoeba, and fungi. There have been reports of fungal keratitis related to contaminated contact lens solution.
- *Fusarium* spp. are frequently associated with eye infections as well as sinusitis, nail infections, and septic arthritis. Neutropenic patients can also have disseminated systemic infections.
- *Fusarium* colonies mature in less than 4 days and start off as white and cottony but rapidly develop a pink to violet center.
- Microscopic examination demonstrates septate hyphae and large canoe-shaped macroconidia with three to five septa.
- Fungal keratitis is currently treated with natamycin for several months. More invasive infections usually require treatment with antifungals, such as amphotericin B, fluconazole, or voriconazole.[11]

82. A. It is standard practice that all yeast and filamentous fungi (molds) are handled and processed under a BSC. Tape or shrink seals are required to seal all agar and broth media to protect against contamination or infection with dimorphic fungi (e.g., *Coccidioides immitis*).
Rationale: Yeast can be handled on the open bench in the general microbiology area; however, molds are always processed under a BSC. Agar plates, not screw-capped agar slants, must be taped or sealed.
B. The use of a BSC is required for processing and handling molds, not yeast. Tape or shrink seals are required when using plated agar media; however, petri plates should not be used if *C. immitis* is suspected.
Rationale: A BSC must be used when processing molds, but yeast cultures can be handled in an open microbiology laboratory. Screw-cap tubes of slanted media are considered safer than agar plates but are not a required safety procedure. If *C. immitis* is suspected, plates must not be used.
C. The required location of the BSC used for handling fungal specimens and cultures is a confined access mycology facility. All agar slants and plates are required to be sealed by tape or shrink seals to prevent contamination.
Rationale: It is recommended, but not required, that a dedicated BSC and separate room be used for mycology specimen and culture workup. Due to the presence of screw caps on agar slants, sealing or taping these is not a standard practice for mycology.
D. Slide cultures of suspect dimorphic fungi, in lieu of wet mount preparations, must be prepared in a BSC located within a confined access room.
Rationale: Standard safety practices require that slide cultures not be prepared for suspected dimorphic fungi. Wet mount preparations, prepared under a BSC, will aid in detecting these molds.
E. Mold species, such as *Aspergillus* and *Candida* species, are less infectious to laboratory workers; therefore, they can be handled and processed outside of a BSC.
Rationale: Candida species do not form airborne spores and can be safely handled without BSC containment precautions; however, *Aspergillus* and other molds should be processed in a BSC to avoid contamination of the laboratory environment and of other specimens.

Major points of discussion
- Accurate data regarding laboratory-acquired mycoses are not available due to a general lack of required reporting to public health agencies. Reporting acquired infections in laboratories is currently required with coccidioidomycosis in California and Arizona, blastomycosis in Louisiana and Wisconsin, and histoplasmosis in Kentucky and Wisconsin.
- Because filamentous fungi produce conidia or spores that can easily become airborne, special safety precautions specific to mycology are required. Examination of molds should be performed in a BSC, not only to prevent contamination of the laboratory environment, but also to avert acquisition of dimorphic fungi, such as *Coccidioides immitis*, *Blastomyces dermatitidis*, and *Histoplasma capsulatum*. Because yeast

do not produce airborne spores, they can be processed on the open workbench.
- Standard safety precautions in mycology require that slide cultures never be prepared if dimorphic fungi are suspected. Slide culture procedures are reserved for the workup of low-virulence fungi. Wet mount preparations are recommended for presumptive identification of dimorphic fungi, and screw-cap tubes of slanted media or plated media can be used to grow nondimorphic molds. However, when the latter are used, oxygen-permeable tape or shrink seals must be used to contain the spores within the plate.
- Although it is recommended that a designated laboratory under negative pressure be used to safely culture and identify molds, it is not a requirement. Handling and processing fungal isolates, including molds, can be safely performed using a certified BSC in the open microbiology laboratory.
- Yeast are routinely identified by commercially prepared biochemical-based assays. Identification of molds includes DNA probe assays for dimorphic fungi, microscopic morphology, and differential or selective media. Molecular methods for identification are rapidly replacing phenotypic assays, such as gene sequencing, nucleic acid amplification, and mass spectrophotometry.[21,36]

83. A. *Aspergillus fumigates.*
Rationale: A. fumigatus has been associated with sinusitis; however, it demonstrates a white reverse color.
B. *Alternaria* spp.
Rationale: Alternaria species can cause sinusitis. This dematiaceous mold is inhibited by cyclohexamide; therefore, it will not grow on Mycosel agar, but it can grow on IMA.
C. *Cryptococcus neoformans.*
Rationale: C. neoformans is a yeast and does not demonstrate mycelial forms.
D. *Fusarium* spp.
Rationale: Fusarium colonies are white and cottony; the reverse is typically a light color.
E. *Mucor* spp.
Rationale: Mucor, a zygomycete, rapidly grows as a white cotton candy–like mold with a white reverse.

Major points of discussion
- Dematiaceous fungi, such as *Alternaria*, can cause cutaneous and subcutaneous infections as well as chronic sinusitis. One of the diagnostic features of this fungal is brown-pigmented hyphae (due to melanin production) that can be observed microscopically in direct unstained specimens.
- Several mold species are associated with allergies. The most common mold allergen sources belong to the taxonomic group fungi imperfecti, which includes *Alternaria* and *Aspergillus* species. Airborne spores of *Alternaria* species are highest during autumn because of the degradation of leaves and other biomaterial.
- *Alternaria* conidia are large and brown, have transverse and longitudinal septations, and can be found singly or in chains.

■ Identification to the species level is difficult based only on macroscopic and microscopic observations. Amplification of the internal transcribed space (ITS) region with pan-fungal primers, followed by sequencing, is a useful molecular method for identifying *Alternaria* species.

■ For chronic sinusitis due to *Alternaria*, amphotericin B is currently the antifungal agent used most frequently, either alone or in combination with flucytosine and/or rifampicin. In most cases, treatment with antifungal agents is combined with surgery.[54]

84. A. India ink examination.
Rationale: The India ink examination is useful for detecting *Cryptococcus neoformans/gattii* in cerebrospinal fluid specimens because the organism has a capsule that excludes the stain.
B. *Aspergillus* antibody EIA.
Rationale: Antibody detection is not useful for diagnosis of acute infection. In addition, many noninfected individuals will have detectable antibodies against *Aspergillus* due to environmental exposure.
C. Galactomannan antigen EIA.
Rationale: This EIA detects *Aspergillus* galactomannan in serum and bronchoalveolar lavage specimens and is used as one component for the diagnosis of invasive aspergillosis.
D. KOH examination.
Rationale: The KOH examination can be used to detect fungal elements directly from specimens. Although hyphae may be observed, this does not aid in the identification of which mold may be present.
E. Calcofluor white examination.
Rationale: Calcofluor white is a fluorescent stain that binds to the cellulose and chitin components of fungi. It is used for direct microscopic examination of specimens. However, it is not specific for *Aspergillus*.

Major points of discussion
■ Blood cultures are rarely positive in patients with invasive aspergillosis. Therefore, a combination of clinical and laboratory parameters is often necessary for diagnosis, including culture of potential fungal metastases, CT scan, chest radiograph, and galactomannan detection.
■ Galactomannan is a fungal cell wall carbohydrate found in serum. Although this antigen can also be detected in cerebrospinal fluid and urine, bronchoalveolar lavage specimens are the only other FDA-approved source for testing.
■ It is recommended that high-risk patients (e.g., neutropenic patients with hematologic malignancies) be tested twice a week to optimize early antigen detection.
■ Some limitations of the assay include false-negative results for patients receiving antifungal therapy and false-positive results for patients with infections due to other molds such as *Penicillium*, *Alternaria*, and *Histoplasma*. In addition, patients who have received piperacillin/tazobactam may have false-positive galactomannan results.
■ Voriconazole is currently the first-line treatment for invasive aspergillosis. Alternative therapies include itraconazole, amphotericin B, caspofungin, micafungin, and posaconazole.[2,56]

85. A. *Paracoccidioides brasiliensis*.
Rationale: Paracoccidioides, a thermally dimorphic fungus, produces septate, branched hyphae with terminal chlamydospores at 25°C.
B. *Blastomyces dermatitidis*.
Rationale: Blastomyces, a thermally dimorphic fungus, produces septate hyphae with conidia at the apex of the conidiophore (resembling a lollipop) at 25°C.
C. *Sporothrix schenckii*.
Rationale: Sporothrix, a rapidly growing thermally dimorphic fungus, produces very narrow hyphae with rosette clusters of conidia at the apex of the conidiophore at 25°C.
D. *Penicillium marneffei*.
Rationale: Penicillium, a rapidly growing, thermally dimorphic fungus, produces septate hyphae with four to five terminal metulae, each with four to six phialides at 25°C.
E. *Histoplasma capsulatum*.
Rationale: Histoplasma, a thermally dimorphic fungus, produces septate hyphae that have large thick walled macroconidia with knobby projections at 25°C. The smooth-walled microconidia are the infectious particles.

Major points of discussion
■ The most common clinical manifestation of histoplasmosis is lung infection. Symptoms can occur 3 to 17 days after exposure and include fever and nonproductive cough. If not treated, the disease can disseminate to other organs and is often diagnosed in bone marrow biopsies. Many people who live in endemic areas inhale the fungus and remain asymptomatic.
■ *H. capsulatum* is most prevalent in the Ohio and Mississippi River valleys and commonly grows in soil contaminated with bat or bird droppings. The fungal spores become airborne when the soil is disturbed, and breathing in the spores can cause infection in the lungs. Histoplasmosis cannot be transmitted from person to person.
■ In tissue sections, *H. capsulatum* can present as a necrotizing granuloma and the small, narrow-based yeast cells are found within histiocytes.
■ A commercially available DNA probe assay can be used to rapidly confirm identification rather than waiting to convert the organism to its yeast form at 37°C.
■ Enzyme immunoassays have been developed to detect *Histoplasma* polysaccharide antigen in urine, serum, and cerebrospinal fluid. This assay is used to diagnose disseminated infection as well as follow response to antifungal therapy.
■ Mild pulmonary histoplasmosis can resolve within 1 month without treatment. Severe cases of acute histoplasmosis are currently treated with itraconazole for up to 3 to 12 months, depending on the severity of the disease and the immune status of the patient.

86. A. Urease test.
Rationale: The urease test is positive for the fungi *Cryptococcus*, *Rhodotorula*, *Candida krusei*, and *Trichophyton mentagrophytes*.
B. Germ tube test.
Rationale: The germ tube test has a very high sensitivity and specificity for *C. albicans*.

C. India ink examination.
Rationale: India ink is useful for identifying *C. neoformans/ gattii* in cerebrospinal fluid specimens because these organisms have a capsule that excludes the stain.
D. Phenol oxidase test.
Rationale: Phenol oxidase is used to identify *C. neoformans/ gattii*. These organisms contain this enzyme in their cell wall, which enables them to convert various amines to melanin, a pigment.
E. Rapid assimilation of trehalose.
Rationale: The rapid assimilation of trehalose test, used to identify *Candida glabrata,* is based on the utilization of trehalose in the presence of cyclohexamide.

Major points of discussion

- *Candida albicans* is the most common *Candida* species isolated from clinical specimens. Infectious processes associated with *C. albicans* include thrush, genital yeast infections, and fungemia, the latter of which is particularly associated with catheters.
- Macroscopically, *C. albicans* is often identified by the presence of filamentous extensions (sometimes referred to as "feet") around the edge of the colonies. The less commonly encountered *C. dubliniensis* can also demonstrate this characteristic.
- For the germ tube test, yeast are suspended in serum and incubated at 35°C to 37°C for 2 hours. A wet mount is examined microscopically for the presence of germ tubes. Germ tubes are hyphae that form directly from the wall of the yeast in a parallel fashion. They differ from pseudohyphae, which have a constriction at the cell wall juncture.
- Cornmeal-Tween agar is often used to demonstrate pseudohyphae with clusters of round blastoconida at the septa, which is characteristic of *C. albicans*.
- Several commercially available systems can identify most species of clinically relevant yeast based on carbohydrate assimilation.

87. A. *Aspergillus flavus.*
Rationale: Colonies of *A. flavus* appear yellow-green to olive. This mold does not cause otomycosis.
B. *Exophiala dermatitidis.*
Rationale: Colonies of *E. dermatitidis* appear black, moist, and yeast-like. This mold does not cause otomycosis.
C. *Aspergillus niger.*
Rationale: Colonies of *A. niger* grow rapidly and have a black surface with a white border. This mold is the primary cause of otomycosis.
D. *Fonsecaea pedrosoi.*
Rationale: *F. pedrosoi* is a slow-growing dematiaceous mold that produces flat, dark green, velvety colonies. This mold does not cause otomycosis.
E. *Epidermophyton floccosum.*
Rationale: *E. floccosum* is a mold that produces colonies that appear folded in the center and grooved radially; that have a brownish-yellow to olive-gray surface. This dermatophyte does not cause otomycosis.

Major points of discussion

- Otomycosis is a superficial fungal infection of the outer ear canal. It is more common in tropical countries. It is typically characterized by a malodorous discharge, inflammation, pruritus, scaling, and severe discomfort.
- *Aspergillus niger*, the most common cause of otomycosis, can also manifest as "fungus balls" in patients with preexisting lung cavities.
- The approach to differentiate among common *Aspergillus* species includes examining colony surface and reverse color, size and appearance of conidiophores, and the presence and distribution pattern of uniseriate or biseriate phialides.
- *A. niger* has septate hyphae, long conidiophores, and biseriate (i.e., vesicles produce sterile cells known as metulae) phialides that radiate around the entire vesicle.
- Otomycosis is treated by debridement followed by topical antifungals such as clotrimazole, miconazole, and tolnaftate.

88. A. *Aspergillus fumigates.*
Rationale: *A. fumigatus* is a filamentous fungus (i.e., mold) that is rarely recovered from blood cultures.
B. *Candida albicans.*
Rationale: *C. albicans* is a yeast that grows within 24 hours on routine bacteriologic media, such as chocolate agar and sheep blood agar.
C. *Candida parapsilosis.*
Rationale: *C. parapsilosis* is a yeast that grows within 24 hours on routine bacteriologic media, such as chocolate agar and sheep blood agar. It is a common cause of fungemia in pediatric patients, particularly those who are immunocompromised.
D. *Malassezia furfur.*
Rationale: *M. furfur* is a yeast that requires long-chain fatty acids for growth. An olive oil overlay on top of the agar surface is necessary for culturing this organism.
E. *Cryptococcus neoformans.*
Rationale: *C. neoformans* is a yeast that grows within 48 hours on routine bacteriologic media, such as chocolate agar and sheep blood agar.

Major points of discussion

- *Malassezia furfur* is a component of the normal skin microbiota in most individuals. Two major risk factors for infection with *M. furfur* are catheter-related fungemia in patients receiving total parenteral nutrition, which is high in lipids, and skin diseases, such as *Pityrosporum* folliculitis, pityriasis (tinea) versicolor, and atopic dermatitis.
- KOH preparations of skin infections with *M. furfur* demonstrate hyphae and spherical yeast cells and demonstrate a "spaghetti and meatball" appearance.
- All *Malassezia* species require long-chain fatty acids for growth, with the exception of *M. pachydermatis*.
- *Malassezia* colonies appear cream colored to yellowish-brown and grow best at 30°C to 35°C.
- Microscopically, *Malassezia* appears as phialides with small collarettes. Identification to the species level is best obtained by using molecular methods such as sequencing.
- For skin infections, oral ketoconazole or itraconazole is commonly used for treatment. For systemic disease, amphotericin B is the drug of choice. Removing the catheter is critical for treating catheter-related infections.

89. A. **Trichophyton rubrum.**
Rationale: T. rubrum is the most common dermatophyte isolated from infected feet and nails. It produces numerous teardrop microconidia and occasional long, thin-walled macroconidia.
B. *Microsporum canis.*
Rationale: M. canis is a dermatophyte that commonly causes scalp and skin infections. Club-shaped microconidia are rare and macroconidia are numerous, spindle shaped, and thick walled.
C. *Trichophyton tonsurans.*
Rationale: T. tonsurans is the primary cause of scalp ringworm in the United States. Microconidia are numerous and vary in shape. Macroconidia are rare, thick walled, and have irregular shapes.
D. *Epidermophyton floccosum.*
Rationale: E. floccosum is a dermatophyte that infects skin and nails. It produces no microconidia and its macroconidia are club shaped, thick walled, and vary in size.
E. *Microsporum gypseum.*
Rationale: M. gypseum is a dermatophyte that does not commonly cause infection. Microconidia are club shaped and macroconidia are numerous, symmetric, and thin walled.

Major points of discussion

- Dermatophytes are filamentous fungi that obtain nutrients from keratinized tissue such as skin, hair, and nails. The clinical manifestation, referred to as ringworm or tinea, is the host response to enzymes produced by the dermatophyte.
- The most common clinical diseases are tinea barbae (infection of the beard area), tinea capitis (infection of the scalp), tinea corporis (usually infection of the trunk of the body), tinea cruris (infection of the groin), tinea pedis (infection of the feet), and tinea unguium (infection of the nails).
- The genera of dermatophytes can be differentiated by the types and microscopic morphologies of the conidia produced (Table 16-10).
- *Trichophyton rubrum* usually has a white to buff surface color and a deep red reverse. It can be differentiated from *T. mentagrophytes* by negative reactions for urease production and in vitro hair perforation.
- Fungal nail infections are often treated with a combination of topical and oral agents. Topical agents include ciclopirox or amorolfine. Oral antifungals include clotrimazole, terbinafine, and itraconazole.

90. A. Routine culture.
Rationale: Culture of the positive blood bottles onto conventional agar media requires at least 24 hours of

incubation and final biochemical identification requires at least one additional day.
B. Chromagar *Candida* culture.
Rationale: Chromagar is differential agar media used for presumptive identification of yeast. The chromogenic substrates in the agar yield characteristic species-specific colony colors, such as for *Candida albicans* (green), *Candida tropicalis* (blue), and *Candida krusei* (pink). It requires at least 24 hours for results.
C. **Peptide nucleic acid fluorescent in situ hybridization.**
Rationale: Peptide nucleic acid fluorescent in situ hybridization uses specific probes to hybridize targeted sequences for identifying *C. albicans*, *C. glabrata*, and *C. tropicalis* within 30 to 90 minutes directly from positive blood cultures.
D. 16S rRNA gene sequencing.
Rationale: 16S rRNA gene sequencing uses specific primers to amplify targeted genetic regions that can be sequenced to identify microorganisms from pure culture, not from blood cultures. Results can be obtained within 2 days.
E. Yeast identification panels.
Rationale: Yeast identification panels contain multiple conventional biochemical tests that are inoculated from pure cultures and not from blood cultures. Results are typically obtained within 1 to 2 days.

Major points of discussion

- *Candida* is the most frequently isolated fungus from blood cultures, and candidemia is the fourth most common cause of hospital-associated bloodstream infections in the United States. *Candida albicans* is the predominant isolate; *C. glabrata* is common among the elderly and *C. parapsilosis* among children. Associated risk factors for candidemia include the use of broad-spectrum antibiotics, central venous catheters, and length of stay in intensive care units.
- Differentiation between *C. albicans* and *C. glabrata* affects patient care by influencing the empiric selection of antifungal therapy. Generally, *C. albicans* is susceptible to fluconazole, whereas *C. glabrata* may be resistant.
- PNA FISH assay uses multicolor labeled fluorescent PNA probes to target specific 26S rRNA sequences of clinically important yeasts, such as *C. albicans* and *C. glabrata*, directly from positive blood culture bottles. When PNA probes hybridize to specific targets, the species is identified by microscopic visualization of the fluorescent cells (e.g., green for *C. albicans*).
- In vitro susceptibility testing for yeast uses broth microdilution technology and requires incubation for 24 to 48 hours for *Candida* and 72 hours for *Cryptococcus neoformans*. Interpretative guidelines for this purpose were established by the Clinical and Laboratory Standards Institute for fluconazole, itraconazole, voriconazole, anidulafungin, caspofungin, micafungin, and flucytosine.
- Invasive *Candida* infections can be treated with lipid formulations of amphotericin B, azoles (e.g., fluconazole), or echinocandins (e.g., caspofungin). *C. glabrata* infections often require echinocandins or amphotericin in lieu of treatment with azoles, which are fungistatic.[24,42,63]

Table 16-10 Characteristics of Dermatophytes

Genus	Macroconidia	Microconidia
Trichophyton	Rare Thin-walled Smooth	Numerous
Microsporum	Numerous Thick-walled Rough	Numerous
Epidermophyton	Numerous Thin- or thick-walled Smooth	Absent

References

1. Aaron L, Saadoun D, Calatroni I, et al. Tuberculosis in HIV-infected patients: a comprehensive review. *Clin Microbiol Infect.* 2004;10:388–398.
2. Aquino VR, Goldani LZ, Pasqualotto AC. Update on the contribution of galactomannan for the diagnosis of invasive aspergillosis. *Mycopathologia.* 2007;163:191–202.
3. Barnes PF, Cave DM. Molecular epidemiology of tuberculosis. *N Engl J Med.* 2003;349:1149–1156.
4. Brotman RB, Klebanoff MA, Nansel TR, et al. Bacterial vaginosis assessed by gram stain and diminished colonization resistance to incident gonococcal, chlamydial and trichomonal genital infection. *J Infect Dis.* 2010;202:1907–1915.
5. Brouqui P, Raoult D. Endocarditis due to rare and fastidious bacteria. *Clin Microbiol Rev.* 2001;14:177–207.
6. Brouwer MC, Tunkel AR, van de Beek D. Epidemiology, diagnosis and antimicrobial treatment of acute bacterial meningitis. *Clin Microb Rev.* 2010;23:467–492.
7. Brown-Elliott BA, Brown JM, Conville PS, Wallace RJ Jr. Clinical and laboratory features of the *Nocardia spp.* based on current molecular taxonomy. *Clin Microbiol Rev.* 2006;19(2):259–82.
8. Brown-Elliott BA, et al. Antimicrobial susceptibility testing, drug resistance mechanisms, and therapy of infections with nontuberculous mycobacteria. *Clin Microbiol Rev.* 2012;25: 545–582.
9. Brown-Elliott BA, Wallace RJ. Clinical and taxonomic status of pathogenic nonpigmented or late-pigmenting rapidly growing mycobacteria. *Clin Microbiol Rev.* 2002;5:716–746.
10. Carapetis JR, Steer AC, Mulholland EK, Weber M. The global burden of group A streptococcal diseases. *Lancet Infect Dis.* 2005;5:685.
11. Centers for Disease Control, Prevention. *Fusarium* keratitis–multiple states. *MMWR.* 2006;55:400–401.
12. Centers for Disease Control, Prevention. Guidelines for preventing the transmission of *Mycobacterium tuberculosis* in health-care settings 2005, *MMWR Recomm Rep.* 2005;54(RR-17):1–141.
13. Centers for Disease Control and Prevention. Prevention of perinatal group B streptococcal disease. *MMWR.* 2010;59 (RR-10):1–32.
14. Centers for Disease Control and Prevention. Report of an Expert Consultation on the Uses of Nucleic Acid Amplification Tests for the Diagnosis of Tuberculosis. Available at www.cdc.gov/tb/ publications/guidelines/amplification_tests/default.htm.
15. Centers for Disease Control, Prevention. Reptile-associated salmonellosis–selected states, 1998-2002. *MMWR.* 2003;52:1206–1209.
16. Centers for Disease Control and Prevention. Sexually transmitted diseases treatment guidelines, 2010. *MMWR.* 2010;59(No. RR-12):1–110.
17. Centers for Disease Control and Prevention. Tattoo-associated nontuberculous mycobacterial skin infections–multiple states, 2011-2012. *MMWR.* 2012;61:653–656.
18. Centers for Disease Control and Prevention. Treatment of Tuberculosis. Available at www.cdc.gov/tb/topic/treatment/ default.htm.
19. Centers for Disease Control and Prevention. Tuberculosis. Available at www.cdc.gov/tb/publications/guidelines/treatment. htm.
20. Centers for Disease Control and Prevention. Tularemia. Available at www.cdc.gov/tularemia/.
21. Chosewood LC, Wilson DE, eds; Centers for Disease Control and Prevention and National Institutes of Health. *Biosafety in microbiological and biomedical laboratories.* 5th ed. Washington, DC: US Department of Health and Human Services; 2006.
22. Clinical and Laboratory Standards Institute. *Methods for dilution antimicrobial susceptibility tests for bacteria that grow aerobically.* M07-A9, (vol 32). Wayne, PA, 2012.
23. Clinical and Laboratory Standards Institute. *Performance standards for antimicrobial susceptibility testing; twenty-first informational supplement.* M100-S21, (vol 31). Wayne, PA, 2012.
24. Clinical and Laboratory Standards Institute. *Reference method for broth dilution antifungal susceptibility testing of yeasts.* M27-A3, (vol 28). Wayne, PA, 2004.
25. Clinical and Laboratory Standards Institute. Quality assurance for commercially prepared microbiological culture media. M22. Wayne, PA, 2004.
26. Congli Y, Caixia Z, Xiuguo H. *Bartonella henselae* infection and its effects on human health. *Rev Med Microbiol.* 2011;10:67–72.
27. Della-Latta P, Jost K, Roberts G, et al. *Mycobacterium tuberculosis: Assessing your laboratory.* Association of Public Health Laboratories, 2009.
28. Department of Health and Human Services. *Biosafety in microbiological and biomedical laboratories.* 5th ed. Washington, DC: US Government Printing Office: 2007.
29. Doganay M, Aygen B. Human brucellosis: an overview. *Int J Infect Dis.* 2003;7:173–182.
30. DuPont HL. Bacterial diarrhea. *N Engl J Med.* 2009;36:1560–1569.
31. Falkinham JO. Epidemiology of infection by nontuberculous mycobacteria. *Clin Microbiol Rev.* 1996;177–215.
32. Farlow J, Wagner DM, Dukerich M, et al. *Francisella tularensis* in the United States. *Emerg Infect Dis.* 2005;11:1835–1841.
33. Ffethers KA, Fairley CK, Hocking JS, et al. Sexual risk factors and bacterial vaginosis: a systematic review and meta-analysis. *Clin Infect Dis.* 2008;47:1426–1435.
34. Field SK. Cowie RL Lung disease due to the more common nontuberculous mycobacteria. *Chest.* 2006;29:1653–1672.
35. Fishbain J, Pelig AY. Treatment of *Acinetobacter* infections. *Clin Infect Dis.* 2010;51:79–84.
36. Schell WA. Mycotic agents of human disease. In Fleming DO, Hunt SL, eds. Biological safety principles and practices, 4th ed. Washington, DC: 2006, American Society of Microbiology.
37. Frank KL, Reichert EJ, Piper KE, Patel R. In vitro effects of antimicrobial agents on planktonic and biofilms forms of *Staphylococcus lugdunensis* clinical isolates. *Antimicrob Agents Chemother.* 2007;51:888.
38. Goering RV. Pulsed field gel electrophoresis: a review of application and interpretation in the molecular epidemiology of infectious disease. *Infect Genet Evol.* 2010;10:866–875.
39. Griffith DE, Aksamit T, Brown-Elliott BA, et al. An Official ATS/ IDSA statement: diagnosis, treatment, and prevention of nontuberculous mycobacterial diseases. *Am J Respir Crit Care Med.* 2007;175:367–416.
40. Gupta K, Hooton TM, Naber KG, et al. International clinical practice guidelines for the treatment of acute uncomplicated cystitis and pyelonephritis in women: a 2010 update by the Infectious Diseases Society of America and the European Society for Microbiology and Infectious Diseases. *Clin Infect Dis.* 2011;52:103–120.
41. Hanssen AM, Johanna U, Ericson S. SCC*mec* in staphylococci: genes on the move. *FEMS Immunol Med Microbiol.* 2006;46:8–20.
42. Heil EL, Daniels LM, Long DM, et al. Impact of a rapid peptide nucleic acid fluorescence in situ hybridization assay on treatment of Candida infections. *Am J Health Syst Pharm.* 2012;69: 1910–1914.
43. Hlavsa MC, Moonan PK, Cowan LS, et al. Human tuberculosis due to *Mycobacterium bovis* in the United States. *Clin Infect Dis.* 2008;47:168–175.
44. Ho P-L, Cheng V C-C, Chu C-M. Antibiotic resistance in community-acquired pneumonia Caused by *Streptococcus pneumoniae*, methicillin-resistant *Staphylococcus aureus* and *Acinetobacter baumannii. Chest.* 2009;136:1119–1127.
45. Huang SS, Septimus E, Kleinman K, et al. Targeted versus universal decolonization to prevent ICU infection. *N Engl J Med.* 2013;368:2255–2265.

46. Iwamoto M, Ayers T, Mahon BE, Swerdlow DL. Epidemiology of seafood-associated infections in the United States. *Clin Microbiol Rev.* 2010;23:399–411.

47. Kambham N. Postinfectious glomerulonephritis. *Adv Anat Pathol.* 2012;19:338–347.

48. Larone DH. *Medically important fungi. a guide to identification.* 5th edition. Washington, DC: ASM Press; 2011: 155-168.

49. Lindeboom JA. Bruijnesteijn van Coppenraet LES, van Soolingen D, Prins JM, Kuijper EJ. Clinical manifestations, diagnosis, and treatment of *Mycobacterium haemophilum* infections. *Clin Microbiol Rev.* 2011;24:701–717.

50. Liu C, Bayer A, Cosgrove SE, et al. Clinical practice guidelines by the Infectious Diseases Society of America for the treatment of methicillin-resistant *Staphylococcus aureus* infections in adults and children. *Clin Infect Dis.* 2011;52:1–38.

51. Munoz-Price LS, Weinstien RA. *Acinetobacter* infection. *N Engl J Med.* 2008;358:1271–1281.

52. Mylonakis E, Paliou M, Hohmann EL, Calderwood SB, Wing EJ. Listeriosis during pregnancy: a case series and review of 222 cases. *Medicine.* 2002;81:260–269.

53. Pappas G, Akritidis N, Bosilkovski M, Tsianos E. Brucellosis. *N Engl J Med.* 2005;52:2325–2336.

54. Pastor FJ, Guarro J. *Alternaria* infections: laboratory diagnosis and relevant clinical features. *Clin Microbiol Infect.* 2008;14:734–746.

55. Paterson D, Bonomo R. Extended spectrum β-lactactamases: a clinical update. *Clin Microbiol Rev.* 2005;18:657–686.

56. Pfeiffer CD, Fine JP, Safdar N. Diagnosis of invasive aspergillosis using a galactomannan assay: a meta-analysis. *Clin Infect Dis.* 2006;42:1417–1427.

57. Poutanen SM, Baron EJ. *Staphylococcus lugdunensis*: a notably distinct coagulase-negative *Staphylococcus. Clin Micro Newslett.* 2001;23:19.

58. Saiman L, O'Keefe M, Graham PL, et al. Hospital transmission of community-acquired methicillin-resistant *Staphylococcus aureus* among postpartum women. *Clin Infect Dis.* 2003;37:1313–1319.

59. Schlaberg R, Huard RC, Della-Latta P. *Nocardia cyriacigeorgica*, an emerging pathogen in the United States. *J Clin Microsc.* 2008;46:265–273.

60. Schlebusch S, Looke DFM. Intraabdominal zygomycosis caused by *Syncephalastrum racemosum* infection successfully treated with partial surgical debridement and high-dose amphotericin B lipid complex. *J Clin Microbiol.* 2005;43:5825–5827.

61. Schlech WF. Foodborne listeriosis. *Clin Infect Dis.* 2000;31:770–775.

62. Scollard DM, Adams LB, Gillis TP, et al. The continuing challenges of leprosy. *Clin Microbiol Rev.* 2006;19:338–381.

63. Shepard JR, Addison RM. Alexander BD, et al. Multicenter evaluation of the *Candida albicans/Candida glabrata* peptide nucleic acid fluorescent in situ hybridization method for simultaneous dual-color identification of *C. albicans* and *C. glabrata* directly from blood culture bottles. *J Clin Microbiol.* 2008;46:50–55.

64. Singh N, Paterson D. *Aspergillus* infections in transplant recipients. *Clin Microbiol Rev.* 2005;18:44–69.

65. Swaminathan S, Alangaden GJ. Treatment of resistant enterococcial urinary tract infections. *Curr Infect Dis Rep.* 2010;12:455–464.

66. Tenover FC, Arbeit RD, Goering PV, et al. Interpreting chromosomal DNA restriction patterns produced by pulsed-field gel electrophoresis: criteria for bacterial strain typing. *J Clin Microbiol.* 1995;33:2233–2239.

67. Versalovic J, Carroll KC, Funke G, et al., eds. *Manual of Clinical Microbiology,* volume 1. Washington, DC: ASM Press.

68. Watkins RR, Lemonovich TL. Diagnosis and management of community-acquired pneumonia in adults. *Am Fam Phys.* 2011;83:1299–1306.

69. Wilkins MJ, et al. Human *Mycobacterium bovis* infection and bovine tuberculosis outbreak, Michigan, 1994-2007. *Emerging Infect Dis.* 2008;14:657–660.

70. Wood N, McIntyre P. Pertussis: review of epidemiology, diagnosis, management and prevention. *Pediatr Respir Rev.* 2008;9:201–212.

71. Wu F, Della-Latta P. Molecular typing strategies. *Semin Perinatol.* 2002;26:357–366.

CHAPTER 17

MICROBIOLOGY: Virology

Susan Whittier, Fann Wu

QUESTIONS

1. Cytomegalovirus (CMV) infection in solid-organ transplant patients is associated with an increased predisposition to allograft rejection, as well as reduced overall patient and allograft survival. To decrease the risk of contracting CMV disease, which one of the following donor/recipient CMV status combinations should be avoided, if at all possible?
   A. Donor negative/recipient positive.
   B. Donor positive/recipient positive.
   C. Donor negative/recipient negative.
   D. Donor positive/recipient negative.
   E. The risk is equal for all donor/recipient matches.

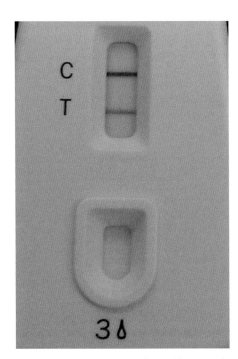

Figure 17-1 Enzyme immunoassay: C is the positive control and T is the sample.

2. A 3-year-old girl presented to the pediatric emergency department (ED) in the autumn, with fever and symptoms consistent with bronchiolitis. A rapid enzyme immunoassay (EIA) was positive for the etiologic agent (Figure 17-1). Which

one of the following microorganisms is most likely to cause this infection?
   A. Parainfluenza.
   B. Rotavirus.
   C. Respiratory syncytial virus (RSV).
   D. *Bordetella pertussis*.
   E. Coronavirus.

3. A 30-year-old immune-competent male patient presented to his physician in the winter with a high fever, headache, myalgias, and nonproductive cough. A chest radiograph revealed a right lower lobe infiltrate. On hospitalization, broad-spectrum antibiotics were instituted, but his symptoms persisted. Which one of the following is the most likely etiologic agent?
   A. *Mycoplasma pneumonia*.
   B. *Streptococcus pneumoniae*.
   C. Influenza A.
   D. Adenovirus.
   E. Parainfluenza.

4. A 47-year-old male kidney transplant patient presented with a low-grade fever, myalgias, and mild gastroenteritis. BK virus was suspected to be the etiologic agent of infection. Which one of the following statements is true regarding BK viruses?
   A. Most individuals have never been exposed to BK virus.
   B. BK virus can remain latent in the kidney and uroepithelial cells.
   C. The assay used for early diagnosis of BK nephropathy is a qualitative (polymerase chain reaction) PCR assay using urine.
   D. Antiviral therapy is used empirically before transplantation.
   E. BK virus is ubiquitous, causing infections in all solid-organ transplant patients.

5. A 28-year-old man was recently diagnosed with HIV-1 infection. His baseline viral load was 204,000 copies/mL and he was started on a highly active antiretroviral therapy (HAART) regimen. One week later, a repeat viral load was 98,000 copies/mL. Which one of the following statements would best describe his condition?
   A. His treatment response was successful because his human immunodeficiency virus type 1 (HIV-1) viral load was significantly reduced.
   B. He has not responded to treatment because his viral load remains unchanged.

C. His HAART regimen should be modified because there was no significant change in viral load.

D. He should continue on HAART and the viral load test should be repeated immediately.

E. He should continue on HAART and his viral load should be measured in 2 to 8 weeks.

6. A 36-year-old woman with a history of intravenous drug abuse was referred for follow-up due to abnormal liver function tests. The result of her hepatitis C virus (HCV) quantitative PCR test was positive. Which one of the following statements best describes the clinical utility of ordering an HCV genotype assay?

A. To confirm the diagnosis of HCV infection.

B. To detect HCV and human immunodeficiency virus coinfection.

C. To monitor antiviral therapy.

D. To predict duration of antiviral therapy.

E. To determine viral load.

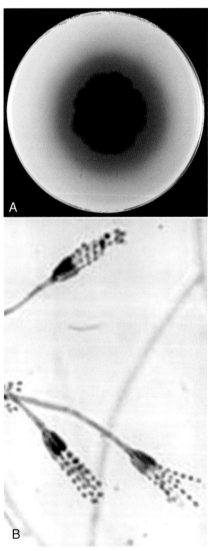

Figure 17-2 **A,** Reverse colony morphology on Sabouraud agar plate. **B,** Wet mount from growth at 30°C (×100).

7. A 32-year-old recent HIV-positive immigrant from Vietnam presented to the ED with fever, weight loss, and lymphadenopathy. Two sets of blood cultures were collected and became positive after 2 days of incubation. The organism demonstrated in Figure 17-2 was recovered after 72 hours of incubation at 30°C. Which one of the following is the etiologic agent?

A. *Penicillium marneffei.*

B. *Aspergillus nidulans.*

C. *Trichophyton rubrum.*

D. *Fusarium solani.*

E. *Cryptococcus neoformans.*

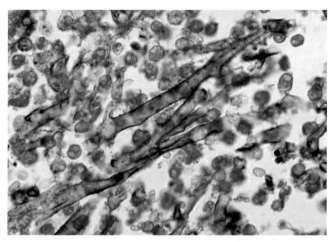

Figure 17-3 Methenemine silver stain of fungal elements.

8. A 13-year-old female bone marrow transplant patient presents with nasal congestion and a severe headache. A needle aspirate from the sinus reveals hyphae by light microscopy (Figure 17-3). Which one of the following infections is highest on the differential diagnosis?

A. Mucormycosis.

B. Aspergillosis.

C. Candidiasis.

D. Mycetoma.

E. Rhinosporidiosis.

9. A 10-year-old boy presents with a 6-month history of progressive hepatomegaly. His mother was positive for chronic hepatitis B virus (HBV) during her pregnancy. Laboratory testing on the child reveals positive HBV surface antigen, negative HBV surface antibody, positive HBV core antibody, and HBV DNA 56,800 IU/mL. Which one of the following statements is true regarding HBV infection?

A. He was exposed to HBV at birth, but the infection was transmitted horizontally.

B. Active replication of HBV is occurring.

C. His liver injury is related to actively replicating HBV in hepatocytes.

D. His HBV core antibody is positive, indicating his infection has cleared.

E. HBV disease is more severe in children than adults.

10. A 25-year-old injection drug user presented to the ED with flulike symptoms, including decreased appetite, fever, fatigue, and headache. He admitted to recent episodes of unprotected sex with both men and women. The patient had a positive HIV 1/2 EIA result; however, the Western blot assay was negative. Which one of the following tests is required to establish a diagnosis?
    A. CD4$^+$ T-cell count.
    B. HIV genotyping.
    C. HIV quantitative PCR.
    D. HIV qualitative PCR.
    E. Human herpesvirus 8 (HHV-8) PCR.

11. A 72-year-old man from Staten Island, New York, presented in the summer with headache, nuchal rigidity, and fever. The diagnosis was made by serology and confirmed by PCR. Which one of the following is the most likely agent of infection?
    A. *Neisseria meningitidis.*
    B. *Cryptococcus neoformans.*
    C. West Nile virus (WNV).
    D. *Naegleria fowleri.*
    E. Parvovirus B19.

12. A 30-year-old man presented to a sexually transmitted disease clinic with a 1-week history of genital lesions. A swab sample of the lesion was collected and transported in viral transport medium to a virology laboratory for herpes virus detection. Same-day detection of herpes simplex viruses (HSV) can be accomplished using which one of the following methods?
    A. The cytopathic changes observed in the cultured cells can distinguish HSV types 1 and 2.
    B. Infected cells can be visualized after staining with virus-specific, fluorescently labeled antibodies.
    C. Shell vial culture followed by the detection of specific HSV proteins in the infected cells using monoclonal antibodies.
    D. Type-specific HSV serological testing.
    E. Reverse transcriptase (RT)-PCR assay for detecting HSV types 1 and 2.

13. Infections by which one of the following viruses is not vaccine preventable?
    A. Mumps virus.
    B. RSV.
    C. Measles virus.
    D. Rotavirus.
    E. Rubella virus.

14. Which one of the following statements regarding the laboratory diagnosis of influenza infection is correct?
    A. Early diagnosis is important because antiviral therapy should be started within 48 hours of the onset of symptoms.
    B. Rapid EIAs are the most sensitive diagnostic tool.
    C. Infected patients shed influenza virus for 24 hours after the onset of symptoms.
    D. Rapid EIAs are available for influenza A, but not influenza B.
    E. If the patient has received an annual influenza vaccine, then infection will be prevented.

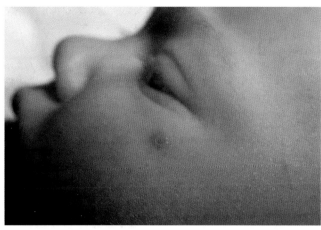

Figure 17-4 Vesiculopustular lesion on the cheek of an 8-month-old girl.

15. An 8-month-old girl presented to the ED with multiple vesiculopustular lesions over her body and a fever of 39°C. One of the lesions was sampled and a diagnosis was made within hours (Figure 17-4). Which one of the following is the etiologic agent in this case?
    A. Varicella zoster virus (VZV).
    B. Coxsackievirus A.
    C. *Streptococcus pyogenes.*
    D. Coxsackievirus B.
    E. Human herpes virus 6 (HHV-6).

16. A 48-year-old woman presented to her physician with an erythematous rash on one side of her body. She also has clusters of small vesicles in the same region. Before the rash appeared, she experienced "burning" pain and the area was tender to palpation. A vesicle was sampled and the laboratory confirmed the diagnosis within 3 hours. Which one of the following is the etiologic agent?
    A. Enterovirus.
    B. Herpes simplex virus.
    C. Parvovirus B19.
    D. Varicella zoster virus (VZV).
    E. Measles virus.

17. A 41-year-old healthy man donated blood at a local Red Cross. A week later, he received a blood screening test report indicating his hepatitis B core antibody (HBcAb) test was positive. He was referred to a liver disease specialist for additional evaluation. Additional test results showed that the patient was hepatitis B surface antigen (HBsAg) negative, hepatitis B surface antibody (HBsAb) positive, and hepatitis anti-core IgM negative. Which one of the following statements best describes the man's current status with regard to hepatitis B virus (HBV)?
    A. Acute HBV infection.
    B. Immune to HBV due to natural infection.
    C. Immune to HBV due to HBV vaccination.
    D. Chronic HBV infection.
    E. Susceptible to HBV infection.

18. Passengers on a cruise ship recently experienced an outbreak of norovirus; 40% of them presented to the medical clinic with vomiting and diarrhea. Which one of the following characteristics of this virus impacts the occurrence and control of outbreaks?

A. Transmission via inhalation of respiratory droplets.
B. Immunity related to prior vaccination.
C. Immunity related to prior infection.
D. Susceptibility of the virus to dilute bleach.
E. Low infectious dose required for infection.

19. Which one of the following viruses is an enveloped, double-stranded DNA virus?
A. Parvovirus B19.
B. Rhinovirus.
C. Rotavirus.
D. Influenza A virus.
E. Herpes simplex virus type 2.

20. A 78-year-old man presented to his physician with a 24-hour history of fever, chills, and severe body aches. A rapid diagnostic test was performed in less than 30 minutes, and oseltamivir was prescribed based on the result. Which one of the following is the etiologic agent of the infection in this patient?
A. RSV.
B. Adenovirus.
C. Influenza A virus.
D. *Haemophilus influenzae.*
E. Parainfluenza virus.

21. A 50-year-old woman presented to her local ED after recently returning from an extended vacation in the Dominican Republic. Her chief complaints included fever, headache, and malaise. She had been bitten by a dog 4 weeks earlier in the Dominican Republic, and the site was still painful. Which one of the following regimens is best for rabies prophylaxis?
A. Chloramphenicol and rabies vaccine.
B. Rabies immune globulin.
C. Ribavirin and rabies vaccine.
D. Rabies vaccine and rabies immune globulin.
E. Rabies vaccine.

22. Which one of the following viruses is an enveloped, single-stranded RNA virus?
A. RSV.
B. Enterovirus 71.
C. Parvovirus B19.
D. Cytomegalovirus.
E. Rotavirus.

23. A 3-month-old girl presents to her pediatrician with a maculopapular rash on her trunk, neck, and arms. Her mother reports that the child had a fever of 103°F 2 days earlier, which has since resolved. She is diagnosed with roseola. Which one of the following is the etiologic agent associated with this disease?
A. Measles virus.
B. Human herpes virus 6.
C. Parvovirus B19.
D. Coxsackievirus.
E. Cytomegalovirus.

24. Which one of the following hepatitis C virus (HCV) genotypes is the most predominant in the United States?
A. Genotype 1.
B. Genotype 2.
C. Genotype 3.
D. Genotype 4.
E. Genotype 5.

25. An astute infection control practitioner observed that three recent admissions for pneumonia were referred from the same long-term care facility. All patients presented with fever, nonproductive cough, and lower lobe infiltrates. Respiratory secretions were collected for bacterial and viral cultures. A rapid amplification assay identified a DNA virus as the etiologic agent, and unnecessary antibiotic therapy was avoided. Which one of the following viruses caused these cases of viral pneumonia?
A. Influenza A.
B. Adenovirus.
C. RSV.
D. Parainfluenza virus.
E. WNV.

26. At a routine well-child visit, it was recommended that a 14-year-old girl receive a vaccine to prevent infection with a sexually transmitted virus and its subsequent sequelae. Which one of the following answers best describes the type(s) of virus(es) that this vaccine protects against?
A. Human papillomavirus types 6, 11, 16, and 18.
B. HIV type 1.
C. Adenovirus serotypes 7, 22, and 43.
D. Herpes simplex virus type 2.
E. Herpes simplex virus type 1.

ANSWERS

1. A. Donor negative/recipient positive.
Rationale: The risk of reactivation of CMV in the recipient is not affected by the seronegative status of the donor.
B. Donor positive/recipient positive.
Rationale: There is a modest risk of CMV super-infection from a seropositive donor to a seropositive recipient.
C. Donor negative/recipient negative.
Rationale: The lack of exposure to CMV in both donor and recipient indicates a lack of exposure to the viral pathogen.
D. Donor positive/recipient negative.
Rationale: Primary CMV infection is most likely to result through viral transmission from a seropositive donor to a recipient that lacks CMV specific immunity.
E. The risk is equal for all donor/recipient matches.

Rationale: CMV seronegative recipients are at very high risk of contracting primary disease if the donor is CMV seropositive.

Major points of discussion

- Serologic testing for anti-CMV IgG is a component of pretransplantation screening for both the organ donor and the recipient. Tests for IgG have higher specificity than IgM assays.
- Approximately 40% to 90% of the general population is CMV seropositive, indicating previous exposure to CMV.
- For the highest-risk patients (i.e., donor positive/recipient negative), prophylaxis is more successful for CMV disease prevention than preemptive therapy.

- Transplant settings associated with the highest risk of CMV disease include heart, lung, and bone marrow transplantation.
- CMV treatment can include intravenous ganciclovir or oral valganciclovir.[13]

2. A. Parainfluenza.
Rationale: Although the clinical symptoms of infection with parainfluenza are similar to those of respiratory syncytial virus, no rapid EIA kits are currently available for its detection.
B. Rotavirus.
Rationale: Rotavirus infections cause diarrhea in children.
C. Respiratory syncytial virus (RSV).
Rationale: RSV is the most frequent cause of bronchiolitis. There are rapid EIA kits for RSV detection.
D. *Bordetella pertussis.*
Rationale: Patients present with paroxysms of coughing and there is no rapid EIA kit to detect this pathogen.
E. Coronavirus.
Rationale: Coronavirus is the etiologic agent of the common cold and presents with rhinitis and cough, not bronchiolitis; no rapid EIA kits are currently available to detect this virus.

Major points of discussion
- RSV is an enveloped, single-stranded RNA virus that belongs to the family of paramyxoviruses.
- RSV is a major cause of bronchiolitis in young children.
- RSV can be rapidly detected directly from respiratory specimens using nucleic acid amplification technology. There are also rapid EIA kits for RSV detection.
- There is no currently no vaccine available to prevent RSV infection.
- Treatment is typically supportive and currently available antiviral agents are not effective.[4]

3. A. *Mycoplasma pneumonia.*
Rationale: The typical presentation for *M. pneumoniae*, which causes "walking" or "atypical" pneumonia, is less severe and would have improved on antibiotics.
B. *Streptococcus pneumoniae.*
Rationale: S. pneumoniae is characterized by a productive cough, and an immunocompetent patient should have responded to antimicrobial therapy.
C. Influenza A.
Rationale: Influenza A is highest on the differential diagnosis in this setting due to the nonproductive cough, severity of presentation, and lack of response to antibiotics.
D. Adenovirus.
Rationale: Adenovirus infections more often present with pharyngitis and bronchiolitis.
E. Parainfluenza.
Rationale: Parainfluenza infections more often present with croup and bronchiolitis.

Major points of discussion
- Influenzae A and B are enveloped, single-stranded RNA viruses belonging to the family Orthomyxoviridae.
- The antiviral agents used to treat influenza A infections are amantadine, rimantadine, and oseltamivir. Oseltamivir is also effective for treating influenza B infections.

- Influenza A destroys the tissue lining of the respiratory tract, inducing inflammation and predisposing the patient to secondary bacterial infections.
- Rapid diagnostic tests for detection of influenza A include EIAs and real-time nucleic acid amplification assays.
- Influenza A has two major surface antigens: hemagglutinin and neuraminidase. Antigenic drifts, due to point mutations in these proteins, necessitate yearly vaccinations. Antigenic shifts can cause pandemics due to major structural changes resulting from genetic reassortment between human and animal influenza A strains.[11]

4. A. Most individuals have never been exposed to BK virus.
Rationale: More than 90% of the population has been infected with BK virus by 10 years of age.
B. BK virus can remain latent in the kidney and uroepithelial cells.
Rationale: BK virus establishes latency in the urogenital tract and reactivates during immunosuppressive therapy.
C. The assay used for early diagnosis of BK nephropathy is a qualitative polymerase chain reaction (PCR) assay using urine.
Rationale: The quantitative BK DNA PCR viral load assay is used for diagnosis and to monitor the response to therapy.
D. Antiviral therapy is used empirically before transplantation.
Rationale: Patients are treated only when BK infection has been diagnosed.
E. BK virus is ubiquitous, causing infections in all solid-organ transplant patients.
Rationale: BK virus can cause infection in either hematopoietic stem cell transplant or kidney transplant patients.

Major points of discussion
- BK virus is a nonenveloped, double-stranded DNA virus in the Polyomavirus family group.
- BK viral infection occurs in 1% to 10% of kidney transplant recipients and typically manifests in the first year following transplantation.
- BK viral load is typically first detected in urine rather than in blood, and the levels of virus in urine can be used to predict viremia.
- The quantitative real-time PCR assay is used to measure viral load in plasma and urine.
- Therapeutic strategies, which often include the antiviral agent cidofovir, can result in good clinical success if BK nephropathy is diagnosed at an early stage.[12]

5. A. His treatment response was successful because his HIV-1 viral load was significantly reduced.
Rationale: A less than threefold reduction in viral load is not considered significant and may be due to biological variation.
B. He has not responded to treatment because his viral load remains unchanged.
C. His HAART regimen should be modified because there was no significant change in viral load.
Rationale: Since the patient has only been on HAART for a week, it is too early to predict the efficacy of the regimen.
D. He should continue on HAART and the viral load test should be repeated immediately.

E. He should continue on HAART and his viral load should be measured in 2 to 8 weeks.
Rationale for B, D, and E: It is recommended that patients have their HIV viral load quantified 2 to 8 weeks post initiation of antiretroviral therapy.[6]

Major points of discussion

■ HIV-1 RNA quantitative tests (i.e., viral load) are used routinely to assess the level of HIV viremia and to assess response to treatment.

■ A combination of several antiretroviral drugs, called HAART, has been very effective in reducing the replication of HIV in the bloodstream.

■ Treatment guidelines recommend that anyone with a viral load in blood of more than 100,000 copies/mL should begin treatment.

■ The Department of Health and Human Services Panel recommended that patients should be tested for HIV viral load 2 to 8 weeks after initiation of antiretroviral therapy and then 3 to 4 months thereafter.

■ Patient testing should be conducted at the same medical laboratory, using the same viral load test and analyzer, due to considerable variation in results using different test methods.

■ Baseline HIV viral load levels should be measured before initiating antiretroviral therapy.

6. A. To confirm the diagnosis of HCV infection.
Rationale: The diagnosis of HCV infection is based on the presence of HCV-specific antibodies and detectable virus in whole blood or plasma.
B. To detect HCV and human immunodeficiency virus coinfection.
Rationale: The HCV genotyping assay only detects HCV genomic targets.
C. To monitor antiviral therapy.
Rationale: The HCV RNA quantitative assay (i.e., HCV viral load) should be performed to monitor antiviral treatment.
D. To predict duration of antiviral therapy.
Rationale: Infection with HCV genotype 1, rather than genotypes 2 or 3, requires a longer course of treatment.
E. To determine viral load.
Rationale: The HCV RNA quantitative assay should be performed to determine the number of viral copies per milliliter of whole blood or plasma.

Major points of discussion

■ There are at least six major HCV genotypes (genotypes 1 to 6).

■ For patients with HCV genotypes 2 and 3, a 24-week course of combination treatment is adequate, whereas for patients with genotype 1, a 48-week course is recommended.

■ HCV genotype 1 (subtypes 1a and 1b) is the most common in the United States, followed by genotypes 2 and 3.

■ Less common HCV genotypes (i.e., genotypes 4 to 6) are beginning to be observed more frequently because of the growing cultural diversity within the United States.

■ HCV genotypes are determined by using direct sequence analysis of the 5′ noncoding regions of the HCV genome, or reverse hybridization analysis using genotype-specific oligonucleotide probes.[8,9]

7. **A. *Penicillium marneffei*.**
Rationale: *P. marneffei* produces a red diffusible pigment and microscopic morphology demonstrates flask-shaped phialides and chains of round conidia.
B. *Aspergillus nidulans*.
Rationale: *A. nidulans* does not produce a diffusible pigment and microscopic morphology demonstrates biseriate phialides and round conidia.
C. *Trichophyton rubrum*.
Rationale: *T. rubrum* does not produce a diffusible pigment and microscopic morphology demonstrates tear-shaped microconidia.
D. *Fusarium solani*.
Rationale: *F. solani* does not produce a diffusible pigment and microscopic morphology demonstrates sickle-shaped septated macroconidia.
E. *Cryptococcus neoformans*.
Rationale: *C. neoformans* is an encapsulated yeast and does not produce a diffusible pigment.

Major points of discussion

■ *P. marneffei*, endemic in Southeast Asia, is a common cause of infections in immunocompromised hosts but can also cause disease in immunocompetent individuals who have traveled to that area.

■ *P. marneffei* demonstrates thermal dimorphism (i.e., mold at 30°C and yeast at 37°C) and growth is inhibited by cyclohexamide.

■ Transmission of *P. marneffei* is most likely airborne, via inhalation of conidia from an environmental reservoir (often associated with exposure to bamboo rats).

■ Other *Penicillium* spp. are not dimorphic and demonstrate septate hyphae in tissue, whereas *P. marneffei* are present in a yeast-like form.

■ *P. marneffei* is typically highly susceptible to miconazole, itraconazole, and ketoconazole but resistant to fluconazole.

8. **A. Mucormycosis.**
Rationale: *Mucor* spp. contain fungal elements that are largely nonseptate with irregular branching.
B. Aspergillosis.
Rationale: *Aspergillus* spp. have hyaline septate hyphae with branching at 45-degree angles.
C. Candidiasis.
Rationale: *Candida* spp. form pseudohyphae that show distinct constrictions at the septa and form budding yeast cells.
D. Mycetoma.
Rationale: Fungi and bacteria causing mycetoma appear as aggregates of intertwined filaments, rather than individual hyphae.
E. Rhinosporidiosis.
Rationale: *Rhinosporidium seeheri* invades mucocutaneous tissue and appears as round mature sporangia containing endospores.

Major points of discussion

■ Zygomycetes are a fungal class that are mostly nonseptate. Most fungi in this class that cause infection belong to the order Mucorales, which includes *Rhizopus*, *Mucor*, *Rhizomucor*, and *Absidia*.

- The hyphae of the Mucorales fungi are nonseptate and branching is nondichotomous, irregular, and sometimes at right angles.
- Mucormycosis can invade the lung, nasal, sinus, brain, and mucous membranes.
- Fungi causing mucormycosis can be differentiated from aspergillosis by the morphology of the hyphae and by the presence of chlamydospores in the hyphae.
- Differential characteristics of commonly encountered pathogens causing mucormycosis include rhizoid production and sporangiophore pigment (see table below).

Characteristics of Representatives of Mucorales

Fungus	Rhizoids	Sporangio-phores	Optimal Growth Temp (°C)	Pathogenicity
Rhizopus	Present	Unbran-ched, brown	45-50, inhibited by cycloheximide	Most common pathogen
Mucor	Absent	Branched, hyaline	≤37	Opportunistic, occasional
Rhizomucor	Few	Branched, dark brown	38-58	Opportunistic, occasional
Absidia (*Lichtheimia*)	Present	Fine branches, hyaline	45-50	Uncommon pathogen

9. A. He was exposed to HBV at birth, but the infection was transmitted horizontally.
Rationale: Mother-to-child vertical transmission at birth plays a very important role in HBV epidemiology.
B. Active replication of HBV is occurring.
Rationale: The presence of HBV DNA in the plasma is a reliable marker of active HBV replication.
C. His liver injury is related to actively replicating HBV in hepatocytes.
Rationale: The HBV replication cycle is not directly cytotoxic to cells. Liver injury is mediated through the immune system.
D. His HBV core antibody is positive, indicating his infection has cleared.
Rationale: HBV core antibody is not a protective antibody. In fact, it is usually present in those chronically infected with HBV.
E. HBV disease is more severe in children than adults.
Rationale: Compared to the disease in adults, HBV infection in children is frequently less severe.

Major points of discussion

- HBV can be vertically transmitted from an infected mother to her child. From 10% to 20% of women seropositive for HBV surface antigen (HBsAg) transmit the virus to their neonates in the absence of immunoprophylaxis. In women who are seropositive for both HBsAg and HBV e-antigen (HBeAg), vertical transmission is approximately 90%.
- The presence of HBV DNA in plasma is a reliable marker of active HBV replication. The level of HBV DNA indicates rapid viral replication in the liver.
- HBV core antibody is not a protective antibody. The presence of antibody to HBsAg is consistent with protection, either through response to infection or vaccine.

- Host immune responses to viral antigens displayed on the surface of infected hepatocytes are the principal determinants of hepatocellular injury.
- HBV is a DNA virus, whereas hepatitis A and C are RNA viruses.[2,7]

10. A. CD4[+] T-cell count.
Rationale: Determination of CD4 cell counts is not used to diagnose HIV infection; these values are helpful in characterizing the patient's level of immune competence after diagnosis and after the implementation of therapy.
B. HIV genotyping.
Rationale: Determination of the HIV genotype is used to guide drug selection and predict resistance.
C. HIV quantitative PCR.
Rationale: The HIV viral load PCR assays are not used to diagnose HIV infection; they can be used as a prognostic tool for monitoring the effectiveness of therapy.
D. HIV qualitative PCR.
Rationale: This assay is very useful for diagnosing acute HIV infection before specific antibodies are detectable by Western blot.
E. Human herpesvirus 8 (HHV-8) PCR.
Rationale: HHV-8 detection by PCR is used to diagnose Kaposi sarcoma, not HIV infection.

Major points of discussion

- The HIV 1/2 EIA antibody screening test has a sensitivity of approximately 99%; confirmatory Western blot testing is required to detect the small number of false-positive EIA results that can occur (~2%).
- For the Western blot to be defined as positive, the following bands must be present: p160/120 or p41 (*env* gene region) and p24 (*gag* gene region).
- HIV-1 RNA and DNA amplification tests are important for the diagnosis of acute or primary infection. There is a window period of up to 6 weeks after exposure before the appearance of HIV antibodies.
- Before the routine use of molecular methods, detection of p24 antigen in serum was used to diagnose acute infection at 1 to 3 weeks postexposure. This analyte has recently been included in an HIV 1/2 antigen-antibody combination screening assay.
- HIV-1 quantitative viral load assays are essential for monitoring antiretroviral treatment response. Because there are variations in detection among the many FDA-cleared assays, it is important that routine monitoring be done using the same assay.[10,16]

11. A. *Neisseria meningitidis.*
Rationale: N. meningitidis causes meningitis and is identified by bacterial culture of the cerebrospinal fluid (CSF) on sheep blood and chocolate agars followed by a latex agglutination test.
B. *Cryptococcus neoformans.*
Rationale: C. neoformans is a cause of fungal meningitis and encephalitis, particularly in AIDS patients. It is identified by direct antigen detection tests and culture.
C. West Nile virus (WNV).
Rationale: WNV causes aseptic meningoencephalitis in individuals exposed to infected mosquitoes and is diagnosed by serology and molecular tests.

D. *Naegleria fowleri.*
Rationale: N. fowleri causes amoebic meningitis and is diagnosed by direct microscopic observation and culture.
E. Parvovirus B19.
Rationale: Parvovirus B19 causes erythema infectiosum (i.e., "fifth disease"), which is a mild illness with a rash, but with no neurologic symptoms. It is diagnosed serologically.

Major points of discussion

- Infected mosquitoes are the vector for human WNV infection. Person-to-person transmission can occur through blood transfusion, organ transplantation, and from mother-to-child via the intrauterine route and breast feeding.
- WNV may cause asymptomatic infection, low grade fever, or neuroinvasive meningitis or encephalitis. The highest incidence of neuroinvasive disease occurs in individuals aged 70 years and older.
- WNV was first detected in North America in 1999 during an epidemic of meningoencephalitis in New York City and has since spread across the continental United States. Case numbers peak in the summer and early autumn. Birds are the hosts that amplify WNV.
- There is currently no WNV vaccine for humans or specific antiviral therapy for WNV. Treatment is purely supportive. Diagnosis of acute WNV infection is based on detecting IgM in serum or CSF. Commercial PCR testing for WNV is also available.
- Prevention measures include the use of mosquito repellents, wearing protective clothing when outdoors, and eliminating standing water where mosquitoes can breed. Vector mosquito control by targeted spraying in areas with new or persistent levels of WNV activity is another potential public health measure.[1,5]

12. A. The cytopathic changes observed in the cultured cells can distinguish HSV types 1 and 2.
Rationale: Although cytopathic effects (CPE) are seen in infected cell cultures, the presence of a specific virus is confirmed by immunofluorescent staining using virus-specific, fluorescently labeled antibodies.
B. Infected cells can be visualized after staining with virus-specific, fluorescently labeled antibodies.
Rationale: The direct fluorescent antibody (DFA) assay can detect HSV directly from the specimen in approximately 2 hours.
C. Shell vial culture followed by the detection of specific HSV proteins in the infected cells using monoclonal antibodies.
Rationale: Although a valuable diagnostic tool, the turnaround time for viral culture is more than 24 hours.
D. Type-specific HSV serological testing.
Rationale: A swab sample is unsuitable for quantifying antibody levels by serological testing.
E. Reverse transcriptase (RT)-PCR assay for detecting HSV types 1 and 2.
Rationale: Herpes virus consists of a relatively large double-stranded, linear DNA genome. RT is unnecessary for detecting HSV by PCR.

Major points of discussion

- HSV-1 and HSV-2 are two members of the herpes virus family that cause disease in humans.
- Most cases of genital herpes are caused by HSV-2, which is spread when an infected person has active lesions that shed the virus.
- Tube culture isolation is the traditional gold standard method for HSV detection. HSV grows readily in a wide variety of cell lines including human fibroblasts and the MRC-5 and A549 cell lines.
- To reduce viral isolation times, centrifugation-enhanced shell vial culture methods are available. The infected cell cultures are stained with HSV type-specific monoclonal antibody reagents to confirm positive results.
- HSV DNA can be detected by many molecular methods, including amplification of the target HSV DNA by PCR.[14]

13. A. Mumps virus.
B. RSV.
Rationale: There is no currently no vaccine for RSV.
C. Measles virus.
D. Rotavirus.
Rationale: Rotavirus vaccinations are given at 2, 4, and 6 months of age.
E. Rubella virus.
Rationale for A, C, and E: The measles/mumps/rubella vaccination series begins at 12 months of age.

Major points of discussion

- Other vaccine-preventable viral infections include varicella zoster virus, hepatitis A and B viruses, poliovirus, and human papillomavirus.
- Vaccines are also available for the following bacteria: *Corynebacterium diphtheriae, Clostridium tetani, Bordetella pertussis, Neisseria meningitidis, Streptococcus pneumoniae,* and *Haemophilus pneumoniae.*
- The influenza vaccine is composed of virus strains predicted to be circulating during the respiratory virus season. Because its composition can change each year, annual vaccination is necessary.
- Infection with RSV does not convey lifelong immunity against subsequent infections by this virus.
- For prophylaxis in high-risk infants, palivizumab, an RSV-directed monoclonal antibody, can be given by monthly injections.

14. A. **Early diagnosis is important because antiviral therapy should be started within 48 hours of the onset of symptoms.**
Rationale: Antiviral therapy is optimal when initiated soon after the onset of symptoms. A typical course is 5 days and can alleviate symptoms and shorten the disease course by 1 to 2 days.
B. Rapid EIAs are the most sensitive diagnostic tool.
Rationale: The sensitivity of rapid EIAs is lower than culture and nucleic acid amplification assays and varies depending on the strain of circulating influenza.
C. Infected patients shed influenza virus for 24 hours after the onset of symptoms.
Rationale: Patients shed influenza virus from the day before symptoms begin through 5 to 10 days after the onset of illness.

D. Rapid EIAs are available for influenza A, but not influenza B.
Rationale: Rapid EIAs and nucleic acid amplification assays are commercially available for both influenza A and B.
E. If the patient had received an annual influenza vaccine, then infection will be prevented.
Rationale: The effectiveness of annual vaccination depends on the circulating influenza strains. Postvaccine immunity can take up to 14 days to occur.

Major points of discussion

- Influenzas A and B are distinguished by two major antigenic differences: the matrix (M) protein and the nucleoprotein (NP). Influenza A viruses are further classified based on two major surface glycoproteins; the hemagglutinin (HA) and neuraminidase (NA).
- For influenza A, there are currently 16 HA subtypes and 9 NA subtypes. H1/H2/H3 and N1/N2 have been associated with widespread human disease.
- Influenza B infects only humans, whereas influenza A infects birds and various mammals. Pigs can act as "mixing vessels" for genetic reassortment between human and avian influenza A strains.
- Antigenic drift is associated with naturally occurring replication mutations in HA and NA. Antigenic shift occurs when RNA segment reassortment occurs between animal and human strains. New strains resulting from antigenic shift have been associated with influenza pandemics.
- The adamantane drugs (amantadine and rimantadine) are approved for influenza A, whereas the neuraminidase inhibitor drugs (zanamivir and oseltamivir) are approved for both influenza A and B. Influenza strain typing is often necessary to guide therapy.

15. A. Varicella zoster virus (VZV).
Rationale: VZV is the causative agent of chickenpox, which is characterized by vesicular lesions that progress to pustules that then become crusted.
B. Coxsackievirus A.
Rationale: Coxsackievirus A infects the skin and mucous membranes and causes herpangina, acute hemorrhagic conjunctivitis, and hand, foot, and mouth (HFM) disease. There is no rapid diagnostic test available.
C. *Streptococcus pyogenes.*
Rationale: S. pyogenes (i.e., "group A strep") can cause a nonbullous impetigo with vesicles, pustules, and sharply demarcated regions of honey-colored crusts. Bacterial culture is used for diagnosis; there is no rapid test available.
D. Coxsackievirus B.
Rationale: Coxsackievirus B is associated with myocarditis and pancreatitis. There is no rapid diagnostic test available.
E. Human herpes virus 6 (HHV-6).
Rationale: HHV-6 causes roseola (i.e. "sixth disease" or exanthema subitum) in children. It is characterized by a febrile illness followed by the development of a maculopapular rash (i.e., not vesicular).

Major points of discussion

- VZV is a member of the herpes virus group. It is an enveloped, double-stranded DNA virus.
- A direct fluorescent antibody stain can be performed on skin scrapings taken from the base of the vesicular lesions. A diagnosis of VZV infection can be made in less than 3 hours.

- VZV lesions are highly contagious; therefore, hospitalized patients are placed on strict infection control precautions.
- Acyclovir is often used to treat immunocompromised children and adults.
- A live, attenuated, varicella vaccine is first administered at 12 months of age. Immunocompromised children may be ineligible for vaccination, because it is a live virus vaccine.

16. A. Enterovirus.
Rationale: Rashes associated with enteroviral infections are not painful and cannot currently be diagnosed by rapid methods.
B. Herpes simplex virus.
Rationale: Herpes simplex virus skin manifestations are vesicular, not erythematous. Rapid diagnosis is available using fluorescent staining of lesion samples.
C. Parvovirus B19.
Rationale: Parvovirus B19 infection is associated with erythema infectiosum (i.e., "fifth disease") and is characterized by a mild rash, typically on the face ("slapped cheek" appearance). No rapid test is available for diagnosis.
D. Varicella zoster virus (VZV).
Rationale: The rash in this case is caused by a reactivation of latent VZV. Rapid diagnosis is available using fluorescent staining of lesion samples.
E. Measles virus.
Rationale: Measles virus causes rubeola and is characterized by a red maculopapular rash that begins at the hairline and spreads to the whole body. No rapid test is available for diagnosis.

Major points of discussion

- Herpes zoster infection (i.e., "shingles") is a reactivation infection of a latent VZV infection. The virus remains dormant in the dorsal root ganglia. The incidence of reactivation increases with advancing age due to declining immunity.
- Skin lesions typically appear in a unilateral dermatome distribution, which is innervated by a specific dorsal root. The rash can be very painful and this discomfort can persist even after the rash has resolved (i.e., postherpetic neuralgia).
- The skin lesions are considered infectious but not to the same degree as primary VZV lesions seen in chickenpox.
- Treatment of this infection with acyclovir can reduce the extent and duration of symptoms and possibly the risk of chronic sequelae (e.g., postherpetic neuralgia).
- A live, attenuated VZV vaccine (Zostavax) has been available in the United States since 2006 for the prevention of VZV infections and its complications in adults older than 50 years.

17. A. Acute HBV infection.
Rationale: The diagnosis of acute HBV infection is based on the presence of both HBsAg and hepatitis anti–core IgM.
B. Immune to HBV due to natural infection.
C. Immune to HBV due to HBV vaccination.
Rationale: Individuals who have been successfully vaccinated against HBV have positive results for HBsAb but not HBcAb.
D. Chronic HBV infection.
Rationale: A positive HBsAg test is indicative of chronic HBV infection.

E. Susceptible to HBV infection.
Rationale for B and E: The presence of both HBsAb and HBcAb indicate that this patient had a prior infection to HBV and is now immune to subsequent HBV infection.

Major points of discussion

- HBV serologic testing involves the measurement of several HBV-specific antigens and antibodies.
- The combinations of different serologic markers are used to identify different phases of HBV infection and to determine whether a patient has acute or chronic HBV infection, is immune to HBV as a result of prior infection or vaccination, or is susceptible to HBV infection.
- All volunteer blood donors are screened for HBV exposure using an HBcAb EIA, HBsAg testing, and, at some blood centers, HBV nucleic acid testing.
- The presence of both HBsAb and HBcAb indicates previous infection with HBV in an undefined time frame.
- The risk of acquiring HBV infection through blood transfusion currently ranges between 1:200,000 and 1:500,000.[15,17]

18. A. Transmission via inhalation of respiratory droplets.
Rationale: Transmission of norovirus is fecal-oral, via contact with contaminated surfaces, or ingestion of contaminated water or food.
B. Immunity related to prior vaccination.
Rationale: There is currently no vaccine available for norovirus.
C. Immunity related to prior infection.
Rationale: Norovirus infection does not lead to lasting immunity.
D. Susceptibility of the virus to dilute bleach.
Rationale: Norovirus is resistant to low levels of chlorine. Concentrated bleach must be used to disinfect surfaces.
E. Low infectious dose required for infection.
Rationale: Ingestion of as few as 10 virus particles can lead to infection.

Major points of discussion

- Norovirus (Norwalk virus), a member of the Caliciviridae family, is a single-stranded RNA virus and is the most common cause of epidemic nonbacterial gastroenteritis in the world.
- Nonenveloped viruses, such as norovirus, survive for longer periods of time on environmental surfaces.
- Symptoms of norovirus infection typically develop 12 to 48 hours after exposure and last for 2 to 3 days.
- Nucleic acid amplification tests (i.e., PCR) are available for diagnosing norovirus infection.
- Oral fluid and electrolyte replacement is recommended for treating norovirus infections.

19. A. Parvovirus B19.
Rationale: Parvovirus B19 is a small, nonenveloped, single-stranded DNA virus.
B. Rhinovirus.
Rationale: Rhinovirus is a small positive-sense, nonenveloped, single-stranded RNA virus.
C. Rotavirus.
Rationale: Rotavirus is a nonenveloped, double-stranded RNA virus.
D. Influenza A virus.
Rationale: Influenza A virus is an enveloped, single-stranded, segmented RNA virus.

E. Herpes simplex virus type 2.
Rationale: Herpes simplex virus type 2, is a large, enveloped, double-stranded DNA virus.

Major points of discussion

- Human parvovirus B19 was first discovered in 1975. It belongs to the *Erythrovirus* genus within the Parvoviridae family. In children, parvovirus B19 causes erythema infectiosum (e.g., "fifth disease").
- Rhinoviruses are small positive-sense, nonenveloped RNA viruses that are the major cause of upper respiratory infections in adults and children.
- Rotavirus is a nonenveloped, double-stranded RNA virus that belongings to the family Reoviridae. It is a worldwide cause of infantile gastroenteritis, accounting for an estimated 600,000 deaths annually.
- Influenza A virus is an enveloped, single-stranded, segmented RNA virus. The envelope is a lipid membrane which is incorporated from the host cell in which the virus multiplies.
- Herpes simplex virus type 2 is an enveloped DNA virus. It belongs to the herpesviruses family and is composed of a relatively large, double-stranded, linear DNA genome. It is the primary cause of genital herpes infections.

20. A. RSV.
Rationale: Although there is a rapid enzyme immunoassay RSV, treatment is typically supportive. Oseltamivir would not be effective.
B. Adenovirus.
Rationale: There is no rapid test available for adenovirus and no antivirals are currently available for treatment.
C. Influenza A virus.
Rationale: A rapid enzyme immunoassay is available for influenzas A and B, and oseltamivir can be used to treat both viruses.
D. *Haemophilus influenza.*
Rationale: H. influenzae is a bacteria and, therefore, would not respond to antiviral therapy.
E. Parainfluenza virus.
Rationale: There is no rapid test available for parainfluenza virus, and no antivirals are available for treatment.

Major points of discussion

- Antiviral therapy for influenza includes neuraminidase inhibitors (i.e., oseltamivir and zanamivir) and amantadine and rimantadine. Neuraminidase inhibitors act directly on the viral proteins, decreasing the virulence of infection.
- Oseltamivir and zanamivir are effective against both influenza A and B. Therapy should be started within 48 hours of symptoms for optimal effectiveness.
- Amantadine is active against influenza A virus and has little or no activity against influenza B virus. The emergence of resistant influenza A strains has limited the utility of this agent.
- Rimantadine inhibits viral replication of influenza A virus H1N1, H2N2, and H3N2 by blocking uncoating of influenza A. The emergence of resistant influenza A strains has limited the utility of this agent.
- Antiviral agents are not currently available for respiratory viral pathogens other than influenza.

21. A. Chloramphenicol and rabies vaccine.
Rationale: Chloramphenicol is not effective against viruses, and the vaccine alone does not offer full protection.
B. Rabies immune globulin.
Rationale: Immune globulin alone is not sufficient because the host will not develop neutralizing antibodies.
C. Ribavirin and rabies vaccine.
Rationale: Ribavirin is not effective against rabies, and the vaccine alone does not offer full protection.
D. Rabies vaccine and rabies immune globulin.
Rationale: The vaccine will generate protective neutralizing antibodies, while the immune globulin provides immediate protection.
E. Rabies vaccine.
Rationale: Vaccine alone is not sufficient because it does not afford immediate protection.

Major points of discussion
- Rabies virus, a member of the Rhabdoviridae family, is an enveloped, bullet-shaped, single-stranded RNA virus.
- Although all mammals are susceptible to rabies, in the United States the majority of cases occur in raccoons, bats, skunks, and foxes.
- Acute symptoms of rabies infection are nonspecific and include fever, headache, and general weakness or discomfort. More specific symptoms emerge as the disease progresses, including confusion, partial paralysis, hallucinations, agitation, hypersalivation, difficulty swallowing, and hydrophobia. Death usually occurs within days of the onset of these advanced symptoms.
- To diagnose human rabies infection, nucleic acid amplification tests can be performed on saliva, serum, cerebrospinal fluid, and skin biopsies of hair follicles at the nape of the neck. Serum and cerebrospinal fluid are also tested for antibodies to rabies virus. Postmortem diagnosis relies on detecting rabies antigens in brain tissue.
- There are no currently available, FDA-approved, antiviral agents for the treatment of rabies. Some guidelines suggest the use of ketamine and amantadine. Alpha-interferon is contraindicated due to its toxicity.

22. **A. RSV.**
Rationale: RSV is an enveloped, single-stranded RNA virus.
B. Enterovirus 71.
Rationale: Enterovirus 71 is a small positive-sense, nonenveloped, single-stranded RNA virus.
C. Parvovirus B19.
Rationale: Parvovirus B19 is a small, nonenveloped, single-stranded DNA virus.
D. Cytomegalovirus.
Rationale: Cytomegalovirus is a large, enveloped, double-stranded DNA virus.
E. Rotavirus.
Rationale: Rotavirus is a nonenveloped, double-stranded RNA virus.

Major points of discussion
- RSV belongs to the family of paramyxoviruses. It is a major cause of bronchiolitis in young children.
- Enterovirus 71, a picornavirus, is a major causative agent of hand, foot, and mouth disease.
- Human parvovirus B19 is a member of the *Erythrovirus* genus within the Parvoviridae family. B19 infection can

lead to a variety of clinical manifestations, including erythema infectiosum in children.
- Cytomegalovirus belongs to the herpesvirus family and is composed of a relatively large double-stranded DNA genome. Primary CMV infection is usually asymptomatic and most infections occur in childhood; however, these infections in immunocompromised patients have greater clinical significance.
- Rotavirus belongs to the family Reoviridae and is a worldwide cause of infantile gastroenteritis, accounting for an estimated 600,000 deaths annually.

23. A. Measles virus.
Rationale: Measles begins with mild to moderate fever, cough, runny nose, red eyes, and sore throat. Two or three days after symptoms begin, small white spots (Koplik's spots) may appear inside the mouth.
B. Human herpes virus 6.
Rationale: Human herpes virus 6 is the etiologic agent of roseola, which is characterized by a high fever; after resolution of the fever, a typical rash then appears.
C. Parvovirus B19.
Rationale: Parvovirus B19, which causes "fifth disease," is characterized by a rash on the cheeks, arms, and legs. The rash first appears on the cheeks and is often referred to as "slapped cheek" rash.
D. Coxsackievirus.
Rationale: The symptoms associated with coxsackievirus infections include sore throat, rash, and blisters.
E. Cytomegalovirus.
Rationale: Although an uncommon disease, CMV mononucleosis can sometimes present with a nonspecific rash.

Major points of discussion
- Roseola infantum, also known as exanthema subitum or "sixth disease" (because it is the sixth rash-causing childhood disease), is a disease of young children, generally younger than 2 years.
- The rash associated with roseola is not itchy, usually lasts a few hours to a few days, begins on the trunk, and then spreads to the arms, legs, and face.
- Roseola is transmitted from person to person through contact with an infected person's respiratory secretions or saliva. Infections occur throughout the year.
- Most children have been exposed to human herpes virus 6 by 2 years of age and develop lifelong immunity.
- Roseola is diagnosed through a medical history and physical exam. No antiviral therapy is currently available.

24. **A. Genotype 1.**
Rationale: Genotype 1 is the most common HCV genotype in the United States (~80%) and the most difficult to treat.
B. Genotype 2.
Rationale: Genotype 2 is the second most common HCV genotype in the United States, accounting for approximately 10% of infections.
C. Genotype 3.
Rationale: Genotype 3 is endemic in southeast Asia and is variably distributed in different countries. This genotype accounts for approximately 6% of infections in the United States.

D. Genotype 4.
Rationale: Genotype 4 is the predominant genotype in the Middle East, Egypt, and Central Africa and is rare in the United States.
E. Genotype 5.
Rationale: Genotype 5 is the predominant genotype in South Africa and is rare in the United States.

Major points of discussion
- HCV is an enveloped RNA virus and has a highly heterogeneous genome.
- A genotype is a viral classification based on the genetic material in the RNA of the virus. There are at least six HCV genotypes.
- Genotype 1 is the most common in the United States and the most refractory to treatment. Knowing the HCV genotype is helpful for physicians in initiating an appropriate treatment plan.
- Genotypes 2 and 3 are associated with more favorable responses. Patients who are infected with HCV genotypes 2 and 3 will have an approximately 80% chance of achieving a sustained viral response with standard therapy.
- In 2011, two new antiviral agents were approved by the FDA for patients infected with HCV genotype 1. Both drugs are inhibitors of the HCV protease. The addition of these new medications resulted in significantly higher rates of sustained virologic response in previously treated patients with chronic HCV genotype 1 infection.[3]

25. A. Influenza A.
Rationale: Influenza A is an RNA virus that can be rapidly detected directly from respiratory specimens using nucleic acid amplification technology.
B. Adenovirus.
Rationale: Adenovirus is a DNA virus that can be rapidly detected directly from respiratory specimens using nucleic acid amplification technology.
C. RSV.
Rationale: RSV is an RNA virus that can be rapidly detected directly from respiratory specimens using nucleic acid amplification technology.
D. Parainfluenza virus.
Rationale: Parainfluenza virus is an RNA virus that can be rapidly detected directly from respiratory specimens using nucleic acid amplification technology.
E. WNV.
Rationale: WNV is a single-stranded RNA flavivirus that is transmitted to humans by a mosquito vector and can cause encephalitis.

Major points of discussion
- Adenoviruses are large, nonenveloped icosahedral viruses and contain a linear double-stranded DNA genome.
- There are more than 40 serotypes of adenovirus that are associated with a wide spectrum of diseases, including upper and lower respiratory tract infections, acute conjunctivitis, and pharyngoconjunctival fever.
- Adenoviruses 40 and 41 are common causes of gastroenteritis in children. A rapid enzyme immunoassay is commercially available to detect these two enteric adenoviruses.
- Adenoviruses grow best in human epithelial cell lines, such as A549 and HeLa cells. Adenoviruses 40 and 41 are currently noncultivatable.
- Currently, there are no antiviral agents for adenovirus and there is no commercially available vaccine, although U.S. military recruits have historically received adenovirus vaccine developed by U.S. Army Medical Research and Material Command.

26. A. Human papillomavirus types 6, 11, 16, and 18.
Rationale: Human papillomavirus is transmitted through sexual contact and can lead to the development of genital warts and cervical carcinoma.
B. HIV type 1.
Rationale: Although HIV type 1 can be transmitted sexually, there is currently no vaccine available.
C. Adenovirus serotypes 7, 22, and 43.
Rationale: Adenoviruses are not sexually transmitted and there is no vaccine currently available.
D. Herpes simplex virus type 2.
Rationale: Although herpes simplex virus type 2 can be transmitted sexually, there is currently no vaccine available.
E. Herpes simplex virus type 1.
Rationale: Although herpes simplex virus type 1 can be transmitted sexually, there is currently no vaccine available.

Major points of discussion
- Human papillomaviruses (HPVs) are small nonenveloped DNA viruses.
- Transmission occurs through direct epithelium-to-epithelium contact and not exposure to body fluids, as is the case for HIV and hepatitis viruses.
- Most HPV infections remain asymptomatic. Low-risk HPV infections can result in the development of benign warts in the anus, cervix, vagina, and vulva and are usually associated with types 6 and 11.
- High-risk HPV infections are associated with invasive cervical carcinoma and are usually types 16 and 18.
- HPV cannot be cultured in vitro and, therefore, detection relies on nucleic acid amplification assays; many such assays are commercially available and are designed to detect high-risk HPV types.
- Two vaccines are currently FDA approved for use in females aged 9 to 26 years: Gardasil (targets types 6, 11, 16, and 18) and Cervarix (targets types 16 and 18). Protection is only provided if vaccination occurs before exposure to HPV.

References

1. 2012 DOHMH Advisory #18. First human case of West Nile virus in NYC 2012. July 30, 2012.

2. American College of Obstetricians and Gynecologists. ACOG Practice Bulletin No. 86: Viral hepatitis in pregnancy. Obstet Gynecol 2007;110:941–956.

3. Bacon BR, Gordon SC, Lawitz E, Marcellin P, Vierling JM, Zeuzem S, Poordad F, Goodman ZD, Sings HL, Boparai N, Burroughs M, Brass CA, Albrecht JK, Esteban R. HCV RESPOND-2 Investigators. Boceprevir for previously treated chronic HCV genotype 1 infection. N Engl J Med 2011;364:1207–1217.

4. Breese Hall C, Weinberg GA, Kwane MK, Blumkin AK, Edwards KM, Staat MA, et al. The burden of respiratory syncytial virus infection in young children. N Engl J Med 2009;360:588–598.

5. Campbell GL, Marfin AA, Lanciotti RS, Gubler DJ. West Nile virus. Lancet Infect Dis 2002;2:519–529.

6. DHHS Panel on Antiretroviral Guidelines for Adults and Adolescents. Guidelines for the use of antiretroviral agents in HIV-1-infected adults and adolescents. Available at aidsinfo.nih.gov/contentfiles/GIChunk/GLChunk_1.pdf.

7. Ganem D, Prince AM. Hepatitis B virus infection–natural history and clinical consequences. N Engl J Med 2004;350:1118–1129.

8. Ghany MG, Nelson DR, Strader DB, Thomas DL, Seeff LB. An update on treatment of genotype 1 chronic hepatitis C virus infection: 2011 practice guideline by the American Association for the Study of Liver Diseases. American Association for Study of Liver Diseases. Hepatology 2011;54:1433–1444.

9. Ghany MG, Strader DB, Thomas DL, Seeff LB. Diagnosis, management, and treatment of hepatitis C: an update. American Association for the Study of Liver Diseases. Hepatology 2009;49:1335–1374.

10. Guidelines for the prevention and treatment of opportunistic infections among HIV-exposed and HIV-infected children. Morb Mortal Wkly Rep MMWR 2009;58:1–166.

11. Harper SA, Bradley JS, Englund JA, File TM, Gravenstrin S, Hayden FG, McGeer AJ, Neuzil KM, Pavia AT, Tapper ML, Uyeki TM, Zimmerman RK. Seasonal influenza in adults and children- diagnosis. treatment, chemoprophylaxis, and institutional outbreak management: Clinical Practice Guidelines of the Infectious Diseases Society of America. Clin Infect Dis 2009;48.

12. Hirsch HH. BK virus: opportunity makes a pathogen. Clin Infect Dis 2005;41:354–360.

13. Kotton CN, Kumar D, Caliendo AM, Asberg A, Chou S, Snydman DR, Allen U, Humar A. International consensus guidelines on the management of cytomegalovirus in solid organ transplantation. Transplantation 2010;89:779–795.

14. Leland DS, Ginocchio CC. Role of cell culture for virus detection in the age of technology. Clin Microbiol Rev 2007;20:49–78.

15. Stramer S. Current risks of transfusion-transmitted agents: a review Arch Pathol Lab Med 2007;131:702–707.

16. Torian LV, Eavery JJ, Punsalang AP, Pirillo RE, Forgione LA, Kent SA, Oleszko WR. HIV type 2 in New York City, 2000-2008. 2010; 51(11):1334-42.

17. Zou S, et al. Current Incidence and residual risk of hepatitis B infection among blood donors in the United States Transfusion 2009;49:1609–1620.

CHAPTER 18

MICROBIOLOGY: Parasitology

Susan Whittier

QUESTIONS

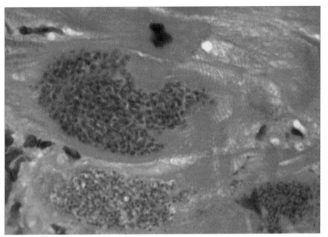

Figure 18-1 Endomyocardial biopsy, H&E stain × 1000).

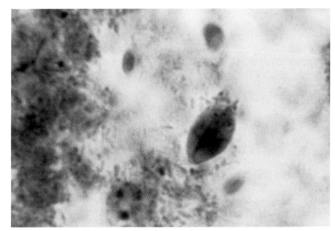

Figure 18-2 Wet mount (×40). The organism is 15 μm long and 10 μm wide. (Courtesy Dr. Mae Melvin, Centers for Disease Control and Prevention.)

1. A 56-year-old female patient presents complaining of fatigue 11 months after receiving a heart transplant. The organ donor emigrated from South America 15 years previously. An endomyocardial biopsy was performed, and the histologic results are shown in Figure 18-1. Which one of the following pathogens is shown?
   A. *Leishmania braziliensis.*
   B. *Listeria monocytogenes.*
   C. *Toxoplasma gondii.*
   D. *Trypanosoma cruzi.*
   E. Cytomegalovirus (CMV).

2. A 14-year-old boy presents to his pediatrician with a 1-week history of abdominal pain, diarrhea, and foul-smelling flatulence. Two weeks before presentation, he was camping with his scout troop and may have ingested water from a nearby stream. Direct examination of a fresh stool sample is shown Figure 18-2. Which one of the following is the etiologic agent causing this patient's illness?
   A. *Cyclospora cayetanensis.*
   B. *Trichomonas hominis.*
   C. *Cryptosporidium parvum.*
   D. *Chilomastix mesnili.*
   E. *Giardia intestinalis.*

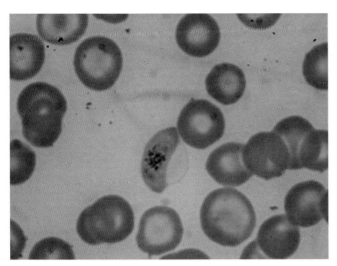

Figure 18-3 Giemsa stain (×1000).

3. Which one of the following is the insect vector responsible for transmitting the organism seen in Figure 18-3?
 A. Tsetse fly.
 B. Anopheline mosquito.
 C. Reduviid bug.
 D. *Ixodes scapularis.*
 E. Black fly.

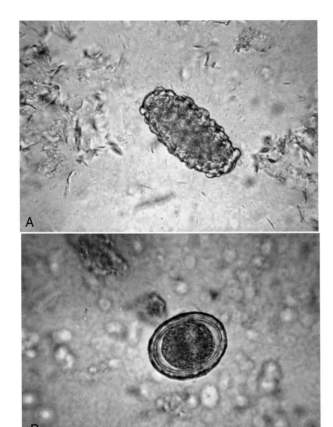

Figure 18-4 **A** and **B,** Structures observed on microscopic examination of a stool specimen (×400).

4. A 6-year-old boy presented with a 1-month history of decreased appetite and abdominal pain. He resides with his parents on a farm in rural South Carolina. No other family members are ill. Microscopic examination of a stool sample is illustrated in Figure 18-4. Which one of the following is the etiologic agent causing his infection?
 A. *Ancylostoma duodenale.*
 B. *Necator americanus.*
 C. *Trichuris trichiura.*
 D. *Enterobius vermicularis.*
 E. *Ascaris lumbricoides.*

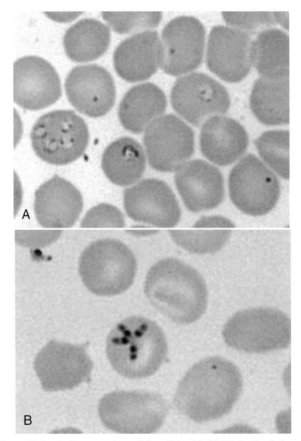

Figure 18-5 **A,** Giemsa stain, peripheral blood (×1000). **B,** Classic form of this parasite.

5. A 12-year-old bone marrow transplant recipient presented to the emergency department with nonspecific influenza-like symptoms, including fever, chills, and myalgia. Initial laboratory test results were consistent with hemolytic anemia. The hematology technologist observed abnormal findings on the smear (Figure 18-5) and referred the slide to the microbiology laboratory. Relevant past medical history includes a blood transfusion 1 month before admission and no recent travel, although his parents confirmed a trip to the Ivory Coast 3 years ago. Which one of the following is the etiologic agent seen in the figure?
 A. *Plasmodium falciparum.*
 B. *Toxoplasma gondii.*
 C. *Plasmodium ovale.*
 D. *Ehrlichia chaffeensis.*
 E. *Babesia microti.*

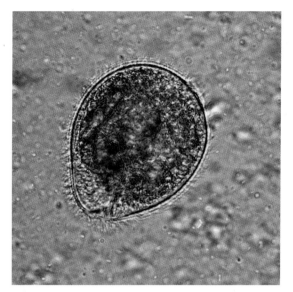

Figure 18-6 Wet mount of stool protozoan ciliate (×400).

6. A 50-year-old pig farmer, a recent immigrant to the United States from Indonesia, presented to his local emergency department with a 3-week history of diarrhea. Examination of his stool demonstrated the ciliated pathogen shown in Figure 18-6. Which one of the following is the etiologic agent?
   A. *Chilomastix mesnili.*
   B. *Enterocytozoon* species.
   C. *Balantidium coli.*
   D. *Iodamoeba bütschlii.*
   E. *Leishmania* species.

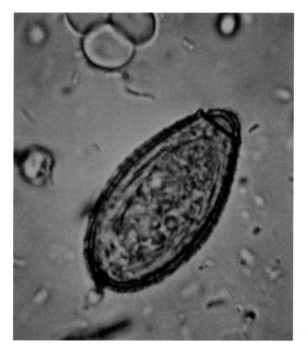

Figure 18-7 Wet mount of stool pathogenic trematode. (×480).

7. A 40-year-old man, recently returned from China, has experienced abdominal discomfort of 1 month's duration. He was subsequently found to have biliary duct obstruction. Stool examination demonstrated the ovum shown in Figure 18-7. Which one of the following trematodes is the etiologic agent of his illness?
   A. *Schistosoma haematobium.*
   B. *Fasciola hepatica.*
   C. *Fasciolopsis buski.*
   D. *Clonorchis sinensis.*
   E. *Paragonimus westermani.*

8. Which one of the following parasites is a liver fluke and infects the biliary ducts of humans?
   A. *Clonorchis* species.
   B. *Paragonimus* species.
   C. *Diphyllobothrium latum.*
   D. *Strongyloides stercoralis.*
   E. *Wuchereria bancrofti.*

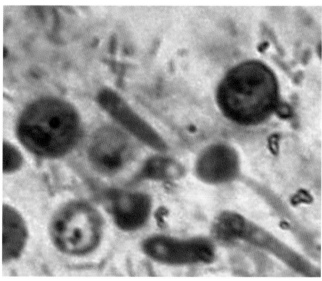

Figure 18-8 Modified acid-fast stain (×1000).

9. A 7-year-old boy presents to his pediatrician with a 5-day history of watery diarrhea, nausea, vomiting, and a low-grade fever. There was no recent travel history, and his other family members were not symptomatic. He had attended a birthday party at an indoor water park 2 weeks before this presentation. Which one of the following is the etiologic agent (shown in Figure 18-8) causing this patient's gastrointestinal disease?
   A. *Cryptosporidium parvum.*
   B. *Isospora belli.*
   C. *Enterocytozoon bienusi.*
   D. *Cyclospora cayetanensis.*
   E. *Giardia intestinalis.*

10. Which one of the following parasites cannot be classified as a helminth?
   A. *Cryptosporidium parvum.*
   B. *Echinococcus granulosis.*
   C. *Taenia solium.*
   D. *Trichuris trichuria.*
   E. *Fasciola hepatica.*

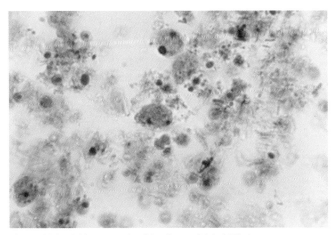

Figure 18-9 Trichrome stain of fecal material (×150).

11. A 4-year-old girl presented to her pediatrician with a 1-week history of abdominal pain and increased bowel movements producing greenish-brown, watery diarrhea. Several children attending her day care center were experiencing similar symptoms. Which one of the following is the etiologic agent shown in Figure 18-9?
   - A. *Dientamoeba fragilis.*
   - B. *Giardia intestinalis.*
   - C. *Cyclospora cayetanensis.*
   - D. *Entamoeba histolytica.*
   - E. *Chilomastix mesnili.*

12. Echinococcosis, or hydatid disease, is an infection by larval tapeworms of the genus *Echinococcus*. Which one of the following statements regarding this infection is correct?
   - A. The life cycle of *Echinococcus multilocularis* includes sheep as the intermediary host and humans as the accidental host.
   - B. The large majority of hydatid cysts occur in the lung through blood dissemination from the intestine.
   - C. *Echinococcus* species are classified as liver and lung trematodes.
   - D. The genus *Echinococcus* contains four species for which humans are an accidental host.
   - E. Immunodiagnostic tests are not useful in diagnosing hydatid disease because of poor sensitivity resulting from the inability of antigen to be released from the cysts.

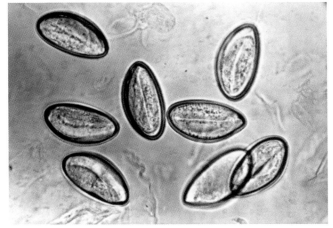

Figure 18-10 Microscopic examination of cellulose tape preparation (×1000).

13. A 4-year-old girl presented with complaints of severe perianal itching. Other children attending her day care setting had similar symptoms. The etiologic agent is shown in Figure 18-10. Which one of the following is the cause of this patient's infection?
   - A. *Enterobius vermicularis.*
   - B. *Ascaris lumbricoides.*
   - C. *Ancylostoma duodenale.*
   - D. *Necator americanus.*
   - E. *Trichuris trichiura.*

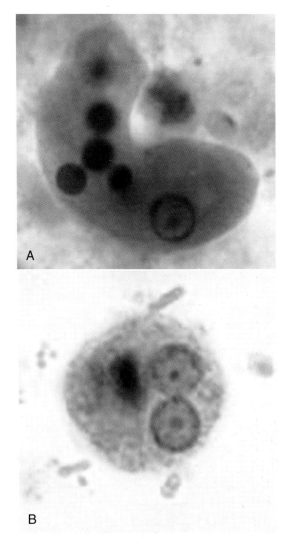

A

B

Figure 18-11 **A** and **B**, Trichrome stain (×100).

14. A 21-year-old female college student presented to the student clinic complaining of a 1-week history of diarrhea and stomach cramps. She had traveled to rural Central America for humanitarian purposes 1 month before presentation. Direct examinations of stained fecal material are shown in Figure 18-11. Which one of the following is the etiologic agent responsible for this patient's gastrointestinal disease?
   - A. *Entamoeba coli.*
   - B. *Blastocystis hominis.*
   - C. *Iodamoeba bütschlii.*
   - D. *Entamoeba histolytica.*
   - E. *Endolimax nana.*

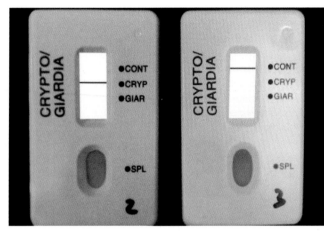

Figure 18-12 Rapid antigen detection results for the patient (left) and a negative control (right).

15. A 40-year-old female patient presented to the emergency department of her local hospital with a 5-day history of watery diarrhea, abdominal cramps, and chills. She had been informed that several family members who also attended a wedding 2 weeks before had similar symptoms, which motivated her to seek medical attention. Stool specimens were collected for bacterial culture, viral studies, and parasitology examinations. A rapid antigen detection test was performed (Figure 18-12). Which one of the following statements provides the best interpretation of these results?
   - A. The patient has cryptosporidiosis.
   - B. The device indicates a false-positive reaction for *Cryptosporidium*.
   - C. The patient may have a dual infection with *Giardia* and *Cryptosporidium*.
   - D. The patient's current diarrheal illness is not due to either *Giardia* or *Cryptosporidium*.
   - E. The test results are inconclusive, and another sample should be tested.

16. Many blood-borne pathogens are transmitted by an insect (vector). Which of the following parasites is not vector transmitted?
   - A. *Toxoplasma gondii.*
   - B. *Plasmodium* species.
   - C. *Leishmania* species.
   - D. *Trypanosoma cruzi.*
   - E. *Babesia microti.*

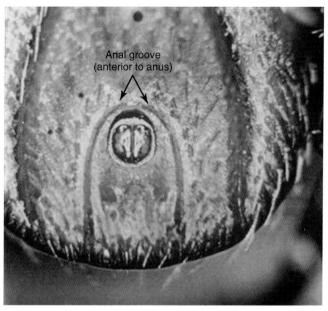

Figure 18-13 Ventral view of ectoparasite.

17. A patient presented to his primary care physician with a rash consistent with erythema migrans. He had removed the ectoparasite, similar to the one shown in Figure 18-13, several days earlier. The patient was prescribed doxycycline and recovered uneventfully. Which one of the following is the most likely infectious disease for which the patient was successfully treated?
   - A. Ehrlichiosis.
   - B. Lyme disease.
   - C. Anaplasmosis.
   - D. Tularemia.
   - E. Rocky Mountain spotted fever.

18. Which one of the following blood collection tubes is optimal for preparing blood smears for the diagnosis of malaria?
   - A. Gold top (serum separator).
   - B. Green top (sodium heparin).
   - C. Gray top (fluoride/oxalate).
   - D. Light blue top (citrate).
   - E. Lavender top (ethylenediaminetetraacetic acid [EDTA]).

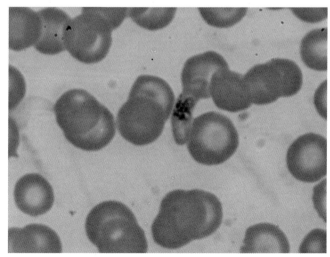

Figure 18-14 Giemsa-stained peripheral blood smear (×1000).

19. A 21-year-old college student presented to his physician with a 2-week history of flu like symptoms, including fever, chills, and malaise. Two months before presentation, he spent 1 week in rural areas of the Dominican Republic as part of a school-based charitable mission. Laboratory tests were ordered, and the technologist reported an unusual observation, which is shown in Figure 18-14. Which one of the following is the best first-line therapy to recommend for this patient?
   A. Intravenous quinidine.
   B. Oral doxycycline.
   C. Intravenous artesunate.
   D. Oral chloroquine.
   E. Oral atovaquone-proguanil.

20. The size of the parasite is critical in distinguishing between parasites in stool that may be morphologically similar. Which one of the following best represents the standard of practice that must be followed to identify parasites accurately in stool specimens?
   A. Examine specimens in preservative only.
   B. Use a calibrated ocular micrometer.
   C. Use an antigen detection test.
   D. Observe the specimen under oil immersion.
   E. Determine the number of ova and cysts per field.

21. A 37-year-old woman presented to the emergency department with a 3-week history of severe headaches and two episodes of seizures. She is a recent immigrant from a rural area of Mexico and was in her usual state of good health until this presentation. Cultures and radiologic examinations were obtained. Computed tomography demonstrated several ring-enhancing cerebral calcifications. Subsequent serologic testing confirmed the diagnosis. Which one of the following is the most likely etiologic agent in this case?
   A. *Nocardia asteroides* complex.
   B. Mixed anaerobic bacterial infection.
   C. *Streptococcus mitis.*
   D. *Taenia solium.*
   E. *Cryptococcus neoformans.*

22. A 50-year-old woman presented to her primary care physician with complaints of a 2-week history of chronic cough and hemoptysis. She had traveled through rural parts of China during the previous month. Stool examinations demonstrated the ovum shown in Figure 18-15. Which one of the following parasites is the most likely etiologic agent of this patient's illness?
   A. *Fasciolopsis buski.*
   B. *Fasciola hepatica.*
   C. *Paragonimus westermani.*
   D. *Diphyllobothrium latum.*
   E. *Clonorchis sinensis.*

23. Which one of the following is not an acceptable practice to ensure stool integrity for morphologic identification of parasites?
   A. Preserve stool in polyvinyl alcohol (PVA).
   B. Refrigerate stool.
   C. Preserve stool in sodium acetate–acetic acid formalin (SAF).
   D. Examine stool immediately.
   E. Preserve stool in ethanol.

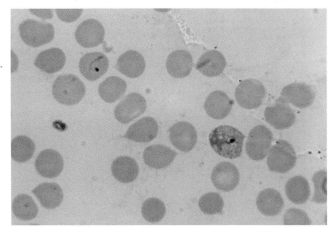

Figure 18-16 Giemsa-stained peripheral blood smear (×1000).

24. A 25-year-old woman presented to her physician with a 2-week history of fever, chills, and headache. Physical examination was significant for splenomegaly. She had recently returned from a 1-month trip to the Philippines where she was staying primarily with relatives in rural areas. Figure 18-16 demonstrates the positive findings of a blood smear preparation. Which one of the following is the most likely etiologic agent in this case?
   A. *Anaplasma phagocytophilum.*
   B. *Plasmodium vivax.*
   C. *Plasmodium falciparum.*
   D. *Ehrlichia chaffeensis.*
   E. *Babesia microti.*

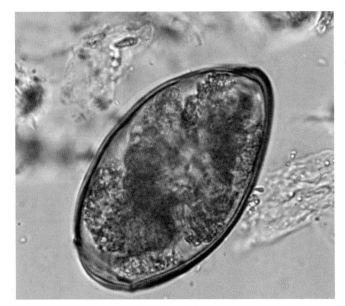

Figure 18-15 Wet mount of stool (×480).

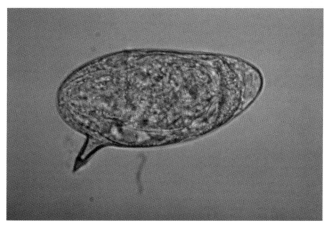

Figure 18-17 Wet mount of stool (×480).

25. An ovum of which one of the following trematodes is shown in Figure 18-17?
   A. *Clonorchis sinensis.*
   B. *Schistosoma mansoni.*
   C. *Fasciola hepatica.*
   D. *Paragonimus westermani.*
   E. *Schistosoma japonicum.*

26. A patient with HIV/AIDS presented to the hospital with a 2-week history of headaches, weakness, and slurred speech. The results of a computed tomography scan with contrast and a magnetic resonance imaging revealed multiple ring-enhancing lesions. Tissue from a brain biopsy was negative on an acid-fast stain. Serodiagnostic tests were positive for the etiologic agent. Which one of the following is the most likely infectious cause of the brain lesions in this patient?
   A. *Toxoplasma gondii.*
   B. *Cryptosporidium parvum.*
   C. *Mycobacterium tuberculosis.*
   D. *Entamoeba histolytica.*
   E. *Balamuthia mandrillaris.*

27. Some parasites are causative agents in transfusion-related infections. Which one of the following parasites is not transmitted by blood transfusion?
   A. *Babesia microti.*
   B. *Trypanosoma cruzi.*
   C. *Toxoplasma gondii.*
   D. *Plasmodium species.*
   E. *Strongyloides stercoralis.*

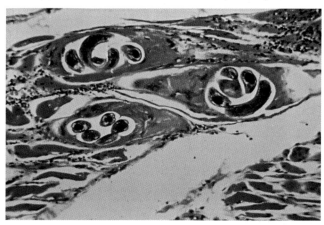

Figure 18-18 Muscle biopsy, H&E stain (×300).

28. Two siblings, 7 and 10 years old, presented to their pediatrician with a 2-day history of fever, facial swelling, and muscle pain. Two weeks earlier, they attended a county fair and consumed pork sandwiches, potato salad, and ice cream. Based on a blood smear, which demonstrated an eosinophilia of 20%, a biopsy was obtained (Figure 18-18). Which one of the following is the most likely etiologic agent for these children's illness?
   A. *Taenia saginata.*
   B. *Wuchereria bancrofti.*
   C. *Trichinella spiralis.*
   D. *Trichomonas hominis.*
   E. *Trichuria trichuria.*

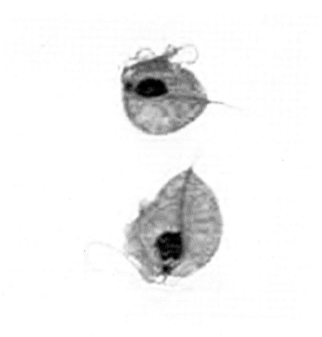

Figure 18-19 Trophozoite with flagella and undulating membrane. The trophozoite is 7 to 23 μm long and 6 to 8 μm wide. The flagella and undulating membrane are present on one side.

29. A 23-year-old woman presented to her doctor with a vaginal discharge that was frothy and malodorous (i.e., "fishy odor"). Which one of the following parasites (Figure 18-19) is the most likely cause of her infection?
   A. *Trichomonas hominis.*
   B. *Gardnerella vaginalis.*
   C. *Treponema pallidum.*
   D. *Mobiluncus species.*
   E. *Trichomonas vaginalis.*

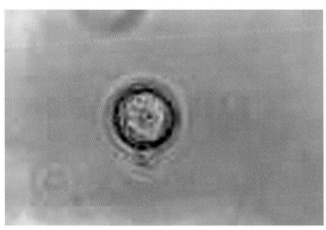

Figure 18-20 Microscopic examination of corneal scraping (×1125).

30. A 19-year-old college student presented to the emergency department complaining of redness, pain, and decreased vision in his left eye. His level of discomfort prevented him from wearing his contact lenses for the previous 2 days. Corneal scrapings were obtained and inoculated on various microbiologic media. Which one of the following is the etiologic agent seen in Figure 18-20?
   A. *Naegleria fowleri*.
   B. Herpes simplex virus.
   C. *Adenovirus*.
   D. *Acanthamoeba*.
   E. *Balamuthia*.

ANSWERS

1. A. *Leishmania braziliensis*.
   Rationale: L. *braziliensis* produces cutaneous lesions.
   B. *Listeria monocytogenes*.
   Rationale: L. *monocytogenes* is a gram-negative bacteria.
   C. *Toxoplasma gondii*.
   Rationale: T. *gondii* cysts appear elongated in tissue, and kinetoplasts are absent.
   D. *Trypanosoma cruzi*.
   Rationale: T. *cruzi* amastigotes and kinetoplasts are demonstrated in this biopsy.
   E. Cytomegalovirus (CMV).
   Rationale: CMV-infected cells contain basophilic cytoplasmic inclusions.

   Major points of discussion
   - The parasite T. *cruzi* is the causative agent of Chagas' disease, also known as American trypanosomiasis.
   - Chagas' disease is endemic in Mexico, South America, and Central America.
   - Vector-borne transmission occurs when the infected triatomine bug (the "kissing bug") takes a blood meal and defecates on the human target. The parasite-infected feces enter through mucous membranes or breaks in the skin.
   - The acute phase of Chagas' disease is often asymptomatic and can last weeks to months. One sign of acute disease is called Romaña's sign, manifested by swelling of the eyelids on the side of the face near the bite wound.
   - In the United States, antiparasitic therapy includes nifurtimox or benznidazole, both of which are available only through the Centers for Disease Control and Prevention (CDC).

2. A. *Cyclospora cayetanensis*.
   Rationale: C. *cayetanensis* is a pathogenic intestinal coccidia characterized by small oocysts that are positive in a modified acid-fast stain and have much thicker walls than C. *parvum*.
   B. *Trichomonas hominis*.
   Rationale: T. *hominis* is a nonpathogenic intestinal flagellate with a single nucleus.

   C. *Cryptosporidium parvum*.
   Rationale: C. *parvum* is a pathogenic intestinal coccidia characterized by small oocysts that are positive in a modified acid-fast stain.
   D. *Chilomastix mesnili*.
   Rationale: C. *mesnili* is a nonpathogenic intestinal flagellate with a single nucleus.
   E. *Giardia intestinalis*.
   Rationale: G. *intestinalis* is a pathogenic intestinal flagellate with two nuclei.

   Major points of discussion
   - G. *intestinalis* (also known as G. *lamblia*) is a protozoan parasite that can be present in diarrheal stool as either a trophozoite or a cyst.
   - The G. *intestinalis* trophozoite is teardrop shaped and has four pairs of flagella, two nuclei, two linear axonemes, and two curved median bodies. The cyst form is oval and contains four nuclei, axenomes, and median bodies.
   - *Giardia* is transmitted by swallowing infectious cysts found in contaminated food or water. Water sources, such as ponds, lakes, and streams, harbor G. *intestinalis* cysts because of fecal contamination by animals and/or humans.
   - Rapid immunochromatographic screening methods are more sensitive than routine ova and parasite examinations. Duodenal aspirates may also be examined for the presence of the parasite.
   - Effective therapy for giardiasis includes metronidazole and nitazoxanide.
   - Hallmark symptoms of giardiasis are explosive watery, foul-smelling diarrhea and flatulence.

3. A. Tsetse fly.
   Rationale: The tsetse fly is the vector responsible for transmitting *Trypanosoma brucei*.
   B. Anopheline mosquito.
   Rationale: The figure demonstrates a gametocyte of P. *falciparum*, a blood parasite transmitted by the female *Anopheles* mosquito.
   C. Reduviid bug.

Rationale: The reduviid bug, a triatomid, is the vector responsible for transmitting *T. cruzi*.
D. *Ixodes scapularis*.
Rationale: I. scapularis is the tick responsible for transmitting *Borrelia burgdorferi*, the causative agent of Lyme disease.
E. Black fly.
Rationale: The black fly is the vector for transmission of *Onchocerca volvulus*, which is associated with river blindness.

Major points of discussion
- Infection with *P. falciparum* is a life-threatening disease requiring rapid identification and determination of the percent parasitemia and immediate notification of the patient's physician.
- For diagnosis, both thick and thin Giemsa-stained blood smears are required, and 200 to 300 oil immersion fields should be examined.
- *P. falciparum* infects all ages of red blood cells (RBCs) and infected RBCs appear to be of normal size.
- The stages of *P. falciparum* observed by direct examination of blood smears are RBCs infected with multiple young trophozoite rings and/or banana-shaped gametocytes.
- In the absence of gametoctyes, the travel history of the patient is critical because babesiosis can mimic *P. falciparum* infection.[8,10]

4. A. *Ancylostoma duodenale*.
Rationale: The *Ancylostoma* (hookworm) egg is oval, thin shelled, and colorless and usually contains 8 to 16 embryonic cells. This egg cannot be distinguished from *N. americanus*.
B. *Necator americanus*.
Rationale: The *Necator* (hookworm) egg is oval, thin shelled, and colorless and usually contains 8 to 16 embryonic cells. This egg cannot be distinguished from that of *A. duodenale*.
C. *Trichuris trichiura*.
Rationale: The *Trichuris* (whipworm) egg is elongated, yellowish brown, and barrel shaped, with colorless polar plugs at each end.
D. *Enterobius vermicularis*.
Rationale: The *Enterobius* (pinworm) egg is elongated, oval, colorless, and flattened on one side.
E. *Ascaris lumbricoides*.
Rationale: The unfertilized *Ascaris* (roundworm) egg is elongated and brown, with a bumpy (i.e., mammillated) shell (Figure 18-4, *A*). The fertilized egg is ovoid and brown with a thick smooth shell (Figure 18-4, *B*).

Major points of discussion
- *A. lumbricoides* is the largest nematode, or roundworm, found in the human intestinal tract. Adult females are 20 to 35 cm long, and adult males are 15 to 30 cm long.
- Infection is primarily acquired by ingestion of fertilized eggs present in the soil. Unfertilized *Ascaris* eggs are noninfectious.
- The life cycle of *Ascaris* includes migration of larvae to the lungs, where they eventually migrate through alveolar walls, up the bronchus, and then are swallowed. Adult worms then develop in the small intestine. Loeffler syndrome is the pulmonary manifestation of the lung phase, which can include cough, dyspnea, and hemoptysis.

- Diagnosis of the pulmonary phase of ascariasis is often made by visualizing larvae in expectorated sputum.
- The drug of choice for treatment of ascariasis is albendazole. Mebendazole, ivermectin, and nitazoxanide are satisfactory alternatives.[5]

5. A. *Plasmodium falciparum*.
Rationale: P. falciparum is characterized by RBCs infected with multiple ring forms. However, *P. falciparum* does not have a dormant liver stage, as with *P. vivax* and *P. ovale* infection, which would recrudesce 3 years after relevant travel.
B. *Toxoplasma gondii*.
Rationale: T. gondii is a protozoan parasite, characterized by crescent-shaped tachyzoites, which can sometimes be observed within Giemsa-stained leukocytes.
C. *Plasmodium ovale*.
Rationale: P. ovale typically demonstrates many developmental stages in peripheral blood and is not characterized by RBCs infected with multiple ring forms.
D. *Ehrlichia chaffeensis*.
Rationale: E. chaffeensis is an intracellular bacterial species that infects mononuclear leukocytes and appears as clusters of bacteria called morulae.
E. *Babesia microti*.
Rationale: B. microti is a protozoan parasite, characterized by RBCs infected with multiple ring forms, and has been transmitted through infected blood products.

Major points of discussion
- *B. microti* is primarily a tick-borne disease, transmitted by the deer tick (*I. scapularis*), which is also the vector for Lyme disease. Tick-borne transmission primarily occurs in the Northeast and upper Midwest regions of the United States.
- Cases of transfusion-related babesiosis are on the rise. Infected blood donors appear healthy, and blood donation protocols do not currently include laboratory test screening for *Babesia*.
- Diagnosis is based on microscopic identification of the organism on Giemsa-stained peripheral blood smears. Findings include RBCs infected with multiple ring forms (early trophozoites), which can sometimes appear as a tetrad or "Maltese cross" (Figure 18-5. *B*) and as extra-erythrocytic trophozoites.
- Typically, the level of parasitemia for babesiosis is only 1% to 2%, but it can be more than 10% in immunocompromised patients, in which case RBC exchange transfusion may be indicated.
- Babesiosis is usually treated with combination therapy, such as atovaquone and azithromycin or clindamycin and quinine.

6. A. *Chilomastix mesnili*.
Rationale: C. mesnili is a flagellated intestinal protozoan.
B. *Enterocytozoon* species.
Rationale: Enterocytozoon species is a microspordium and an obligate intracellular parasite. It is neither ciliated nor flagellated.
C. *Balantidium coli*.
Rationale: B. coli is the only ciliated parasite that infects humans.
D. *Iodamoeba bütschlii*.

Rationale: I. bütschlii is an intestinal ameba that moves sluggishly by means of cytoplasmic protrusions called pseudopods.
E. *Leishmania* species.
Rationale: Leishmania is a hemoflagellate that circulates in the bloodstream or may be present in lymph nodes or muscle.

Major points of discussion

- *B. coli* is the largest protozoan and the only ciliate that infects humans. The surface of the parasite is covered with short cilia. The trophozoite measures 70 μm in length and 45 μm in width.
- *B. coli* infection is usually limited to the intestines and is ingested in fecally contaminated food or water. Individuals who have close contact with pigs are commonly infected.
- *B. coli* is best identified using wet mounts of stool because the parasite does not stain adequately. They can be seen and identified under low or high power because of their large size.
- The symptoms associated with balantidiasis include diarrhea, dysentery, and abscess formation.
- The treatment of choice for balantidiasis is tetracycline, although metronidazole and iodoquinol can be used as alternatives.

7. A. *Schistosoma haematobium.*
Rationale: The egg of *S. haematobium* is 112 to 170 μm in length, has a yellow-brown shell, and has a distinct ~~lateral~~ spine. *terminal*
B. *Fasciola hepatica.*
Rationale: The egg of *F. hepatica* is 130 to 150 μm in length, has a yellow-brown shell, and has an operculum but no opercular shoulders.
C. *Fasciolopsis buski.*
Rationale: The egg of *F. buski* is 130 to 140 μm in length, has a transparent shell, and has an operculum with no opercular shoulders at the narrower end.
D. *Clonorchis sinensis.*
Rationale: The egg of *C. sinensis,* or the liver fluke, is 20 to 35 μm in length, has a thick yellow-brown shell, and has an operculum with opercular shoulders.
E. *Paragonimus westermani.*
Rationale: The egg of *P. westermani,* or the lung fluke, is 80 to 120 μm in length, has a thick brown-yellow shell, and has an operculum with opercular shoulders.

Major points of discussion

- *C. sinensis,* also known as the liver fluke or Oriental liver fluke, is found throughout Asia, including China, Japan, Korea, and Taiwan.

- *C. sinensis* miracidia are ingested by freshwater snails, which are the first intermediate host.
- Cercariae are released from the snail host and encyst (referred to as metacercariae) in the skin of freshwater fish or on vegetation, which are the second intermediate hosts.
- The most serious complication of infections with *C. sinensis* is cholangiocarcinoma, or cancer of the bile duct.
- Praziquantel is the drug of choice for treating infections with *C. sinensis.*

8. A. *Clonorchis* species.
Rationale: The trematode *C. sinensis* causes biliary infection and is known as the Chinese or Oriental liver fluke.
B. *Paragonimus* species.
Rationale: Paragonimus species is a lung fluke.
C. *Diphyllobothrium latum.*
Rationale: D. latum is an intestinal cestode or tapeworm.
D. *Strongyloides stercoralis.*
Rationale: S. stercoralis is an intestinal nematode (i.e., a roundworm).
E. *Wuchereria bancrofti.*
Rationale: W. bancrofti is a filarial nematode (i.e., a roundworm) that causes elephantiasis.

Major points of discussion

- *Clonorchis* species, *Opisthorchis* species, and *Fasciola hepatica* are trematodes that parasitize the bile ducts of humans, often resulting in biliary obstruction.
- Liver flukes are associated with neoplasia of the bile duct and cholangiocarcinoma, in particular, in elderly patients.
- The laboratory diagnosis of *C. sinensis* is made by examining multiple stool specimens and comparing the size and morphology of the eggs (Table 18-1).
- The source of infection with liver flukes is uncooked fish or water plants. The reservoir hosts for *C. sinensis* and *Opisthorchis* species include dogs, cats, and other mammals that ingest fish. The most common definitive hosts for *F. hepatica* are sheep and other herbivores that ingest aquatic plants.
- The drug of choice for treating trematode infections is praziquantel.[7]

9. A. *Cryptosporidium parvum.*
Rationale: C. parvum oocysts are round and small (1 to 3 μm) and are positive in a modified acid-fast stain.
B. *Isospora belli.*
Rationale: I. belli oocysts are positive in a modified acid-fast stain but are much larger (20 to 33 μm long and 10 to 19 μm wide) than those in Figure 18-8.

Table 18-1

Trematode	Common Name	Foodborne Source	Definitive Host	Egg Size (μm)	Presence of Embryo in Egg
Clonorchis sinensis	Chinese liver fluke	Uncooked freshwater fish	Fish-eating mammals (e.g., dogs and cats)	12-19 × 28-35	Yes
Opisthorchis species	*O. viverrini* = Southeast Asian liver fluke; *O. felineus* = cat liver fluke	Uncooked freshwater fish	Fish-eating mammals (e.g., dogs and cats)	11-17 × 19-30	Yes
Fasciola hepatica	Sheep liver fluke	Uncooked aquatic plants	Sheep and other herbivores	63-90 × 130-150	No

C. *Enterocytozoon bienusi.*
Rationale: *E. bienusi* are small microsporidia (2 to 7 μm long and 1.5 to 5 μm wide), not positive in an acid-fast stain, and best visualized using a modified trichrome stain.
D. *Cyclospora cayetanensis.*
Rationale: *C. cayetanensis* oocysts are positive in a modified acid-fast stain but are larger (8 to 10 μm) than those in Figure 18-8 and have a thick wall.
E. *Giardia intestinalis.*
Rationale: *G. intestinalis* cysts are much larger (11 to 14 μm long and 7 to 10 μm wide) than those pictured Figure 18-8 and are not positive in a modified acid-fast stain.

Major points of discussion

- *C. parvum* has a protective outer shell that enables it to survive outside the body for extended periods of time and makes it very resistant to chlorine-based disinfectants.
- In the United States, *C. parvum* is one of the most common causes of waterborne disease (recreational water and drinking water) in humans.
- Rapid antigen detection assays are commercially available for the diagnosis of cryptosporidiosis directly from stool specimens.
- Infections with *C. parvum* may be self-limited in patients with a normal immune system.
- In severely immunocompromised individuals, extraintestinal infections can also occur, primarily affecting the lungs.
- Nitazoxanide can be used to treat diarrhea caused by *C. parvum* in people with healthy immune systems; however, the effectiveness in immunocompromised individuals is unclear.

10. A. *Cryptosporidium parvum.*
Rationale: *C. parvum* is an intestinal coccidian, not a helminth (i.e., worm).
B. *Echinococcus granulosis.*
Rationale: *E. granulosis* is a tissue cestode, or tapeworm.
C. *Taenia solium.*
Rationale: *T. solium* is an intestinal cestode, or tapeworm.
D. *Trichuris trichuria.*
Rationale: *T. trichuria* is an intestinal nematode, or roundworm.

E. *Fasciola hepatica.*
Rationale: *F. hepatica* is a trematode, commonly called the liver fluke.

Major points of discussion

- Parasites are classified as protozoa (single-celled organisms) and helminths (multicellular organisms).
- Intestinal protozoa include the flagellates, amebae, coccidian, and ciliates. Diagnosis of infections (other than coccidian) is based on microscopic examinations of stool for trophozoites and cysts.
- Detection of coccidian often requires special stains, such as a modified acid-fast stain (for *Cryptosporidium*) or a modified trichrome stain (for microsporidia).
- Helminths include the nematodes, cestodes, and trematodes. Infections are diagnosed detecting eggs, larvae, or adult worms in stool. Nematodes are the most prevalent helminths that cause infections in humans.
- Characteristics of helminth eggs used for identification include size, shape, color, and shell thickness (Table 18-2).[7]

11. A. *Dientamoeba fragilis.*
Rationale: The trophozoite of *D. fragilis*, a pathogenic intestinal flagellate, can have one or two nuclei and three to five granules of nuclear chromatin.
B. *Giardia intestinalis.*
Rationale: *G. intestinalis* is a pathogenic intestinal flagellate whose trophozoites are characterized by two nuclei, peripheral chromatin, and flagella.
C. *Cyclospora cayetanensis.*
Rationale: *C. cayetanensis* is a pathogenic intestinal coccidian characterized by small, modified acid-fast-stain–positive oocysts; it does not have a trophozoite stage.
D. *Entamoeba histolytica.*
Rationale: The trophozoite of *E. histolytica*, a pathogenic intestinal ameba, has one nucleus with an even distribution of chromatin on the nuclear membrane and a small central karyosome.
E. *Chilomastix mesnili.*
Rationale: *C. mesnili* is a nonpathogenic intestinal flagellate that has a single nucleus and a distinct oral groove close to the nucleus.

Table 18-2 Helminth Characteristics

Helminth Classification	Morphology	Reproductive System	Example	Egg Size (μm)	Egg Morphology
Trematodes (flukes)	Dorsoventrally flat worms with oral and ventral suckers	Hermaphroditic	*Clonorchis sinensis*	28-35 × 12-19	Embryonated, operculated
			Fasciola hepatica	130-150 × 63-90	Unembryonated, operculated
Cestodes (tapeworms)	Proglottids (egg-producing units) develop from scolices	Hermaphroditic	*Taenia* species	30-47 diameter	Embryonated, striated shell
			Diphyllobothrium latum	58-75 × 40-50	Operculated, knob at opposite end of operculum, unembryonated
Nematodes (roundworms, hookworms)	Bilaterally symmetrical with functional digestive tracts	Separate sexes (males smaller than females)	*Trichuris trichiura*	50-54 × 20-23	Barrel-shaped, thick shell with polar plugs
			Enterobius vermicularis	70-85 × 60-80	Embryonated, thick shell, football-shaped

Table 18-3 Helminth Characteristics

Feature	*Giardia intestinalis*	*Dientamoeba fragilis*
Shape	Pear-shaped	Ameboid
Size	10-20 μm long, 5-15 μm wide	5-15 μm
Nuclei (#)	2	1-2
Peripheral chromatin	Yes	No
Median bodies (#)	Yes (2)	No
Flagella (#)	Yes (4 pair)	No
Sucking disk	Yes	No

Major points of discussion

- The life cycle of *D. fragilis* does not include a cyst stage. The morphology of *D. fragilis* can be differentiated from that of *G. intestinalis*, as described in Table 18-3.
- The mode of transmission is through fecal-oral spread and sometimes through coinfected eggs of *E. vermicularis* (pinworm).
- Disease is more common in children; adults are typically asymptomatically colonized.
- Examination of a single stool sample has a sensitivity of 50%; multiple samples (up to 6) are necessary to optimize detection.
- Common treatment strategies for *D. fragilis* infection include metronidazole, iodoquinol, and paromomycin.

12. A. The life cycle of *Echinococcus multilocularis* includes sheep as the intermediary host and humans as the accidental host.
Rationale: Sheep are the intermediary host with *E. granulosus* infections; mice, squirrels, voles, and shrews are intermediary hosts with *E. multilocularis*.
B. The large majority of hydatid cysts occur in the lung through blood dissemination from the intestine.
Rationale: The organ that is mainly infected in hydatid disease is the liver, primarily the right lobe.
C. *Echinococcus* species are classified as liver and lung trematodes.
Rationale: *Echinococcus* species are tissue cestodes or tapeworms. Trematodes are flukes.
D. The genus *Echinococcus* contains four species for which humans are an accidental host.
Rationale: Infections by *E. granulosus* are the most common, but *E. multilocularis*, *E. vogeli*, and *E. oligarthrus* also infect humans.
E. Immunodiagnostic tests are not useful in diagnosing hydatid disease because of poor sensitivity resulting from the inability of antigen to be released from the cysts.
Rationale: Serologic tests aid in the diagnosis of echinococcosis; immunoblot assays are particularly useful.

Major points of discussion

- Transmission of hydatid disease is known to occur between dogs and sheep in parts of Utah, Arizona, New Mexico, California, and other Western states.
- Immunoblot assays using specific antibodies that recognize the hydatid antigens are very specific as confirmatory tests. Enzyme-linked immunosorbent assay methods using monoclonal antibodies are highly sensitive as a screen to diagnose human hydatid disease.

- If hydatid cyst fluid is obtained, examination using light or fluorescent microscopy may reveal hydatid scolices, daughter cysts, or hooks.
- Surgical removal of cysts can be risky because of fluid spillage, which causes intraperitoneal seeding of infection during the procedure.
- Treatment for cystic echinococcosis includes surgery, puncture-aspiration-injection-respiration, and chemotherapy with albendazole or mebendazole.

13. A. *Enterobius vermicularis*.
Rationale: The *Enterobius* (pinworm) egg is elongated, oval, colorless, and flattened on one side.
B. *Ascaris lumbricoides*.
Rationale: The unfertilized *Ascaris* (roundworm) egg is elongated and brown with a bumpy (i.e., mammillated) shell, whereas the fertilized egg is ovoid and brown with a thick, smooth shell.
C. *Ancylostoma duodenale*.
Rationale: The *Ancylostoma* (hookworm) egg is oval, thin shelled, and colorless and usually contains 8 to 16 embryonic cells. This egg cannot be distinguished from that of N. americanus.
D. *Necator americanus*.
Rationale: The *Necator* (hookworm) egg is oval, thin shelled, and colorless and usually contains 8 to 16 embryonic cells. This egg cannot be distinguished from that of A. duodenale.
E. *Trichuris trichiura*.
Rationale: The *Trichuris* (whipworm) egg is elongated, yellow-brown, and barrel shaped and has colorless polar plugs at each end.

Major points of discussion

- The nematode, or pinworm, *E. vermicularis*, is the most common helminthic infection in the United States. Humans are the only known host of this parasite.
- Disease is initiated when infective eggs are ingested, which hatch in the intestine and develop into adult worms. Approximately 1 month later, gravid females migrate nocturnally out of the anus and deposit eggs on the skin of the perianal region. The eggs become infective within hours.
- Self-infection typically occurs when young children scratch their itchy, perianal area while sleeping and transfer infective eggs to their mouth. Person-to-person transmission can also occur through handling contaminated clothing or bed linens.
- Eggs are collected in the morning, before defecation, by pressing transparent adhesive tape (the "Scotch tape test") on the perianal skin and then microscopically examining the tape when placed on a slide.
- The drug of choice for *Enterobius* infection is pyrantel pamoate.

14. A. *Entamoeba coli*.
Rationale: E. coli is nonpathogenic, it does not ingest RBCs in the trophozoite form, and the cyst contains up to eight nuclei.
B. *Blastocystis hominis*.

Rationale: B. hominis, which is occasionally pathogenic, does not demonstrate a true trophozoite form. Cysts and ameboid forms may be observed in fecal preparations.
C. *Iodamoeba bütschlii.*
Rationale: I. bütschlii is nonpathogenic, it does not ingest RBCs in the trophozoite form, and the cyst contains a single nucleus and a large glycogen vacuole.
D. *Entamoeba histolytica.*
Rationale: Figure 18-11, A shows an *E. histolytica* trophozoite with ingested RBCs in the cytoplasm. Figure 18-11, B shows a thin-walled *E. histolytica* cyst containing two nuclei and a chromatoidal bar.
E. *Endolimax nana.*
Rationale: E. nana is nonpathogenic, it does not ingest RBCs in the trophozoite form, and the oval cyst contains four nuclei.

Major points of discussion
■ Infection with *E. histolytica* is associated with the ingestion of contaminated food or water and is most prevalent in tropical and subtropical regions.
■ The liver is the most common site of extraintestinal *E. histolytica* disease.
■ Microscopically, *E. histolytica* cannot be differentiated from the nonpathogenic *E. dispar* unless trophozoites with ingested RBCs are present.
■ Rapid antigen detection assays are commercially available, some of which can distinguish *E. histolytica* from *E. dispar.*
■ Treatment for *E. histolytica* gastrointestinal disease includes paromomycin or iodoquinol for cyst forms and metronidazole or tinidazole for trophozoites.

15. A. The patient has cryptosporidiosis.
Rationale: It cannot be determined whether the patient has cryptosporidiosis because the control line on the device used for the patient's sample is not present, indicating a quality control failure.
B. The device indicates a false-positive reaction for *Cryptosporidium.*
Rationale: It cannot be determined whether the patient's result is a true positive or a false positive because the control line is not present, indicating a quality control failure.
C. The patient may have a dual infection with *Giardia* and *Cryptosporidium.*
Rationale: There is no indication that the *Giardia* antigen was detected. In addition, it cannot be determined whether the patient has cryptosporidiosis because the control line is not present, indicating a quality control failure.
D. The patient's current diarrheal illness is not due to either *Giardia* or *Cryptosporidium.*
Rationale: This cannot be determined because the control line on the device used for the patient's sample is not present, indicating a quality control failure.
E. The test results are inconclusive, and another sample should be tested.
Rationale: The control line on the device used for the patient's sample is not present, indicating a quality control failure. Therefore, these results cannot be interpreted appropriately. The test should be repeated.

Major points of discussion
■ Rapid antigen detection assays typically include a control line, which indicates that all reagents have been added and the test result is valid.
■ For gastrointestinal disease, rapid antigen detection tests are available for *Clostridium difficile, Giardia, Cryptosporidium, E. histolytica,* rotavirus, and adenovirus 40/41.
■ External controls, either provided by the manufacturer or previously characterized patient samples, are used for quality control purposes when new lot numbers or shipments of kits are received.
■ Patient results cannot be released if there is a failure in any aspect of the quality control process.
■ Kit components cannot be exchanged between lot numbers or within kits of the same lot number. Extra devices or reagents must be discarded.

16. A. *Toxoplasma gondii.*
Rationale: T. gondii is not vector borne. It is transmitted congenitally and through exposure to cat feces and eating undercooked meat.
B. *Plasmodium* species.
Rationale: Malaria is contracted through the bite of the Anopheles mosquito.
C. *Leishmania* species.
Rationale: Leishmaniasis is associated with phlebotomine sand flies.
D. *Trypanosoma cruzi.*
Rationale: Chagas' disease is contracted by the bite of the triatomine or kissing bug.
E. *Babesia microti.*
Rationale: The *Ixodes* (hard-bodied) tick is the vector for babesiosis.

Major points of discussion
■ In 2010, more than 200 million cases of malaria occurred worldwide, and about 650,000 people died, most (91%) in the African region. Only *Anopheles* mosquitoes support the sporogenic development of *Plasmodium* species, and the female mosquito can remain infective for life (Table 18-4).
■ The *Anopheles gambiae* mosquito has a predominant role in transmitting *P. falciparum.*
■ Little is known about the prevalence of *Babesia* in malaria-endemic countries, where misidentification as *Plasmodium* probably occurs. In Europe, most reported cases of babesiosis are due to *B. divergens* and occur in splenectomized patients. In the United States, *B. microti* is the agent most frequently identified (Northeast and Midwest) and it can occur in nonsplenectomized individuals.
■ The World Health Organization estimates the worldwide prevalence of leishmaniasis to be about 12 million cases, with an annual mortality of about 60,000 individuals.
■ Hard- and soft-bodied ticks are ectoparasites, distinguished by the presence or absence of a dorsal plate that covers the insect's surface. *Dermacentor* (dog tick) has white markings on the dorsal plate, and *Ixodes* (deer tick) does not.[7,11]

Table 18-4 Vector-Borne Parasites

Parasite	Disease	Vector	Endemic Areas
Babesia microti	Babesiosis	*Ixodes scapularis* (black-legged, hard-bodied tick; deer tick)	Northeast and upper Midwest United States
Leishmania	Leishmaniasis (cutaneous, mucocutaneous, and visceral)	*Phlebotomus* and *Lutzomyia* (female sand flies)	Afro-Eurasia (*Phlebotomus*) Western hemisphere (*Lutzomyia*)
Plasmodium species	Malaria	Female *Anopheles* mosquitoes	Tropical and subtropical regions, including sub-Saharan Africa, Asia, Mexico, and Central and South America
Trypanosoma cruzi	Chagas' disease (American trypanosomiasis)	*Triatoma infestans* *Rhodnius prolixus* *Triatomine*, kissing or reduviid bugs	Mexico and South and Central America
Trypanosoma brucei gambiense *Trypanosoma brucei rhodesiense*	African trypanosomiasis (sleeping sickness)	*Glossina* vectors (tsetse flies)	*T. brucei gambiense*: Western Africa *T. brucei rhodesiense*: Eastern Africa

17. A. Ehrlichiosis.
Rationale: *E. chaffeensis* is associated with human monocytic ehrlichiosis and the *Amblyomma* tick vector, which has a posterior anal groove.
B. Lyme disease.
Rationale: Early localized Lyme disease, caused by the spirochete *B. burgdorferi*, presents with erythema migrans and is transmitted by the *Ixodes* tick, which has an anterior anal groove (as seen in Figure 18-13).
C. Anaplasmosis.
Rationale: *Anaplasma phagocytophilum* is associated with human granulocytic anaplasmosis and does not present with a rash, although it is transmitted by the *Ixodes* tick.
D. Tularemia.
Rationale: The most common form of tularemia is caused by *Francisella tularensis*, which are small gram-negative bacilli. It is an ulceroglandular infection that is transmitted by the *Dermacentor* or *Amblyomma* tick, both of which have posterior anal grooves.
E. Rocky Mountain spotted fever.
Rationale: Rocky Mountain spotted fever, which is caused by the spirochete *Rickettsia rickettsii*, presents with a petechial rash on the palms and soles. It is transmitted by the *Dermacentor* tick, which has a posterior anal groove.

Table 18-5

Characteristic	Hard Tick	Soft Tick
Scutum present	Yes	No
Festoons present	Sometimes	No
Mouth parts visible (dorsal view)	Yes	No

Table 18-6

Characteristic	*Ixodes* (Deer Tick)	*Dermacentor* (Dog Tick)	*Amblyomma* (Lone Star Tick)
Festoons present	No	Yes	Yes
Scutum	Plain	Ornate with colored markings	Ornate (females have a distinct white spot)
Anal groove	Anterior	Posterior	Posterior

Major points of discussion

- Ticks are divided into two main families: soft ticks (Argasidae) and hard ticks (Ixodidae). Their distinguishing characteristics are summarized in Table 18-5.
- Features of the three most common species of hard ticks are outlined in Table 18-6.
- Female ticks are associated with a higher transmission of Lyme disease. Therefore, if gender differentiation is requested, the scutum, or dorsal shield, is smaller in female ticks compared with male ticks.
- The likelihood of acquiring Lyme disease from an infected tick correlates with the length of time of tick attachment and the amount of blood ingested by the tick.
- The use of molecular amplification techniques for detecting *B. burgdorferi* in ticks may be useful for local epidemiologic purposes but these techniques are not recommended for clinical management of patients presenting with presumptive Lyme disease.[12]

18. A. Gold top (serum separator).
Rationale: This tube type is used for serum measurements in chemistry and for serology testing.
B. Green top (sodium heparin).
Rationale: This tube type is used for plasma measurements in chemistry.
C. Gray top (fluoride/oxalate).
Rationale: This tube type inhibits glycolysis and is used for glucose measurements.
D. Light blue top (citrate).
Rationale: This tube type is used for coagulation testing.
E. Lavender top (ethylenediaminetetraacetic acid (EDTA).
Rationale: This tube type is used for performing complete blood cell counts and for preparing blood smears for malaria diagnosis, which must be prepared from anticoagulated blood.

Major points of discussion

- EDTA is preferred over heparin as an anticoagulant because heparin may cause morphologic distortion and hinder diagnosis.
- Infection with *P. falciparum* can rapidly progress to severe malaria; therefore, all requests for malaria diagnosis are considered STAT, and positive results are reported as a critical value.

- One set of negative blood smears does not rule out malaria; several specimens should be examined over a 36-hour time frame.
- Plasmodial species are detected and identified by examining Giemsa-stained thin and thick blood smears.
- Examination of thick smears is considered the gold standard for detection because a larger volume of blood is used. Thin smears are necessary for speciation of malarial parasites.[7]

19. A. Intravenous quinidine.
Rationale: This antiparasitic agent is one component of a regimen used to treat severe malaria, which can be characterized by mental status changes, organ failure, and generalized convulsions.
B. Oral doxycycline.
Rationale: This antimicrobial is often paired with quinine to treat patients who acquired malaria in chloroquine- and mefloquine-resistant regions.
C. Intravenous artesunate.
Rationale: This antiparasitic drug is available from the CDC on a compassionate use basis to treat severe malaria.
D. Oral chloroquine.
Rationale: The banana-shaped gametocyte seen in Figure 18-14 is diagnostic for *P. falciparum*. The Dominican Republic is categorized as an area with chloroquine-sensitive malarial parasites of this type.
E. Oral atovaquone-proguanil.
Rationale: This antiparasitic approach is used to treat patients who acquired malaria in chloroquine- and mefloquine-resistant regions.

Major points of discussion
- Definitive identification of an infecting *Plasmodium* species incorporates microscopic observations, determination of percent parasitemia, severity of illness, travel history, and compliance with malarial prophylaxis.
- *P. falciparum* is characterized microscopically by RBCs infected with multiple ring forms and, less commonly, by the presence of banana-shaped gametocytes.
- Infection with *P. falciparum* can be rapidly life threatening; therefore, whole blood specimens require immediate processing and rapid notification of clinicians so that appropriate therapy can be initiated as quickly as possible.
- The processing and interpretation of peripheral blood smears for parasites requires the preparation of both thick and thin smears, examination of 200 to 300 low-power microscopic fields, and determination of percent parasitemia for positive samples.
- Chloroquine-resistant *P. falciparum* is common throughout Africa, South America, and Southeast Asia.[3]

20. A. Examine specimens in preservative only.
Rationale: The size of a parasite can be determined from either a wet preparation of fresh stool or a permanently stained slide.
B. Use a calibrated ocular micrometer.
Rationale: The microscope used to measure the size of the parasite must be calibrated for each objective and eyepiece pair (e.g., for low power, high power, and oil immersion).

C. Use an antigen detection test.
Rationale: It is recommended that positive parasite antigen detection results by morphology be confirmed by another method, but they are not considered routine practice for ova and parasite identification.
D. Observe the specimen under oil immersion.
Rationale: The type of ocular used to determine parasite size is chosen by the examiner based on ease of measurement.
E. Determine the number of ova and cysts per field.
Rationale: Quantifying the number of parasites per microscopic field is only critical to determine the percent parasitemia in malaria cases. It is not used when examining stool specimens for ova and parasites.

Table 18-7

		Entamoeba histolytica (µm)	*Entamoeba hartmanii* (µm)
Trophozoite	Wet mount	Length <12	Length <12
	Stool preservative	Length >10	Length >10
Cyst	Wet mount	Diameter ≥11	Diameter ≤9
	Stool preservative	Diameter ≥8	Diameter ≤8

Major points of discussion
- At times, parasite size can be the only way to distinguish between similar parasites, for example, to distinguish between *E. histolytica* and *E. hartmanii*. Examination can be from wet mounts or stools in preservative (Table 18-7).
- Ocular micrometers must be calibrated each year for each objective and eyepiece.
- Fresh stool specimens should be examined within 30 minutes of collection to optimize detection of trophozoites. If this time recommendation cannot be met, the stool must be placed in fixative.
- Each analyst should be tested for competency in ocular calibration each year.
- The calibrated measurements should be conspicuously posted near the microscope.

21. A. *Nocardia asteroides* complex.
Rationale: Brain abscesses, rather than calcified lesions, are the hallmark of nocardial disease, and no serologic testing is available.
B. Mixed anaerobic bacterial infection.
Rationale: Brain abscesses, rather than calcified lesions, are the hallmark of bacterial disease, and no serologic testing is available.
C. *Streptococcus mitis*.
Rationale: Brain abscesses, rather than calcified lesions, are the hallmark of streptococcal disease, and no serologic testing is available.
D. *Taenia solium*.
Rationale: Neurocysticercosis, one of the leading causes of adult-onset seizures, is associated with the ingestion of *T. solium* eggs.
E. *Cryptococcus neoformans*.
Rationale: Brain lesions associated with *C. neoformans* are not calcified, and antigen, rather than antibody, detection would support the diagnosis.

Major points of discussion

- *T. solium* taeniasis is acquired through ingesting undercooked infected pork, which contains cysticerci. Patients are often asymptomatic and may pass proglottids or, more rarely, eggs in their stool.
- Cysticercosis is acquired through ingesting *T. solium* eggs, which are shed in the feces of a human tapeworm carrier. Oncospheres hatch in the intestine and migrate to striated muscles and other tissues, including the brain, which results in neurocysticercosis.
- Examination of gravid proglottids can help differentiate *T. solium* from *T. saginata* (beef tapeworm). India ink is injected into the proglottids to observe the uterine branches. *T. solium* has 7 to 13 branches, whereas *T. saginata* has 15 to 20.
- *Taenia* eggs are difficult to distinguish from each other. Both *T. solium* and *T. saginata* eggs are round, yellow-brown, and thick shelled.
- For neurocysticercosis, surgical removal of the cysticerci is preferred and is often accompanied by treatment with praziquantel or niclosamide.[6]

22. A. *Fasciolopsis buski.*
Rationale: The egg of *F. buski* is 130 to 140 μm in length, has a transparent shell, and has an operculum with no opercular shoulders at the narrow end.
B. *Fasciola hepatica.*
Rationale: The egg of *F. hepatica* is 130 to 150 μm in length, has a yellow-brown shell, and has an operculum but no opercular shoulders.
C. *Paragonimus westermani.*
Rationale: The egg of *P. westermani,* or the lung fluke, is 80 to 120 μm in length, has a thick brown-yellow shell, and an operculum with opercular shoulders.
D. *Diphyllobothrium latum.*
Rationale: The egg of *D. latum,* which is a cestode, is 58 to 75 μm in length, has a yellow-brown shell, and has an operculum but no opercular shoulders.
E. *Clonorchis sinensis.*
Rationale: The egg of *C. sinensis,* or the liver fluke, is 20 to 35 μm in length, has a thick yellow-brown shell, and has an operculum with opercular shoulders.

Major points of discussion

- *P. westermani,* also known as the lung fluke, occurs primarily in Asia, including China, the Philippines, Japan, Vietnam, South Korea, Taiwan, and Thailand.
- *P. westermani* miracidia are ingested by freshwater snails, which are the first intermediate host.
- Cercariae are released from the snail host and encyst (referred to as metacercariae) in the gills of crabs and crayfish, which are the second intermediate hosts.
- The infection is transmitted to humans by the ingestion of raw or undercooked crab or crayfish. The larval stages of the parasite are released, migrate within the body, and end up in the lungs. After 6 to 10 weeks, the larvae mature into adult flukes.
- *Paragonimus* eggs can be found in feces and sputum. Pulmonary paragonimiasis is often misdiagnosed as tuberculosis.
- Praziquantel is the drug of choice for treating infections with *P. westermani.*

23. A. Preserve stool in polyvinyl alcohol (PVA).
Rationale: PVA is a preservative that permits preparation of a permanent stain, which is highly recommended for parasite examination.
B. Refrigerate stool.
Rationale: Stool can be refrigerated for up to 3 hours after collection to examine for morphologic identification.
C. Preserve stool in sodium acetate–acetic acid formalin (SAF).
Rationale: The SAF fixative can be used to preserve stool integrity and permits preparation of a permanent stain for microscopic examination.
D. Examine stool immediately.
Rationale: If fresh stools are examined and stained immediately upon collection, preservatives are not needed.
E. Preserve stool in ethanol.
Rationale: Ethanol is used for DNA extraction and not for morphologic examination.

Major points of discussion

- Preservatives are used to ensure stool integrity from the time of collection to morphologic examination. These preservatives are purchased in kit format and commonly include one of the following: sodium acetate–acetic acid formalin (SAF), PVA, or merthiolate (thimerosal) iodine formalin (MIF).
- With the use of stool preservative kits, delivery time to the laboratory is then not a critical factor in terms of maintaining morphologic integrity of the parasites.
- The advantages of examining fresh stool include the ability to see motile trophozoite forms of intestinal protozoa. However, liquid stool should be examined within 30 minutes, soft stool within 1 hour, and formed stool within 24 hours of passage.
- The disadvantages of using formalin alone as a fixative include the inability to preserve the parasite morphology for a satisfactory, permanent, stained smear. In addition, 5% formalin can only be used to preserve protozoan cysts, whereas 10% formalin is reserved for helminth ova and larvae.
- It is recommended that at least three stool specimens be examined to rule out parasitic infection, one per day or one every other day.[7]

24. A. *Anaplasma phagocytophilum.*
Rationale: *A. phagocytophilum* is an intracellular bacterial species that infects granulocytes and appears as clusters of bacteria called morulae.
B. *Plasmodium vivax.*
Rationale: *P. vivax*–infected cells demonstrate delicate ring forms with stippling in the cytoplasm (Schüffner dots) and ameboid trophozoites, both of which can be seen in Figure 18-16.
C. *Plasmodium falciparum.*
Rationale: *P. falciparum* is characterized by RBCs infected with multiple ring forms or banana-shaped gametocytes. Other life cycle stages are not typically present.
D. *Ehrlichia chaffeensis.*
Rationale: *E. chaffeensis* is an intracellular bacterial species that infects mononuclear leukocytes and appears as clusters of bacteria called morulae.
E. *Babesia microti.*

Rationale: B. microti is a protozoan parasite characterized by RBCs infected with multiple ring forms (sometimes seen in a tetrad or Maltese cross form).

Major points of discussion

- *P. vivax* is a predominant cause of malaria in Asia. In the Philippines, *P. vivax* accounts for 30% of disease and the remainder is *P. falciparum*.
- *P. vivax* and *P. ovale* can demonstrate a dormant stage, referred to as hypnozoites, which persist in the liver. Relapses can occur years after the initial infection.
- *P. vivax* has a predilection for young red blood cells and infected cells are enlarged.
- Mature *P. vivax* schizonts have 12 to 24 merozoites.
- Because chloroquine resistance is common in the Philippines, therapeutic choices include atovaquone-proguanil, doxycycline, or mefloquine.
- *Ehrlichia*, *Anaplasma*, and *Babesia* are transmitted through the bites of infected ticks, whereas *Plasmodium* species are transmitted through the female *Anopheles* mosquito.[3]

25. A. *Clonorchis sinensis*.
Rationale: The egg of *C. sinensis,* or the liver fluke, is 20 to 35 μm in length, has a thick yellow-brown shell, and has an operculum with opercular shoulders.
B. *Schistosoma mansoni*.
Rationale: The egg of *S. mansoni* is 114 to 180 μm in length, has a thin yellow-brown shell, and has a large lateral spine projecting near one end.
C. *Fasciola hepatica*.
Rationale: The egg of *F. hepatica* is 130 to 150 μm in length, has a yellow-brown shell, and has an operculum but no operculum shoulders.
D. *Paragonimus westermani*.
Rationale: The egg of *P. westermani,* or the lung fluke, is 80 to 120 μm in length, has a thick brown-yellow shell, and has an operculum with opercular shoulders.
E. *Schistosoma japonicum*.
Rationale: The egg of *S. japonicum* is 55 to 85 μm in length, has a yellowish shell, and may have a small lateral spine at one end.

Major points of discussion

- The eggs of the three most common *Schistosoma* species can be differentiated based on size and the location of the spine: *S. mansoni* (114 to 180 μm long, large lateral spine), *S. haemotobium* (112 to 170 μm long, terminal spine), and *S. japonicum* (55 to 85 μm long, may or may not have small lateral spine).
- *S. mansoni* and *S. japonicum* eggs are found in feces, whereas *S. haemotobium* eggs are found in urine.
- All schistosomes that infect humans use freshwater aquatic snails as an intermediate host.
- Infective larvae (i.e., cercariae) in contaminated freshwater sources penetrate the skin and sometimes cause dermatitis (swimmer's itch).
- Praziquantel is the drug of choice for treating schistosomiasis.

26. **A. *Toxoplasma gondii*.**
Rationale: T. gondii is a protozoan parasite that is the most common cause of ring-enhancing central nervous system

lesions in HIV-infected patients. Serologic tests for immunoglobulin G antibodies help in the diagnosis of toxoplasmic encephalitis in immunosuppressed patients.
B. *Cryptosporidium parvum*.
Rationale: Immunosuppressed patients are at risk for contracting infections with *Cryptosporidium* species. The parasite is a partially acid-fast, intestinal protozoan. Antigen detection tests are diagnostic from stool specimens.
C. *Mycobacterium tuberculosis*.
Rationale: M. tuberculosis is an acid-fast pathogen. No serologic tests are currently available for diagnosis of extrapulmonary or pulmonary tuberculosis.
D. *Entamoeba histolytica*.
Rationale: Cerebral amebiasis is an extremely rare cause of brain abscess. It might be considered in patients with known amebiasis or secondary infection from hepatic or pulmonary involvement.
E. *Balamuthia mandrillaris*.
Rationale: B. mandrillaris is a free-living ameba that can cause amebic encephalitis. Neuroimaging tests show nonenhancing, space-occupying lesions.

Major points of discussion

- In addition to patients with HIV/AIDS, organ transplant recipients are also at high risk of developing toxoplasmosis. Most HIV/AIDS patients with toxoplasmic encephalitis test positive for pathogen-specific immunoglobulin G (IgG) antibodies in their serum.
- *T. gondii* is a protozoan parasite that is transmitted to humans through ingestion of oocysts from the feces of cats, the definitive host, or from consuming undercooked or raw meat.
- There are three stages in the life cycle of *T. gondii*: tachyzoites (i.e., trophozoites) that destroy infected cells during acute illness, bradyzoites that multiply in tissue cysts, and sporozoites in oocysts.
- Human transplacental infections can be fatal for the fetus, especially in the first trimester of pregnancy. Congenitally acquired toxoplasmosis can have serious sequelae, including cerebral calcifications and hydrocephalus in infected infants.
- Immunodiagnostic tests are critical in determining infection in pregnant women, patients with chorioretinitis, and immune-compromised hosts. Immunocompetent women who are seropositive for pathogen-specific IgG antibodies are considered immune; however, seronegative individuals are at risk for infection. To diagnose acute infection, IgM and IgG serodiagnostic tests should be performed.
- *T. gondii* infections are treated with pyrimethamine (with or without sulfadiazine) in pregnant women with acute infection, congenitally infected neonates, immunosuppressed individuals, and patients with acute or recurrent ocular disease.[2,3]

27. A. *Babesia microti*.
Rationale: B. microti is an infectious agent that is transmitted by blood transfusions in the United States. The continued increase in transfusion-associated babesiosis is due in part to the expansion of the endemic range of the parasite.
B. *Trypanosoma cruzi*.

Rationale: Chagas' disease can be transmitted by blood transfusions, particularly in endemic areas. *T. cruzi* parasites can be identified in the acute phase of infection.

C. *Toxoplasma gondii.*

Rationale: *T. gondii* can be contracted by transfusion of granulocytes, although transmission is rarely seen in the United States. There are no reports of transmission of toxoplasmosis by packed RBC transfusions.

D. *Plasmodium species.*

Rationale: Globally, malaria is the most common parasite transmitted by transfusion; however, this is rarely seen in the United States because of low prevalence and the strict exclusion criteria used when enrolling volunteer blood donors. Infections can be transmitted by transfusions of whole blood, RBCs, leukocytes, plasma, and platelets.

E. **Strongyloides stercoralis.**

Rationale: The larvae of *S. stercoralis* enter the cutaneous blood vessels and invade the lungs. Although they can cause serious infections in immune-compromised hosts, there have been no reports of transfusion-transmitted infections.

Major points of discussion

- U.S. blood collection centers are able to screen for *T. cruzi* (Chagas' disease). The blood center will attempt to notify the donor if results are positive.
- Potential blood donors who have been diagnosed with malaria cannot donate blood for 3 years after treatment, and they must be free of symptoms.
- The incidence of blood transfusion–transmitted parasitic infections is lower than that of bacterial and viral infections.
- Although transfusion-related Lyme disease has not been reported in the published literature, donors with a history of this disease must have undergone a full course of antibiotic treatment and must be asymptomatic before donating blood.
- A comprehensive donor history questionnaire is completed in an effort to capture those donors with travel history or risk factors that would indicate high risk for transmission of blood-borne pathogens.[9,10]

28. A. *Taenia saginata.*

Rationale: The tapeworm *T. saginata* is acquired through ingestion of poorly cooked infected beef and does not demonstrate an extraintestinal life cycle in humans.

B. *Wucheria bancrofti.*

Rationale: Infection with the filarial worm *W. bancrofti* is diagnosed by detecting microfilariae in blood.

C. **Trichinella spiralis.**

Rationale: Acquisition of the tissue nematode *T. spiralis* is associated with consumption of poorly cooked infected pork. Striated muscle is a common site to find encapsulated larvae.

D. *Trichomonas hominis.*

Rationale: The flagellate *T. hominis* does not have an extraintestinal life cycle.

E. *Trichuria trichuria.*

Rationale: The nematode *T. trichuria* does not have an extraintestinal life cycle.

Major points of discussion

- Trichinellosis is acquired by ingesting meat containing encysted *Trichinella* larvae. Gastric acid and pepsin lead

to release of the larvae, which then invade the small bowel mucosa, where they develop into adult worms. After 1 week, the females release larvae that migrate to the striated muscles, where they encyst.

- All stages of *T. spiralis* development (i.e., adult and larval stages) occur in a single host, and there is no egg stage.
- The sylvatic cycle, involving infected predator/scavenging animals, is most common in bear, moose, and wild boar. Hunters can acquire infection from ingesting undercooked game meat.
- The first few days of symptoms are gastrointestinal, but by 2 weeks, they include muscle pain, fever, and facial swelling (particularly periorbital edema).
- *Trichinella* antibodies can be detected by an enzyme immunoassay 3 to 5 weeks after infection.
- Prompt treatment with albendazole or mebendazole is recommended to kill the adult worms before they release larvae.

29. A. *Trichomonas hominis.*

Rationale: *T. hominis* is a nonpathogenic parasite that is present in the intestinal tract and not the urogenital system.

B. *Gardnerella vaginalis.*

Rationale: *G. vaginalis* is a bacterium and not a parasite. It is associated with bacterial vaginosis.

C. *Treponema pallidum.*

Rationale: *T. pallidum* is the causative agent of syphilis. It is a spiral-shaped bacterium, not a parasite.

D. *Mobiluncus species.*

Rationale: Members of the genus *Mobiluncus* are nonpathogenic, anaerobic bacteria that increase in number in women with bacterial vaginosis.

E. **Trichomonas vaginalis.**

Rationale: *T. vaginalis* is a flagellated parasite that causes vaginitis accompanied by frothy discharge with a fishy odor.

Major points of discussion

- *T. vaginalis* is a protozoan parasite with only a trophozoite stage. It is characterized by four to five flagella and an undulating membrane, which are responsible for its motility. It is transmitted sexually, and its presence in children is highly suggestive of sexual abuse.
- Trichomoniasis presents with an elevated vaginal pH, an amine odor, and frothy or milky discharge. In men, *T. vaginalis* is detected most commonly from urine and urethral specimens.
- Culture is the gold standard for diagnosis of trichomoniasis. Pouches with specific growth media are inoculated, incubated for 2 to 5 days, and flagellated. *T. vaginalis* are viewed microscopically. Wet mount preparations of vaginal discharge for observing the motile parasite are highly insensitive. Nucleic acid amplification tests are commercially available, have high sensitivity, and have a rapid turnaround time to results.
- Only about 5% of women with trichomoniasis present with "strawberry cervix" (i.e., colpitis macularis), but when seen, it is highly specific for this infection. This presentation results from microscopic, punctate petechiae on the cervix.
- Metronidazole or tinidazole are the treatments of choice for trichomoniasis.

30. A. *Naegleria fowleri.*

Rationale: The cyst of *N. fowleri,* a free-living ameba, has a smooth, thick double wall. The organism is associated with primary amebic meningoencephalitis, not keratitis.

B. Herpes simplex virus.

Rationale: Herpes simplex virus, the most common cause of viral keratitis, cannot be visualized by routine microscopy; it requires cell culture or direct staining with fluorescently labeled monoclonal antibodies.

C. *Adenovirus.*

Rationale: Adenovirus, the most common cause of viral conjunctivitis, cannot be visualized by routine microscopy. Adenovirus requires cell culture followed by staining with fluorescently labeled monoclonal antibodies.

D. *Acanthamoeba.*

Rationale: The cyst of *Acanthamoeba,* a free-living ameba, has a wrinkled double wall and is a well-characterized cause of keratitis and corneal ulceration.

E. *Balamuthia.*

Rationale: Although the cyst of *Balamuthia* looks similar to *Acanthamoeba*, this free-living ameba is associated with granulomatous amebic encephalitis, not keratitis.

Major points of discussion

- *Acanthamoeba* are ubiquitous in the environment and are most commonly associated with the following infections: keratitis (usually associated with improper disinfection of contact lenses), granulomatous amebic encephalitis in immunocompromised patients, and a disseminated infection that involves the skin and/or lungs.

- *Acanthamoeba* has two life cycle stages: trophozoites and cysts. Although both stages can gain entry into the body, trophozoites are the infective form.

- The *Acanthamoeba* trophozoite is large (15 to 25 μm), has no flagella, and produces filiform pseudopodia. In contrast, *N. fowleri* does have a flagellate stage of its life cycle.

- *Acanthamoeba* can be cultured on non-nutrient agar plates with Page's saline and an overlaid growth of *Escherichia coli*, which serves as a food source.

- Successful treatment of keratitis depends on early diagnosis and combination therapy, including propamidine, miconazole nitrate, and neomycin. Surgical intervention is often necessary.[1]

References

1. Bharathi MJ, Ramakrishnan R, Meenakshi R, et al. Microbiological diagnosis of infective keratitis: comparative evaluation of direct microscopy and culture results. Br J Ophthalmol 2006;90:1271–1276.
2. Calderaro A, Peruzzi S, Piccolo G, et al. Laboratory diagnosis of *Toxoplasma gondii* infection. Int J Med Sci 2009;6:135–136.
3. Centers for Disease Control, Prevention. Guidelines for prevention and treatment of opportunistic infections among HIV-exposed and infected children. MMWR Recomm Rep 2009;58 (RR-11):1–176.
4. Centers for Disease Control, Prevention. Malaria surveillance—United States 2010. MMWR Morb Mortal Wkly Rep 2012;61 (2):1–22.
5. Forbes BA, Sahm DF, Weissfeld AS, editors: *Bailey & Scott's Diagnostic Microbiology*, 12th ed. St. Louis: Elsevier: 2007.
6. Garcia HH, DelBrutto OH, Nash TE, et al. New concepts in the diagnosis and management of neurocysticercosis *(Taenia solium).* Am J Trop Med Hyg 2005;72:39.
7. Garcia LS. Diagnostic Medical Parasitology. 5th ed. Washington, DC: ASM Press: 2007.
8. Herwaldt BL, Linden JV, Bosserman E, et al. Transfusion-associated babesiosis in the United States: a description of cases. Ann Intern Med 2011;155:509–519.
9. Kaur P, Basu S. Transfusion-transmitted infections: existing and emerging pathogens. J Postgrad Med 2005;51:146–151.
10. Lux JZ, Weiss D, Linden JV, et al. Transfusion-associated babesiosis after heart transplant. Emerg Infect Dis 2003;9:116–119.
11. Patterson FC, Winn WC. Practical identification of hard ticks in the parasitology laboratory. Pathol Case Rev 2003;8:187–198.
12. Wormser G, Dattwyler RJ, Shapiro ED, et al. Clinical assessment, treatment, and prevention of Lyme disease, human granulocytic anaplasmosis, and babesiosis: clinical practice guidelines by the Infectious Diseases Society of America. Clin Infect Dis 2006; 43(9):1089–1134.

CHAPTER 19

TRANSFUSION MEDICINE: Blood Collection, Immunohematology, and Transfusion Services

Eldad A. Hod, Richard O. Francis, Suzanne A. Arinsburg, Jeffrey S. Jhang, Yvette C. Tanhehco, Joseph (Yossi) Schwartz, Steven L. Spitalnik

QUESTIONS

Blood Collection and Donor Issues

1. Blood components are currently tested for which one of the following infectious diseases?
   - A. Malaria.
   - B. Syphilis.
   - C. Babesia.
   - D. Dengue virus.
   - E. Chikungunya virus.

2. Which one of the following is the approximate current estimated residual risk of hepatitis B virus (HBV) transmission from blood transfusion?
   - A. 1:8,000 to 1:10,000.
   - B. 1:80,000 to 1:100,000.
   - C. 1:800,000 to 1:1,000,000.
   - D. 1:8,000,000 to 1,000,000,000.
   - E. HBV has not been transmitted by blood transfusion in the past 10 years.

3. Which one of the following is true regarding the manufacturing of cryoprecipitate from fresh frozen plasma (FFP)?
   - A. FFP is thawed and centrifuged at 20°C to 24°C and the precipitate is frozen at –18°C within 1 hour of preparation.
   - B. FFP is thawed and centrifuged at 20°C to 24°C and the precipitate is frozen at –1°C to 6°C within 1 hour of preparation.
   - C. FFP is thawed and centrifuged at 1°C to 6°C and the precipitate is frozen at –18°C within 1 hour of preparation.
   - D. FFP is thawed and centrifuged at 1° to 6°C and the precipitate is frozen at –18°C within 2 hours of preparation.
   - E. FFP is thawed and centrifuged at 20°C to 24°C and the precipitate is frozen at –18°C within 2 hours of preparation.

4. Which one of the following patients should receive irradiated red blood cells (RBCs)?
   - A. A 35-year-old male patient with human immunodeficiency virus (HIV).
   - B. A 22-year-old man with hemophilia and a joint bleed.
   - C. A 50-year-old woman with metastatic breast cancer.
   - D. A 45-year-old female patient after a bone marrow transplant.
   - E. An 8-year-old girl after a motor vehicle accident.

5. Which one of the following is the mechanism by which irradiation of blood components prevents transfusion-associated graft-versus-host disease?
   - A. Inactivation of B-lymphocytes.
   - B. Inactivation of T-lymphocytes.
   - C. Inactivation of plasma cells.
   - D. Inactivation of granulocytes.
   - E. Inactivation of macrophages.

6. Which one of the following is true regarding blood component labeling?
   - A. Labeling can occur at any time during the manufacturing process.
   - B. Labeling should occur before all manufacturing steps.
   - C. Labeling should occur before a product is placed on hold.
   - D. Labeling should occur after all infectious disease testing is completed.
   - E. Labeling should occur after all blood component modifications (i.e., irradiation, leukoreduction) are completed.

7. Which one of the following is the most common cause of filter failure during leukoreduction?
   - A. Hereditary elliptocytosis.
   - B. Sickle cell trait.
   - C. Thalassemia.
   - D. Hereditary spherocytosis.
   - E. Glucose-6-phosphate dehydrogenase deficiency.

8. Which one of the following is the U.S. Food and Drug Administration (FDA)-approved shelf-life of RBCs stored in citrate-phosphate-dextrose-adenine-one (CPDA-1) and additive solution-3 (AS-3)?
   - A. 21 days.
   - B. 35 days.
   - C. 42 days.
   - D. 56 days.
   - E. 112 days.

9. Which one of the following is correct regarding the rejuvenation of RBCs?

A. RBCs collected in citrate-phosphate-dextrose (CPD) may be rejuvenated up to 3 days after expiration and then frozen for up to 10 years.

B. RBCs collected in AS-1 may be rejuvenated up to 3 days after expiration and then frozen for up to 3 years.

C. RBCs collected in CPD may be rejuvenated up to 42 days after collection and then frozen for up to 3 years.

D. RBCs collected in AS-1 may be rejuvenated up to 42 days after collection and then frozen up to 10 years.

E. RBCs collected in CPD or AS-1 may be rejuvenated at any time up to their expiration date and then frozen up to 10 years.

10. The nurse calls to inform you that a 22-year-old male patient with acute lymphoblastic leukemia has a hemoglobin of 6 g/dL (reference range, 13.3 to 16.2 g/dL). You decide to order 2 U RBCs. Which one of the following RBC unit modifications should be specified in your order to ensure that the patient receives the appropriate blood?

A. Leukoreduced.

B. Leukoreduced and irradiated.

C. Leukoreduced, irradiated, and washed.

D. Leukoreduced, irradiated, washed, and hemoglobin S–negative.

E. This patient can receive unmodified random donor RBCs.

11. Which one of the following is correct regarding prestorage leukoreduction?

A. Leukoreduction increases the risk of human leukocyte antigen (HLA) alloimmunization.

B. Leukoreduction increases the incidence of febrile nonhemolytic transfusion reactions.

C. Leukoreduction prevents transfusion-associated graft-versus-host disease.

D. Leukoreduction reduces the risk of cytomegalovirus (CMV) transmission.

E. Leukoreduction prevents transfusion-related acute lung injury.

12. Which one of the following patients is the best candidate for intraoperative blood recovery?

A. A 40-year-old man undergoing hip replacement for a hip fracture after a motor vehicle accident.

B. A 38-year-old woman undergoing laparotomy for lysis of adhesions secondary to metastatic colon cancer.

C. A 65-year-old man undergoing colectomy for bowel rupture.

D. A 75-year-old woman undergoing coronary artery bypass grafting.

E. A 34-year-old pregnant woman with placenta previa.

13. Which one of the following is true regarding granulocyte transfusions?

A. Granulocytes are effective only at yields greater than 5×10^6 cells/kg.

B. Granulocyte yields are greatest after donor stimulation with corticosteroids.

C. Granulocytes should always be leukoreduced.

D. Granulocytes should never be irradiated.

E. Granuloctyes should be transfused within 24 hours of collection.

14. During a whole blood donation by a 25-year-old woman, 350 mL of blood is collected. Which one of the following statements about the unit is true?

A. The unit must be discarded because of an insufficient volume collected.

B. The amount of anticoagulant in the collection bag *must* be adjusted.

C. No additional labeling or processing steps other than standard procedures are required.

D. The RBCs from the unit can be used for transfusion, but plasma and platelet components may not.

E. The unit may be used only for research purposes.

15. An 18-year-old male arrives at a mobile blood drive reporting that he would like to donate blood but that he received the hepatitis B vaccine yesterday. Which one of the following is the deferral period for this prospective donor given his history of recent vaccination and his report that he feels well today?

A. 2 weeks.

B. 4 weeks.

C. 21 days.

D. 12 months.

E. None.

16. A 36-year-old man presents to a blood drive at his workplace for a whole blood donation. During the evaluation he reveals that approximately 2 weeks ago he spent approximately 24 hours in jail for public drunkenness. Which one of the following is the deferral period for this prospective donor?

A. None.

B. 4 months.

C. 12 months.

D. 3 years.

E. Permanent.

17. A 58-year-old woman presents for whole blood donation. She reports that she completed a course of warfarin anticoagulation for pulmonary embolism approximately 4 days ago. Which one of the following is the correct deferral period from the time of her last warfarin dose?

A. 7 days.

B. 14 days.

C. 1 month.

D. 6 months.

E. Permanently.

18. A unit of RBCs was issued to the intensive care unit and returned unused to the blood bank. At which one of the following temperature ranges should the component have been maintained for it to be suitable for reissue?

A. 1°C to 10°C.

B. 1°C to 6°C.

C. 20°C to 24°C.

D. –18°C or less.

E. 30°C to 37°C.

19. A 54-year-old woman presents to her local blood donation site for autologous donation for an upcoming hip replacement surgery. How many days before the anticipated surgery date (date of expected transfusion) must the collections be completed?

A. 2 days.

B. 3 days.

C. 28 days.

D. 56 days.

E. 112 days.

Blood Bank Regulations

20. A sample for pretransfusion testing is received by the transfusion service for a 48-year-old woman scheduled to undergo laparoscopic cholecystectomy in 1 week. Which of the

following comments on the requisition form can extend the expiration time of the type and screen?

A. "No history of transfusion or pregnancy in the past 90 days."
B. "Patient has a history of a negative antibody screen."
C. "No history of transfusion or pregnancy in the past 30 days."
D. "Pregnancy and transfusion history unknown."
E. "Patient is older than 40 years of age."

21. A type and screen sample was received by your transfusion service and discarded because it was improperly labeled. Which one of the following samples is properly labeled for pretransfusion testing?

A. A sample labeled at the nursing station with a label containing the patient's full name, hospital identification number, date of collection, and the phlebotomist's initials.
B. A sample labeled at the patient's bedside with a label containing the patient's full name, hospital identification number, date of collection, and the phlebotomist's initials.
C. A sample labeled at the patient's bedside with a label containing the hospital identification number, patient diagnosis, phlebotomist's initials, and date of collection.
D. A sample labeled at the patient's bedside with a label containing the patient's full name, hospital identification number, patient's location, and the date of collection.
E. A sample labeled at the patient's bedside with a label containing the patient's full name, hospital identification number, the phlebotomist's initials, and patient's date of birth.

22. The pretransfusion testing has been completed for a patient for whom 2 U RBCs have been ordered. In which one of the following situations is it acceptable to use a computer (i.e., electronic) crossmatch for release of these units instead of an immediate-spin (IS) or anti-human globulin (AHG) crossmatch?

A. The patient has a history of an anti-K antibody, which is currently not detected, and no new clinically significant antibodies.
B. A warm autoantibody of unknown clinical significance is currently detected and underlying alloantibodies have been ruled out.
C. The patient has no history of alloantibodies or autoantibodies and the antibody screen is currently negative.
D. The patient has a newly positive antibody screen and the antibody has been identified as anti-RhD due to passive transfer from Rh immune globulin.
E. The patient has no history of clinically significant antibodies and currently an anti-E antibody has been identified.

23. A shipment of RBC units has arrived at your transfusion service. Which one of the following confirmatory tests must be performed before these units can be made available for transfusion?

A. Confirmatory Rh typing of Rh-positive units.
B. Confirmatory ABO typing of only group O RBC components.
C. Confirmatory testing for weak D.
D. Direct antiglobulin testing.
E. Confirmatory ABO typing of all RBC components.

24. Which one of the following is a benefit of International Society of Blood Transfusion (ISBT) 128 standard labeling?

A. Increased ability to transfer blood components between different facilities.
B. Faster processing of different blood components.
C. Uniformity of labeling allowing better traceability of blood components.
D. Improved use of autologous or directed donations.
E. Allows for use of a computerized crossmatch for all transfusions.

25. While on your blood bank rotation, you observe that all blood products are visually inspected before release. Which one of the following types of activities is this considered to be?

A. Quality assurance.
B. Quality control.
C. Quality management.
D. Quality indicator.
E. Quality improvement.

26. Ten units of cryoprecipitate were thawed but not pooled for a patient who is suspected of having disseminated intravascular coagulation (DIC). Which one of the following are the correct storage temperature and expiration of these thawed units?

A. 20°C to 24°C, 6 hours.
B. 20°C to 24°C, 4 hours.
C. 30°C to 37°C, 30 minutes.
D. 1°C to 6°C, 24 hours.
E. 1°C to 6°C, 5 days.

Immunohematology

27. A type and screen is performed on a sample received from a 45-year-old male patient. The results of the type and screen and initial red cell antibody panel are shown in Tables 19-1 through 19-3. Pretreatment of selected panel red cells with ficin, trypsin, or dithiothreitol (DTT) does not change the reactivity pattern shown in the red cell antibody panel and testing of the patient's red cells with *Ulex europaeus* lectin is negative (no agglutination). These findings are consistent with the presence of which one of the following antibodies?

A. Anti-k.
B. Warm autoantibody.
C. Anti-H.
D. Anti-Fy3.
E. Anti-Kp^b.

Table 19-1

Front Type		Back Type		RhD Typing
Anti-A	Anti-B	A1 cells	B cells	Anti-D
0	0	4+	4+	4+

Table 19-2 Antibody Screen

	Immediate Spin	37°C	AHG
Screening cell I	4+	4+	4+
Screening cell II	4+	4+	4+

Table 19-3

Panel Cell	D	C	c	E	e	K	k	Kp^a	Kp^b	Js^a	Js^b	Jk^a	Jk^b	Fy^a	Fy^b	M	N	S	s	AHG	Check Cells
											Antibody Panel									Test Method	
1	+	+	−	−	+	+	+	0	+	0	+	0	+	+	+	+	+	+	+	4+	
2	+	+	−	−	+	0	+	0	+	0	+	+	+	0	+	+	0	+	+	4+	
3	+	0	+	+	0	0	+	0	+	0	+	+	+	+	+	+	0	0	+	4+	
4	+	0	+	0	+	0	+	0	+	0	+	+	+	0	0	+	+	0	0	4+	
5	0	+	+	0	+	0	+	0	+	0	+	0	+	0	+	+	+	0	+	4+	
6	0	0	+	+	+	+	+	0	+	0	+	0	+	+	0	+	0	+	+	4+	
7	0	0	+	0	+	0	+	0	+	0	+	+	+	0	+	0	+	0	+	4+	
8	0	0	+	0	+	0	+	0	+	0	+	+	0	+	0	+	+	+	+	4+	
9	0	0	+	0	+	+	+	0	+	0	+	+	0	+	0	0	+	0	+	4+	
10	0	0	+	0	+	0	+	0	+	0	+	0	+	+	0	0	+	+	+	4+	
11	+	0	+	0	+	0	+	0	+	0	+	+	+	0	0	+	+	+	0	4+	
Patient's cells																				0	2+

28. Which one of the following is the probability that a random donor unit will be compatible with a patient with the results of the red cell antibody panel and selected cell panel shown in Tables 19-4 and 19-5?

A. 2%.
B. 23%.
C. 50%.
D. 85%.
E. 91%.

Table 19-4

Panel Cell	D	C	c	E	e	K	k	Kp^a	Kp^b	Js^a	Js^b	Jk^a	Jk^b	Fy^a	Fy^b	M	N	S	s	AHG	Ficin	Check cells
1	+	+	0	0	+	+	+	0	+	0	+	0	+	+	+	+	+	+	+	3+	4+	
2	+	+	0	0	+	0	+	0	+	0	+	+	+	0	+	+	0	+	+	1+	3+	
3	+	0	+	+	0	0	+	0	+	0	+	+	0	+	+	+	0	0	+	0	0	2+
4	+	0	+	0	+	0	+	0	+	0	+	+	+	0	0	+	+	0	0	1+	3+	
5	0	+	+	0	+	0	+	0	+	0	+	+	0	+	0	+	+	+	0	+	2+	4+
6	0	0	+	+	+	+	+	0	+	0	+	+	0	+	+	0	+	0	+	+	3+	4+
7	0	0	+	0	+	0	+	0	+	0	+	+	+	0	0	+	0	+	0	0	0	2+
8	0	0	+	0	+	0	+	0	+	0	+	+	0	+	0	+	+	+	+	0	0	2+
9	0	0	+	0	+	+	+	0	+	0	+	+	0	+	0	0	+	0	+	1+	1+	
10	0	0	+	0	+	0	+	0	+	0	+	0	+	+	0	0	+	+	+	2+	4+	
11	+	0	+	0	+	0	+	0	+	0	+	+	+	0	0	+	+	+	0	1+	3+	
Patient's cells																				0		2+

Table 19-5

Panel Cell	D	C	c	E	e	K	k	Kp^a	Kp^b	Js^a	Js^b	Jk^a	Jk^b	Fy^a	Fy^b	M	N	S	s	AHG	Ficin
1	+	+	0	0	+	0	+	0	+	0	+	+	0	0	+	0	+	0	+	0	2+
2	+	+	0	0	+	0	+	+	+	0	+	+	0	0	+	+	0	+	0	0	2+
3	+	0	+	+	0	0	+	0	+	0	+	+	0	+	+	+	0	0	+	0	2+
4	+	0	+	0	+	0	+	0	+	0	+	+	+	0	0	+	+	0	0		
5	0	+	+	0	+	0	+	0	+	0	+	+	+	0	+	0	+	0	+		
6	0	0	+	+	+	0	+	0	+	0	+	+	0	+	+	+	+	+	+	0	2+
7	0	0	+	0	+	+	+	0	+	0	+	+	+	0	+	+	+	0	+		
8	0	0	+	0	+	0	+	0	+	0	+	+	+	+	0	0	+	0	+		
9	+	0	+	+	+	+	+	0	+	0	+	+	0	0	+	+	+	+	+	1+	
10	+	0	+	+	0	0	+	0	+	0	+	0	+	0	+	+	+	0	+		
11	+	+	0	0	+	0	+	0	+	0	+	+	0	+	0	+	+	0	+	0	2+
12	0	0	+	0	+	+	+	0	+	0	+	0	+	+	0	+	0	+	0		
13	0	0	+	0	+	0	+	0	+	+	+	+	0	0	0	+	0	+		0	2+
14	0	0	+	0	+	0	+	0	+	0	+	0	+	0	+	+	+	0	+		
15	0	0	+	0	+	0	+	0	+	+	+	+	+	+	0	+	+	0	+		
16	0	0	+	0	+	0	+	0	+	0	+	0	+	+	+	+	+	+	+		

29. A 36-year-old woman in the second trimester of pregnancy is admitted to labor and delivery for abdominal pain. The patient has the blood typing results shown in Table 19-6. The red cell antibody screen is positive, and an antibody against the D antigen is identified in the patient's plasma. Assuming no Rh-immunoglobulins have been administered to this patient, which one of the following is the best explanation for these results?
    A. Rh positive with an anti-D autoantibody.
    B. Partial D phenotype with an anti-D autoantibody.
    C. Rh positive with an anti-D alloantibody.
    D. Partial D phenotype with an anti-D alloantibody.
    E. Weak D phenotype with an anti-D alloantibody.

Table 19-6

	Forward Typing			Reverse Type	
Anti-A	Anti-B	Anti-D	Anti-D+AHG	A1 cells	B cells
0	4+	0	2+	4+	0

30. A 32-year-old woman is admitted to the intensive care unit with severe burns after a motor vehicle accident. She types as blood group B. She has DIC and has been requiring multiple units of plasma and platelets. The blood bank has an insufficient supply of group B plasma and platelets. Which one of the following will be compatible for this patient?
    A. Group O plasma and group B platelets.
    B. Group A plasma and group AB platelets.
    C. Group AB plasma and group A platelets.
    D. Group O plasma and group A platelets.
    E. Group A plasma and group B platelets.

31. A 46-year-old woman has seven biological children, and she reports that there is only one father for all seven children. Two of the offspring are group O, two are group A, two are group B, and one is group AB. Which one of the following choices show the possible phenotypes of the mother and father, respectively?
    A. AB and A.
    B. AB and B.
    C. AB and AB.
    D. A and B.
    E. None; nonpaternity.

32. A 58-year-old man has a history of pneumonia due to *Mycoplasma* infection. Following treatment, the patient's hemoglobin decreases from 15.2 g/dL (reference range, 13.3 to 16.2 g/dL) to 8.1 g/dL. The type and screen shows a cold reacting antibody. This antibody is most likely against which one of the following antigens?
    A. I.
    B. i.
    C. P.
    D. Le^a.
    E. A.

33. Serologic testing of a patient's red cells showed an Fy(a–b–) Duffy antigen phenotype. Which one of the following is the most likely race/ethnicity of this patient?
    A. White.
    B. Black.
    C. Asian/Pacific Islander.
    D. Native American.
    E. Inuit.

34. A patient's antibody screen is positive and an antibody panel is performed. Six of 10 panel cells are reactive when tested using polyethylene glycol (PEG) and the indirect antiglobulin test (IAT). A ficin-treated panel is tested, resulting in no reactivity in all red cells tested. These findings are most consistent with antibodies to which of the following red cell antigens?
    A. Rh.
    B. Kell.
    C. Duffy.
    D. Lewis.
    E. Kidd.

35. A 26-year-old pregnant woman in the third trimester carrying a fetus with hemolytic disease of the fetus and newborn is admitted to the hospital for an intrauterine transfusion. Which one of the following antibodies would be the most likely cause of the hemolytic disease?
    A. P1.
    B. i.
    C. I.
    D. S.
    E. Le^a.

36. Kell antigens are destroyed by sulfhydryl reagents such as dithiothreitol (DTT; ZZAP) and mercaptoethanol (ME). This suggests that which one of the following elements of the Kell antigen structure is very important for its stability?
    A. Cysteine residues.
    B. N- and/or O-glycans.
    C. Zinc binding site.
    D. Kx antigen.
    E. Dombrock antigen.

37. Which one of the following Lewis phenotypes can produce anti-Le^a antibodies?
    A. Le(a+b–).
    B. Le(a+b+).
    C. Le(a–b+).
    D. Le(a–b–).

38. Antibodies against which one of the following antigens of the MNSs blood group system are generally considered clinically insignificant and ignored for transfusion purposes?
    A. En^a.
    B. M.
    C. S.
    D. s.
    E. U.

39. Which one of the following is the highest incidence antigen in the Rh blood group system?
    A. D.
    B. C.
    C. c.
    D. E.
    E. e.

40. What is the modified Wiener terminology for someone with the Fisher-Race genotype Dce/dce?
    A. R_1/r.
    B. R_2/r.
    C. R_1/r'.
    D. R_z/r'.
    E. R_0/r.

41. What is the risk of giving leukoreduced RhD-positive RBCs to an RhD-negative patient with a negative red cell antibody screen who is not a female of reproductive age?
    A. Acute intravascular hemolysis.
    B. Increased risk of a febrile transfusion reaction.
    C. Inability to receive future RBC transfusions.
    D. Anaphylactic reaction due to naturally occurring IgE antibodies to the RhD antigen.
    E. Potential alloimmunization to RhD.

42. Which one of the following antigens is part of a blood group collection rather than a blood group system?
    A. Diego.
    B. Cartwright.
    C. Colton.
    D. Dombrock.
    E. Cost.

43. A 44-year-old male patient with thalassemia major and hepatitis C is found to have a positive direct antiglobulin test (DAT) on pretransfusion testing. He receives 2 U RBCs every 3 weeks. His hemoglobin and hematocrit are as expected based on previous pretransfusion labs. No reaction is seen on the red cell antibody screen or the eluate. Which one of the following is the most likely significance of the positive DAT in this patient?
    A. Delayed serologic transfusion reaction.
    B. Delayed hemolytic transfusion reaction.
    C. Drug-induced hemolytic anemia.
    D. Nonspecific uptake of immunoglobulin.
    E. Laboratory analytical error.

44. Which one of the following is characteristic of naturally occurring antibodies?
    A. Usually are antibodies of the IgG subtype.
    B. React optimally at 37°C.
    C. Require antihuman globulin for agglutination.
    D. Do not readily fix complement and are associated with extravascular hemolysis.
    E. Do not cross the placenta.

45. A 72-year-old man is admitted for a fracture of the right radius. His hemoglobin is found to be 6.2 g/dL (reference range, 13.2 to 16.2 g/dL). A transfusion is ordered and the blood bank type and screen results are as shown in Table 19-7. A peripheral blood smear is provided in Figure 19-1. Which one of the following tests can resolve the ABO discrepancy?
    A. Saline replacement technique.
    B. Chloroquine treatment of red cells.
    C. Addition of rabbit erythrocyte stroma.
    D. Prewarm all reagents to 37°C.
    E. Cold autoadsorption.

Table 19-7

Front Type		Back Type		RhD Typing
Anti-A	Anti-B	A1 cells	B cells	Anti-D
4+	0	2+	4+	2+

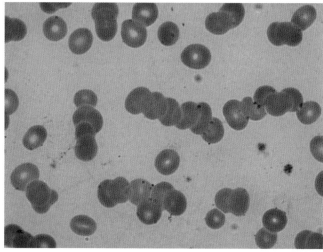

Figure 19-1 Stacked RBCs on a peripheral blood smear from a patient with an ABO discrepancy.

The blood bank received an order for a RBC transfusion for a 72-year-old patient with a hemoglobin of 6.0 g/dL, coronary artery disease, chest pain, shortness of breath, and tachycardia and a positive antibody screen with the red cell antibody panel shown in Table 19-8. Use this scenario to answer the following two questions.

Table 19-8

Panel Cell	D	C	c	E	e	K	k	Kp^a	Kp^b	Js^a	Js^b	Jk^a	Jk^b	Fy^a	Fy^b	M	N	S	s	AHG	Eluate
																				Test Method	
1	+	+	−	−	+	+	+	0	+	0	+	0	+	+	+	+	+	+	+	4+	4+
2	+	+	−	−	+	0	+	0	+	0	+	+	+	0	+	+	0	+	+	4+	4+
3	+	0	+	+	0	0	+	0	+	0	+	+	+	+	+	+	0	0	+	4+	4+
4	+	0	+	0	+	0	+	0	+	0	+	+	+	0	0	+	+	0	0	4+	4+
5	0	+	+	0	+	0	+	0	+	0	+	0	+	0	+	+	+	0	+	4+	4+
6	0	0	+	+	+	+	+	0	+	0	+	0	+	+	0	+	0	+	+	4+	4+
7	0	0	+	0	+	0	+	0	+	0	+	+	+	0	+	0	+	0	+	4+	4+
8	0	0	+	0	+	0	+	0	+	0	+	+	0	+	0	+	+	+	+	4+	4+
9	0	0	+	0	+	+	+	0	+	0	+	+	0	+	0	0	+	0	+	4+	4+
10	0	0	+	0	+	0	+	0	+	0	+	0	+	+	0	0	+	+	+	4+	4+
11	+	0	+	0	+	0	+	0	+	0	+	+	+	0	0	+	+	+	0	4+	4+
Patient's cells																				4+	

46a. Which one of the following antibodies is present in the plasma of this patient and fully explains the results of the red cell antibody panel testing shown in Table 19-8?

A. Warm autoantibody.

B. Anti-D alloantibody.

C. Multiple alloantibodies to the following antigens: C, E, K, Fy^a, S.

D. Alloantibody to a high-prevalence antigen.

E. Alloantibody to a low-prevalence antigen.

46b. After further testing, the blood bank sends up a unit of packed RBCs and the physician taking care of the patient returns the unit because the unit was incompatible on full crossmatch. Which one of the following is the most appropriate response?

A. This is a laboratory error; the blood bank will initiate an investigation and reissue a crossmatch-compatible unit.

B. This is the correct RBC unit, but rituximab should be administered first to prevent a hemolytic transfusion reaction.

C. A full crossmatch should not have been performed; the blood bank will release an electronically crossmatch-compatible red cell unit.

D. The transfusion should be delayed until crossmatch-compatible antigen-negative units are identified.

E. Crossmatch-incompatible RBCs are the only option and the transfusion should not be delayed.

47. A type and screen is performed on a sample received from a currently stable 65-year-old female patient with history of transfusion. The results of the type and screen are shown in Tables 19-9 and 19-10. Which one of the following is the next step in the workup of this patient?

A. Direct antiglobulin test.

B. Antibody panel.

C. Eluate.

D. Nothing; the antibody screen is negative.

E. Repeat the antibody screen.

Table 19-9

	D	C	c	E	e	K	k	Jk^a	Jk^b	Fy^a	Fy^b	M	N	S	s	Le^a	Le^b	Anti-human Globulin	Check Cells
					Antibody Screen													Test Method	
Cell I	+	+	0	0	+	+	+	+	0	+	0	0	+	0	+	+	0	0	0
Cell II	+	0	+	+	0	0	+	0	+	+	+	+	+	+	+	0	+	0	0

Table 19-10

Front Type		Back Type		RhD Typing
Anti-A	Anti-B	A1 cells	B cells	Anti-D
0	0	4+	4+	4+

Table 19-11

	D	C	c	E	e	K	k	Jk^a	Jk^b	Fy^a	Fy^b	M	N	S	s	Le^a	Le^b	Anti-human Globulin	Check Cells
																		Antibody Screen	**Test Method**
Cell I	+	+	0	0	+	+	+	+	0	+	0	0	+	0	+	+	0	0	2+
Cell II	+	0	+	+	0	0	+	0	+	+	+	+	+	+	+	0	+	0	2+

Table 19-12

Front Type		Back Type		RhD Typing
Anti-A	Anti-B	A1 cells	B cells	Anti-D
4+	4+	0	0	2+

48. A 72-year-old female patient undergoing hip surgery has the type and screen results shown in Tables 19-11 and 19-12. Previous typing is consistent with these results and she has no history of a positive antibody screen. Two units of RBCs are ordered before the start of surgery in case the surgeon encounters significant bleeding. Assuming all crossmatching methods are technically possible at this hospital, which of the following would be the most appropriate and efficient crossmatch to perform before release of the units?
   A. No crossmatch is necessary; any two units may be released.
   B. Electronic crossmatch.
   C. Immediate spin crossmatch.
   D. Full AHG crossmatch in tube.
   E. Full AHG crossmatch in solid phase.

49. What is the significance of a positive DAT?
   A. The patient is experiencing a delayed hemolytic transfusion reaction.
   B. The patient is hemolyzing red cells.
   C. The patient has an autoantibody.
   D. The patient has antibody or complement bound to circulating red cells.
   E. The patient has an alloantibody to a red cell antigen.

Table 19-13

	Direct Antiglobulin Test	
	Test	Check Cells
Anti-IgG	0	2+
Anti-C3b	4+	

50. A previously healthy 5-year-old boy manifests hemoglobinuria 4 days after a measles/mumps/rubella (MMR) vaccine. The results of a DAT are shown in Table 19-13. An eluate performed is nonreactive. Further testing is performed, and the patient's serum causes hemolysis in tubes first incubated in ice and then at 37°C but not in tubes maintained at 37°C or 4°C throughout. These findings are consistent with which one of the following conditions?
   A. Paroxysmal cold hemoglobinuria.
   B. Paroxysmal nocturnal hemoglobinuria.
   C. Delayed hemolytic transfusion reaction.
   D. Warm autoimmune hemolytic anemia.
   E. Cold autoimmune hemolytic anemia.

51. Which one of the following factors promotes agglutination in the identification of an anti-D alloantibody?
   A. Temperature less than 30°C.
   B. Low pH (pH 2).
   C. Decreasing incubation time.
   D. Lowering the salt concentration.
   E. Decreasing the serum/red cell ratio.

52. A 54-year-old man is going to the operating room for a liver transplant. Per your hospital protocol, the blood bank crossmatches 20 packed red cell units in preparation for the case. The patient has a history of prior alloimmunization with an antibody to the E antigen of the Rh blood group system on current and previous testing. On crossmatching 20 E antigen–negative units, 1 U is found to be incompatible. Repeat testing of this unit confirms that it is E antigen negative and that it is indeed crossmatch incompatible. Which one of the following is the most appropriate explanation for this finding, and what should be done with this unit?
   A. This is likely a nonspecific finding due to the patient's liver disease. This unit may be used for this patient in the operating room.
   B. In addition to the anti-E antibody, the patient has an antibody to a low-prevalence antigen. The incompatible unit can be reissued to another patient, and another unit should be crossmatched for this patient.
   C. The patient does not have an anti-E antibody and a repeat antibody screen and full red cell phenotype should be performed. Surgery should be delayed until the nature of the patient's antibody is resolved.
   D. In addition to the anti-E antibody, the patient has a warm autoantibody. Because this is an autoantibody, the incompatible unit may be transfused in this patient.
   E. In addition to the anti-E antibody, the patient has an antibody to a high-prevalence antigen. The incompatible unit should be discarded from inventory because it contains a high-prevalence antigen.

53. A 1-day-old infant born at 39 weeks to a 29-year-old woman G2P1 is noted to have yellow sclera. Laboratory tests on the cord blood reveal that the infant is type A Rh positive, direct antiglobulin test positive, and has a hemoglobin of 6 g/dL (reference range, 14.7 to 18.6 g/dL). The mother is type O Rh positive and the red cell antibody screen is negative. Hemolytic disease of the fetus and newborn (HDFN) is suspected. Which one of the following maternal antibodies is most likely cause of the anemia and jaundice in this infant?

A. Anti-D.
B. Anti-K.
C. Anti-c.
D. Anti-A.
E. Anti-A,B.

54. A 45-year-old female patient presented to the emergency department 6 days ago with upper gastrointestinal bleeding that necessitated the transfusion of 2 U crossmatch-compatible blood. Her pretransfusion red cell alloantibody screen was negative. Her hemoglobin is dropping. A new red cell alloantibody screen is positive and an anti-Fy^a antibody is identified. The attending physician is not sure if bleeding or hemolysis is causing the drop in hemoglobin. Which one of the following sets of laboratory tests should be ordered for this patient?
A. Complete blood cell count, direct and indirect bilirubin, and haptoglobin.
B. Complete blood cell count, direct and indirect bilirubin, haptoglobin, and lactate dehydrogenase.
C. Complete blood cell, direct and indirect bilirubin, haptoglobin, lactate dehydrogenase, direct antiglobulin test, and urinalysis.
D. Complete blood cell count, direct and indirect bilirubin, haptoglobin, lactate dehydrogenase, direct antiglobulin test, urinalysis, and ionized calcium.
E. Complete blood cell count, direct and indirect bilirubin, haptoglobin, lactate dehydrogenase, direct antiglobulin test, urinalysis, and potassium.

55. The Kleihauer-Betke test is used to quantitate the extent of fetal maternal hemorrhage. Which one of the following is the basis of this test?
A. Fetal hemoglobin is more resistant to hypotonic saline.
B. Fetal hemoglobin forms rosettes around Rh-positive cells.
C. Fetal hemoglobin is less soluble than hemoglobin A.
D. Fetal hemoglobin is resistant to acid treatment.
E. Fetal hemoglobin is less dense than hemoglobin A.

56. The patient with blood bank testing results shown in Tables 19-14 through Tables 19-16 has an antibody to which one of the following blood group antigen systems?
A. Rh.
B. Kell.
C. Kidd.
D. Duffy.
E. MNS.

Table 19-14

						Antibody Screen												Test Method	
	D	C	c	E	e	K	k	Jk^a	Jk^b	Fy^a	Fy^b	M	N	S	s	Le^a	Le^b	Anti-human Globulin	Check Cells
Cell I	+	+	0	0	+	+	+	+	0	+	0	0	+	0	+	+	0	2+	
Cell II	+	0	+	+	0	0	+	0	+	0	+	+	0	+	0	0	+	0	2+

Table 19-15

							Antibody Panel												Test Method		
Panel Cell	D	C	c	E	e	K	k	Js^a	Js^b	Jk^a	Jk^b	Fy^a	Fy^b	M	N	S	s	PEG-AHG	Ficin	Check Cells
1	+	+	0	0	+	+	+	0	+	0	+	+	+	0	+	+	+	0	0	2+
2	+	+	0	0	+	0	+	0	+	(+)	+	0	+	+	0	+	+	1+	2+	
3	+	0	+	+	0	0	+	0	+	(+)	+	+	+	0	0	0	+	1+	2+	
4	+	0	+	0	+	0	+	0	+	(+)	+	0	0	+	+	0	0	1+	2+	
5	0	+	+	0	+	0	+	0	+	0	+	0	+	+	+	0	+	0	0	2+
6	0	0	+	+	+	+	+	0	+	0	+	+	0	+	0	+	0	0	0	2+
7	0	0	+	0	+	0	+	0	+	(+)	+	0	+	0	+	0	+	1+	2+	
8	0	0	+	0	+	0	+	0	+	(+)	0	+	0	+	0	+	0	2+	3+	
9	0	0	+	0	+	+	+	0	+	(+)	0	+	0	0	+	0	+	2+	3+	
10	0	0	+	0	+	0	+	0	+	0	+	+	0	0	+	0	+	0	0	2+
11	+	0	+	0	+	0	+	0	+	0	+	0	0	+	+	+	0	0	0	2+
Patient's cells																		0		2+

Table 19-16

Front Type		Back Type		RhD Typing
Anti-A	Anti-B	A1 cells	B cells	Anti-D
0	4+	4+	0	4+

57. A 28-year-old sickle cell patient has the blood bank results shown in the panel (Tables 19-17, 19-18, and 19-19). A full phenotype of this patient reveals that he is D+, C–, c+, E–, e+, K–, k+, Jk^a+, Jk^b+, Fy^a–, Fy^b–, M+, N+, S–, and s–. Which one of the following antibodies is most likely present?

A. Anti-Fy3.

B. Anti-k.

C. Anti-Js^b.

D. Anti-Kp^a.

E. Anti-U.

Table 19-17

Front Type		Back Type		RhD Typing
Anti-A	Anti-B	A1 cells	B cells	Anti-D
0	0	4+	4+	4+

Table 19-18

	D	C	c	E	e	K	k	Jk^a	Jk^b	Fy^a	Fy^b	M	N	S	s	Le^a	Le^b	Anti-human Globulin	Check Cells
Cell I	+	+	0	0	+	+	+	+	0	+	0	0	+	0	+	+	0	2+	
Cell II	+	0	+	+	0	0	+	0	+	0	+	+	0	+	0	0	+	2+	

Antibody Screen (antigen columns); *Test Method* (Anti-human Globulin, Check Cells).

Table 19-19

Panel Cell	D	C	c	E	e	K	k	Kp^a	Kp^b	Js^a	Js^b	Jk^a	Jk^b	Fy^a	Fy^b	M	N	S	s	PEG-AHG	Check Cells
1	+	+	0	0	+	+	+	0	+	0	+	0	+	+	+	0	+	+	+	2+	
2	+	+	0	0	+	0	+	0	+	0	+	+	+	0	+	+	0	+	+	2+	
3	+	0	+	+	0	0	+	0	+	0	+	+	+	+	+	0	0	0	+	2+	
4	+	0	+	0	+	0	+	+	+	0	+	+	+	0	+	+	+	0	0	0	2+
5	0	+	+	0	+	0	+	0	+	0	+	0	+	0	+	+	+	0	+	2+	
6	0	0	+	+	+	+	+	0	+	0	+	0	+	+	0	+	0	+	0	2+	
7	0	0	+	0	+	0	+	0	+	0	+	+	+	0	+	0	+	0	+	2+	
8	0	0	+	0	+	0	+	0	+	0	+	+	0	+	0	+	0	+	0	2+	
9	0	0	+	0	+	+	+	0	+	0	+	+	0	+	0	0	+	0	+	2+	
10	0	0	+	0	+	0	+	0	+	0	+	0	+	+	0	0	+	0	+	2+	
11	+	0	+	0	+	0	+	0	0	0	+	0	+	0	0	+	+	+	0	2+	
Patient's cells																				0	2+

Antibody Screen (antigen columns); *Test Method* (PEG-AHG, Check Cells).

58. A 28-year-old woman G3P2 is admitted for delivery at 38 weeks of gestation. Routine type and screen results are shown in Tables 19-20, 19-21, and 19-22. Assuming this patient has a history of receiving only standard of care, which one of the following is the most likely cause of this result?
A. Sensitization to RhD from a prior pregnancy.
B. Sensitization to a non-Rh antigen from a prior pregnancy.
C. Passively acquired RhD antibodies.
D. Naturally occurring antibodies of pregnancy.
E. Warm autoantibodies.

Table 19-20

Front Type		Back Type		Rh(D) Typing
Anti-A	Anti-B	A1 cells	B cells	Anti-D
4+	0	0	4+	0

Table 19-21

	Antibody Screen																	Test Method	
	D	C	c	E	e	K	k	Jkᵃ	Jkᵇ	Fyᵃ	Fyᵇ	M	N	S	s	Leᵃ	Leᵇ	Anti-human Globulin	Check Cells
Cell I	+	+	0	0	+	+	+	+	0	+	0	0	+	0	+	+	0	1+	
Cell II	+	0	+	+	0	0	+	0	+	+	+	+	+	+	+	0	+	1+	

Table 19-22

	Antibody Panel																	Test Method		
Panel Cell	D	C	c	E	e	K	k	Jsᵃ	Jsᵇ	Jkᵃ	Jkᵇ	Fyᵃ	Fyᵇ	M	N	S	s	PEG-AHG	Ficin	Check Cells
1	+	+	0	0	+	+	+	0	+	0	+	+	+	+	+	+	+	1+	2+	
2	+	+	0	0	+	0	+	0	+	+	+	0	+	+	0	+	+	1+	2+	
3	+	0	+	+	0	0	+	0	+	+	+	+	+	+	0	0	+	1+	2+	
4	+	0	+	0	+	0	+	0	+	+	+	0	0	+	+	0	0	1+	2+	
5	0	+	+	0	+	0	+	0	+	0	+	0	+	+	+	0	+	0	0	2+
6	0	0	+	+	+	+	+	0	+	0	+	+	0	+	0	+	0	0	0	2+
7	0	0	+	0	+	0	+	0	+	+	+	0	+	0	+	0	+	0	0	2+
8	0	0	+	0	+	0	+	0	+	+	0	+	0	+	0	+	0	0	0	2+
9	0	0	+	0	+	+	+	0	+	+	0	+	0	0	+	0	+	0	0	2+
10	0	0	+	0	+	0	+	0	+	0	+	+	0	0	+	+	+	0	0	2+
11	+	0	+	0	+	0	+	0	+	+	+	0	0	+	+	+	0	1+	2+	
Patient's cells																		0		2+

59. In general, which one of the following is the difference in the reactivity of IgM and IgG antibodies?
A. IgM antibodies and IgG antibodies frequently cause acute intravascular hemolysis.
B. IgM antibodies and IgG antibodies cannot cause acute intravascular hemolysis.
C. IgM antibodies frequently cause extravascular hemolysis, and IgG antibodies frequently cause intravascular hemolysis.
D. IgM antibodies can cause intravascular hemolysis, and IgG antibodies can cause extravascular hemolysis.
E. IgM antibodies and IgG antibodies frequently cause extravascular hemolysis.

Table 19-23

Forward Typing				Reverse Type	
Anti-A	Anti-B	Anti-D	Weak D	A1 Cells	B Cells
0	4+	0	2+	4+	0

60. You are the technologist testing units at a blood donor center. The blood typing results for a 26-year-old female donor are shown in Table 19-23. After reviewing the results, which one of the following labels should be placed on the red cell unit?
A. Group O, Rh negative.
B. Group A, Rh negative.
C. Group A, Rh positive.
D. Group B, Rh negative.
E. Group B, Rh positive.

Blood Component Therapy

61. A 20-year-old man presents to the emergency department with multiple gunshot wounds to the abdomen and profuse bleeding from his wounds. His hemoglobin is 5 g/dL (reference range, 13.3 to 16.2 g/dL). The trauma team requests 4 U RBCs to transfuse immediately. Which one of the following red cell units should be transfused?
    A. Group O, uncrossmatched RBCs.
    B. Group O, IS crossmatched RBCs.
    C. Type-specific, uncrossmatched RBCs.
    D. Type-specific, IS crossmatched RBCs.
    E. Type-specific, fully crossmatched RBCs.

62. A 38-year-old woman G2P1 presents at 16 weeks of gestation to the obstetrics clinic at your hospital. She is found to be type O Rh negative with a positive red cell antibody screen. Anti-D is identified in the patient's plasma. Which one of the following is the next step in this patient's management?
    A. Give RhIG (RhoGAM) at a dose of 300 µg.
    B. Determine the anti-D antibody titer.
    C. Perform a middle cerebral artery Doppler.
    D. Perform cordocentesis to obtain fetal blood for hemoglobin determination.
    E. Perform an intrauterine transfusion.

63. A 32-year-old type O, Rh-negative woman G2P1 delivered a type O Rh-positive infant. The rosette test is positive and the Kleihauer-Betke shows 1.5% fetal cells. Which one of the following is the correct dose of RhIG for this patient?
    A. 1 vial of RhIG.
    B. 2 vials of RhIG.
    C. 3 vials of RhIG.
    D. 4 vials of RhIG.
    E. 5 vials of RhIG.

64. Which one of the following should be used first for the treatment of minor bleeding in a patient with uremia and a normal platelet count and normal hemoglobin?
    A. Platelets.
    B. Fresh frozen plasma.
    C. Desmopressin acetate (DDAVP).
    D. Cryoprecipitate.
    E. Factor VIII.

65. A 54-year-old man is receiving RBCs for postoperative anemia. He was admitted for elective three-vessel coronary artery bypass graft surgery. He is also receiving fluids. Which one of the following fluids can be transfused in the same line as the RBCs?
    A. Lactated Ringer's solution.
    B. 5% albumin.
    C. Normal saline.
    D. 5% dextrose.
    E. Vancomycin.

66. Which one of the following is an appropriate indication for platelet transfusion?
    A. Platelet count = 21,000/µL; 12-year-old with acute myelocytic leukemia, stable, no bleeding.
    B. Platelet count = 31,000/µL; patient bleeding during laparoscopic colectomy.
    C. Platelet count = 6,000/µL; 12-year-old with immune thrombocytopenia, stable, no bleeding.
    D. Platelet count = 61,000/µL; patient having femoral vein catheter placement.
    E. Platelet count = 110,000/µL; patient after evacuation of a subdural hematoma.

Table 19-24

	Patient	Reference Range	Units
White blood cell count	7.6	3.04-9.06	$\times 10^9$/L
Hemoglobin	14.5	13.3-16.2	g/dL
Hematocrit	45.0	38.8-46.4	%
Platelets	254	165-415	$\times 10^9$/L
Prothrombin time (PT)	12.8	12.7-15.4	seconds
Activated partial thromboplastin time (aPTT)	27	26.3-39.4	seconds
Fibrinogen	245	233-496	mg/dL

Table 19-25

	Patient	Reference Range	Units
White blood cell count	8.9	3.04-9.06	$\times 10^9$/L
Hemoglobin	11.6	13.3-16.2	g/dL
Hematocrit	35	38.8-46.4	%
Platelets	120	165-415	$\times 10^9$/L
PT	18	12.7-15.4	seconds
aPTT	38	26.3-39.4	seconds
Fibrinogen	135	233-496	mg/dL

67. A 54-year-old male patient underwent coronary artery bypass graft surgery. His preoperative labs are shown in Table 19-24. Postoperatively, he continues to have drainage of about 100 mL/h of serosanguinous fluid from his chest tube. His postoperative labs are shown in Table 19-25. Which one of the following is the most likely cause of his bleeding?
    A. Insufficient reversal of heparin.
    B. Platelet dysfunction secondary to cardiopulmonary bypass.
    C. Disseminated intravascular coagulation.
    D. Surgical lesion.
    E. Platelet refractoriness.

Table 19-26

	Patient	Reference Range	Units
White blood cell count	6.8	3.04-9.06	$\times 10^9$/L
Hemoglobin	13.4	13.3-16.2	g/dL
Hematocrit	36.0	38.8-46.4	%
Platelets	345	165-415	$\times 10^9$/L
PT	12.4	12.7-15.4	seconds
aPTT	28	26.3-39.4	seconds
Fibrinogen	266	233-496	mg/dL

Table 19-27

	Patient	Reference Range	Units
White blood cell count	7.8	3.04-9.06	$\times 10^9$/L
Hemoglobin	9.9	13.3-16.2	g/dL
Hematocrit	31.0	38.8-46.4	%
Platelets	101	165-415	$\times 10^9$/L
PT	13	12.7-15.4	seconds
aPTT	39	26.3-39.4	seconds
Fibrinogen	126	233-496	mg/dL

68. A 73-year-old female patient underwent aortic valve repair using cardiac bypass. Her preoperative laboratory results are shown in Table 19-26. Postoperatively, she continues to have about 300 mL/h output from her chest tube. Her postoperative laboratory results are shown in Table 19-27. Which one of the following is the next step in the management of this patient?
    A. Return to the operating room to look for a surgical cause of her bleeding.
    B. Transfuse 1 dose of single-donor apheresis platelets.
    C. Transfuse 4 U fresh frozen plasma.
    D. Transfuse 10 U cryoprecipitate.
    E. Transfuse 2 U RBCs.

69. Cryoprecipitate-reduced plasma has decreased levels of which one of the following factors?
    A. Factor V.
    B. Thrombin.
    C. von Willebrand factor.
    D. Protein S.
    E. Plasminogen.

70. Which one of the following is an FDA-approved indication for recombinant activated factor VII?
    A. Prevention of bleeding during invasive procedures in hemophilia A patients with factor VIII inhibitors.
    B. Correction of an elevated international normalized ratio (INR) in a patient taking warfarin with an intracranial bleed.
    C. Treatment of hemorrhage in a patient undergoing liver transplantation.
    D. Treatment of hemorrhage in a patient with disseminated intravascular coagulation.
    E. Treatment of hemorrhage in a patient receiving aspirin therapy with a lower gastrointestinal tract bleed.

71. A 54-year-old patient has persistent oozing after three-vessel coronary artery bypass graft surgery. The oozing is attributed to the effect of residual heparin. Which one of the following is the best product to reverse the effects of heparin in this patient?
    A. Fresh frozen plasma.
    B. Recombinant activated factor VII.
    C. Platelets.
    D. Cryoprecipitate.
    E. Protamine sulfate.

72. A 25-year-old man presents to the emergency department after blunt trauma to his abdomen. He has received 15 U RBCs, 7 U plasma, and 5 doses of single donor apheresis platelets. The surgeon calls to request recombinant activated factor VII. Which one of the following steps should be taken next in the management of this patient?
    A. Give platelets and cryoprecipitate before recombinant activated factor VII at a dose of 90 μg/kg.
    B. Give RBCs and cryoprecipitate before recombinant activated factor VII at a dose of 90 μg/kg.
    C. Give plasma and cryoprecipitate before giving recombinant activated factor VII at a dose of 90 μg/kg.
    D. Give platelets and RBCs before giving recombinant activated factor VII at a dose of 90 μg/kg.
    E. Give recombinant activated factor VII at a dose of 90 μg/kg.

73. Which one of the following is the proposed mechanism for the increased platelet requirements in patients on extracorporeal membrane oxygenation (ECMO) circuits?
    A. Increased consumption secondary to disseminated intravascular coagulopathy.
    B. Increased consumption secondary to mucosal bleeding from anticoagulation.
    C. Increased clearance secondary to heparin-induced thrombocytopenia.
    D. Increased clearance secondary to platelet activation and adherence to tubing and the membrane oxygenator.
    E. Increased clearance secondary to increased capillary leak.

74. A 64-year-old man is about to undergo a laparoscopic colon resection for diverticulitis. His current platelet count is 100×10^9/L (reference range 165-415 $\times 10^9$/L). The surgeon is requesting one dose of single-donor apheresis platelets. Which one of the following is the best recommendation regarding the transfusion needs of this patient?
    A. Recommend platelets to ensure hemostasis during the procedure.
    B. Recommend platelets because of his decreased platelet count.
    C. Do not recommend platelets since his current platelet count is sufficient.
    D. Do not recommend platelets since they may promote inflammation in this patient.
    E. Only recommend platelets if the patient develops moderate bleeding.

75. Which one of the following is the half-life of recombinant activated factor VII in adults?
    A. 30 minutes.
    B. 2 hours.
    C. 4 hours.
    D. 6 hours.
    E. 8 hours.

Table 19-28

	Patient	Reference Range	Units
Hemoglobin	12.2	13.3-16.2	g/dL
Hematocrit	36.9	38.8-46.4	%
Platelets	278	165-415	$\times 10^9$/L
Factor IX	20	50-150	%

76. A 42-year-old man presents to the emergency department with spontaneous bleeding into his knee. The patient has a history of severe hemophilia B. He is on factor IX prophylactic therapy at home. He weighs 75 kg. Laboratory results are as shown in Table 19-28. The hematologist on call asks you to calculate the appropriate loading dose of factor IX. The final factor IX level should be 100%. Which one of the following is the correct dose for this patient?
A. 1,500 IU.
B. 3,000 IU.
C. 4,500 IU.
D. 6,000 IU.
E. 7,500 IU.

Table 19-29

	Patient	Reference Range	Units
Hemoglobin	10.3	13.3-16.2	g/dL
Hematocrit	31.2	38.8-46.4	%
Platelets	376	165-415	$\times 10^9$/L
Factor VIII	3	50-150	%

77. A 35-year-old man presents to the emergency department with bleeding after a tooth extraction. The patient has a history of moderate hemophilia A. He is not using factor VIII prophylactic therapy because of noncompliance. He weighs 85 kg. Laboratory results are as shown in Table 19-29. The hematologist on call asks you to calculate the appropriate loading dose of factor VIII. The final factor VIII level should be 100%. Which one of the following is the correct dose for this patient?
A. 3400 IU.
B. 5100 IU.
C. 5673 IU.
D. 5848 IU.
E. 7396 IU.

78. A 56-year-old male patient with chronic lymphocytic leukemia is suspected of being refractory to platelet transfusions. The patient received 1 dose of apheresis platelets for a morning platelet count of 7,000/μL. His 1-hour posttransfusion platelet count is 10,000/μL. He weighs 105 kg and is 1.9 m in height. His body surface area is 2.35 m². Assuming there are 3.0×10^{11} platelets/dose, which one of the following is his corrected count increment (CCI)?
A. 1,900 platelets $\times$ m²/μL.
B. 2,350 platelets $\times$ m²/μL.
C. 3,830 platelets $\times$ m²/μL.
D. 4,737 platelets $\times$ m²/μL.
E. 7,833 platelets $\times$ m²/μL.

79a. The hematology resident calls you requesting HLA-matched platelets for a 22-year-old male patient with acute lymphoblastic leukemia. The patient's platelet count does not seem to increase appropriately after platelet transfusions. The patient is stable and not bleeding. Which one of the following steps should be taken next in the management of this patient?
A. Order HLA-matched platelets.
B. Order crossmatched platelets.
C. Order a platelet antibody screen.
D. Order 1-hour posttransfusion platelet counts.
E. Order a platelet drip of 1 dose of single donor apheresis platelets transfused over 4 hours.

79b. Which one of the following clinical symptoms would most likely suggest a nonimmune cause for the platelet refractoriness in this patient?
A. Splenic infarction.
B. Localized infection.
C. Aspirin therapy.
D. Obesity.
E. Antibiotic therapy.

Table 19-30

	Patient	Reference Range	Units
White blood cell count	4.26	3.54-9.06	$\times 10^9$/L
Hemoglobin	10.9	13.3-16.2	g/dL
Hematocrit	31.5	38.8-46.4	%
Platelet count	389	165-415	$\times 10^9$/L
PT	14.2	12.7-15.4	seconds
aPTT	28.5	26.3-39.4	seconds
Fibrinogen	75	233-496	mg/dL

80. Preoperative lab tests in a 45-year-old female patient undergoing hysterectomy secondary to dysfunctional uterine bleeding are show in Table 19-30. Which one of the following products should be given before surgery?
A. Fresh frozen plasma.
B. Cryoprecipitate-depleted plasma.
C. Cryoprecipitate.
D. Platelets.
E. RBCs.

81. A 25-year-old male patient presented to the emergency department with severe bleeding after a motor vehicle accident. He received multiple units of RBCs, platelets, and fresh frozen plasma to treat the acute hemorrhage. In the intensive care unit (ICU), it is noted that he has persistent oozing from multiple sites. His fibrinogen is noted to be 50 g/dL (reference range, 233 to 496 g/dL). The ICU physician would like to increase the patient's fibrinogen to 150 mg/dL. The patient weighs 83 kg and his hematocrit is 40.0% (reference range, 38.8% to 46.4%). Which one of the following is the correct number of units of cryoprecipitate needed to achieve the desired fibrinogen level?
A. 7 U.
B. 9 U.
C. 10 U.
D. 14 U.
E. 21 U.

Table 19-31

	Patient	Reference Range	Units
White blood cell count	9.81	3.54-9.06	$\times 10^9$/L
Hemoglobin	8.2	13.3-16.2	g/dL
Hematocrit	24.8	38.8-46.4	%
Platelet count	256	165-415	$\times 10^9$/L
PT	14.3	12.7-15.4	seconds
aPTT	27.0	26.3-39.4	seconds

82. An 80-year-old male patient is brought to the emergency department after falling and hitting his head. Computed tomography scan reveals a subdural hemorrhage causing a midline shift. The patient's family reports that the patient is taking aspirin and warfarin. His lab test results are as shown in Table 19-31. Which one of the following products do you recommend?
   A. Platelets.
   B. Fresh frozen plasma.
   C. RBCs.
   D. Cryoprecipitate.
   E. Granulocytes.

83. A 17-year-old male patient with no significant past medical history presents to his primary care physician with petechiae on his face and easy bruising. Routine laboratory tests are significant for a platelet count of 5×10^9/L (reference range $165\text{-}415 \times 10^9$/L). Which one of the following steps should be taken next in the management of this patient?
   A. Transfuse one dose of single-donor apheresis platelets.
   B. Corticosteroids.
   C. Therapeutic plasmapheresis.
   D. Thrombopoietin.
   E. Rituximab.

84. In which one of the following clinical conditions are platelet transfusions absolutely contraindicated in the absence of life-threatening bleeding?
   A. Immune thrombocytopenia.
   B. History of allergic reactions to platelets.
   C. Platelet refractoriness.
   D. Neonatal alloimmune thrombocytopenia.
   E. Thrombotic thrombocytopenic purpura.

Table 19-32

	Reference Range	Units
White blood cell count	3.54-9.06	x10^9/L

85. Which one of the following patients is the best candidate for granulocyte transfusions (Table 19-32)?
   A. An 85-year-old female patient with a history of cardiac disease, hypertension, and metastatic breast carcinoma currently hospitalized with urosepsis, WBC 20.2×10^9/L.
   B. A 10-year-old boy with acute lymphoblastic leukemia with disseminated CMV infection, WBC 0.4×10^9/L.

   C. A 45-year-old female patient with acute myelogenous leukemia after unrelated allogeneic hematopoietic stem cell transplant and documented engraftment failure, WBC 0.2×10^9/L.
   D. A 62-year-old female patient with chronic lymphocytic leukemia with staphylococcal sepsis receiving antibiotic therapy, WBC 2.0×10^9/L.
   E. A 5-year-old boy ith neuroblastoma after autologous hematopoietic stem cell transplant with disseminated candidiasis unresponsive to antifungal therapy, WBC 0.1×10^9/L.

86. An otherwise healthy full-term neonate born to a 30-year-old healthy woman G2P1 is found to have an intracranial hemorrhage 1 hour after delivery. The pregnancy was unremarkable. Which one of the following should be at the top of your differential diagnosis?
   A. Idiopathic thrombocytopenic purpura.
   B. Thrombotic thrombocytopenic purpura.
   C. Neonatal alloimmune thrombocytopenia.
   D. Congenital CMV infection.
   E. Hemolytic disease of the fetus and newborn.

Table 19-33

	Patient	Reference Range	Units
White blood cell count	7.81	3.54-9.06	$\times 10^9$/L
Hemoglobin	10.5	13.3-16.2	g/dL
Hematocrit	31.1	38.8-46.4	%
Platelet count	7	165-415	$\times 10^9$/L

87. A 55-year-old woman with severe nasal and gum bleeding 1 week after a hysterectomy for endometrial carcinoma presents to her physician. She received 2 U RBCs postoperatively for symptomatic anemia. Her current lab test results are shown in Table 19-33. Which one of the following is the most likely diagnosis?
   A. Transfusion-related acute lung injury.
   B. Posttransfusion purpura.
   C. Transfusion-associated graft-versus-host disease.
   D. Platelet refractoriness.
   E. HLA alloimmunization.

88. A 75-year-old patient with a history of a deep venous thrombosis 3 months earlier and taking warfarin presents to the emergency department with new-onset shortness of breath. His current INR is 9. There is no evidence of bleeding and the patient is hemodynamically stable. Which one of the following is the most appropriate course of action?
   A. Hold warfarin therapy.
   B. Hold warfarin therapy and give oral vitamin K.
   C. Hold warfarin therapy and give intramuscular vitamin K.
   D. Hold warfarin therapy and give intravenous vitamin K and fresh frozen plasma.
   E. Hold warfarin therapy and give intravenous vitamin K and recombinant activated factor VII.

Table 19-34

	Patient	Reference Range	Units
White blood cell count	6.21	3.54-9.06	$\times 10^9$/L
Hemoglobin	11.3	13.3-16.2	g/dL
Hematocrit	34	38.8-46.4	%
Platelet count	75	165-415	$\times 10^9$/L
PT	16	12.7-15.4	seconds
aPTT	40.1	26.3-39.4	seconds
Fibrinogen	134	233-496	mg/dL

89. A 45-year-old female with hepatitis C in stable condition needs to have a liver biopsy. Her preprocedure labs are shown in Table 19-34. The interventional radiologist wants to transfuse 2 U fresh frozen plasma before the procedure. Which one of the following is the best recommendation?
    A. Transfuse 4 to 6 U fresh frozen plasma to correct her coagulopathy.
    B. Transfuse 10 U cryoprecipitate to provide additional fibrinogen.
    C. Transfuse 1 dose of single-donor apheresis platelets to correct her thrombocytopathy.
    D. Transfuse 2 U RBCs to correct the anemia.
    E. No transfusion is needed at this time.

90. Which one of the following is the rationale behind early transfusion of plasma products in severe hemorrhage?
    A. Treatment of early and profound coagulopathy.
    B. Prevention of hypothermia.
    C. Improved oxygen delivery to the tissues.
    D. To provide volume replacement.
    E. To facilitate healing.

Table 19-35

	Patient	Reference Range	Units
White blood cell count	6.11	3.54-9.06	$\times 10^9$/L
Hemoglobin	6.1	13.3-16.2	g/dL
Hematocrit	21.8	38.8-46.4	%
Platelet count	345	165-415	$\times 10^9$/L
PT	120	12.7-15.4	seconds
aPTT	28.0	26.3-39.4	seconds
INR	>9		

91. A 75-year-old patient with a history of a deep venous thrombosis 3 months ago who is taking warfarin presents to the emergency department with an acute gastrointestinal bleed. His lab test results are shown in Table 19-35. Which one of the following is the most appropriate course of action?
    A. Hold warfarin therapy.
    B. Hold warfarin therapy and give oral vitamin K.
    C. Hold warfarin therapy and give intramuscular vitamin K.
    D. Hold warfarin therapy and give intravenous vitamin K and fresh frozen plasma.
    E. Hold warfarin therapy and give intravenous vitamin K and recombinant activated factor VII.

Adverse Reactions

92. A 75-year-old male patient received 4 U RBCs to treat anemia secondary to lower gastrointestinal tract bleeding. He complains of perioral tingling and numbness toward the end of the last unit. Which one of the following is the most likely cause of these symptoms?
    A. The citrate in the anticoagulant solution.
    B. The dextrose in the anticoagulant solution.
    C. Monobasic sodium phosphate in the anticoagulant solution.
    D. The mannitol in the additive solution.
    E. The adenine in the additive solution.

93. Which one of the following is an adverse event associated with the use of recombinant activated factor VII?
    A. Transfusion-related acute lung injury.
    B. Increased transfusion requirements.
    C. Thromboembolic events.
    D. Viral transmission.
    E. Hemolysis.

94. A patient develops sudden back pain, fever, and red urine 10 minutes into the transfusion of a unit of RBCs. Which one of the following should be on the top of your differential diagnosis?
    A. Febrile nonhemolytic transfusion reaction.
    B. Transfusion-related acute lung injury.
    C. Acute hemolytic transfusion reaction.
    D. Anaphylactic transfusion reaction.
    E. Transfusion-related sepsis.

95. A stable 35-year-old white male patient develops urticaria and acute dyspnea requiring emergent intubation 15 minutes into the transfusion of 1 U fresh frozen plasma. His pretransfusion vital signs are heart rate (HR), 70 beats/min; respiratory rate (RR), 18/min; blood pressure (BP), 125/80 mm Hg; temperature (T), 36.8°C; and O_2 saturation, 99% on room air. Postreaction vital signs are HR, 130 beats/min; RR, 30/min; BP, 90/50 mm Hg; T, 36.8°C; and O_2 saturation, 75% on room air. He had a similar reaction to plasma in the past, also requiring intubation. Which of the following should be at the top of your differential diagnosis as a cause of the transfusion reaction?
    A. Acute hemolytic transfusion reaction.
    B. Anaphylactic transfusion reaction.
    C. Transfusion-associated circulatory overload.
    D. Transfusion-related acute lung injury.
    E. Transfusion-related sepsis.

96. According to expert opinion, which one of the following is the pathophysiology of a febrile nonhemolytic transfusion reaction (FNHTR) after transfusion of a prestorage leukoreduced blood component?
    A. Passive transfusion of cytokines or recipient cytokine response to transfusion.
    B. Passive transfusion of anti-HLA antibodies for which the patient has the cognate antigen.
    C. Passive transfusion of biologically active lipids.
    D. Passive transfusion of cells carrying an RBC antigen for which the patient makes an alloantibody.
    E. Passive transfusion of plasma proteins to which the recipient makes IgE antibodies.

97. According to the Canadian Consensus Conference definition, which one of the following is part of the diagnostic criteria for transfusion-related acute lung injury (TRALI)?
    A. Onset of symptoms within 24 hours of transfusion.
    B. Presence of fever.
    C. Leukopenia.
    D. No evidence of left atrial hypertension.
    E. Presence of irreversible lung injury.

98. A 63-year-old man presents to the emergency department with acute mental status changes after falling and hitting his head. He takes warfarin for a deep venous thrombosis diagnosed 3 months ago. His INR is 6.0 (target, 2.5 to 3.5). Transfusion of fresh frozen plasma is started to reverse his INR. Thirty minutes into his transfusion he develops acute dyspnea, tachycardia, and hypotension. His temperature remains stable. Chest radiograph shows bilateral pulmonary infiltrates. Which one of the following should be on the top of your differential diagnosis for the cause of his acute dyspnea?
    A. Transfusion-related circulatory overload.
    B. Transfusion-related acute lung injury.
    C. Anaphylaxis.
    D. Acute hemolytic transfusion reaction.
    E. Transfusion-related sepsis.

99. A 32-year-old man with β-thalassemia major receives a transfusion every 2 weeks to maintain a hemoglobin of 10 g/dL (13.3-16.2 g/dL). He takes an iron chelator to prevent iron overload. Which one of the following is the mechanism by which transfusion-induced iron overload occurs?
    A. Increased iron from transfused RBCs leads to production of non–transferrin-bound iron.
    B. Increased iron from transfused RBCs leads to decreased hepcidin levels.

C. Increased iron from transfused RBCs leads to increased expression of ferroportin.
D. Increased iron from transfused RBCs leads to decreased hemosiderin.
E. Increased iron from transfused RBCs leads to decreased transferrin saturation.

100. Which one of the following is most commonly associated with transfusion-transmitted sepsis after transfusion of RBCs?
    A. *Staphylococcus aureus.*
    B. *Streptococcus bovis.*
    C. *Pseudomonas aeruginosa.*
    D. *Yersinia enterocolitica.*
    E. *Bacillus cereus.*

101a. A 20-year-old man with acute lymphoblastic leukemia develops rigors, a temperature of 40°C, and severe hypotension 15 minutes after the start of a transfusion. His pretransfusion vital signs are heart rate, 85 beats/min; blood pressure, 110/70 mm Hg; respiratory rate, 20/min; and temperature, 37.5°C. Which one of the following should be on the top of your differential diagnosis list for the cause of his symptoms?
    A. Septic transfusion reaction.
    B. Transfusion-related acute lung injury.
    C. Transfusion-associated circulatory overload.
    D. Anaphylactic transfusion reaction.
    E. Delayed hemolytic transfusion reaction.

101b. Which one of the following products did the patient most likely receive?
    A. RBCs.
    B. Platelets.
    C. Fresh frozen plasma.
    D. Cryoprecipitate.
    E. Granulocytes.

102. A platelet transfusion for a 5 year-old girl is stopped after one half of the unit has been transfused because of a fever (temperature from 99.4°F to 101.0°F) and hemoglobinuria. The front and back type results from a pretransfusion and a posttransfusion sample are provided in Tables 19-36 through 19-39. Which one of the following is the most likely diagnosis?

A. Delayed serologic transfusion reaction.
B. Delayed hemolytic transfusion reaction.
C. Acute hemolytic transfusion reaction.
D. Febrile nonhemolytic transfusion reaction.
E. Rh disease.

Table 19-36 Pretransfusion ABO Typing

Front Type		Back Type		RhD Typing
Anti-A	Anti-B	A1 cells	B cells	Anti-D
4+	0	0	4+	4+

Table 19-37 ABO Typing

Front Type		Back Type		RhD Typing
Anti-A	Anti-B	A1 cells	B cells	Anti-D
4+	0	1+	4+	4+

Table 19-38 Pretransfusion Antibody Screen

	Antibody Screen																	Test Method	
	D	C	c	E	e	K	k	Jk^a	Jk^b	Fy^a	Fy^b	M	N	S	s	Le^a	Le^b	Anti-human Globulin	Check Cells
Cell I	+	+	0	0	+	+	+	+	0	+	0	0	+	0	+	+	0	0	2+
Cell II	+	0	+	+	0	0	+	0	+	+	+	+	+	+	+	0	+	0	2+

Table 19-39 Post-transfusion Antibody Screen

	Antibody Screen																	Test Method	
	D	C	c	E	e	K	k	Jk^a	Jk^b	Fy^a	Fy^b	M	N	S	s	Le^a	Le^b	Anti-human Globulin	Check Cells
Cell I	+	+	0	0	+	+	+	+	0	+	0	0	+	0	+	+	0	0	2+
Cell II	+	0	+	+	0	0	+	0	+	+	+	+	+	+	+	0	+	0	2+

Table 19-40

Panel Cell	D	C	c	E	e	K	k	Kp^a	Kp^b	Js^a	Js^b	Jk^a	Jk^b	Fy^a	Fy^b	M	N	S	s	Eluate	Check Cells
1	+	+	−	−	+	+	+	0	+	0	+	0	+	+	+	+	+	+	+	2+	
2	+	+	−	−	+	0	+	0	+	0	+	+	+	0	+	+	0	+	+	0	2+
3	+	0	+	+	0	0	+	0	+	0	+	+	+	+	+	+	0	0	+	0	2+
4	+	0	+	0	+	0	+	0	+	0	+	+	+	0	0	+	+	0	0	0	2+
5	0	+	+	0	+	0	+	0	+	0	+	0	+	0	+	+	+	0	+	0	2+
6	0	0	+	+	+	+	+	0	+	0	+	0	+	+	0	+	0	+	+	2+	
7	0	0	+	0	+	0	+	0	+	0	+	+	+	0	+	0	+	0	+	0	2+
8	0	0	+	0	+	0	+	0	+	0	+	+	0	+	0	+	+	+	+	0	2+
9	0	0	+	0	+	+	+	0	+	0	+	+	0	+	0	0	+	0	+	2+	
10	0	0	+	0	+	0	+	0	+	0	+	0	+	+	0	0	+	+	+	0	2+
11	+	0	+	0	+	0	+	0	+	0	+	+	+	0	0	+	+	+	0	0	2+
Patient's cells																				Mixed Field	

Table 19-41

Test	Direct Antiglobulin Test
Anti-IgG	Mixed field positive
Anti-C3d	0

103. A 42-year-old male patient was transfused for traumatic injury 1 week before the direct antiglobulin test and eluate testing shown in Tables 19-40 and 19-41. Currently, the patient is stable with normal total bilirubin, lactate dehydrogenase, and haptoglobin levels. Which one of the following is most consistent with these findings?

A. Delayed serologic transfusion reaction.
B. Delayed hemolytic transfusion reaction.
C. Acute hemolytic transfusion reaction.
D. Presence of a warm autoantibody.
E. Presence of a cold autoantibody.

104. A 68-year-old man with myelodysplastic syndrome is receiving a transfusion with the first of 2 U RBCs. After infusion of approximately 100 mL of the product, the patient develops chills, his temperature increases to 101°F (initial temperature, 98.7°F), and he complains of lower back pain. The transfusion is stopped and the remainder of the unit of RBCs is returned to the blood bank for evaluation. According to AABB standards, which one of the following should be included in the evaluation of a suspected hemolytic transfusion reaction?

A. Repeat Rh determination.
B. Indirect antiglobulin test.
C. Review and interpretation by the medical director.
D. Serum haptoglobin.
E. Complete blood cell count.

ANSWERS

BLOOD COLLECTION AND DONOR ISSUES

1. A. Malaria.
Rationale: Currently, there is no FDA-approved test to screen blood donors for malaria.
B. Syphilis.
Rationale: A serologic test for syphilis is performed on all blood components.
C. Babesia.
D. Dengue virus.
E. Chikungunya virus.
Rationale: Currently, there is no FDA-approved test to screen blood donors for babesia, dengue virus, or chikungunya virus.

Major points of discussion

■ All allogeneic blood donations are tested for the HBV surface antigen (HBsAG), anti-hepatitis B virus core (HBc) antibody, HBV DNA, anti-hepatitis C virus antibody, hepatitis C virus RNA, anti-HIV-1/2, HIV-1 RNA, anti-human T lymphocyte virus (HTLV) I/II antibody, a serologic test for syphilis, and West Nile virus RNA.

■ Currently, the FDA recommends that all blood donors be screened one time for antibodies to *Trypanosoma cruzi*.

■ Currently, there is no FDA-approved test to detect babesia in blood donors. Potential blood donors who have a history of babesia infection are indefinitely deferred from blood donation.

■ Both nucleic acid amplification and serologic tests to detect past or present babesia infection are in development.

■ Donors who have traveled to malaria risk areas are deferred for 1 year. Donors who either lived in an endemic area or who have had malaria are deferred for 3 years.[5]

2. A. 1:8,000 to 10,000.
   B. 1:80,000 to 100,000.
   Rationale: This is not the current estimated residual risk.
   C. 1:800,000 to 1,000,000.
   Rationale: This is the approximate current residual risk of HBV transmission.
   D. 1:8,000,000 to 1,000,000,000.
   Rationale: This is not the current estimated residual risk.
   E. HBV has not been transmitted by blood transfusion in the past 10 years.
   Rationale: HBV has been transmitted via blood transfusion in the past 10 years.

Major points of discussion
■ HBV is a double-stranded DNA virus of the Hepadnaviridae family.
■ It is transmissible through both cellular and noncellular blood components and many plasma derivatives.
■ All blood donors are screened for HBV with enzyme immunoassays or chemiluminescence assays for the HBsAg and the anti-HBc antibody.
■ HBV nucleic acid amplification tests (NATs) are FDA-approved for screening blood donors.
■ HBV NAT testing may significantly reduce the window period before seroconversion and detect occult infection in HBsAg and anti-HBc antibody–negative donors.

3. A. Fresh frozen plasma (FFP) is thawed and centrifuged at 20°C to 24°C and the precipitate is frozen at –18°C within 1 hour of preparation.
   B. FFP is thawed and centrifuged at 20°C to 24°C and the precipitate is frozen at –1°C to 6°C within 1 hour of preparation.
   C. FFP is thawed and centrifuged at 1°C to 6°C and the precipitate is frozen at –18°C within 1 hour of preparation.
   D. FFP is thawed and centrifuged at 1°C to 6°C and the precipitate is frozen at –18°C within 2 hours of preparation.
   E. FFP is thawed and centrifuged at 20°C to 24°C and the precipitate is frozen at –18°C within 2 hours of preparation.
   Rationale: FFP is thawed and centrifuged at at 1°C to 6°C and the precipitate is frozen at –18°C within 1 hour of preparation to make cryoprecipitate.

Major points of discussion
■ Cryoprecipitate is the cold insoluble protein that forms when fresh frozen plasma is thawed and centrifuged at 1°C to –6°C.
■ The precipitate is resuspended in 10 to 15 mL of plasma.
■ Cryoprecipitate must be refrozen within 1 hour of preparation.
■ It may be stored at –18°C for up to 1 year after the collection date.
■ Cryoprecipitate contains factor VIII, fibrinogen, factor XIII, von Willebrand factor, and fibronectin.
■ According to the AABB standards, cryoprecipitate must have at least 80 IU of factor VIII and 150 mg of fibrinogen.

4. A. A 35-year-old male patient with human immunodeficiency virus (HIV).

B. A 22-year-old man with hemophilia and a joint bleed.
C. A 50-year-old woman with metastatic breast cancer.
Rationale: Irradiated cellular blood components are usually not indicated for patients with HIV, hemophilia, and nonhematologic malignancies
D. A 45-year-old female patient after a bone marrow transplant.
Rationale: After a bone marrow transplant, patients are severely immunocompromised and are at risk for transfusion-associated graft-versus-host disease.
E. An 8-year-old girl after a motor vehicle accident.
Rationale: Irradiated cellular blood components are not indicated for immunocompetent children.

Major points of discussion
■ Cellular blood components are irradiated to prevent transfusion-associated graft-versus-host disease (TA-GvHD).
■ Severely immunocompromised patients or patients who are homozygous for an HLA haplotype of the donor are at risk for developing TA-GvHD.
■ At-risk populations include patients with hematologic malignancies, recipients of peripheral hematopoietic stem cell or marrow transplants, those undergoing fludarabine therapy or intrauterine transfusions, neonates (particularly premature neonates or those undergoing whole blood exchange), and recipients of directed donations from family members.
■ Signs and symptoms of TA-GvHD include maculopapular rash, fever, diarrhea, and marrow aplasia.
■ Symptoms are usually noted 7 to 10 days after transfusion in adults and about 28 days after transfusion in neonates.

5. A. Inactivation of B-lymphocytes.
Rationale: B cells are not involved in the pathogenesis of TA-GvHD.
B. Inactivation of T-lymphocytes.
Rationale: Irradiation inactivates immunocompetent T cells, thereby preventing engraftment and proliferation.
C. Inactivation of plasma cells.
Rationale: Plasma cells are not found in cellular blood components.
D. Inactivation of granulocytes.
Rationale: Granulocytes are not involved in the pathogenesis of TA-GvHD.
E. Inactivation of macrophages.
Rationale: Macrophages are not found in cellular blood components.

Major points of discussion
■ Cellular components may be irradiated to prevent TA-GvHD.
■ TA-GvHD occurs when donor-derived immunocompetent T-lymphocytes engraft in the host, proliferate, and attack host tissues.
■ Irradiation is the only method known to eliminate the risk of TA-GvHD.
■ Blood components may be irradiated using gamma rays or x-rays at a dose of at least 25 Gy to the center of the bag and 15 Gy to the periphery of the bag.

6. A. Labeling can occur at any time during the manufacturing process.
B. Labeling should occur before all manufacturing steps.
C. Labeling should occur before a product is placed on hold.
D. Labeling should occur after all infectious disease testing is completed.
E. Labeling should occur after all blood component modifications (i.e., irradiation, leukoreduction) are completed.
Rationale: Labeling should occur after confirmation that all infectious disease testing is nonreactive or results are negative.

Major points of discussion
- The Code of Federal Regulations (CFR) has requirements for the labeling of blood components.
- Blood components should only be labeled after the following have taken place:
  - All donation records have been reviewed and compared with all past records for accuracy and consistency.
  - All holds are resolved.
  - Infectious disease test results are confirmed to be negative or nonreactive.
  - All quality control processes for both the product and all equipment, supplies, and reagents used in manufacturing have been completed and reviewed.

7. A. Hereditary elliptocytosis.
B. Sickle cell trait.
Rationale: About 50% of RBC units from donors with sickle cell trait fail to filter appropriately.
C. Thalassemia.
D. Hereditary spherocytosis.
E. Glucose-6-phosphate dehydrogenase deficiency.
Rationale for A, C, D, and E: This is not a frequent cause of filter failure.

Major points of discussion
- RBCs and platelets may be leukoreduced to decrease the number or leukocytes in the final transfused component. This decreases the risk of febrile nonhemolytic transfusion reactions, HLA alloimmunization, and transfusion-transmitted CMV.
- The final leukocyte count must be less than 5×10^6/unit of RBCs or platelets in the United States.
- No standards exist for the number of residual leukocytes in plasma units in the United States.
- RBCs may be leukoreduced before storage or at the bedside.
- Prestorage leukoreduction is performed within 5 days of collection by allowing RBCs to flow through a leukoreduction filter via gravity.
- Leukoreduction of RBCs from donors with sickle cell trait leads to prolonged filtration times and higher post-leukoreduction leukocyte counts.

8. A. 21 days.
Rationale: This is the shelf-life for RBCs collected in CPD or CP2D.
B. 35 days.
Rationale: This is the shelf-life for RBCs collected in CPDA-1.

C. 42 days.
Rationale: This is the shelf-life of RBCs collected in anticoagulant with a preservative solution.
D. 56 days.
Rationale: This is the deferral period between whole blood donations.
E. 112 days.
Rationale: This is the deferral period after a 2-U apheresis red cell donation.

Major points of discussion
- Whole blood is collected in an anticoagulant solution.
- Anticoagulant solutions consist of varying concentrations of citrate, phosphate, and dextrose. Adenine may or may not be included.
- Anticoagulant solutions improve red cell function by decreasing loss of 2,3-diphosphoglycerate (2,3-DPG), which is necessary for release of oxygen to the tissues.
- Levels of 2,3-DPG in an RBC unit decrease 2 weeks after collection, but levels return to normal 24 hours after transfusion.
- Additive solutions, AS-1, AS-2, and AS-3, increase the shelf-life of RBCs by providing additional saline, adenine, and dextrose. AS-1 and AS-3 also contain mannitol.

9. **A. RBCs collected in citrate-phosphate-dextrose (CPD) may be rejuvenated up to 3 days after expiration and then frozen for up to 10 years.**
Rationale: RBCs collected in CPD or CPDA-1 may be rejuvenated up to 3 days after expiration and then frozen for up to 10 years.
B. RBCs collected in AS-1 may be rejuvenated up to 3 days after expiration and then frozen for up to 3 years.
Rationale: RBCs collected in AS-1 cannot be rejuvenated after their initial expiration date.
C. RBCs collected in CPD may be rejuvenated up to 42 days after collection and then frozen for up to 3 years.
Rationale: RBCs collected in CPD may be rejuvenated after their expiration date and then frozen for up to 10 years.
D. RBCs collected in AS-1 may be rejuvenated up to 42 days after collection and then frozen up to 10 years.
Rationale: RBCs collected in AS-1 can only be frozen for up to 3 years
E. RBCs collected in CPD or AS-1 may be rejuvenated at any time up to their expiration date and then frozen up to 10 years.
Rationale: The conditions for rejuvenation and storage for RBCs collected in CPD and AS-1 are not the same.

Major points of discussion
- RBCs stored in AS-1 may be rejuvenated up to the original 42-day expiration date and then frozen for up to 3 years.
- The FDA has not approved the use of rejuvenation solutions for RBCs collected or stored in other preservative or additive solutions
- RBCs that have been rejuvenated must be washed to remove all of the rejuvenation solution before release for transfusion.

10. A. Leukoreduced.
B. Leukoreduced and irradiated.
Rationale: This patient should receive leukoreduced products to reduce the likelihood of CMV transmission and decrease

the risk of HLA alloimmunization, but this is not sufficient modification for this patient's clinical needs. This patient also requires irradiated cellular components to prevent TA-GVHD.

C. Leukoreduced, irradiated, and washed.

D. Leukoreduced, irradiated, washed, and hemoglobin S–negative.

Rationale: This patient does not require washed products since he does not have a history of multiple severe, progressive allergic/anaphylactic transfusion reactions or documented IgA deficiency with anti-IgA antibodies. Furthermore, this patient does not require hemoglobin S–negative RBCs.

E. This patient can receive unmodified random donor RBCs.

Rationale: This patient is immunocompromised and should not receive unmodified RBC units.

Major points of discussion

■ Leukoreduction reduces the incidence of febrile nonhemolytic transfusion reactions, the risk of HLA alloimmunization, and the risk of CMV transmission.

■ Irradiation of cellular blood products prevents transfusion-associated graft-versus-host disease.

■ All severely immunocompromised patients, including those with hematologic malignancies, hematopoietic stem cell transplant recipients, fludarabine therapy recipients, premature neonates, recipients of intrauterine transfusions, neonate recipients of whole blood exchange, and recipients of directed donations and HLA-matched transfusions, require irradiated blood products.

■ Irradiated RBC units expire 28 days after irradiation or the original expiration date of the unit, whichever comes first.

■ Washed RBCs are indicated for patients with a history of multiple severe, progressive allergic/anaphylactic transfusion reactions or documented IgA deficiency with anti-IgA antibodies.

■ Washing can decrease the RBC mass up to 20% and changes the expiration to 24 hours after washing because an open system is created.

■ Hemoglobin S–negative units may be chosen for neonates and patients with sickle cell disease due to the deleterious effects of hemoglobin S in these patient populations.

11. A. Leukoreduction increases the risk of human leukocyte antigen (HLA) alloimmunization.

Rationale: Leukoreduction decreases the risk of HLA alloimmunization.

B. Leukoreduction increases the incidence of febrile nonhemolytic transfusion reactio

Rationale: Leukoreduction decreases the incidence of febrile nonhemolytic transfusion reactions.

C. Leukoreduction prevents transfusion-associated graft-versus-host disease.

Rationale: Irradiation is the only method shown to eliminate the risk of transfusion-associated graft-versus-host disease.

D. Leukoreduction reduces the risk of cytomegalovirus (CMV) transmission.

Rationale: Leukoreduction reduces the risk of CMV transmission by removing the white cells that harbor CMV.

E. Leukoreduction prevents transfusion-related acute lung injury.

Rationale: Leukoreduction is not a reliable method to prevent transfusion-related acute lung injury.

Major points of discussion

■ RBCs and platelets can be leukoreduced to remove the white blood cells from the final product.

■ AABB standards require that products labeled as leukoreduced have less than 5×10^6 leukocytes/unit.

■ Products that are leukoreduced before storage should be leukoreduced within 5 days of collection.

■ Prestorage leukoreduction prevents the accumulation of leukocyte-generated cytokines in stored blood components.

■ Leukoreduction has been shown to decrease the risk of HLA alloimmunization, decrease the risk of CMV transmission, and decrease the incidence of febrile nonhemolytic transfusion reactions.

12. A. A 40-year-old man undergoing hip replacement for a hip fracture after a motor vehicle accident.

Rationale: There is a potential risk of fat emboli when bone fragments are in the operative field.

B. A 38-year-old woman undergoing laparotomy for lysis of adhesions secondary to metastatic colon cancer.

Rationale: Metastatic cancer cells have been found in salvaged blood, and the risk of increased spread is unknown.

C. A 65-year-old man undergoing colectomy for bowel rupture.

Rationale: Intraoperative blood recovery is not recommended from contaminated sites, including the bowel, because of the risk of bacteremia/sepsis.

D. A 75-year-old woman undergoing coronary artery bypass grafting.

Rationale: There is no contraindication to intraoperative blood salvage for this patient.

E. A 34-year-old pregnant woman with placenta previa.

Rationale: The affects of amniotic fluid within salvaged blood are not fully known.

Major points of discussion

■ The use of intraoperative blood recovery may decrease the need for allogeneic transfusions.

■ Blood lost during surgery is collected using low-pressure suction into a collection chamber and can be reinfused during or after the surgery.

■ Citrate is added as an anticoagulant.

■ Unwashed salvaged blood contains free hemoglobin; activated coagulation factors and platelets; cellular debris; other tissue contaminants, including tissue factor; and contaminants from the operative field.

■ Salvaged blood can be washed to decrease the risks associated within reinfusion of free hemoglobin, activated coagulation factors and platelets, and fibrin degradation products. Additionally, surgical field contaminants, including saline and irrigant solutions, are removed.

■ The risks of intraoperative blood recovery are low with infrequent complications, especially when washed salvaged blood is used.

■ The theoretical risks of the introduction of fat, amniotic fluid, and cancer cells into salvaged blood and the effects of such are not known.

- Use of intraoperative blood recovery in highly contaminated areas such as the bowel is not recommended.
- However, the use of intraoperative blood recovery in patients who do not accept allogeneic blood components, such as Jehovah's Witnesses, can be lifesaving despite the risks outlined here.

13. A. Granulocytes are effective only at yields greater than 5×10^6 cells/kg.
Rationale: The minimum effective granulocyte dose is 1×10^{10} cells/kg.
B. Granulocyte yields are greatest after donor stimulation with corticosteroids.
Rationale: Granulocyte yields are greatest after donor stimulation with corticosteroids and granulocyte colony-stimulating factor (G-CSF).
C. Granulocytes should always be leukoreduced.
Rationale: Granulocytes should never be leukoreduced as most granulocytes would be filtered out.
D. Granulocytes should never be irradiated.
Rationale: Granulocytes should always be irradiated because of the risk of transfusion-associated graft-versus-host disease.
E. Granuloctyes should be transfused within 24 hours of collection.
Rationale: According to AABB standards, granulocytes expire 24 hours after collection.

Major points of discussion
- Granulocytes can be prepared from whole blood but are generally collected through apheresis.
- Granulocytes are collected from donors who have been stimulated with corticosteroids to increase the yield.
- Stimulation with G-CSF and corticosteroids further improves the yield; however, G-CSF is not yet approved for donor stimulation and is not routinely used by donor centers.
- Granulocyte yields less than 1×10^{10} cells/kg are generally considered to be ineffective.
- Granulocytes are stored between 20° and 24°C and expire 24 hours after collection.
- Granulocytes are collected using hydroxyethyl starch during apheresis to sediment the RBCs and further separate the RBC and granulocyte layers during centrifugation.
- The final granulocyte product will still contain a significant number of RBCs and should be ABO compatible.
- Granulocytes should be collected from cytomegalovirus (CMV)-negative donors when the recipient is CMV negative to prevent transfusion transmission.
- Transfusing granulocytes through microaggregate or leukoreduction filters is contraindicated.

14. A. The unit must be discarded because of an insufficient volume collected.
Rationale: RBCs can be prepared from the collected whole blood; it does not have to be discarded.
B. The amount of anticoagulant in the collection bag *must* be adjusted.
Rationale: Because the volume collected is greater than 300 mL, the amount of anticoagulant does not have to be adjusted.

C. No additional labeling or processing steps other than standard procedures are required.
Rationale: The unit should be labeled "Red Blood Cells Low Volume."
D. The RBCs from the unit can be used for transfusion, but plasma and platelet components may not.
Rationale: Platelet and plasma components should not be used because of the abnormal anticoagulant/plasma ratio.
E. The unit may be used only for research purposes.
Rationale: The RBCs can be used for transfusion, provided that they are properly labeled.

Major points of discussion
- The AABB standards state that for blood collection, the volume of the collected blood should be proportional to the amount of anticoagulant/preservative solution that is in the collection container.
- In the United States, the volume of blood collected during routine phlebotomy is either 450 mL ± 10% (405 to 495 mL) or 500 mL ± 10% (450 to 550 mL).
- If 300 to 404 mL of whole blood is collected into an anticoagulant volume intended for 450 ± 10%, or if 333 to 449 mL of whole blood is collected into an anticoagulant volume intended for 500 mL ± 10%, RBCs prepared from the unit should be labeled "Red Blood Cells Low Volume."
- No other components should be made from this low-volume collection.
- If the collection volume is less than 300 mL, the amount of anticoagulant must be proportionally decreased.[1]

15. A. 2 weeks.
Rationale: The deferral period after receipt of live attenuated viral and bacterial vaccines for measles (rubeola), mumps, polio (Sabin/oral), typhoid (oral), and yellow fever is 2 weeks.
B. 4 weeks.
Rationale: The deferral period after receipt of live attenuated viral and bacterial vaccines for German measles (rubella) and chickenpox (varicella zoster) is 4 weeks.
C. 21 days.
Rationale: This is the deferral period for recipients of the smallpox vaccine who do not have postvaccination complications.
D. 12 months.
Rationale: This is the deferral period following receipt of unlicensed vaccines.
E. None.
Rationale: This is the deferral period following receipt of toxoids; synthetic or killed viral, bacterial, or rickettsial vaccines (includes hepatitis B vaccine); recombinant vaccines; and intranasal live attenuated flu vaccine.

Major points of discussion
- Blood donor deferral following immunization varies depending on the type of vaccine that is administered.
- Vaccines with no deferral if the donor is symptom-free and afebrile are as follows:
  - Toxoids; or synthetic or killed viral, bacterial, or rickettsial vaccines: anthrax, cholera, diphtheria, hepatitis A, hepatitis B, influenza, Lyme disease, paratyphoid, pertussis, plague, pneumococcal polysaccharide, polio (Salk/injection), rabies, Rocky Mountain spotted fever, tetanus, typhoid (by injection).

● Recombinant vaccine: human papillomavirus.
● Intranasal live attenuated flu vaccine.
■ Live attenuated viral and bacterial vaccines with a 2-week deferral are measles (rubeola), mumps, polio (Sabin/oral), typhoid (oral), and yellow fever.
■ Live attenuated viral and bacterial vaccines with a 4-week deferral are German measles (rubella) and chickenpox (varicella zoster).
■ Unlicensed vaccines have a 12-month deferral unless otherwise indicated by the medical director of the blood collection agency.
■ Deferral for smallpox vaccination according to FDA guidance includes the following:
  ● Donors without vaccine complications should be deferred until after the vaccination scab has separated spontaneously or for 21 days after vaccination, whichever is the later date. If the scab was removed before separating spontaneously, the FDA recommends deferring the donor for 2 months after vaccination.
  ● Donors with vaccine complications should be deferred until 14 days after all vaccination complications have completely resolved.
  ● Symptomatic contacts of recipients of smallpox vaccine should also be deferred based on the following:
    ○ History of localized skin lesions without other symptoms:
      ● If the scab separated spontaneously and is no longer present, the donor does not need to be deferred based on prior exposure to a vaccine recipient;
      ● If the scab was removed, it is recommended that the donor be deferred for 3 months from the date of vaccination of the recipient with whom the contact occurred. If the date is not known but could have been within the past 3 months, it is recommended that the donor be deferred for 2 months from the present time.
    ○ History of complications of vaccinia infection acquired through close contact with a vaccine recipient: Defer until 14 days after all vaccine complications have completely resolved.
  ● Complications of smallpox vaccine include[8]:
    ○ Eczema vaccinatum
    ○ Generalized vaccinia
    ○ Progressive vaccinia
    ○ Postvaccinial encephalitis
    ○ Vaccinial keratitis

16. A. None.
Rationale: Because his period of incarceration (24 hours) was less than 72 consecutive hours, the donor is not deferred based on being in a correctional institution.
B. 4 months.
Rationale: This is the current deferral period for a donor for whom at least one donation has been positive for West Nile virus by nucleic acid amplification testing (NAT).
C. 12 months.
Rationale: This is the deferral period that would have applied to this donor had he been incarcerated for more than 72 consecutive hours.
D. 3 years.
Rationale: This is the deferral period for prospective donors who had a diagnosis of malaria (3 years after becoming

asymptomatic) or who have lived for at least 5 years in a malaria-endemic region (3 years after departure from malaria-endemic area).
E. Permanent.
Rationale: A donor with a confirmed positive test for hepatitis B surface antigen (HBsAg) would be permanently deferred.

Major points of discussion
■ Prospective donors who by report or physical examination are believed to be at increased risk of having an infectious disease are deferred for various periods.
■ Reasons for a permanent deferral from donation: confirmed positive test for HBsAg and use of etretinate (Tegison).
■ Reasons for indefinite deferral:
  ● History of viral hepatitis after the 11th birthday
  ● Repeatedly reactive test for anti-HBc on more than one occasion
  ● Repeatedly reactive test for HTLV on more than one occasion
  ● Present or past clinical laboratory evidence of infection with HIV, hepatitis C virus, or HTLV
  ● History of babesiosis or Chagas disease
  ● Evidence or obvious signs of parenteral drug abuse
  ● Administration of nonprescription drugs using a needle
  ● Risk of variant Creutzfeldt-Jakob disease (as defined in most recent FDA guidance)
■ Reasons for a 3-year deferral include diagnosis of malaria (3 years after becoming asymptomatic) and living for at least 5 years in a malaria-endemic area (3 years after departure from area).
■ Reasons for a 12-month deferral:
  ● Travel to an area where malaria is endemic
  ● Exposure to blood via mucous membranes
  ● Penetration of skin with instrument/object contaminated with blood or body fluids that is not from the donor (includes tattoos or permanent make-up unless applied by a state-regulated entity with sterile needles and ink that has not been reused)
  ● Sexual contact or lived with an individual who has acute or chronic hepatitis B; has symptomatic hepatitis C; or is symptomatic for any other viral hepatitis
  ● Sexual contact with an individual with HIV infection or who is at high risk of HIV infection
  ● Incarceration in a correctional institution for more than 72 consecutive hours
  ● Diagnosis of syphilis or gonorrhea (must have completed treatment)
  ● Reactive screening test positive for syphilis and no confirmatory test was performed
  ● Confirmed positive test for syphilis[1]

17. A. 7 days.
Rationale: Donors who have been taking warfarin are eligible to donate 7 days after their last dose.
B. 14 days.
Rationale: This is the deferral period for donors who have been treated with clopidogrel or ticlopidine.
C. 1 month.
Rationale: This is the deferral period for donors who have been treated with finasteride or isotretinoin.
D. 6 months.

Rationale: This is the deferral period for donors who have been treated with dutasteride.
E. Permanently.
Rationale: This is the deferral period for donors who have been treated with etretinate.

Major points of discussion

- The blood donation deferral period for prospective donors varies based on the medication being considered:
  - Permanent deferral: etretinate.
  - Indefinite deferral: bovine insulin manufactured in the United Kingdom (bovine spongiform encephalopathy risk).
- Deferral for 3 years after last dose: acitretin.
- Deferral for 12 months after last dose: hepatitis B immune globulin.
- Deferral for 6 months after last dose: dutasteride.
- Deferral for 1 month after last dose: finasteride and isotretinoin.
- Donors who are taking medications that irreversibly inhibit platelet function should not be used as the sole source of platelets.
- Antiplatelet agents:
  - Aspirin and piroxicam: defer for 2 full days after last dose.
  - Clopidogrel and ticlopidine: defer for 14 days after last dose.
- Warfarin: defer for 7 days after the last dose.[1]

18. A. 1°C to 10°C.
Rationale: Temperature at which the RBCs should be maintained during transportation.
B. 1°C to 6°C.
Rationale: Temperature at which the RBCs should be stored while in the blood bank.
C. 20°C to 24°C.
Rationale: Temperature at which platelets should be stored and transported.
D. –18°C or less.
Rationale: Temperature at which cryoprecipitate and plasma are stored.
E. 30°C to 37°C.
Rationale: Temperature at which cryoprecipitate and plasma are thawed.

Major points of discussion

- AABB standards provide criteria for the reissue of blood, blood components, tissue, and derivatives that have been returned to the blood bank or transfusion service.
- The container closure should not be disturbed.
- The appropriate temperature should be maintained and this temperature will vary based on the type of product.
- For RBC components, at least one sealed segment of continuous donor tubing should have remained attached to the container. Removed segments can be reattached only after ensuring that the tubing identification numbers on the removed segments and container are identical.
- It is recorded that the product was inspected and is acceptable for reissue.[1]

19. A. 2 days.
Rationale: This is the interval between procedures for platelet donors.

B. 3 days.
Rationale: This is the time period between the last autologous donation and anticipated time of transfusion as defined by the AABB standards.
C. 28 days.
Rationale: This is the minimum period that must lapse between plasmapheresis collections for "infrequent" plasma donors.
D. 56 days.
Rationale: This is the deferral period following donation of a unit of whole blood.
E. 112 days.
Rationale: This is the deferral period following 2-U RBC apheresis donation.

Major points of discussion

- The requirements for autologous blood donation are not as strict as for allogeneic donation.
- Autologous donation requires an order from the patient's physician.
- The autologous donor should have hemoglobin 11 g/dL or greater or hematocrit 33% or greater.
- All autologous collections should be completed more than 72 hours (3 days) before the time of anticipated surgery or transfusion.
- The unit should be reserved only for autologous transfusion.
- In contrast to units collected for autologous transfusion, directed donor units can be transferred to the general inventory if not used.
- An autologous donor should be deferred if he or she has a medical condition for which there is a risk of bacteremia.

BLOOD BANK REGULATIONS

20. A. "No history of transfusion or pregnancy in the past 90 days."
Rationale: If the history of no transfusion or pregnancy during the past 3 months (90 days) is certain, the risk of new alloantibody formation is low.
B. "Patient has a history of a negative antibody screen."
Rationale: This statement does not indicate that the patient has not been pregnant or had a transfusion in the past 3 months (90 days).
C. "No history of transfusion or pregnancy in the past 30 days."
Rationale: The requirement is that there has not been pregnancy or transfusion for 3 months (90 days), not 1 month (30 days).
D. "Pregnancy and transfusion history unknown."
Rationale: When the pregnancy and transfusion history are unknown, the sample for pretransfusion testing must not be older than 3 days at the time of intended transfusion.
E. "Patient is older than 40 years of age."
Rationale: The age of the patient is not important in determining the expiration date of the type and screen.

Major points of discussion

- For pretransfusion testing, if there is a history of pregnancy or transfusion within the past 3 months, or if the pregnancy or transfusion histories are uncertain, the sample used for testing cannot be more than 3 days old at the time of intended transfusion. The rationale is that recent transfusion or pregnancy can cause production of unexpected RBC antibodies.

- Historically, the selection of 3 days as the expiration interval was arbitrary.
- The day of collection of the sample is counted as day zero.
- There is no requirement for a pretransfusion sample to be less than 3 days old for patients who have not been pregnant or had transfusions in the past 3 months (90 days).
- If the history of no transfusion or pregnancy over the past 3 months is certain, the length of time a pretransfusion sample is valid for testing is determined based on the manufacturer's instructions for sample acceptability for the test being performed.

21. A. A sample labeled at the nursing station with a label containing the patient's full name, hospital identification number, date of collection, and the phlebotomist's initials.
Rationale: The sample should be labeled at the patient's bedside.
B. A sample labeled at the patient's bedside with a label containing the patient's full name, hospital identification number, date of collection, and the phlebotomist's initials.
Rationale: This sample was labeled at the patient's bedside, has two unique patient identifiers, indicates the date the sample was collected, and identifies the phlebotomist.
C. A sample labeled at the patient's bedside with a label containing the hospital identification number, patient diagnosis, phlebotomist's initials, and date of collection.
Rationale: This sample does not have two unique patient identifiers.
D. A sample labeled at the patient's bedside with a label containing the patient's full name, hospital identification number, patient's location, and the date of collection
Rationale: The phlebotomist for this sample is not identified.
E. A sample labeled at the patient's beside with a label containing the patient's full name, hospital identification number, the phlebotomist's initials, and patient's date of birth.
Rationale: The date of collection is not indicated.

Major points of discussion
- Blood samples for pretransfusion testing must be labeled with enough information to provide unique identification of the patient from whom the blood is drawn.
- Two independent, unique identifiers (name, date of birth, medical record number) should be used.
- Completed labels should be attached to the specimen tube at the patient's bedside after the specimen is collected.
- A procedure must be established to identify the date the sample was collected, as well as the individual who collected the specimen from the patient.
- The transfusion service should only accept specimens that are fully and legibly labeled.
- Upon receipt of a specimen for pretransfusion testing, the transfusion service should confirm that identifying information on the specimen label is in agreement with identifying information on the request for testing. If the information does not agree or, if there are doubts, a new sample should be obtained.
- The patient sample and a segment from red cell–containing components are to be retained by the transfusion service in the refrigerator for at least 7 days after transfusion.

22. A. The patient has a history of an anti-K antibody, which is currently not detected, and no new clinically significant antibodies.
Rationale: For a computer crossmatch to be used, there must not be a history of clinically significant antibodies.
B. A warm autoantibody of unknown clinical significance is currently detected and underlying alloantibodies have been ruled out.
Rationale: For a computer crossmatch to be used, the current antibody screen must be negative.
C. The patient has no history of alloantibodies or autoantibodies and the antibody screen is currently negative.
Rationale: It is acceptable to omit the IS or AHG crossmatches and use a computer crossmatch if the current antibody screen is negative for clinically significant antibodies and there is no history of clinically significant antibodies.
D. The patient has a newly positive antibody screen and the antibody has been identified as anti-RhD due to passive transfer from Rh immune globulin.
Rationale: Although the positive antibody screen is due to passive transfer of antibodies, a computer crossmatch cannot be used.
E. The patient has no history of clinically significant antibodies and currently an anti-E antibody has been indentified.
Rationale: The current antibody screen is positive; therefore, a computer crossmatch cannot be used.

Major points of discussion
- Before issuing an RBC unit, either a serologic or computer crossmatch must be performed. A serologic crossmatch consists of testing a sample of the recipient's serum or plasma against a sample of donor RBCs from an attached segment on the donor unit to determine if there is ABO compatibility and clinically significant antibodies to RBC antigens present on donor cells.
- The serologic methods used for crossmatch include the IS or AHG crossmatch.
- AHG crossmatch must be performed for patients with a positive antibody screen or a history of a clinically significant antibody.
- A computerized crossmatching system or IS crossmatch may be used for patients with a negative antibody screen and no history of clinically significant antibodies.
- For a computer system to be used to detect ABO incompatibility, it must meet several requirements:
  - The computer system must be validated on site to ensure only ABO-compatible whole blood or RBC components have been selected.
  - Two determinations of the recipient's ABO group are made, one on a current sample and the second by the one of the following methods: (1) retesting the same sample, (2) testing a second current sample, (3) comparison with previous records.
  - The computer system contains the unit number, component name, ABO group and Rh type of the component; confirmed donor unit ABO group; two unique recipient identifiers; recipient's ABO group, Rh type and antibody screen results; and interpretation of compatibility.
  - A method exists to verify correct entry of data before the release of blood or blood components.

- The computer system contains logic to alert the user to discrepancies between the donor ABO group and Rh type on the unit label and those determined by blood group confirmatory tests, as well as to alert the user to ABO incompatibility between the recipient and donor unit.

23. A. Confirmatory Rh-typing of Rh-positive units.
Rationale: Confirmatory Rh-typing of Rh-negative units is required, not Rh-positive units.
B. Confirmatory ABO typing of only group O RBC components.
Rationale: Confirmatory ABO typing must be done on *all* RBC components.
C. Confirmatory testing for weak D.
Rationale: Weak D testing, if necessary, is performed at the time of donation and there is no requirement to confirm at the transfusion service.
D. Direct antiglobulin testing.
Rationale: Direct antiglobulin testing of donor units is not performed before transfusion.
E. Confirmatory ABO typing of all RBC components.
Rationale: Confirmatory ABO typing is performed as a measure to prevent transfusion of ABO-incompatible RBCs.

Major points of discussion
- The ABO group of all RBC units and the Rh-type of RBC units labeled as Rh-negative must be confirmed using a serologic test by the transfusing facility. The purpose of these measures is to prevent the transfusion of mislabeled, ABO- and Rh-incompatible RBCs.
- Confirmatory testing is performed on a sample from an attached segment. The unit itself is not entered.
- Confirmatory testing for weak D is not required.
- Discrepancies must be resolved before the unit can be issued.
- The facility that collected blood with discrepant results should be notified.

24. A. Increased ability to transfer blood components between different facilities.
Rationale: The ISBT 128 standard does not address the transfer of blood components between facilities.
B. Faster processing of different blood components.
Rationale: The ISBT 128 standard does not affect the speed of processing or manufacturing.
C. Uniformity of labeling allowing better traceability of blood components.
Rationale: The ISBT 128 standard is a uniform international system of labeling.
D. Improved use of autologous or directed donations.
Rationale: ISBT does not affect blood component use.
E. Allows for use of a computerized crossmatch for all transfusions.
Rationale: A full crossmatch is required for all patients with a history of alloantibodies to red cell antigens.

Major points of discussion
- The ISBT 128 standard is an international FDA-approved uniform bar code labeling system.
- The AABB required that all institutions implement the ISBT 128 standard by May 1, 2008.

- The ISBT 128 standatd allows for improved traceability and transfer of components between institutions though uniformity of labeling and improved bar coding.
- The ISBT 128 standard allows for improved traceability, auditing, and inventorying of blood components within institutions.
- The ISBT 128 standard allows for more detailed encoding of information regarding each individual component.

25. A. Quality assurance.
Rationale: Quality assurance activities do not involve performance of a process.
B. Quality control.
Rationale: The outcome of this process gives information about whether the product should be issued.
C. Quality management.
Rationale: The means by which the goals of a quality program are met.
D. Quality indicator.
Rationale: Used to track progress and attainment of quality goals.
E. Quality improvement.
Rationale: Used to achieve higher levels of performance.

Major points of discussion
- The goal of quality assurance (QA) is to ensure that a blood product meets defined standards and requirements. QA activities include record reviews, quality indicator monitoring, and internal assessments.
- Quality control (QC) activities provide feedback to staff to let them know that they should continue because conditions are acceptable or if the process should be stopped because something is wrong. Examples of QC activities are reagent QC, visual inspections, clerical checks, measurements of parameters of blood components including cell counts and volume, and equipment monitoring.
- Quality management (QM) includes the processes, procedures, and overall structure that ensure that the goals of an organization's quality program are met. QM includes strategic planning, quality planning, implementation, evaluation, and resource allocation.
- Quality indicators are used to track progress toward quality goals and objectives.
- Quality improvements are the means by which higher levels of performance are reached by an organization by removing existing deficiencies in the process, product, or service or through creating better features that add value.

26. **A. 20°C to 24°C, 6 hours.**
Rationale: These are the conditions for unpooled thawed single units.
B. 20°C to 24°C, 4 hours.
Rationale: These are the conditions for pooled units (open system).
C. 30°C to 37°C, 30 minutes.
Rationale: The product is thawed at 30°C to 37°C but stored at 20°C to 24°C.
D. 1°C to 6°C, 24 hours.
Rationale: These are the conditions for plasma frozen within 8 or 24 hours (after thawing).
E. 1°C to 6°C, 5 days.
Rationale: This is the regulation for storage of thawed plasma.

Major points of discussion

- Cryoprecipitate is made by thawing FFP at 1°C to 6°C, collecting the cryoprecipitate, and freezing it at –18°C or less within 1 hour.
- When stored at –18°C or less, the expiration of cryoprecipitate is 12 months from the date of original collection.
- Before issue, the frozen cryoprecipitate is thawed at 37°C, and if unpooled (single unit, closed system), should be stored at 20°C to 24°C for up to 6 hours.
- If multiple units of cryoprecipitate are pooled (open system) after thawing, the product should be stored at 20°C to 24°C for up to 4 hours.
- If Rh-positive and Rh-negative units are pooled together, the pooled unit should be labels as "Rh positive" or "pooled Rh."

IMMUNOHEMATOLOGY

27. A. Anti-k.
    B. Warm autoantibody.
    Rationale: The autocontrol would be expected to be positive in the presence of a warm autoantibody behaving as a panagglutinin. In addition, warm autoantibodies are typically of the IgG isotype and are unlikely to cause agglutination of screening cells at "Immediate Spin."
    C. Anti-H.
    Rationale: The patient's red cells do not react with *U. europaeus* lectin, suggesting that the patient's red cells do not express the H antigen and, therefore, the patient expresses the Bombay O_h phenotype.
    D. Anti-Fy3.
    Rationale: This is a rare antibody that reacts with all red cells except those with the Fy(a–b–) phenotype. Since there are Fy(a–b–) cells present on the antibody panel in the tables, antibodies against Fy3 are ruled out.
    E. Anti-Kp^b.
    Rationale for A and E: k and Kp^b are high-prevalence antigens of the Kell blood group system that are sensitive to DTT; thus, pretreatment of panel red cells with DTT would be expected to decrease the reactivity with the patient's plasma.

Major points of discussion

- There are two different fucosyltransferase enzymes (FUT1 and FUT2) that are capable of synthesizing the H antigen. FUT1 (H gene) is responsible for synthesizing the H antigen on type 2 oligosaccharide chains found on red cell glycoproteins and glycolipids. FUT2 (Secretor gene) is responsible for synthesizing H-and Le^b antigens on type 1 oligosaccharide chains found on mucins in secretions and on glycolipids in plasma and on red cells.
- Bombay O_h individuals are homozygous for nonfunctional H (*hh*) and secretor (*sese*) genes. The anti-H produced by these individuals is predominantly of the IgM isotype and can cause clinically significant acute hemolytic transfusion reactions.
- The amount of H antigen on red cells is greatest on O RBCs and least on A1B RBCs.

- The extracellular domain of the glycoprotein expressing Kell antigens is extensively folded by disulfide bonding; thus, Kell antigens are sensitive to DTT.
- Unlike Fy^a and Fy^b, the Fy3 epitope is protease resistant.

28. A. 2%.
    Rationale: This is the approximate probability that a random donor unit is compatible for a patient with an anti-e antibody.
    B. 23%.
    Rationale: This patient has an antibody against Jk^b and K. The prevalence of Jk^b-negative individuals is approximately 25% and of K-negative individuals is approximately 90%. Thus, the probability that a random donor unit will be compatible with these two antibodies is equal to the multiplication of the respective prevalences or $0.25 \times 0.90 = 0.23$, or 23%.
    C. 50%.
    Rationale: This is the approximate probability that a random donor unit is compatible for a patient with an anti-S antibody.
    D. 85%.
    Rationale: This is the approximate probability that a random donor unit is compatible for a patient with an anti-D antibody.
    E. 91%.
    Rationale: This is the approximate probability that a random donor unit is compatible for a patient with an anti-K antibody.

Table 19-42

Antigen	Percent Compatible
D	15
C	30
c	20
E	70
e	02
K	91
k	<0.1
Fy^a	35
Fy^b	20
Jk^a	25
Jk^b	25
M	20
N	25
S	50
s	10

Major points of discussion

- To calculate the number of units that need to be screened to find *n* compatible units, divide *n* by the probability of finding one compatible unit. For example, 44 U RBCs will have to be screened to find 10 compatible units for this patient (10/0.23 = 44).
- Most RhD-negative individuals are also negative for the C and E antigens (ce/ce phenotype); thus, RhD-negative units will typically be compatible with patients who have an anti-C or anti-E in plasma.
- To calculate the probability that a random donor unit is compatible for a patient with multiple

alloantibodies, multiply the probability of compatibility for each antigen for which the patient has an antibody against.

- Table 19-42 shows the approximate probability that a random donor unit is compatible (i.e., the probability that the donor unit is antigen-negative).
- Enzymes such as ficin and papain **DiMiNish** expression of Duffy, M, and N antigens, enhance expression of Rh and Kidd antigens, and do not affect K antigens.[12]

29. A. Rh positive with an anti-D autoantibody.
Rationale: Autoantibodies with strictly anti-D specificity are not typically observed.
B. Partial D phenotype with an anti-D autoantibody
Rationale: Individuals with a partial D phenotype can make alloantibodies to the part of the D antigen they do not express. Thus, these antibodies would be alloantibodies, not autoantibodies.
C. Rh positive with an anti-D alloantibody.
Rationale: Rh-positive individuals do not make anti-D alloantibodies.
D. Partial D phenotype with an anti-D alloantibody.
Rationale: The presence of an anti-D antibody implies that the patient is a partial D and has made an alloantibody to the part of the D antigen she does not express.
E. Weak D phenotype with an anti-D alloantibody.
Rationale: Patients who are weak D are not expected to make anti-D alloantibodies.

Major points of discussion
- The patient's red cells react with anti-D only when antihuman globulin is added, suggesting that the patient is either a weak D or a partial D. The patient is not Rh positive.
- Many partial D phenotypes are due to hybrid genes in which parts of *RHD* are replaced by *RHCE*.
- The vast majority of D-negative individuals have a deletion of the *RHD* gene.
- *RHD* and *RHCE* are in close physical proximity on the chromosome and are 97% identical.
- The Rh haplotype influences the level of D antigen expression with more D expressed on red cells lacking the C antigen.
- Donor blood must be tested for weak D and must be labeled Rh positive if the test is positive. This is done to avoid immunizing Rh-negative recipients with weak D red cells.

30. A. Group O plasma and group B platelets.
B. Group A plasma and group AB platelets.
C. Group AB plasma and group A platelets.
Rationale: Neither group AB nor B plasma contains B antibodies and would be compatible with this patient. Platelets do not have to be ABO matched.
D. Group O plasma and group A platelets.
Rationale for A and D: Group O plasma contains antibodies to the B antigen on the patient's red cells.
E. Group A plasma and group B platelets.
Rationale for B and E: Group A plasma contains antibodies to the B antigen on the patient's red cells.

Major points of discussion
- ABO compatible platelets should be provided when possible. ABO-incompatible platelets may be cleared from the circulation at a faster rate. Rarely, high-titer anti-A or anti-B antibodies present in the plasma of platelet units are responsible for acute hemolytic transfusion reactions.
- Anti-A and anti-B antibodies of the IgM isotype are predominant in individuals who are blood group B and A, respectively. IgG is the major isotype in group O individuals. Group O individuals can make anti-A, anti-B, and anti-A,B antibodies.
- Group O red cells are the universal donor cells and AB plasma is the universal donor plasma component. Thus, O red cells and AB plasma are typically in the most limited supply.
- ABO antigens are also present on platelets, leukocytes, and endothelial cells. Thus, ABO-incompatible solid organ transplants can result in hyperacute rejection.
- Reverse- or back-typing is not necessary in infants less than 4 months of age, because anti-A and anti-B antibodies do not develop until 3 to 6 months of age.

31. A. AB and A.
B. AB and B.
C. AB and AB.
Rationale: Because A and B are dominant to O, if one parent is group AB, there cannot be children who are group O.
D. A and B.
E. None; nonpaternity.
Rationale: If each parent is heterozygous (AO and BO), then there is a 25% chance of having a child with each of the four blood groups (A, B, O, and AB).

Major points of discussion
- The ABO, H, Lewis, I, and P blood group systems are carbohydrate antigen systems present on glycoproteins and glycolipids on the red cell membrane.
- Enzymes known as glycosyltransferases are responsible for adding specific sugars to specific oligosaccharide chains on glycolipids and glycoproteins.
- The Bombay phenotype results from absence of the H antigen. This can be detected by type O individuals who have absent reactivity with the anti-H lectin, *U. europaeus*.
- Subgroups of A and B exist that differ both quantitatively and qualitatively. The most common subgroups of A are A1 and A2 and they can be differentiated with the lectin *Dolichos biflorus*. A2 individuals can make anti-A1 antibodies.
- The H antigen is synthesized by fucosyltransferases (FUT). FUT1 (H gene) fucosylates type 2 chain oligosaccharides to form the type 2 chain H. FUT2 (Secretor gene) fucosylates type 1 chain oligosaccharides to form the type 1 chain H and Le[b].

32. **A. I.**
B. i.
Rationale: Autoantibodies to the I antigen are common and are associated with *Mycoplasma* infections. Autoantibodies to the i antigen are uncommon and are associated with infectious mononucleosis. These are typically IgM

antibodies that can fix complement and cause cold autoimmune hemolytic anemia.

C. P.

Rationale: The P antigen is a high-frequency antigen associated with paroxysmal cold hemoglobinuria (PCH).

D. Le^a.

Rationale: Antibodies against the Le^a antigen are generally naturally occurring and of IgM isotype but are generally not considered clinically significant.

E. A.

Rationale: Antibodies against the A antigen are naturally occuring and are found in people who are blood group O or B but not blood group A or AB. Anti-A antibodies do not cause autoimmune hemolytic anemia.

Major points of discussion

- The I gene codes for a glycosyltransferase enzyme that converts the linear i antigen into the branched I antigen.
- Adults have increased I antigen with reciprocal decreased i antigen; thus, plasma containing anti-I typically shows weaker or no agglutination with cord RBCs.
- Cold autoantibodies may interfere with blood typing, resulting in ABO typing discrepancies.
- Cold autoadsorption of serum can be performed to remove strong cold autoantibodies that interfere with testing.
- The Donath-Landsteiner test is used to demonstrate an anti-P autoantibody present in PCH.

33. A. White.

B. Black.

Rationale: Depending on geographic location, approximately two thirds of blacks have the Fy(a–b–) Duffy antigen phenotype.

C. Asian/Pacific Islander.

D. Native American.

E. Inuit.

Rationale for A, C, D, and E: The Fy(a–b–) Duffy antigen phenotype is rare in whites, Asians, Native Ameicans, and Inuits.

Major points of discussion

- The Duffy antigen is a receptor for *Plasmodium vivax*; thus, the Fy(a–b–) Duffy antigen phenotype confers protection in areas where *P. vivax* is endemic.
- The mutation resulting in the Fy(a–b–) Duffy antigen phenotype found in blacks disrupts the binding site for the erythroid-specific GATA-1 transcription factor; thus, Duffy is expressed in other tissues but not on red cells. Furthermore, the Fy^b antigen is typically encoded by this gene, so these individuals do not make anti-Fy^b.
- Anti-Fy3 antibodies can be made in rare individuals who have an inactivating mutation in the *DARC* gene (which encodes Duffy) and lack Duffy expression on red cells and in tissues.
- Fy^a and Fy^b antigens on red cells are susceptible to proteases such as ficin and papain; however, Fy3 is not.
- Anti-Fy^a antibodies are more common than anti-Fy^b antibodies; however, both can cause acute or delayed hemolytic transfusion reactions and hemolytic disease of the fetus and newborn.

34. A. Rh.

B. Kell.

Rationale: Expression of Kell antigens on red cells is unaffected by enzyme treatment.

C. Duffy.

Rationale: Expression of Duffy antigens (Fy^a and Fy^b) on red cells is destroyed by enzyme treatment.

D. Lewis.

E. Kidd.

Rationale for A, D, and E: Expression of Rh, Lewis (Le^a and Le^b), or Kidd (Jk^a and Jk^b) antigens on red cells is enhanced by enzyme treatment.

Major points of discussion

- Although ficin and papain destroy the Fy^a and Fy^b antigens, Fy3 is resistant to enzyme treatment.
- The Duffy antigen is also known as the Duffy Antigen Receptor for Chemokines (DARC), because it is a receptor for a variety of chemokines. It is also a receptor for *P. vivax*.
- People of African descent who are Fy(a–b–) typically express the Duffy antigen in tissues, just not on red cells.
- Fy(a–b–) is very common in people of African descent but rare in Caucasians.
- Anti-Fy3 antibodies react with all red cells, except those that are Fy(a–b–).

35. A. P1.

Rationale: Anti-P1 is a commonly encountered, naturally occurring IgM antibody; thus, it does not cross the placenta and cause hemolytic disease of the fetus and newborn.

B. i.

Rationale: Anti-i is an uncommon cold agglutinin and is primarily of IgM isotype. Although fetal red cells express i antigens, these antibodies do not cross the placenta and are not associated with hemolytic disease of the fetus and newborn.

C. I.

Rationale: Anti-I is a naturally occurring antibody associated with cold agglutinin disease and typically of IgM isotype. In addition, I antigens are poorly expressed on fetal red cells; thus, anti-I antibodies are not associated with hemolytic disease of the fetus and newborn.

D. S.

Rationale: Anti-S antibodies are typically IgG antibodies that can cross the placenta and have been implicated in severe and fatal cases of hemolytic disease of the fetus and newborn.

E. Lea.

Rationale: Lewis antibodies are naturally occurring antibodies and are typically of IgM isotype; thus, they do not cross the placenta. In addition, Lewis antigens are not expressed on fetal red cells; thus, anti-Lewis antibodies are not associated with hemolytic disease of the fetus and newborn.

Major points of discussion

- Because the I antigen is poorly expressed on cord RBCs, cord cells are used for testing for the presence of anti-I antigen. If an anti-I antibody is present, there should be no reaction when the serum is reacted with cord cells.

- Lewis blood group antigens are glycosphingolipids that are passively adsorbed onto red cell membranes; they are not synthesized by red cells.
- Antibodies to the Kell antigen cause hemolytic disease of the fetus and newborn but also suppress fetal erythropoiesis.
- Historically, hemolytic disease of the fetus and newborn due to anti-D was very common; however, with the use of Rh immune globulin, the incidence due to anti-D has been greatly reduced and now ABO hemolytic disease of the fetus and newborn is the most common cause.
- Group O mothers typically have the highest titers of IgG anti-A and anti-B antibodies; thus, group A and B infants born to group O mothers are expected to have the most severe disease.

36. **A. Cysteine residues.**
    Rationale: Sulfhydryl reagents reduce disulfide bonds to produce free sulfhydryl (–SH) groups. There are multiple disulfide bonds between cysteine residues in the extracellular domain of the Kell antigen.
    B. N- and/or O-glycans.
    Rationale: Glycans are carbohydrate chains that are attached to certain amino acids such as asparagine (N-glycans) and serine/threonine (O-glycans). These structures are not affected by sulfhydryl reagents.
    C. Zinc binding site.
    Rationale: Although the Kell antigen has a zinc binding site, it is not affected by sulfhydryl reagents.
    D. Kx antigen.
    Rationale: Absence of the Xk protein, which carries the Kx antigen, leads to weakened Kell expression and the McLeod syndrome. Although Xk and Kell form a complex linked by a single disulfide bond, the Kx antigen is not the sulfhydryl reagent–sensitive structure that is important for Kell antigen stability.
    E. Dombrock antigen.
    Rationale: The Dombrock blood group system is distinct from Kell and not responsible for Kell stability.

Major points of discussion
- ZZAP contains both proteases and DTT, so it destroys both Kell antigens and other antigens sensitive to proteases.
- The McLeod syndrome results from deletion of a part of the X chromosome that includes the *XK* gene. It may also result in deletion of the region on chromosome X responsible for causing chronic granulomatous disease (CGD).
- The McLeod syndrome is an X-linked disorder associated with acanthocytosis and other cardiac, neurologic, muscular, and psychiatric symptoms.
- The K antigen of the Kell blood group system has a relatively low prevalence of less than 10%. The antithetical antigen, k (cellano), has high prevalence in all populations.
- Kell antigens are resistant to enzymes such as ficin and papain.
- Other antigens in the Kell blood group system include Kp^a, Kp^b, Js^a, and Js^b.

37. A. Le(a+b–).
    B. Le(a+b+).

Rationale: Individuals who are Le(a+b+) or Le(a+b–) express the Le^a antigen so would not produce anti-Le^a antibodies.
C. Le(a–b+).
Rationale: Individuals who are Le(a–b+) also make a small amount of Le^a antigen so would not produce anti-Le^a antibodies.
D. Le(a–b–).
Rationale: Only individuals who are Le(a–b–) can produce anti-Le^a antibodies.

Major points of discussion
- Pregnant women who are LeLe or Lele often have decreased levels of Lewis antigens on their red cells, some of whom transiently type as Le(a–b–).
- Because of a developmental delay in full expression of Lewis antigens on red cells, neonates type as Le(a–b–).
- Antibodies against Lewis antigens are usually naturally occurring IgM antibodies.
- Individuals who are Le(a+b–) rarely make anti-Le^b antibodies.
- Lewis antibodies are generally cold reactive and are not considered clinically significant.

38. A. En^a.
    Rationale: Antibodies to En^a may be made by very rare individuals who lack all or part of glycophorin A (which encodes the M and N antigens). Although very rare, these antibodies have caused severe hemolytic transfusion reactions and hemolytic disease of the fetus and newborn and should not be ignored.
    B. M.
    Rationale: Anti-M is a naturally occurring antibody that is typically not active at 37°C and is not considered clinically significant in most cases. It is generally ignored in transfusion practice unless it is active at 37°C.
    C. S.
    D. s.
    Rationale: Anti-s and anti-S are clinically significant IgG antibodies.
    E. U.
    Rationale: Relatively rare individuals who lack a region of glycophorin B (which encodes S and s) lack the high-prevalence U antigen. Anti-U antibodies are clinically significant.

Major points of discussion
- M and N are antithetical antigens found on glycophorin A (GPA).
- S and s are antithetical antigens found on glycophorin B (GPB).
- GPA is restricted to cells of erythroid origin; thus, it is commonly used as an erythroid marker.
- Lack of the high-prevalence U antigen is more common in people of African descent.
- On a red cell antibody panel, antibodies against the U or En^a antigens would react with all of the panel red cells. These are high-prevalence antigens and compatible blood is difficult to find.
- Anti-N is also a rare naturally occurring antibody that is typically not active at 37°C and is not considered clinically significant in most cases. It is generally ignored in transfusion practice unless it is active at 37°C.

39. A. D.
Rationale: Approximately 85% of random RBCs are D antigen positive.
B. C.
Rationale: Approximately 70% of random RBCs are C antigen positive.
C. c.
Rationale: Approximately 80% of random RBCs are c antigen positive.
D. E.
Rationale: Approximately 30% of random RBCs are E antigen positive.
E. e.
Rationale: Approximately 98% of random RBCs are e antigen positive.

Major points of discussion
- The most common Rh-negative Fisher-Race haplotype is ce.
- The most common Rh-positive Fisher-Race haplotype in whites is DCe and in blacks is Dce.
- Notice that all of the common haplotypes described above include e, which is the highest-frequency antigen found in the Rh system.
- One gene codes for the D antigen and a second gene codes for the CE antigens.
- The frequency of the Rh antigens varies by race/ethnicity (for example, RhD-positive is more common in Asian populations).

40. A. R_1/r.
Rationale: This represents the genotype DCe/dce.
B. R_2/r.
Rationale: This represents the genotype DcE/dce.
C. R_1/r'.
Rationale: This represents the genotype DCe/dCe.
D. R_z/r'.
Rationale: This represents the genotype DCE/dCe.
E. R_0/r.
Rationale: This represents the genotype Dce/dce.

Major points of discussion
- Rh nomenclature includes both the Weiner and the Fisher-Race systems.
- Weiner terminology allows for the description of the genes present on each chromosome separately.
- A capital R is used to indicate that D is present and a lowercase r is used to indicate that D is absent. The addition of numbers or letters indicates the presence of the C/c genes and the E/e genes.
- R_0 and r are used to indicate that ce is present: designated Dce and dce, respectively. R_1 or r' indicates that C is present: designated DCe and dCe, respectively. R_2 or r'' is used to indicate that E is present: designated DcE and dce, respectively. R_z and r^y are used to indicate that CE is present: designated DCE and dCE, respectively.
- The most common Rh-negative Wiener haplotype is r.
- The most common Rh-positive Wiener haplotype in whites is R_1 and in blacks is R_0.
- When performing panel testing for patients with anti-D, it is difficult to rule out antibodies to the C and E antigens because the Wiener genotypes r'/r' and r''/r'' are rare and are typically not present as panel cells.

- Treatment of red cells with enzymes such as ficin or papain enhance expression of Rh antigens.
- D is the most immunogenic Rh antigen.

41. A. Acute intravascular hemolysis.
Rationale: The antibody screen is negative; thus, if there is hemolysis, it would be a delayed hemolytic transfusion reaction.
B. Increased risk of a febrile transfusion reaction.
C. Inability to receive future RBC transfusions.
Rationale: Although RhD is highly immunogenic, this patient may not develop an anti-D antibody. Furthermore, if an antibody is produced, the patient would still be able to receive compatible RhD-negative blood.
D. Anaphylactic reaction due to naturally occurring IgE antibodies to the RhD antigen.
Rationale for B and D: There is minimal risk of an acute reaction to RhD-positive blood in an RhD-negative individual.
E. Potential alloimmunization to RhD.
Rationale: RhD is the most immunogenic red cell antigen; thus, the biggest concern in this situation is alloimunization to RhD with the potential of a subsequent delayed hemolytic transfusion reaction.

Major points of discussion
- Approximately 15% of the population is RhD negative. Most of these individuals will also have the phenotype rr (based on the modified Weiner terminology) or ce/ce.
- Patients with sickle cell disease treated with long-term transfusions frequently have transfusion with phenotypically matched blood to prevent alloimmunization. However, there are no standard guidelines for whether to transfuse phenotypically matched red cells in antibody screen–negative patients and, if so, which antigens to match for (e.g., many centers match only for Rh and Kell).
- Recipients with weak D type may, in fact, be partial D. Thus, a weak D patient should be transfused with RhD-negative blood.
- Rh immunoglobulin given during pregnancy to RhD-negative women and within 72 hours of delivery can prevent most cases of alloimmunization to RhD.
- If the RhD-negative platelet supply is limited, RhD-positive platelets may be given to an RhD-negative patient. Platelets do not express the Rh antigen, but there may be a small amount of red cells contaminating the platelet unit. Thus, one dose of Rh immunoglobulin can be given in these situations to prevent alloimmunization.
- One 300-μg dose of Rh immunoglobulin covers 15 mL of RBCs (30 mL of whole blood).

42. A. Diego.
Rationale: The antigens of the Diego blood group system are located on band 3, a major red cell membrane glycoprotein.
B. Cartwright.
Rationale: Also known as the Yt system, Yt^a and Yt^b are antithetical antigens on acetylcholinesterase, a GPI-linked enzyme found on red cell membranes.
C. Colton.
Rationale: The Colton blood group antigens are expressed on aquaporin-1, a water channel on red cell membranes.

D. Dombrock.
Rationale: The Dombrock blood group system is composed of five antigens. Of these, antibodies to Do[a] and Do[b] have been implicated in acute and delayed hemolytic transfusion reactions.
E. Cost.
Rationale: Although Cost antigens are present on red cells, they are not considered part of a blood group system; rather they are considered part of a blood group collection (the Cost collection).

Major points of discussion

- A blood group *system* consists of one or more antigens controlled at a single gene locus, or by two or more very closely linked homologous genes with little or no observable recombination between them.
- There are currently 31 blood group antigen systems.
- Some antigens are low-prevalence antigens with a very low frequency in the population. Although these antigens may not be detected on antibody panels (because they are so rare that they are not present on most antibody panels), potential transfusion reactions can be avoided by performing a full crossmatch before release of the blood product.
- Band 3 is a red cell anion exchanger and is important for attachment of the red cell membrane to the cytoskeleton.
- Because acetylcholinesterase is a GPI-linked protein, expression of the Cartwright antigens is absent or decreased on red cells from patients with PCH.[10]

43. A. Delayed serologic transfusion reaction.
Rationale: A positive DAT with a red cell alloantibody identified in the eluate in the absence of laboratory evidence of hemolysis would suggest a delayed serologic transfusion reaction.
B. Delayed hemolytic transfusion reaction.
Rationale: A positive DAT with a red cell alloantibody identified in the eluate and laboratory evidence of hemolysis would suggest a delayed hemolytic transfusion reaction.
C. Drug-induced hemolytic anemia.
Rationale: There is no medication history and no evidence of hemolysis in the case presented.
D. Nonspecific uptake of immunoglobulin.
Rationale: Many patients have positive DATs with negative eluates. Most are not clinically significant, and it is not useful to pursue this workup. A history of hepatitis C may suggest the presence of cirrhosis and a "polyclonal gammopathy" with nonspecific uptake of these immunoglobulins.
E. Laboratory analytical error.
Rationale: Errors are always a possibility in laboratory testing. However, a history of hepatitis C suggests increased levels of immunoglobulins.

Major points of discussion

- A positive DAT and negative eluate can be seen with passively acquired isohemagglutinins from incompatible plasma transfusions. For example, transfusion of group O platelets to a group A patient can result in coating of the patient's A red cells with anti-A antibodies from the platelet transfusion. Eluate testing is routinely performed on screening cells, which are group

O. Therefore, the eluate will be negative in this scenario. If the eluate were tested against group A1 cells, it would be positive in this situation.
- The differential for a positive DAT and negative eluate include passively acquired isohemagglutinins (e.g., ABO-incompatible bone marrow transplant, transfusion of ABO-incompatible platelets), drug-induced hemolytic anemia, PCH (Donath-Landsteiner antibody), and nonspecific immunoglobulin uptake.
- Laboratory evidence of hemolysis includes a drop in hemoglobin and hematocrit or lack of an expected rise in the hemoglobin after transfusion, increased lactate dehydrogenase (LDH), decreased haptoglobin, increased indirect bilirubin, and blood on urine dipstick with no red cells on microscopic examination.
- A negative eluate is expected in drug-induced hemolytic anemia unless the offending drug is included in the testing.
- Hepatitis C is associated with mixed cryoglobulinemia (polyclonal IgG with monoclonal IgM). Therapeutic plasma exchange is effective at removing cryoglobulins and is indicated in symptomatic patients as adjunctive therapy.[2]

44. A. Usually are antibodies of the IgG subtype.
Rationale: Naturally occurring antibodies are usually of the IgM subtype.
B. React optimally at 37°C.
Rationale: Naturally occurring antibodies are usually IgM antibodies, which react best at 4°C.
C. Require antihuman globulin for agglutination.
Rationale: Naturally occurring antibodies are usually of the IgM subtype and can agglutinate without antihuman globulin.
D. Do not readily fix complement and are associated with extravascular hemolysis.
Rationale: Naturally occurring antibodies are usually of the IgM subtype, which can readily fix complement and are associated with intravascular hemolysis.
E. Do not cross the placenta.
Rationale: Naturally occurring antibodies are typically IgM antibodies that do not cross the placenta.

Major points of discussion

- Although multivalent IgM molecules readily agglutinate RBCs without antihuman globulin, some IgG antibodies against high-density antigens can also directly agglutinate RBCs.
- Treating IgM antibodies with sulfhydryl reagents such as DTT abolishes agglutinating activity and can aid in detection of coexisting IgG antibodies.
- Cold agglutinin syndrome is usually caused by IgM autoantibodies that bind to red cells and fix complement in the peripheral circulation where the temperature is cooler. As the red cells circulate to warmer parts of the body, the IgM autoantibodies dissociate, leaving the complement behind.
- IgM cold-reactive agglutinins associated with hemolysis usually have a high titer and wide thermal amplitude (i.e., they are reactive at >30°C).
- Naturally occurring anti-A and anti-B antibodies do not develop until 3 to 6 months of age. However, IgG

anti-A and anti-B antibodies can cross the placenta and remain in the infant's circulation after birth, especially in mothers who are type O and have higher titers of IgG anti-A and anti-B antibodies. This can result in ABO HDFN.

45. A. Saline replacement technique.
Rationale: The typing results show an unexpected antibody on the back type (anti-A) due to rouleaux. This can be resolved by washing away plasma, replacing with saline, and then checking for agglutination.
B. Chloroquine treatment of red cells.
Rationale: Chloroquine is used to weaken antigens, such as HLA on red cells (Bg antigens) or platelets. It does not resolve rouleaux.
C. Addition of rabbit erythrocyte stroma.
Rationale: Rabbit erythrocyte stroma is added to remove cold autoanti-I and -IH from plasma.
D. Prewarm all reagents to 37°C.
Rationale: Prewarming is performed when an interfering cold autoantibody is present.
E. Cold autoadsorption.
Rationale: Cold autoadsorption is performed to remove interfering cold autoantibodies.

Major points of discussion
■ Rouleaux formation is caused by excess proteins in the plasma that cause red cells to stack on top of each other ("stack of coins").
■ Causes of excess protein in plasma that cause rouleaux include lymphoproliferative disorders (e.g., multiple myeloma), liver disease, inflammation (e.g., infection), cancer, and connective tissue disorders.
■ The erythrocyte sedimentation rate (ESR) is increased in the setting of rouleaux because the red cells that are stuck together settle faster.
■ In this case, a subgroup of A with anti-A1 formation should be considered. A2 subgroup can be determined using *Dolichos biflorus* lectin, which will agglutinate A1 cells but not A2 cells. In addition, the patient's plasma should be tested against both A1 and A2 cells. Plasma from a patient who is blood type A2 with anti-A1 should agglutinate only A1 red cells.
■ Acquired anti-A1 can result from transfusion of incompatible plasma containing products (e.g., type O red cells, type B or O platelets).

46a. A. Warm autoantibody.
Rationale: The antibody reacts with all panel cells with equal strength and the autologous control is positive. The eluate testing is consistent with a panagglutinin. These findings are consistent with the presence of a warm autoantibody.
B. Anti-D alloantibody.
Rationale: An anti-D alloantibody does not explain why Rh-negative panel cells are reactive.
C. Multiple alloantibodies to the following antigens: C, E, K, Fyª, S.
Rationale: The presence of alloantibodies does not explain the positive autocontrol.
D. Alloantibody to a high-prevalence antigen.
Rationale: This would explain the positive reactivity to all panel cells but would not explain the positive autologous control.

E. Alloantibody to a low-prevalence antigen
Rationale: Most panel cells and the autocontrol should be negative if there is an alloantibody to a low-prevalence antigen.

46b. A. This is a laboratory error; the blood bank will initiate an investigation and reissue a crossmatch-compatible unit.
B. This is the correct RBC unit, but rituximab should be administered first to prevent a hemolytic transfusion reaction.
Rationale: Rituximab may be used in the setting of a chronic warm autoimmune hemolytic anemia; however, it would not be beneficial in the acute setting to prevent a hemolytic transfusion reaction
C. A full crossmatch should not have been performed; the blood bank will release an electronically crossmatch-compatible red cell unit.
Rationale: A full crossmatch must be performed in all cases in which there is a positive antibody screen. An electronic crossmatch cannot be performed in this case.
D. The transfusion should be delayed until crossmatch-compatible antigen-negative units are identified
Rationale for A and D: The red cell antibody panel is consistent with the presence of a warm autoantibody, in which case, all potential red cell units would be crossmatch incompatible.
E. Crossmatch-incompatible RBCs are the only option and the transfusion should not be delayed.
Rationale: The patient has cardiac risk factors and symptomatic anemia; thus, transfusion should not be delayed. In the presence of a warm autoantibody, all red cells units will be crossmatch incompatible but should survive in circulation similarly to the patient's autologous red cells.

Major points of discussion
■ Transfused crossmatch-incompatible red cells to a patient with a warm autoimmune hemolytic anemia will survive as well as the patient's autologous red cells.
■ In nonemergent situations, a warm autoadsorption of the plasma sample should be performed to exclude the presence of underlying alloantibodies.
■ A warm autoantibody will interfere with full red cell phenotyping of the patient because some commercial phenotyping reagents (e.g., for the Duffy antigen) are polyclonal IgG reagents that have to be tested using anti-human globulin. In this setting, the red cells should first be treated to remove the warm autoantibody (e.g., ethylenediamine tetraacetic acid [EDTA] glycine acid [EGA] treatment), followed by phenotypic testing; otherwise, false-positive results will be obtained from the anti-human globulin reacting with the warm autoantibody.
■ In a patient with a history of recent transfusion, the presence of a positive autologous control should alert you to the possibility of a delayed hemolytic/serologic transfusion reaction.
■ In the setting of a delayed hemolytic/serologic transfusion reaction, the eluate is helpful in demonstrating the alloantibody coating the circulating transfused incompatible red cells.

47. A. Direct antiglobulin test.
Rationale: This should be done for the workup of hemolysis or if the autologous control is positive.
B. Antibody panel.
Rationale: An antibody panel would be the next step if the antibody screen is positive.
C. Eluate.
Rationale: An eluate is performed if the direct antiglobulin test is positive using anti-IgG to determine the specificity of the antibodies that are binding circulating red cells.
D. Nothing; the antibody screen is negative.
Rationale: The antibody screen is not necessarily negative in this case because the check cells are negative.
E. Repeat the antibody screen.
Rationale: The check cells are negative, suggesting a problem in the antibody screen testing. The next step should be to repeat the antibody screen.

Major points of discussion
- Check cells are red cells that are coated with IgG antibodies. They are added to verify negative results obtained at the anti-human globulin stage.
- Causes of false-negative results with check cells include inadequate cell washing, delay in adding the anti-human globulin reagent following washing, and failure to add the anti-human globulin.
- Inadequate washing may lead to false-negative results with check cells because inadequate washing can leave free plasma antibodies behind. Anti-human globulin preferentially binds to free antibodies in solution rather than antibodies on red cells. Thus, if there are free antibodies left over as a result of inadequate washing, this will block function of the anti-human globulin reagent, preventing agglutination.
- If there is significant delay in adding the anti-human globulin reagent, IgG antibodies can fall off from sensitized red cells incubated in saline. Thus, these free IgG antibodies can block function of the anti-human globulin reagent, preventing agglutination.
- Check cells are not required in all testing methods. For example, gel testing systems do not use check cells. Each manufacturer will specify controls that must be used with a specific method.

48. A. No crossmatch is necessary; any two units may be released.
Rationale: Although the patient is type AB and should be compatible with all ABO types, a crossmatch must be performed before transfusion.
B. Electronic crossmatch.
Rationale: The patient does not have a history of red cell antibodies and the current red cell screen is negative. Assuming the blood bank computer system meets the requirements for an electronic crossmatch, this would be the most efficient choice requiring the least amount of technical work.
C. Immediate spin crossmatch.
Rationale: This would be the most efficient choice if an electronic crossmatch were not possible.
D. Full AHG crossmatch in tube.
E. Full AHG crossmatch in solid phase.
Rationale: A full crossmatch is more time-consuming and is unnecessary in a patient without a history of red cell antibodies and with a negative antibody screen.

Major points of discussion
- A crossmatch must be performed unless emergency release red cell units are requested.
- An immediate spin crossmatch can be used as the sole crossmatching method only if the patient has a negative antibody screen and no history of red cell antibodies.
- An immediate spin crossmatch is used to ensure the absence of ABO incompatibility.
- A full crossmatch should include a 37°C incubation of a sample of red cells from the attached segment of the unit to be transfused, the patient's serum or plasma, and the addition of AHG. This can be performed using tube testing, column agglutination, or solid-phase systems.
- For patients with a positive antibody screen (either historically or currently) or an alloantibody to a low-prevalence antigen, the full crossmatch will prevent transfusion of incompatible red cells not identified in red cell antibody testing due to the low prevalence of the incompatible antigen.

49. A. The patient is experiencing a delayed hemolytic transfusion reaction
Rationale: Patients with a delayed hemolytic transfusion reaction may have a positive DAT, but the differential diagnosis for a positive DAT is much broader than a delayed hemolytic transfusion reaction.
B. The patient is hemolyzing red cells.
Rationale: Laboratory evidence of hemolysis includes a drop in hemoglobin and hematocrit or lack of an expected rise in the hemoglobin after transfusion, increased LDH, decreased haptoglobin, increased indirect bilirubin, and blood on urine dipstick with no red cells on microscopic examination.
C. The patient has an autoantibody.
Rationale: In a recently transfused patient, a positive DAT can be due to presence of an alloantibody binding to transfused incompatible red cells. Thus, a positive DAT is not specific for the presence of an autoantibody.
D. The patient has antibody or complement bound to circulating red cells.
Rationale: A DAT tests for the presence of IgG antibodies and/or complement on circulating red cells.
E. The patient has an alloantibody to a red cell antigen.
Rationale: A DAT can also indicate the presence of a circulating autoantibody, among other causes. Furthermore, alloantibodies will not be detected using a DAT unless the patient has had a recent transfusion with incompatible red cells.

Major points of discussion
- The differential diagnosis of a positive DAT includes autoantibodies, hemolytic transfusion reactions, drug-induced hemolytic anemia, hemolytic disease of the fetus and newborn, passively acquired antibodies (from transfusion of plasma containing components, intravenous immunoglobulin, Rh immunoglobulin), nonspecific adsorbtion of antibodies, passenger lymphocyte syndrome, and complement activation.

- A DAT should be perfomed in a patient presenting with hemolysis and should be performed when investigating a transfusion reaction.
- The DAT must be performed on washed red cells; otherwise, the immunoglobulins and complement that are present in plasma can neutralize the anti-IgG and anti-C3d reagents.
- Some blood banks initially use a polyspecific reagent containing both anti-IgG and anti-C3d when performing a DAT. If this test is positive, it is followed by testing with monospecific reagents to differentiate between immunoglobulin and complement coating the red cells.
- Warm-reactive IgM antibodies can cause false-positive DATs. To control for this, red cells should be tested with an inert negative control reagent such as 6% albumin or saline. If agglutination is observed with the negative inert control reagent, the DAT result is invalid.

50. A. Paroxysmal cold hemoglobinuria.
Rationale: The clinical scenario (live attenuated viral vaccine), DAT results, and findings from the described Donath-Landsteiner test are highly suggestive of a diagnosis of paroxysmal cold hemoglobinuria.
B. Paroxysmal nocturnal hemoglobinuria.
Rationale: Paroxysmal nocturnal hemoglobinuria is caused by a defective *PIG-A* gene leading to absence of GPI-linked proteins such as CD55 (decay accelerating factor) and CD59 (membrane inhibitor of reactive lysis) on red cells, making the cells more prone to complement-mediated lysis. The Donath-Landsteiner test described in the question would not be expected to yield a positive result in this setting.
C. Delayed hemolytic transfusion reaction.
Rationale: A history of transfusion is not given for this patient.
D. Warm autoimmune hemolytic anemia.
Rationale: The DAT is expected to be positive for IgG antibodies, and the eluate is expected to be positive and behave as a panagglutinin in cases of warm autoimmune hemolytic anemia.
E. Cold autoimmune hemolytic anemia.
Rationale: Although a positive DAT to complement components is expected only in cases of cold autoimmune hemolytic anemia, the positive Donath-Landsteiner test is diagnostic of a different entity and not seen with IgM cold-reactive antibodies.

Major points of discussion
- The biphasic hemolysin in PCH is typically against the high-prevalence P antigen. It is caused by a complement-activating IgG antibody that binds red cells at cooler temperatures (found in the extremities), fixes complement, then dissociates from the red cells at warmer temperatures. Because the IgG typically dissociates at 37°C, routine direct antiglobulin testing shows only complement binding the red cells with a negative eluate. However, the Donath-Landsteiner test will expose the presence of a biphasic hemolysin that binds red cells at 4°C and causes hemolysis at 37°C.
- Although transfusion of patients with PCH is rarely necessary, if hemolysis is significant, transfusion should not be withheld. Because of the rarity of P antigen–negative units (i.e., p or P^k phenotypes), P antigen–positive blood should be transfused.

- PCH is associated with syphilis and viral infections and is typically a self-limiting condition.
- The P1 antigen is a member of neolacto-family glycosphingolipid antigens, while the P^k and P antigens are globo-glycosphingolipids. Anti-P1 is a commonly encountered cold autoantibody. It can be inhibited by hydatid cyst fluid or pigeon egg substance, both of which contain P1 substance.
- Rare individuals with the p phenotype can produce anti-PP1P^k. This condition is associated with early spontaneous abortions, and this antibody can cause potent hemolytic transfusion reactions.

51. A. Temperature less than 30°C.
Rationale: Clinically significant IgG alloantibodies typically react optimally at 37°C.
B. Low pH (pH 2).
Rationale: Physiologic pH is optimal for detecting most clinically significant alloantibodies.
C. Decreasing incubation time.
Rationale: Although excessive incubation times may decrease reactivity, in general, increased incubation time enhances alloantibody reactivity.
D. Lowering the salt concentration.
Rationale: Use of an enhancing solution, such as low–ionic strength saline solution (LISS), promotes antigen-antibody interactions by decreasing the shielding effect of Na$^+$ and Cl$^-$ ions.
E. Decreasing the serum/red cell ratio.
Rationale: Weak antibodies can be diluted by decreasing the serum/red cell ratio. This ratio is often increased to enhance reactivity.

Major points of discussion
- Commonly used enhancing solutions include albumin (22%), LISS, and PEG solutions.
- PEG may also enhance warm autoantibody reactivity; thus, testing using saline or LISS solutions may be preferred in the presence of autoantibodies.
- Solid-phase technology is similar to an enzyme-linked immunosorbent assay (ELISA). Wells are precoated with red cells or red cell membranes of known phenotype and incubated with patient serum or plasma. Unbound antibodies are washed off and the remaining antibodies are detected using anti-IgG antibodies.
- Column agglutination uses a column composed of gel or glass beads to trap agglutinated red cells and prevent them from reaching the bottom of the column on centrifugation.
- For patients who have had recent transfusions in whom a red cell phenotype is obscured by the transfused red cells, molecular methods exist for obtaining a molecularly defined red cell phenotype. Although this testing is useful in certain situations, it is not currently used in routine practice.

52. A. This is likely a nonspecific finding due to the patient's liver disease. This unit may be used for this patient in the operating room.
Rationale: An incompatible unit should not be transfused into this patient with a history of alloantibodies. Nineteen out of 20 units are compatible and should be transfused if needed.

B. In addition to the anti-E antibody, the patient has an antibody to a low-prevalence antigen. The incompatible unit can be reissued to another patient, and another unit should be crossmatched for this patient.
Rationale: Antibodies to low-prevalence antigens are typically identified as a nonspecific positive result on an antibody panel or at the full crossmatch stage of testing. Because the incompatible antigen is of low prevalence, very few red cells in inventory will be positive for this antigen and further screening will identify compatible units. Furthermore, this unit can be re-issued to another patient who does not have this specific antibody.
C. The patient does not have an anti-E antibody and a repeat antibody screen and full red cell phenotype should be performed. Surgery should be delayed until the nature of the patient's antibody is resolved.
Rationale: Most of the units (19/20) were crossmatch compatible with this patient; thus, surgery should proceed without delay. The nature of this specific antibody may never be resolved, however, an attempt to identify it with selected antibody panels can be performed.
D. In addition to the anti-E antibody, the patient has a warm autoantibody. Because this is an autoantibody, the incompatible unit may be transfused in this patient.
Rationale: If the patient had an autoantibody, it would have been seen on pretransfusion testing, not at the crossmatch step. In addition, in the presence of a warm autoantibody, all fully crossmatched units would be expected to be incompatible.
E. In addition to the anti-E antibody, the patient has an antibody to a high-prevalence antigen. The incompatible unit should be discarded from inventory because it contains a high-prevalence antigen.
Rationale: If the patient had an antibody to a high-prevalence antigen, then almost all of the 20 crossmatched units would be crossmatch incompatible. Almost all units contain high-prevalence antigens. Fortunately, most patients do not make antibodies to these high-prevalence antigens because they express them too.

Major points of discussion
- It is difficult to phenotype red cells for antigens of low prevalence because commercial phenotyping reagents do not exist. Thus, it is impossible to order antigen-negative units and the crossmatch is used to rule out an incompatibility due to such an antibody.
- Other possible explanations for the scenario described in this case are that the incompatible unit was mistyped and was ABO incompatible, had a positive direct antiglobulin test, or was polyagglutinable.
- Identifying the specificity of an antibody to a low-prevalence antigen is not necessary and is often only of academic interest.
- Some antibodies to low-prevalence antigens can cause hemolytic disease of the fetus and newborn; however, routine red cell screening tests on the mother's plasma will likely be negative. Testing the father's red cells with the mother's plasma can be helpful in these cases. Furthermore, reacting an eluate from the newborn to the father's red cells can also help implicate an antibody to a low-prevalence antigen as the probable cause of hemolysis.

- When a patient has an antibody to a low-prevalence antigen, virtually all red cells are compatible. Conversely, when a patient has an antibody to a high-prevalence antigen, virtually all red cells are incompatible.

53. A. Anti-D.
Rationale: The mother is Rh positive and cannot make anti-D.
B. Anti-K.
Rationale: An antibody to the Kell antigen can lead to HDFN. However, it is not the most likely etiology because the maternal red cell antibody screen is negative. HDFN due to antibodies against antigens in the Kell system suppressess erythropoiesis and presents with a more profound anemia. Kell antigens are present on erythropoietic precursor cells in the bone marrow. Hemolysis is less commonly seen.
C. Anti-c.
Rationale: Anti-c antibodies are a common cause of HDFN, although it is not the most likely cause, particularly with a negative maternal antibody screen.
D. Anti-A.
Rationale: Anti-A antibodies are usually IgM and cannot cross the placenta.
E. Anti-A,B.
Rationale: Anti-A,B antibodies are usually IgG and can cross the placenta. Anti-A,B antibodies cause ABO HDFN.

Major points of discussion
- HDFN is most commonly due to ABO incompatibility.
- Group O mothers have naturally occurring high-titer anti-A,B antibodies that are IgG antibodies and can cross the placenta into the fetal circulation.
- Anti-A,B antibodies readily bind to both A and B antigens on fetal cells, leading to increased destruction.
- Group A neonates tend to be more severely affected, particularly in Caucasian populations, because of the increased RBC expression of the A antigen compared with the B antigen.
- ABO HDFN tends to be clinically mild since A and B antigens are poorly expressed on fetal and neonatal RBCs, and tissue and soluble antigens neutralize some of the antibody.
- Exchange transfusions are rarely needed.
- In these cases, the infant's direct antiglobulin test will be positive, and the eluate will be positive only if group A and B RBCs are included in the panel.

54. A. Complete blood ell ccount, direct and indirect bilirubin, and haptoglobin.
B. Complete blood cell count, direct and indirect bilirubin, haptoglobin, and lactate dehyrogenase.
Rationale: These tests are part of the workup but do not constitute the full workup for hemolysis.
C. Complete blood cell count, direct and indirect bilirubin, haptoglobin, lactate dehydrogenase, direct antiglobulin test, and urinalysis.
Rationale: These are the laboratory tests that should be ordered for diagnosis of hemolysis.
D. Complete blood cell count, direct and indirect bilirubin, haptoglobin, lactate dehydrogenase, direct antiglobulin test, urinalysis, and ionized calcium.

Rationale: Ionized calcium does not provide any information in the workup of hemolysis.

E. Complete blood cell count, direct and indirect bilirubin, haptoglobin, lactate dehydrogenase, direct antiglobulin test, urinalysis, and potassium.

Rationale: A potassium level does not provide any information in the workup of hemolysis.

Major points of discussion

- The first step in the management of any transfusion reaction is to immediately stop the transfusion.
- An acute hemolytic transfusion reaction must always be ruled out.
- Blood samples and all bags and tubing from recently transfused product(s) should be sent to the blood bank for a visual inspection for hemoglobinemia, repeat type and screen on the patient, repeat type on transfused products, and a direct antiglobulin test.
- If hemolysis is present, indirect bilirubin and lactate dehydrogenase should be elevated. Haptoglobin is decreased in intravascular hemolysis and may not be affected in extravascular hemolysis unless the hemolysis is brisk.
- Urinalysis is sent to detect hemoglobinuria, which is seen with intravascular hemolysis or brisk extravascular hemolysis.
- Clerical checks must be completed to ensure that the correct unit was transfused to the correct patient and all laboratory samples were drawn and labeled appropriately. Clerical error is the most common cause of hemolytic transfusion reactions.
- In this patient, the direct antiglobulin test would be expected to be positive with anti-Fy^a in the eluate if Fy^a-positive RBCs were transfused.
- Anti-Fy^a antibodies may drop below the level of detection, increasing the risk for anamnestic reactions and delayed hemolytic transfusion reactions.
- The hemolysis seen with anti-Fy^a is usually extravascular.
- One would expect to see a decrease in hemoglobin and hematocrit, elevated lactate dehydrogenase and indirect bilirubin, and a positive direct antiglobulin test result with anti-Fy^a in the eluate. The transfused donor RBCs should be typed for Fy^a antigen.

55. A. Fetal hemoglobin is more resistant to hypotonic saline.
Rationale: Sickle cells (hemoglobin SS) are more resistant than hemoglobin AA cells to hypotonic saline. This technique is used to phenotype the RBCs of a patient with sickle cell anemia who was recently transfused.
B. Fetal hemoglobin forms rosettes around Rh-positive cells.
Rationale: In the fetal screen or rosette test, Rh D-positive indicator cells form rosettes around Rh D–positive fetal cells incubated with anti-D.
C. Fetal hemoglobin is less soluble than hemoglobin A.
Rationale: Sickle hemoglobin S is less soluble than hemoglobin A in solutions that decrease the amount of oxygen present. This is the basis for the hemoglobin S solubility test.
D. Fetal hemoglobin is resistant to acid treatment.
Rationale: Hemoglobin F in fetal cells is resistant to acid elution and these cells will stain pink on a smear of

maternal blood. Maternal red cells that are hemoglobin AA will appear as "ghosts" since the hemoglobin elutes with acid treatment.
E. Fetal hemoglobin is less dense than hemoglobin A.
Rationale: Reticulocytes can be separated from mature RBCs by centrifugation because they are less dense.

Major points of discussion

- When an Rh-negative woman delivers an Rh-positive infant, the presence of fetal maternal hemorrhage is detected by the fetal screen or rosette test.
- Rosette test: Maternal blood is incubated with anti-D. If Rh-positive fetal RBCs are present, they will become coated with the anti-D. Rh-positive indicator RBCs are added. The anti-D coated fetal cells will form rosettes around the indicator cells. These rosettes can be identified under the microscope.
- The rosette test can detect a minimum of about 10 mL of fetal maternal hemorrhage.
- If the rosette test is positive, then a Kleihauer-Betke test is run to quantify the amount of fetal maternal hemorrhage.
- Kleihauer-Betke test: Fetal hemoglobin is more resistant than hemoglobin A (adult hemoglobin) to acid elution. A slide with maternal blood is exposed to acid. Under the microscope, the maternal cells will appear pale or like ghosts and the fetal cells will be pink. The fetal cells and maternal cells are counted for a total of 2000 cells. The result is given as the percent fetal cells present.
- This percent can be used to calculate the dose of RhIG needed to prevent maternal alloimmunization to the D antigen.
- The quantity of fetal cells within the maternal circulation is calculated using the following formula: fetal cells × maternal blood volume (mL) total cells counted = fetal hemorrhage (mL).
- The dose of RhIG is calculated as number of vials = fetal hemorrhage (mL)/30 mL. If the calculated dose is a decimal 0.5 or greater, then round up. Then an additional vial is added due to inaccuracy of the tests.

56. A. Rh.
Rationale: Alloantibodies to the D, C, c, E, and e antigens of the Rh blood group system are not observed on this panel.
B. Kell.
Rationale: Alloantibodies to the K, k, Kp^a, Kp^b, Js^a, and Js^b antigens of the Kell blood group system are not observed on this panel.
C. Kidd.
Rationale: The antibody panel shows an alloantibody to Jk^a of the Kidd blood group system.
D. Duffy.
Rationale: Alloantibodies to the Fy^a and Fy^b antigens of the Duffy blood group system are not observed on this panel.
E. MNS.
Rationale: Alloantibodies to the M, N, S, and s antigens of the MNS blood group system are not observed on this panel.

Major points of discussion

- Some Kidd antibodies can bind complement, leading to intravascular hemolysis.

- Kidd antibodies are dangerous because they have a tendency to drop to undetectable levels in plama. Thus, pretransfusion testing can miss the presence of a Kidd antibody and subsequent exposure results in a strong anamnestic response.
- Red cells that are homozygous for an antigen may react more strongly with a particular antibody than red cells that are heterozygous for the antigen (as demonstrated by the panel in this question). This effect is termed the dosage effect and is typically observed with antibodies to the Rh, MNS, Kidd, Duffy, and Lutheran blood group systems.
- The Kidd antigens are located on a membrane protein responsible for urea transport.
- After the ABO and Rh systems, antibodies to antigens of the Kell blood group system are the most common and are commonly associated with hemolytic transfusion reactions and hemolytic disease of the fetus and newborn.

57. A. Anti-Fy3.
Rationale: Panel red cell No. 11 is Fy3-negative (both Fy^a and Fy^b negative) and reacts, while panel red cell No. 4 is Fy3-positive and does not react. Thus, the patient is unlikely to have an anti-Fy3 alloantibody.
B. Anti-k.
Rationale: Panel red cell No. 4 is k-positive and does not react; thus, the patient is unlikely to have an anti-k alloantibody. The patient is also k-positive and, therefore, cannot make an alloantibody to the k antigen.
C. Anti-Js^b.
Rationale: Panel red cell No. 4 is Js^b-positive and does not react; thus, the patient is unlikely to have an anti-Js^b alloantibody.
D. Anti-Kp^a.
Rationale: Kp^a is a low-prevalence antigen and panel red cell No. 4 is Kp^a-positive; thus, the patient does not have an anti-Kp^a alloantibody.
E. Anti-U.
Rationale: Rare individuals of predominantly African descent have the S–s–U– phenotype and can make antibodies to the high-prevalence U antigen.

Major points of discussion
- The S, s, and U antigens are located on the transmembrane glycoprotein, glycophorin B.
- The M and N antigens are located on the transmembrane glycoprotein, glycophorin A.
- Approximately 2% of blacks are S–s– and lack the high-prevalence antigen U. Anti-U, anti-S, and anti-s antibodies are clinically significant and can cause fatal hemolytic transfusion reactions and hemolytic disease of the fetus and newborn.
- Antibodies to the M and N antigens are typically IgM, are not active at 37°C, and are rarely clinically significant.
- Rare individuals that lack all or part of glycophorin A can make antibodies to the high-prevalence En^a antigen. These antibodies are clinically significant and can cause severe hemolytic transfusion reactions and hemolytic disease of the fetus and newborn.

58. A. Sensitization to RhD from a prior pregnancy.
Rationale: Standard of care is to administer Rh immune globulin at 28 weeks of gestation; this effectively prevents sensitization to the RhD antigen.
B. Sensitization to a non-Rh antigen from a prior pregnancy.
Rationale: The antibody panel in not consistent with presence of an antibody to a non-Rh antigen.
C. Passively acquired RhD antibodies.
Rationale: This result is most likely caused by the presence of anti-RhD alloantibodies from administration of Rh immune globulin at 28 weeks of gestation.
D. Naturally occurring antibodies of pregnancy.
Rationale: RhD antibodies are not naturally occurring.
E. Warm autoantibodies.
Rationale: The autocontrol is negative on the red cell panel.

Major points of discussion
- Rh immune globulin is made from human plasma of RhD-immunized individuals.
- In a pregnant RhD-negative woman, Rh immune globulin should be administered at 28 weeks of gestation and within 72 hours of delivery of an RhD antigen–positive baby. Additional doses should be provided following invasive procedures such as amniocentesis or abortions.
- A dose of 300 μg of Rh immune globulin is sufficient to suppress 30 mL of whole blood (15 mL of RBCs).
- The appropriate dose of Rh immune globulin to administer following delivery depends on the amount of fetal maternal hemorrhage detected. This can be measured using the rosette test, the Kleihauer-Betke test, or by flow cytometry.
- The mechanism of action of Rh immune globulin is still unknown.

59. A. IgM antibodies and IgG antibodies frequently cause acute intravascular hemolysis.
B. IgM antibodies and IgG antibodies cannot cause acute intravascular hemolysis.
C. IgM antibodies frequently cause extravascular hemolysis, and IgG antibodies frequently cause intravascular hemolysis.
D. IgM antibodies can cause intravascular hemolysis, and IgG antibodies can cause extravascular hemolysis.
E. IgM antibodies and IgG antibodies frequently cause extravascular hemolysis.
Rationale: IgM, which is multivalent, can fix complement and cause acute intravascular hemolysis. IgG, which only has two Fab sites, is less efficient at fixing complement and causes extravascular hemolysis.

Major points of discussion
- General characteristics of IgM red cell antibodies: five immunoglobin molecules covalently bound; total of 10 Fab binding sites; cause agglutination at room temperature; antibodies can fix complement and cause intravascular hemolysis; most are not reactive at 37°C; and are distributed intravascularly.
- General characteristics of IgG red cell antibodies: two Fab binding sites; do not cause agglutination at room temperature; require antihuman globulin to

show agglutination; are much less efficient than IgM in fixing complement; cause extravascular hemolysis (decreased red cell survival due to clearance by reticuloendothelial system); and are distributed intravascularly and extravascularly.

- IgG-coated red cells are cleared by macrophages via the Fc receptor.
- IgM antibody reactivity can be abolished using sulfhydryl agent such as DTT.
- Naturally occurring antibodies to ABO antigens are predominantly IgM antibodies. However, anti-A and anti-B antibodies can also be IgG subclass, particularly in individuals who are group O who may have high-titer anti-A, anti-B, or anti-A,B IgG antibodies.

60. A. Group O, Rh negative
B. Group A, Rh negative.
C. Group A, Rh positive.
D. Group B, Rh negative.
E. Group B, Rh positive.
Rationale: The forward and reverse typing is consistent with blood group B and the anti-D testing is suggestive of a weak or a partial D phenotype; thus, the unit should be labeled Rh positive.

Major points of discussion

- Blood centers must test donors for weak D phenotype, because if labeled as Rh negative, units from these donors can cause alloimmunization to the RhD antigen in transfusion recipients.
- Weak D testing is not required for transfusion recipients because it is perfectly safe to consider a weak D individual as RhD-negative for transfusion purposes.
- Infants whose mothers are candidates for Rh immune globulin should be tested for the weak D phenotype.
- DVI is the most common partial D phenotype in whites; DIIIa is the most common in blacks.
- Individuals with the partial D phenotype can make alloantibodies to the RhD antigen; individuals with the weak D phenotype will not.

BLOOD COMPONENT THERAPY

61. A. Group O, uncrossmatched RBCs.
Rationale: This patient is severely anemic due to an acute drop in hemoglobin and needs immediate resuscitation with RBCs.
B. Group O, IS crossmatched RBCs.
Rationale: An immediate spin is used to double check ABO compatibility. This patient needs emergent transfusion and cannot wait for an immediate spin crossmatch to be completed.
C. Type-specific, uncrossmatched RBCs.
Rationale: This patient is severely anemic and requires emergent transfusion. Performing an ABO type and providing type-specific RBCs will cause unnecessary delay.
D. Type-specific, IS crossmatched red blood cel
Rationale: This patient is severely anemic and requires emergent transfusion. Performing an ABO type and providing type-specific immediate: spin crossmatched RBCs will cause unnecessary delay.
E. Type-specific, fully crossmatched RBCs.

Rationale: This patient is severely anemic and requires emergent transfusion. Unless the patient has RBC alloantibodies, a full crossmatch is not necessary, although in emergent situations, random units may have to be provided.

Major points of discussion

- Uncrossmatched group O RBCs may be required for immediate transfusion in emergent situations.
- Blood banks should have a protocol by which uncrossmatched group O RBCs may be released.
- Units can be crossmatched at a later time to ensure compatibility.
- Blood should be drawn as soon as possible so that the blood bank can start a type and screen. This will allow type-specific RBCs to be provided as soon as possible and for the timely determination of the presence of RBC alloantibodies.
- If a patient has RBC alloantibodies and requires emergent transfusion, antigen-negative units may not always be immediately available.
- If possible, antigen-negative units should be provided.
- If it not possible to provide antigen-negative units, the transfusion service should discuss the risks and benefits of transfusion versus other therapies.
- The clinical team should monitor the patient for signs of hemolysis.

62. A. Give RhIG (RhoGAM) at a dose of 300 μg.
Rationale: RhIG is not indicated in this patient since she has already made anti-D. RhIG is given to Rh-negative women at 28 weeks of gestation and postdelivery to prevent the formation of anti-D.
B. Determine the anti-D antibody titer.
Rationale: This is the next step in management. If the titer of anti-D is 8 or less, than titers should be determined every 4 to 6 weeks. If the critical titer of 16 or 32 is reached, then fetal middle cerebral artery Dopplers should be performed.
C. Perform a middle cerebral artery Doppler.
Rationale: This is performed when the mother's anti-D has reached a critical titer.
D. Perform cordocentesis to obtain fetal blood for hemoglobin determination.
Rationale: This is performed after it is determined by middle cerebral artery Doppler that the infant has an increase in cardiac output and is anemic.
E. Perform an intrauterine transfusion.
Rationale: This would not be performed until it is established that the fetus is anemic and requires transfusion.

Major points of discussion

- ABO and Rh typing and antibody screen/antibody identification are performed at the first prenatal visit.
- Antibodies to antigens in the Rh, Kell, and Duffy systems are the most common causes of HDFN; however, there are many reports of other IgG antibodies causing HDFN.
- If a clinically significant antibody is identified, paternal expression should be determined.
- Serologic testing should be performed first to determine whether the father expresses the antigen and whether he is homozygous or heterozygous. Fetal tissue may be obtained via chronionic villus sampling, amniocentesis, or cordocentesis for molecular typing.

- The maternal antibody titer should be determined during the first trimester, if possible, to establish a baseline.
- For anti-D, the critical titer is 16 or 32 at antihuman globulin phase. If the titer is less than or equal to 8, maternal samples should be drawn every 4 to 6 weeks to determine the antibody titer. Often, previous frozen maternal samples are run simultaneously with new samples to account for differences in technique between technologists. A twofold increase in the titer is considered clinically significant.
- A titer of 16 or 32 is considered clinically significant for most other antigens as well. However, Kell antigens are expressed on erythropoietic precursor cells and HDFN due to Kell antibodies can suppress erythropoiesis. A titer of 8 is generally considered clinically significant for antibodies directed against antigens in the Kell system.
- If the mother has a clinically significant titer, the fetus may be monitored with middle cerebral artery Dopplers. An increase in cardiac output due to fetal anemia will be detected as an increase in middle cerebral artery peak blood flow velocity.
- Fetal samples may be drawn via cordocentesis for direct measurement of the hemoglobin and hematocrit, and intrauterine transfusions may be provided. Red blood cells for intrauterine transfusion should be irradiated, leukoreduced or cytomegalovirus negative, hemoglobin S negative, and lack the offending antigen(s).
- Prior to the use of middle cerebral artery Dopplers, the clinical status of the fetus would be monitored by amniocentesis for mothers with critical titers. The change in the optical density (OD) of the amniotic fluid is proportional to the bilirubin concentration. The optical densities would be plotted on a graph (Liley's system) of OD versus weeks of gestation to determine the severity of disease.

63. A. 1 vial of RhIG.
B. 2 vials of RhIG.
C. 3 vials of RhIG.
Rationale: These doses are not sufficient to prevent alloimmunization to the D antigen.
D. 4 vials of RhIG.
Rationale: This is the correct dose as calculated by $1.5\% \times$ 5,000 mL (estimated maternal whole blood volume) = 75 mL fetal whole blood. 75 mL/30 mL (amount of fetal whole blood covered by 1 vial of RhIG) = 2.5 vials; 2.5 vials are rounded up to 3 vials. One additional vial is added for a total of 4 vials due to the inaccuracy of the Kleihauer-Betke test.
E. 5 vials of RhIG.
Rationale: This dose is more than is required to prevent alloimmunization to the D antigen.

Major points of discussion
- Pregnant women who are Rh negative who are pregnant with an Rh-positive fetus are at risk for becoming alloimmunized to the D antigen. If the father and mother are both Rh negative, there is no risk for alloimmunization.
- Rh immunoglobulin (RhIG) is administered at 28 weeks of gestation, postdelivery of an Rh-positive newborn, or at any time there is risk of fetal maternal hemorrhage

(amniocentesis, cordocentesis, version procedure, maternal abdominal trauma).
- One dose of RhIG is 300 μg and will prevent alloimmunization to 30 mL of fetal whole blood or 15 mL of fetal RBCs.
- After delivery, or if fetal maternal hemorrhage is suspected, a rosette test is performed to detect the presence of Rh-positive fetal RBCs.
- If the rosette test is positive, 300 μg of RhIG should be given.
- A Kleihauer-Betke test or flow cytometry is performed next to quantitate the extent of the fetal maternal hemorrhage and more accurately dose RhIG.
- After the percentage fetal RBCs within the maternal circulation is determined, the quantity of fetal cells within the maternal circulation is calculated using the following formula: fetal cells × maternal blood volume (mL)/total cells counted = fetal hemorrhage (mL).
- The dose of RhIG is calculated as number of vials = fetal hemorrhage (mL)/30 mL. If the calculated dose is a decimal 0.5 or greater, then round up. Then an additional vial is added due to inaccuracy of the tests.

64. A. Platelets.
Rationale: The uremic toxins in these patients will also affect exogenous platelets. Platelets should only be provided when clinically necessary.
B. Fresh frozen plasma.
Rationale: Fresh frozen plasma has not been demonstrated to improve hemostasis in uremic patients.
C. Desmopressin acetate (DDAVP).
Rationale: This is a first-line agent to improve hemostasis in uremic patients by inducing the release of endogenous von Willebrand factor from endothelial cells.
D. Cryoprecipitate.
Rationale: Cryoprecipitate can be useful in controlling uremic bleeding, but it is not a first-line agent due to the risks of allogeneic transfusions.
E. Factor VIII.
Rationale: Factor VIII has not been demonstrated to improve hemostasis in uremic patients.

Major points of discussion
- Uremia is associated with a bleeding diathesis with mucocutaneous bleeding, easy bruising, and bleeding in association with injury or invasive procedures.
- The cause of bleeding in these patients is multifactorial with dysfunction in platelet-platelet interactions and platelet-endothelium interactions and thrombocytopenia.
- These patients also present with thrombotic complications.
- Patients exhibit dysfunction in platelet aggregation and secretion.
- Platelets in uremic patients demonstrate decreased binding of von Willebrand factor and fibrinogen.
- The defects seen are partially reversible by removal of uremic toxins by dialysis.
- DDAVP is one of the first-line agents to improve hemostasis in uremic patients. It can be used both prophylactically before invasive procedures and in the treatment of active bleeding.

- DDAVP induces the release of endogenous von Willebrand factor from endothelial cells, leading to improvements in hemostasis.
- Cryoprecipitate can also be used to provide additional von Willebrand factor, but it is not a first-line treatment due to the risks associated with allogeneic transfusions.
- Correction of anemia in these patients also improves hemostasis.[4]

65. **A. Lactated Ringer's solution.**
Rationale: The calcium in lactated Ringer solution will bind to the citrate in the RBCs, potentially leading to clot formation.
B. 5% albumin.
Rationale: The FDA has not approved the addition of 5% albumin to blood components.
C. Normal saline.
Rationale: Per AABB standards, only normal saline may be infused in the same line as a blood component.
D. 5% dextrose.
Rationale: The FDA has not approved the addition of 5% dextrose to blood components
E. Vancomycin.
Rationale: No drugs or medications may be infused along with a blood component per AABB Standards.

Major points of discussion
- Only normal saline (0.9% sodium chloride) may be administered in the same line as a blood component.
- All other drugs, medications, and solutions must be infused through a separate line, ideally at a separate location.
- The FDA must approve the use of any drug or solution in this manner.
- Documentation must be available to demonstrate safety before the administration of any drug or solution in the same line as a blood component.
- The blood component must not be adversely affected by the addition of the drug or solution.

66. **A. Platelet count = 21,000/μL; 12-year-old with acute myeloid leukemia (AML), stable, no bleeding.**
Rationale: This patient does not require a platelet transfusion, and should be stable with a platelet count above 10,000/μL.
B. Platelet count = 31,000/μL; patient bleeding during laparoscopic colectomy.
Rationale: Bleeding with a platelet count less than 50,000/μL is an indication for platelet transfusion.
C. Platelet count = 6,000/μL; 12-year-old with immune thrombocytopenia, stable, no bleeding.
Rationale: Stable nonbleeding patients with immune thrombocytopenia do not require platelet transfusions.
D. Platelet count = 61,000/μL; patient having femoral vein catheter placement.
Rationale: A platelet count greater than 50,000/μL is considered to be hemostatic for patients about to undergo a surgical procedure.
E. Platelet count = 110,000/μL; patient postevacuation of a subdural hematoma.
Rationale: A platelet count above 100,000/μL is considered to be sufficient for neurosurgical patients.

Major points of discussion
- Currently accepted platelet transfusion triggers are:
  - 10,000/μL for stable nonbleeding patients
  - 50,000/μL for patients who are bleeding or about to undergo a surgical procedure
  - 100,000/μL for patients with intracerebral, intraocular, and pulmonary bleeding
- Ideally, platelet transfusion therapy should be tailored to the individual patient's needs.
- One dose (one bag) of single donor apheresis platelets is expected to increase the platelet count by 30,000/μL to 60,000/μL.

67. **A. Insufficient reversal of heparin.**
Rationale: The PTT is within the reference range, so the effects of heparin have been reversed.
B. Platelet dysfunction secondary to cardiopulmonary bypass.
Rationale: Platelets are activated by contact with the cardiopulmonary bypass circuit leading to dysfunction.
C. Disseminated intravascular coagulation.
Rationale: There is no evidence of disseminated intravascular coagulation in this patient.
D. Surgical lesion.
Rationale: Surgical lesions usually lead to greater serosanginous drainage than seen in this patient or frank bleeding.
E. Platelet refractoriness.
Rationale: There is no evidence of platelet refractoriness in this patient since the platelet count is near the normal reference range.

Major points of discussion
- Bleeding post cardiopulmonary bypass is not uncommon.
- Contact with the bypass tubing leads to activation of platelets and impaired function.
- Complement, coagulation factors, and the fibrinolytic system are also activated, leading to further activation of platelets.
- Consequently, these patients require platelet transfusion therapy based on clinical, not laboratory, findings.
- Postoperative bleeding of 100 mL/h is most likely due to the dysfunction associated with cardiopulmonary bypass and not a surgical lesion.

68. **A. Return to the operating room to look for a surgical cause of her bleeding.**
Rationale: Output of 300 mL/h is likely due to a surgical lesion.
B. Transfuse 1 dose of single donor apheresis platelets.
Rationale: Platelet dysfunction can lead to postoperative bleeding in this patient, but this quantity of postoperative bleeding is more likely due to a surgical lesion. Platelet count is surgically hemostatic.
C. Transfuse 4 U fresh frozen plasma.
Rationale: PT and aPTT are within the reference range, and fresh frozen plasma transfusion is not indicated.
D. Transfuse 10 U cryoprecipitate.
Rationale: The fibrinogen level is greater than 100 mg/dL and is sufficient for hemostasis in this patient.

E. Transfuse 2 U RBCs.
Rationale: There is no evidence of a lack of oxygen delivery in this patient.

Major points of discussion
- Cardiopulmonary bypass is associated with bleeding due to both surgical and nonsurgical causes.
- About 50% of postoperative bleeding in these patients is due to surgical causes.
- These patients often require platelet and plasma support due to activation of platelets and the coagulation and fibrinolytic systems.
- Plasma therapy in these patients should be guided by appropriate coagulation testing.
- Platelet counts do not reflect platelet function, and the patient's clinical status should guide platelet transfusion decisions.

69. A. Factor V.
Rationale: Factor V levels are equivalent to that found in FFP.
B. Thrombin.
Rationale: Thrombin levels are equivalent to that found in FFP.
C. von Willebrand factor.
Rationale: Levels are reduced in cryoprecipitate-reduced plasma.
D. Protein S.
Rationale: Protein S levels are equivalent to that found in FFP.
E. Plasminogen.
Rationale: Plasminogen levels are equivalent to that found in FFP.

Major points of discussion
- Cryoprecipitate-reduced plasma is the supernatant left over after cryoprecipitate production.
- It has decreased levels of von Willebrand factor antigen and activity.
- Ultralarge von Willebrand multimers are removed from cryoprecipitate-reduced plasma during manufacture of cryoprecipitate.
- The only therapeutic use of cryoprecipitate-reduced plasma is in the treatment of thrombotic thrombocytopenic purpura.
- It may also be used in the manufacture of albumin, intravenous immunoglobulin, and clotting factor concentrates other than factor VIII.

70. A. Prevention of bleeding during invasive procedures in hemophilia A patients with factor VIII inhibitors.
Rationale: This is one of the FDA-approved indications for the use of recombinant activated factor VII.
B. Correction of an elevated international normalized ratio (INR) in a patient on warfarin with an intracranial bleed.
C. Treatment of hemorrhage in a patient undergoing liver transplantation.
D. Treatment of hemorrhage in a patient with disseminated intravascular coagulation.
E. Treatment of hemorrhage in a patient on aspirin therapy with a lower gastrointestinal tract bleed.
Rationale: This is not an FDA-approved use of recombinant activated factor VII.

Major points of discussion
- Recombinant activated factor VII is FDA approved for the following indications:
  - Treatment of acute bleeding in patients with hemophilia A or B with inhibitors to factor VIII or factor IX, respectively.
  - Treatment of acute bleeding in patients with acquired hemophilia.
  - Prevention of bleeding in surgical interventions or invasive procedures in patients with hemophilia A or B and inhibitors to factor VIII or factor IX, respectively.
  - Prevention of bleeding in surgical interventions or invasive procedures in patients with acquired hemophilia.
  - Treatment of acute bleeding in patients with congenital factor VII deficiency.
  - Prevention of bleeding in surgical interventions or invasive procedures in patients with congenital factor VII deficiency.
- Recombinant factor VII is most commonly used for non–FDA-approved indications (off-label use).

71. A. Fresh frozen plasma.
Rationale: Fresh frozen plasma should not be used to reverse the effects of heparin.
B. Recombinant activated factor VII.
Rationale: Recombinant activated factor VII should not be used to reverse heparin.
C. Platelets.
Rationale: Platelet transfusion will have no effect on heparin.
D. Cryoprecipitate.
Rationale: Cryoprecipitate should not be used to reverse the effects of heparin.
E. Protamine sulfate.
Rationale: Protamine rapidly reverses the effects of heparin.

Major points of discussion
- Unfractionated heparin binds to antithrombin and accelerates the inactivation of thrombin and factor Xa, preventing fibrin formation.
- Protamine sulfate binds to and neutralizes heparin.
- Protamine must be dosed carefully since it can have an anticoagulant effect resulting in hemorrhage.
- Protamine can also be used to reverse the effects of low-molecular-weight heparins, but it only partially reverses anti-Xa activity.
- Fresh frozen plasma provides an additional source of antithrombin, thereby potentially increasing the anticoagulant effects of heparin.

72. A. Give platelets and cryoprecipitate before recombinant activated factor VII at a dose of 90 µg/kg.
Rationale: This patient has received more platelets than is necessary compared with the quantity of other products given.
B. Give RBCs and cryoprecipitate before recombinant activated factor VII at a dose of 90 µg/kg.
Rationale: Additional RBCs may be needed, but this patient needs optimization of other products first.
C. Give plasma and cryoprecipitate before giving recombinant activated factor VII at a dose of 90 µg/kg.

Rationale: This patient has not received enough plasma compared with the quantity of RBCs transfused. It is important to ensure that enough thrombin and fibrinogen are present as a substrate before giving recombinant activated factor VII.

D. Give platelets and RBCs before giving recombinant activated factor VII at a dose of 90 μg/kg.

Rationale: Product utilization needs to be optimized for this patient before the administration of additional RBCs and platelets.

E. Give recombinant activated factor VII at a dose of 90 μg/kg.

Rationale: It is important to ensure that enough thrombin and fibrinogen are present as a substrate before giving recombinant activated factor VII.

Major points of discussion

■ Increasing evidence supports the use of a high ratio of RBCs:platelets:plasma in massively transfused patients.

■ The use of high ratios of RBCs:platelets:plasma has been associated with improved survival.

■ Different definitions of massive transfusion have been used, but the two most common are transfusion of 10 U or more of RBCs or replacement of a patient's blood volume in 24 hours or less.

■ The patient in this question has received too many platelet doses and not enough plasma based upon current evidence.

■ Recombinant activated factor VII complexes with tissue factor to activate factor X to factor Xa and factor IX to factor IXa.

■ The activation of these factors leads to activation of the common pathway of coagulation and formation of a fibrin plug.

■ For this to occur, sufficient quantities of substrate must be present.

■ This patient needs additional plasma and cryoprecipitate to help ensure efficacy of recombinant activated factor VII.

73. A. Increased consumption secondary to disseminated intravascular coagulopathy.

Rationale: Patients may develop disseminated intravascular coagulopathy while on ECMO circuits, but it is not the cause of increased platelet requirements for most patients on ECMO.

B. Increased consumption secondary to mucosal bleeding from anticoagulation.

Rationale: This does not cause an increase in platelet requirements during ECMO.

C. Increased clearance secondary to heparin-induced thrombocytopenia.

Rationale: Heparin is used to anticoagulate the ECMO circuit, but not every patient will develop heparin-induced thrombocytopenia, which is caused by antibodies to heparin complexed with platelet factor 4.

D. Increased clearance secondary to platelet activation and adherence to tubing and the membrane oxygenator.

Rationale: Platelet contact with the surface of the tubing leads to activation.

E. Increased clearance secondary to increased capillary leak.

Rationale: Capillary leak syndrome can develop in patients on ECMO, but it is not the cause of increased platelet requirements for most patients on ECMO.

Major points of discussion

■ Cardiopulmonary bypass and ECMO circuits lead to widespread activation of the hemostatic system.

■ Platelet contact with the tubing in these circuits leads to activation.

■ The increase in free radicals produced by high oxygen tension leads to further platelet activation.

■ Platelet aggregation and function are impaired during the course of ECMO treatment.

■ Platelet transfusions are required to maintain platelet counts above 100,000/μL.

74. A. Recommend platelets to ensure hemostasis during the procedure.

B. Recommend platelets due to his decreased platelet count.

Rationale: The platelet count ($>50 \times 10^9$/L) is sufficient to maintain adequate hemostasis during this procedure.

C. Do not recommend platelets because his current platelet count is sufficient.

Rationale: The patient's platelet count ($>50 \times 10^9$/L) is sufficient for hemostasis in this clinical setting.

D. Do not recommend platelets since they may promote inflammation in this patient.

Rationale: Platelets should not promote inflammation in this patient.

E. Only recommend platelets if the patient develops moderate bleeding.

Rationale: The platelet count should be sufficient if moderate bleeding develops.

Major points of discussion

■ Without evidence of platelet dysfunction, a platelet count of 100×10^9/L should be sufficient to maintain hemostasis in a patient undergoing abdominal surgery.

■ The transfusion trigger for a patient with bleeding or about to undergo a surgical procedure is 50×10^9/L.

■ In patients with platelet dysfunction, such as patients on aspirin therapy, the decision to transfuse should be based on the patient's clinical status and not the platelet count.

■ Platelet units can have several hundred milliliters of plasma, so plasma compatible units should be used if possible.

■ Platelets do not express the D antigen, but a small dose of RBCs that may be sufficient to induce alloimmunization may be present. Rh-compatible units should be transfused if possible.

75. A. 30 minutes.
B. 2 hours.

Rationale: The half-life of recombinant activated factor VII in adults is approximately 2 hours.

C. 4 hours.
D. 6 hours.
E. 8 hours.

Rationale for A, C, D, and E: These are not the half-life of recombinant activated factor VII in adults.

Major points of discussion

- Recombinant activated factor VII is a lyophilized powder that is reconstituted in a histidine diluent and administered as an intravenous slow bolus injection over 3 to 5 minutes.
- After administration, recombinant activated factor VII complexes with tissue factor and activates factor X to factor Xa and factor IX to factor IXa. This leads to the formation of a fibrin plug and local hemostasis.
- Thrombin generation in response to recombinant activated factor VII is dose dependent.
- PT and aPTT show no direct correlation with the efficacy of recombinant activated factor VII in achieving hemostasis.
- The PT will shorten in most patients, but the clinical significance of this is unknown.
- A dose of approximately 90 μg/kg is recommended, but doses ranging from 35 to 120 μg/kg have been demonstrated to be effective in clinical trials.

76. A. 1,500 IU.
B. 3,000 IU.
C. 4,500 IU.
D. 6,000 IU.
Rationale: This is the correct dosage for this patient calculated using dose required (IU) = weight (kg) × desired factor IX increase (IU/dL) × 1 IU/kg.
E. 7,500 IU.
Rationale for A, B, C, and E: These are not the correct dosages for this patient.

Major points of discussion

- Hemophilia B is a sex-linked recessive genetic disorder leading to a deficiency in factor IX.
- Patients have a prolonged activated partial thromboplastin time, normal prothrombin time, and decreased factor IX activity.
- Hemophilia B is divided clinically into three groups: mild, greater than 5% factor IX activity; moderate, 1% to 5% factor IX activity; and severe, less than 1% factor IX activity.
- Treatment involves administration of factor IX concentrates to prevent and manage bleeding episodes.
- The factor IX dose is calculated using this formula: dose required (IU) = weight (kg) × desired factor IX increase (IU/dL) × 1 IU/kg.
- Factor IX does not remain in the intravascular space. About 50% of the administered factor IX will distribute to the extravascular space.
- Factor IX should be dosed every 24 hours due to the in vivo half-life of factor IX.

77. A. 3,400 IU.
B. 5,100 IU.
C. 5,673 IU.
Rationale: This is the correct dosage for this patient calculated using dose required (IU) = weight (kg) × desired factor VIII increase (IU/dL) × [1 – hematocrit (%)].
D. 5,848 IU.
E. 7,396 IU.
Rationale for A, B, D, and E: This is not the correct dosage for this patient.

Major points of discussion

- Hemophilia A is an X-linked recessive genetic disorder leading to a deficiency in factor VIII.
- Patients have a prolonged activated partial thromboplastin time, normal prothrombin time, and decreased factor VIII activity.
- Hemophilia A is divided clinically into three groups: mild-greater than 5% factor VIII activity, moderate, 1% to 5% factor VIII activity, and severe, less than 1% factor VIII activity.
- Treatment involves administration of factor VIII concentrates to prevent and manage bleeding episodes.
- The factor VIII dose is calculated using this formula: Dose required (IU) = weight (kg) × desired factor VIII increase (IU/dL) × (1 – hematocrit).
- Factor VIII should be dosed every 12 hours due to the in-vivo half-life of factor VIII.[6]

78. A. 1,900 platelets × m^2/μL.
B. 2,350 platelets × m^2/μL.
Rationale: This is the corrected count increment as calculated by the formula: CCI = [body surface area (m^2) × (post platelet count – pre platelet count) × 10^{11}]/number of platelets transfused.
C. 3,830 platelets × m^2/μL.
D. 4,737 platelets × m^2/μL.
E. 7,833 platelets × m^2/μL.
Rationale for A, C, D, and E: This is not the corrected count increment.

Major points of discussion

- Platelet refractoriness is a common problem in multiply transfused patients.
- A CCI is calculated to determine whether a patient is responding appropriately to platelet transfusions.
- A CCI is calculated using a pretransfusion platelet count and a platelet count obtained 10 to 60 minutes posttransfusion.
- The formula is: CCI = [body surface area (m^2) × (post platelet count – pre platelet count) × 10^{11}]/number of platelets transfused.
- Many institutions define platelet refractoriness as two CCIs of less than 5,000 platelets × m^2/μL; however, some institutions use 7,500 platelets × m^2/μL.
- If the patient appears to be refractory, but the CCI is greater than 5,000 or 7,500 platelets × m^2/μL, then nonimmune causes should be considered.
- A platelet antibody screen can be ordered to determine if the patient has anti HLA antibodies, anti-platelet antibodies, or a combination of both.
- Anti–class I HLA antibodies are the most common cause of immune platelet refractoriness.
- Nonimmune causes include fever, sepsis, antibiotics, disseminated intravascular coagulation, and splenomegaly.

79a. A. Order HLA-matched platelets.
Rationale: HLA-matched platelets are not appropriate therapy at this time since the presence of an anti-HLA antibody has not been established.
B. Order crossmatched platelets.

Rationale: Crossmatched platelets are not appropriate therapy at this time since the presence of anti-platelet antibodies has not been established.

C. Order a platelet antibody screen.

Rationale: A platelet antibody screen should be ordered after it is determined that an immune cause of platelet refractoriness is likely present.

D. Order 1-hour posttransfusion platelet counts.

Rationale: A 1-hour posttransfusion platelet count will allow you to calculate a corrected count increment. This will help you to establish whether platelet clearance is due to an immune or non-immune cause.

E. Order a platelet drip of 1 dose of single-donor apheresis platelets transfused over 4 hours.

Rationale: This is not indicated and will not likely increase the platelet count.

79b. A. Splenic infarction.

Rationale: Splenic infarction is not associated with platelet refractoriness.

B. Localized infection.

Rationale: Sepsis, but not localized infections, is associated with platelet refractoriness.

C. Aspirin therapy.

Rationale: Aspirin causes irreversible platelet dysfunction but does not cause platelet refractoriness.

D. Obesity.

Rationale: Obese patients may require more doses of platelets to see the desired increment in platelet count because of their increased body surface area.

E. Antibiotic therapy.

Rationale: Multiple antibiotics have been associated with refractoriness to platelet transfusions.

Major points of discussion

- Platelet refractoriness is a common issue and may be due to immune or nonimmune causes.
- Nonimmune causes include fever, sepsis, antibiotics, disseminated intravascular coagulation, and splenomegaly.
- Patients receiving multiple RBC or platelet transfusions may develop anti–class I HLA antibodies, anti-platelet antibodies, or a combination of both.
- A CCI calculated using a 1-hour posttransfusion platelet count of less than 5000 platelets $\times$ m^2/µL indicates a likely immune cause of refractoriness.
- The CCI is calculated using the following formula: CCI = [body surface area (m^2) $\times$ (post platelet count – pre platelet count) $\times 10^{11}$]/number of platelets transfused.
- A platelet antibody screen will detect the presence of anti–class I HLA antibodies, anti-platelet antibodies, or a combination of both.
- The patient's plasma is mixed with a panel of platelets to determine reactivity.
- Anti–class I HLA antibody reactivity is destroyed with chloroquine.
- Depending on the antibody specificity seen, HLA-matched platelets or crossmatched platelets may be used.
- Some institutions will do a trial of ABO-matched platelets as platelets express ABH antigens and an improvement in the posttransfusion increment may be seen.

80. A. Fresh frozen plasma.

Rationale: Fresh frozen plasma is not indicated in this patient since the PT and aPTT are within the reference ranges and the patient does not have evidence of a coagulopathy.

B. Cryoprecipitate-depleted plasma.

Rationale: The only clinical indication for cryoprecipitate-depleted plasma is thrombotic thrombocytopenic purpura.

C. Cryoprecipitate.

Rationale: Cryoprecipitate is indicated for this patient since she has documented hypofibrinogenemia.

D. Platelets.

Rationale: Platelets are not indicated for this patient since her platelet count is within the reference range and there is no evidence of a thrombocytopathy.

E. RBCs.

Rationale: Red blood cells are not indicated, as there is no evidence of reduced oxygen-carrying capacity in this patient.

Major points of discussion

- Cryoprecipitate is most commonly used to replace fibrinogen due to increased losses or consumption.
- Each unit of cryoprecipitate must have a minimum of 150 mg of fibrinogen and 80 IU of factor VIII.
- Cryoprecipitate also contains factor XIII, von Willebrand factor, and fibronectin.
- Patients with fibrinogen levels less than 100 mg/dL are considered to have hypofibrinogenemia.
- The PT and aPTT may start to prolong at fibrinogen levels of less than 100 mg/dL.

81. A. 7 U.

B. 9 U.

C. 10 U.

D. 14 U.

Rationale: This is the correct dose based on the formula: Dose (units) = [post-fibrinogen (mg/dL) – pre-fibrinogen (mg/dL) $\times$ plasma volume]/250 mg/unit using (1 – hematocrit) $\times$ 0.7 dL/kg $\times$ body mass (kg) to calculate the plasma volume.

E. 21 U.

Rationale for A, B, C, and E: These are not the correct doses.

Major points of discussion

- Each unit of cryoprecipitate must have a minimum of 150 mg of fibrinogen, although the average unit has approximately 250 mg.
- Usually a dose of 10 U of cryoprecipitate is administered, but an exact dose can be calculated for fibrinogen replacement.
- The formula for calculating the number of units of cryoprecipitate needed is: Dose (units) = [post-fibrinogen (mg/dL) – pre-fibrinogen (mg/dL) $\times$ plasma volume]/250 mg/unit.
- Plasma volume is calculated as (1 – hematocrit) $\times$ 0.7 dL/kg $\times$ body mass (kg).
- Each unit is 10 to 15 mL.
- The units can be pooled in the blood bank or at the patient's bedside.
- Once pooled, they expire after 4 hours instead of 6 hours for unpooled units.

- Patients with congenital afibrinogenemia or dysfibrinogenemia may require routine fibrinogen replacement therapy. The FDA has approved an intravenous fibrinogen concentrate for this purpose.

82. A. Platelets.
Rationale: This patient took aspirin, which is an irreversible inhibitor of platelet function. Since this patient presents with bleeding, platelet transfusion would be indicated.
B. Fresh frozen plasma.
Rationale: FFP is not indicated since the PT is in the reference range. The patient is likely not taking the warfarin prescribed.
C. RBCs.
Rationale: Red blood cells are not indicated since the patient is not showing symptoms of anemia.
D. Cryoprecipitate.
Rationale: Cryoprecipitate is not indicated since the PT and aPTT are within the reference range.
E. Granulocytes.
Rationale: Granulocytes are not indicated since the patient is not neutropenic and does not have a documented infection unresponsive to antibiotic therapy.

Major points of discussion
- Aspirin irreversibly inhibits platelet cyclooxygenase, preventing the production of thromboxane A_2.
- Thromboxane A_2 activates platelets and is a potent aggregating agent.
- Aspirin therapy can lead to an increased risk of bleeding in some patients.
- For most patients, one dose of single-donor apheresis platelets would be sufficient to correct the thrombocytopathy.
- Other than correcting the thrombocytopathy in this patient, the patient's clinical status and laboratory values should guide the decision to transfuse.
- Despite the history of warfarin therapy, fresh frozen plasma is not indicated in this patient since his PT is within the reference range.

83. A. Transfuse one dose of single-donor apheresis platelets.
Rationale: Platelets are not indicated in the treatment of this patient, as they would likely be rapidly cleared.
B. Corticosteroids.
Rationale: Corticosteroids are the first-line treatment for immune thrombocytopenia.
C. Therapeutic plasmapheresis.
Rationale: Immune thrombocytopenia is a category IV indication for plasmapheresis. Current evidence demonstrates that plasmapheresis is ineffective and should not be used.
D. Thrombopoietin.
Rationale: Thrombopoietin is not a first-line treatment for immune thrombocytopenia.
E. Rituximab.
Rationale: Rituximab is not a first-line treatment for immune thrombocytopenia.

Major points of discussion
- Immune thrombocytopenia (ITP) is the most likely cause of isolated thrombocytopenia in an otherwise healthy patient.

- It is defined as an isolated platelet count less than 100×10^9/L.
- Patients may present with petechiae/purpura, bruising, or mucosal bleeding, but many patients are asymptomatic.
- ITP is due to accelerated destruction of platelets by antiplatelet antibodies. There is increased clearance of antibody-coated platelets by the spleen.
- Additionally, there is evidence of decreased production of platelets by megakaryocytes in the bone marrow.
- Corticosteroids, intravenous immunoglobulin, and anti-Rho(D) immune globulin (WinRho) are the first-line agents for the treatment of ITP.
- Splenectomy, rituximab, and thrombopoietin receptor agonists are second-line therapies.
- In the absence of severe bleeding, ITP is considered a relative contraindication for platelet transfusion since the patient's antiplatelet antibodies will rapidly clear the transfused platelets.

84. A. Immune thrombocytopenia.
Rationale: In the absence of significant bleeding, platelet transfusions are not indicated in these patients since antiplatelet antibodies will rapidly clear transfused platelets. However, transfusion of platelets is not harmful to these patients.
B. History of allergic reactions to platelets.
Rationale: Premedication may be given to ameliorate allergic symptoms in these patients. Platelet transfusions should be provided if clinically necessary.
C. Platelet refractoriness.
Rationale: These patients may not respond appropriately to random donor platelets, and transfusing human leukocyte antigen–matched or crossmatched platelets should be considered.
D. Neonatal alloimmune thrombocytopenia.
Rationale: Platelet transfusions are often indicated in the treatment of neonatal alloimmune thrombocytopenia to prevent intracranial hemorrhage. Antigen-negative platelets may need to be provided, but random donor platelets have been shown to be beneficial in many cases.
E. Thrombotic thrombocytopenic purpura.
Rationale: Transfusion of platelets in patients with thrombotic thrombocytopenic purpura is contraindicated in the absence of life-threatening bleeding or surgery due to the potential thrombotic effect.

Major points of discussion
- Thrombotic thrombocytopenic purpura (TTP) is a thrombotic microangiopathy characterized by profound thrombocytopenia and microangiopathic hemolytic anemia due to the production of anti-ADAMTS13 (a disintegrin and metalloproteinase with a thrombospondin type 1 motif, member 13) antibodies causing a deficiency in ADAMTS13.
- TTP is classically described as the pentad of microangiopathic hemolytic anemia, thrombocytopenia, fever, renal disease, and neurologic dysfunction; the presence of microangiopathic hemolytic anemia and thrombocytopenia is sufficient evidence to initiate treatment.
- ADAMTS13 is a metalloprotease that cleaves ultralarge von Willebrand factor multimers.

- Deficiency in ADAMTS13 due to the presence of an inhibitor leads to activation of platelets by ultralarge von Willebrand factor multimers and the formation of multiple thromboses within the microvasculature and hemolytic anemia.
- Platelet transfusion is contraindicated in these patients as the transfused platelets may contribute to the formation of additional thromboses.
- Platelet transfusions should be provided to these patients in the setting of life-threatening bleeding or surgery.
- For similar reasons, platelet transfusions are contraindicated in patients with heparin-induced thrombocytopenia in the absence of limb- or life-threatening bleeding or surgery.

85. A. An 85-year-old female patient with a history of cardiac disease, hypertension, and metastatic breast carcinoma currently hospitalized with urosepsis, WBC 20.2×10^9/L.
Rationale: Granulocytes would not be indicated in this patient since her bone marrow is responding appropriately to the infection.
B. A 10-year-old boy with acute lymphoblastic leukemia with disseminated CMV infection, WBC 0.4×10^9/L.
Rationale: Granulocyte transfusions are not indicated in the treatment of viral infections.
C. A 45-year-old female patient with acute myelogenous leukemia after unrelated allogeneic hematopoietic stem cell transplant and documented engraftment failure, WBC 0.2×10^9/L.
Rationale: Granulocyte transfusions should only be given to patients with documented bacterial or fungal infections and expected bone marrow recovery.
D. A 62-year-old female patient with chronic lymphocytic leukemia with staphylococcal sepsis on antibiotic therapy, WBC 2.0×10^9/L.
Rationale: Granulocyte transfusions should only be given to patients who are severely neutropenic with absolute neutrophil counts less than 500/μL.
E. A 5-year-old boy with neuroblastoma after autologous hematopoietic stem cell transplant with disseminated candidiasis unresponsive to antifungal therapy, WBC 0.1×10^9/L.
Rationale: This patient is a candidate for granulocyte transfusions.

Major points of discussion
- Granulocyte transfusions have been reported to be successful in the treatment of bacterial and fungal infections in severely neutropenic patients who are unresponsive to antibiotic or antifungal therapy.
- Granulocyte transfusions should only be considered in patients with temporary severe neutropenia and bone marrow recovery is expected.
- The absolute neutrophil count of recipients should be less than 500/μL.
- Patients with chronic granulomatous disease and deep-seated abscesses or fungal infections unresponsive to antibiotic/antifungal therapy are also considered candidates for granulocyte transfusion therapy.
- Granulocyte transfusions are given once daily until the patient recovers.

- Granulocyte transfusions should be ABO-compatible and irradiated.
- Granulocytes should be CMV negative when provided to CMV-negative patients.
- Granulocyte transfusions and amphotericin administration should be spaced out temporally due to the increase in respiratory reactions.
- Doses less than 1×10^{10} cells/kg are generally ineffective.
- Donors are stimulated with corticosteroids with or without costimulation with granulocyte-colony stimulating factor (G-CSF) to achieve higher yields.

86. A. Idiopathic thrombocytopenic purpura.
Rationale: Idiopathic thrombocytopenic purpura (ITP) is unlikely without a history of ITP or bleeding in the mother. Neonates with thrombocytopenia secondary to maternal ITP have a low risk of bleeding.
B. Thrombotic thrombocytopenic purpura.
Rationale: Congenital thrombotic thrombocytopenic purpura (TTP) or Upshaw-Schulman syndrome is not the most likely diagnosis.
C. Neonatal alloimmune thrombocytopenia.
Rationale: Neonatal alloimmune thrombocytopenia (NAIT) is the most common cause of early-onset severe neonatal thrombocytopenia and intracranial hemorrhage in an otherwise healthy full-term neonate.
D. Congenital CMV infection.
Rationale: Congenital CMV can cause neonatal thrombocytopenia, but it is not the most likely diagnosis.
E. Hemolytic disease of the fetus and newborn.
Rationale: HDFN can cause severe anemia but would not be expected to cause thrombocytopenia and hemorrhage.

Major points of discussion
- NAIT is the most common cause of thrombocytopenia (platelet count <50,000/μL) in an otherwise healthy neonate.
- NAIT is due to maternal anti-platelet antibodies that react to a paternally inherited fetal platelet antigen.
- NAIT most commonly occurs due to incompatibility in human platelet antigen (HPA)-1a.
- Only 2% of whites are negative for HPA-1a, and HPA-1a negative mothers may be exposed to the foreign antigen during pregnancy.
- The neonate may present with petechiae, purpura, or bleeding, but most cases are asymptomatic.
- Intracranial hemorrhage is the most severe consequence of NAIT and may occur in up to 10% of cases. The vast majority of cases of intracerebral hemorrhage secondary to NAIT occur in utero.
- Alloimmunization is thought to occur during the first incompatible pregnancy with subsequent fetuses/neonates being affected; however, recent data demonstrate that NAIT may present in the first incompatible pregnancy as well.
- Diagnosis is confirmed by identification of a maternal antibody directed against a paternally inherited fetal platelet antigen using either serologic tests or platelet genotyping.
- Washed maternal platelets may be used to provide antigen-negative transfusions, but random platelets have been shown to be effective especially in emergent settings.

87. A. Transfusion-related acute lung injury.
Rationale: Transfusion-related acute lung injury presents with hypoxemia within 6 hours of transfusion.
B. Post-transfusion purpura.
Rationale: Rapid onset of severe thrombocytopenia approximately 10 days after transfusion is compatible with posttransfusion purpura.
C. Transfusion-associated graft-versus-host disease.
Rationale: Pancytopenia, not just thrombocytopenia, would be expected with transfusion-associated graft-versus-host disease.
D. Platelet refractoriness.
Rationale: This patient is not receiving platelet transfusions at this time.
E. HLA alloimmunization.
Rationale: The patient may be alloimmunized to HLA antigens but that would not be the cause of her thrombocytopenia in this setting.

Major points of discussion
- Post-transfusion purpura (PTP) is an uncommon posttransfusion complication.
- PTP occurs in patients who are alloimmunized to platelet antigens, most commonly to HPA-1a.
- PTP most commonly occurs after the transfusion of RBCs but may also occur after platelet and plasma transfusions.
- The platelets in the transfused product along with autologous platelets are destroyed leading to thrombocytopenia.
- The mechanism by which autologous platelets are destroyed is unknown, but it is thought that the preformed anti-platelet antibody has some autoreactivity that develops after reexposure to the foreign platelet antigen.
- Patients typically present with severe thrombocytopenia (platelet counts <10,000/μL) and bleeding.
- The thrombocytopenia is typically self-limiting and lasts approximately 2 weeks.
- The treatment of choice is intravenous immunoglobulin infusions, but the efficacy of this treatment is unknown.
- It is suggested that future transfusions should be matched for the foreign antigen as recurrences, though rare, have been reported.

88. A. Hold warfarin therapy.
Rationale: For a patient with an INR of 9, holding warfarin therapy is not sufficient treatment.
B. Hold warfarin therapy and give oral vitamin K.
Rationale: This is the recommended treatment for a patient with an INR greater than 5 without significant bleeding.
C. Hold warfarin therapy and give intramuscular vitamin K.
Rationale: Intramuscular administration of vitamin K is not recommended due to the significant risk of hematoma.
D. Hold warfarin therapy and give intravenous vitamin K and fresh frozen plasma.
Rationale: Fresh frozen plasma would not be indicated at an INR of 9 in the absence of bleeding.
E. Hold warfarin therapy and give intravenous vitamin K and recombinant activated factor VII.
Rationale: Recombinant activated factor VII would not be indicated in this patient due to the absence of significant bleeding.

Major points of discussion
- A patient with an INR of 9 is at risk of developing significant bleeding. Warfarin therapy should be immediately stopped and oral vitamin K should be administered.
- Warfarin inhibits the synthesis of the vitamin K–dependent clotting factors (II, VII, IX, and X) by inhibiting gamma carboxylation.
- Replacement of vitamin K will allow for repletion of the vitamin K–dependent clotting factors and correction of the INR.
- Fresh frozen plasma may be used to replace vitamin K–dependent clotting factors and to reverse the INR in patients on warfarin with bleeding.
- The use of fresh frozen plasma to correct mildly elevated INRs prophylactically before interventional procedures is not recommended.
- Prothrombin complex concentrates and recombinant activated factor VII are only recommended in the presence of significant bleeding and very elevated INRs.

89. A. Transfuse 4 to 6 U fresh frozen plasma to correct her coagulopathy.
Rationale: Transfusion of plasma to correct the mild elevations in the PT and aPTT before interventions/surgery is not indicated.
B. Transfuse 10 U cryoprecipitate to provide additional fibrinogen.
Rationale: The patient has sufficient fibrinogen for hemostasis in the absence of significant bleeding or consumption.
C. Transfuse 1 dose of single-donor apheresis platelets to correct her thrombocytopathy.
Rationale: There is no evidence of thrombocytopathy in this patient at this time.
D. Transfuse 2 U RBCs to correct the anemia.
Rationale: There is no evidence of symptomatic anemia necessitating transfusion of RBCs.
E. No transfusion is needed at this time.
Rationale: This patient should be hemostatic with her current laboratory values.

Major points of discussion
- The PT and aPTT are not good predictors of bleeding during surgical interventions.
- These tests may be elevated when patients have mild deficiencies in multiple clotting factors that are not associated with an increased bleeding risk. As such, plasma transfusion in not indicated in this patient.
- Furthermore, transfusion of plasma to correct a mildly elevated PT or aPTT produces little change in the laboratory value being treated.
- If plasma transfusion is indicated, a dose of 10 to 20 mL/kg should be provided to have a clinical effect.
- Due to the short half-life of certain clotting factors, plasma transfusions should be given immediately before the intervention to provide the desired hemostatic effect.

90. **A. Treatment of early and profound coagulopathy.**
Rationale: Coagulopathy during massive transfusion can occur very rapidly and current evidence supports transfusion of high ratios of plasma to RBCs.

B. Prevention of hypothermia.
Rationale: Plasma transfusions will not prevent hypothermia.
C. Improved oxygen delivery to the tissues.
Rationale: Red blood cell not plasma transfusions increase oxygen delivery to the tissues.
D. To provide volume replacement.
Rationale: Plasma transfusions should never be used as volume replacement.
E. To facilitate healing.
Rationale: Transfusion of plasma does not facilitate healing.

Major points of discussion

- Patients with severe hemorrhage necessitating massive transfusion often present with early and profound coagulopathy.
- Administration of colloids and RBC products further exacerbate dilutional and consumptive coagulopathy.
- Coagulopathy is further worsened by hypothermia, acidosis, hepatic impairment from hemorrhagic shock, and disseminated intravascular coagulation induced by tissue injury.
- Early transfusion of plasma products helps to correct the early coagulopathy seen in severely injured patients and improves mortality.
- Reduced hemorrhage by treating early coagulopathy helps to prevent the "bloody vicious cycle."
- The "bloody vicious cycle" is the development of hypothermia, coagulopathy, and acidosis induced by hemorrhage. Each of these factors further worsens the other two, often leading to rapid death.
- Some studies support the administration of blood products in a ratio that mimics whole blood.
- The best ratio of RBCs to platelets to plasma is debatable at present, but higher ratios are associated with better outcomes and improved mortality.
- Many hospitals have implemented massive transfusion protocols dictating how RBCs, plasma, platelets, cryoprecipitate, and sometimes recombinant activated factor VII should be transfused to massively bleeding patients.
- Different definitions of massive transfusion have been used, but the two most common are transfusion of greater than or equal to 10 U RBCs or replacement of a patient's blood volume in 24 hours or less.[13]

91. A. Hold warfarin therapy.
Rationale: Warfarin therapy should be held, but this is not sufficient treatment for this clinical scenario.
B. Hold warfarin therapy and give oral vitamin K.
Rationale: Warfarin therapy should be held and vitamin K should be administered, but oral vitamin K alone is not sufficient treatment for this clinical scenario.
C. Hold warfarin therapy and give intramuscular vitamin K.
Rationale: Intramuscular administration of vitamin K is not recommended due to the significant risk of hematoma.
D. Hold warfarin therapy and give intravenous vitamin K and fresh frozen plasma.
Rationale: This is appropriate therapy for this patient.
E. Hold warfarin therapy and give intravenous vitamin K and recombinant activated factor VII.

Rationale: Warfarin therapy should be held and intravenous vitamin K should be administered, but an immediate source of clotting factors should be provided. The use of recombinant activated factor VII is not indicated for the severity of bleeding in this patient.

Major points of discussion

- A patient with an INR of 9 with significant bleeding as seen in this patient necessitates immediate reversal of warfarin therapy.
- For this patient, intravenous vitamin K and fresh frozen plasma will correct the clotting factor deficiencies.
- Warfarin inhibits the synthesis of the vitamin K–dependent clotting factors (II, VII, IX, and X) by inhibiting gamma carboxylation.
- The use of prothrombin complex concentrates or recombinant activated factor VII are more commonly used in the setting of very significant bleeding.
- Both prothrombin complex concentrates and recombinant activated factor VII have a low risk of thrombosis.
- After administration of appropriate therapy to reverse warfarin, the INR should be closely monitored.
- Intravenous vitamin K may need to be readministered every 12 hours to continually replace clotting factors with shorter half-lives.

ADVERSE REACTIONS

92. **A. The citrate in the anticoagulant solution.**
Rationale: Citrate binds to free calcium ions, and can cause hypocalcemia. Symptoms of hypocalcemia include perioral tingling and numbness.
B. The dextrose in the anticoagulant solution.
Rationale: Dextrose is added as an energy source for the RBCs and does not cause the symptoms described.
C. Monobasic sodium phosphate in the anticoagulant solution.
Rationale: The addition of phosphate helps to maintain 2,3-DPG levels and does not cause the symptoms described.
D. The mannitol in the additive solution
Rationale: Mannitol allows for an increase in storage time by decreasing hemolysis and does not cause the symptoms described.
E. The adenine in the additive solution
Rationale: Adenine is added to increase the ATP levels needed for RBC survival and does not cause the symptoms described.

Major points of discussion

- Mild hypocalcemia typically presents with numbness and tingling in the perioral area and the fingers and toes, muscle tremors, and hypotension.
- Severe hypocalcemia can lead to tetany, refractory hypotension, seizures, syncope, and cardiac arrhythmias.
- Citrate is used as an anticoagulant and buffer in blood components.
- Citrate is rapidly metabolized by the liver to bicarbonate.
- Citrate binds free calcium ions, leading to hypocalcemia.

■ Hypocalcemia usually occurs during massive transfusion, therapeutic plasmapheresis, and in patients with liver dysfunction from underlying liver disease or hypothermia.
■ The increase in bicarbonate from citrate metabolism can lead to metabolic alkalosis.[13]

93. A. Transfusion-related acute lung injury.
Rationale: There is no plasma in recombinant activated factor VII; therefore, there is no risk of TRALI.
B. Increased transfusion requirements.
Rationale: The use of recombinant activated factor VII has been shown to reduce blood use in some studies.
C. Thromboembolic events.
Rationale: Thrombosis is a major concern when using recombinant activated factor VII.
D. Viral transmission.
Rationale: Recombinant activated factor VII is not human derived.
E. Hemolysis.
Rationale: Hemolysis is not a known adverse event associated with the use of recombinant activated factor VII.

Major points of discussion
■ Although rare, thromboembolic events are the major adverse event seen with recombinant activated factor VII use.
■ Thromboembolic events reported include cerebral vascular accidents, myocardial infarction, pulmonary embolism, deep vein thrombosis, thrombosis at the injection site, bowel infarction, and other arterial thromboses. Some of these events have been fatal.
■ Other reported adverse events include disseminated intravascular coagulopathy, pruritis, urticaria, hypersensitivity reactions, hypotension, nausea, vomiting, fever, injection site reactions, hemorrhage, headache, and thrombophlebitis.
■ It is unknown whether all of these adverse events were directly related to the administration of recombinant activated factor VII or related to the underlying disease process.
■ Rare cases of neutralizing antibody formation have been reported in patients with factor VII deficiency treated with recombinant activated factor VII.

94. A. Febrile nonhemolytic transfusion reaction.
Rationale: This may be a febrile nonhemolytic transfusion reaction, but other more important causes of these symptoms must be ruled out.
B. Transfusion-related acute lung injury.
Rationale: Dyspnea or hypoxemia is the presenting symptom of transfusion-related acute lung injury, which is not present in this patient.
C. Acute hemolytic transfusion reaction.
Rationale: The signs and symptoms are most likely associated with an acute hemolytic transfusion reaction.
D. Anaphylactic transfusion reaction.
Rationale: Urticaria and angioedema are the presenting symptoms, which are not present in this patient.
E. Transfusion-related sepsis.
Rationale: Acute onset of fever is a presenting symptom, but the back pain and red urine seen in this patient are

better explained by other diagnoses that must be ruled out first.

Major points of discussion
■ Acute hemolytic transfusion reactions (AHTRs) are rare but important causes of transfusion reactions.
■ They are the third most common cause of transfusion-related fatalities.
■ AHTRs may be due to the transfusion of ABO or non-ABO incompatible blood or may be nonimmune in origin.
■ There are many causes of nonimmune acute hemolysis, including improper storage conditions, infusion through a small-bore needle, blood warmer or rapid infuser malfunction, and infusion in the same line as other incompatible solutions (e.g., hypotonic saline).
■ Presenting signs and symptoms range from fever, chills, rigors, and back or flank pain to red urine, shock, hypotension, and disseminated intravascular coagulation.
■ If any transfusion reaction is suspected, the transfusion should be stopped immediately. The bag, tubing, and a blood and urine sample should be sent to the laboratory for analysis. Supportive care should be administered.
■ AHTRs are due to the interaction of a preformed antibody to a foreign RBC antigen in the transfused product resulting in complement activation and hemolysis.
■ AHTRs are most commonly due to clerical errors leading to improper patient identification, improper specimen labeling, and improper unit identification.[7]

95. A. Acute hemolytic transfusion reaction.
Rationale: This reaction would be accompanied by signs and symptoms of hemolysis, which are not provided for this patient.
B. Anaphylactic transfusion reaction.
Rationale: These reactions can be characterized by urticaria and angioedema as seen in this patient.
C. Transfusion-associated circulatory overload.
Rationale: Transfusion-associated circulatory overload is characterized by acute pulmonary edema due to volume overload. Although there is acute dyspnea, other evidence of volume overload including hypertension, jugular venous distention, or peripheral edema are not noted in this patient.
D. Transfusion-related acute lung injury.
Rationale: Transfusion-related acute lung injury is less likely due to the presence of urticaria and a similar past reaction.
E. Transfusion-related sepsis.
Rationale: These reactions are typically associated with hypotension, which is not present, and fever; in addition, sepsis is unlikely to occur multiple times in the same patient. Urticaria would not be present.

Major points of discussion
■ There is a wide spectrum of allergic reactions that can be seen in response to transfusion of blood components.
■ Mild allergic reactions are typically characterized by urticaria.

- More severe allergic or anaphylactic reactions are accompanied by angioedema with dyspnea and wheezing. Hypotension and shock can occur. Fever is not present.
- These reactions are due to preformed IgE antibody in the recipient to a protein found in the donor's plasma.
- Patients with absolute IgA deficiency may form anti-IgA antibodies which may lead to anaphylactic reactions.
- However, the vast majority of anaphylactic reactions are not due to anti-IgA antibodies in IgA deficient patients.

96. **A. Passive transfusion of cytokines or recipient cytokine response to transfusion.**
    Rationale: The cause of residual febrile nonhemolytic transfusion reactions is not known, but they may be due to platelet-derived factors and the production of cytokines by the recipient in response to the transfusion.
    B. Passive transfusion of anti–human leukocyte antigen (HLA) antibodies for which the patient has the cognate antigen.
    Rationale: TRALI is due to the passive transfusion of anti-HLA antibodies.
    C. Passive transfusion of biologically active lipids.
    Rationale: TRALI can occur from the transfusion of biologically active lipids.
    D. Passive transfusion of cells carrying an RBC antigen for which the patient makes an alloantibody.
    Rationale: Acute or delayed hemolytic transfusion reactions are due to RBC alloantibodies to foreign RBC antigens in transfused RBCs.
    E. Passive transfusion of plasma proteins to which the recipient makes IgE antibodies.
    Rationale: Allergic transfusion reactions are due to activation of mast cells after IgE antibodies bind to donor plasma proteins.

Major points of discussion
- FNHTRs are defined by an increase in body temperature by 1°C above 37°C.
- Other symptoms include chills, rigors, headache, nausea, vomiting, and changes in respiratory rate, heart rate, and blood pressure.
- FNHTR is a diagnosis of exclusion, and all other causes of fever must be ruled out.
- Fever can be a presenting symptom of much more serious transfusion reactions, including acute hemolytic reactions and transfusion-related sepsis, or may be unrelated to the transfusion.
- Transfused white blood cells that interact with anti-neutrophil or anti-HLA antibodies in the recipient along with transfused leukocyte-derived cytokines were responsible for the vast majority of FNHTRs before prestorage leukoreduction.
- The incidence of FNHTRs decreased dramatically after the introduction of prestorage leukoreduction. However, bedside leukoreduction does not prevent

the transfusion of elaborated cytokines produced during storage.

97. A. Onset of symptoms within 24 hours of transfusion.
    Rationale: Onset of symptoms must be within 6 hours of transfusion.
    B. Presence of fever.
    Rationale: Fever may or may not be present, but it is not part of the Canandian Consensus Conference definition of TRALI.
    C. Leukopenia.
    Rationale: Leukopenia may or may not be present, but it is not part of the Canandian Consensus Conference definition of TRALI.
    D. No evidence of left atrial hypertension.
    Rationale: This is part of the Canadian Consensus Conference definition of TRALI.
    E. Presence of irreversible lung injury.
    Rationale: This is not part of the Canadian Consensus Conference definition of TRALI, but the acute lung injury associated with TRALI is usually transient.

Major points of discussion
- TRALI is characterized by acute lung injury associated with transfusion.
- The Canadian Consensus Conference defined TRALI as new-onset acute lung injury meeting the following criteria:
  - Acute onset.
  - Hypoxemia defined as Pao_2/Fio_2 300 or less, oxygen saturation less than 90% on room air, or other evidence of hypoxemia.
  - Bilateral infiltrates on frontal chest radiograph.
  - No evidence of left atrial hypertension.
  - Onset of symptoms within 6 hours of transfusion.
  - No preexisting lung injury and no temporal or alternative risk factor for acute lung injury.
- Possible TRALI was defined as above with the presence of an alterative risk factor for acute lung injury.
- Accompanying symptoms may include dyspnea, fever, chills, hypertension, and hypotension.
- Symptoms usually improve within 48 to 96 hours.
- Transfusion of any plasma-containing blood component can be associated with TRALI. The greater the amount of plasma, the higher the risk (e.g., plasma more than RBCs).
- TRALI is currently understood as a two-hit model in which a preexisting event (trauma, surgery, infection, transfusion) causes the elaboration of biologically active compounds leading to priming and sequestration of neutrophils and activation of the pulmonary endothelium. The transfusion of biologically active mediators, anti-HLA antibodies, or anti-neutrophil antibodies activates the primed neutrophils. These events lead to endothelial damage in the lung and consequent pulmonary capillary leak syndrome and pulmonary edema.[11]

98. A. Transfusion-related circulatory overload.
    Rationale: Transfusion-related circulatory overload (TACO) presents with hypertension, not hypotension.
    B. Transfusion-related acute lung injury.

Rationale: This signs and symptoms meet the Canadian Consensus Conference definition of transfusion-related acute lung injury.

C. Anaphylaxis.

Rationale: Evidence of an allergic reaction including urticaria and angioedema are not present.

D. Acute hemolytic transfusion reaction.

Rationale: Signs and symptoms of hemolysis are not present.

E. Transfusion-related sepsis.

Rationale: Transfusion-related sepsis usually presents with fever, which is not seen in this patient.

Major points of discussion

- The patient described shows evidence of new-onset acute lung injury with hypoxemia, bilateral infiltrates on chest radiograph, no evidence of left atrial hypertension with no preexisting lung injury or alternative risk factor for acute lung injury within 6 hours of transfusion and, therefore, meets the Canadian Consensus Conference criteria for TRALI.
- TRALI must occur within 6 hours of transfusion but usually occurs within 2 hours of transfusion.
- TRALI must be differentiated from TACO, which may be difficult at times.
- Both present with dyspnea as the predominant symptom.
- TACO is due to cardiogenic pulmonary edema, while TRALI is due to noncardiogenic pulmonary edema.
- The absence of left atrial hypertension is included in the definition of TRALI to help with this distinction, although in practice, this proves to be difficult.
- Evidence of an anti-HLA or an anti-neutrophil antibody in the donor with the cognate antigen in the recipient provides support for a diagnosis of TRALI.
- Donors with an anti-HLA or anti-neutrophil antibody who have been implicated in a case of TRALI are deferred from future donations.[11]

99. **A. Increased iron from transfused RBCs leads to production of non–transferrin-bound iron.**

Rationale: Uptake of non–transferrin-bound iron along with uptake of transferrin bound iron leads to cellular damage by iron catalyzed production of reactive oxygen species.

B. Increased iron from transfused RBCs leads to decreased hepcidin levels.

Rationale: Hepcidin levels in chronically transfused patients are expected to be high to prevent additional iron absorption into the circulation.

C. Increased iron from transfused RBCs leads to increased expression of ferroportin.

Rationale: Ferroportin is internalized and degraded in response to the increased hepcidin levels expected in chronically transfused patients.

D. Increased iron from transfused RBCs leads to decreased hemosiderin.

Rationale: Hemosiderin deposition within tissues would be increased due to the excess iron.

E. Increased iron from transfused RBCs leads to decreased transferrin saturation.

Rationale: The transferrin saturation is expected to be increased in patients with iron overload.

Major points of discussion

- Males and nonmenstruating females have no effective mechanism to excrete excess iron and only about 1 to 2 mg are lost per day by sloughing of skin and small intestinal cells.
- Iron levels are regulated by the 25–amino acid hormone hepcidin, which prevents absorption of iron from duodenal enterocytes and prevents iron recycling from macrophages.
- Senescent RBCs are cleared by macrophages in the reticuloendothelial system. The enzyme heme oxygenase-1 releases ferrous iron from heme, also releasing biliverdin and carbon monoxide in the process.
- Under normal conditions, iron circulates in plasma bound to transferrin. Cells possess transferrin receptors on their membrane, which allows them to internalize iron.
- Non–transferrin-bound iron is taken up by the liver, pancreatic beta cells, cardiomyocytes, and other tissues leading to the generation of reactive oxygen species and subsequent DNA and cellular damage.
- Each unit of RBCs contains approximately 200 to 250 mg of iron.
- Chronically transfused patient populations, including patients with thalassemia, sickle cell disease, and other chronic anemias, are at the greatest risk of developing transfusion-induced iron overload.

100. A. *Staphylococcus aureus.*

Rationale: *S. aureus* is one of the most common contaminants in platelet products.

B. *Streptococcus bovis.*

Rationale: *S. bovis* has been implicated in cases of platelet-associated transfusion-transmitted sepsis.

C. *Pseudomonas aeruginosa.*

Rationale: *P. aeruginosa* has been implicated in RBC-associated transfusion-transmitted sepsis.

D. *Yersinia enterocolitica.*

Rationale: *Y. enterocolitica* is associated with approximately 46% to 56% of cases of RBC-associated transfusion-transmitted sepsis.

E. *Bacillus cereus.*

Rationale: *B. cereus* has been implicated in cases of platelet-associated transfusion-transmitted sepsis.

Major points of discussion

- Red blood cell–associated transfusion-transmitted sepsis is estimated to occur in about 1:250,000 RBC transfusions.
- Gram-negative organisms, mostly Enterobacteriaceae, are the primary cause of RBC-associated transfusion-transmitted sepsis.
- *Yersinia enterocolitica* accounts for approximately 46% to 56% of cases.
- *Serratia* spp., *Pseudomonas* spp., *Campylobacter* spp., and *Enterobacter* spp. have also been implicated.
- The overall fatality rate is high due to the transfusion of preformed bacterial endotoxin and the consequent rapid onset of septic shock.[3,9]

101a. **A. Septic transfusion reaction.**
Rationale: These reactions have a broad range of clinical severity ranging from mild fever and chills to fatal reactions.
B. Transfusion-related acute lung injury.
Rationale: According the Canadian Consensus Conference definition of TRALI, dyspnea must be one of the presenting symptoms.
C. Transfusion-associated circulatory overload.
Rationale: Dyspnea is one of the presenting symptoms.
D. Anaphylactic transfusion reaction.
Rationale: Fever is not usually present.
E. Delayed hemolytic transfusion reaction.
Rationale: These reactions occur more than 24 hours after the start of transfusion but are generally recognized 3 to 10 days after transfusion. Clinical and laboratory evidence of hemolysis is seen.

101b. A. RBCs.
Rationale: Red blood cells are the second most commonly bacterially contaminated product, although contamination and resultant septic reactions are relatively rare.
B. Platelets.
Rationale: Transfusion-associated bacteremia/sepsis is estimated at 1:60,000 platelet transfusions.
C. Fresh frozen plasma.
Rationale: Fresh frozen plasma is rarely associated with transfusion-transmitted sepsis.
D. Cryoprecipitate.
Rationale: Cryoprecipitate is rarely associated with transfusion-transmitted sepsis.
E. Granulocytes.
Rationale: Transfusion-transmitted sepsis associated with granulocyte transfusion has not been reported to date.

Major points of discussion
- Bacteremia or sepsis is the most common transfusion-transmitted infection today.
- Transfusion-transmitted sepsis is most commonly associated with platelet transfusions as they are stored at room temperature, which facilitates bacterial growth.
- These reactions may be very serious and even fatal.
- The most common sources of bacterial contamination are superficial and deep-rooted skin flora and subclinical infections in donors.
- Gram-positive bacteria, including coagulase-negative *Staphylococcus* spp., *Staphylococcus aureus*, *Streptococcus* spp., and *Bacillus cereus*, are the most common contaminants.
- Gram-negative contaminants are less common in platelets but are more often associated with fatal reactions secondary to endotoxemic shock.
- All platelet products are currently cultured before release to decrease the risk of transfusion-transmitted sepsis.
- Transfusion-transmitted sepsis has also been associated with the transfusion of RBCs; however, this is rare as the refrigerated storage temperature limits growth of most bacteria.

- Gram-negative organisms, mostly Enterobacteriaceae, are the primary cause of RBC–associated transfusion-transmitted sepsis, and *Yersinia enterocolitica* accounts for approximately 46% to 56% of cases.
- Transfusion-transmitted sepsis may present with fever, chills, hypotension, disseminated intravascular coagulation, renal failure, and frank shock during or shortly after a transfusion.

102. A. Delayed serologic transfusion reaction.
Rationale: The described reaction is acute and shows evidence of hemolysis.
B. Delayed hemolytic transfusion reaction.
Rationale: The described reaction to platelets is acute.
C. Acute hemolytic transfusion reaction.
Rationale: The patient developed an ABO-typing discrepancy from passive transfusion of anti-A antibodies in the platelet unit accompanied by evidence of hemolysis (hemoglobinuria and fever).
D. Febrile nonhemolytic transfusion reaction.
Rationale: There is evidence of hemolysis (hemoglobinuria and fever), so this should not be called a non-hemolytic reaction.
E. Rh disease.
Rationale: There is no evidence of an antibody to the Rh D antigen.

Major points of discussion
- Platelets do not have to be ABO-matched for transfusion; thus, this case represents a blood group A transfusion recipient transfused a blood group B or O platelet unit.
- Transfusion of even a small amount of plasma containing potent anti-A antibodies can induce hemoglobinuria. Thus, this reaction can even occur from transfusion of group O red cells, which contain less plasma than platelet units.
- Acute hemolysis is triggered by binding of antibodies that can fix complement. Activation of complement results in lysis of red cells with release of free hemoglobin into the circulation.
- The signs and symptoms of acute hemolytic transfusion reactions vary from none to the "feeling of impending doom," flushing, fever and chills, pain at the infusion site, flank/back pain, nausea, vomiting, disseminated intravascular coagulation, renal failure, shock, and death.
- Free hemoglobin is bound in the circulation by haptoglobin; free heme by hemopexin.

103. **A. Delayed serologic transfusion reaction.**
Rationale: The eluate is consistent with the presence of an alloantibody to the K antigen of the Kell blood group system; however, there is no evidence of hemolysis.
B. Delayed hemolytic transfusion reaction.
C. Acute hemolytic transfusion reaction.
Rationale: There is no evidence of hemolysis; thus, these are not hemolytic reactions.
D. Presence of a warm autoantibody
Rationale: Although the direct antiglobulin test is positive, it is a mixed field reaction and the eluate is consistent with the presence of an alloantibody to the K antigen of the Kell blood group system.

E. Presence of a cold autoantibody.
Rationale: The direct antiglobulin test is positive for IgG with a mixed field reactivity pattern. No evidence of IgM autoantibodies is provided.

Major points of discussion

- A mixed field reaction implies that there are two phenotypically distinct populations of RBCs in the circulation. In this case, the transfused cells that are K antigen positive are circulating with bound antibody, while the patient's red cells are not K antigen positive and, thus, are not circulating with bound alloantibody.
- A delayed serologic transfusion reaction refers to signs of a new alloantibody to circulating transfused RBCs without signs of hemolysis.
- Delayed serologic transfusion reactions are more common than delayed hemolytic transfusion reactions (i.e., most alloantibodies do not cause symptoms of hemolysis).
- Laboratory evidence of hemolysis in plasma includes: free hemoglobin, increased bilirubin, increased lactate dehydrogenase, decreased haptoglobin. Hemoglobin and urobilinogen may be seen in urine samples.
- When a patient develops a new alloantibody to a red cell antigen, all future transfusions should "honor" this alloantibody and only antigen-negative units should be provided.

104. A. Repeat Rh determination.
Rationale: The ABO group determination should be repeated.
B. Indirect antiglobulin test.
Rationale: Direct antiglobulin test should be performed.

C. Review and interpretation by the medical director.
Rationale: This is required per AABB Standards.
D. Serum haptoglobin.
Rationale: A serum haptoglobin may be useful but is not a part of the initial evaluation.
E. Complete blood count.
Rationale: A complete blood count is not required by AABB Standards.

Major points of discussion

- According to AABB Standards, the blood bank or transfusion service is to have policies, processes, and procedures for evaluating and reporting suspected transfusion reactions.
- These steps include speedy evaluation, review of clerical information by the blood bank or transfusion service, and notification of the blood bank or transfusion service medical director.
- The evaluation of a suspected hemolytic transfusion reaction should include the following:
  - Inspection of the posttransfusion reaction serum for evidence of hemolysis (use pretransfusion sample for comparison).
  - Repeat ABO group determination on the posttransfusion blood sample.
  - Direct antiglobulin test on the posttransfusion blood sample (if positive, compare to most recent pretransfusion sample).
  - Blood bank or transfusion service should have a process for indicating under what circumstances additional testing should be performed and what that testing should be.
  - Review and interpretation by the medical director.[1]

References

1. AABB. Standards for blood banks and transfusion services. 27th ed. Bethesda, MD: AABB: 2011.
2. Arinsburg SA, Skerrett DL, Kleinert D, Giardina PJ, Cushing MM. The significance of a positive DAT in thalassemia patients. Immunohematology 2010;26:87–91.
3. Blajchman MA, Beckers EAM, Dickmeiss E, Lin L, Moore G, Muylle L. Bacterial detection of platelets: current problems and possible resolutions. Transfus Med Rev 2005;18:195–204.
4. Boccardo P, Remuzzi G. Platelet dysfunction in renal failure. Semin Thromb Hemost 2004;30:579–589.
5. Candotti D, Allain JP. Transfusion-transmitted hepatitis B virus infection. J Hepatol 2009;51:798–809.
6. Corash L. Bacterial contamination of platelet components: potential solutions to prevent transfusion-transmitted sepsis. Exp Rev Hematol 2011;4:509–525.
7. Fatalities reported to FDA following blood collection and transfusion: annual summary for fiscal year 2010. Available at www.fda.gov/downloads/BiologicsBloodVaccines/SafetyAvailability/ReportaProblem/TransfusionDonationFatalities/UCM254860.pdf/.
8. FDA. Guidance for industry: recommendations for deferral of donors and quarantine and retrieval of blood and blood products in recent recipients of smallpox vaccine (Vaccinia virus) and certain contacts of smallpox vaccine recipients, 2002. Available at www.fda.gov/downloads/BiologicsBloodVaccines/GuidanceComplianceRegulatoryInformation/Guidances/Blood/ucm080319.pdf/.
9. Guinet F, Carniel E, Leclercq A. Transfusion-transmitted Yersinia enterocolitica sepsis. Clin Infect Dis 2011;53:583–591.
10. ISBT. Blood group terminology. Available at www.isbtweb.org/working-parties/red-cell-immunogenetics-and-blood-group-terminology/blood-group-terminology/.
11. Kleinman D, Caulfield T, Chan P, et al. Toward an understanding of transfusion-related acute lung injury: statement of a consensus panel. Transfusion 2004;44:1774–1789.
12. Reid MA, Lomas-Francis C. The blood group antigen facts book. 2nd ed. London, UK: Elsevier; 2007.
13. Sihler KC, Napolitano LM. Massive transfusion: new insights. Chest 2009;136:1654–1667.

CHAPTER 20

TRANSFUSION MEDICINE:
Therapeutic Apheresis

Suzanne A. Arinsburg, Joseph (Yossi) Schwartz, Eldad A. Hod, Richard O. Francis, Jeffrey S. Jhang, Yvette C. Tanhehco, Steven L. Spitalnik

QUESTIONS

1. Which type of apheresis procedure is best indicated to decrease recipient antibody titers in ABO-incompatible solid organ transplants?
   A. Leukapheresis.
   B. Erythrocytapheresis.
   C. Thrombocytapheresis.
   D. Plasmapheresis.
   E. Low-density lipoprotein (LDL) apheresis.

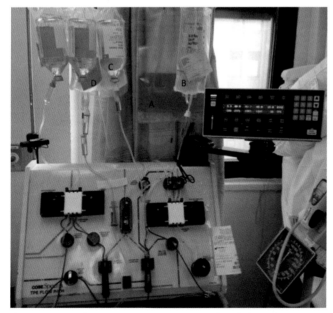

Figure 20-1 Apheresis instrument setup. An apheresis instrument is currently arranged for a patient treatment. Individual fluid bags are labeled as *A* to *D*.

2a. The instrument shown in Figure 20-1 is being used to perform which one of the following procedures?
   A. Plasmapheresis.
   B. Plateletpheresis.
   C. Red blood cell (RBC) exchange.
   D. Leukapheresis.
   E. Stem cell collection.

2b. Which labeled container in Figure 20-1 contains the most fibrinogen?
   A. A
   B. B
   C. C
   D. D
   E. None of the labeled containers contains measurable amounts of fibrinogen.

3. Which statement best describes the use of therapeutic plasma exchange (TPE) for the desensitization of renal transplant candidates with a positive living donor kidney crossmatch due to donor-specific human leukocyte antigen (HLA) antibodies?
   A. TPE is considered to be first-line therapy.
   B. TPE is considered to be second-line therapy.
   C. The benefit of TPE is unclear.
   D. TPE is ineffective.
   E. TPE has never been tried in this setting.

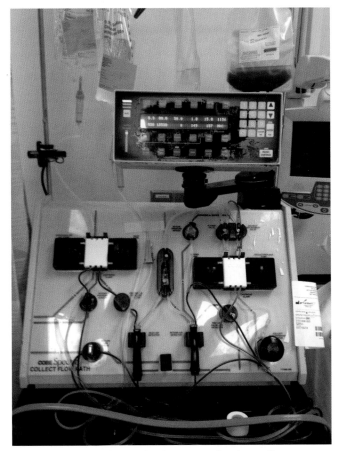

Figure 20-2 Apheresis procedure in progress. Continuous-flow centrifugation apheresis instrument performing the procedure described in Question 4.

Table 20-1A Pretransfusion

Peak Name	Calibrated Area (%)	Area (%)	Retention Time (min)	Peak Area
F	0.5	—	1.04	7948
Unknown	—	0.7	1.25	11,244
P2	—	2.1	1.34	34,608
Unknown	—	0.4	1.52	6679
P3	—	2.1	1.71	35,027
Ao	—	49.1	2.51	810,899
A2	3.8	—	3.67	73,296
S-window	—	40.7	4.47	673,295

Table 20-1B Posttransfusion

Peak Name	Calibrated Area (%)	Area (%)	Retention Time (min)	Peak Area
Unknown	—	0.0	0.97	960
F	0.5	—	1.06	10,143
Unknown	—	1.1	1.19	23,938
P2	—	3.0	1.32	63,982
Unknown	—	0.5	1.49	9939
P3	—	3.2	1.69	68,798
Ao	—	59.7	2.43	1,281,729
A2	3.3	—	3.62	80,883
S-window	—	25.3	4.42	543,615
Unknown	—	2.9	4.77	62,402

Table 20-1C Transfused Unit

Peak Name	Calibrated Area (%)	Area (%)	Retention Time (min)	Peak Area
Unknown	—	0.1	0.99	1189
F	0.2	—	1.07	4114
Unknown	—	2.4	1.19	42,931
P2	—	3.3	1.34	59,935
Unknown	—	0.5	1.51	9350
P3	—	4.3	1.71	77,946
Ao	—	66.3	2.46	1,195,915
A2	1.4	—	3.63	28,874
D-window	—	0.4	4.07	8042
S-window	—	0.7	4.59	12,300
Unknown	—	20.1	4.77	362,012

4. A 53-year-old 70-kg man with a history of acute myelogenous leukemia (AML) is admitted with shortness of breath and headache and a white blood cell (WBC) count of 120×10^9/L (reference range 3.54 to 9.06×10^9/L), hemoglobin of 6.5 g/dL (reference range 13.3 to 16.2 g/dL), and a platelet count of 50×10^9/L (reference range 165 to 415×10^9/L). The procedure shown in Figure 20-2 is initiated. Which one of the following choices is the most appropriate volume of blood to be processed?
   - A. 2.5 to 5 L.
   - B. 5 to 7.5 L.
   - C. 7.5 to 10 L.
   - D. 10 to 15 L.
   - E. 15 to 20 L.

5. A 45-year-old man with sickle cell anemia is scheduled to undergo knee replacement surgery. His preoperative hemoglobin level is 6.0 g/dL (reference range 13.3 to 16.2 g/dL) with a hemoglobin S level of 80%. He is currently not receiving any therapy for sickle cell anemia. Which one of the following preoperative management options is indicated?
   - A. No specific therapy is indicated.
   - B. Begin hydroxyurea and delay surgery until the maximum tolerated dose (MTD) is achieved.

   - C. Transfuse 4 U of RBCs.
   - D. Perform an exchange transfusion, setting the end hemoglobin to 10.0 g/dL and the fraction of cells remaining to 0.3.
   - E. Perform an exchange transfusion, setting the end hemoglobin to 10.0 g/dL and the fraction of cells remaining to 0.6.

6. A 22-year-old patient with sickle cell anemia receives an exchange transfusion with 4 U banked RBCs. Pre- and postprocedure hemoglobin quantification by high-performance liquid chromatography (HPLC) is shown in

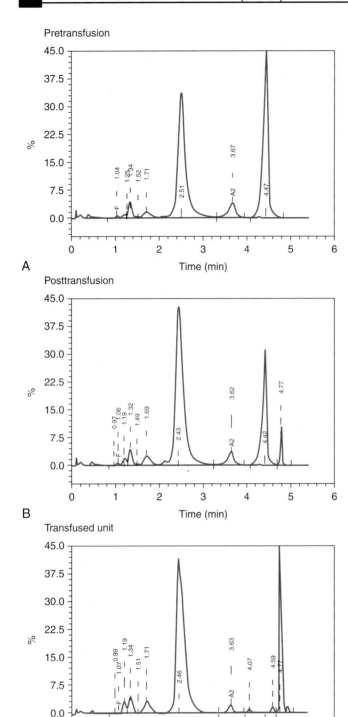

Pretransfusion

A

Posttransfusion

B

Transfused unit

C

Figure 20-3 Hemoglobin quantification by HPLC. **A,** Patient sample preprocedure. **B,** Patient sample postprocedure. **C,** Sample from a transfused unit. Results of hemoglobin quantification by HPLC on preprocedure and postprocedure patient samples and on a transfused unit.

Figure 20-3 and Table 20-1. Hemoglobin quantification from one of the units the patient received is shown. Hemoglobin Hasharon has a retention time of 4.77 minutes. In which one of the following scenarios would transfusion of the implicated unit shown in the figure result in the *least* amount of circulating hemoglobin Hasharon in the patient after the procedure?

A. The unit was the first of the four used for the exchange.
B. The unit was the second of the four used for the exchange.
C. The unit was the third of the four used for the exchange.
D. The unit was the fourth of the four used for the exchange.
E. The order of use of the units would not affect the postprocedure percentage of circulating hemoglobin Hasharon.

7. A 13-year-old 50-kg boy with sickle cell anemia is admitted to your hospital with cough, headache, wheezing, O_2 saturation of 70% on nonrebreather mask, and multilobar pulmonary infiltrates on chest radiograph. The patient is in the intensive care unit (ICU) and is about to be intubated. His hemoglobin level is 8.5 g/dL (reference range 12.8 to 16.0 g/dL) with a hemoglobin S level of 80%. What is the optimal management option if available immediately?
   A. Transfuse 2 U RBCs.
   B. Hydroxyurea 20 mg/kg.
   C. Manual exchange using 6 U RBCs.
   D. Automated RBC exchange (RCE) transfusion, setting the end hematocrit to 30% and the fraction of RBCs remaining to 0.3.
   E. Partial automated RCE transfusion, setting the end hemoglobin to 12.0 g/dL and the fraction of cells remaining to 0.6.

8. Therapeutic apheresis is a first-line treatment for which one of the following disorders?
   A. Warm autoimmune hemolytic anemia.
   B. Hyperviscosity with monoclonal gammopathy.
   C. Bleeding with coagulation factor inhibitors.
   D. Thrombosis with antiphospholipid antibody syndrome.
   E. Bleeding with posttransfusion purpura.

9. Which one of the following rationales for use of therapeutic leukocytapheresis in the treatment of hyperleukocytosis associated with leukemia is best supported by current evidence?
   A. To improve the efficacy of chemotherapy by decreasing the overall tumor burden.
   B. To improve long-term mortality in patients with acute myeloid leukemia.
   C. To prevent leukostasis and the resultant complications in patients with chronic myelogenous leukemia.
   D. To treat complications associated with leukostasis in patients with acute myeloid leukemia.
   E. To prevent tumor lysis syndrome in patients with acute lymphoblastic leukemia.

10. RBC exchange (RCE) is a category II indication for the treatment of severe malaria. Which one of the following statements regarding RCE for the treatment of malaria is true?
   A. RCE can be used in conjunction with antimalarial therapy to treat uncomplicated malaria when available.
   B. Antimalarial therapy should be held until after the RCE is completed.
   C. There is a high risk of RBC antigen alloimmunization in these patients and RCE should be avoided.
   D. A minimum of two RCEs should be performed to decrease the parasitemia significantly.
   E. RCE is used only for severe malaria in conjunction with antimalarial therapy.

11. Which one of the following patients is the best candidate for therapeutic plateletpheresis based on current evidence?
    A. A 65-year-old man with essential thrombocythemia and a history of myocardial infarction with a platelet count of 400×10^9/L.
    B. A 20-year-old man status post-splenectomy for a traumatic splenic laceration with a platelet count of 1000×10^9/L.
    C. A 45-year-old woman with ovarian carcinoma, a history of thromboembolism, and a platelet count of 750×10^9/L.
    D. A 70-year-old man with chronic myelogenous leukemia, a history of myocardial infarction, and a platelet count of 750×10^9/L.
    E. A 57-year-old woman with chronic myelogenous leukemia and acute hemorrhage, and a platelet count of 750×10^9/L.

12. The American Society for Apheresis (ASFA) periodically publishes guidelines, using an evidence-based approach, regarding the use of therapeutic apheresis in clinical practice. Based on the 2013 ASFA guidelines, there are four categories describing the indications for therapeutic apheresis. Which one of the following is the best description of a category III indication by the ASFA 2013 guidelines?
    A. Disorders for which apheresis is accepted as first-line therapy, either as a primary stand-alone treatment or in conjunction with other modes of treatment.
    B. Disorders for which apheresis is accepted as second-line therapy, either as a stand-alone treatment or in conjunction with other modes of treatment.
    C. The optimal role of apheresis is not established; decision making should be individualized.
    D. Disorders in which published evidence demonstrates or suggests that apheresis is ineffective or harmful. Institutional review board (IRB) approval is desirable if apheresis treatment is undertaken in these circumstances.
    E. Disorders that, based on the available evidence, should never be treated with apheresis.

13. Thrombotic thrombocytopenic purpura (TTP) is a category I indication for TPE. Which one of the following statements best describes the rationale behind its efficacy?
    A. TPE has an immunomodulatory effect by decreasing ADAMTS13 autoantibody production by plasma cells.
    B. TPE removes B cells from the circulation, thereby decreasing ADAMTS13 autoantibody production.
    C. TPE removes ADAMTS13 autoantibody and replaces ADAMTS13 protease activity.
    D. TPE removes ADAMTS13 protease activity and replaces platelets.
    E. TPE provides ultra-large von Willebrand multimers to the patient.

14. Fresh frozen plasma (FFP) is an appropriate replacement fluid during therapeutic apheresis for which one of the following indications?
    A. Renal transplantation with antibody-mediated rejection.
    B. Acute chest syndrome in sickle cell disease.
    C. Acute inflammatory demyelinating polyradiculopathy (i.e., Guillain-Barré syndrome).
    D. Phytanic acid storage disease (i.e., Refsum disease).
    E. TTP.

15. Excellent vascular access is important during apheresis procedures due to the high-flow rates required by the instrumentation. Which one of the following statements is true?

A. Femoral venous access is preferred for long-term treatment due to the ease of catheter placement.
B. Subclavian venous access has the highest rate of infection and should only be used emergently.
C. Peripheral venous access is preferred for all procedures when possible.
D. Arteriovenous (AV) fistulas should never be accessed for apheresis procedures.
E. Carotid artery access is preferred for apheresis procedures because it allows the highest flow rates.

16. A 54-year-old man with a new diagnosis of chronic inflammatory demyelinating polyradiculoneuropathy (CIDP) has been referred to you for TPE. What would be the best course of treatment for this patient?
    A. Perform TPE 2 to 3 times per week using albumin as replacement until improvement is seen.
    B. Perform TPE 1 to 2 times per month using albumin as replacement until improvement is seen.
    C. Perform TPE 2 to 3 times per week using FFP as replacement until improvement is seen.
    D. Perform TPE 1 to 2 times per month using FFP as replacement until improvement is seen.
    E. Recommend corticosteroids or intravenous immunoglobulin (IVIg), both of which are more efficacious.

17. TPE is a first-line therapy for which one of the following indications?
    A. Rheumatoid arthritis.
    B. Diarrhea-associated hemolytic uremic syndrome.
    C. Posttransfusion purpura.
    D. Cryoglobulinemia.
    E. Pemphigus vulgaris.

18. You are called to consult on a 33-year-old male patient admitted for hemoptysis and hematuria. Renal biopsy demonstrated crescent formation and linear deposits of IgG along the glomerular basement membrane (GBM). Laboratory testing reveals the presence of anti-GBM antibodies, but anti-neutrophil cytoplasmic antibodies (ANCAs) are not detected. Based on these findings, which one of the following statements is true?
    A. A combination of TPE, cyclophosphamide, and steroids is the treatment of choice.
    B. TPE should be reserved for patients who are dialysis dependent.
    C. Chronic immunosuppression and repeated courses of TPE are required to prevent relapse.
    D. TPE is ineffective in patients who present with diffuse alveolar hemorrhage.
    E. Plasma is the only replacement fluid to be used due to the high risk of diffuse alveolar hemorrhage.

19. Which statement regarding hematopoietic progenitor cell (HPC) collection is true?
    A. The number of CD34$^+$ cells usually decreases during the procedure.
    B. CD34$^+$ cells are found within the mononuclear cell layer during the procedure.
    C. CD34$^+$ cell counts peak after 7 days of granulocyte colony-stimulating factor (G-CSF) administration.
    D. Patients are not at a higher risk of citrate toxicity during large-volume leukapheresis.
    E. HPCs are not found in the peripheral blood of healthy individuals.

20. A 35-year-old female patient presents to her primary care physician complaining of "foamy" urine and bilateral lower extremity edema. She has a history of fatigue, a malar rash, diffuse myalgias, and arthralgias. Physical exam is remarkable for a blood pressure of 155/100 mm Hg and 3+ bilateral lower extremity pitting edema. Her urinalysis is remarkable for showing a specific gravity of 5.0, blood of 3+, protein of 4+, 12 to 16 RBCs per high-power field, rare hyaline casts, and 3 RBCs casts. Which one of the following is the most appropriate course of treatment?
    A. TPE every other day for five treatments using albumin as replacement.
    B. Corticosteroid therapy and an angiotensin-converting enzyme inhibitor (ACEI).
    C. Corticosteroid therapy and TPE every other day for five treatments using albumin as replacement.
    D. Corticosteroid therapy, ACEI, and TPE every other day for five treatments using albumin as replacement.
    E. Corticosteroid therapy, cyclophosphamide, ACEI, and TPE every other day for five treatments using albumin as replacement.

21. Which statement is true regarding the use of TPE in the treatment of myasthenia gravis?
    A. Antibodies against the acetylcholine receptor must be present for TPE to be effective.
    B. Response to TPE is rapid and symptoms usually improve within 1 to 7 days.
    C. Immunosuppressive medications should be held until after the course of TPE is completed.
    D. TPE is less effective than IVIg and should only be used to treat refractory patients.
    E. Use of TPE prior to thymectomy should be avoided due to the removal of coagulation factors.

22. Which statement about heart transplantation in adults is true?
    A. Extracorporeal photopheresis (ECP) is used prophylactically to prevent acute cellular rejection.
    B. Transplantation across ABO types is easily managed with TPE and immunosuppression.
    C. TPE is a first-line therapy for acute cellular rejection.
    D. FFP is the replacement fluid of choice during TPE due to the high incidence of coagulopathy.
    E. Acute antibody-mediated rejection is most commonly seen in this setting.

23. Plerixafor is a mobilization agent used in combination with G-CSF to collect hematopoietic stem cells. Which one of the following best describes the mechanism of action of plerixafor?
    A. Increased production of HPCs in the bone marrow.
    B. Decreased destruction of HPCs in the peripheral blood.
    C. Increased release of HPCs from the bone marrow.
    D. Increased maturation of HPCs in the bone marrow.
    E. Increased activation of HPCs in the peripheral blood.

24. For which one of the following renal diseases is TPE considered a first-line treatment?
    A. Focal segmental glomerulosclerosis.
    B. Antibody-mediated rejection of a renal allograft.
    C. Diarrhea-associated hemolytic uremic syndrome.
    D. Immune complex–induced rapidly progressive glomerulonephritis.
    E. Myeloma kidney.

25. For which one of the following is TPE indicated in the setting of solid organ transplantation?
    A. To decrease RBC alloantibody titers.
    B. To decrease donor-specific anti-HLA titers.
    C. To decrease donor-specific anti–human platelet antigen (HPA) antibody titers.
    D. To decrease complement levels.
    E. To decrease donor-specific anti–human neutrophil antigen (HNA) antibody titers.

26. A 34-year-old woman presents to your hospital with fever and the new onset of mental status changes. She is found to be anemic, with a hemoglobin of 8.2 g/dL (reference range 12.0 to 15.8 g/dL) and thrombocytopenic, with a platelet count of 7×10^9/L (reference range 165 to 415×10^9/L), and with a few schistocytes identified on a peripheral blood smear. Which one of the following statements is the best course of action?
    A. Transfuse 1 U RBCs and 1 dose of single-donor apheresis platelets.
    B. Transfuse 10 U cryoprecipitate.
    C. Transfuse 2 U plasma.
    D. Initiate a series of plasmapheresis procedures.
    E. Perform a whole blood exchange.

27. Which statement is true regarding ASFA guidelines for therapeutic apheresis?
    A. Category I indications include diseases and syndromes for which apheresis is the primary treatment.
    B. Category II indications include diseases and syndromes for which apheresis is the primary treatment in conjunction with another treatment modality.
    C. Category III indications include diseases and syndromes for which apheresis is a second-line therapy.
    D. Category IV indications include diseases and syndromes for which apheresis is the last line of treatment.
    E. Category V indications include diseases and syndromes for which apheresis is ineffective or harmful.

28. The ASFA periodically publishes guidelines, using an evidence-based approach, regarding the use of therapeutic apheresis in clinical practice. Based on the 2013 ASFA guidelines, there are four categories describing the indications for therapeautic apheresis. According to the 2013 ASFA guidelines, which one of the following is the correct category for severe malaria?
    A. Disorder for which apheresis is accepted as first-line therapy, either as a primary stand-alone treatment or in conjunction with other modes of treatment.
    B. Disorder for which apheresis is accepted as second-line therapy, either as a primary stand-alone treatment or in conjunction with other modes of treatment.
    C. The optimal role of apheresis is not established; decision making should be individualized.
    D. Disorder in which published evidence demonstrates or suggests that apheresis is ineffective or harmful.
    E. Disorder for which approval for a research study is required from an IRB.

29. The ASFA periodically publishes guidelines, using an evidence-based approach, regarding the use of therapeutic apheresis in clinical practice. Based on the 2013 ASFA guidelines, there are four categories describing the indications for therapeautic apheresis. According to the 2013 ASFA guidelines, which one of the following is the correct category for hematopoietic stem cell

transplant-associated thrombotic microangiopathy?

A. Disorder for which apheresis is accepted as first-line therapy, either as a primary stand-alone treatment or in conjunction with other modes of treatment.

B. Disorder for which apheresis is accepted as second-line therapy, either as a primary stand-alone treatment or in conjunction with other modes of treatment.

C. The optimal role of apheresis is not established; decision making should be individualized.

D. Disorder in which published evidence demonstrates or suggests that apheresis is ineffective or harmful.

E. Disorder for which approval for a research study is required from an IRB.

30. In the context of therapeutic plasmapheresis, which one of the following is a characteristic of an "ideal solute"?

A. It equilibrates between the intravascular and extravascular spaces.

B. It is synthesized during the time frame of the plasmapheresis procedure.

C. It is catabolized during the time frame of the plasmapheresis procedure.

D. It is completely intravascular.

E. It is an IgG antibody.

ANSWERS

1. A. Leukapheresis.
Rationale: The selective removal of WBCs is not indicated in this setting.
B. Erythrocytapheresis.
Rationale: The selective removal of RBCs is not indicated in this setting.
C. Thrombocytapheresis.
Rationale: The selective removal of platelets is not indicated in this setting.
D. Plasmapheresis.
Rationale: The selective removal of plasma is indicated in this setting.
E. Low-density lipoprotein (LDL) apheresis.
Rationale: The selective removal of LDL is not indicated in this setting.

Major points of discussion

■ High-titer recipient IgM isohemagglutinins may cause hyperacute rejection of ABO-incompatible solid organ allografts.

■ Peritransplant plasmapheresis in conjunction with immunosuppression and/or IVIg may lower antibody titers and prevent hyperacute rejection of ABO-incompatible solid organ allografts.

■ The replacement fluid for plasmapheresis is albumin, FFP, or a combination of the two, depending on the presence or absence of a coagulopathy.

■ The goal of plasmapheresis is to reduce anti-A and/or anti-B antibody titers to a level low enough to prevent hyperacute rejection. Titers of 4 to 16 have been used for kidney transplantation and titers of 8 to 64 for liver transplantation.

■ The number of peritransplant plasmapheresis procedures depends on the initial isohemagglutinin titer.

2a. A. Plasmapheresis.
Rationale: The picture represents a standard setup for a plasmapheresis procedure using albumin and saline for replacement fluids.
B. Plateletpheresis.
Rationale: Hints that this is not a plateletpheresis include the absence of platelets in the collection bag and the use of multiple albumin bottles for replacement fluid, which would be unnecessary for a plateletpheresis procedure.
C. Red blood cell (RBC) exchange.

Rationale: The collection bag would be filled with RBCs in an RBC exchange.
D. Leukapheresis.
Rationale: Hints that this is not a leukapheresis include the absence of WBCs in the collection bag and the use of multiple albumin bottles for replacement fluid, which would be unnecessary for a leukapheresis procedure.
E. Stem cell collection.
Rationale: Hints that this is not a stem cell collection include the absence of cells in the collection bag and the use of multiple albumin bottles for replacement fluid, which would be unnecessary for a stem cell collection procedure.

2b. A. A
Rationale: This is the collection bag, which is expected to contain roughly the amount of fibrinogen as in plasma.
B. B
Rationale: This is the saline replacement bag containing normal saline.
C. C
Rationale: This is a bottle of albumin being used as replacement fluid.
D. D
Rationale: This is a bag of citrate, which is used for anticoagulation during the procedure. Although the citrate label is difficult to see in this figure, the only container expected to have appreciable fibrinogen in a plasmapheresis procedure is the collection bag, unless FFP is used as replacement fluid.
E. None of the labeled containers contains measurable amounts of fibrinogen.
Rationale: The collection bag in a plasmapheresis procedure contains plasma, which contains fibrinogen as an "ideal solute."

Major points of discussion

■ Apheresis procedures are also used to collect double RBC products, platelets, and granulocytes from healthy donors.

■ The efficiency of the apheresis procedure decreases as the procedure progresses.

■ Blood component separation can be accomplished by centrifugation or filtration. In a continuous-flow centrifugation device, blood is separated by density and the resulting layers can be removed selectively (e.g., plasma, platelets, leukocytes, RBCs). Filtration devices, which are less commonly used, separate plasma from cells using a microporous filter.

■ Selective absorption using affinity columns exist for removing specific components from plasma, such as LDLs or immunoglobulins.

■ Photopheresis is a procedure in which the WBC layer is collected and treated with 8-methoxypsoralen and ultraviolet light. This crosslinks DNA and induces apoptosis. It was initially developed for treating cutaneous T-cell lymphoma; however, it is currently used in treating organ rejection (heart and lung) and graft-versus-host disease.

3. A. TPE is considered to be first-line therapy.
   B. TPE is considered to be second-line therapy.
   C. The benefit of TPE is unclear.
   D. TPE is ineffective.
   E. TPE has never been tried.
   Rationale: TPE for the desensitization of renal transplant candidates with a positive living donor kidney crossmatch caused by donor-specific HLA antibodies is considered to be second-line therapy, either as a standard treatment or in conjunction with other modes of treatment.

Major points of discussion

■ The ASFA has published evidence-based guidelines for the use of therapeutic apheresis in various disorders.

■ Each disorder is assigned a category (i.e., I to IV) and strength of recommendation.

■ TPE has been shown to be a second-line therapy, either alone or in conjunction with other immunosuppressive therapy, to desensitize patients with a positive crossmatch to a living donor kidney caused by donor-specific HLA antibodies.

■ Immunosuppressive medications, either alone or in combination with therapeutic plasmapheresis, high-dose IVIg, and/or rituximab, can be used to prevent and treat antibody-mediated rejection.

■ Patients may develop anti-HLA antibodies through prior transfusions, pregnancies, and/or transplantation.

■ Removal of donor-specific HLA antibodies prior to transplantation could enable a negative crossmatch and prevent hyperacute/acute rejection.

■ Posttransplant immunosuppression can prevent loss of the organ caused by an anamnestic response.[8]

4. A. 2.5 to 5 L.
   B. 5 to 7.5 L.
   C. 7.5 to 10 L.
   D. 10 to 15 L.
   E. 15 to 20 L.
   Rationale: 1.5 to 2 total blood volumes should be processed in a leukapheresis procedure.

Major points of discussion

■ Hyperleukocytosis may lead to symptoms of leukostasis; these symptoms include central nervous system manifestations, such as headache or altered mental

status, and pulmonary manifestations, such as hypoxemia, dyspnea, diffuse alveolar hemorrhage, and respiratory failure.

■ The total blood volume in adults can be estimated as 70 mL/kg; thus, a 70-kg adult will have a approximately 5-L total blood volume.

■ RBCs should not be transfused in patients with leukostasis until cytoreduction is achieved to prevent further increases in whole blood viscosity.

■ The leukapheresis procedure is expected to lower the WBC count by 30% to 60%. The procedure is not more effective because WBCs are not "ideal solutes."

■ Studies suggest that prompt treatment of leukostasis with leukapheresis only reduces the risk of early death in this setting.

5. A. No specific therapy is indicated.
   Rationale: There are increased complications for sickle cell patients undergoing surgery; thus, some form of therapy to reduce the hemoglobin S percentage is warranted.
   B. Begin hydroxyurea and delay surgery until the maximum tolerated dose (MTD) is achieved.
   Rationale: Although hydroxyurea is useful for increasing hemoglobin F levels and reducing sickle cell anemia–related complications, this surgery does not have to be delayed until hydroxyurea takes effect.
   C. Transfuse 4 U RBCs.
   Rationale: This approach will bring the patient's hemoglobin S level to approximately 50%. Evidence suggests that conservative management raising hemoglobin to 10 g/dL is as effective as exchange transfusions, with fewer side effects.
   D. Perform an exchange transfusion, setting the end hemoglobin to 10.0 g/dL and the fraction of cells remaining to 0.3.
   Rationale: Although this is an appropriate choice, and some physicians will opt for an exchange transfusion prior to surgery, the evidence suggests that conservative management is as effective with fewer side effects.
   E. Perform an exchange transfusion, setting the end hemoglobin to 10.0 g/dL and the fraction of cells remaining to 0.6.
   Rationale: Simple transfusion would be as effective in lowering the hemoglobin S level and is associated with less risk to the patient.

Major points of discussion

■ Perioperative complications, such as acute chest syndrome, are common in patients with sickle cell anemia.

■ In a landmark, multicenter, randomized control study, conservative management consisting of transfusion to a hemoglobin of 10 g/dL was as effective as RCE but associated with fewer transfusion-related complications.

■ The fraction of RBCs remaining refers to how many of the original circulating RBCs remain after the exchange procedure. The lower the fraction, the larger is the volume to be processed and the longer the length of the procedure. A setting of 0.3 is most commonly used as it provides a good balance between the volume of blood required for the procedure and the desired decrease in circulating hemoglobin S levels.

■ In general, sickle cell anemia patients are not transfused to hemoglobin levels above 10.0 g/dL to prevent increased viscosity, which is associated with higher hemoglobin levels in the presence of sickle erythrocytes.

■ Chronic RCEs are useful for preventing severe manifestations of sickle cell anemia, such as stroke and acute chest syndrome.[10]

6. **A. The unit was the first of the four used for the exchange.**
B. The unit was the second of the four used for the exchange.
C. The unit was the third of the four used for the exchange.
D. The unit was the fourth of the four used for the exchange.
E. The order of use of the units would not affect the postprocedure percentage of circulating hemoglobin Hasharon.
Rationale: The apheresis procedure is a continuous exchange procedure; thus, RBCs exchanged in the beginning of the procedure are removed as the procedure progresses.

Major points of discussion

■ Most therapeutic apheresis procedures use continuous flow centrifugation in which blood is withdrawn and returned continuously. In this setting, blood returned to the patient can be subsequently removed as the procedure progresses. Thus, it is not practically possible to remove 100% of the original patient RBCs in an exchange procedure.

■ Blood transfused into patients with sickle cell anemia should be tested for hemoglobin S trait and only transfused if negative. However, blood is not routinely tested for other hemoglobinopathies and it is not uncommon to observe other variant hemoglobins present in the transfused individuals.

■ "Ideal solutes" are those that are predominantly intravascular and can be removed effectively by the apheresis procedure. A single plasma volume exchange will remove approximately 63% of an ideal solute. A double plasma volume exchange will remove approximately 86% of an ideal solute, and a triple plasma volume exchange will remove 95% of an ideal solute.

■ Examples of molecules or cells that approximate ideal solutes include fibrinogen, IgM antibodies, and RBCs. IgG antibodies and leukemic WBCs are not ideal solutes.

■ The ASFA publishes the guidelines for TPE. The evidence and lack of evidence for these procedures are reviewed periodically by a committee in charge of setting the guidelines.

7. A. Transfuse 2 U RBCs.
Rationale: This would increase the patient's hemoglobin level to more than 10 g/dL, which is associated with increased viscosity.
B. Hydroxyurea 20 mg/kg.
Rationale: Although hydroxyurea is useful for increasing hemoglobin F and reducing sickle cell anemia–related complications, this is inappropriate for the treatment of acute chest syndrome.
C. Manual exchange using 6 U RBCs.
Rationale: If an automated exchange were not available, a manual exchange would be an appropriate option.

D. Automated RBC exchange (RCE) transfusion, setting the end hematocrit to 30% and the fraction of RBCs remaining to 0.3.
Rationale: The appropriate settings for an automated exchange would result in a hematocrit of no greater than 30% (i.e., a hemoglobin no greater than 10 g/dL) and hemoglobin S level less than 30%.
E. Partial automated RCE transfusion, setting the end hemoglobin to 12.0 g/dL and the fraction of cells remaining to 0.6.
Rationale: A partial exchange would not reduce the hemoglobin S to less than 30%. Furthermore, the total hemoglobin should not be raised above 10 g/dL.

Major points of discussion

■ Complications of sickle cell anemia include stroke, acute chest syndrome, pain crises, splenic sequestration, hepatopathy, and priapism.

■ Chronic transfusion (simple and/or exchange) therapy is effective in primary and secondary prevention of stroke in patients with sickle cell anemia.

■ The risks of RCE include all the risks of transfusions, such as febrile nonhemolytic transfusion reactions, hemolytic transfusion reactions (delayed/acute), allergic reactions, and transfusion-transmitted infections.

■ RBC units destined for patients with sickle cell anemia should be screened for sickle trait. Thus, patients with sickle cell anemia should receive only sickle-negative blood.

■ The goal of chronic transfusion therapy for sickle cell anemia patients is to maintain the percentage of hemoglobin S at less than 30%. This has been shown to reduce the incidence of stroke and other disease manifestations, such as pain crises and acute chest syndrome.[1]

8. A. Warm autoimmune hemolytic anemia.
Rationale: This is a category III indication for TPE. Prednisone is the treatment of choice.
B. Hyperviscosity with monoclonal gammopathy.
Rationale: This is a category I indication for TPE.
C. Bleeding with coagulation factor inhibitors.
Rationale: This is a category III indication for TPE.
D. Thrombosis with antiphospholipid antibody syndrome.
Rationale: This is a category II indication for TPE. TPE may be used in combination with anticoagulants, corticosteroids, and/or IGIg.
E. Bleeding with posttransfusion purpura.
Rationale: This is a category III indication for TPE. High-dose IVIg is the treatment of choice.

Major points of discussion

■ Hyperviscosity resulting from monoclonal gammopathy can lead to neurologic dysfunction, bleeding diathesis, and retinopathy.

■ Hyperviscosity causes an increased shear stress in the microvasculature, leading to endothelial damage.

■ Hypervolemia may also occur, leading to respiratory compromise, congestive heart failure, and coma.

■ This is most common in monoclonal gammopathies with IgM paraproteins.

■ There is a logarithmic increase in serum viscosity with increases in the monoclonal protein.

■ TPE is a category I indication to prophylactically decrease paraprotein levels in patients taking rituximab with IgM greater than 5000 mg/dL, or in the treatment of symptomatic hyperviscosity syndrome caused by monoclonal gammopathy.

9. A. To improve the efficacy of chemotherapy by decreasing the overall tumor burden.
Rationale: This is not an indication for the use of leukocytapheresis.
B. To improve long-term mortality in patients with acute myeloid leukemia.
Rationale: Leukocytapheresis has not been shown to improve long-term mortality in acute myeloid leukemia.
C. To prevent leukostasis and the resultant complications in patients with chronic myelogenous leukemia.
Rationale: Currently, leukocytapheresis is not recommended for the treatment of chronic myelogenous leukemia.
D. To treat complications associated with leukostasis in patients with acute myeloid leukemia.
Rationale: Leukocytapheresis is a category I recommendation for the treatment of leukostasis in patients with acute myeloid leukemia.
E. To prevent tumor lysis syndrome in patients with acute lymphoblastic leukemia.
Rationale: Leukocytapheresis has not been shown to be more effective than chemotherapy and supportive care in these patients and is considered a category III indication for prophylaxis for hyperleukocytosis.

Major points of discussion
■ The use of leukocytapheresis is a category I indication for the treatment of hyperleukocytosis and a category III indication for prophylaxis for complications of leukostasis from hyperleukocytosis.
■ Leukocytapheresis should be considered in the treatment of patients with acute myeloid leukemia and a WBC count more than 100×10^9/L and patients with acute lymphoblastic leukemia and a WBC count more than 400×10^9/L.
■ Leukostasis can lead to organ and tissue dysfunction and ischemia resulting from obstruction of the microvasculature.
■ Leukocytapheresis has been shown to improve the pulmonary and neurologic complications seen with leukostasis in acute leukemia.
■ Induction chemotherapy should not be delayed for leukocytapheresis to be completed.
■ From 1.5 to 2 total blood volumes should be processed.
■ Reductions in the WBC count and blast count cannot be predicted reliably because additional marginated leukemic cells may be released into the circulation and leukemic blasts may not be as efficiently removed by centrifugation as expected.

10. A. RCE can be used in conjunction with antimalarial therapy to treat uncomplicated malaria when available.
Rationale: RCE is not indicated in the treatment of uncomplicated malaria.
B. Antimalarial therapy should be held until after the RCE is completed.

Rationale: Antimalarial therapy is the primary treatment and should be started immediately.
C. There is a high risk of RBC antigen alloimmunization in these patients and RCE should be avoided.
Rationale: These patients are not at any increased risk for RBC alloimmunization.
D. A minimum of two RCEs should be performed to decrease the parasitemia significantly.
Rationale: One or two treatments may be performed.
E. RCE is used only for severe malaria in conjunction with antimalarial therapy.
Rationale: RCE may be used to treat severe malaria (i.e., parasitemia >10%, renal or pulmonary complications, or cerebral involvement).

Major points of discussion
■ RCE is a category II indication for the treatment of severe malaria with parasitemia more than 10%, pulmonary or renal complications, or cerebral malaria.
■ Severe cases may be complicated by severe anemia, pulmonary edema, seizures, shock, disseminated intravascular coagulopathy, renal failure, metabolic derangements, coma, and death.
■ Antimalarial therapy should not be postponed but should be started immediately.
■ Most severe cases are due to *Plasmodium falciparum*.
■ From 1 to 2 RBC volumes should be processed using donor RBCs as the replacement fluid.
■ Complications of RCE for malaria include any complication associated with RBC transfusion and apheresis procedures.
■ These complications include transfusion reactions, RBC alloimmunization, hypocalcemia, hypovolemia, bleeding, and infection.

11. A. A 65-year-old man with essential thrombocythemia and a history of myocardial infarction with a platelet count of 400×10^9/L.
Rationale: This patient has a normal platelet count (reference range 165 to 415×10^9/L) and therapeutic plateletpheresis is not indicated.
B. A 20-year-old man status post-splenectomy for a traumatic splenic laceration with a platelet count of 1000×10^9/L.
C. A 45-year-old woman with ovarian carcinoma, a history of thromboembolism, and a platelet count of 750×10^9/L.
Rationale: The efficacy of therapeutic plateletpheresis in the treatment of secondary thrombocytosis has not been proven and has been given a category III recommendation. Medical management with hydroxyurea should be considered first.
D. A 70-year-old man with chronic myelogenous leukemia, a history of myocardial infarction, and a platelet count of 750×10^9/L.
Rationale: Therapeutic plateletpheresis is not a first-line therapy for this patient. A trial of hydroxyurea should be considered first to lower this patient's platelet count.
E. A 57-year-old woman with chronic myelogenous leukemia and acute hemorrhage, and a platelet count of 750×10^9/L.
Rationale: This patient is the best candidate for therapeutic plateletpheresis due to her acute hemorrhage. Symptomatic

thrombocytosis is a category II indication for therapeutic plateletpheresis.

Major points of discussion

■ Therapeutic plateletpheresis has a category II recommendation for the treatment of symptomatic thrombocytosis and a category III recommendation for the treatment of secondary thrombocytosis or prophylaxis for complications associated with thrombocytosis.

■ Thrombocytosis may be primary or secondary.

■ Primary thrombocytosis is seen in myeloproliferative disorders, including essential thrombocythemia and chronic myelogenous leukemia. Complications of thrombocytosis, such as thrombosis and hemorrhage, may be seen in these patients.

■ Risk factors for thrombosis and hemorrhage in these patients include patient age older than 60 years, a history of cardiovascular disease, and a history of thrombosis.

■ Secondary thrombocytosis can be associated with multiple disorders, including malignancy, splenectomy, infection, and chronic inflammation. Complications of thrombocytosis are rarely seen in these patients.

■ Medical management to decrease the platelet count using hydroxyurea, anagrelide, or interferon alfa should be considered prior to therapeutic plateletpheresis. Plateletpheresis is usually used only in rare cases.

■ From 1.5 to 2 total blood volumes are usually processed in one procedure; the decrease in platelet count cannot be reliably predicted based on the processed blood volume. Treatment should be guided by intraprocedure platelet counts.[8]

12. A. Disorders for which apheresis is accepted as first-line therapy, either as a primary stand-alone treatment or in conjunction with other modes of treatment.
Rationale: This is the description of a category I indication.
B. Disorders for which apheresis is accepted as second-line therapy, either as a stand-alone treatment or in conjunction with other modes of treatment.
Rationale: This is the description of a category II indication.
C. The optimal role of apheresis is not established; decision making should be individualized.
Rationale: This is the description of a category III indication.
D. Disorders in which published evidence demonstrates or suggests that apheresis is ineffective or harmful.
Institutional review board (IRB) approval is desirable if apheresis treatment is undertaken in these circumstances.
Rationale: This is the description of category IV indication.
E. Disorders that, based on the available evidence, should never be treated with apheresis.
Rationale: There is no such category described in the ASFA guidelines.

Major points of discussion

■ The ASFA guidelines provide an important evidence-based tool for the practice of therapeutic apheresis.

■ In the 2013 ASFA guidelines, the descriptions of the various categories were simplified compared with previous versions of the guidelines. Changes in these descriptions include the addition of the strength of the recommendation, which allowed categorization to be

better aligned with the strength of the evidence and the quality of the relevant publications in the literature.

■ The definition of category III reflects the individual character of the decision-making process for diseases in this category.

■ The recommendation grade and the individual patient's clinical circumstances should guide whether or not therapeutic apheresis is included in the treatment plan for category III indications.

■ Other professional organizations in other fields (e.g., neurology) also prepare consensus guidelines regarding the indications for therapeutic apheresis. These may not always agree with those promulgated by the ASFA.[8]

13. A. TPE has an immunomodulatory effect by decreasing ADAMTS13 autoantibody production by plasma cells.
Rationale: TPE has not been shown to have an effect on antibody production by plasma cells in this setting.
B. TPE removes B cells from the circulation, thereby decreasing ADAMTS13 autoantibody production.
Rationale: TPE does not remove significant numbers of B cells from the circulation.
C. TPE removes ADAMTS13 autoantibody and replaces ADAMTS13 protease activity.
Rationale: Based on the available evidence, this is the current rationale for the efficacy of TPE in the treatment of TTP.
D. TPE removes ADAMTS13 protease activity and replaces platelets.
Rationale: TPE does not replace platelets.
E. TPE provides ultra-large von Willebrand multimers to the patient.
Rationale: TPE does not provide ultra-large von Willebrand multimers to the patient.

Major points of discussion

■ TTP is classically characterized by a pentad of clinical findings: thrombocytopenia, microangiopathic hemolytic anemia (MAHA), mental status changes, renal failure, and fever.

■ In practice, thrombocytopenia and MAHA (noted as anemia with schistocytes or fragmented RBCs on peripheral blood smear and an elevation in lactate dehydrogenase) without other clinical explanations (i.e., disseminated intravascular coagulation) are sufficient to diagnose TTP and initiate treatment.

■ TPE should be started as soon as possible due to the high mortality rate associated with TTP.

■ TTP is associated with a severe deficiency in ADAMTS13 (i.e., *ad*isintergrin *a*nd *m*etalloproteinase with a *t*hrombospondin type 1 motif, member 13) enzyme activity, which cleaves ultra-large von Willebrand multimers.

■ The majority of idiopathic cases of TTP are due to an autoantibody against ADAMTS13.

■ Congenital TTP (i.e., Upshaw-Schulman syndrome) is associated with somatic mutations in the *ADAMTS13* gene that lead to a severe decrease in ADAMTS13 activity.

■ TPE is thought to remove the autoantibody and replace ADAMTS13 protease activity, which is found in FFP.

■ FFP or cryoprecipitate-reduced plasma should be used as the replacement fluid to provide a source of ADAMTS13.

14. A. Renal transplantation with antibody-mediated rejection.
B. Acute chest syndrome in sickle cell disease.
Rationale: Sickle hemoglobin-negative RBCs should be used to replace the patient's sickle RBCs.
C. Acute inflammatory demyelinating polyradiculopathy (i.e., Guillain-Barré syndrome).
D. Phytanic acid storage disease (i.e., Refsum disease).
Rationale for A, C, and D: Albumin is the appropriate replacement fluid in these cases.
E. TTP.
Rationale: FFP or cryoprecipitate-reduced plasma is the appropriate replacement fluid in this case.

Major points of discussion
■ During TPE, the patient's plasma is removed and must be replaced with some replacement fluid to maintain oncotic pressure.
■ Five percent albumin, with or without normal saline, is the most commonly used replacement fluid.
■ Five percent albumin will maintain normal oncotic pressure with a minimal risk of allergic reaction and infectious disease transmission.
■ FFP is used as a replacement fluid in patients with TTP, coagulation factor deficiencies, or other bleeding risks.
■ FFP is associated with an increased risk of allergic reactions, infectious disease transmission, other transfusion reactions, and citrate toxicity due to anticoagulation with citrate.
■ In TTP, FFP or cryoprecipitate-reduced plasma is used to replace ADAMTS13 protease activity.
■ Patients who undergo daily plasmapheresis with albumin replacement may become deficient in fibrinogen (most common) or other coagulation factors; in this setting, FFP may be used in conjunction with albumin as a replacement fluid.
■ RBCs are used as a replacement product in RCE procedures.

15. A. Femoral venous access is preferred for long-term treatment due to the ease of catheter placement.
Rationale: Femoral access is typically only used as a temporary site because it limits patient mobility and can be complicated by infection.
B. Subclavian venous access has the highest rate of infection and should only be used emergently.
Rationale: Femoral venous access is complicated more often by infection than subclavian venous access.
C. Peripheral venous access is preferred for all procedures when possible.
Rationale: The catheter is the greatest risk factor for adverse events during a trial of apheresis and should be avoided when possible.
D. Arteriovenous (AV) fistulas should never be accessed for apheresis procedures.
Rationale: AV fistulas may be used for apheresis procedures as long as the nursing staff members are adequately trained in their use.
E. Carotid artery access is preferred for apheresis procedures because it allows the highest flow rates.
Rationale: The carotid artery is never accessed for therapeutic apheresis procedures.

Major points of discussion
■ Excellent venous access must be established for apheresis procedures due to the high whole blood flow rates.
■ Peripheral veins are the first choice for venous access due to the low risk of adverse events. However, most patients' peripheral veins are not adequate to withstand multiple repetitive apheresis procedures.
■ Central venous catheters must have a double lumen to allow for blood draw and return. They must be staggered (proximal and distal port) to prevent mixing of returned and drawn blood. They also must be firm enough to prevent collapse due to high pressure.
■ Central venous access may be complicated by infection, hemorrhage, thrombosis, pneumothorax, and arrhythmias.
■ Femoral venous access
  ● Advantages: Ease of insertion, may be placed at the bedside, easier to control hemorrhage
  ● Disadvantages: Increased risk of infection, risk of femoral artery puncture, increased risk of thrombosis, limited patient mobility
■ Subclavian/internal jugular access
  ● Advantages: Long-term placement, lower risk of infection
  ● Disadvantages: Hemothorax, pneumothorax, cardiac arrhythmias, more difficult to place, requires radiographic confirmation of correct placement

16. A. **Perform TPE 2 to 3 times per week using albumin as replacement until improvement is seen.**
Rationale: This is the recommended course of TPE for the treatment of CIDP.
B. Perform TPE 1 to 2 times per month using albumin as replacement until improvement is seen.
Rationale: TPE should be performed more often initially until improvement is noted. Then treatment can be tapered.
C. Perform TPE 2 to 3 times per week using FFP as replacement until improvement is seen.
D. Perform TPE 1 to 2 times per month using FFP as replacement until improvement is seen.
Rationale: FFP is not an appropriate replacement fluid for this patient. Additionally, TPE should be performed more often initially until improvement is noted. Then treatment can be tapered.
E. Recommend corticosteroids or intravenous immunoglobulin (IVIg), both of which are more efficacious.
Rationale: TPE, corticosteroids, and IVIg have been shown to be equally effective for the treatment of CIDP.

Major points of discussion
■ CIDP is a progressive and/or relapsing symmetric sensorimotor disorder characterized by symmetrical muscle weakness that may be accompanied by numbness and paresthesias.
■ It is thought to be due to a B-cell and T-cell autoimmune process, possibly mediated by autoantibodies recognizing myelin-associated glycolipid antigens, leading to demyelination of peripheral nerves.
■ CIDP is a category I indication for TPE according to the ASFA guidelines published in 2013.
■ From 1 to 1.5 total plasma volumes are removed using albumin, with or without saline, as the replacement fluid.

- TPE is usually performed 2 to 3 times per week until symptom improvement is noted. Treatment may then be tapered.
- Relapse may be seen with discontinuation of treatment and maintenance therapy is often necessary.[8]

17. A. Rheumatoid arthritis.
Rationale: TPE is not recommended for the treatment of rheumatoid arthritis.
B. Diarrhea-associated hemolytic uremic syndrome.
Rationale: TPE is not recommended for the treatment of diarrhea-associated hemolytic uremic syndrome and is a category IV indication.
C. Posttransfusion purpura.
Rationale: TPE is indicated for the treatment of posttransfusion purpura only in patients who are refractory to IVIg treatment and have persistent profound thrombocytopenia. This is a category III indication for TPE.
D. Cryoglobulinemia.
Rationale: TPE is a first-line treatment for cryoglobulinemia.
E. Pemphigus vulgaris.
Rationale: TPE is not recommended for the treatment of pemphigus vulgaris and is a category IV indication.

Major points of discussion
- Cryoglobulins are immunoglobulins that precipitate at low temperatures.
- There are three types of cryoglobulins:
  1. Type I cryoglobulins are single monoclonal proteins, usually IgG or IgM. These are usually seen in Waldenström's macroglobulinemia, multiple myeloma, and lymphoproliferative disorders.
  2. Type II cryoglobulins are monoclonal proteins, usually IgM, with a polyclonal component, usually IgG. These "mixed" cryoglobulins are usually associated with hepatitis C.
  3. Type III cryoglobulins are polyclonal immunoglobulins, usually IgG or IgM. Commonly, a polyclonal anti-IgG IgM forming precipitating immune complexes is seen. These are usually associated with hepatitis C, autoimmune diseases, and inflammatory conditions.
- The immunoglobulins and immune complexes precipitate in areas of the body exposed to lower temperatures, thereby causing small-vessel damage.
- TPE can be used to decrease cryoglobulin levels.
- TPE is used most often to treat severe cryoglobulinemia in patients with renal impairment, vasculitis, and/or neuropathy.
- Severe, symptomatic cryoglobulinemia is a category I indication for TPE according to the ASFA guidelines published in 2013.
- Cryoglobulinemia secondary to hepatitis C is a category II indication for TPE according to the ASFA guidelines published in 2013.[2,8]

18. A. **A combination of TPE, cyclophosphamide, and steroids is the treatment of choice.**
Rationale: See Major Points of Discussion.
B. TPE should be reserved for patients who are dialysis dependent.
Rationale: TPE is not effective for renal dysfunction once patients are dialysis dependent and should be used only if diffuse alveolar hemorrhage is present.

C. Chronic immunosuppression and repeated courses of TPE are required to prevent relapse.
Rationale: Relapses are not typically seen in patients who are ANCA negative, and treatment can be discontinued once remission is achieved.
D. TPE is ineffective in patients who present with diffuse alveolar hemorrhage.
Rationale: Approximately 90% of patients with diffuse alveolar hemorrhage respond to TPE and it is a category I indication for TPE.[8]
E. Plasma is the only replacement fluid to be used due to the high risk of diffuse alveolar hemorrhage.
Rationale: Albumin may be used in patients without evidence of coagulopathy or diffuse alveolar hemorrhage. If diffuse alveolar hemorrhage is present, plasma may be used as replacement at the end of the procedure to maintain levels of coagulation factors, particularly fibrinogen.

Major points of discussion
- Rapidly progressive glomerulonephritis (RPGN) is a kidney disease with rapid loss of renal function and a decrease in the glomerular filtration rate of at least 50%. Histologically, crescent formation is seen in at least 50% of glomeruli.
- RPGN is separated into three categories based on immunofluorescence staining on renal biopsy. The clinical presentation, response to treatment, and prognosis differ among the three categories.
- The three categories are anti-GBM antibody disease (Goodpasture disease), immune complex disease, and pauci-immune disease.
- Anti-GBM disease is characterized by linear deposits of IgG along the GBM and is caused by an autoantibody to collagen type IV.
- From 10% to 40% of affected patients may have detectable ANCA.
- Clinically, these patients may present with renal manifestations, including hematuria, oliguria, and anuria, and pulmonary manifestations, including cough, hemoptysis, and diffuse alveolar hemorrhage.
- Without treatment, anti-GBM disease is rapidly progressive with a high mortality rate. A combination of TPE, cyclophosphamide, and steroids is the treatment of choice and should be started as early as possible.
- Anti-GBM disease that is dialysis independent or accompanied by diffuse alveolar hemorrhage is a category I indication for TPE based on the ASFA guidelines published in 2013.
- The renal dysfunction in patients with anti-GBM disease who are dialysis dependent is unresponsive to TPE and the renal damage is irreversible. This is a category IV indication for TPE.

19. A. The number of CD34[+] cells usually decreases during the procedure.
Rationale: In most cases, the number of CD34[+] cells increases during the procedure, thereby allowing more CD34[+] cells to be collected than appears based on calculations using preprocedure CD34[+] cell counts. The marrow is thought to release additional HPCs into the circulation during the time frame of the procedure.
B. CD34[+] cells are found within the mononuclear cell layer during the procedure.

Rationale: A leukapheresis-type procedure is performed, focusing on collecting mononuclear cells.

C. CD34$^+$ cell counts peak after 7 days of granulocyte colony-stimulating factor (G-CSF) administration.

Rationale: CD34$^+$ cell counts usually peak on day 5 after 4 days of G-CSF mobilization. WBC counts will continue to rise.

D. Patients are not at a higher risk of citrate toxicity during large-volume leukapheresis.

Rationale: The increased time and volume of blood processed increases the risk of citrate toxicity.

E. HPCs are not found in the peripheral blood of healthy individuals.

Rationale: HPCs are found in low numbers in the peripheral blood (<1%).

Major points of discussion

- HPCs are present in both the bone marrow and the peripheral blood in adults.
- Peripheral blood–derived HPCs are easier to collect and lead to more rapid engraftment compared with bone marrow–derived HPCs.
- Administration of hematopoietic cytokines, such as G-CSF, is required to cause a transient increase of circulating HPCs in the peripheral blood.
- Large-volume leukapheresis (LVL) is usually performed to collect adequate numbers of CD34$^+$ cells in the fewest number of procedures possible.
- From 15 to 40 L of blood may be processed during LVL.
- Patients undergoing LVL are at increased risk of citrate toxicity and thrombocytopenia.

20. A. TPE every other day for five treatments using albumin as replacement.

B. Corticosteroid therapy and an angiotensin-converting enzyme inhibitor (ACEI).

Rationale: This is appropriate therapy for this patient.

C. Corticosteroid therapy and TPE every other day for five treatments using albumin as replacement.

D. Corticosteroid therapy, ACEI, and TPE every other day for five treatments using albumin as replacement.

E. Corticosteroid therapy, cyclophosphamide, ACEI, and TPE every other day for five treatments using albumin as replacement.

Rationale for A, C, D, and E: This patient has systemic lupus erythematosus and currently presents with lupus nephritis. These are not appropriate therapies for this patient.

Major points of discussion

- Lupus nephritis is a category IV indication for TPE according to the ASFA 2013 guidelines.
- TPE has not been shown to demonstrate any benefit in treating lupus nephritis.
- Corticosteroid therapy is used in patients with clinically significant renal disease. Cyclophosphamide or other immunosuppressive agents may be used in severe cases or in patients who are unable to tolerate corticosteroid therapy.
- Hypertension should be treated aggressively in these patients.
- Severe systemic lupus erythematosus is a category II indication for TPE according to the ASFA 2013 guidelines.[8]

21. A. Antibodies against the acetylcholine receptor must be present for TPE to be effective.

Rationale: TPE is effective for both seropositive and seronegative patients.

B. Response to TPE is rapid and symptoms usually improve within 1 to 7 days.

Rationale: See Major Points of Discussion.

C. Immunosuppressive medications should be held until after the course of TPE is completed.

Rationale: Immunosuppressive medications should be initiated during the course of TPE. These medications are typically given immediately after, and not prior to, TPE to prevent their removal since TPE can clear protein-bound drugs from the circulation, such as IVIg.

D. TPE is less effective than IVIg and should only be used to treat refractory patients.

Rationale: TPE has been shown to be equally effective as, if not more effective than, IVIg.

E. Use of TPE prior to thymectomy should be avoided due to the removal of coagulation factors.

Rationale: TPE is commonly used prior to thymectomy with improved outcomes in most studies. Most coagulation factor levels are normal within 1 to 2 days after TPE.

Major points of discussion

- Myasthenia gravis is an autoimmune disease most commonly caused by antibodies against the acetylcholine receptor (anti-AChR) on the muscle cell motor endplate at the neuromuscular junction. The acetylcholine receptors on the muscle are then unresponsive to impulses sent by presynaptic nerves, leading to weakness and fatigue in skeletal muscles.
- Anti-AChR antibodies are detectable in 80% to 90% of patients. These antibodies can block impulses sent by afferent nerves, decrease the number of available receptors at the motor endplate, or lead to cellular damage.
- Antibodies against the muscle-specific receptor tyrosine kinase (anti-MusK) are found in approximately 50% of patients without identifiable anti-AChR antibodies.
- Myasthenia gravis may be treated with cholinesterase inhibitors, immunosuppressive medications, TPE, and IVIg.
- There is an increased incidence of thymomas in patients with myasthenia gravis. Thymectomy can produce disease remission or improvement in patients both with and without thymomas.
- Myasthenia gravis (moderate and severe) and pre-thymectomy are category I indications for using TPE according to the ASFA guidelines published in 2013.
- TPE should consist of 1 to 1.5 total plasma volumes using albumin, with or without saline, as replacement fluid.[8]

22. A. **Extracorporeal photopheresis (ECP) is used prophylactically to prevent acute cellular rejection.**

Rationale: Prophylaxis for acute cellular rejection after heart transplantation is a category I indication for extracorporeal photopheresis.

B. Transplantation across ABO types is easily managed with TPE and immunosuppression.

Rationale: ABO-incompatible heart transplantation is associated with high rates of hyperacute rejection and early graft failure and is generally avoided in adults.

C. TPE is a first-line therapy for acute cellular rejection.

Rationale: TPE is not used to treat acute cellular rejection.
D. FFP is the replacement fluid of choice during TPE due to the high incidence of coagulopathy.
Rationale: FFP and/or albumin may be used as a replacement fluid.
E. Acute antibody-mediated rejection is most commonly seen in this setting.
Rationale: Acute cellular rejection is more common in this setting.

Major points of discussion

- ABO or major HLA incompatibility can lead to hyperacute rejection and cardiac allograft failure.
- ABO-incompatible heart transplantation in adults is avoided but may be performed in children up to 40 months of age.
- ABO-incompatible heart transplantation is more successful in young children and infants due to lower anti-A and anti-B antibody titers and the relative immaturity of their immune systems.
- ABO antigens are expressed on endothelial cells.
- ECP may be used to prevent (category I indication) or treat (category II indication) acute cellular rejection in heart transplantation.
- ECP uses ultraviolet light in the presence of a psoralen to induce DNA damage, leading to immunomodulation, destruction of allograft-specific T-cell populations, and induction and expansion of regulatory T cells. The exact mechanism by which ECP affects the immune system is currently unknown.
- TPE may be used to treat acute antibody-mediated cardiac allograft rejection (category III indication), but the efficacy is not conclusively documented at this time.

23. A. Increased production of HPCs in the bone marrow.
B. Decreased destruction of HPCs in the peripheral blood.
C. Increased release of HPCs from the bone marrow.
D. Increased maturation of HPCs in the bone marrow.
E. Increased activation of HPCs in the peripheral blood.
Rationale: By enhancing their release from the bone marrow, plerixafor leads to leukocytosis and increased hematopoietic stem cell counts in the peripheral blood.

Major points of discussion

- HPCs are present in the bone marrow and peripheral blood in adults.
- CD34$^+$ HPCs are present in very small quantities (<1%) in the peripheral blood.
- Administration of hematopoietic cytokines causes transient increases of HPCs in the peripheral blood.
- Plerixafor is a reversible inhibitor of stromal cell–derived factor-1 binding to its chemokine receptor (i.e., CXCR-4).
- Binding of stromal cell–derived factor-1 to CXCR-4, along with interactions with other adhesion molecules, leads to trafficking and adhesion of HPCs to the stem cell niche within the bone marrow.
- Plerixafor is administered after four daily doses of G-CSF, 10 to 11 hours prior to the start of collection, and every subsequent day with G-CSF for a maximum of four doses after the start of collection.

- Peripheral blood–derived HPCs are easier to collect and lead to more rapid engraftment compared with bone marrow–derived HPCs.
- Plerixafor is FDA approved for use in combination with G-CSF for the mobilization of autologous HPCs for peripheral blood collection and subsequent autologous transplantation in patients with multiple myeloma or non-Hodgkin lymphoma.[9]

24. A. Focal segmental glomerulosclerosis.
Rationale: TPE is a second-line treatment or category II indication for desensitization prior to renal transplantation in the setting of a living donor with a positive crossmatch caused by donor-specific HLA antibody(ies).
B. Antibody-mediated rejection of a renal allograft.
Rationale: TPE has been shown to be a first-line therapy, either alone or in conjunction with other immunosuppressive therapy, to treat this type of rejection.
C. Diarrhea-associated hemolytic uremic syndrome.
Rationale: Published evidence suggests that TPE is ineffective in this setting.
D. Immune complex–induced rapidly progressive glomerulonephritis.
Rationale: Published evidence is insufficient to establish a definitive benefit for TPE in this setting.
E. Myeloma kidney.
Rationale: TPE is considered a second-line therapy, either as a standard treatment or in conjunction with other modes of treatment.

Major points of discussion

- Antibody-mediated rejection is a category I indication for TPE based on the ASFA guidelines published in 2013.
- Antibody-mediated rejection of renal allografts is due to either preformed or de novo donor-specific antibodies.
- Patients with antibody-mediated renal allograft rejection should start immunosuppressive therapy to limit antibody production prior to starting TPE.[8]

25. A. To decrease RBC alloantibody titers.
Rationale: The use of TPE to decrease RBC alloantibody titers is not recommended in this setting.
B. To decrease donor-specific anti-HLA antibody titers.
Rationale: TPE has been used for decreasing donor-specific HLA antibody titers in solid organ transplants.
C. To decrease donor-specific anti–human platelet antigen (HPA) antibody titers.
Rationale: Although TPE may decrease donor-specific anti-HPA antibody titers, it has not been recommended specifically for this purpose.
D. To decrease complement levels.
Rationale: The use of TPE to decrease complement levels is not recommended in this setting.
E. To decrease donor-specific anti–human neutrophil antigen (HNA) antibody titers.
Rationale: The use of TPE to decrease anti-HNA antibody titers is not recommended in this setting.

Major points of discussion

- High-titer recipient isohemagglutinins (i.e., anti-ABO antibodies) or HLA antibodies may cause hyperacute rejection of solid organ transplants.

- Peritransplant TPE in conjunction with immunosuppression and/or IVIg may lower antibody titers and prevent hyperacute rejection.
- The replacement fluid for plasma exchange is albumin, FFP, or a combination of the two, depending on the presence or absence of coagulopathy.
- The goal of TPE in this setting is to reduce antibody titers to a low enough level to prevent hyperacute rejection. Acceptable titers for transplantation depend on the type of organ being transplanted and type of antibodies present.
- The number of peritransplant plasma exchange procedures depends on the initial antibody titers.
- The use of TPE to treat antibody-mediated rejection in the setting of renal transplantation is a category I indication based on ASFA guidelines published in 2013.[8]

26. A. Transfuse 1 U RBCs and 1 dose of single-donor apheresis platelets.
Rationale: This patient does not require an RBC transfusion, and platelet transfusions should be avoided in this setting in the absence of life-threatening bleeding.
B. Transfuse 10 U cryoprecipitate.
Rationale: This patient does not need cryoprecipitate in this setting.
C. Transfuse 2 U plasma.
Rationale: If plasmapheresis is unavailable, then transfusion of FFP is the next-best course of action until plasmapheresis can be performed.
D. Initiate a series of plasmapheresis procedures.
Rationale: This is the first-line therapy for patients with TTP and should be initiated as soon as possible.
E. Perform a whole blood exchange.
Rationale: Although this would provide new plasma and would remove autoantibodies, this is not the best course of treatment for this patient.

Major points of discussion
- Plasmapheresis is the first-line therapy for TTP and is a category I indication according to the ASFA guidelines published in 2013.
- TTP is a characterized by a pentad of clinical findings: thrombocytopenia, MAHA, mental status changes, renal failure, and fever.
- This patient most likely has TTP based on her presenting signs and symptoms: fever, thrombocytopenia, MAHA, and mental status changes.
- The presence of these findings in the absence of another clinical explanation is sufficient to start plasmapheresis emergently due to the high mortality of untreated TTP.
- If plasmapheresis is not available, plasma should be transfused to replace ADAMSTS13, the metalloproteinase that cleaves ultra-large von Willebrand multimers, which is deficient in TTP patients.
- Plasmapheresis should be performed daily until the platelet count is greater than 150×10^9/L and lactate dehydrogenase (LDH) levels are close to normal values for 2-3 consecutive days.[6,8]

27. **A. Category I indications include diseases and syndromes for which apheresis is the primary treatment.**
Rationale: See Major Points of Discussion.

B. Category II indications include diseases and syndromes for which apheresis is the primary treatment in conjunction with another treatment modality.
Rationale: Category II indications includes diseases and syndromes for which apheresis is a second-line therapy.
C. Category III indications include diseases and syndromes for which apheresis is a second-line therapy.
Rationale: Category III indications include diseases and syndromes for which the efficacy of apheresis has not been established.
D. Category IV indications include diseases and syndromes for which apheresis is the last line of treatment.
Rationale: Category IV indications include diseases and syndromes for which apheresis is ineffective or harmful.
E. Category V indications include diseases and syndromes for which apheresis is ineffective or harmful.
Rationale: There is no category V defined in these guidelines.

Major points of discussion
- The ASFA issues guidelines are based on current evidence for the use of therapeutic apheresis.
- Four categories are used to define the indications for apheresis for diseases and syndromes.
- The strength of the recommendation for the use of apheresis is described, as well as based on the quality of the evidence that is currently available.
- Category I indications include disorders for which apheresis is a first-line therapy, either alone or in conjunction with other treatment modalities (e.g., TTP).
- Category II indications include disorders for which apheresis is a second-line therapy, either alone or in conjunction with other treatment modalities (example: ABO-incompatible hematopoietic cell transplant).
- Category III indications include disorders for which the efficacy and role of apheresis has not been established (example: sepsis with multiorgan failure).
- Category IV indications include disorders for which apheresis is ineffective or harmful (e.g., schizophrenia).[8]

28. A. Disorder for which apheresis is accepted as first-line therapy, either as a primary stand-alone treatment or in conjunction with other modes of treatment.

Rationale: This is the description of a category I indication.
B. Disorder for which apheresis is accepted as second-line therapy, either as a primary stand-alone treatment or in conjunction with other modes of treatment.
Rationale: This is the description of a category II indication. Severe malaria is a category II indication for the use of RBC exchange (i.e., erythrocytapheresis). Antimalarial antimicrobial therapy is the first-line approach for treating malaria.
C. The optimal role of apheresis is not established; decision making should be individualized.
Rationale: This is the description of a category III indication.
D. Disorder in which published evidence demonstrates or suggests that apheresis is ineffective or harmful.
E. Disorder for which approval for a research study is required from an IRB.
Rationale: These are part of the description of a category IV indication.

Major points of discussion

■ The ASFA guidelines provide an important evidence-based tool for the practice of therapeutic apheresis.

■ In the 2013 ASFA guidelines, the descriptions of the various categories were amended and simplified in comparison to previous editions of the guidelines. Changes in the descriptions of the categories included the addition of the strength of the recommendation, which allowed categorization to be better aligned with the strength of the evidence and the quality of the relevant publications in the literature.

■ The current description of category II is disorders for which apheresis is accepted as second-line therapy, either as a stand-alone treatment or in conjunction with other modes of treatment. For severe malaria, the recommendation grade is 2B, which is a weak recommendation supported only by moderate quality evidence, such as controlled trials.

■ RCE (automatic or manual) in severely ill patients with high levels of parasitemia (i.e., >10%) is believed to improve the rheological properties of the blood and to reduce levels of parasite-derived toxins, hemolytic metabolites, and cytokines. It is an adjunct therapy to the use of specific anti-malarial agents.[3,5,8]

29. A. Disorder for which apheresis is accepted as first-line therapy, either as a primary stand-alone treatment or in conjunction with other modes of treatment.
Rationale: This is the description of a category I indication.
B. Disorder for which apheresis is accepted as second-line therapy, either as a primary stand-alone treatment or in conjunction with other modes of treatment.
Rationale: This is the description of a category II indication.
C. The optimal role of apheresis is not established; decision making should be individualized.
Rationale: This is the description of a category III indication. Thrombotic microangiopathy: hematopoietic stem cell transplant–associated is a category III indication for the use of plasmapheresis. It should be considered as salvage therapy for selected patients with persistent/progressive thrombotic microangiopathy despite resolution of infections and graft-versus-host disease.
D. Disorder in which published evidence demonstrates or suggests that apheresis is ineffective or harmful.
E. Disorder for which approval for a research study is required from an IRB.
Rationale: These are part of the description of category IV indications.

Major points of discussion

■ The ASFA guidelines provide an important evidence-based tool for the practice of therapeutic apheresis.

■ In the 2013 ASFA guidelines, the descriptions of the various categories were amended and simplified compared with the previous editions of the guidelines. Changes in the descriptions of the categories included the addition of the strength of the recommendation, which allowed categorization to be better aligned with the strength of the evidence and the quality of the relevant publications in the literature.

■ The current definition of category III reflects the individual character of the decision-making process for diseases in this category. The recommendation grade and individual patient's clinical circumstances should guide inclusion of therapeutic apheresis in the treatment plan for category III indications. The current description of category III is as follows: Disorders in which the optimum role of apheresis is not established and decision making should be individualized. For transplantation-associated thrombotic microangiopathy, the recommendation grade is 2C.

■ Although a consensus statement by the Bone Marrow and Transplant Clinical Trials Network Toxicity Committee recommends that therapeutic plasmapheresis not be considered as a standard of care for this entity, some patients do respond and treatment decisions should be individualized for patients with persistent transplantation-associated thrombotic microangiopathy.[4,7,8]

30. A. It equilibrates between the intravascular and extravascular spaces.
Rationale: An ideal solute resides only in the intravascular space.
B. It is synthesized during the time frame of the plasmapheresis procedure.
Rationale: Ideal solutes are not rapidly synthesized and there is no net synthesis during the time frame of the procedure.
C. It is catabolized during the time frame of the plasmapheresis procedure.
Rationale: Ideal solutes are not rapidly catabolized and there is no net catabolism during the time frame of the procedure.
D. It is completely intravascular.
Rationale: Plasmapheresis directly removes soluble substances only from the intravascular space.
E. It is an IgG antibody.
Rationale: IgG antibodies are predominantly extravascular; thus, these are less efficiently removed by plasmapheresis.

Major points of discussion

■ For practical purposes, the intravascular compartment is considered an isolated system that can be depleted of its soluble contents by the exchange of patient plasma with a replacement fluid.

■ The synthetic rate, fractional catabolic rate, and intercompartmental movement of an ideal solute are balanced in a steady state and proceed much slower than the actual removal of plasma from the intravascular space.

■ IgM is 76% intravascular, whereas IgG is only 45% intravascular. Thus, plasmapheresis is much more efficient at removing IgM antibodies.

■ Fibrinogen and IgM approximate the characteristics of a soluble ideal solute; IgG does not behave as an ideal solute. For cytapheresis (e.g., erythrocytapheresis, leukapheresis), RBCs, which travel in the laminar flow, approximate the characteristics of a cellular "ideal solute," whereas leukocytes, which can marginate, do not behave as ideal solutes.

■ After a 1–plasma volume exchange, approximately 37% of an ideal solute will still remain in the circulation.[11]

References

1. Adams RJ, McKie VC, Hsu L, et al. Prevention of a first stroke by transfusions in children with sickle cell anemia and abnormal results on transcranial Doppler ultrasonography. N Engl J Med 1998;339:5–11.
2. Berkman EM, Orlin JB. Use of plasmapheresis and partial plasma exchanges in the management of patients with cryoglobulinemia. Transfusion 1980;20:171–178.
3. Burchard GD, Kröger J, Knobloch J, et al. Exchange blood transfusion in severe falciparum malaria: retrospective evaluation of 61 patients treated with, compared to 63 patients treated without, exchange transfusion. Trop Med Int Health 1997;2:733–740.
4. Ho VT, Cutler C, Carter S, et al. Blood and marrow transplant clinical trials network toxicity committee consensus summary: thrombotic microangiopathy after hematopoietic stem cell transplantation. Biol Blood Marrow Transplant 2005;11:571–575.
5. Powell VI, Grima K. Exchange transfusion for malaria and Babesia infection. Transfus Med Rev 2002;16:239–250.
6. Rock GA, Shumak KH, Buskard NA, et al. Comparison of plasma exchange with plasma infusion in the treatment of thrombotic thrombocytopenic purpura. Canadian Apheresis Study Group N Engl J Med 1991;325:393–397.
7. Ruutu T, Barosi G, Benjamin RJ, et al. Diagnostic criteria for hematopoietic stem cell transplant-associated microangiopathy: results of a consensus process by an International Working Group. Haematologica 2007;92:95–100.
8. Schwartz J, Winters JL, Padmanabhan A, et al. Guidelines on the use of therapeutic apheresis in clinical practice-evidence-based approach from the Writing Committee of the American Society for Apheresis: the sixth special issue. J Clin Apheresis 2013;28:145–284.
9. Tanhehco YC, Vogl DT, Stadtmauer EA, et al. The evolving role of plerixafor in hematopoietic progenitor cell mobilization. Transfusion 2013;53:2314–2326.
10. Vichinsky EP, Haberkern CM, Neumayr L, et al. A comparison of conservative and aggressive transfusion regimens in the perioperative management of sickle cell disease. N Engl J Med 1995;333:206–213.
11. Weinstein R. Basic principles of therapeutic blood exchange. In McLeod BC, Szczepiorkoski Z, Weinstein R, et al., eds. Apheresis: principles and practice. 3rd ed. Bethesda, MD: AABB Press, 2010.

CHAPTER 21

TRANSFUSION MEDICINE: Cellular Therapy

Joseph (Yossi) Schwartz, Yvette C. Tanhehco, Suzanne A. Arinsburg, Jeffrey S. Jhang, Eldad A. Hod, Richard O. Francis, Steven L. Spitalnik

QUESTIONS

1. Which one of the following tests is most likely to be routinely performed as part of the quality control of hematopoietic progenitor cell (HPC) products?
   A. Immature platelet fraction.
   B. Dye exclusion viability assay.
   C. *Acanthamoeba* culture.
   D. Mac-1 enumeration.
   E. Dimethyl sulfoxide (DMSO) concentration.

2. Which one of the following is an advantage of using peripheral blood–derived HPCs instead of bone marrow–derived or cord blood–derived HPCs for an allogeneic transplant?
   A. Lower incidence of graft-versus-host disease (GVHD).
   B. More rapid engraftment.
   C. Lower T-cell content.
   D. Less stringent human leukocyte antigen (HLA) matching.
   E. Mobilization with a growth factor, chemotherapy, or adhesion molecule antagonist is not required.

3. Which one of the following is the most common adverse effect of plerixafor+granulocyte colony-stimulating factor (G-CSF) mobilization for peripheral blood HPC collection?
   A. Gastrointestinal symptoms.
   B. Blindness.
   C. Diffuse redness of the skin.
   D. Dysuria.
   E. Seizures.

4. Which of one of the following is an immediate adverse event following an autologous, peripheral blood HPC infusion?
   A. Bronchospasm.
   B. Jaundice.
   C. Infertility.
   D. Mucositis.
   E. Splenic enlargement.

5. Which one of the following sites is the most optimal for harvesting bone marrow?
   A. Sternum.
   B. Posterior iliac crest.
   C. Anterior iliac crest.
   D. Femur.
   E. Ribs.

6. Which one of the following preharvest peripheral blood cell counts best predicts the yield of a peripheral blood HPC collection by apheresis?
   A. CD34$^+$ cells.
   B. Total nucleated cells.
   C. Total mononuclear cells.
   D. Polymorphonuclear cells.
   E. CD38$^+$ cells.

7. Which one of the following solutions is used to cryopreserve HPCs?
   A. Glycerol+DMSO+autologous plasma.
   B. Glycerol+Adsol.
   C. Glycerol+autologous plasma.
   D. DMSO+Adsol.
   E. DMSO+autologous plasma.

8. Which one of the following is the most common adverse effect of mobilizing HPCs with G-CSF?
   A. Bone pain.
   B. Bronchospasm.
   C. Jaundice.
   D. Splenic enlargement.
   E. Sweet syndrome.

9. Samples for transmissible disease testing of allogeneic HPC donors must be collected within:
   A. 1 day.
   B. 7 days.
   C. 14 days.
   D. 30 days.
   E. 60 days.

10. Which one of the following doses is generally considered the minimum number of stem cells required for a single transplant?
    A. 2×10^{10} CD3$^+$ cells/kg.
    B. 3×10^8 CD38$^+$ cells/kg.
    C. 2×10^6 CD34$^+$ cells/kg.
    D. 2×10^6 CD34$^+$ cells/mL.
    E. 3×10^7 CD38$^+$ cells/mL.

11a. For which one of the following disorders is plerixafor specifically approved for use by the U.S. Food and Drug Administration (FDA)?

A. Multiple myeloma and Hodgkin lymphoma.

B. Non-Hodgkin lymphoma and Hodgkin lymphoma.

C. Acute leukemia and multiple myeloma.

D. Multiple myeloma and non-Hodgkin lymphoma.

E. Acute leukemia and healthy donors.

11b. Which one of the following is the mechanism of action of plerixafor?

A. Stimulates stem cell proliferation.

B. Antagonizes C-X-C chemokine receptor type 4 (CXCR4).

C. Acts as a ligand for the c-kit (CD117) receptor.

D. Induces shedding of membrane bound stem cell factor (SCF).

E. Irreversibly inhibits thymidylate synthase.

12. An A-negative patient with a negative antibody screen received a stem cell transplant from a B-positive donor 1 week ago. If the patient requires transfusion, which one of the following types of packed red blood cells should the patient receive?

A. A–

B. A+

C. B–

D. B+

E. O–

13. An A-positive patient has a history of anti-K antibodies. The patient receives an O-positive stem cell transplant from a donor who had a negative antibody screen 2 weeks ago. Which one of the following types of red cells should be provided?

A. O–

B. O+ plus K–

C. A–

D. A+ plus K–

E. AB+ plus K–

14. Which one of the following is the best predictor of poor stem cell mobilization?

A. Age less than 5 years.

B. Etoposide mobilization.

C. Radiotherapy.

D. Male gender.

E. Fewer than 20 CD34$^+$ cells/μL peripheral blood preharvest count.

15. Which one of the following statements about informed consent for the collection of umbilical cord blood (UCB) hematopoietic stem cells for public cord blood banking is true?

A. Informed consent to collect UCB must be obtained from the mother and father of the infant.

B. Informed consent to collect UCB is obtained from the mother because of the infant's inability to give consent and because her blood needs to be tested for transmissible diseases.

C. Informed consent should be obtained from the father to perform transmissible disease testing on his blood to improve the safety of the UCB.

D. Informed consent for UCB collected is required for UCB collected in utero, but not when collected ex utero.

E. Informed consent for UCB is required because the mother and father both require HLA typing.

16. Which one of the following is a requirement for shipping cryopreserved products according to the Foundation for the Accreditation of Cellular Therapy (FACT) standards?

A. Liquid nitrogen dry shippers have to be validated to maintain a temperature of –150°C or less for at least 48 hours past the time of delivery to the transplant facility.

B. Liquid nitrogen dry shippers have to be validated to maintain a temperature of –196°C or less for at least 48 hours past the time of delivery to the transplant facility.

C. Liquid nitrogen dry shippers have to be validated to maintain a temperature of –150°C or less for at least 24 hours past the time of delivery to the transplant facility.

D. Liquid nitrogen dry shippers have to be validated to maintain a temperature of –196°C or less for at least 24 hours past the time of delivery to the transplant facility.

E. Liquid nitrogen dry shippers have to be validated to maintain a temperature of –150°C or less until the time of delivery to the transplant facility.

17. Which one of the following HLA loci is most commonly matched for in unrelated allogeneic peripheral blood–derived HPC transplants?

A. HLA-A, -B, and -C.

B. HLA-DR, -DQ, and -DP.

C. HLA-A, -B, -DR, and -DQ

D. HLA-A, -C, -DR, -DQ, and -DP.

E. HLA-A, -B, -C, -DR, and -DQ.

18. Which one of the following types of red blood cells should be given to a patient who is O+ with a negative antibody screen after receiving an A+ stem cell transplant 2 days ago?

A. A–

B. A+

C. B–

D. B+

E. O+

19. A patient receives an ABO blood group major mismatched HPC transplant. Which one of the following events may be attributed to this type of ABO incompatibility?

A. An acute hemolytic reaction at the time of HPC transplant due to the infusion of incompatible plasma containing anti-A and/or anti-B antibodies.

B. Delayed red blood cell engraftment.

C. Delayed hemolysis due to the production of anti-A and/or anti-B antibodies by donor lymphocytes.

D. An increased risk for posttransplant Epstein-Barr virus infection.

E. Transplant-associated thrombotic microangiopathy.

20. A patient receives an ABO blood group minor mismatched HPC transplant. Which one of the following adverse events may be attributed to this type of ABO incompatibility?

A. An acute hemolytic reaction at the time of HPC infusion due to the presence of incompatible red blood cells in the donor product.

B. Delayed red blood cell engraftment.

C. Delayed hemolysis due to the production of anti-A and/or anti-B antibodies by donor lymphocytes.

D. An increased risk for posttransplant Epstein-Barr virus infection.

E. Transplant-associated thrombotic microangiopathy.

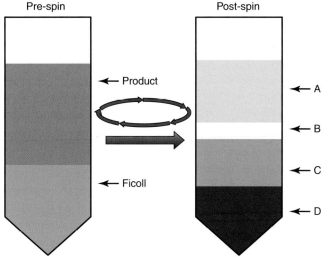

Pre-spin | Post-spin

← Product

← A

← B

← C

← Ficoll

← D

Figure 21-1 The tube on the left contains Ficoll on the bottom and the bone marrow product layered on top. After centrifugation, the contents of the conical tube separate into four parts shown on the right.

21. A 12-year-old boy with sickle cell disease is undergoing an ABO-mismatched bone marrow transplant. The donor is blood group type A and the recipient is type O. Density gradient centrifugation with Ficoll is used to deplete the product of red cells. As shown in Figure 21-1, which one of the following layers contains the granulocytes?
   A. A
   B. B
   C. C
   D. D

ANSWERS

1. A. Immature platelet fraction.
   Rationale: Cell counts, including total nucleated cell count, viable CD34$^+$ cells, CD3$^+$ T cells, and red cells, are routinely determined as part of the quality control of HPC products. The immature platelet fraction is not part of routine cell enumeration.
   B. Dye exclusion viability assay.
   Rationale: Dye exclusion (e.g., trypan blue, 7-amino-actinomycin D [7-AAD]) or metabolic viability assays (e.g., tetrazolium reduction) are part of the quality control of HPC products.
   C. *Acanthamoeba* culture.
   Rationale: Although *Acanthamoeba* has been identified in contact lens solutions, it is not a routine test for the quality control of HPC products
   D. Mac-1 enumeration.
   Rationale: CD34$^+$ cell enumeration is performed as part of the quality control of HPC products. Macrophage enumeration using the Mac-1 marker is not performed.
   E. Dimethyl sulfoxide (DMSO) concentration.
   Rationale: DMSO is most often used as the cryoprotectant for HPC products. Although there are maximum limits to the amount of DMSO that should be infused in the product, DMSO concentrations are not measured directly from the product.

   Major points of discussion
   ■ The total nucleated cell count is determined by automated procedures and is used to calculate the number of nucleated cells per kilogram of recipient body weight.
   ■ Cell viability is determined by using dye exclusion reagents such as trypan blue dye, fluorescent dyes such as acridine orange and propidium iodide, and 7-AAD.
   ■ HPC products are tested for bacterial and fungal contamination that may have occurred during collection or processing. HPC products can also be

contaminated when patients are bacteremic or septic during the collection.
   ■ A positive culture result of stem cells collected from bone marrow harvesting does not necessarily lead to immediate discard of the product. Since these cells are "irreplaceable," they are often transplanted because of emergency need.
   ■ The CD34 antigen is used to evaluate the "quality" of HPC products. The percentage of CD34$^+$ cells in the product is determined by flow cytometry and is used to calculate the CD34$^+$ cell dose. This is expressed as the number of CD34$^+$ cells per kilogram of recipient body weight.

2. A. Lower incidence of graft-versus-host disease (GVHD).
   Rationale: HPCs collected from peripheral blood have the highest incidence of chronic GVHD among the three sources of HPCs (i.e., peripheral blood, bone marrow, cord blood).
   B. More rapid engraftment.
   Rationale: HPCs obtained from peripheral blood lead to more rapid neutrophil and platelet engraftment in patients compared with HPCs obtained from bone marrow and cord blood. Rapid engraftment is important because short engraftment times are associated with fewer infections, fewer transfusions, shorter hospital stays, and lower cost. HPCs obtained from cord blood have the longest time to engraftment. HPCs from the bone marrow engraft faster than cord blood–derived HPCs but slower than peripheral blood–derived HPCs.
   C. Lower T-cell content.
   Rationale: HPCs collected from peripheral blood have a higher T-cell content compared with HPCs from bone marrow and cord blood. Higher T-cell content increases the risk of GVHD.
   D. Less stringent human leukocyte antigen (HLA) matching.

Rationale: The HLA type of the donor must be closely matched to the recipient for both peripheral blood– and bone marrow–derived HPCs. The requirements are less restrictive for cord blood–derived HPCs.

E. Mobilization with a growth factor, chemotherapy, or adhesion molecule antagonist is not required.

Rationale: A low level of HPCs is present in the circulation; however, mobilization with a growth factor, chemotherapy, adhesion molecule (e.g., CXCR4) antagonist, or a combination of the three is necessary to obtain sufficient HPCs from the peripheral blood for transplantation.

Major points of discussion

- HPCs for allogeneic transplantation can be obtained from three different sources: bone marrow, peripheral blood, and cord blood.
- Bone marrow–derived HPCs can provide an adequate number of CD34+ HPCs for transplantation and this source is associated with less chronic GVHD compared with peripheral blood–derived HPCs; however, they are more difficult to obtain (e.g., requires anesthesia) and are associated with longer neutrophil and platelet engraftment times.
- Transplantation of peripheral blood–derived HPCs is associated with shorter engraftment times. They are also easier to collect; however, growth factors, chemotherapy, and/or CXCR4 antagonists are necessary to mobilize the HPCs into the circulation.
- Cord blood–derived HPCs are associated with the lowest incidence of chronic GVHD and have a less-restrictive HLA-matching requirement; however, they contain fewer HPCs and have the longest time to engraftment.
- The time to engraftment is an important consideration when selecting an HPC source. Shorter engraftment times are associated with fewer infections, fewer transfusions, shorter hospital stays, and lower cost.

3. **A. Gastrointestinal symptoms.**

Rationale: The two most commonly reported adverse effects of plerixafor administration are (1) gastrointestinal symptoms such as diarrhea, nausea, vomiting, abdominal pain, and flatulence and (2) injection site erythema. Other adverse effects reported in 5% or more patients who received plerixafor + G-CSF in phase III trials include bone pain, headache, and paresthesias.

B. Blindness.

Rationale: Blindness was not reported as an adverse effect in phase III trials of plerixafor + G-CSF in patients with multiple myeloma and non-Hodgkin's lymphoma.

C. Diffuse redness of the skin.

Rationale: Injection site erythema is a commonly reported adverse effect of plerixafor administration. Redness of the skin is a less common side effect.

D. Dysuria.

Rationale: Dysuria is not a common side effect of plerixafor. Gastrointestinal symptoms are more common.

E. Seizures.

Rationale: Seizures are not a common side effect of plerixafor. Gastrointestinal symptoms are more common.

Major points of discussion

- Plerixafor is a small bicyclam molecule that is a reversible inhibitor of stromal cell–derived factor-1 binding to its receptor CXCR4.
- Plerixafor is indicated in combination with G-CSF to mobilize HPCs from the marrow to the peripheral blood in patients with multiple myeloma and non-Hodgkin lymphoma undergoing autologous transplantation.
- Plerixafor is administered subcutaneously after 4 days of G-CSF at a dose of 240 µg/kg approximately 11 hours prior to collection by apheresis. The dose can be repeated for up to 4 additional days with G-CSF.
- Variability exists in the interval between plerixafor administration and apheresis collection at different institutions. Studies in normal donors suggest there is sustained release of stem cells from 4 to 20 hours after administration of plerixafor with peak release between 10 and 14 hours after administration.
- The most common ($\geq$5%) adverse effects reported in phase III trials of plerixafor + G-CSF are diarrhea, nausea, vomiting, abdominal pain, flatulence, fatigue, injection site erythema, injection site pruritus, bone pain, headache, and paresthesia.[3,4]

4. **A. Bronchospasm.**

Rationale: Mild allergic to anaphylactic reactions, possibly due to DMSO, can be seen with HPC infusions.

B. Jaundice.

Rationale: Jaundice can be seen in acute GVHD of the liver, which is not seen with autologous HPC transplantation.

C. Infertility.

Rationale: Infertility can result from high-dose chemotherapy, but it is not a side effect of HPC infusion.

D. Mucositis.

Rationale: Mucositis is a common adverse effect of chemotherapy. It is not an immediate adverse event associated with HPC infusion.

E. Splenic enlargement.

Rationale: Splenic enlargement and rupture can occur in allogeneic donors and patients after receiving G-CSF. It is not associated with HPC infusion.

Major points of discussion

- Adverse events associated with HPC product infusions include nausea, diarrhea, flushing, bradycardia, hypertension, hypotension, and abdominal pain. In addition, mild allergic to anaphylactic reactions, possibly due to DMSO, can be seen.
- Treatment of the adverse effects of HPC infusion includes slowing, but not halting, the infusion until the symptoms pass.
- Premedicating with antihistamines can prevent hypotensive and allergic reactions. Adequate hydration and alkalinization of the urine prior to the infusion may reduce the risk of renal complications from free hemoglobin released by red cell lysis during cryopreservation.
- The total volume of HPC product infused should not contain more than 1 g/kg DMSO per day.
- HPC products can be washed prior to infusion to reduce DMSO infusion–related toxicities.

5. A. Sternum.
   B. Posterior iliac crest.
   Rationale: This site provides the most practical and productive site for marrow collection.
   C. Anterior iliac crest.
   D. Femur.
   E. Ribs.
   Rationale for A, C, D, and E: These sites may be used because they have red marrow, which consists of hematopoietic tissue, but the posterior iliac crest is the most practical and productive site for marrow collection.

Major points of discussion

- Bone marrow harvests are performed with the patient under general anesthesia.
- Red marrow, which contains hematopoietic tissue, is found mainly in flat bones such as the pelvis, sternum, skull, ribs, vertebrae, and scapulae. It can also be found in the epiphyseal ends of long bones such as the femur and humerus. By adolescence, active marrow is usually found only in the cavities of these axial bones.
- The posterior iliac crest is the most optimal site for bone marrow aspirations in adults, children, and most infants because it is easily accessible, produces a high yield, and causes the least discomfort to the patient compared with other sites.
- The anterior iliac crest may be used for bone marrow aspirations in adults when access to the posterior iliac crest is limited due to difficulty with positioning, morbid obesity, skin diseases, or previous irradiation.
- The greater trochanter of the femur, individual vertebral bodies, or ribs may be used for bone marrow aspirations. Obtaining bone marrow from these sites may require surgical consultation and computed tomography guidance.
- Obtaining bone marrow from a site that has been previously irradiated should be avoided because it is likely to have less overall cellularity.

6. **A. CD34⁺ cells.**
   Rationale: CD34 is a surrogate marker for HPCs. Higher levels of circulating peripheral blood CD34⁺ cells prior to the start of collection are associated with higher product yields.
   B. Total nucleated cells.
   Rationale: Total nucleated or white blood cell counts are not as predictive as the CD34⁺ cell count in determining the success of a peripheral blood HPC collection.
   C. Total mononuclear cells.
   Rationale: Total mononuclear cell counts are not used to predict peripheral blood stem cell harvest yields.
   D. Polymorphonuclear cells.
   Rationale: Polymorphonuclear cell counts or neutrophil counts are not used to predict peripheral blood stem cell harvest yields.
   E. CD38⁺ cells.
   Rationale: CD38 is a marker of cell activation. It is not used to predict peripheral blood stem cell harvest yields.

Major points of discussion

- CD34 is a cell surface glycoprotein that acts as a surrogate marker of HPCs.

- The number of CD34⁺ cells in the peripheral blood is measured prior to the start of apheresis collection. Apheresis collection commences when the number of CD34⁺ cells is at or above a prespecified threshold (e.g., >20 CD34⁺ cells/μL).
- The dose of stem cells for transplantation is based on the number of CD34⁺ cells/kg recipient body weight.
- Pluripotent hematopoietic stem cells are CD34⁺CD38⁻.
- The cellular content of HPCs obtained from peripheral blood differs significantly from those obtained from bone marrow.

7. A. Glycerol+DMSO+autologous plasma.
   B. Glycerol+Adsol.
   C. Glycerol+autologous plasma.
   D. DMSO+Adsol.
   E. DMSO+autologous plasma.
   Rationale: Glycerol is a cryopreservative solution for red blood cells. Adsol is an additive solution for red blood cells collected in citrate-phosphate-dextrose. DMSO and autologous plasma or another source of protein comprises the cryopreservative solution used for HPCs.

Major points of discussion

- Peripheral blood–derived HPC products can be stored for up to 48 hours without cryopreservation before infusion, according to National Marrow Donor Program guidelines.
- HPC products can be stored at 4°C to 15°C overnight before processing without compromising graft quality and engraftment.
- Cryopreservation of HPCs involves suspending the cells in a solution composed of DMSO (10% final concentration) and autologous plasma or another source of protein.
- Controlled-rate freezing (1° to 2°C/min to –30°C to –50°C, 2° to 10°C/min to –90°C) is used to cryopreserve products in cryopreservation medium.
- Cryopreserved products may be stored in a mechanical freezer at less than –70°C or in liquid nitrogen freezers (liquid phase at –196°C or vapor phase at <–150°C) for several years without compromising cell viability.

8. **A. Bone pain.**
   Rationale: The most commonly reported adverse effects of G-CSF mobilization are bone pain, myalgia, headache, and fatigue (>50%).
   B. Bronchospasm.
   Rationale: Allergic reactions (e.g., hives, erythema, bronchospasm, anaphylaxis) can be seen with G-CSF mobilization, but they are not as common as bone pain.
   C. Jaundice.
   Rationale: Liver changes are not a common side effect of G-CSF.
   D. Splenic enlargement.
   Rationale: Enlargement of the spleen can be seen with G-CSF treatment but is rare. Activities that can lead to traumatic splenic rupture should be avoided.
   E. Sweet syndrome.
   Rationale: Drug-induced febrile neutrophilic dermatosis is rare.

Major points of discussion

- G-CSF is the principal hematopoietic growth factor used for HPC mobilization.
- G-CSF is usually administered once a day by subcutaneous injection in doses ranging from 5 to 20 μg/kg/day.
- G-CSF is associated with the release of metalloproteases that are hypothesized to cleave at least one receptor–ligand pair that tethers stem cells to the bone marrow stroma.
- G-CSF causes a predictable increase in circulating CD34$^+$ stem cells and other leukocytes. Peripheral blood stem cell collection can usually begin about 3 to 4 days after the first dose.
- Symptoms reported with G-CSF administration include bone pain, myalgia, headache, fatigue, insomnia, flu-like symptoms, nausea, sweats, anorexia, fever, chills, emesis, and allergic reactions.[6]

9. A. 1 day.
   B. 7 days.
   C. 14 days.
   D. 30 days.
   E. 60 days.
   Rationale: Infectious disease testing of HPC donors should be performed within 30 days of collection.

Major points of discussion

- A cell therapy processing laboratory must have standard operating procedures for the storage of untested or infectious products.
- Infectious disease testing of HPC donors should be performed within 30 days before collection.
- Infectious disease testing of HPC products includes HIV 1 and 2, hepatitis C, hepatitis B, HTLV 1 and 2, cytomegalovirus, and *Treponema pallidum*. Although not required by the FDA, testing for West Nile virus and Chagas disease is commonly included.
- HPC products can be stored in the vapor phase of liquid nitrogen or placed inside another plastic bag that is sealed before storage to minimize the risk of cross-contamination among HPC products.
- HPC products from allogeneic donors who are confirmed to be HIV positive are not used. However, other positive disease markers do not necessarily prohibit the use of collections from a particular donor.

10. A. 2×10^{10} CD3$^+$ cells/kg.
   B. 3×10^8 CD38$^+$ cells/kg.
   C. 2×10^6 CD34$^+$ cells/kg.
   D. 2×10^6 CD34$^+$ cells/mL.
   E. 3×10^7 CD38$^+$ cells/mL.
   Rationale: 2×10^6 CD34$^+$ cells/kg recipient body weight is generally considered the minimum number of stem cells required for a single transplant. CD3 is a T-cell marker; CD34 is a stem cell marker; and CD38 is a marker found on B cells and natural killer cells.

Major points of discussion

- CD34 is a cell surface glycoprotein that is used as a surrogate marker for hematopoietic stem cells.
- Long-term hematopoietic restoration will occur with as few as 1×10^6 CD34$^+$ cells/kg recipient body weight.

- 2×10^6 CD34$^+$ cells/kg recipient body weight is generally accepted as the minimum dose for a single transplant to ensure reliable engraftment.
- Larger doses of infused CD34$^+$ cells increase the speed of engraftment. Infusion of 5×10^6 CD34$^+$ cells/kg recipient body weight results in faster engraftment compared with infusion of 2×10^6 CD34$^+$ cells/kg recipient body weight.
- Other factors aside from infused CD34$^+$ cell dose that affect the speed of engraftment after autologous transplantation include the type and extent of previous myelotoxic therapy and ease of hematopoietic stem cell mobilization.
- Higher doses of infused CD34$^+$ stem cells in allogeneic transplantation are associated with a higher frequency and severity of chronic, but not usually acute, GVHD in some related donor myeloablative transplants.

11a. A. Multiple myeloma and Hodgkin lymphoma.
   B. Non-Hodgkin lymphoma and Hodgkin lymphoma.
   C. Acute leukemia and multiple myeloma.
   Rationale: Plerixafor is not approved for patients with acute leukemia because it has the ability to mobilize leukemic cells, but it is approved for use in patients with multiple myeloma.
   D. Multiple myeloma and non-Hodgkin lymphoma.
   Rationale for A, B, and D: Plerixafor is approved for use in patients with multiple myeloma and non-Hodgkin lymphoma based on two pivotal phase III trials. It is not approved for use in patients with Hodgkin lymphoma.
   E. Acute leukemia and healthy donors.
   Rationale: Plerixafor is not approved for healthy donors or for use in patients with acute leukemia because it has the ability to mobilize leukemic cells.

11b. A. Stimulates stem cell proliferation.
   Rationale: G-CSF and granulocyte-monocyte colony-stimulating factor (GM-CSF) work through this mechanism.
   B. Antagonizes C-X-C chemokine receptor type 4 (CXCR-4).
   Rationale: Plerixafor is a CXCR-4 antagonist.
   C. Acts as a ligand for the c-kit (CD117) receptor.
   Rationale: SCF binds c-kit. It is not clinically used as a mobilization regimen.
   D. Induces shedding of membrane-bound stem cell factor (SCF).
   Rationale: Osteoclast metalloproteinase MMP-9 induces shedding of SCF cytokine into the bone marrow. It is not clinically used as a mobilization regimen.
   E. Irreversibly inhibits thymidylate synthase.
   Rationale: 5-Fluorouracil is used as a chemotherapeutic agent.

Major points of discussion

- Plerixafor reversibly inhibits stromal cell–derived factor-1 binding to its receptor CXCR-4.
- Plerixafor in combination with G-CSF is used to mobilize HPCs to the peripheral blood in patients with multiple myeloma and non-Hodgkin lymphoma undergoing collection for autologous transplantation.
- Plerixafor is administered subcutaneously after 4 days of G-CSF at a dose of 240 μg/kg approximately

11 hours prior to collection by apheresis. It can be repeated for up to 4 additional days with G-CSF. Studies on intravenous administration of plerixafor have been performed. Variability exists in the interval between plerixafor administration and apheresis collection at different institutions. Studies in normal donors suggest there is sustained release of stem cells from 4 to 20 hours after administering plerixafor with peak release between 10 and 14 hours after administration.

- Plerixafor is being studied to support mobilization in other conditions such as Hodgkin lymphoma.
- Plerixafor can mobilize leukemic cells, so it is not FDA approved for use in patients with acute leukemia. However, studies using plerixafor to delocalize leukemic stem cells out of their protective niche and away from their protective signals to make them more vulnerable to chemotherapy agents are under way.
- Plerixafor is not FDA approved for use in healthy donors for allogeneic transplantation. However, studies have shown that it is safe in family or volunteer HPC donors.[1,3-5,7]

12. A. A–
B. A+
Rationale for A and B: The passenger anti-B antibodies in the stem cell graft would hemolyze type A red blood cells.
C. B–
D. B+
Rationale for C and D: The patient's anti-B antibodies would hemolyze type B red blood cells.
E. O–
Rationale: Type O red blood cells are compatible with both the patient's and donor's plasma and would not be hemolyzed.

Major points of discussion
- Patients undergoing HPC transplantation frequently require transfusion support.
- ABO incompatibility generally does not disqualify a potential stem cell donor because pluripotent and early committed HPCs lack ABO antigens.
- A major ABO incompatibility occurs when the recipient has antibodies against blood group antigens present on the surface of the donor's red blood cells (e.g., type O recipient and type A, B, or AB donor). An acute hemolytic transfusion reaction can result when the product is infused. Red cell reduction of the product prior to the transplant is useful.
- A minor ABO incompatibility occurs when the donor has antibodies against blood group antigens present on the recipient's red blood cells (e.g., type AB recipient and type A donor). Plasma reduction of the product is useful.
- A bidirectional ABO incompatibility occurs when both major and minor incompatibilities are present (e.g., type A recipient and type B donor).

13. A. O–
B. O+ plus K–
C. A–
D. A+ plus K–
E. AB+ plus K–
Rationale: This is a minor ABO-incompatible transplant and the recipient has not engrafted. The red blood cells should

be compatible with both the donor and recipient plasma. Because the patient has a history of anti-K antibodies, K– red blood cells should be given.

Major points of discussion
- Patients undergoing HPC transplantation frequently require transfusion support.
- Red blood cell engraftment may take up to 6 weeks.
- ABO incompatibility is not a contraindication when selecting potential stem cell donors because pluripotent and early committed HPCs lack ABO antigens.
- A minor ABO incompatibility occurs when donor antibodies against blood group antigens present on the recipient's red blood cells are introduced.
- Removing plasma from the product, which contains the donor isohemagglutinins, may minimize hemolysis in a minor ABO-incompatible stem cell transplant.

14. A. Age less than 5 years.
Rationale: Age greater than 60 years is a predictor of poor stem cell mobilization.
B. Etoposide mobilization.
Rationale: More than three prior chemotherapy cycles was found to predict poor stem cell mobilization.
C. Radiotherapy.
Rationale: Previous radiotherapy is a predictor of poor stem cell mobilization.
D. Male gender.
Rationale: Female gender is a predictor of lower yields.
E. Fewer than 20 CD34$^+$ cells/μL peripheral blood preharvest count.
Rationale: More than 20 CD34$^+$ cells/μL would predict a good yield.

Major points of discussion
- On average, 5% to 10% of patients undergoing non-plerixafor mobilization fail to reach the accepted minimum of 2×10^6 CD34$^+$ cells/kg. Up to 46% are considered poor mobilizers.
- Predictors of poor mobilization include age greater than 60 years, progressive disease, severe bone marrow involvement, type of disease (e.g., non-Hodgkin lymphoma), number of prior chemotherapy cycles and/ or radiotherapy, type of chemotherapy (e.g., methotrexate and lenalidomide), and previously failed mobilization attempts.
- Options for poor mobilizers include remobilization, addition of plerixafor to a mobilization with G-CSF with or without chemotherapy, and bone marrow harvest.
- Combined plerixafor and G-CSF mobilization significantly increases the efficacy of remobilization in patients with a previous failed mobilization attempt; it has a success rate of greater than 60%.
- Remobilization with plerixafor results in timely and stable engraftment with rare and/or manageable side effects in most patients.

15. A. Informed consent to collect UCB must be obtained from the mother and father of the infant.
B. Informed consent to collect UCB is obtained from the mother because of the infant's inability to give consent and because her blood needs to be tested for transmissible diseases.

Rationale: See Major Points of Discussion.

C. Informed consent should be obtained from the father to perform transmissible disease testing on his blood to improve the safety of the UCB.

Rationale for A and C: Informed consent from the father is not necessary and will not add to the safety of the UCB. Only the mother's consent is required.

D. Informed consent for UCB collected is required for UCB collected in utero, but not when collected ex utero.

Rationale: UCB that is collected in utero is less costly than UCB that is collected ex utero because dedicated UCB bank collection personnel are not needed on site. Informed consent is required for both types of collections.

E. Informed consent for UCB is required because the mother and father both require HLA typing.

Rationale: UCB for allogeneic transplantation must be typed for HLA class I (A and B loci) and class II (DRB1 loci). HLA-C and DQB loci typing are recommended as well. The mother and father are not routinely typed.

Major points of discussion

- The first reported use of umbilical cord blood as a source of hematopoietic stem cells was in 1972.[8]
- Informed consent must be obtained from the mother for the collection, processing, testing, storage, and medical use of UCB.
- To ensure that the UCB does not harbor genetic or transmissible diseases, the mother's medical history is obtained through an interview or review of her medical record.
- UCB cannot be obtained from mothers who have first-degree relatives with a history of malignancy or parents who have been treated with chemotherapy.
- UCB with sickle cell or thalassemia trait may occasionally be stored if they have unique HLA types needed for transplantation.

16. **A. Liquid nitrogen dry shippers have to be validated to maintain a temperature of –150°C or less for at least 48 hours past the time of delivery to the transplant facility.**
B. Liquid nitrogen dry shippers have to be validated to maintain a temperature of –196°C or less for at least 48 hours past the time of delivery to the transplant facility.
C. Liquid nitrogen dry shippers have to be validated to maintain a temperature of –150°C or less for at least 24 hours past the time of delivery to the transplant facility.
D. Liquid nitrogen dry shippers have to be validated to maintain a temperature of –196°C or less for at least 24 hours past the time of delivery to the transplant facility.
E. Liquid nitrogen dry shippers have to be validated to maintain a temperature of –150°C or less until the time of delivery to the transplant facility.

Rationale: Liquid nitrogen dry shippers should be validated to maintain a temperature of –150°C or less for at least 48 hours past the time of delivery to the transplant facility.

Major points of discussion

- Cryopreserved HPC units are usually transported to transplant facilities in portable liquid nitrogen "dry" shipping containers. These dry shippers are insulated containers that absorb liquid nitrogen into the vessel wall to create an ultracold environment.
- FACT requires that liquid nitrogen dry shipping containers be validated to maintain a temperature of –150°C or less for at least 48 hours past the time of delivery to the transplant facility.
- AABB (formerly the American Association of Blood Banks) and FACT require continuous monitoring of the temperature in the dry shippers during shipment.
- The shipping container should include the name, address, and phone number of the shipping and receiving facilities; the phrases "Medical Specimen," "Do Not X-Ray," and "Do Not Irradiate" (if applicable); and biohazard labels (as appropriate).
- Detailed records need to be maintained that include the identity of the shipping facility, date and time the unit was shipped and received, courier, and contents of each shipping container.

17. A. HLA-A, -B, and -C.
B. HLA-DR, -DQ, and -DP.
C. HLA-A, -B, -DR, and -DQ.
D. HLA-A, -C, -DR, -DQ, and -DP.
E. HLA-A, -B, -C, -DR, and -DQ.

Rationale: Stem cell transplant donors and recipients are typed for their HLA-A, -B, -C, -DR, and -DQ alleles. In some cases, HLA-DP may be typed as well.

Major points of discussion

- HLA compatibility between the donor and recipient is important for engraftment and to minimize GVHD in allogeneic transplants.
- Donors and recipients are typed for HLA class I (A, B, and C loci) and class II (DR, DQ, and sometimes DP) alleles.
- The goal of bone marrow stem cell and peripheral blood stem cell transplantation is to match the HLA-A, -B, -C, and -DRB1 alleles of the prospective donor and recipient.
- Umbilical cord blood stem cells have less-stringent HLA-matching criteria (HLA-A, -B, and -DRB1 alleles) between donor and recipient.
- Molecular techniques are used to determine the HLA type of the donor and recipient for optimal assessment of class I and class II allele compatibility.

18. A. A–
B. A+

Rationale: The patient's anti-A antibodies would hemolyze type A red blood cells.

C. B–
D. B+

Rationale: Type B red blood cells would be hemolyzed by the patient's and donor's passenger anti-B antibodies.

E. O+

Rationale: Type O red blood cells are compatible with both the patient's and donor's isoagglutinins and would not be hemolyzed.

Major points of discussion

- Patients undergoing HPC transplantation frequently require transfusion support.

- ABO incompatibility does not disqualify potential stem cell donors because pluripotent and early committed HPCs lack ABO antigens.
- A major ABO incompatibility occurs when the recipient has antibodies against blood group antigens present on the surface of the donor's red blood cells.
- Major ABO incompatibility poses two challenges. First, there is a potential for acute intravascular hemolysis when ABO-incompatible donor red blood cells are infused with the graft to the recipient. Second, there could be continued production of circulating ABO antibodies by the recipient directed against donor red blood cells and erythroid progenitors produced by the engrafted HPCs, which could lead to pure red cell aplasia in severe cases.
- Red blood cell depletion removes incompatible red blood cells from the graft to minimize the risk of hemolysis during infusion.

19. A. An acute hemolytic reaction at the time of HPC transplant due to the infusion of incompatible plasma containing anti-A and/or anti-B antibodies.
Rationale: This is a complication of an ABO minor-mismatched HPC transplant.
B. Delayed red blood cell engraftment.
Rationale: This is a potential adverse consequence of a major ABO incompatibility due to anti-A and/or anti-B antibody production by residual recipient plasma cells that survived the preparative conditioning regimen.
C. Delayed hemolysis due to the production of anti-A and/or anti-B antibodies by donor lymphocytes.
Rationale: This phenomenon, due to passenger lymphocyte syndrome, is a complication of an ABO minor-mismatched HPC transplant.
D. An increased risk for posttransplant Epstein-Barr virus infection.
E. Transplant-associated thrombotic microangiopathy.
Rationale: These complications are not related to whether the HPC transplantation is mismatched for the ABO blood group.

Major points of discussion
- Although the earliest HPCs do not express the A and/or B antigens, more committed cells of the erythroid lineage express these antigens.
- Delayed red blood cell engraftment is a potential adverse consequence of a major ABO incompatibility.
- Delayed engraftment is due to production anti-A and/or anti-B antibodies by residual plasma cells in the recipient that survive the preparative conditioning regimen.
- In the context of a major ABO-mismatched HPC transplant, an acute hemolytic reaction at the time of HPC infusion may also occur due to the presence of ABO-incompatible red blood cells in the donor product and circulating anti-A and/or anti-B antibodies in the recipient.
- Red blood cells can be depleted from the donor product in the setting of a major ABO mismatched HPC transplant, typically by performing simple red cell depletion, density gradient red cell depletion, or CD34 selection.[2]

20. A. An acute hemolytic reaction at the time of HPC infusion due to the presence of incompatible red blood cells in the donor product.
Rationale: This is a complication of an ABO major-mismatched HPC transplant.
B. Delayed red blood cell engraftment.
Rationale: This is a potential adverse consequence of a major ABO incompatibility due to anti-A and/or anti-B antibody production by residual recipient plasma cells that survived the preparative conditioning regimen.
C. Delayed hemolysis due to the production of anti-A and/or anti-B antibodies by donor lymphocytes.
Rationale: This phenomenon can occur due to the passenger lymphocyte syndrome.
D. An increased risk for posttransplant Epstein-Barr virus infection.
E. Transplant-associated thrombotic microangiopathy.
Rationale: These complications are not related to whether the HPC transplantation is mismatched for the ABO blood group.

Major points of discussion
- Transplantation of a minor mismatched ABO blood group HPC product can result in delayed hemolysis due to the passenger lymphocyte syndrome. This is caused by viable B-lymphocytes present in the HPC product that produce anti-A and/or anti-B isoagglutinins directed against residual red blood cells in the recipient.
- The passenger lymphocyte syndrome can also be seen in solid organ transplants (e.g., liver and kidney) when there is a minor ABO blood group mismatch (e.g., transplantation of an organ from a blood group O donor into a blood group A recipient).
- Hemolysis due to the passenger lymphocyte syndrome can also be seen with antibodies against non-ABO blood group antigens. For example, following transplantation from an Rh(D)– donor with anti-D antibodies into an Rh(D)+ recipient. However, these cases are unusual and the degree of hemolysis is usually mild and well compensated.
- A hemolytic transfusion reaction at the time of HPC transplantation due to infusion of incompatible plasma containing anti-A and/or anti-B is another complication of ABO minor-mismatched HPC transplantation. Nonetheless, the hemolysis seen in this case is typically much less dramatic than that seen in ABO major-mismatched transplants.
- Depleting the plasma from HPC product can prevent hemolysis at the time of infusion due to a minor incompatibility.[2]

21. A. A.
Rationale: The uppermost layer contains plasma and platelets.
B. B.
Rationale: This layer contains the peripheral blood mononuclear cells, which is the layer containing the stem cells. After washing this layer, these cells are used for the transplant.
C. C.

Rationale: The Ficoll separates the erythrocytes from the peripheral blood mononuclear cells.
D. D.
Rationale: This layer contains both the red cells and the granulocytes.

Major points of discussion

- Approximately half of all HPC transplants are ABO mismatched.
- ABO-mismatched transplants can be major, minor, or bidirectional mismatches.
- Major mismatches occur when the donor red cells are incompatible with the recipient plasma. This occurs with type A, B, or AB donors and type O recipients. Major mismatches are also seen in A or B recipients receiving a product from an AB or B donor or an AB or A donor, respectively.
- Major ABO mismatches are at risk for immediate hemolysis at the time of infusion. Red cell depletion of the product is the most common way to prevent this. In addition, delayed engraftment or pure red cell aplasia can be complications of major mismatches.
- Red cell depletion can be performed by simple centrifugation or density-gradient centrifugation by manual, semi-automated, or automated methods. Manual density gradient centrifugation depletes over 95% of red cells while recovering 50% to 70% of the mononuclear cells.
- Minor mismatches occur when the donor plasma is incompatible with the recipient red cells, such as with a type O donor and a type A, B, or AB recipient. In addition, minor mismatches can occur with a type A or B donor and AB recipient.
- Minor mismatches are at risk for immediate hemolysis that can be prevented with plasma depletion. In addition, passenger lymphocyte syndrome and delayed hemolytic transfusion reactions can be complications of minor mismatches.
- Bidirectional mismatches occur when a major and minor mismatch occur simultaneously, such as in a type A donor and type B recipient or a type B donor and type A recipient. These products are both depleted of red cells and plasma prior to transplantation.[2]

References

1. Cashen A, Lopez S, Gao F, et al. A phase II study of plerixafor (AMD3100) plus G-CSF for autologous hematopoietic progenitor cell mobilization in patients with Hodgkin lymphoma. Biol Blood Marrow Transplant 2008;14:1253–1261.
2. Daniel-Johnson J, Schwartz J. How do I approach ABO-incompatible hematopoietic progenitor cell transplantation? Transfusion 2011;51:1143–1149.
3. DiPersio JF, Micallef IN, Stiff PJ, et al. Phase III prospective randomized double-blind placebo-controlled trial of plerixafor plus granulocyte colony-stimulating factor compared with placebo plus granulocyte colony-stimulating factor for autologous stem-cell mobilization and transplantation for patients with non-Hodgkin's lymphoma. J Clin Oncol 2009;27:4767–4773.
4. DiPersio JF, Stadtmauer EA, Nademanee A, et al. Plerixafor and G-CSF versus placebo and G-CSF to mobilize hematopoietic stem cells for autologous stem cell transplantation in patients with multiple myeloma. Blood 2009;113:5720–5726.
5. Lemery SJ, Hsieh MM, Smith A, et al. A pilot study evaluating the safety and CD34+ cell mobilizing activity of escalating doses of plerixafor in healthy volunteers. Br J Haematol 2011;153:66–75.
6. Pulsipher MA, Chitphakdithai P, Miller JP, et al. Adverse events among 2408 unrelated donors of peripheral blood stem cells: Results of a prospective trial from the National Marrow Donor Program. Blood 2009;113:3604–3611.
7. Tavor S, Petit I. Can inhibition of the SDF-1/CXCR4 axis eradicate acute leukemia? Semin Cancer Biol 2010;20:178–185.
8. Ende M, Ende N. Hematopoietic transplantation by means of fetal (cord) blood. A new method. Va Med Mon (1918) 1972;99:276–280.

CHAPTER 22

MOLECULAR PATHOLOGY

Mahesh M. Mansukhani, Peter L. Nagy, Ali Naini, Vimla Aggarwal

QUESTIONS

1. Mutations in which one of the following genes is associated with familial amyotrophic lateral sclerosis (ALS)?
   A. Glutathione reductase (*GSR*).
   B. Catalase (*CAT*).
   C. Glutathione peroxidase (*GPX*).
   D. Manganese-superoxide dismutase (*SOD2*).
   E. Copper/zinc superoxide dismutase (*SOD1*).

2. Which one of the following represents the central dogma of molecular biology?
   A. DNA → protein → RNA.
   B. DNA → RNA → protein.
   C. RNA → protein → DNA.
   D. RNA → DNA → protein.
   E. Protein → RNA → DNA.

Cystic fibrosis screening results obtained from an otherwise asymptomatic 34-year-old pregnant woman show compound heterozygosity for two mutations in the *CFTR* gene: delF08 (c.F508del) and R117H; in addition, her two intron 8 alleles are 7T/9T. These results are confirmed by repeat testing on the original blood tube. Use this scenario to answer the following two questions.

3a. Which one of the following is the best next step to pursue?
   A. Perform DNA sequencing with long-range polymerase chain reaction (PCR) to determine whether the 7T allele variant is on the same allele as the R117H mutation.
   B. Ask for another blood sample from the patient because the current result "does not make sense."
   C. Test the patient's blood relatives to determine whether the 7T variant is on the same allele as the R117H mutation.
   D. Schedule the patient for a chorionic villous sampling to ensure that the fetus is not affected.
   E. Screen the patient's reproductive partner for *CFTR* gene mutations.

3b. The patient's reproductive partner (i.e., the father of the fetus), who is asymptomatic, is screened with the standard panel. Which one of the following statements best describes the risk for this couple having a child affected by cystic fibrosis?
   A. Highest if the father is a non-Jewish Caucasian because the condition is most common among Caucasians.
   B. Lowest if the father is an Ashkenazi Jew because of the high detection rate among Ashkenazi Jews.
   C. Highest if the father is of Hispanic origin because of the combination of a high carrier rate and a low detection rate among Hispanics.
   D. Lowest if the father is of East Asian origin because of the low carrier rate among Asians.
   E. Can be reduced significantly if the father is of East Asian origin by using an extended panel to include East Asian–specific mutations.

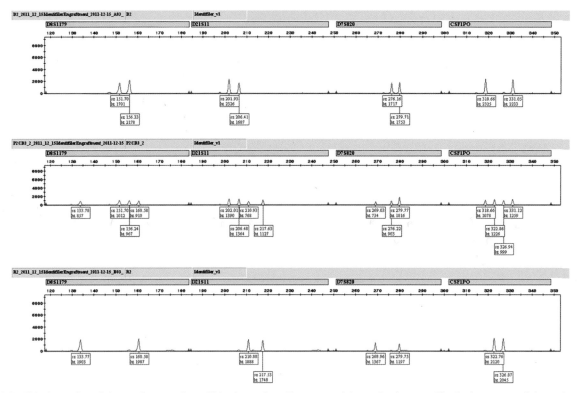

Figure 22-1 This electrophoresis image shows a subset of identity markers. The top panel shows the donor profile; the bottom panel shows the recipient's pretransplantation profile; and the middle panel shows the current sample from the transplant recipient.

4. These results are from the peripheral blood of a child with acute lymphocytic leukemia who underwent an allogeneic hematopoietic stem cell transplantation 1 year previously. Which one of the following statements regarding the results shown in Figure 22-1 is true?
   A. If the transplantation had been performed a year ago, this is an ideal result.
   B. The results are concerning because of the high proportion of recipient DNA in the sample.
   C. The results are concerning because of the low proportion of recipient DNA in the sample.
   D. The results are concerning because of the high proportion of donor DNA in the sample.
   E. This is not the appropriate test to perform in this setting.

5. Cystic fibrosis is caused by mutations in the gene encoding for the cystic fibrosis transmembrane conductance regulator (CFTR) protein. The ΔF508 deletion is a common mutation. Which one of the following patient populations in the United States has the highest prevalence of the ΔF508 deletion?
   A. Caucasians.
   B. African Americans.
   C. Asians.
   D. Ashkenazi Jews.
   E. Hispanics.

6. The prevalence of cystic fibrosis in the United States varies in different populations. Which one of the following statements regarding prevalence is true?
   A. Highest in both the Caucasian and Ashkenazi Jewish populations.
   B. Highest in both the Caucasian and African American populations.

   C. Highest in both the Caucasian and Hispanic populations.
   D. Highest in both the Caucasian and Asian populations.
   E. Highest in both the Caucasian and Native American populations

7. Which one of the following statements best describes the current approach used to screen newborns for cystic fibrosis in the United States?
   A. Measurement of immunoreactive trypsinogen and DNA analysis.
   B. Measurement of both immunoreactive trypsinogen and pancreatitis-associated protein.
   C. Measurement of both immunoreactive trypsinogen and serum amylase.
   D. Measurement of both immunoreactive trypsinogen and serum chloride.
   E. Measurement of both immunoreactive trypsinogen and nasal potential difference.

8. A positive immunoreactive trypsinogen result, along with one DNA mutation, is found when screening a newborn for cystic fibrosis. Which one of the following is the appropriate next step in the management of this patient?
   A. Make the diagnosis of cystic fibrosis, as recommended by the Cystic Fibrosis Foundation.
   B. Perform additional genetic and sweat chloride testing to exclude or confirm the diagnosis of cystic fibrosis.
   C. Repeat the immunoreactive trypsinogen and DNA assays to confirm the abnormal results.
   D. Measure serum and urine chloride to exclude or confirm the diagnosis of cystic fibrosis.
   E. Measure serum amylase, lipase, and trypsin to exclude or confirm the diagnosis of cystic fibrosis.

9. The two strands of DNA that compose the double helix are held together by which one of the following?
   A. Sulfhydryl bonds.
   B. Hydrogen bonds.
   C. Phosphodiester bonds.
   D. Nitrogen bonds.
   E. Carbon bonds.

10. Which one of the following is correct for the human genome?
    A. It has a haploid copy number.
    B. Nucleated cells contain 22 chromosomes.
    C. Consists of DNA, which has a circular structure.
    D. Contains 3×10^9 base pairs of DNA.
    E. Contains 100,000 protein-coding genes.

11. Which one of the following pathologic conditions is caused by mitochondrial DNA (mtDNA) rearrangement?
    A. Leber's hereditary optic neuropathy (LHON).
    B. Mitochondrial encephalomyopathy, lactic acidosis, and strokelike episodes (MELAS).
    C. Myoclonus epilepsy and ragged red fibers (MERRF).
    D. Kearns-Sayre syndrome (KSS).
    E. Neuropathy, ataxia, and retinitis pigmentosa (NARP).

12. Which one of the following is the best method for detecting mtDNA rearrangements?
    A. Sanger cycle sequencing.
    B. Restriction fragment-length polymorphism (RFLP) analysis.
    C. Amplification refractory mutation system–polymerase chain reaction (ARMS-PCR).
    D. Real-time PCR.
    E. Southern blot analysis.

13. Which one of the following methods is best used to detect multiple mtDNA deletions in a very small muscle biopsy taken from a 7-year-old male patient?
    A. RFLP analysis.
    B. Southern blotting with a radiolabeled probe.
    C. Long-range PCR and gel electrophoresis.
    D. Sequencing by capillary electrophoresis.
    E. Single-stranded conformation polymorphism (SSCP).

14. Mutation in which one of the following genes causes mtDNA depletion?
    A. Mitochondrial tRNA lysine *(MT-TK)*.
    B. Mitochondrial tRNA leucine 1 *(MT-TL1)*.
    C. Mitochondrial tRNA tryptophan (*MT-TW*).
    D. Mitochondrial tRNA isoleucine *(MT-TI)*.
    E. mtDNA polymerase gamma *(POLG)*.

15. Which of the following methods is best used for accurate determination of mtDNA copy number?
    A. Southern blot analysis with radiolabeled probes.
    B. Southern blot analysis with fluorescence detection.
    C. Real-time PCR with TaqMan probes.
    D. Sanger sequencing of the whole mitochondrial genome.
    E. Next-generation sequencing of the whole mitochondrial genome.

16. Which one of the following mutations is associated with MELAS, maternally inherited progressive external ophthalmoplegia (MI-PEO), and maternally inherited diabetes and deafness (MIDD)?

A. An adenine-to-guanine transition at nucleotide 3243 position (3243A>G) in mitochondrial tRNA Leu$^{(UUR)}$ (*MTTL1*).
B. An adenine-to-guanine transition at nucleotide 8344 position (8344A>G) in mitochondrial tRNA Lys (*MTTK*).
C. A thymidine-to-cytosine transition at nucleotide 8993 position (8993T>C) in mitochondrial ATPase 6 (*MTATP6*).
D. A thymidine-to-cytosine transition at nucleotide 9176 position (9176T>C) in mitochondrial ATPase 6 (*MTATP6*).
E. A guanine-to-adenine at nucleotide 1178 position (11778G>A) in mitochondrial subunit ND4 of complex I (*MTND4*).

17. Mutations in which one of the following genes cause mitochondrial isolated myopathy?
    A. Complex I subunit *ND4* gene.
    B. Complex I subunit *ND1* gene.
    C. Cytochrome *b* (*cyt b*) gene.
    D. Cytochrome *c* oxidase subunit 1 (*COX1*) gene.
    E. Succinate dehydrogenase *(SDHA)* gene.

18. Which one of the following statements is correct?
    A. All respiratory chain proteins are encoded by mtDNA.
    B. Sperm do not contain mtDNA.
    C. All mtDNA-encoded proteins are components of the respiratory chain.
    D. mtDNA is independent of nuclear DNA (nDNA) and does not require nDNA gene products for its function.
    E. All mtDNA in the zygote is derived from sperm.

19. A 17-year-old boy presents with severe gastrointestinal dysmotility, progressive external ophthalmoplegia (PEO), cachexia, and peripheral neuropathy, a clinical phenotype consistent with mitochondrial neurogastrointestinal encephalomyopathy (MNGIE). A muscle biopsy revealed neurogenic changes and cytochrome *c* oxidase (COX)-deficient fibers reflecting mitochondrial myopathy. He was referred to your molecular pathology laboratory for diagnosis confirmation. Which one of the following tests is best used to confirm the diagnosis of MNGIE?
    A. Thymidine phosphorylase (TP) activity in peripheral blood leukocytes.
    B. Mitochondrial respiratory chain complex I activity.
    C. Mitochondrial respiratory chain complex II activity.
    D. Mitochondrial respiratory chain complex IV activity.
    E. ATPase activity in peripheral blood leukocytes.

20. Which one of the following forms of inheritance is associated with mtDNA-related disorders?
    A. Autosomal recessive.
    B. Autosomal dominant.
    C. Maternal.
    D. X-linked recessive.
    E. X-linked dominant.

21. A change in the nucleotide sequence of the DNA is best known as which of the following?
    A. Mutation.
    B. Polymorphism.
    C. Genotype.
    D. Allele.
    E. Rare variant.

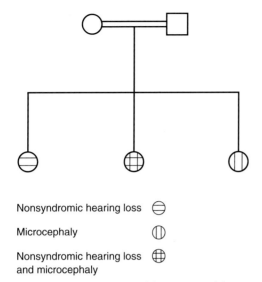

Figure 22-2 Note the consanguinity of the parents and the apparently independent segregation of disease phenotypes in the children.

Nonsyndromic hearing loss

Microcephaly

Nonsyndromic hearing loss and microcephaly

The clinical geneticist at your institution requests your help in formulating a diagnostic approach for a family he is following. The parents are healthy cousins and have three children: one with microcephaly, one with deafness, and one with both conditions. The pedigree for this family is shown in Figure 22-2. Use this scenario to answer the following 12 questions.

22a. Which one of the following best describes the scenario that is most consistent with this clinical situation?

- A. This is a mitochondrial disease. The mother is a healthy carrier, and the disease manifests in the children differentially because of heteroplasmy.
- B. This is an autosomal dominant deafness syndrome with low penetrance and variable expressivity.
- C. This is a family with two mutations that cause two separate disorders, each inherited in an autosomal recessive manner.
- D. This is manifestation of a "mutator" syndrome that causes frequent mutations in the germline of the parents; thus, healthy parents have multiple affected children.
- E. This situation is due to maternal consumption of genetically modified produce during each pregnancy.

22b. Which one of the following is the best next step to take for this case?

- A. You recommend comparative genomic hybridization microarray studies to identify large structural chromosomal defects.
- B. You recommend comparative genomic hybridization microarray studies to identify regions of homozygosity between the siblings affected by the same disease. This will allow you to narrow the list of genes known to cause the conditions observed in this family.
- C. You propose targeted testing for all mutations known to cause deafness and microcephaly using Sanger sequencing.
- D. You propose full genome sequencing because you suspect that the changes responsible for the phenotypes observed are in noncoding regions of the human genome.
- E. You recommend targeted testing for the most common point mutations associated with deafness and microcephaly.

22c. The targeted sequencing fails to diagnose the cause(s) of deafness and microcephaly in this family. The parents decide to have more children. In your discussions with your clinical geneticist colleagues, which one of the following recommendations is the best advice?

- A. The family should be advised that, because they already have three affected children, they have a good chance of producing a healthy child.
- B. The family should be advised not to consider additional children because the risk for having additional affected children is uncertain.
- C. The family should be advised that the risk for having an affected child is one in four for microcephaly or deafness, whereas the chances of having a child with both disorders is one in eight, without providing any further recommendations.
- D. The family should be advised about the possibility of further genetic testing in case the parents are interested in pursuing prenatal diagnosis or in vitro fertilization.
- E. The family should be advised that there are no further diagnostic options available for them, and they should consider adoption.

22d. You raise the possibility to your clinical colleagues of using Next-Gen sequencing to help establish a molecular diagnosis for the condition(s) affecting this family. They ask about the difference between Next-Gen sequencing and traditional Sanger sequencing. Which one of the following is the best response?

- A. It is still experimental, whereas Sanger sequencing is currently available.
- B. It involves sequencing a single molecule, instead of many copies of the same molecule.
- C. It can provide megabases worth of nucleotide sequence, whereas Sanger sequencing is only practical for sequencing, at maximum, a few kilobases.
- D. It is based on irreversible termination of extension on a subpopulation of the templates.
- E. Interpretation of the data obtained is much more straightforward.

22e. During your explanation of Next-Gen sequencing, you use the phrase "sequence capture." Your clinical colleagues ask you about the meaning of this term. Which one of the following is the best answer to this question?

- A. It refers to a process in which sequence changes known to cause specific disease phenotypes are detected.
- B. The human genome contains a great deal of noncoding DNA, the role of which is not clearly established in disease. To limit the cost of clinical testing by sequencing, it is practical to focus on certain segments of the genome that have previously been shown to be associated with human disease. Upon sequencing the full genome, these segments are computationally identified and analyzed, whereas the data from noncoding regions of the genome are left in a non–human-readable form; this is sequence capture.
- C. It refers to the laboratory procedure that selects fragments of diagnostic interest from human genomic DNA for sequence analysis.
- D. It refers to the method of data collection from the sequencer.
- E. It refers to the fact that sequences slowly leak out of the reaction chamber of the sequencer, and they need to be prevented from contaminating the instrument by capturing them using a secondary container that is replaced regularly.

22f. The parents decide to pursue further genetic testing. You explain to your clinical colleagues that, in this case, full exome sequencing is probably the best next step. You mention that alternatives would include sequencing all genes implicated in deafness and microcephaly, or full genome sequencing. They ask you to explain your rationale. Which one of the following justifications is *not* correct?

A. Full exome sequencing is the best approach because the number of genes implicated in both microcephaly and deafness is large, and there are numerous, as yet unidentified, genes that can cause these phenotypes.

B. Full exome sequencing is less expensive than full genome sequencing, and most known pathogenic mutations are within exons or at intron-exon junctions.

C. Analysis of a full exome dataset is less complex than that of a full genome sequencing dataset.

D. Sequencing only known genes and loci would be effective if the patients in this family had a mutation previously identified in other families, but it would not detect private mutations specific to this family.

E. Exome sequencing provides the most even and reliable sampling of the coding regions of the human genome, even if expense is not a consideration.

22g. You and your colleagues decide to proceed with the exome sequencing approach. They ask you which members of the family should be tested. Which one of the following is the most reasonable answer under these circumstances?

A. Both parents and all three children should be sequenced.

B. Only the parents should be sequenced.

C. The parents, one child with deafness, and one child with microcephaly should be sequenced.

D. Only the child with both microcephaly and deafness should be sequenced.

E. Only the three siblings should be sequenced. There is no need to sequence the parents.

22h. The decision is made to sequence the three siblings. Which one of the following best describes the requirements that need to be satisfied before testing can commence?

A. The patients must be older than 18 years.

B. Both parents must sign an informed consent form, and the children must sign an assent form.

C. At least one parent must sign an informed consent form. The children with microcephaly are exempt from signing the assent form; assent only needs to be obtained from the deaf child.

D. You must confirm that the parents' insurance will cover the cost of testing.

E. You have to obtain U.S. Food and Drug Administration (FDA) approval for the method to be used.

22i. All administrative hurdles are now cleared. The sequencing is performed. The results indicate the presence of approximately 40,000 single-nucleotide polymorphisms (SNPs) in each sample. The data analysis software allows for filtering the identified mutations based on various criteria. Which one of the following filtering approaches is *not* correct?

A. All known mutations (i.e., previously detected in other "healthy" individuals) should be excluded from the search for the cause of the disease.

B. Mutations that do not cause amino acid changes, frame shifts, transcriptional stops, or splicing defects should be removed in the initial analysis.

C. Emphasis should be placed on mutations for which any one patient is homozygous.

D. Mutations that are present in a homozygous form in all three siblings should be excluded as the cause of both deafness and microcephaly.

E. The children with deafness should be homozygous for the same mutation; similarly, the children with microcephaly should be homozygous for the same mutation.

22j. Several mutations were found in homozygous form in each sibling. Which one of the following web-based resources is *not* useful in identifying the mutations responsible for the patients' conditions?

A. Online Mendelian Inheritance in Man (OMIM): http://www.ncbi.nlm.nih.gov/omim

B. University of Santa Cruz web browser: http://genome.ucsc.edu

C. dbSNP database: http://www.ncbi.nlm.nih.gov/SNP/

D. 1000 genome database: http://www.1000genomes.org

E. Leiden database: http://www.dmd.nl

22k. Analysis of the three exome-sequencing datasets is completed, and clearly disruptive homozygous mutations in genes previously implicated in microcephaly and deafness are identified, which are in agreement with the expected phenotypes seen in each sibling. Which one of the following is required before the results can be reported?

A. The exome sequencing must be repeated.

B. The sequencing data must be reanalyzed using another analysis software program.

C. The identity of the samples and the correctness of the mutations must be confirmed using an alternative method.

D. The mutations must be confirmed to be absent in 400 healthy control samples.

E. You must confirm that the mutations have never been seen previously in any population sampled.

22l. The parents return several months later to request preimplantation testing for the mutations identified in the affected siblings as part of an in vitro fertilization effort. Which one of the following is the best strategy to pursue for this testing?

A. Following full genome amplification, the exome sequencing has to be repeated on cells derived from all embryos.

B. Following whole genome amplification, the DNA from each embryo has to be genotyped for the mutations identified in the three siblings with deafness and/or microcephaly.

C. Following whole genome amplification, all embryos have to be tested for aneuploidy using a microarray methodology.

D. The embryos with the pathogenic mutations need to be preserved for future diagnostic test development.

E. Embryos that are carriers for either the deafness or microcephaly mutations can be implanted with their normal counterparts because they would also result in normal children and would improve the chances of successful implantation.

23. Which one of the following answers best describes what a PCR includes?

A. Denaturation, digestion, detection.

B. Denaturation, annealing, amplification.

C. Digestion, annealing, amplification.

D. Denaturation, annealing, labeling.

E. Denaturation, annealing, digestion.

24. When designing primers for PCR, which one of the following is the best approach?
    A. Choose primers that show significant complementarity to each other, especially at the 3′ ends.
    B. Ensure that the forward and reverse primers have a melting temperature (Tm) that differs by at least 5°C.
    C. Choose primers that are complementary to the same DNA strand.
    D. Choose primers that have a GC content of at least 90% to ensure strong binding.
    E. Check that the primers used to amplify genomic human DNA are validated against variant databases (e.g., dbSNP) to avoid primer–binding-site polymorphisms.

25. Which one of the following statements about controls for PCR or reverse-transcriptase PCR (RT-PCR) is true?
    A. When setting up a PCR, one should always add a template to the no-DNA control first to avoid accidentally contaminating it.
    B. When setting up a PCR, one should add a template to the test samples first, followed by the no-DNA control, and then add the normal and abnormal controls.
    C. When setting up an RT-PCR, in addition to a no-template (i,e., no RNA) control, one should set up a no-RT control for each RNA sample being tested to test for directly amplifiable RNA.
    D. When setting up a PCR following an RT reaction, one should set up a separate no-template control in addition to the product of the no-RNA RT reaction.
    E. The use of deoxyuridine triphosphate (dUTP) in PCR with uracil-*N*-glycosylase to prevent PCR contamination is of no value for RT-PCR because RNA contains uracil.

26a. A DNA test was performed on a child with severe developmental delay, especially language delay, and an apparently "happy" disposition with inappropriate laughter. PCR of bisulfite-treated DNA with melting curve analysis of an *SNRPN* exon 1 amplicon showed only an unmethylated allele. Which one of the following statements is correct?
    A. Only a maternal allele is present; this is consistent with a diagnosis of Angelman syndrome.
    B. Only the paternal allele is present; this is consistent with a diagnosis of Angelman syndrome.
    C. Only the paternal allele is present; this is consistent with Prader-Willi syndrome.
    D. Only the maternal allele is present; this is consistent with Prader-Willi syndrome.
    E. Only one allele is present. Parental testing to determine the parent of origin of the missing allele will distinguish between Prader-Willi and Angelman syndromes.

26b. Which one of the following statements is true about the inheritance of Prader-Willi and Angelman syndromes?
    A. Prader-Willi syndrome and Angelman syndrome are caused by different mutations in the same gene.
    B. Inactivating mutations in *UBE3A* will cause Prader-Willi syndrome only if present on the paternal allele.
    C. Inactivating mutations in *UBE3A* will cause Prader-Willi syndrome only if present on the maternal allele.

    D. Inactivating mutations of *UBE3A* cause Angelman syndrome when present on the maternal allele.
    E. Inactivating mutations of *UBE3A* cause Angelman syndrome only when present on the paternal allele.

26c. Which one of the following statements is true about genomic imprinting?
    A. Contrary to classic Mendelian genetics, the parent of origin affects the expression of most genes in higher mammals.
    B. All imprinted loci in placental mammals show expression from only the maternal allele.
    C. All imprinted loci in placental mammals show expression from only the paternal allele.
    D. Most cases of Angelman syndrome and Prader-Willi syndrome are caused by imprinting defects.
    E. Beckwith-Wiedemann syndrome, Russell-Silver syndrome, and transient neonatal diabetes mellitus type 1 are linked to imprinted loci.

27. Which one of the following statements regarding RNA transcription and processing is true?
    A. RNA polymerase I, which synthesizes most messenger RNAs (mRNAs), is recruited to promoters by bound transcription factors.
    B. Promoters, which are recognized by RNA polymerase, include the TATA box, usually at the -25 position; the GC box that can function in either orientation; and the CAAT box that is usually located at the -80 position.
    C. Enhancers, which are always in close proximity to promoters, increase transcription activity of the associated gene.
    D. Noncoding genes are always transcribed by RNA polymerase II.
    E. The primary transcript of polypeptide-encoding RNAs often contains introns and exons. Introns are characterized by 5′AG and a 3′GU.

28. Which one of the following statements is true regarding sequencing for genetic variants?
    A. Genomic DNA is a better template to evaluate the presence and effect of deep intronic variants, as these are not present in mRNA or complementary DNA (cDNA).
    B. The smaller a deletion, the more likely it is to be missed by Sanger sequencing after DNA PCR .
    C. Nonsense mutations in the first exon may be missed when performing cDNA sequencing.
    D. Sequencing of the entire coding region of a gene will identify virtually all significant mutations in a gene.
    E. When a missense mutation in a gene known to be associated with a condition is seen in a symptomatic individual, the mutation is most likely to be significant.

29. Which one of the following neurologic diseases is caused by a triplet repeat expansion in the coding region of the involved gene?
    A. Fragile X.
    B. Friedreich ataxia.
    C. Spinocerebellar ataxia type 8 (SCA8).
    D. Myotonic dystrophy.
    E. Huntington disease.

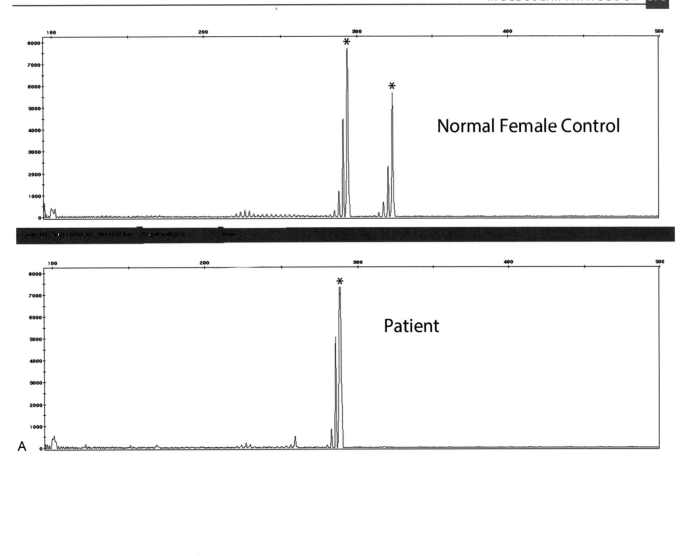

Figure 22-3 Images of a fragile X capillary electrophoresis (**A**) and a Southern blot (**B**). **A**, The capillary electrophoresis shows a single normal FMR1 allele. **B**, In the Southern blot, the first 4 lanes are digested with EcoR1, and the last four are the same samples digested with EcorR1 and Eag1. The lower band in these lanes represents a double digest with EcorR1 and Eag1. Methylated and unmethylated alleles in this case are indicated by a single and double asterisk, respectively.

30a. Figure 22-3 shows the results of PCR (i.e., capillary electrophoresis) and Southern blot tests for the *FMR1* CGG repeat expansion associated with fragile X syndrome. Which one of the following statements regarding the PCR result is true?

    A. Only one allele is seen on the capillary electrophoresis image. Therefore, this must be from a male.

B. The pretest risk for an expansion is higher in a woman with an affected nephew (brother's son).

C. In a male with mental retardation, the capillary electrophoresis result shown provides strong evidence against fragile X syndrome.

D. In a girl with developmental delay, the capillary electrophoresis alone excludes *FMR1*-associated mental retardation.

E. In a mother of a boy with developmental delay, the PCR result rules out an *FMR1* expansion as the basis for the child's condition.

30b. Which of the following statements is true about Southern blot tests and/or the results shown in Figure 22-3?

A. The results of the capillary electrophoresis and Southern blot test, taken together, are consistent with a normal male.

B. Southern blot texting is more reliable than PCR in excluding fragile X tremor ataxia syndrome (FXTAS).

C. Southern blot testing is more reliable then PCR in excluding *FMR1*-associated premature ovarian failure.

D. The Southern blot test result adds little to the PCR, which is more sensitive and reliable.

E. In a woman undergoing carrier testing, this result is strong evidence against her carrying a premutation or full mutation.

31. A 60-year-old man is being evaluated for placement of a coronary artery stent. His physician plans to start him on regimen of a clopidogrel after the procedure. Pharmacogenomic testing of which one of the following genes would be most useful for predicting whether he is a poor metabolizer?

A. *CYP2C19*.

B. *CYP2D6*.

C. *CYP2C9*.

D. *VKORC1*.

E. *TPMT*.

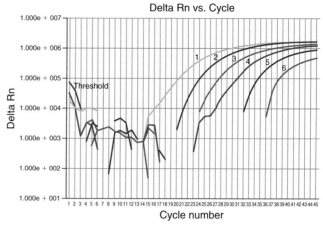

Figure 22-4 Serial monitoring for minimal residual disease by reverse-transcription quantitative PCR. *BCR-ABL1* transcript levels were measured in the laboratory from time point 1 (i.e., at diagnosis) to time point 6 (i.e., the current sample).

32. A 65-year-old man with chronic myeloid leukemia is being treated with imatinib. His *BCR-ABL1* mRNA transcript levels are being monitored by a laboratory that uses an RT-PCR. Figure 22-4 shows the patient's *BCR-ABL1* transcript levels as measured in the laboratory from time point 1 (i.e., at diagnosis) to time point 6 (i.e., the current sample). Which one of the following is the best next step?

A. Test for *BCR-ABL1* kinase domain mutations.

B. Perform a bone marrow biopsy for pathology and cytogenetics.

C. Switch the patient to a second-generation tyrosine kinase inhibitor (TKI).

D. Repeat this quantitative PCR assay in 3 to 6 months.

E. Consider sending the patient for an urgent allogeneic stem cell transplantation.

ANSWERS

1. A. Glutathione reductase (*GSR*).
Rationale: The *GSR* gene encodes the glutathione reductase protein, a nicotine adenine disphosphonucleotide, reduced (NADPH)-dependent enzyme, which maintains glutathione in a reduced form. Its deficiency has been associated with hemolytic crisis but not with ALS.
B. Catalase (*CAT*).
Rationale: CAT encodes catalase, which detoxifies hydrogen peroxide. Catalase deficiency has only been reported to cause progressive oral gangrene.
C. Glutathione peroxidase (*GPX*).
Rationale: GPX encodes the glutathione peroxidase protein, which functions in hydrogen peroxide detoxification and has not been associated with ALS.
D. Manganese-superoxide dismutase (*SOD2*).
Rationale: SOD2 encodes manganese-containing superoxide dismutase, a mitochondrial protein that is part of antioxidant machinery in this organelle. Mutations in this gene have not been associated with ALS.
E. **Copper/zinc superoxide dismutase (*SOD1*).**
Rationale: Mutations in *SOD1*, which is located on chromosome 21 and encodes Cu/Zn-superoxide dismutase, cause ALS in approximately 20% of familial ALS cases.

Major points of discussion

- ALS is a progressive, late-onset motor neuron disease caused by selective premature degeneration and death of upper and lower motor neurons in the motor cortex, brainstem, and spinal cord.

- The disease starts in adult life, typically between 50 and 60 years of age.

- The ensuing progressive paralysis is typically fatal within 3 to 5 years of clinical onset, usually as the result of failure of the respiratory system.

- ALS is one of the more prevalent adult-onset neurodegenerative diseases, with an incidence of 1 to 2 per 100,000 in most populations. The incidence is much higher in the Pacific island of Guam and the Kii Peninsula of Japan, possibly because of consumption of an environmental toxin, β-methylamino-L-alanine.

- The cause of ALS is unknown in most cases, and these cases are referred to as sporadic ALS (SALS).

- Approximately 10% of ALS cases are inherited in a dominant manner and are referred to as familial ALS (FALS).

- To date, mutations in 12 genes have been reported to cause FALS. Among these, *SOD1* mutations, which are transmitted in a dominant fashion, account for approximately 20% of all familial ALS forms and about 2% of all ALS cases.[3,5,6]

2. A. DNA → protein → RNA.
  B. DNA → RNA → protein.
  C. RNA → protein → DNA.
  D. RNA → DNA → protein.
  E. Protein → RNA → DNA.
  Rationale: DNA is transcribed into RNA, and the RNA is translated into protein.

Major points of discussion

■ The information between DNA, RNA, and protein is related.

■ The genetic information coded by the DNA determines the sequences of the amino acids in the encoded proteins.

■ First RNA is synthesized from the DNA template through a process called *transcription*.

■ This RNA, carrying the coded information in a form called *messenger RNA*, is translated to determine the sequence of the amino acids in the protein. mRNA is decoded by *transfer RNA* (tRNA) on cellular ribosomes to produce amino acid sequences or proteins in the process called *translation*.

■ This flow of information is referred to as the central dogma of molecular biology.

3a. A. Perform DNA sequencing with long-range polymerase chain reaction (PCR) to determine whether the 7T allele variant is on the same allele as the R117H mutation.
  Rationale: In this instance, the 7T allele is almost certainly in linkage with the R117H mutation.
  B. Ask for another blood sample from the patient because the current result "does not make sense."
  Rationale: This result can be seen in a 34-year-old. The CFTR protein containing the R117H mutation will have some function.
  C. Test the patient's blood relatives to determine whether the 7T variant is on the same allele as the R117H mutation.
  Rationale: This is not necessary because in this instance the 7T allele is almost certainly associated with the R117H mutation.
  D. Schedule the patient for a chorionic villous sampling to ensure that the fetus is not affected.
  Rationale: This is premature because it would depend on whether the father is a cystic fibrosis carrier.
  E. Screen the patient's reproductive partner for *CFTR* gene mutations.
  Rationale: This patient is at least a cystic fibrosis carrier, and she might develop lung disease later in life. However, the most important step is to ensure that the father is not a carrier.

3b. A. Highest if the father is a non-Jewish Caucasian because the condition is most common among Caucasians.
  Rationale: Although Caucasians are likely to have the highest carrier rate, the standard panel has the highest detection rate among Caucasians.
  B. Lowest if the father is an Ashkenazi Jew because of the high detection rate among Ashkenazi Jews.

Rationale: The detection rate of the standard American College of Medical Genetics panel is even higher among Ashkenazi Jews.
  C. Highest if the father is of Hispanic origin because of the combination of a high carrier rate and a low detection rate among Hispanics.
  Rationale: The residual risk is lower among Hispanics than East Asians.
  D. Lowest if the father is of East Asian origin because of the low carrier rate among Asians.
  Rationale: Asians have the highest residual risk because of the low detection rate.
  E. Can be reduced significantly if the father is of East Asian origin by using an extended panel to include East Asian–specific mutations.
  Rationale: Extended panels do not help with East Asian populations because of the high percentage of private mutations.

Major points of discussion

■ Cystic fibrosis (Online Mendelian Inheritance in Man [OMIM] #219700) is an autosomal recessive condition that results from loss-of-function mutations in both alleles of the *CFTR* gene on 7q31.3, an adenosine triphosphate (ATP)-binding cassette family member with 1480 amino acids, encoded by 27 exons. It is one of the most common fatal autosomal recessive conditions among Caucasians, with a prevalence of approximately 1 in 2500 to 3000 live births and a carrier frequency of 1 in 25. The carrier rate is approximately 1 in 46 among Hispanic Americans, 1 in 65 among African Americans, and 1 in 90 among Asian Americans.

■ The disease is characterized by recurrent pulmonary infections resulting from failure to eliminate viscous secretions, with or without pancreatic insufficiency; increased sweat chloride as the result of excessive salt loss; neonatal meconium ileus in 10% to 20% of infants; chronic sinusitis; congenital bilateral absence of vas deferens; and liver disease. The average overall survival of individuals with cystic fibrosis is 30 years.

■ More than 1000 mutations are known in the *CFTR* gene, with most representing infrequent (<0.1%) or private mutations. The most common mutation, delF508, accounts for 30% to 70% of mutations, depending on race. When performing carrier screening, the American College of Medical Genetics recommends testing for the 23 most common variants, each of which has a frequency of more than 0.1% among cystic fibrosis patients; this panel has a detection rate of 94.04% among Ashkenazi Jews; 88.29% among non-Hispanic Caucasians; 64.46% among African Americans; 71.72% among Hispanic Americans; and 48% among Asian Americans.

■ When a test result for these mutations is negative, it reduces the risk of being a carrier, but does not eliminate it. The residual risk is 1 in 384 for Ashkenazi Jews; 1 in 206 for non-Hispanic Caucasians; 1 in 171 for African Americans; 1 in 203 for Hispanic Caucasians; and 1 in 183 for Asian Americans. Residual risks should be reported.

■ Clinical tests include genotyping tests that check for specific mutations; mutation scanning assays; direct DNA sequencing assays; and tests for large deletions or

rearrangements. Together they may still miss some mutations, and tests such as sweat chloride analysis may be needed to confirm the diagnosis.
- The R117H mutation is a variant that acts as a severe disease-causing mutation only when it is on the same allele as a 5T intron 8 polymorphism that results in increased alternate splicing, excluding exon 9, with reduced full-length mature mRNA. The longer alleles (7T and 9T) are associated with increased full-length transcript and a milder reduction in function due to R117H. Individuals with a 7T on the same allele as the R117H mutation, along with a severe mutation on the opposite allele, may develop lung disease later in life (in the sixth, and even seventh, decade). The 5T allele itself may be associated with congenital absence of the vas deferens.
- When the R117H mutation is seen with a 5T variant in an individual, testing of family members may be needed to determine on which allele the 5T variant is located. The 5T allele by itself may be associated with congenital absence of vas deferens, either when it occurs as a homozygous variant or when it occurs with other *CFTR* mutations. Because of this association, many tests report the 5T/7T and 9T results only when there is an R117H mutation.[24,35]

4. A. If the transplantation had been performed a year ago, this is an ideal result.
Rationale: This is not an ideal result. The presence of a high proportion of recipient DNA 1 year after transplantation would be indicative of either graft failure or relapse of the acute leukemia.
B. The results are concerning because of the high proportion of recipient DNA in the sample.
Rationale: The presence of a high proportion of recipient DNA is indicative of either graft failure or relapse of the acute leukemia.
C. The results are concerning because of the low proportion of recipient DNA in the sample.
Rationale: Recipient DNA is present in a high proportion in this sample, and as such, is very concerning. The presence of a high proportion of recipient DNA is indicative of either graft failure or relapse of the acute leukemia.
D. The results are concerning because of the high proportion of donor DNA in the sample.
Rationale: A high proportion of donor DNA in the sample would be a reassuring finding.
E. This is not the appropriate test to perform in this setting.
Rationale: This is the standard test performed in this type of post-transplantation setting.

Major points of discussion
- Chimerism testing using polymorphic short tandem repeat (STR) loci (microsatellite loci) is now standard in the post–bone marrow transplantation setting.
- Testing is most commonly performed using multiplex marker kits that use up to 16 STR loci as identity markers.
- For each informative locus (at least one allele differing between donor and recipient), it is possible to determine the proportions of donor and recipient DNA using peak heights or peak areas corresponding to recipient and donor alleles.

- After hematopoietic stem cell transplantations for malignancies such as acute lymphocytic leukemia, the recipient's bone marrow should be repopulated primarily by donor cells.
- A drop in donor DNA percentage or an increase in recipient DNA percentage may indicate relapse or impending relapse.
- The results shown here for this patient demonstrate an almost equal proportion of donor and recipient cells, indicating either graft failure or relapse of the acute leukemia.[4]

5. **A. Caucasians.**
Rationale: The ΔF508 deletion is found in approximately 72% of the Caucasian population in the United States.
B. African Americans.
Rationale: The ΔF508 deletion is found in approximately 44% of the African American population.
C. Asians.
Rationale: The ΔF508 deletion is found in approximately 39% of the Asian American population.
D. Ashkenazi Jews.
Rationale: The ΔF508 deletion is found in approximately 31% of the Ashkenazi Jewish population.
E. Hispanics.
Rationale: The ΔF508 deletion is found in approximately 54% of the Hispanic population.

Major points of discussion
- Deletion of the phenylalanine at position 508 of the *CFTR* gene is the most common mutation in the European Caucasian population of patients with cystic fibrosis.
- There are more than 1800 known mutations of the *CFTR* gene.
- The American College of Medical Genetics and Genomics recommends that at least 23 different mutations be evaluated when testing for cystic fibrosis. Some testing programs detect more than 40 mutations.
- Different ethnic populations have different *CFTR* gene mutations. In locales with a diverse patient population, the selection of the *CFTR* mutations to be tested will affect the number of cystic fibrosis cases that are detected.
- Some *CFTR* mutations that are detected may not be clinically significant.[2,13]

6. **A. Highest in both the Caucasian and Ashkenazi Jewish populations.**
B. Highest in both the Caucasian and African American populations.
C. Highest in both the Caucasian and Hispanic populations.
D. Highest in both the Caucasian and Asian populations.
E. Highest in both the Caucasian and Native American populations.
Rationale: Caucasian and Ashkenazi Jewish populations have the highest prevalence cystic fibrosis.

Major points of discussion
- The prevalence of cystic fibrosis in the Caucasian population is about 1:3000.
- The prevalence of cystic fibrosis in the African American population is about 1:15,000.
- The prevalence of cystic fibrosis in the Hispanic population is about 1:9000.

- The prevalence of cystic fibrosis in the Asian population is about 1:35,000.
- The prevalence of cystic fibrosis is higher in the Caucasian than in the African American, Hispanic, and Asian populations.
- The prevalence of cystic fibrosis in the Ashkenazi Jewish population is about 1:2300 and is similar to the prevalence in the Caucasian population.
- The prevalence of cystic fibrosis in the Native American population is believed to be about 1:10,000.

7. **A. Measurement of immunoreactive trypsinogen and DNA analysis.**
   Rationale: This is currently the most common procedure used to screen newborns for cystic fibrosis in the United States.
   B. Measurement of both immunoreactive trypsinogen and pancreatitis–associated protein.
   Rationale: This procedure is used in Europe for screening newborns for cystic fibrosis.
   C. Measurement of both immunoreactive trypsinogen and serum amylase.
   Rationale: Serum amylase, a marker for pancreatitis, is not used to screen for cystic fibrosis.
   D. Measurement of both immunoreactive trypsinogen and serum chloride.
   Rationale: Serum chloride is not used to screen for cystic fibrosis.
   E. Measurement of both immunoreactive trypsinogen and nasal potential difference.
   Rationale: Measurement of nasal potential difference is a manual, time-consuming test that can be used to diagnose cystic fibrosis. However, it is not a screening procedure.

Major points of discussion
- Trypsinogen is produced in the pancreas and transported to the intestine, where it is activated to form the enzyme trypsin. In cystic fibrosis, thick mucus can obstruct the pancreatic ducts and prevent trypsinogen from reaching the intestine. Therefore, blood levels of immunoreactive trypsinogen will usually be elevated in newborns with cystic fibrosis.
- There are a considerable number of false-positive immunoreactive trypsinogen results. A positive immunoreactive trypsinogen result triggers the performance of a DNA mutation analysis.
- A negative immunoreactive trypsinogen result in a patient with cystic fibrosis, although rare, can be obtained and does not routinely trigger a DNA mutation analysis. If cystic fibrosis is suspected, the patient should undergo genetic testing or have a sweat chloride measurement.
- In the nasal potential difference method, the active transport of ions, mainly sodium and chloride, across the respiratory epithelium generates a potential difference that can be measured. The abnormal sodium and chloride transport in the respiratory epithelia of patients with cystic fibrosis can be measured and used to diagnose patients with this disease.
- Sweat conductivity and sweat osmolality are screening tests for cystic fibrosis. A positive result must be confirmed by sweat chloride measurements.[2,13]

8. A. Make the diagnosis of cystic fibrosis, as recommended by the Cystic Fibrosis Foundation.
   Rationale: This result cannot be used to diagnose cystic fibrosis.
   B. Perform additional genetic and sweat chloride testing to exclude or confirm the diagnosis of cystic fibrosis.
   Rationale: This is the recommended approach.
   C. Repeat the immunoreactive trypsinogen and DNA assays to confirm the abnormal results.
   Rationale: Immunoreactive trypsinogen and DNA testing are usually not repeated.
   D. Measure serum and urine chloride to exclude or confirm the diagnosis of cystic fibrosis.
   Rationale: These tests are not used to assess patients for cystic fibrosis.
   E. Measure serum amylase, lipase, and trypsin to exclude or confirm the diagnosis of cystic fibrosis.
   Rationale: These tests are not used to assess patients for cystic fibrosis.

Major points of discussion
- A positive immunoreactive trypsinogen result is followed by DNA mutation analysis. Detection of one mutation cannot be used to diagnose cystic fibrosis. Follow-up testing by measuring sweat chloride and extended DNA analysis are used to confirm the diagnosis of cystic fibrosis.
- A positive immunoreactive trypsinogen result followed by detection of two disease-causing mutations is strongly suggestive of cystic fibrosis. In this case, an elevated sweat chloride result will confirm the diagnosis of cystic fibrosis.
- A positive immunoreactive trypsinogen result followed by a negative DNA mutation result requires another blood sample to be taken 3 weeks later and the immunoreactive trypsinogen and DNA mutation assays repeated.
- A negative immunoreactive trypsinogen result with a negative DNA mutation result in a second blood sample suggests that the positive immunoreactive trypsinogen result obtained in the first sample was a false-positive result.
- Serum amylase, lipase, trypsin, chloride, and urine chloride testing are not recommended in the evaluation of cystic fibrosis.[2,13]

9. A. Sulfhydryl bonds.
   Rationale: There are no sulfhydryl (-SH) groups in the DNA double helix. In proteins, the disulfide bonds are formed between the thiol groups of cysteine residues.
   B. Hydrogen bonds.
   Rationale: Two strands of the DNA are held together by hydrogen bonds to form a duplex.
   C. Phosphodiester bonds.
   Rationale: The 3′,5′-phosphodiester bonds link the adjacent nucleotides in a DNA polynucleotide chain.
   D. Nitrogen bonds.
   Rationale: These are not involved in maintaining the DNA double helix.
   E. Carbon bonds.
   Rationale: Carbon bonds do not hold together the two strands of the double helix.

Major points of discussion

- The DNA molecule has a linear backbone consisting of alternating sugar residues and phosphate groups.
- The sugar residues are linked by a 3′,5′-phosphodiester bond, in which a phosphate group links the 3′ carbon atom of one sugar to the 5′ carbon atom of the next sugar in the sugar-phosphate backbone.
- The two strands of DNA are held together by hydrogen bonds to form a duplex.
- Hydrogen bonding occurs between the laterally opposed complementary base pairs on the two strands of the DNA duplex.
- The stability of the DNA double helix is maintained by hydrogen bonding between the A-T and G-C base pairs.
- The individual hydrogen bonds are weak, but the two strands of the double helix are held together by many hydrogen bonds.
- Hydrogen bonding also permits formation of DNA-RNA duplexes and double-stranded RNA.

10. A. It has a haploid copy number.
    Rationale: Except for the gametes (which are haploid), all nucleated cells are diploid.
    B. Nucleated cells contain 22 chromosomes.
    Rationale: The number of chromosomes in a nucleated cell is 46, which is double the number found in the gametes (23 chromosomes).
    C. Consists of DNA, which has a circular structure.
    Rationale: The human genome consists of DNA, which has a double helix structure.
    D. Contains 3×10^9 base pairs of DNA.
    Rationale: This is the correct answer.
    E. Contains 100,000 protein coding genes.
    Rationale: The number of protein-coding genes in the human genome is approximately 20,000.

Major points of discussion

- The human genome is organized into 46 chromosomes in the nucleus.
- Each human chromosome consists of a single, continuous DNA double helix.
- The nuclear genome consists of 46 DNA molecules, totaling approximately 6 billion nucleotides.
- Each nucleated cell in the body carries its own copy of the genome, which by current estimates contains approximately 20,000 protein-coding genes.
- The genes are encoded in the DNA of the genome. The DNA is a double helix structure, which was elucidated by James Watson and Francis Crick in 1953.

11. A. Leber's hereditary optic neuropathy (LHON).
    Rationale: LHON is most often caused by missense point mutations in genes encoding complex I subunits.
    B. Mitochondrial encephalomyopathy, lactic acidosis, and strokelike episodes (MELAS).
    Rationale: To date, all cases of MELAS have been reported to be caused by point mutations in several mitochondrial tRNA genes or genes encoding subunits of the respiratory chain.
    C. Myoclonus epilepsy and ragged red fibers (MERRF).
    Rationale: MERRF is most often caused by mutations in mitochondrial lysine tRNA.
    D. Kearns-Sayre syndrome (KSS).
    Rationale: KSS is caused by a single deletion in mitochondrial DNA.

E. Neuropathy, ataxia, and retinitis pigmentosa (NARP).
Rationale: NARP is associated predominantly with a point mutation in the *ATPASE6* gene.

Major points of discussion

- To date, hundreds of different pathogenic deletions of 2 to 10 kb have been reported. These deletions invariably delete several tRNA genes. Large-scale mitochondrial DNA duplications are also associated with these disorders, and deleted and duplicated mtDNA coexist in these patients.
- The only novel sequence in the duplicated mtDNA, compared with wild type, is at the boundary of the duplicated region, which is the same as the boundary present in the deleted DNA, indicating that the two mtDNAs (i.e., duplicated and deleted) originated through a common mechanism.
- Far more patients harbor deleted mtDNA compared with duplicated mtDNA; because of this, and because it is technically difficult to differentiate duplicated mtDNA from deleted mtDNA, the importance of duplicated mtDNA in clinical disease has not been fully recognized.
- Large-scale partial deletions of mtDNA have been well documented in patients with PEO and KSS. However, the size and location of the deletion, and the proportion of deleted DNA, differ among patients and do not appear to correlate with disease severity.
- Interestingly, although different patients with KSS harbor different deleted mtDNAs, which cause the loss of different genes, all patients have fundamentally the same clinical presentation.[12,25,33]

12. A. Sanger cycle sequencing.
    Rationale: Direct sequencing of mtDNA is rarely used for detecting mtDNA rearrangements.
    B. Restriction fragment-length polymorphism (RFLP) analysis.
    Rationale: RFLP analysis is commonly used to detect mtDNA point mutations.
    C. Amplification refractory mutation system–PCR (ARMS-PCR).
    Rationale: ARMS-PCR can only be used to detect known mutations.
    D. Real-time PCR.
    Rationale: In the context of mtDNA analysis, real-time PCR is used to determine mtDNA copy number.
    E. Southern blot analysis.
    Rationale: Southern blot analysis is regarded as the gold standard for detecting mtDNA rearrangements.

Major points of discussion

- Several diseases associated with large-scale rearrangements of mtDNA have been described. These could be caused by either deletions or duplications. PEO and KSS are the two well-known syndromes caused by single deletions of mtDNA.
- Direct sequencing of the whole mitochondrial genome using Sanger sequencing to detect rearrangements is very labor intensive and time consuming. In addition, it cannot determine heteroplasmy level. Next-generation sequencing not only can accurately determine the break points of the deleted segment but it also can determine the heteroplasmy level. This methodology is not yet in

routine use but may become the future method of choice for mtDNA analysis.

- RFLP methodology, which refers to the difference between the sizes of fragments produced by a restriction enzyme, is a very useful technique to detect known mtDNA point mutations. This method has the advantage of being able to determine the heteroplasmy level of the mutation.

- ARMS-PCR is accurate and convenient for detecting known point mutations in mtDNA. However, it cannot detect new mutations or determine heteroplasmy level.

- Southern blotting is the method of choice for mtDNA rearrangement analysis. It can easily detect mtDNA duplications or deletions and can also estimate their level of heteroplasmy. The two major inherent disadvantages of this method are that it (1) it requires a relatively large amount of DNA (5 to 10 µg) and (2) has a long turnaround time (2 to 3 days).[11,17,25]

13. A. RFLP analysis.
Rationale: RFLP analysis is best used to detect known point mutations in mtDNA.
B. Southern blotting with a radiolabeled probe.
Rationale: Southern blots needs large amounts of DNA (5 µg or more).
C. Long-range PCR and gel electrophoresis.
Rationale: mtDNA multiple deletions can be quickly detected by long-range PCR on small biopsy specimens.
D. Sequencing by capillary electrophoresis.
Rationale: Multiple deletions are extremely difficult to detect by conventional sequencing.
E. Single-stranded conformation polymorphism (SSCP).
Rationale: SSCP can best detect nucleotide variations in small PCR-amplified fragments and should not be used to detect multiple deletions in mtDNA.

Major points of discussion

- Deleted mtDNA can be transmitted by Mendelian inheritance in disorders characterized by PEO. The autosomal dominant form of this disease (AD-PEO) primarily affects muscle, whereas the autosomal recessive form (AR-PEO) usually involves multiple systems. *[handwritten: progressive ext. ophthalmoplegia]*

- The mechanism causing mtDNA deletions is unclear. In muscle morphology, marked accumulation of mitochondria in cytochrome c (COX)-deficient fibers (COX-negative ragged red fibers) is the common finding. It appears that each individual fiber contains a clonal expansion of a single deletion event.

- It has been reported that mutations in the heart/skeletal muscle isoform of the adenine nucleotide translocator (ANT1), which exchanges adenosine diphosphate and ATP across the mitochondrial inner membrane, causes mtDNA multiple deletions associated with cardiomyopathy.

- Long-range PCR is commonly used to provide rapid and reliable exclusion of rearrangements in tissue. PCR amplification and electrophoresis of normal mtDNA produces a single large band on the gel. The appearance of additional smaller bands represents multiple mtDNA deletions.

- Long-range PCR is very sensitive and may detect rearrangements that are not at clinically significant levels. For example, very low levels of deleted mtDNA, which cannot be detected by regular Southern blotting, are detected by long-range PCR. Therefore, it is crucial

that the age of the patient is taken into account when interpreting the results. Further investigation is always recommended before issuing a final report on positive results.[11,17,25]

14. A. Mitochondrial tRNA lysine *(MT-TK).*
Rationale: Mutations in *MT-TK* are associated with MERRF syndrome.
B. Mitochondrial tRNA leucine 1 *(MT-TL1).*
Rationale: Mutations in *MT-TL1* most commonly cause MELAS.
C. Mitochondrial tRNA tryptophan *(MT-TW).*
Rationale: Mutations in *MT-TW* have been associated with dementia and chorea (DEMCHO) but not depletion.
D. Mitochondrial tRNA isoleucine *(MT-TI).*
Rationale: Mutations in *MT-TI* are most commonly associated with cardiomyopathy.
E. mtDNA polymerase gamma *(POLG).*
Rationale: POLG is one of the nine genes with mutations that have been reported to cause mtDNA depletion.[8,17,32]

Major points of discussion

- mtDNA depletion syndrome (MDS) is an autosomal disease first described in 1991. It is phenotypically heterogeneous and caused by a severe drop in mtDNA copy number in affected tissues. Unlike other respiratory chain disorders, MDS may manifest solely in a specific organ; this makes molecular diagnosis a challenge if the affected tissue cannot be sampled by biopsy.

- Muscle and liver were originally reported to be affected by MDS, but now it is divided into three clinical categories: myopathic MDS (OMIM #609560), encephalomyopathic MDS (OMIM #612073 and OMIM #612075), and hepatocerebral MDS (OMIM #251880).

- To date, mutations in at least nine genes have been associated with MDS. Four genes are involved in deoxyribonucleotide triphosphate (dNTP) metabolism: thymidine kinase 2 *(TK2)*, associated with myopathic MDS, deoxyguanosine kinase *(DGUOK)*, associated with hepatocerebral MDS, polymerase gamma *(POLG)* also with hepatocerebral MDS, and, more specifically, Alper syndrome; and succinate-CoA ligase, adenosine diphosphate (ADP)-forming β-subunit *(SUCLA2)*, associated with encephalomyopathic MDS.

- Human DNA polymerase is composed of two subunits, a 140-kDa catalytic subunit encoded by *POLG* on chromosome 15q25, and a 55-kDa accessory subunit encoded by *POLG2* on chromosome 17q23-24. The catalytic subunit of mtDNA polymerase gamma, encoded by *POLG1*, is the only DNA polymerase found in mitochondria, which is responsible for DNA replication and repair. Mutations in *POLG* can cause mtDNA depletion or multiple mtDNA deletions. To date, more than 120 variants have been associated with different pathologic phenotypes (http://tools.niehs.nih.gov/polg/).

- Because of the heterogeneous nature of its clinical phenotype, definitive diagnosis of MDS is a daunting task. Based on clinical presentation of the patient, one or more genes can be selected for sequencing. For example, if the presentation is predominantly myopathic, then *TK2* sequencing may be considered first, whereas if the presentation is mainly hepatocerebral, sequencing *DGOUK* should be considered first.

15. A. Southern blot analysis with radiolabeled probes.
Rationale: Southern blot with radiolabeled probe detection is valuable for evaluating mtDNA rearrangements, such as deletions or duplications.
B. Southern blot analysis with fluorescence detection.
Rationale: Southern blot analysis with a fluorescence detection system is very sensitive for qualitative, but not quantitative, evaluation of mtDNA.
C. Real-time PCR with TaqMan probes.
Rationale: Real-time PCR accompanied by TaqMan probe technology is highly sensitive and accurate and is currently available for determining mtDNA copy number.
D. Sanger sequencing of the whole mitochondrial genome.
Rationale: Direct sequencing of mtDNA detects sequence variation but cannot determine mtDNA copy number.
E. Next-generation sequencing of the whole mitochondrial genome.
Rationale: Next-generation sequencing of the mitochondrial genome can determine any base-pair variation with a high level of accuracy but it does not determine copy number.

Major points of discussion

- Traditionally, estimating mtDNA copy number relied on Southern blotting approaches. This involves using two labeled probes, one specific for mtDNA and one specific for a nuclear gene, usually a housekeeping gene, such as glyceraldehyde diphosphate dehydrogenase (GAPDH) or β-globulin. In this method, mtDNA is linearized after digestion with an endonuclease enzyme, such as *PvuII*, and then transferred to a nylon membrane. After autoradiography, the intensity of bands corresponding to mtDNA and the nuclear gene is measured by densitometry. This method is very labor intensive, time consuming, and expensive. Furthermore, it is semi-quantitative and only allows an estimate of mtDNA content.
- mtDNA can also be quantified by PCR. Competitive PCR is one approach, which involves introduction of a serially diluted competitive template into the tissue extract. mtDNA quantitation is achieved by radiometric comparison of the relative amounts of the two products.
- In recent years, the development of quantitative real-time PCR (qPCR) technology has significantly improved the estimation of mtDNA copy number in clinical specimens, such as blood and tissue. qPCR assays are extremely sensitive and can detect only a few copies, or even a single copy, of target DNA in a clinical specimen.
- Two chemistries, TaqMan and SYBR green, are most commonly used. Assays based on TaqMan chemistry have the advantage of being capable of simultaneously quantifying more than one target in a sample. SYBR-based qPCR assays, although more convenient than TaqMan-based assays, are less accurate because SYBR green can bind to DNA molecules other than the target. Therefore, highly optimized PCR conditions are a prerequisite for successful application of this approach.
- Two approaches are used to calculate mtDNA in qPCR assays. (1) The first calculation uses a standard curve, in which known amounts of DNA are used to construct the standard curve from which the copy number of the unknown sample is delineated. (2) Another approach uses relative quantification, in which the relative copy number of target DNA to a reference DNA, amplified simultaneously, is calculated. The advantage of the latter method is that it obviates the need for a standard curve. However, when the latter method is used, it is imperative to ensure that the efficiencies of target and reference amplification are very similar.

16. A. An adenine-to-guanine transition at nucleotide 3243 position (3243A>G) in mitochondrial tRNA Leu$^{(UUR)}$ (*MTTL1*).
Rationale: This mutation is the most common cause of MELAS. It is also associated with MI-PEO and MIDD.
B. An adenine-to-guanine transition at nucleotide 8344 position (8344A>G) in mitochondrial tRNA Lys (*MTTK*).
Rationale: This mutation is the most common cause of MERRF but has not been associated with MELAS, MI-PEO, or MIDD.
C. A thymidine-to-cytosine transition at nucleotide 8993 position (8993T>C) in mitochondrial ATPase 6 (*MTATP6*).
Rationale: This mutation is the most common cause of NARP but has not been associated with MELAS, PEO, or MIDD.
D. A thymidine-to-cytosine transition at nucleotide 9176 position (9176T>C) in mitochondrial ATPase 6 (*MTATP6*).
Rationale: This mutation, similar to 8993T>C, is associated with NARP (i.e., maternally inherited Leigh disease) but has not been associated with MELAS, PEO, or MIDD.
E. A guanine-to-adenine at nucleotide 1178 position (11778G>A) in mitochondrial subunit ND4 of complex I (*MTND4*).
Rationale: This mutation is commonly associated with LHON but has not been associated with MELAS, PEO, or MIDD.

Major points of discussion

- MELAS is the most common maternally inherited mitochondrial disorder. The 3243A>G mutation in tRNA Leu$^{(UUR)}$ is present in approximately 80% of patients with typical MELAS phenotype. Other mutations in the same gene (e.g., 3271T>C and 3252A>G) also cause this disease.
- Morphologically, most ragged red fibers are COX positive, which is in contrast to other mitochondrial syndromes involving tRNA mutations that are devoid of COX activity. Moreover, ragged red fibers are most visible in the vasculature, which shows an intense histochemical reactivity for succinate dehydrogenase.
- MI-PEO, which is phenotypically similar to the sporadic form of the disease, is also associated with the 3243A>G mutation. It has also been associated with mutations in other mitochondrial tRNAs, including tRNA asparagine, tRNA lysine, and tRNA tyrosine. Unlike in MELAS, the ragged red fibers found in MI-PEO are COX negative.
- MERRF is characterized by myoclonus, generalized seizures, ataxia, and myopathy with ragged red fibers. Again, unlike in MELAS, these ragged red fibers are devoid of COX activity. The most common mutation associated with MERRF is an A>G transition at nucleotide 8344 (8344A>G) in tRNA lysine, which is found in most cases. Another mutation in the same gene (8356T>C) is also a rare cause of the disease. The 8344A>G mutation can be reliably detected by analyzing blood samples.
- Mutations in the *MTATP6* gene at position 8993, predominantly a T>G transversion, account for more

than 50% of NARP cases. Another mutation at the same position associated with NARP is a T > C transition, converting leucine to proline at position 156. A high load of these two mutations (8993T > G/C) can also cause maternally inherited Leigh disease.[10,25,34]

17. A. Complex I subunit *ND4* gene.
Rationale: Mutations in *ND4* are associated with LHON, MELAS, and Leigh syndrome (LS).
B. Complex I subunit *ND1* gene.
Rationale: Mutations in *ND1* cause MELAS, LHON, and MELAS/LHON overlap but not isolated myopathy.
C. Cytochrome b (*cyt b*) gene.
Rationale: Mutations in myogenic stem cells, presumably occurring after germ-layer differentiation, cause isolated myopathy. To date, most known mutations in *cyt b* occur in this category.
D. Cytochrome *c* oxidase subunit 1 (*COX1*) gene.
Rationale: *COX1* mutations are associated with multisystem disorders, sideroblastic anemia, and sensorineuronal hearing loss.
E. Succinate dehydrogenase *(SDHA)* gene.
Rationale: Succinate dehydrogenase, encoded by *SDHA*, is a nuclear gene; its mutations do not cause isolated mitochondrial myopathy.

Major points of discussion

- Mutations in the mitochondrial genome cause a wide variety of clinical syndromes. Mutations in messenger RNAs (mRNAs) affect specific proteins of the respiratory chain, whereas mutations in mitochondrial tRNAs affect the general synthesis of mitochondrial proteins.
- Mitochondrial disorders, such as NARP, maternally inherited LS, or LHON, are caused by mutations in different subunits of five complexes.
- Although mutations in mitochondrial tRNA genes affect the synthesis of all mitochondrially encoded proteins, mutations in different tRNA genes produce different clinical phenotypes. For example, mutations in tRNA lysine cause MERRF, whereas mutations in tRNA isoleucine cause cardiomyopathy.
- Mutations in rRNA genes, which also affect general protein synthesis, cause deafness or cardiomyopathy. The A > G transition mutation in the 12S rRNA gene at nt-1555 causes maternally inherited deafness but usually through interaction with aminoglycoside drugs, such as gentamycin, kanamycin, and streptomycin.
- Although a relatively large number of mtDNA mutations have been associated with LHON, only four mutations, all located in the complex I gene, are considered primary, pathogenic mutations.[9,11]

18. A. All respiratory chain proteins are encoded by mtDNA.
Rationale: The mitochondrial respiratory chain consists of about 75 protein subunits organized in five separate complexes. Only 13 of these are encoded by mtDNA, the rest by nuclear DNA.
B. Sperm do not contain mtDNA.
Rationale: Sperm contain thousands of mitochondria in each cell, each containing 5 to 10 copies of mtDNA.
C. All mtDNA-encoded proteins are components of the respiratory chain.

Rationale: mtDNA encodes 13 proteins that are incorporated into mitochondrial respiratory chain complexes.
D. mtDNA is independent of nuclear DNA (nDNA) and does not require nDNA gene products for its function.
Rationale: mtDNA functions under the overarching control of nDNA because it requires several nDNA-encoded proteins for its maintenance and proper functioning.
E. All mtDNA in the zygote is derived from sperm.
Rationale: All mitochondria and, therefore, all mtDNA in the zygote are derived from the ovum.

Major points of discussion

- The mitochondrial respiratory chain is composed of about 75 multiprotein subunits organized in five separate complexes embedded in the inner mitochondrial membrane. Thirteen of these subunits are encoded by mtDNA: seven in complex I, one in complex III, three in complex IV, and two in ATP synthase or complex V.
- Human mtDNA is a 16-kb circular, double-stranded molecule that contains 37 genes: 2 rRNA, 22 tRNA, and 13 structural genes encoding subunits of the mitochondrial respiratory chain.
- All eukaryotic cells contain many copies of mtDNA, which, at division, distribute randomly among daughter cells. In normal tissues, all copies of mtDNA are identical (homoplasmy). Disease-causing mutations usually affect some, but not all, mtDNA. Therefore, in this case, cells and tissues harbor both wild-type and mutant mtDNA, a condition known as heteroplasmy. A minimal amount of mutant mtDNA must be present before there is a manifestation of respiratory dysfunction and appearance of clinical symptoms; this is known as the *threshold effect*.
- The threshold in tissues such as brain, muscle, heart, and endocrine glands with high oxidative energy demand is low compared with other tissues. Therefore, these tissues are especially vulnerable to respiratory chain dysfunction.
- Because mitochondria are randomly distributed at cell division, the proportion of mutant and wild-type mtDNA in daughter cells may change, and the phenotype may change accordingly. This phenomenon, called *mitotic segregation*, explains the age-related variability of clinical features frequently observed in mtDNA-related disorders.[9,11,18]

19. A. Thymidine phosphorylase (TP) activity in peripheral blood leukocytes.
Rationale: MNGIE is caused by TP deficiency, the activity of which is easily measured in peripheral blood leukocytes.
B. Mitochondrial respiratory chain complex I activity.
Rationale: Complex I activity of the respiratory chain remains unaltered in TP deficiency.
C. Mitochondrial respiratory chain complex II activity.
Rationale: Complex II activity of the respiratory chain remains unaltered in TP deficiency.
D. Mitochondrial respiratory chain complex IV activity.
Rationale: Although the mosaic pattern of COX-deficient fibers is a common histologic finding in MNGIE, it is not specific for MNGIE, and the same pattern may be observed in other mitochondrial myopathies.
E. ATPase activity in peripheral blood leukocytes.
Rationale: ATPase activity levels in blood leukocytes are not informative because they are not altered in MNGIE.

Major points of discussion

- MNGIE is an autosomal recessive mitochondrial disorder characterized by PEO, severe gastrointestinal dysmotility, cachexia, and peripheral neuropathy. Brain magnetic resonance imaging scans are consistent with leukoencephalopathy. The age at clinical onset is in the late teens, and the disease is usually fatal by 40 years of age.
- Neurogenic changes and the presence of ragged red fibers and occasional COX-deficient fibers observed on muscle morphology provide further evidence for neuropathy and mitochondrial myopathy. Abnormalities of intestinal smooth muscle and the enteric nervous system are common findings in histologic studies of the gastrointestinal system.
- MNGIE, which is mapped to chromosome 22q13.32, is caused by mutations in the *TP* gene. The disease is transmitted in a recessive pattern, and affected individuals are either homozygotes or compound heterozygotes.
- Human TP catabolizes the dephosphorylation of thymidine to thymine. Its expression level and activity are significantly increased in certain tumors. TP is widely expressed in human tissues, including the brain, peripheral nerves, spleen, lung, bladder, and gastrointestinal system. Paradoxically, skeletal muscle has no TP activity despite the fact that this tissue is usually affected by MNGIE.
- Various mitochondrial abnormalities, such as decreased mitochondrial respiratory chain activity, ragged red fibers, and multiple deletions, are common findings. However, these are inconsistent and nonspecific. The definitive diagnosis is made by quantifying TP activity in peripheral blood leukocytes and determining plasma thymidine levels because TP levels in leukocytes decrease by more than 90% in MNGIE and plasma thymidine levels are about 50-fold higher than normal. Molecular studies in TP deficiency include sequencing all 10 exons of the gene to search for known and novel mutations.[15,20,25]

20. A. Autosomal recessive.
    B. Autosomal dominant.
    Rationale: mtDNA inheritance does not follow Mendelian genetics rules.
    C. Maternal.
    Rationale: A unique feature of mitochondria (and all mtDNAs) is that they are inherited only from the mother. Therefore, a mother harboring an mtDNA point mutation passes it on to all of her children, but only her daughters transmit it to their progeny.
    D. X-linked recessive.
    E. X-linked dominant.
    Rationale: mtDNA is not a constituent of the X chromosome.

Major points of discussion

- In eukaryotic cells, mitochondria are the only organelles other than the nucleolus that contain their own DNA and the machinery for synthesizing RNA and proteins. There are hundreds to thousands of mitochondria per cell, each containing five mtDNA molecules on average. Human mtDNA is a 16,569-bp, double-stranded molecule containing 37 genes.
- Of more than 1500 different proteins found in mitochondria, only 13 are encoded by mtDNA. The rest are encoded by nDNA and imported from the cytoplasm.

- Mutations in mtDNA lead to respiratory chain diseases. Many of these disorders involve brain and skeletal muscle and are also known as *mitochondrial encephalomyopathies*. Because the respiratory chain is under dual genetic control, the proteins that make up the respiratory chain involve both Mendelian and mitochondrial genetics.
- The prevalence of mitochondrial disease is about 10 to 15 cases per 100,000 individuals, which is similar to other neurologic disorders such as ALS and the muscular dystrophies.
- Mitochondrial genetics differs from Mendelian genetics in three major aspects: maternal inheritance, heteroplasmy, and mitotic segregation. Although paternal mtDNA enters the oocyte at fertilization, these molecules are destroyed during early development, and only mitochondria contributed by oocytes repopulate the embryo. Therefore, if a mother carries an mtDNA point mutation, she will pass it on to all of her children.[10,11,14]

21. A. Mutation.
    Rationale: See Major Points of Discussion.
    B. Polymorphism.
    Rationale: When a change in DNA sequence (i.e., a variant) is so common that it is present at more than a 1% frequency in the general population, the variant is known as polymorphism.
    C. Genotype.
    Rationale: This refers to the genetic constitution of an individual.
    D. Allele.
    Rationale: This refers to one of the two or more forms of a gene.
    E. Rare variant.
    Rationale: Alleles with a frequency of less than 1% are called rare variants.

Major points of discussion

- Alleles are alternative forms of the same gene or DNA sequence.
- The genotype refers to the genetic constitution of an individual or the alleles present at one locus.
- Mutation is a change in DNA sequence, including base-pair substitution, insertion, and deletion. Mutations originate by one of two basic mechanisms: errors introduced during DNA replication or failure to repair after DNA damage.
- A mutation may lead to complete loss of expression of the gene or to formation of a variant protein with altered properties.
- Some mutations are not deleterious and have no phenotypic effect, either because the change does not alter the amino acid sequence of the polypeptide or, even if it does, the resulting change in the encoded amino acid sequence does not alter the functional properties of the protein. Therefore, not all mutations have clinical consequences. During evolution, the influx of nucleotide variation ensures genetic diversity and individuality.
- Many deleterious mutations that lead to genetic disease are rare variants; however, there is no simple correlation between allele frequency and the effect of the allele on health. Many rare variants appear to have no deleterious effect, whereas some variants common enough to be polymorphisms are known to predispose to serious diseases.

22a. A. This is a mitochondrial disease. The mother is a healthy carrier, and the disease manifests in the children differentially because of heteroplasmy.
Rationale: Deafness and microcephaly can both be caused by mitochondrial dysfunction. Relatively common and maternally inherited, aminoglycoside-induced nonsyndromic deafness is caused by the A1555G mutation in mtDNA, whereas microcephaly in the Old Order Amish population is autosomal recessive due to a c.530G > C transversion in SLC25A19. There is no mutation in mtDNA known to cause both deafness and microcephaly.
B. This is an autosomal dominant deafness syndrome with low penetrance and variable expressivity.
Rationale: The two deaf children show an equally severe phenotype, as do the two microcephalic children; thus, variable expressivity is not likely. In addition, having three affected children in three births is not consistent with low penetrance.
C. This is a family with two mutations that cause two separate disorders, each inherited in an autosomal recessive manner.
Rationale: This is the most probable scenario because the parents are both healthy, and the disorders manifest early with identical phenotypes and clearly segregate, as expected with a Mendelian autosomal recessive model.
D. This is manifestation of a "mutator" syndrome that causes frequent mutations in the germline of the parents; thus, healthy parents have multiple affected children.
Rationale: Hereditary nonpolyposis colon cancer (HNPCC) is caused by a defect in DNA mismatch repair (MMR) genes. However, such patients do not have children with microcephaly or deafness.
E. This situation is due to maternal consumption of genetically modified produce during each pregnancy.
Rationale: There is no confirmed scientific evidence that genetically modified produce causes human disease.

22b. A. You recommend comparative genomic hybridization microarray studies to identify large structural chromosomal defects.
Rationale: Although developmental delay and mental retardation are associated with loss of chromosomal segments that can be identified using microarray technologies, most known causes of microcephaly and deafness are due to single-nucleotide changes present at low allele frequencies in the population.
B. You recommend comparative genomic hybridization microarray studies to identify regions of homozygosity between the siblings affected by the same disease. This will allow you to narrow down the list of genes that are known to cause the conditions observed in this family.
Rationale: Although this approach will narrow the regions that harbor the disease-causing genes, the resolution is not high enough based on six observed meiotic events.
C. You propose targeted testing for all mutations known to cause deafness and microcephaly using Sanger sequencing.
Rationale: Sanger sequencing is most cost effective when used to identify mutations in high-probability gene targets. Unfortunately, both microcephaly and deafness can be caused by many low-frequency alleles.
D. You propose full genome sequencing because you suspect that the changes responsible for the phenotypes observed are in noncoding regions of the human genome.

Rationale: Full genome sequencing is still not cost effective for screening for mutations in candidate genes. As new technologies appear, this approach may become more widely used.
E. You recommend targeted testing for the most common point mutations associated with deafness and microcephaly.
Rationale: ASPM (locus name MCPH5; chromosome 1q31) accounts for 37% to 54% of cases of microcephaly. *GJB2* (which encodes connexin 26) and *GJB6* (which encodes connexin 30) account for about 50% of autosomal recessive nonsyndromic hearing loss. It would be most sensible to first test these three genes for mutations.

22c. A. The family should be advised that, because they already have three affected children, they have a good chance of producing a healthy child.
Rationale: The chance of having an affected child with either disease is one in four, whereas having a child affected with both diseases is one in eight. Already having children with the disease does not alter the risk for future children.
B. The family should be advised not to consider additional children because the risk for having additional affected children is uncertain.
Rationale: The risk can be calculated with certainty. The chance of having an affected child with either disease is one in four, whereas having a child affected with both diseases is one in eight. Already having children with the disease does not alter the risk for future children.
C. The family should be advised that the risk for having an affected child is one in four for microcephaly or deafness, whereas the chances of having a child with both disorders is one in eight, without providing any further recommendations.
Rationale: The parents should be informed that preimplantation screening for affected embryos can improve their chances of having a healthy child.
D. The family should be advised about the possibility of further genetic testing in case the parents are interested in pursuing prenatal diagnosis or in vitro fertilization.
Rationale: The introduction of high-throughput sequencing into clinical practice allows for the simultaneous screening of a large number of disease-causing genes. After the disease-causing mutation is identified, targeted testing of the embryos for the deleterious mutations would be feasible.
E. The family should be advised that there are no further diagnostic options available for them, and they should consider adoption.
Rationale: High-throughput sequencing provides a powerful tool for identifying rare disease-causing mutations.

22d. A. It is still experimental, whereas Sanger sequencing is currently available.
Rationale: Next-Gen sequencing is currently available using multiple platforms from companies such as Roche, Illumina, and Applied Biosystems. Multiple academic and commercial entities currently offer Next-Gen sequencing for clinical diagnostic purposes.
B. It involves sequencing a single molecule, instead of many copies of the same molecule.

Rationale: Currently available commercial systems (e.g., from Roche, Illumina, and Applied Biosystems) all sequence multiple copies of the same molecule. Many thousands of independent clones are sequenced simultaneously. Instruments that work by sequencing single molecules, such as those commercially available from Pacific Biosystems, may soon become sufficiently reliable for clinical use.

C. It can provide megabases worth of nucleotide sequence, whereas Sanger sequencing is only practical for sequencing, at maximum, a few kilobases.
Rationale: The output of the HiSeq 2500 from Illumina in a single run is approximately 1 terabase (Tb), which corresponds to more than 100 times the size of the human diploid genome.

D. It is based on irreversible termination of extension on a subpopulation of the templates.
Rationale: Sanger sequencing uses irreversible termination of synthesis. At each cycle, fluorescently labeled dideoxynucleotides are mixed in with normal, unlabeled deoxynucleotides and are incorporated in a small percentage of extension products, which are irreversibly terminated. The length and color of the various terminated DNA molecules are then determined, and the sequence is derived from these data. In contrast, the principle of the Illumina instrument is based on reversible termination of synthesis. Fluorescently labeled nucleotides are added together in each extension cycle. No unlabeled nucleotides are present. Incorporation of specific nucleotides is detected simultaneously based on the color of the hundreds of thousands of extended products corresponding to different sequencing reactions. The fluorescent tag interfering with extension is then removed, and a new cycle of extension begins. The Roche and Applied Biosystems instruments use incorporation of unlabeled single nucleotides added one at a time in successive cycles. Incorporation is detected by coupled photochemistry in the Roche instrument (pyrosequencing) and by pH measurements in the Applied Biosystems instrument.

E. Interpretation of the data obtained is much more straightforward.
Rationale: Interpretation of Next-Gen datasets requires sophisticated computational algorithms and large amounts of computing and data storage capacity.

22e. A. It refers to a process in which sequence changes known to cause specific disease phenotypes are detected.
Rationale: Detection of sequence variations, neutral or pathogenic, is a process that occurs after the region of interest is sequenced and compared with a reference sequence that is considered normal.

B. The human genome contains a great deal of noncoding DNA, the role of which is not clearly established in disease. To limit the cost of clinical testing by sequencing, it is practical to focus on certain segments of the genome that have previously been shown to be associated with human disease. Upon sequencing the full genome, these segments are computationally identified and analyzed, whereas the data from noncoding regions of the genome are left in a non-human-readable form; this is sequence capture.
Rationale: It is a process that takes place before sequencing, not after the sequence is obtained. Regions of interest are either amplified using PCR-based or other locus-specific amplification methods, or captured using hydrogen bonding between complementary RNA or DNA baits; the DNA library created from the sample can then be analyzed.

C. It refers to the laboratory procedure that selects fragments of diagnostic interest from human genomic DNA for sequence analysis.
Rationale: Site-specific amplification-based methods are more suitable for smaller (e.g., up to 200 kb) genomic regions, whereas hybridization-based methods are more appropriate for capturing regions in the 100-kb to 100-Mb range.

D. It refers to the method of data collection from the sequencer.
Rationale: Sequence capture is a biochemical process based on amplification by synthesis or hydrogen bond formation between complementary strands on nucleic acids.

E. It refers to the fact that sequences slowly leak out of the reaction chamber of the sequencer, and they need to be prevented from contaminating the instrument by capturing them using a secondary container that is replaced regularly.
Rationale: Sequences are recorded interpretations of data obtained from the observation of chemical reactions taking place during sequencing. They are not a physical substance.

22f. A. Full exome sequencing is the best approach because the number of genes implicated in both microcephaly and deafness is large, and there are numerous, as yet unidentified, genes that can cause these phenotypes.
Rationale: Full exome sequencing will provide a comprehensive list of mutations in annotated protein-coding genes. Because, in this case, we are looking for homozygosity for two nontolerated/disruptive mutations, the chances that the cause of the disease can be determined with certainty are good.

B. Full exome sequencing is less expensive than full genome sequencing, and most known pathogenic mutations are within exons or at intron-exon junctions.
Rationale: With currently available technology, full genome sequencing is approximately 10 times more expensive than full exome sequencing.

C. Analysis of a full exome dataset is less complex than that of a full genome sequencing dataset.
Rationale: The size of the dataset is approximately 50 times larger for a full genome sequencing experiment. Interpretation is also more difficult because there is currently no good method for predicting the pathogenicity of mutations present in non–protein-coding regions of the genome.

D. Sequencing only known genes and loci would be effective if the patients in this family had a mutation previously identified in other families, but it would not detect private mutations specific to this family.
Rationale: Although there are many known cases of deafness and microcephaly, there are also many regions implicated in the pathogenesis of these diseases, where the genes involved are not yet identified.

E. Exome sequencing provides the most even and reliable sampling of the coding regions of the human genome, even if expense is not a consideration.
Rationale: With currently available capture reagents, even at 100-fold medium coverage depth, approximately 10% of the regions targeted are not sufficiently sampled (at least

10-fold coverage). At 200-fold coverage, this is reduced to approximately 5%.

22g. A. Both parents and all three children should be sequenced.
Rationale: The key to finding the cause of the diseases is to look for homozygosity for disruptive mutations in the affected children. Once such differences are found, they can be verified to be heterozygous in the parents using a targeted sequencing approach.
B. Only the parents should be sequenced.
Rationale: Sequencing the parents would not be sufficient to identify the disease-causing allele(s) because the parents share about 25% of their genome.
C. The parents, one child with deafness, and one child with microcephaly should be sequenced.
Rationale: The power of the analysis is provided by comparing the three siblings; that is, the six underlying meiotic events.
D. Only the child with both microcephaly and deafness should be sequenced.
Rationale: Valuable extra information can be gained from the children who are affected only with one disease because they should be homozygous only for one set of disruptive mutations.
E. Only the three siblings should be sequenced. There is no need to sequence the parents.
Rationale: The key to finding the causes of these diseases is to identify homozygosity for disruptive mutations in the affected children. After such differences are found, they can be verified to be heterozygous in the parents using a targeted sequencing approach.

22h. A. The patients must be older than 18 years.
Rationale: Patients younger than 18 years need to sign an assent document, which explains to them, at their level of comprehension, the reasons for testing and the events associated with testing. Consent is signed by the parent or legal guardian. Testing can only be performed for conditions that are either present or will manifest before age 18 years.
B. Both parents must sign an informed consent form, and the children must sign an assent form.
Rationale: The signature of one parent is sufficient, and the children with microcephaly might be so severely affected that the assent document cannot be explained to them and they cannot sign it. There should be a court document assigning the decision-making capacity to the parent or legal guardian.
C. At least one parent must sign an informed consent form. The children with microcephaly are exempt from signing the assent form; assent only needs to be obtained from the deaf child.
Rationale: The signature of one parent is sufficient, and the children with microcephaly might be so severely affected that the assent document cannot be explained to them and they cannot sign it. There should be a court document assigning the decision-making capacity to the parent or legal guardian.
D. You must confirm that the parents' insurance will cover the cost of testing.
Rationale: Prior insurance clearance is not required for testing to be performed; however, it is important to explain to the patients the amount that they might be billed for, in case insurance does not cover the testing expenses.

E. You have to obtain U.S. Food and Drug Administration (FDA) approval for the method to be used.
Rationale: Most tests in molecular pathology are developed and validated by the laboratories themselves. The College of American Pathologists (CAP) is the agency that supervises the performance characteristics of such tests. In some states, New York for example, the state authorities need to provide written approval for performing the test based on a submitted written validation summary.

22i. **A. All known mutations (i.e., previously detected in other "healthy" individuals) should be excluded from the search for the cause of the disease.**
Rationale: Disease-causing alleles are often present in carriers who are "healthy" and who participate as healthy controls in genotyping and sequencing projects mapping human genetic diversity. Thus, SNPs that have been observed previously should not be excluded from the analysis.
B. Mutations that do not cause amino acid changes, frame shifts, transcriptional stops, or splicing defects should be removed in the initial analysis.
Rationale: This will decrease the number of SNPs evaluated to approximately 1000 per sample.
C. Emphasis should be placed on mutations for which any one patient is homozygous.
Rationale: Because we are trying to determine the molecular cause of two independently segregating disease phenotypes based on an autosomal recessive mode of inheritance, the affected children have to be homozygous for either or both of the disease-causing mutations.
D. Mutations that are present in a homozygous form in all three siblings should be excluded as the cause of both deafness and microcephaly.
Rationale: Because only two of the three children have deafness and microcephaly, respectively, any mutation that is present in a homozygous form in all three children is, by definition, not the cause of either condition.
E. The children with deafness should be homozygous for the same mutation; similarly, the children with microcephaly should be homozygous for the same mutation.
Rationale: The unaffected child for either condition should be either wild-type or heterozygous for the SNPs that are thought to cause the deafness or the microcephaly.

22j. A. Online Mendelian Inheritance in Man (OMIM): http://www.ncbi.nlm.nih.gov/omim
Rationale: OMIM is a comprehensive compendium of human genes and genetic phenotypes. It contains information on all known Mendelian disorders and on more than 12,000 genes. It focuses on the relationship between phenotype and genotype and is updated daily, and its entries contain links to other resources.
B. University of Santa Cruz web browser: http://genome.ucsc.edu
Rationale: This site contains the reference sequence and working draft assemblies for a large collection of genomes, as well as coding and noncoding RNAs and epigenetic modifications. The site also displays currently curated SNPs and highlights known pathogenic SNPs in red.
C. dbSNP database: http://www.ncbi.nlm.nih.gov/SNP/

Rationale: This database is curated by the National Center for Biotechnology Information (NCBI) and provides tools to search for all previously detected SNPs. It provides data concerning allele frequencies for most common SNPs in various ethnic populations.

D. 1000 genome database: http://www.1000genomes.org
Rationale: Because full genome sequences are compared, genomic deletions and rearrangements are also included in the list of genetic polymorphisms. This is a work in progress, and its usefulness will increase as more genome sequences are added and analyzed.

E. Leiden database: http://www.dmd.nl
Rationale: This database is specifically designed for scientists performing research and/or diagnosis in the setting of Duchenne and Duchenne-like muscular dystrophies (e.g., Duchenne, Becker, limb-girdle). Although some additional databases about various disease groups are linked to this site, it has a somewhat limited disease-specific focus.

22k. A. The exome sequencing must be repeated.
Rationale: Verification of mutations identified using high-throughput sequencing is more economically done using a targeted sequencing approach.

B. The sequencing data must be reanalyzed using another analysis software program.
Rationale: All mutations identified by the software of choice are visually verified. Observing the coverage depth, the quality of the alignments, and the individual reads allows one to judge the level of certainty of a specific mutation call. Using an alternative alignment method would be appropriate, if one wanted to evaluate the overall accuracy of the mutation-calling algorithm during validation of the test.

C. The identity of the samples and the correctness of the mutations must be confirmed using an alternative method.
Rationale: It is vital that results are confirmed to belong to the relevant patient. This is ensured by genotyping DNA from the original sample using an alternative method, such as SNP microarray studies, and comparing the genotyping and sequencing results. The presence of the pathogenic mutation also needs to be confirmed using targeted sequencing.

D. The mutations must be confirmed to be absent in 400 healthy control samples.
Rationale: Disease-causing mutations are often family or clan specific and might not be present in controls from even ethnically matched populations.

E. You must confirm that the mutations have never been seen previously in any population sampled.
Rationale: Disease-causing alleles are often present in carriers who are "healthy" and participate as healthy controls in genotyping and sequencing projects mapping human genetic diversity. Thus, SNPs that have been observed previously should not be excluded from the analysis.

22l. A. Following full genome amplification, the exome sequencing has to be repeated on cells derived from all embryos.
Rationale: After a disease-causing mutation has been identified with certainty, a targeted sequencing approach is more appropriate.

B. Following whole genome amplification, the DNA from each embryo has to be genotyped for the mutations identified in the three siblings with deafness and/or microcephaly.
Rationale: Whole genome amplification is required because the DNA content of the cell consists of two copies only and the chances that the site-specific PCR will not work at such a low template level is possible. In addition, there is a potential risk of cross-contamination from other sources. Whole genome amplification using random primers decreases the chance of false-negative, as well as false-positive, results.

C. Following whole genome amplification, all embryos have to be tested for aneuploidy using a microarray methodology.
Rationale: Because we are looking for specific changes, genome-wide microarray testing is not required. Microarray testing for aneuploidy has not been shown to improve the chances of children being born with such conditions. This is because most aneuploid fetuses are spontaneously aborted early during pregnancy.

D. The embryos with the pathogenic mutations need to be preserved for future diagnostic test development.
Rationale: There is no medical need to preserve the embryos. DNA from such embryos could be preserved for potential use as positive controls in future studies.

E. Embryos that are carriers for either the deafness or microcephaly mutations can be implanted with their normal counterparts because they would also result in normal children and would improve the chances of successful implantation.
Rationale: Because the number of embryos generated is typically not limiting, there is no pressure to use carrier embryos.

Major points of discussion
■ Differences between Sanger sequencing and high-throughput (Next-Gen) sequencing:
● Sanger sequencing uses irreversible termination of synthesis. At each cycle, fluorescently labeled dideoxynucleotides are mixed with normal, unlabeled deoxynucleotides and are incorporated in a small percentage of extension products, which are irreversibly terminated. The length and color of the various terminated DNA molecules are then determined, and the sequence is derived from these data.
● The principle of the currently most successful Next-Gen sequencing instrument, from Illumina, is based on reversible termination of synthesis. Fluorescently labeled nucleotides are added in each extension cycle. No unlabeled nucleotides are present. Incorporation of specific nucleotides is detected simultaneously based on the color of the hundreds of thousands of extended products corresponding to different sequencing reactions. The fluorescent tag interfering with extension is then removed, and a new cycle of extension begins. The Roche and Applied Biosystems instruments use incorporation of unlabeled single nucleotides added one at a time in successive cycles. Incorporation is detected by coupled photochemistry in the Roche instrument (pyrosequencing) and by pH measurements in the Applied Biosystems instrument.

- Methods of sequence capture:
  - The human genome contains a great deal of noncoding DNA, the roles of which are not clearly established. To limit the cost of clinical testing by sequencing, it is practical to focus on certain segments of the genome that were previously shown to be associated with human disease. Sequence capture is a process that selectively enriches for regions of interest either through PCR-based selective amplification or selective retention based on hybridization between complementary RNA or DNA baits; the DNA library created from the sample can then be analyzed.
  - Site-specific amplification-based methods are more suitable for smaller (e.g., <200 kb) genomic regions, whereas hybridization-based methods are more appropriate for capturing regions in the 100-kb to 100-Mb range.
- *SNP filtering.* Full exome sequencing, depending on the exact capture reagent used and the depth of sequencing applied, can result in identifying 40,000 to 100,000 SNPs in a given sample. The data analysis software allows for filtering the mutations found based on various criteria. The easiest approach simply screens the SNP list generated by the analysis software for known disease-causing mutations. Next, one can focus on mutations in genes that have been previously implicated in disease pathogenesis. Among these mutations, one must prioritize mutations in exon-intron junctions that result in altered splicing, nonsense mutations (introduction of a STOP codon), and nonconserved missense mutations. The latter category is the most problematic. Algorithms have been developed to predict the expected severity of a given missense mutation. These rely on the chemical nature of the amino acid changed, its evolutionary conservation, and its position in the 3D structure of the protein (http://www.gen2phen.org/wiki/tools-predicting-overal-functional-consequences-snps). Such predictions, although generally correct, must be applied with caution for any specific mutation. To assign pathogenicity to a previously unseen missense mutation requires either documenting its higher prevalence in an ethnically matched control population or following its segregation with the disease phenotype in the family. For dominant mutations, which result in a phenotype even in the presence of a single mutant allele, this is difficult because it is rare to have a sufficient number of family members that can be tested. Establishing pathogenicity for loss-of-function mutations is easier. In such cases, both alleles must have the mutation to result in a phenotype. The number of disruptive SNPs that are present in homozygous form is much lower. If one removes genes, such as olfactory receptor genes and genes responsible for the immunologic diversity, only a few such mutations remain to evaluate.
- The World Wide Web is replete with extremely useful websites relating to human genetic diversity and disease-causing mutations. Some of the most important entry points into this web of resources are listed below.
- Online Mendelian Inheritance in Man (OMIM): http://www.ncbi.nlm.nih.gov/omim
  - **UCSC web browser:** http://genome.ucsc.edu
  - **dbSNP database:** http://www.ncbi.nlm.nih.gov/projects/SNP
  - **1000 genome database:** http://www.1000genomes.org
  - **Leiden database:** http://www.dmd.nl
- Next-Gen sequencing will have a profound effect on medicine. It is probable that the availability of this technology in the clinic will result in the generation of hundreds of thousands of datasets. Although screening these datasets for known pathogenic mutations will provide genetic diagnosis for a significant portion of the individuals tested, it will also result in an explosion of disease-causing mutation discovery and, ultimately, better understanding of human biology. This raises important questions about the use of genomic information for improving our analytical abilities by cataloging human genetic diversity while maintaining individual privacy. Additional ethical questions relating to reporting incidental findings must be addressed and continuously reassessed as our understanding of the genetic predictors of human disease improves.[19,21,31]

23. A. Denaturation, digestion, detection.
Rationale: Digestion and detection are not the basic steps in PCR.
B. Denaturation, annealing, amplification.
Rationale: The three steps of PCR include denaturation of DNA to convert it from double-stranded DNA to single-stranded DNA by heating; binding (annealing) of oligonucleotide primers that are complementary to the DNA sequence; and synthesis of the new DNA strands that are complementary to the target DNA strand (amplification).
C. Digestion, annealing, amplification.
Rationale: The PCR reaction does not include DNA digestion.
D. Denaturation, annealing, labeling
Rationale: A standard PCR reaction does not include labeling.
E. Denaturation, annealing, digestion.
Rationale: The PCR reaction does not include DNA digestion.

Major points of discussion
- PCR is a standard method for analyzing DNA and RNA samples in research and clinical laboratories.
- This procedure produces millions of copies of a short segment of DNA through repeated cycles of (1) denaturation, (2) annealing, and (3) amplification.
- It is an alternative to cloning for generating millions of copies of a sequence of DNA. It is extremely sensitive (i.e., allows amplification of minute amounts of target DNA, including DNA from a single cell), rapid, and robust (e.g., can be used with DNA isolated from degraded tissues and formalin-fixed samples).
- PCR (1) is used to generate a sufficient quantity of DNA to perform a test (e.g., sequence analysis, mutation scanning) or (2) may be a test by itself (e.g., allele-specific amplification, trinucleotide repeat quantification).
- A wide variety of PCR approaches are used for specific applications, including RT-PCR and real-time PCR (also called quantitative PCR or qPCR).

24. A. Choose primers that show significant complementarity to each other, especially at the 3' ends.
Rationale: Primers should not show significant complementarity, especially at their 3' ends, to avoid primer-dimer formation.

B. Ensure that the forward and reverse primers have a melting temperature (Tm) that differs by at least 5° C.
Rationale: Primers should, ideally, have a Tm that differs by less than 5°C.
C. Choose primers that are complementary to the same DNA strand.
Rationale: Primers should be complementary to opposite strands. (Note that because DNA sequences are always written in the 5'-to-3' direction, and because DNA strands are antiparallel, each PCR primer, as written, is the "reverse complement" of the strand that it binds.)
D. Choose primers that have a GC content of at least 90% to ensure strong binding.
Rationale: PCR primers should ideally have a GC content in the 60% to 70% range. However, this may vary depending on the target and application.
E. Check that the primers used to amplify genomic human DNA are validated against variant databases (e.g., dbSNP) to avoid primer–binding-site polymorphisms.
Rationale: This should always be done to avoid problems with allelic dropout; in particular, polymorphisms should especially be avoided toward the 3' ends of the primers.

Major points of discussion
- The design of PCR primers to amplify human genomic targets has been simplified with the completion of the human genome project. Commonly available freeware, such as Primer3, which can design primers according to specifications, and Primer-BLAST (http://www.ncbi.nlm.nih.gov/tools/primer-blast/), which is based on this algorithm, can further determine the specificity of the primers.
- Primers are generally chosen to have a melting temperature of between 52°C and 65°C (ideally between 52°C and 58°C), to be 18 to 22 nucleotides in length, and to have a GC content of approximately 60% to 70%.
- The primers should not show self-complementarity, or self-priming; they should also not be complementary to each other, especially at their 3' ends and should, ideally, have a similar Tm.
- The presence of pseudogenes, gene-family members with high homology to the target, and gene duplications can each complicate efforts to design specific primers and may require testing of multiple primer pairs.
- Primer–binding-site polymorphisms, especially at the 3' end of the primer, can result in failure to amplify an allele, with resulting failure to detect any mutation(s) that may be on the same allele. A web-based service to check for this is available from the National Genetics Reference Laboratory (NGRL) at Manchester (www.ngrl.org.uk/Manchester/).[29]

25. A. When setting up a PCR, one should always add a template to the no-DNA control first to avoid accidentally contaminating it.
B. When setting up a PCR, one should add a template to the test samples first, followed by the no-DNA control, and then add the normal and abnormal controls.
Rationale: The template should be added last.
C. When setting up an RT-PCR, in addition to a no-template (i.e., no RNA) control, one should set up a no-RT control for

each RNA sample being tested to test for directly amplifiable RNA.
Rationale: This control is performed to check for directly amplifiable DNA.
D. When setting up a PCR following an RT reaction, one should set up a separate no-template control, in addition to the product of the no-RNA RT reaction.
Rationale: The additional no-template control will distinguish between contamination of the RT step (the additional control will show no contamination) and of the PCR step; both controls will show contamination.
E. The use of deoxyuridine triphosphate (dUTP) in PCR with uracil-*N*-glycosylase to prevent PCR contamination is of no value for RT-PCR because RNA contains uracil.
Rationale: The dUTP with uracil-*N*-glycosylase works well with both DNA-PCR and RT-PCR.

Major points of discussion
- Contamination of PCR reactions can result from carryover contamination of the PCR product, cross-contamination with template, or (especially when dealing with microorganisms) environmental contamination (including from laboratory personnel).
- Physical controls include separate pre- and post-PCR areas with separate sets of instruments. Procedural approaches to minimizing contamination include ultraviolet irradiation of equipment and surfaces, cleaning of surfaces with bleach or other nucleic acid–damaging agents, autoclaving when possible, the use of single-use aliquots of reagents, and the use of disposable containers when possible.
- An enzymatic approach to preventing cross-contamination is the use of dUTP in PCR to partially substitute for thymidine. The resulting double-stranded DNA product will contain uracil and can be treated with uracil-*N*-glycosylase so the PCR product will not be able to act as a template.
- In addition, the use of proper negative controls is necessary to detect contamination. This includes using a template control (or multiple controls when testing for microorganisms), which must always be set up and capped last to maximize the chances of detecting contamination occurring at any time during reaction setup.
- When performing RT-PCR, a no-RT control is needed to detect DNA amplification. In addition, a separate negative control is required for the PCR step to detect DNA contamination occurring at this step. The use of single-tube RT-PCR, whenever possible, obviates this issue.[29]

26a. A. Only a maternal allele is present; this is consistent with a diagnosis of Angelman syndrome.
Rationale: The maternal *SNRPN* allele is methylated.
B. Only the paternal allele is present; this is consistent with a diagnosis of Angelman syndrome.
C. Only the paternal allele is present; this is consistent with Prader-Willi syndrome.
Rationale: Absence of the maternal allele at this locus is the most common cause of Angelman syndrome.
D. Only the maternal allele is present; this is consistent with Prader-Willi syndrome.
Rationale: The maternal *SNRPN* allele is methylated.

E. Only one allele is present. Parental testing to determine the parent of origin of the missing allele will distinguish between Prader-Willi and Angelman syndromes.
Rationale: The absence of a methylated allele at this locus is consistent with Angelman syndrome.

26b. A. Prader-Willi syndrome and Angelman syndrome are caused by different mutations in the same gene.
Rationale: These two clinically distinct conditions are not caused by the same gene; however, the same deletion on chromosome 15 will cause Prader-Willi syndrome when on the paternal allele and Angelman syndrome when on the maternal allele.
B. Inactivating mutations in *UBE3A* will cause Prader-Willi syndrome only if present on the paternal allele.
C. Inactivating mutations in *UBE3A* will cause Prader-Willi syndrome only if present on the maternal allele.
Rationale: Inactivating mutations of *UBE3A* cause Angelman syndrome when present on the maternal allele.
D. Inactivating mutations of *UBE3A* cause Angelman syndrome when present on the maternal allele.
Rationale: *UBE3A* is mainly expressed from the maternal allele. Therefore, inactivating mutations of *UBE3A* causes Angelman syndrome.
E. Inactivating mutations of *UBE3A* cause Angelman syndrome only when present on the paternal allele.
Rationale: The paternal *UBE3A* allele is methylated, and only the maternal allele is expressed. Therefore, only mutations in the maternal allele cause Angelman syndrome.

26c. A. Contrary to classic Mendelian genetics, the parent of origin affects the expression of most genes in higher mammals.
Rationale: There are only a limited number of imprinted loci in the genome.
B. All imprinted loci in placental mammals show expression from only the maternal allele.
C. All imprinted loci in placental mammals show expression from only the paternal allele.
Rationale: Some imprinted loci are paternally imprinted and maternally expressed, whereas others are maternally imprinted and paternally expressed.
D. Most cases of Angelman syndrome and Prader-Willi syndrome are caused by imprinting defects.
Rationale: Although these diseases involve an imprinted locus, most cases result from deletions or uniparental disomy. Primary imprinting defects are rare.
E. Beckwith-Wiedemann syndrome, Russell-Silver syndrome, and transient neonatal diabetes mellitus type 1 are linked to imprinted loci.
Rationale: In addition to Prader-Willi syndrome and Angelman syndrome, these are some conditions that involve imprinted loci.

Major points of discussion
- Genomic imprinting is a form of epigenetic inheritance in which certain loci are marked differently (usually with DNA methylation, but also with histone modifications, and so on) in maternal and paternal alleles, resulting in differential expression of the two alleles. Therefore, the mutation's effect is affected by parent of origin, unlike classic Mendelian inheritance.

- Maternally imprinted genes are paternally expressed, and paternally imprinted genes are maternally expressed.
- The clinically distinct Prader-Willi and Angelman syndromes involve the same locus on 15q11-13; a deletion of this locus on the paternal chromosome causes Prader-Willi syndrome and on the maternal chromosome causes Angelman syndrome.
- The imprinted domain in this locus contains a number of centromeric genes that are paternally expressed and maternally imprinted, and two telomeric genes that are maternally expressed, including *UBE3A*.
- Approximately 70% of cases of Prader-Willi syndrome and Angelman syndrome are caused by a de novo large deletion in this locus: Prader-Willi syndrome in the paternal and Angelman syndrome in the maternal allele. About 25% to 30% of cases of Prader-Willi syndrome are caused by maternal uniparental disomy and 1% to 2% of cases of Angelman syndrome by paternal uniparental disomy. These have a recurrence rate of less than 1%.
- Approximately 1% of cases of Prader-Willi syndrome and 2% to 4% of cases of Angelman syndrome are caused by an imprinting defect. When these are the result of an inherited imprinting center deletion (rare), the recurrence risk in siblings is 50%.
- Approximately 2% to 5% of cases of Angelman syndrome are caused by inactivating mutations of *UBE3A* in a maternal allele; if this mutation is present in the mother, the recurrence risk in siblings is 50%.
- The *SNRPN* promoter is methylated and inactive in the maternal allele and unmethylated and active in the paternal allele; this is the basis for Southern blot testing with a methylation-sensitive enzyme and an *SNRPN* probe, or methylation-specific/-sensitive PCR testing. Additional tests include testing for *UBE3A* mutations and testing for small interstitial deletions of the imprinting center. The latter two are important because of the high recurrence risk in siblings. Less than 1% of cases of Prader-Willi syndrome, but almost 15% to 20% of cases of Angelman's syndrome, have no identifiable molecular cause.
- Other genetic conditions that involve imprinted loci include Beckwith-Wiedemann syndrome, an overgrowth syndrome involving imprinted loci on 11p15.5; Russell-Silver syndrome with growth retardation, relative macrocephaly, and a "triangular face," associated with maternal uniparental disomy of chromosome 7 or hypomethylation of 11p15.5 and/or other imprinted loci; and transient neonatal diabetes mellitus type 1, involving imprinted genes on chromosome 6q24.
- Imprinted loci have been identified on human chromosomes 6, 7, 11, 14, and 15; about 60 imprinted human genes are known.[7,35]

27. A. RNA polymerase I, which synthesizes most messenger RNAs (mRNAs), is recruited to promoters by bound transcription factors.
Rationale: This describes RNA polymerase II.
B. Promoters, which are recognized by RNA polymerase, include the TATA box, usually at the -25 position; the GC box that can function in either orientation; and the CAAT box that is usually located at the -80 position.
Rationale: See Major points of discussion.

C. Enhancers, which are always in close proximity to promoters, increase transcription activity of the associated gene.
Rationale: Enhancers can be anywhere in relation to the transcription start site.
D. Noncoding genes are always transcribed by RNA polymerase II.
Rationale: Noncoding genes may be transcribed by any of the three RNA polymerases.
E. The primary transcript of polypeptide-encoding RNAs often contains introns and exons. Introns are characterized by 5'AG and a 3'GU.
Rationale: They are characterized by 5'GU and a 3'AG.

Major points of discussion

- In eukaryotic cells, three classes of RNA polymerase transcribe most genes. RNA polymerase I is localized to the nucleolus and transcribes ribosomal RNA genes (e.g., 28S, 18S, and 5.8S rRNAs) from a single transcript. RNA polymerase II transcribes all polypeptide-coding genes and some noncoding RNAs, including microRNAs (miRNAs); RNA polymerase III transcribes a few other small RNAs.
- RNA polymerase II recognizes three promoter sites:
  - The TATA box, usually in the -25 position (25 bases upstream of the transcription start site), usually a TATAAA or similar sequence, in genes with restricted expression (either temporal restriction or restriction to a specific cell type).
  - The GC box, usually for housekeeping genes.
  - The CAAT box, usually in the -80 position.
- Primary transcripts of most RNAs have multiple introns. In DNA, introns are characterized by a 5'GT and a 3'AG, which are splice donor and acceptor sites, respectively (GU and AG in RNA, respectively). Adjacent sequences are also highly conserved. In addition, there is a conserved branch site sequence toward the 3' end of the intron, which is situated less than 20 nucleotides from a polypyrimidine tract separated by two bases from the splice acceptor AG. In a minority of cases, the splice donor may be an AU and the acceptor an AC.
- RNA transcripts undergo 5' capping with 7-methylguanine and polyadenylation at the 3' end. The 3' polyadenylation site is usually separated from the stop codon by a sequence of variable length, called the 3'-untranslated region (3'UTR). There may be a sequence upstream of the first translated codon, which is called the 5'UTR. The 3'UTR may contain sequences complementary to one or more miRNAs, which may regulate mRNA translation.
- Polypeptides are encoded by mRNA, with each amino acid encoded by a triplet codon. The first translated codon is invariably an ATG and encodes a methionine. The last coding triplet is followed by one of three stop codons, which are followed by the 3'UTR. This translation takes place on ribosomes.[30]

28. A. Genomic DNA is a better template to evaluate the presence and effect of deep intronic variants, as these are not present in mRNA or complementary DNA (cDNA).
Rationale: Most DNA sequencing tests will miss deep intronic variants, and their effects cannot be easily evaluated. Nonetheless, if deep intronic variants affect splicing, they will show with cDNA sequencing.
B. The smaller a deletion, the more likely it is to be missed by Sanger sequencing after DNA PCR.
Rationale: Large deletions are more likely to be missed by DNA PCR sequencing.
C. Nonsense mutations in the first exon may be missed when performing cDNA sequencing.
Rationale: Nonsense-mediated decay can lead to loss of the mutant transcript.
D. Sequencing of the entire coding region of a gene will identify virtually all significant mutations in a gene.
Rationale: This is not always the case, and deep intronic mutations and large deletions and rearrangements can account for a large percentage of mutations in some genes (e.g., *NF1*).
E. When a missense mutation in a gene known to be associated with a condition is seen in a symptomatic individual, the mutation is most likely to be significant.
Rationale: This is not necessarily true; the identified mutation could be a neutral nonsynonymous variant.

Major points of discussion

- DNA sequencing is considered the gold standard for mutation detection. The most common approach to DNA sequencing (i.e., amplification of the coding sequence of a gene, along with adjacent introns, the 5'UTR and 3'UTR, followed by dideox terminator sequencing), will detect most point mutations in the coding sequencing. as well as splice acceptor and donor site mutations and small insertions and deletions. Heterozygous large deletions, if they span a primer-binding site, will not be detected because of failure to amplify the mutant allele. In addition, rearrangements and deep intronic mutations will not be detected unless specifically sought.
- cDNA sequencing, performed after reverse transcription of RNA, will detect the effect of intronic mutations on the final transcript. However, in addition to the general lability of RNA, cDNA sequencing can only be performed on cells that express the gene. In addition, the phenomenon of "nonsense-mediated decay" should be guarded against. RNAs that have nonsense mutations within the first exon are released early from the ribosome and are degraded, resulting in sequencing of only the normal allele.
- With modern methods, DNA base calling is performed by software. Sequences should be of high quality, and to ensure both sensitivity and specificity, sequencing both strands of each segment is recommended.
- When a missense mutation is found, interpretive reports should indicate the certainty that the mutation is or is not deleterious. The American College of Medical Genetics and Genomics recommends a set of interpretive categories.
- The American College of Medical Genetics and Genomics categories include the following:
  1. Known sequence variation that is a recognized cause of the disorder.
  2. A previously unreported sequence variation that is expected to cause the disorder (e.g., mutations of the initiation codon; splice junctions; frame-shift mutations).
  3. A previously unreported sequence variant that may or may not cause the condition (e.g.,

nonconservative substitution of an evolutionarily conserved residue).

4. A previously unreported variant that is probably not causative of the disease.
5. A previously reported variation that is known not to be causative of the disease.
6. A variation that is not expected to be causative of a disease but is associated with a clinical syndrome in population studies.

■ The sequence variation should be related to a reference sequence in a public database such as GenBank. If available, the reference sequence should be obtained from the National Center for Biotechnology Information Reference Sequence Database.

■ When two variants are found in a gene, it cannot be assumed that they are on separate alleles. Family testing should be recommended. When performing family testing, the risk for detection of unsuspected nonpaternity should be considered.[23]

29. A. Fragile X.
Rationale: Fragile X is caused by a CGG expansion in the 5′-UTR of the *FMR* gene.
B. Friedreich ataxia.
Rationale: Friedreich ataxia is caused by the expansion of GAA repeats in intron 1 of the *FA* gene.
C. Spinocerebellar ataxia type 8 (SCA8).
Rationale: SCA8 is caused by the expansion of CTG repeats in the 5′-UTR of the *SCA8* gene.
D. Myotonic dystrophy.
Rationale: Myotonic dystrophy is caused by the expansion of CTG repeats in the 3′-UTR of the *DM* gene.
E. Huntington disease.
Rationale: Huntington disease is caused by the expansion of CAG repeats in the first exon of the *huntingtin* (*htt*) gene, leading to the expansion of a polyglutamine tract in the huntingtin protein.

Major points of discussion

■ Huntington disease (HD) is a progressive neurodegenerative disorder with midlife onset, characterized by involuntary choreic movements and psychiatric disorders. It affects about 1 in 10,000 individuals. The symptoms result from the selective loss of neurons in the caudate nucleus and putamen.

■ A rapid progressive variant of HD, which presents with rigidity and intellectual decline before the age of 20 years, occurs in about 5% of affected patients.

■ The HD gene is large (11 kb), contains 67 exons, and is on the short arm of chromosome 4 (4p16.3). The encoded protein, huntingtin (htt), consists of 3136 amino acid residues with a molecular weight of 350 kDa. The mutation associated with clinical manifestations of the disease is expansion of an unstable CAG repeat encoding a polyglutamine tract in the first exon of the *htt* gene.

■ The range of repeat length in the unaffected population varies from 6 to 35 repeats.

■ Normal alleles are defined as alleles with no more than 26 CAG repeats.

■ Alleles with 27 to 35 repeats are defined as mutable normal. These alleles have not been convincingly associated with the HD phenotype, but they can be meiotically unstable in sperm, and pathologic expansion of the paternally derived allele in this size range has been described.

■ HD alleles with reduced penetrance are defined as alleles with 36 to 39 CAG repeats.

■ HD alleles with full penetrance are defined as alleles with at least 40 CAG repeats.

■ CAG-repeat expansion mutations account for more than 99% of cases of HD. Therefore, tests that effectively detect and measure the CAG repeat in the *htt* gene have more than 99% sensitivity.

■ With regard to specificity, the absence of HD pathology has not been documented in any individual with an HD allele size of at least 40 repeats who died, disease-free, after living up to or past the normal life expectancy. Thereforc, positive results are 100% specific.[1,16,27]

30a. A. Only one allele is seen on the capillary electrophoresis image. Therefore, this must be from a male.
Rationale: Whereas a normal male will show a single normal allele, this result may also be seen when a woman has two identical alleles or one normal allele and one expanded allele that fails to amplify.
B. The pretest risk for an expansion is higher in a woman with an affected nephew (brother's son).
Rationale: The affected nephew must have inherited the expanded allele from his mother; therefore, this woman will have a risk equal to that of the general population.
C. In a male with mental retardation, the capillary electrophoresis result shown provides strong evidence against fragile X syndrome.
Rationale: More than 99% of fragile X mental retardation is caused by *FMR1* CGG expansions. Although rare cases of mosaicism or other inactivating *FMR1* mutations may be missed by this test, the result shown excludes most cases of fragile X mental retardation in males.
D. In a girl with developmental delay, the capillary electrophoresis alone excludes *FMR1*-associated mental retardation.
Rationale: The result shows only one allele; a full expansion of the second allele, which can be associated with mental retardation in girls, may be missed by this test.
E. In a mother of a boy with developmental delay, the PCR result rules out an *FMR1* expansion as the basis for the child's condition.
Rationale: The woman may have an expansion that is not detected by PCR.

30b. A. The results of the capillary electrophoresis and Southern blot test, taken together, are consistent with a normal male.
Rationale: Both methylated and unmethylated, nonexpanded alleles are seen on the Southern blot analysis, consistent with two X chromosomes (XX female, or XXY male).
B. Southern blot texting is more reliable than PCR in excluding fragile X tremor ataxia syndrome (FXTAS).
Rationale: FXTAS is associated with premutations, which are better assessed by PCR.
C. Southern blot testing is more reliable then PCR in excluding *FMR1*-associated premature ovarian failure.

Rationale: Premature ovarian failure is associated with premutations.

D. The Southern blot test result adds little to the PCR, which is more sensitive and reliable.

Rationale: Large expansions may be missed by PCR. Therefore, the Southern blot test confirms that the woman is not a carrier.

E. In a woman undergoing carrier testing, this result is strong evidence against her carrying a premutation or full mutation.

Rationale: Both the capillary electrophoresis and Southern blot test show normal results. Together, they have a high negative predictive value for *FMR1* repeat expansions.

Major points of discussion

- Fragile X syndrome, the most common inherited cause of mental retardation, is associated with an expansion of a CGG repeat in the 5′-UTR of the *FMR1* gene on chromosome Xq27.3, with resulting hypermethylation, loss of transcription, and absence of the protein in males. All males and many females with a full mutation show developmental delay.

- Definitions: normal alleles (~5 to 44, most commonly 29 or 30, repeats); intermediate or "gray-zone" alleles (~45 to 54 repeats) carry no risk for expansion to full mutations in the next generation, but future generations or distant relatives may have expansions; premutations (~55 to ~200 to 230 repeats) carry an increased risk for expansion to full mutations with maternal transmission; full mutations (>200 or >230 repeats) are usually fully hypermethylated.

- PCR with primers flanking the repeat can measure the number of repeats; very large repeats may fail to amplify. Southern blot analysis following restriction enzyme digestion with two enzymes (one methylation-sensitive) identifies expansions and the methylation status of alleles; this is the gold standard.

- In approximately 40% of women who show a single band by PCR with flanking primers, a "repeat-primed" PCR that binds to the CGG repeats and can detect the presence of expanded alleles that fail to amplify with flanking primers will distinguish between true homozygotes and the rare woman who carries a very large second allele.

- "Size mosaicism," or the presence of alleles of different sizes, occurs most commonly in males with (unmethylated) premutation and (methylated) full-mutation alleles; this can complicate analysis in rare cases. Therefore, a very clean background on the Southern blot test is critically important.

- Women with premutation alleles have an increased risk for premature ovarian failure or early menopause. This does not change the protein sequence and requires transcription of the allele (full mutations are not associated with this risk). This implies RNA toxicity. Similarly, males (and some females) with premutation alleles develop FXTAS during adulthood.

- Prenatal testing is available for this disorder. When testing chorionic villous samples, methylation analysis of the allele, to distinguish premutations from full mutations, can be misleading because of absent/incomplete methylation of extraembryonic tissue.

- The FMRP protein regulates the translation of proteins in polyribosomes and at dendrites. Deregulated translation of proteins in neurons is the basis of the phenotype expressed in this disorder. Some of the targets regulated by FMRP are genes known to be associated with autism spectrum disorder.[22,26]

31. A. CYP2C19.

Rationale: CYP2C19 loss-of-function alleles appear to be associated with higher rates of recurrent cardiovascular events in patients receiving clopidogrel.

B. CYP2D6.

Rationale: Tamoxifen is metabolized by CYP2D6 to the more potent endoxifen.

C. CYP2C9.

D. VKORC1.

Rationale: The clinical pharmacogenetic tests relevant for warfarin use are CYP2C9 and VKORC1.

E. TPMT.

Rationale: TPMT testing is recommended before starting treatment with azathioprine.

Major points of discussion

- Clopidogrel is an antiplatelet agent that is used for secondary prophylaxis of acute neurologic and cardiovascular events (i.e., stroke and myocardial infarction, respectively).

- Clopidogrel is a prodrug and is converted by *CYP2C19* to its active metabolite, which then inhibits the platelet $P2Y_{12}$ (i.e., ADP) receptor.

- *CYP2C19* loss-of-function alleles (e.g., *CYP2C19*2*) appear to be associated with higher rates of recurrent cardiovascular events in patients receiving clopidogrel. If the patient is a poor metabolizer, an alternate $P2Y_{12}$ inhibitor may be indicated.

- Pharmacogenomic testing is not recommended for all patients receiving clopidogrel.

- Testing is recommended when there is recurrent stent thrombosis despite compliance with taking medications and when dual-antiplatelet therapy is otherwise indicated.

32. A. Test for *BCR-ABL1* kinase domain mutations.

Rationale: *BCR-ABL1* kinase domain mutation analysis is recommended when quantitative PCR rises and/or when there is suboptimal response to imatinib.

B. Perform a bone marrow biopsy for pathology and cytogenetics.

Rationale: Bone marrow analysis by pathology and cytogenetics is performed at the time of diagnosis of chronic myelogenous leukemia (CML).

C. Switch the patient to a second-generation tyrosine kinase inhibitor (TKI).

Rationale: The sample at time point 1 has the highest amount of *BCR-ABL1* mRNA, whereas the sample at time point 6 has the least. Therefore, the transcript level has decreased progressively. A second-generation TKI (e.g., dasatinib and nilotinib) is approved for the treatment of imatinib-intolerant or -resistant patients.

D. Repeat this quantitative PCR assay in 3 to 6 months.

Rationale: A major molecular response is defined as a 3-log reduction in transcript level. Monitoring should be repeated in 3 to 6 months using this type of quantitative PCR assay.

E. Consider sending the patient for an urgent allogeneic stem cell transplantation.

Rationale: Allogeneic stem cell transplantation should be considered for patients with imatinib or second-generation TKI resistance.

Major points of discussion

- Real-time quantitative PCR is usually the molecular method of choice for monitoring minimal residual disease for CML.
- In a real-time PCR assay, a positive reaction is detected by accumulation of a fluorescent signal.
- The cycle threshold (Ct) is defined as the number of cycles needed for the fluorescent signal to cross a defined threshold. Therefore, Ct levels are inversely proportional to the amount of target nucleic acid in the sample (i.e., the lower the Ct, the higher the amount of target nucleic acid in the sample).
- A major molecular response (MMR) in CML is a 3-log reduction (i.e., 1000 times) in the level of *BCR-ABL1* transcript. Because each cycle approximately doubles the transcript, an increase in the Ct by approximately 10 cycles ($2^{10} = 1024$) would be approximately a 3-log reduction.
- *BCR-ABL1* kinase domain mutation analysis is recommended both in the case of MMR with increasing quantitative PCR on serial PCR and an increasing quantitative PCR that crosses a defined threshold. It should also be considered if MMR is not achieved.[28]

References

1. American College of Medical Genetics/American Society of Human Genetics: Huntington's Disease Genetic Testing Working Group. Am J Hum Genet 1998;62:1243–1247.
2. American College of Obstetricians and Gynecologists. Committee Opinion No. 486. Update on carrier screening for cystic fibrosis. Obstet Gynecol 2011;117:1028–1031.
3. Anderson P, Al-Chalabi A. Clinical genetics of amyotrophic lateral sclerosis: what do we really know? Nat Rev 2011;7:603–615.
4. Bader P, Willasch A, Klingebiel T. Monitoring of post-transplant remission of childhood malignancies: is there a standard? Bone Marrow Transplant 2008;42(Suppl 2):S31–4.
5. Barber S, Shaw P. Oxidative stress in ALS: key role in motor neuron injury and therapeutic target. Free Radic Biol Med 2010;48:629–641.
6. Boillee S, Vande Velde C, Cleveland D. ALS: a disease of motor neurons and their nonneuronal neighbors. Neuron 2006;52:39–59.
7. Buiting K. Prader-Willi syndrome and Angelman syndrome. Am J Med Genet Part C Semin Med Genet 2010;154C:365–376.
8. Copeland WC. Inherited mitochondrial diseases of DNA replication. Annu Rev Med 2008;59:131–146.
9. DiMauro S, Hirano M. Pathogenesis and treatment of mitochondrial disorders. Adv Exp Med Biol 2009;652:139–170.
10. DiMauro S, Schon E. Mitochondrial DNA mutations in human disease. Am J Med Genet 2001;106:18–26.
11. DiMauro S, Schon E. Mitochondrial respiratory-chain diseases. N Engl J Med 2003;348:2656–2668.
12. Edmond JC. Mitochondrial disorders. Int Ophthalmol Clin 2009;16:1178–1184.
13. Farrell PM, Rosenstein BJ, White TB, et al. Guidelines for diagnosis of cystic fibrosis in newborns through older adults: Cystic Fibrosis Foundation Consensus Report. J Pediatr 2008;153:S4–S14.
14. Greaves L, Reeve A, Taylor R, et al. Mitochondrial DNA and disease. J Pathol 2012;226:274–286.
15. Hirano M, Silvestri G, Blake D, et al. Mitochondrial neurogastrointestinal encephalomyopathy (MNGIE): clinical, biochemical and genetic features of an autosomal recessive mitochondrial disorder. Neurology 1994;44:721–727.
16. Huntington's Disease Collaborative Research Group. A novel gene containing a trinucleotide repeat that is expanded and unstable on Huntington's disease chromosomes. Cell 1993;72:971–983.
17. Kirshnan K, Blackwood J, Reeve A, et al. Detection of mitochondrial DNA variation in human cells. In: Barnes MR, Breen G, eds. Genetic Variation: Methods in Molecular Biology. Totowa, NJ: Humana, 2010:227–257.
18. Lehninger A, Nelson D, Cox M. Principles of Biochemistry. 2nd ed. New York: World Publishers; 1993.
19. Metzker ML. Sequencing technologies: the next generation. Nat Rev Genet 2010;11(1):31–46.
20. Nishino I, Spinazzola A, Hirano M. Thymidine phosphorylase gene mutations in MNGIE, a human mitochondrial disorder. Science 1999;283:689–692.
21. Parla JS, Iossifov I, Grabill I, et al. A comparative analysis of exome capture. Genome Biol 2011;12:R97.
22. Pirozzi F, Tabolacci E, Neri G. The FRAXopathies: definition, overview, and update. Am J Med Genet A 2011;155A:1803–1816.
23. Richards CS, Bale S, Bellissimo DB. et al; Molecular Subcommittee of the ACMG Laboratory Quality Assurance Committee. ACMG recommendations for standards for interpretation and reporting of sequence variations: Revisions 2007. Genet Med 2008;10:294–300.
24. Richards CS, Bradley LA, Amos J, et al. Standards and guidelines for *CFTR* mutation testing. Genet Med 2002;4:379–391.
25. Schon E, Hirano H, DiMauro S. Molecular genetic basis of the mitochondrial encephalomyopathies. In: Schapira AH, DiMauro S (eds). Mitochondrial Disorders in Neurology, Boston: Butterworth Heinemann, 2002:69–113.
26. Sherman S, Pletcher BA, Driscoll DA. Fragile X syndrome: diagnostic and carrier testing. Genet Med 2005;7:584–587.
27. Shoulson I, Young A. Milestones in Huntington disease. Mov Disord 2011;26:1127–1133.
28. Soverini S, Hochhaus A, Nicolini FE, et al. BCR-ABL kinase domain mutation analysis in chronic myeloid leukemia patients treated with tyrosine kinase inhibitors: recommendations from an expert panel on behalf of European LeukemiaNet. Blood 2011;118 (5):1208–1215.
29. Stirling D. Quality control in PCR. Methods Mol Biol 2003;226:21–24.
30. Strachan T, Read A. Human Molecular Genetics. 4th ed. New York: Garland Science, 2011.
31. Su Z, Ning B, Fang H, et al. Next-generation sequencing and its applications in molecular diagnostics. Expert Rev Mol Diagn 2011;11(3):333–343.
32. Suomalainen A, Isohanni P. Mitochondrial DNA depletion syndromes: many genes, common mechanisms. Neuromuscul Disord 2010;20:429–437.
33. Thorburn DR, Dahl HH. Mitochondrial disorders: genetic, counseling, prenatal diagnosis and reproductive options. Am J Med Genet 2001;106:102–114.
34. Tylor RW, Schaefer AM, Barron MJ, et al. The diagnosis of mitochondrial muscle disease. Neuromuscul Disord 2004;14:235–245.
35. Watson MS, Cutting GR, Desnick RJ, et al. Cystic fibrosis population carrier screening: 2004 revision of American College of Medical Genetics mutation panel. Genet Med 2004;6(5):387–391.
36. Weksberg R. Imprinted genes and human disease. Am J Med Genet Part C Semin Med Genet 2010;154C:317–320.

CHAPTER 23

CYTOGENETICS

Vundavalli V. Murty, Vaidehi Jobanputra, Brynn Levy

QUESTIONS

1. Array comparative genomic hybridization (aCGH) or chromosomal microarray analysis (CMA) would yield a normal result for which cytogenetic abnormality?
   A. 46,XY,inv(11)(p13;q21).
   B. 45,XY,der(13;21)(q10;q10),+21.
   C. 47,XY,+mar.
   D. 46,XY,del(7)(q11.2;q11.2).
   E. 46,XY,add(11)(q23).

2. A bone marrow specimen was submitted for cytogenetics analysis from a 3-month-old boy presenting with a white blood cell count of 289,700/μL, a hemoglobin of 6.4 g/dL, and a platelet count of 17,000/μL. The bone marrow aspirate smear was highly cellular with many blasts. Chromosome analysis showed simple karyotypic changes (Figure 23-1, A). The karyotype is described as 46,XY,t(2;19)(q23;q13.4),t(4;11) (q21;q23). Based on the breakpoint at 11q23, fluorescence in situ hybridization (FISH) analysis was performed using a myeloid/lymphoid leukemia (MLL) gene dual-color break-apart probe (Figure 23-1, B). The MLL gene was rearranged with the 4q21 locus, consistent with t(4;11)(q21; q23). Based on this karyotype and FISH analysis, which statement represents the most likely diagnosis and prognosis?
   A. Burkitt lymphoma (BL) with a poor prognosis.
   B. Myelodysplastic syndrome (MDS) with a good prognosis.
   C. Acute lymphoblastic leukemia (ALL) with a poor prognosis.
   D. ALL with a good prognosis.
   E. Acute promyelocytic leukemia (APL) with a good prognosis.

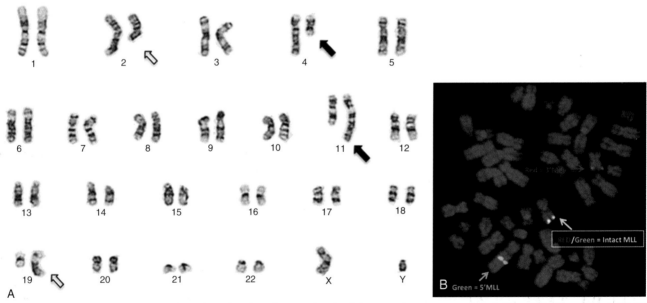

Figure 23-1 **A,** Karyotype showing two balanced translocations. One translocation is between chromosome regions 4q21 and 11q23, resulting in t(4;11) (q21;q23) (*solid arrows*). The second translocation is between chromosome regions 2q23 and 19q13.4, resulting in t(2;19)(q23;q13.4) (*open arrows*). The karyotype is described as 46,XY,t(2;19)(q23;q13.4),t(4;11)(q21;q23). **B,** A metaphase showing FISH hybridization using a dual-color break-apart probe of the myeloid/lymphoid leukemia (*MLL*) gene mapped to 11q23. One copy of the intact *MLL* gene (red+green=yellow) is present and the second copy of *MLL* is rearranged (i.e., separation of green and red).

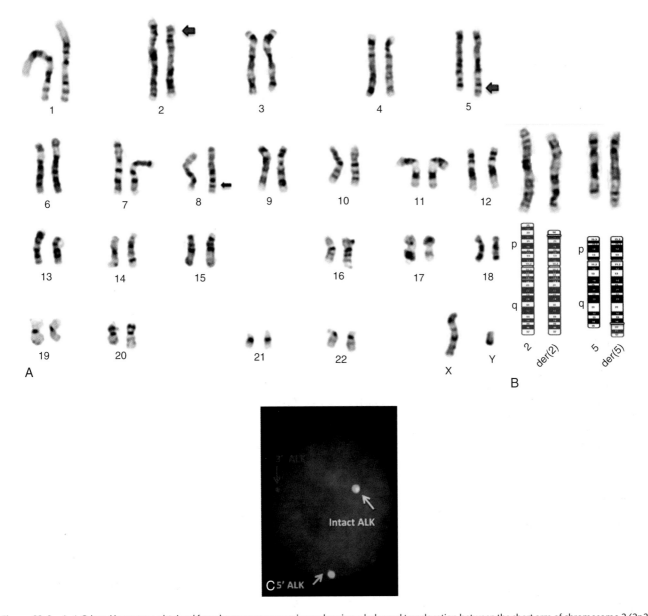

Figure 23-2 **A,** A G-band karyotype obtained from bone marrow specimen showing a balanced translocation between the short arm of chromosome 2 (2p23; map position of anaplastic lymphoma kinase [*ALK*] gene) and the long arm of chromosome 5 (5q35) (*red arrows*). Another abnormality seen, as an addition on 8q24 (*black arrow*). This karyotype is described as 46,XY,t(2;5)(p23;q35),add(8)(q24). **B,** The balanced translocation between chromosome regions 2p23 and 5q35. G-banding (top) and ideogram (bottom) of chromosomes 2 and 5 with normal chromosomes are shown on the left and rearranged chromosomes are shown on the right in each pane. *p,* short arm; *q,* long arm. Chromosome 2 is shown in red and chromosome 5 is in black. The translocation breakpoints on der(2) and der(5) are indicated. **C,** Interphase FISH analysis showing the rearrangement using an ALK break-apart probe. The yellow arrow shows the unrearranged gene. Green and red arrows indicate the rearranged ALK gene as the 3' end is displaced from the 5' end of the gene.

3. A bone marrow sample from a 13-year-old boy was submitted for cytogenetic workup to rule out non-Hodgkin lymphoma (NHL). The bone marrow aspirate showed a marked increase in lymphoid cells with sizes ranging from small to large, containing cleaved nuclei with multiple nucleoli. These abnormal cells had a coarsely reticular to fine chromatin and a small-to-moderate amount of blue-gray agranular cytoplasm. Flow cytometric analysis, after preferential gating for CD45 bright cells, showed a predominant lymphoid population that expresses CD45, CD16/56, CD7, CD13, HLA-DR, CD30, and CD25. No CD43, or surface or cytoplasmic CD3, or αβ or γδ T-cell receptors (TCRs) were identified in these atypical lymphocytes. Chromosome analysis (Figure 23-2, *A*) showed a simple karyotype consisting of a balanced translocation with breakpoints at chromosome regions 2p23 and 5q34, resulting in the t(2;5)(p23;q35) translocation (Figure 23-2, *B*) and an abnormal chromosome 8. FISH analysis using an anaplastic lymphoma kinase (ALK) break-apart probe was positive for rearrangement (Figure 23-2, *C*). Based on the morphologic, flow cytometric, and cytogenetic findings, what is the most likely diagnosis in this case?

A. Natural killer (NK)-cell leukemia and lymphoma.
B. Anaplastic large cell lymphoma (ALCL).
C. Hepatosplenic T-cell lymphoma.
D. T-cell prolymphocytic leukemia (T-PLL).
E. Angioimmunoblastic T-cell lymphoma.

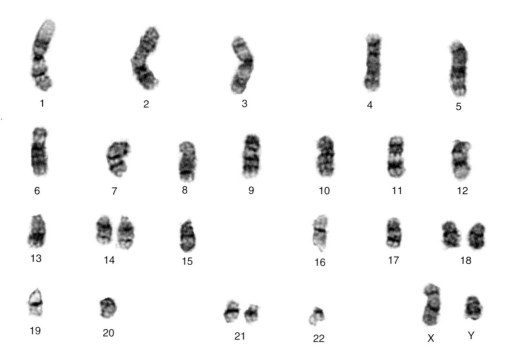

Figure 23-3 Karyotype showing near-haploid chromosomes with loss of one copy of homologues of all autosomes except 14, 18, and 21. This karyotype is described as 27<1N>,XY,+14,+18,+21.

4. A bone marrow specimen from a 6-year-old boy with suspected acute leukemia was submitted for chromosome analysis. Histological examination of the bone marrow biopsy revealed complete replacement of normal cells with small to medium-sized immature blast cells (86%) with high mitotic activity. Flow cytometry analysis of the marrow in the CD45-negative gate showed immature precursor cells positive for CD19, HLA-DR, CD34, CD10, TdT, and CD22. Chromosome analysis showed loss of one copy of most of the autosomes, as shown in the Figure 23-3. This karyotype is described as 27<1 N>,XY,+14, +18,+21. Based on this karyotype, combined with the morphology and flow cytometry findings, which one of the following statements describes the most likely diagnosis and prognosis in this case?

A. BL, predicting a poor prognosis.
B. MDS, predicting a good prognosis.
C. ALL, predicting a poor prognosis.
D. ALL, predicting a good prognosis.
E. APL, predicting a good prognosis.

5. Bone marrow biopsy from a 40-year-old man with acute myeloid leukemia (AML) shows a preponderance of hypergranular promyelocytes and bundles of Auer rods. Which one of the following is the most likely karyotype in his bone marrow metaphase cells?

A. 46,XY,(8;21)(q22;q22).
B. 46,XY,inv(16)(p13q22).
C. 46,XY,t(4;11)(q21;q23).
D. 46,XY,t(15;17)(q24;q21).
E. 46,XY,inv(3)(q21q26).

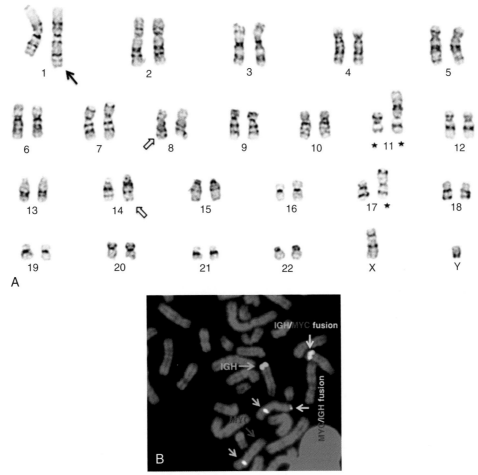

Figure 23-4 **A,** The G-band karyotype of the bone marrow sample shows a translocation between 14q32 (map position of the immunoglobulin heavy chain [*IGH*] gene) and 8q24 (map position of the *MYC* gene), resulting in the reciprocal translocation t(8;14) (*open arrows*). Other abnormalities seen include a trisomy 1q duplication (*solid arrow*) and chromosome 11p, 11q, and 17p abnormalities (*asterisks*). **B,** FISH analysis showing the *IGH/MYC* translocation. Yellow arrow shows rearranged fusion genes, with green arrows indicating a normal *IGH* gene. A normal *MYC* gene (orange) and centromere 8 (aqua) are also shown.

6. A 13-year-old boy presented with a previous history of an autologous hematopoietic stem cell transplant as therapy for BL and currently has a mildly hypocellular bone marrow. Immunohistochemical staining was positive for CD19, negative for CD34, and positive for Epstein-Barr virus. The bone marrow specimen was submitted for cytogenetic workup. Chromosome analysis (Figure 23-4, *A*) showed a complex karyotype that included a translocation between chromosome regions 14q32 and 8q24, resulting in t(8;14), a duplication of 1q, and other structural abnormalities. FISH analysis using an *IGH/MYC* translocation probe confirmed the t(8;14) translocation (Figure 23-4, *B*). Based on this karyotype, what is the most likely diagnosis of this lymphoma?

   A. BL.
   B. Hodgkin disease.
   C. Multiple myeloma.
   D. Mucosa-associated lymphoid tissue (MALT) lymphoma.
   E. Marginal zone lymphoma (MZL).

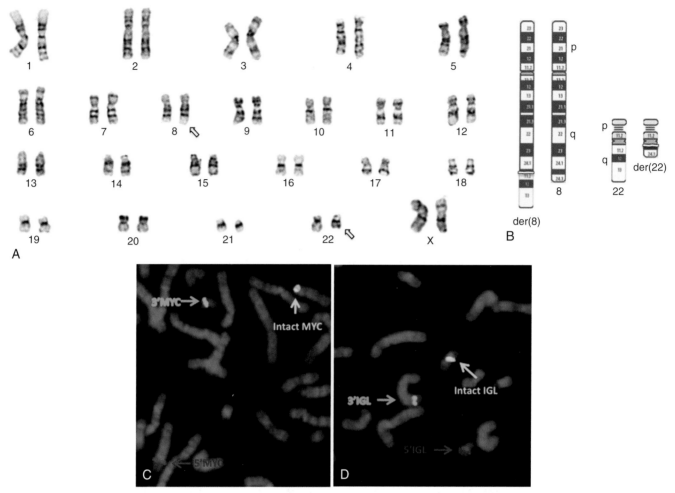

Figure 23-5 **A,** The G-band karyotype of the bone marrow sample showed a translocation between 8q24 (map position of the *MYC* gene) and 22q11.2 (map position of *IGL*, the immunoglobulin λ light chain gene), resulting in a reciprocal t(8;22) translocation (*arrows*). **B,** Ideogram showing the t(8;22)(q24;q11.2) translocation. Normal chromosomes are shown inside and the translocated chromosomes [der(8) and der(22)] outside. p, short arm; q, long arm. **C** and **D,** FISH analysis showing results with the *MYC* (**C**) and *IGL* (**D**) break-apart probes. Yellow arrows show unrearranged genes; green and red arrows indicate rearranged genes.

7. A 66-year-old woman with a history of end-stage renal disease (ESRD) treated with a renal transplant 3 years previously currently presented with acute renal failure and thrombocytopenia. A bone aspirate showed trilinear hematopoiesis with maturation and extensive marrow involvement by abnormal lymphoid cells. Immunohistochemical staining showed that this population was CD20$^+$, CD10$^+$, and CD43$^-$. Flow cytometric analysis of the bone marrow showed the abnormal population to be CD10$^+$, CD19$^+$, CD20$^+$, CD38$^+$, CD5$^-$, sIgM$^+$, and λ-restricted. The bone marrow specimen was submitted for cytogenetic workup. Chromosome analysis (Figure 23-5, *A*) showed a translocation between chromosome regions 8q24 and 22q11.2, resulting in a t(8;22) translocation. FISH analysis using *MYC* and *IGL* break-apart probes were positive (Figure 23-5, *C* and *D*), confirming the t(8;22) translocation. Based on the morphologic, immunohistochemical, flow cytometric, and cytogenetic observations in this case, what is the most likely diagnosis?

   A. BL.
   B. MZL.
   C. Multiple myeloma.
   D. MALT lymphoma.
   E. AML.

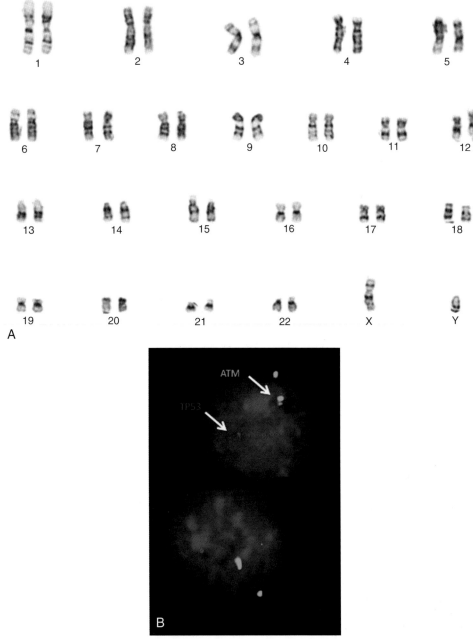

Figure 23-6 **A,** G-banded karyotype showing a normal male karyotype. **B,** Dual-color interphase FISH analysis of *ATM* (11q22) in green and *TP53* (17p13) in red. Loss of one red signal is seen in 55% of the cells analyzed.

8. A blood sample from a patient diagnosed with chronic lymphocytic leukemia (CLL) was submitted for cytogenetic workup. Based on the karyotype and FISH images shown in Figure 23-6, and the corresponding FISH data, which one of the following interpretations is correct regarding the prognosis of CLL in this patient?

A. The karyotype predicts a good prognosis.

B. The two copies of the ataxia-telangiectasia mutated (*ATM*) gene by interphase FISH predict a good prognosis.

C. The G-band karyotype and FISH together do not predict any particular prognosis.

D. Heterozygous deletion of the *TP53* gene predicts a poor prognosis.

E. Heterozygous deletion of the *TP53* gene predicts a good prognosis.

9. What is the best estimate of the incidence of chromosome abnormalities in spontaneous abortions according to recent cytogenetic studies on the products of conception from first-trimester miscarriages?
   A. 10% to 15%.
   B. 15% to 30%.
   C. 30% to 45%.
   D. 60% to 70%.
   E. 75% to 80%.

10. Which statement best describes how cytogenetic analysis routinely identifies chromosomes?
    A. Their specific bar code, the size of the centromere, and the amount of heterochromatin.
    B. The size of the chromosome, the banding pattern, and the length of the telomere.
    C. The length of the telomere, the location of the centromere, and their specific bar code.
    D. The position of the centromere, the size of the chromosome, and the banding pattern.
    E. The location of the heterochromatin, their specific bar code pattern, and the location of the centromere.

11. Which essential amino acid needs to be added to cell culture medium just prior to use?
    A. L-Isoleucine.
    B. L-Lysine.
    C. L-Valine.
    D. L-Leucine.
    E. L-Glutamine.

12. Chromosome analysis, performed on a patient's products of conception (POC), shows 10 cells with a 69,XXY karyotype and 10 cells with a 46,XX karyotype. Which is the most appropriate interpretation of this result?

A. This result indicates a sample mix-up in the laboratory with the POC being triploid and the normal female cells coming from another specimen in the laboratory.
B. The 69,XXY cells are an artifact of tissue culture and the POC contains only normal female cells.
C. The POC has a 69,XXY karyotype and the cells with the 46, XX karyotype are maternal in origin.
D. This is a twin pregnancy: One twin has a 69,XXY karyotype and the other twin has a 46,XX karyotype.
E. This represents true triploidy mosaicism; the fetus has two cell lines (69,XXY and 46,XX).

13. A bone marrow sample from a 53-year-old male patient with a history of anemia, leukocytosis, and thrombocytosis was submitted for cytogenetic workup. Morphologic analysis of a bone marrow core biopsy showed a myeloproliferative neoplasm with myelofibrosis. Flow cytometric analysis showed a phenotype of CD34$^+$, HLA-DR$^+$, CD117$^+$, CD13$^{+/-}$, and CD33$^{+/-}$ in 1% of the nucleated cells. Based on these observations, a diagnosis of a low-grade myeloid neoplasm was rendered. Karyotype analysis identified a deletion of the long arm of chromosome 20 [del(20)(q11.22)] as the sole abnormality (Figure 23-7). Based on the karyotypic change of del(20q), which one of the following interpretations regarding the diagnosis and/or prognosis is correct?
A. Deletion 20q as the sole abnormality is *not* associated with myeloid neoplasms, such as MDS or AML.
B. Deletion 20q as the sole abnormality is associated with MDS and predicts a good prognosis.
C. Deletion 20q as the sole abnormality is diagnostic of a specific subtype of AML and predicts a poor prognosis.
D. Deletion 20q as the sole abnormality predicts a poor prognosis in MDS.
E. Deletion 20q in a complex karyotype predicts a good prognosis in MDS.

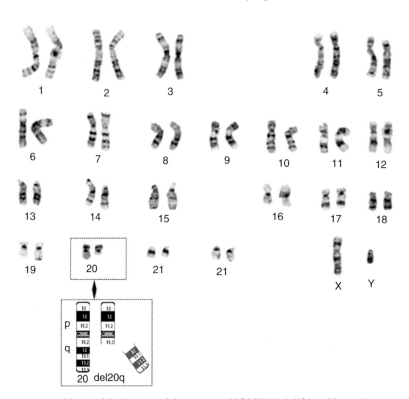

Figure 23-7 G-banded karyotype showing deletion of the long arm of chromosome 20 [del(20)(q1.2)] (small box). Diagrammatic representation of deletion 20q is shown in the larger inset box. The deleted region of 20q is shown as the broken and displaced part in red.

14. During a genetic counseling session, a couple report that a third cousin has Down syndrome. There is no other family history of Down syndrome. Which one of the following statements describes the most likely risk for this couple to have a child with Down syndrome?
   A. Low, because the couple already has six children and none of them have Down syndrome.
   B. High, as most Down syndrome cases are inherited.
   C. The same as the age-related risk of the mother.
   D. High, because the mother of the child with Down syndrome was 22 when the child was born.
   E. Low, because the cousin is on the father's side of the family.

15. A woman has an amniocentesis for prenatal chromosome diagnosis because she is a carrier of a Robertsonian translocation. Her karyotype is 45,XX,der(13;21)(q10;q10). Interphase FISH on the uncultured cells from the amniotic fluid sample shows the following signal pattern in 50 nuclei examined:
   Probe set A: 2 Red, 3 Green
   Probe set B: 2 Aqua, 1 Green, 1 Red
The probe sets (A and B) used for detection of aneuploidy in this FISH assay are as follows:
   Probe set A:
      Locus-specific probe for chromosome 21q22.13 region: Red
      Locus-specific probe for chromosome 13q14 region: Green
   Probe set B:
      Centromeric probe for chromosome 18: Aqua
      Centromeric probe for the X chromosome: Green
      Centromeric probe for the Y chromosome: Red
This observed signal pattern in the cells from the amniotic fluid sample is most consistent with which one of the following karyotypes?
   A. 46,XY.
   B. 45,XY,der(13;21)(q10;q10).
   C. 46,XY,der(13;21)(q10;q10),+21.
   D. 46,XY,der(13;21)(q10;q10),+13.
   E. 46,XY,der(13;21)(q10;q10),+18.

16. A 63-year-old female patient presented with lymphadenopathy. A submandibular lymph node was excised and a portion submitted for cytogenetic workup. Histologically, the lymph node showed scattered lymphoid follicles and increased numbers of large centroblast-like cells. Immunohistochemical staining was positive for CD20, CD79a, and CD10, and negative for cyclin D1 and MUM1. Cytogenetic analysis (Figure 23-8) showed a complex karyotype that included a translocation between chromosome regions 14q32 and 18q21, resulting in t(14;18). Based on the karyotype observation of t(14;18) and the other chromosome changes, what is the most likely diagnosis of this neoplastic disorder?
   A. BL.
   B. HL.
   C. Multiple myeloma.
   D. MALT lymphoma.
   E. Follicular lymphoma (FL).

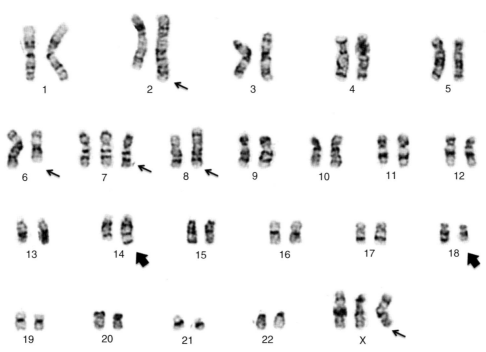

Figure 23-8 The G-band karyotype of the lymph node sample showed a translocation between 14q32 (map position of the immunoglobulin heavy chain (*IGH*) gene) and 18q21 (map position of the *BCL2* gene), resulting in reciprocal translocation t(14;18) (*large arrows*). Other abnormalities seen are trisomy X, 2q triplication, deletion of the long arm of chromosome 6, trisomy 7, and an addition on the short arm of chromosome 8 (*small arrows*).

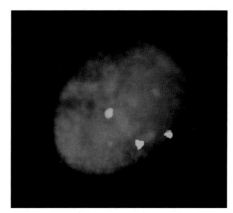

Figure 23-9 Interphase FISH using probes specific for chromosomes X, Y, and 18. The figure shows a representative FISH image from an analysis performed on cells prepared from amniotic fluid. The image shows the FISH signals from a commercial panel of CEP probes for the centromeric regions of chromosomes X, Y, and 18. The X chromosome is represented in green, the Y chromosome in red, and chromosome 18 in aqua.

Figure 23-9 shows a representative FISH image from an analysis performed on cells prepared from amniotic fluid. The image shows the FISH signals from a commercial panel of chromosome enumeration (CEP) for the centromeric regions of chromosomes X, Y, and 18. The X chromosome is represented in green, the Y chromosome in red, and chromosome 18 in aqua.

17a. If all the remaining chromosomes are normal, what is the predicted karyotype based on this hybridization pattern?
   A. 46,XX.
   B. 47,XXY.
   C. 47,XX,+18.
   D. 47,XY,+18.
   E. 46,XY.

17b. What is the correct International System for Human Cytogenetic Nomenclature (ISCN) designation for this image?
   A. ish(DXZ1x1,DYZ3x1,D18Z1 × 2).
   B. 46,XX.ish(CEP-X,CEP-Y)x1,(CEP-18) × 2.
   C. 46. nuc ish(CEP X,Y,18,18).
   D. nuc ish(DXZ1x1,DYZ3x1,D18Z1 × 2).
   E. nuc ish(X,Y,18,18).

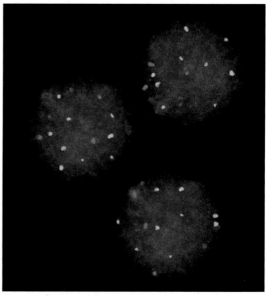

Figure 23-10 The figure shows a representative FISH image from an analysis performed on cells prepared from chorionic villi. The FISH assay used a commercial panel of probes specific for chromosomes 13 (red), 16 (aqua), 18 (purple), 21 (green), and 22 (yellow).

18. Figure 23-10 shows a representative FISH image from an analysis performed on cells prepared from chorionic villi obtained from a 10-week gestational-aged fetus with anomalies observed by ultrasound. The signals correspond to the following chromosomes as follows: chromosome 13 (red), chromosome 16 (aqua), chromosome 18 (purple), chromosome 21 (green), and chromosome 22 (yellow). Which one of the following is the most likely diagnosis based on the observed hybridization pattern?
   A. A fetus with triploidy.
   B. A fetus with tetraploidy.
   C. A fetus with trisomy 13, trisomy 16, trisomy 18, trisomy 21, and trisomy 22.
   D. A fetus with malignant transformation.
   E. Uncertain, because the multiple signals observed are more likely an indication of assay failure. A repeat FISH analysis is indicated.

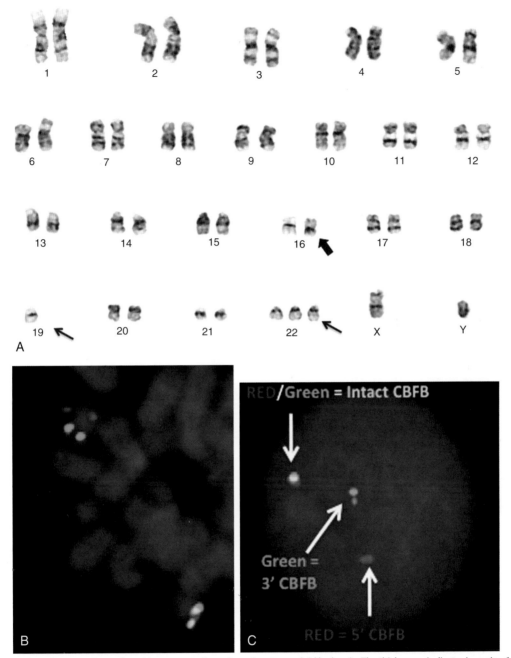

Figure 23-11 **A,** Karyotype from a patient referred for cytogenetic workup of acute myeloid leukemia. The thick arrow indicates inversion 16; the thin arrows indicate monosomy 19 and trisomy 22. **B,** FISH analysis using a dual-color, break-apart probe for core-binding factor beta (*CBFB*), mapped to 16q22. **C,** FISH analysis of the *CBFB* break-apart probe on an interphase cell.

19. A sample from a patient with a suspected myeloid disorder and with an abnormal eosinophil component was submitted for cytogenetic workup. Karyotype analysis identified inv(16) (p13.1q22) (Figure 23-11, *A*). FISH analysis using a core-binding factor subunit β (*CBFB*) break-apart probe showed rearrangement of this gene (Figure 23-11, *B, C*). Based on the karyotypic change of inv(16) and rearrangement of the *CBFB* locus by FISH, which one of the following interpretations regarding diagnosis and prognosis is correct?

A. Inversion 16 and *CBFB* gene rearrangement are *not* diagnostic of any subtype of acute myeloblastic leukemia (AML).

B. Inversion 16 and *CBFB* gene rearrangement are diagnostic of a specific subtype of AML and predict a good prognosis.

C. Inversion 16 and *CBFB* gene rearrangement are diagnostic of a specific subtype of AML and predict a poor prognosis.

D. Inversion 16 and *CBFB* gene rearrangement are diagnostic of a specific subtype of AML, but have no prognostic value.

E. Inversion 16 and *CBFB* gene rearrangement are diagnostic of ALL.

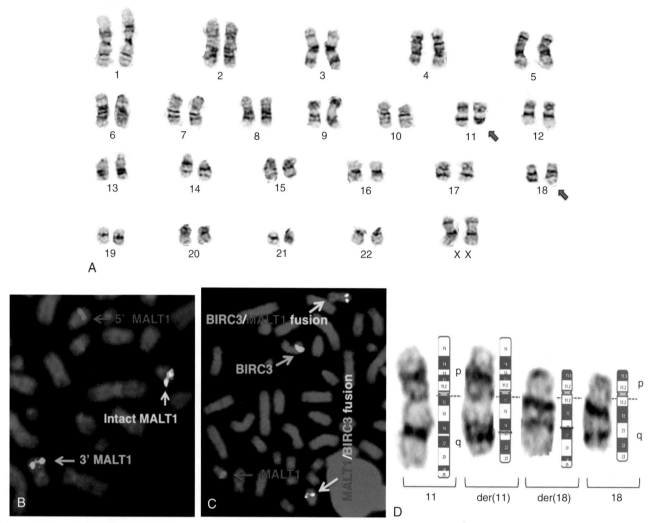

A

Figure 23-12 **A,** The G-band karyotype showing a translocation between 11q21 (map position of the mucosa-associated lymphoid tissue lymphoma translocation gene 1 [*MALT1*]) and 18q21 (the map position of baculoviral IAP repeat containing 3 gene [*BIRC3*]), resulting in the reciprocal translocation t(11;18)(q21;q21) (*arrows*). **B,** FISH analysis using a *MALT1* break-apart probe, which is positive for rearrangement (*red and green arrows*). The yellow arrow shows the intact *MALT1* copy. **C,** FISH analysis using a *MALT1/BIRC3* dual-color, dual-fusion probe, which is positive for the t(11;18)(q21;q21) translocation. Yellow arrows indicate rearranged fusion genes, the red arrow indicates the normal *MALT1* gene, and the green arrow indicates the normal *BIRC3* gene. **D,** G-band (left) and ideogram (right) of chromosomes 11 and 18 illustrate the t(11;18)(q21;q21) translocation. Normal chromosomes 11 (*blue*) and 18 (*red*) are shown at the margins of this panel and the translocated chromosomes (derivative 11 and derivative 18) are shown in the center. *p,* short arm; *q,* long arm. Lines on der(11) and der(18) indicate the translocation breakpoint junctions.

20. A bone marrow specimen was submitted for cytogenetic workup of a 55-year-old woman who presented with a hypercellular bone marrow with trilineage hematopoiesis, along with a focal interstitial lymphoplasmacytic infiltrate. The patient had a previous history of lymphoma of the small bowel. Immunohistochemical stains showed predominantly CD3-positive T cells and rare CD20-positive B cells. Chromosome analysis (Figure 23-12, *A*) showed a translocation between chromosome regions 11q21 and 18q21, resulting in a t(11;18) translocation. FISH analysis, using both a *MALT1* break-apart probe and a *MALT/BIRC3* translocation probe, showed 5% of cells with this rearrangement, thereby confirming the t(11;18) translocation. Based on the karyotype identification of t(11;18) and FISH positivity of *MALT1/BRIC3* rearrangement, what is the most likely diagnosis of this lymphoma?

    A. BL.

    B. HL.

    C. FL.

    D. MALT lymphoma.

    E. Splenic marginal zone lymphoma (SMZL).

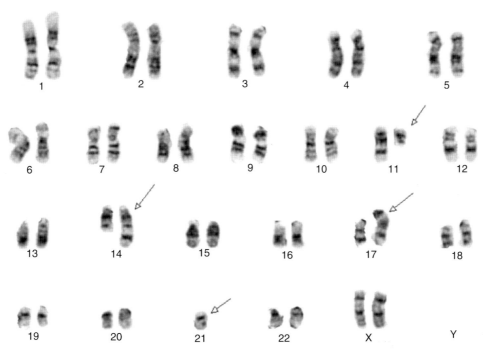

Figure 23-13 G-banded karyotype analysis showing 46,XX,t(11;14)(q13;q32),i(17)(q10),-21. There is a translocation involving breakpoints at 11q13 (the map position of the *cyclin D1* gene) and 14q32 (the map position of the *IHC* gene). The long arrows indicate the 11:14 translocation; the short arrows indicate isochromosome 17 and monosomy 21.

21. A peripheral blood sample from a 72-year-old female patient with lymphocytosis was submitted for cytogenetic workup for a suspected lymphoma. G-banding karyotype analysis was performed (Figure 23-13), which showed a balanced translocation between chromosomes 11q13 and 14q32, an isochromosome of the long arm of chromosome 17, and loss of chromosome 21. The presence of t(11;14) is a characteristic feature of which one of the following types of lymphoma?
   A. BL.
   B. Mantle cell lymphoma.
   C. MZL.
   D. MALT lymphoma.
   E. Diffuse large B-cell lymphoma.

A female child with dysmorphic features, mild mental retardation, a ventricular septal defect, ocular coloboma, preauricular skin tags and pits, and anal atresia has a cytogenetic workup that shows a supernumerary marker chromosome (SMC), 47,XX,+mar (Figure 23-14). Single-nucleotide polymorphism (SNP) microarray analysis is ordered and reveals that the SMC derives from chromosome 22. The extra genomic material appears to be present in a total of four copies, indicating that the SMC is an inversion duplication of the 22p11.2-22q11.21 region, including the *TBX1* gene.

22a. The patient's karyotype and clinical features are most consistent with which one of the following clinical diagnoses?
   A. DiGeorge syndrome.
   B. Cat-eye syndrome.
   C. Angelman syndrome.
   D. Charcot-Marie-Tooth syndrome type 1A.
   E. Beckwith-Wiedemann syndrome.

22b. Precise identification of the origin of marker chromosomes derived from chromosome 22 using commercial centromeric FISH probes is not possible because of which one of the following reasons?
   A. Most markers derived from chromosome 22 are mosaic.
   B. Commercial chromosome 22 probes are not approved by the Food and Drug Administration (FDA).
   C. Chromosomes 14 and 22 share common α-satellite sequences.
   D. There are no commercial probes for chromosome 22.
   E. Most markers derived from chromosome 22 also contain chromosomal sequences from chromosome 18.

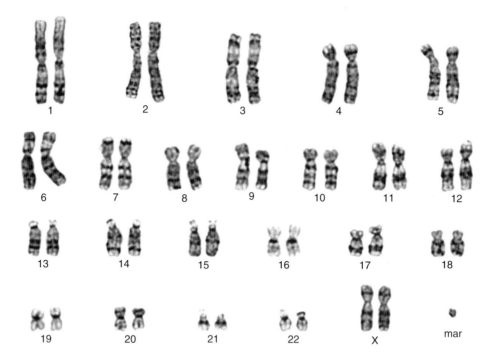

Figure 23-14 Male karyotype showing an SMC. 47,XX,+mar.

An amniocentesis specimen of a 24-year-old woman is found to have a de novo supernumerary marker chromosome (SMC). FISH studies indicate that this marker chromosome is derived from chromosome 15, because the probe for the centromere of chromosome 15 hybridized brightly to the marker chromosome. Results of FISH studies using the small nuclear ribonucleoprotein polypeptide N (*SNRPN*) probe, which hybridizes to the 15q11.2 region, were negative. Additional molecular studies reveal biparental inheritance of the normal chromosome 15 homologues.

23a. Which is the best estimate of the overall risk of an abnormal pregnancy outcome associated with these findings?
  A. Not significantly increased over the background risk of 3% to 4%.
  B. High, because chromosome 15 contains imprinted genes.
  C. Negligible, because there are no imprinted genes on chromosome 15.
  D. High, because the marker chromosome likely resulted from a rescue of a trisomy 15 fetus.
  E. Unclear, because further molecular testing is required before accurate risk assessment can be made.

23b. Which chromosomal characteristic is the most likely cause of the clinical features of the majority of cases of Prader-Willi syndrome (PWS)?
  A. A balanced translocation between the short arms of chromosomes 4 and 5.
  B. An unbalanced translocation that always involves the proximal long arm of chromosome 22.
  C. An insertion of extra chromosomal material into the distal long arm region of chromosome 17.
  D. A duplication of chromosomal material at the proximal region of the long arm of chromosome 7.
  E. A deletion on the proximal region of the long arm of chromosome 15.

24. Which method can best detect a small deletion on the short arm of chromosome 17 associated with Smith-Magenis syndrome (SMS)?
  A. A whole chromosome paint probe specific for chromosome 17.
  B. Spectral karyotyping (SKY) using multicolor chromosome paint probes for all chromosomes.
  C. A locus-specific FISH probe for the commonly deleted region on chromosome 17.
  D. A centromere 17–specific FISH probe.
  E. A subtelomeric probe for the short arm of chromosome 17.

25a. A dysmorphic male child with lissencephaly (i.e., "smooth brain" with pachygyria, incomplete or absent gyration of the cerebrum) has the following karyotype: 46,XY,der(17)t(15;17)(p11.2;p13.3). Which one of the following statements best describes the child's karyotype?
  A. The karyotype shows a balanced translocation between the short arms of chromosomes 15 and 17.
  B. The karyotype shows an unbalanced translocation between the short arms of chromosomes 15 and 17, which results in partial trisomy of 15p and partial monosomy of 17p.
  C. The karyotype shows an unbalanced translocation between the short arms of chromosomes 15 and 17, which results in partial monosomy of 15p and partial trisomy of 17p.
  D. The karyotype shows an unbalanced derivative chromosome 17 resulting from a translocated insertion of short arm material from chromosome 15p at band p13.3 into 17p11.2.
  E. The karyotype shows an unbalanced derivative chromosome 17 resulting from a translocated insertion of short arm material from chromosome 15p at band p11.2 into 17p13.3.

25b. Which clinical diagnosis is most consistent with this patient's karyotype and clinical features?
  A. Sotos syndrome.
  B. SMS.

C. Cri-du-chat syndrome.
D. DiGeorge syndrome.
E. Miller-Dieker syndrome.

25c. Which statement best describes the phenotype associated with the following karyotype: 46,XY,der(17)t(15;17) (p11.2;p13)?

A. A sequence-based mutation because the karyotype is balanced.
B. The missing genetic material from the short arm of chromosome 15 and the extra genetic material from the short arm of chromosome 17.
C. The extra genetic material from the short arm of chromosome 15 and the missing genetic material from the short arm of chromosome 17.
D. Only the missing genetic material from the short arm of chromosome 17.
E. Only the extra genetic material from the short arm of chromosome 15.

26. A bone marrow specimen from an 89-year-old male patient with paraproteinemia was submitted to the cytogenetics laboratory. The findings in the hematopathology laboratory identified CD5-positive cells and κ-restriction of the neoplastic cells. Chromosome analysis performed on the bone marrow showed a complex karyotype with both copies of chromosome 14 rearranged at the 14q32 band, as shown in Figure 23-15, *A*. The karyotype was described as follows:

45, X,–Y,trp(1)(q22q31),add(12)(q13),ins(13:?)(q14;?), t(14;20)(q32;q11.2),add(14)(q32)[10]/46,XY[10].

Based on the cytogenetic breakpoint at 14q32, FISH analysis was performed using a *IGH* dual-color break-apart probe and *IGH* was found to be rearranged, as shown in Figure 23-15, *B*. Based on the results of these analyses, what is the best interpretation?

A. BL.
B. MZL.
C. Multiple myeloma, possibly with good prognosis.
D. Multiple myeloma, possibly with poor prognosis.
E. MALT lymphoma.

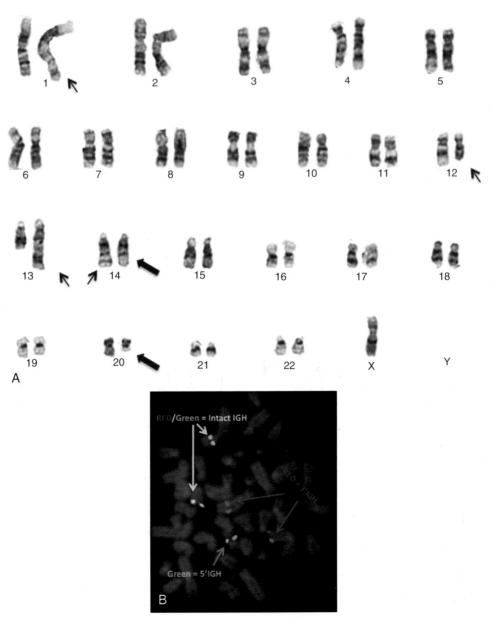

Figure 23-15 **A,** Karyotypic identification of complex clonal chromosome abnormalities, which include a balanced translocation between 14q32 and 20q11.2 [t(14;20)(q32;q11.2)] (*large arrows*). Other karyotypic changes *(small arrows)* include the following: 1q duplication, deletion at 12q15, abnormal 13q, and addition at 14q32. **B,** FISH analysis using a *IGH* dual-color break-apart probe that was positive for rearrangement (*red and green arrows*). The yellow arrows show intact *IGH*. The green and red arrows show the 5′ and 3′ portions of the *IGH* translocation.

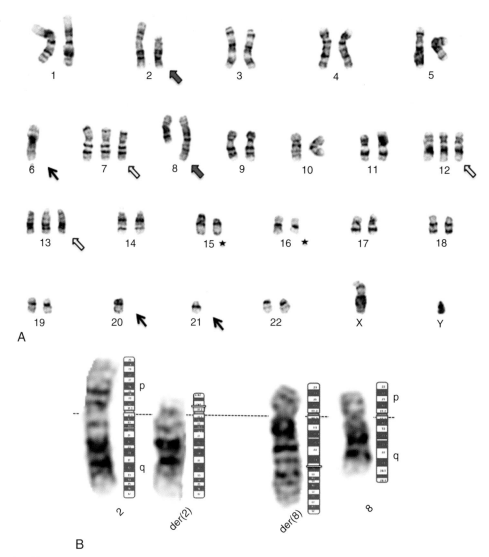

Figure 23-16 **A,** The G-band karyotype of a jejunal biopsy showing complex karyotypic alterations, including a translocation between 8q24 (map position of the *MYC* gene) and 2p11.2 (map position of *IGK*, the immunoglobulin kappa light chain gene), resulting in a reciprocal translocation t(2;8) (*red arrows*). Chromosome gains are shown in the open arrows, losses in black arrows, and deletions by asterisks. **B,** G-banding (left) and ideogram (right) of chromosomes 2 and 8 illustrate the t(2;8)(p11.2;q24) translocation. Normal chromosomes 2 (*red*) and 8 (*blue*) are shown at the margins and the translocated chromosomes (derivative 2 and derivative 8) are shown in the center. *p,* short arm; *q,* long arm. Dotted lines on der(2) and der(8) indicate the translocation breakpoints.

27. A 75-year-old male patient presented with an intestinal obstruction and perforation secondary to the presence of a jejunal mass, which was submitted for cytogenetic workup. Microscopic analysis of the jejunal mass showed a dense and diffuse proliferation of large lymphoid cells spanning the entire thickness of the small bowel wall. Immunohistochemistry showed that these cells were CD20$^+$, CD79a$^+$, CD10$^+$, Bcl6$^+$, CD5$^-$, and MUM1$^-$. The proliferation rate was approximately 70% as determined by Ki-67 immunostaining, and Epstein-Barr virus–encoded small RNA (EBER) was negative by in situ hybridization. Flow cytometric analysis, after preferential gating of CD45 bright cells, showed a κ-restricted B-cell population with the phenotype of CD19$^+$, CD20$^+$, CD10$^+$, cytoplasmic CD79a$^+$, CD34$^-$, CD5$^-$, CD23$^-$, HLA-DR$^+$, CD38$^+$, CD52$^+$, CD43$^{-/+}$, sIgM$^+$. Chromosome analysis (Figure 23-16, *A*) showed a complex karyotype, including a translocation between chromosome regions 8q24 and 2p11.2, resulting in t(2;8), several gains of chromosomes, losses of chromosomes, and deletions of chromosomes. Based on the morphologic, immunohistochemical, flow cytometric, and cytogenetic observation of the t(2;8) translocation associated with a complex karyotype, what is the most likely diagnosis of this neoplasm?

A. High-grade B-cell non-Hodgkin lymphoma (B-NHL).
B. MZL.
C. Multiple myeloma.
D. MALT lymphoma.
E. HL.

28. Which one of the following chromosome abnormalities is associated with a poor prognosis in patients with MDS?
   A. 46,XY,del(5)(q13q33).
   B. 47,XY,+8.
   C. 46,XY,del(20)(q11.2q13.3).
   D. 45,X,-Y.
   E. 46,XY,del(7)(q11.2q36).

29. Deletions of chromosomes 1p and 19q are of diagnostic and prognostic significance in which one of the following types of tumors of the nervous system?
   A. Astrocytomas.
   B. Medulloblastomas.
   C. Meningiomas.
   D. Oligodendrogliomas.
   E. Ependymomas.

30. A right kidney mass obtained after partial nephrectomy from a 55-year-old male patient was submitted for cytogenetic workup. Karyotype analysis showed gains of chromosomes 3, 7, 12, 16, and 17, and loss of the Y chromosome (Figure 23-17). Based on the karyotypic gains of these chromosomes, what is the most likely diagnosis?
   A. Chromophobe-type renal cell carcinoma (RCC).
   B. Renal oncocytoma.
   C. Papillary RCC.
   D. Conventional clear cell RCC.
   E. Renal angiomyolipoma.

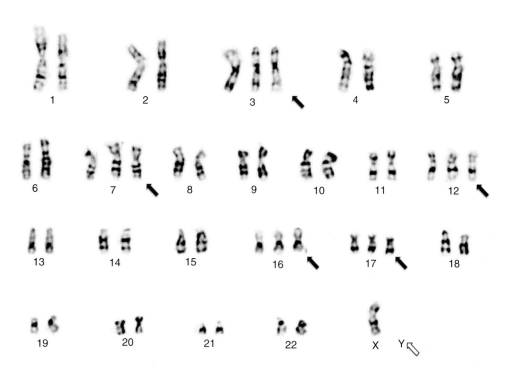

Figure 23-17 Chromosome analysis shows a hyperdiploid karyotype with a gain of chromosomes 3, 7, 12, 16, and 17 (*solid arrows*) and a loss of the Y chromosome (*open arrow*). The karyotype is reported as 50,X,-Y,+3,+7,+12,+16,+17[20].

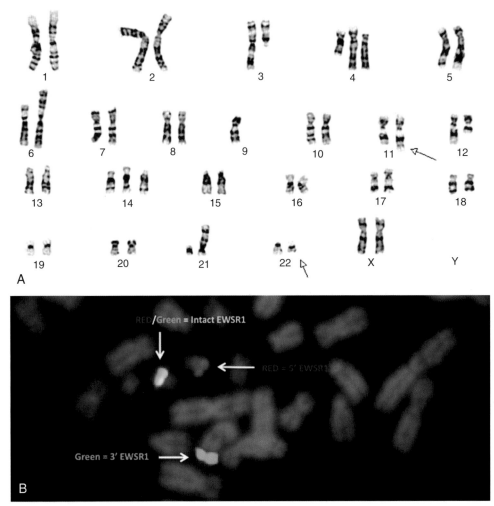

Figure 23-18 **A,** Karyotype showing complex chromosome abnormalities, including a balanced translocation between chromosome regions 11q24 and 22q12, as indicated by the arrows. This translocation is described as t(11;22(q24;q12). **B,** Partial metaphases showing FISH analysis using a dual-color break-apart probe of the EWSR1 gene mapped to 22q12. One copy of the intact gene (red+green=yellow) is present, and the second copy of *EWSR1* is rearranged (i.e., separation of green and red).

31. A 16-year-old girl presented with a right shoulder mass, which was submitted for cytogenetic workup. The findings in surgical pathology identified tumor cells that were positive for CD99, beta-catenin, vimentin, and synaptophysin. Chromosome analysis performed after short-term cell culture showed a highly abnormal karyotype, as shown in Figure 23-18, *A*. Based on the breakpoint at 22q12, FISH analysis was performed using an *EWSR1* dual-color break-apart probe. Based on the karyotype and FISH analysis, what is the most likely diagnosis of this tumor?
    A. Embryonal rhabdomyosarcoma.
    B. Primitive neuroectoderal tumor.
    C. Giant cell tumor of bone.
    D. Lipoma.
    E. Alveolar rhabdomyosarcoma.

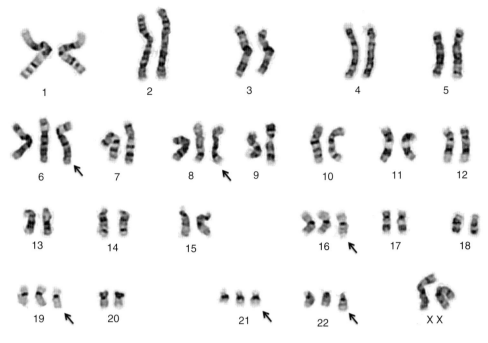

Figure 23-19 Karyotype showing high hyperdiploidy with gain of chromosomes 6, 8, 16, 19, 21, and 22 (indicated by arrows). The karyotype is described as 52,XX,+6,+8,+16,+19,+21,+22[15].

32. A bone marrow specimen from a 10-month-old female infant with persistent fever, but no significant past medical history, and suspicion of acute leukemia, was submitted for chromosome analysis. Histological examination of a bone marrow biopsy revealed complete replacement of normal hematopoietic elements with atypical, small- to medium-sized lymphocytes with irregular nuclear contours, dispersed chromatin, indistinct nucleoli, and little to no cytoplasm. Numerous mitotic figures were seen. Flow cytometric analysis of the marrow after exclusion of the CD45-negative to dim gate, showed a phenotype of $CD19^+$, $CD79a^+$, $CD22^+$, $CD10^+$, $CD20^-$, $CD34^+$ (partial), $CD117^-$, HLA-DR$^+$, $CD43^+$, $CD38^+$, $CD52^+$, and TdT$^+$. Chromosome analysis showed a gain of specific chromosomes (Figure 23-19). This karyotype is described as 52,XX,+6,+8,+16,+19,+21,+22[15]/46,XX[5]. Based on this karyotype, combined with the morphological and flow cytometric findings, which statement best describes the most likely diagnosis and prognosis in this case?

   A. Chronic myeloid leukemia (CML), predicting a poor prognosis.
   B. MDS, predicting a good prognosis.
   C. Pre-B-cell ALL (pre-B ALL), predicting a poor prognosis.
   D. Pre-B ALL, predicting a good prognosis.
   E. AML, predicting a good prognosis.

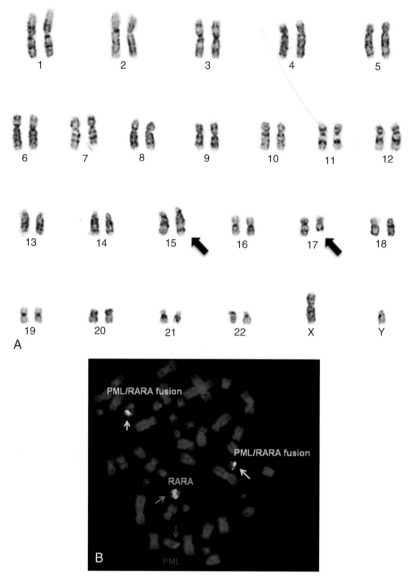

Figure 23-20 **A,** G-banded karyotype showing translocation between 15q22 and 17q21 (*arrows*) resulting in t(15;17)(q22;q21). **B,** FISH analysis using a *PML/RARA* dual-color, dual-fusion probe on a metaphase preparation. The *PML* probe on 15q22 is labeled with an orange fluorochrome and the *RARA* probe on 17q21 is labeled with a green fluorochrome. The hybridization pattern of the two fused signals is shown using yellow arrows (reciprocal translocation between *PML* and *RARA*), suggestive of a rearrangement between chromosomes 15q22 and 17q21. The normal *PML* locus on 15q22 is shown by the red arrow and the normal *RARA* locus is shown by the green arrow.

33. A sample from an 11-year-old boy with a history of easy bruising, pancytopenia, and blasts on peripheral smear was submitted for cytogenetic analysis. The karyotype analysis identified t(15;17)(q22;q21) (Figure 23-20, *A*); FISH analysis using promyelocytic leukemia *(PML)* and retinoic acid receptor alpha *(RARA)* gene probes showed rearrangement between these genes (Figure 23-20, *B*). Based on the karyotypic identification of 46,XY,t(15;17)(q22;q21) and the FISH identification of rearrangement between the *PML* and *RARA* loci, which statement is correct?

A. The t(15;17)(q22;q21) translocation is commonly seen in MDS.
B. The t(15;17)(q22;q21) translocation is diagnostic of CML.
C. The t(15;17)(q22;q21) translocation is diagnostic of APL but does not predict treatment outcome.
D. The chromosomal translocation (15;17)(q22;q21) is *not* associated with acute myelocytic leukemia.
E. The t(15;17)(q22;q21) translocation is diagnostic of APL and predicts a favorable treatment outcome.

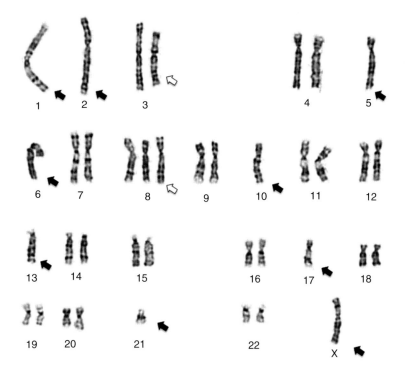

Figure 23-21 Chromosome analysis shows a hypodiploid karyotype with loss of chromosomes 1, 2, 5, 6, 10, 13, 17, 21, and the Y chromosome (*solid arrows*). Open arrows indicate a trisomy 8 and abnormal chromosomes 3 and 8. The karyotype is reported as 38,X,-Y,-1,-2,t(3;8)(p21.3;p12),-5,-6, +8,-10,-13,-17,-21[20].

34. A portion of a kidney mass obtained after radical nephrectomy from a 73-year-old male patient was submitted for cytogenetic workup. Karyotype analysis showed the loss of chromosomes 1, 2, 5, 6, 10, 13, 17, 21, and the Y chromosome (Figure 23-21). In addition, a t(3;8)(p21.3;p12) and trisomy 8 were identified. Based on the karyotypic loss of chromosomes, what is the most likely diagnosis?
   A. Chromophobe-type RCC.
   B. Renal oncocytoma.
   C. Papillary RCC.
   D. Conventional clear cell RCC.
   E. Renal angiomyolipoma.

35. Deletion of the short arm of chromosome 3 is a characteristic finding in which one of the following types of RCC?
   A. Clear cell RCC.
   B. Papillary RCC.
   C. Chromophobe RCC.
   D. Mucinous tubular and spindle cell carcinoma.
   E. Oncocytoma.

36. What is the correct ISCN 2009 nomenclature for a female carrier of a balanced Robertsonian translocation involving chromosomes 13 and 21?
   A. 45,XX,t(13;21)(p10;p10).
   B. 45,XX,der(13;21)(q10;q10).
   C. 46,XX,t(13;21)(p10;q10).
   D. 46,XX,der(13),t(13;21)(p10;p10).
   E. 46,XX,der(13;21)(q10;p10).

37. A solid tumor from a 25-year-old patient shows a translocation (X;18)(p11.2;q11.2). This is a characteristic finding in which setting?
   A. Synovial sarcoma.
   B. Desmoplastic small round cell tumor.
   C. Embryonal rhabdomyosarcoma.
   D. Alveolar rhabdomyosarcoma.
   E. Myxoid liposarcoma.

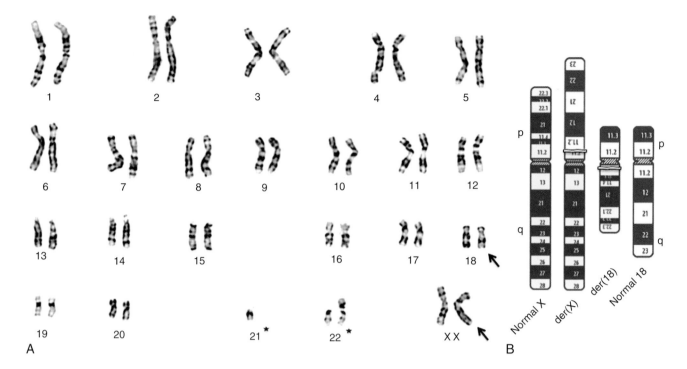

Figure 23-22 **A,** G-band karyotype showing a balanced translocation between chromosome regions Xp11.2 and 18q11.2 (*arrows*). This translocation is described as t(X;18)(p11.2;q11.2). Additional abnormalities seen in this patient are shown by asterisks. **B,** Diagrammatic illustration of t(X;18)(p11.2;q11.2). Normal G-band ideograms of chromosomes X and 18 are shown at the margins, and the derivative chromosomes X and 18 resulting from the t(X;18) translocation are shown in center. *p,* short arm; *q,* long arm. Chromosome X is shown in blue and chromosome 18 in red. Lines on der(X) and der(18) indicate the translocation breakpoints.

38. A lung nodule resection of a metastatic tumor from a 25-year-old female patient was submitted for cytogenetic workup of a soft tissue neoplasm. The findings in surgical pathology identified tumor cells composed of intersecting highly cellular bundles of spindle shaped cells. Immunohistochemical stains were positive for EMA, ESO-1, and PDGFR-β and negative for HMB-45, S100, cytokeratin, HHF35F, and c-*kit*. Chromosome analysis performed after short-term cell culture showed an abnormal karyotype (Figure 23-22, *A*). Based on the breakpoints at Xp11.2 and 18q11.2, including other abnormalities, the karyotype was described as 46,X,t(X;18)(p11.2;q11.2),der(21;22)(q10;q10)[12]/46,XX[8]. Based on the t(X;18) translocation identified by karyotype analysis, which one of the following is the most likely diagnosis?
   A. Embryonal rhabdomyosarcoma.
   B. Alveolar rhabdomyosarcoma.
   C. Primitive neuroectoderal tumor.
   D. Synovial sarcoma.
   E. Myxoid liposarcoma.

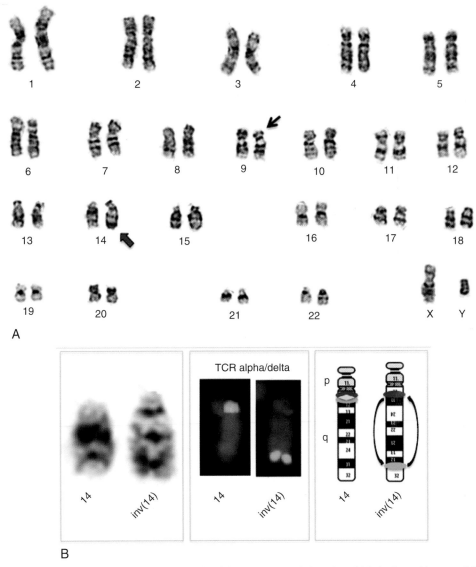

Figure 23-23 **A,** The G-band karyotype obtained from peripheral blood shows a paracentric inversion of 14q (*red arrow*) between 14q11.2 (map position of the TCR α/δ gene) and 14q32 (map position of the T-cell leukemia/lymphoma *1* [*TCL1*] gene) and deletion on short arm of chromosome 9 (*black arrow*). This karyotype is described as 46,XY,del(9)(p22),inv(14)(q11.2q32). **B,** Illustration of the paracentric inversion of the long arm of chromosome 14. G-banded chromosome 14 (*left*), TCR α/δ dual-color break-apart probe rearrangement (*middle*) and ideogram of chromosome 14 (*right*), showing a normal chromosome on the left and the rearranged chromosome on the right in each box. *p*, short arm; *q*, long arm. The fused yellow signal of the left chromosome 14 in the middle box is the normal *TCR α/δ* gene and the separation of red and green on the right chromosome is rearranged. In the right box, the fused red-green signal (i.e., yellow) is normal and the rearrangement results in separation of red from green, as shown in the ideogram. The curved arrows indicate the inversion rearrangement.

39. A peripheral blood sample from a 52-year-old male patient was submitted for cytogenetic workup to rule out lymphoma. Flow cytometric analysis, after preferential gating for CD45 bright cells, showed a predominant population of small CD4+ T cells with the following phenotype: CD3+, CD4+, CD8−, CD2+, CD7+, CD5+, TCR-αβ+, CD43+, CD38+, CD25−, and CD52+. The peripheral blood cells were negative for B-cell markers, myeloid markers, and immaturity markers. Chromosome analysis (Figure 23-23, *A*) showed a simple karyotype consisting of a paracentric inversion of the long arm of chromosome 14, involving regions between q11.2 and q32, resulting in inv(14)(q11.2q32) (Figure 23-23, *B*) and a deletion on the short arm of chromosome 9p22 [del(9)(p22)]. Based on the flow cytometric findings and the cytogenetic observation of inv(14)(q11.2q32), what is the most likely diagnosis of this lymphoma?

  A. BL.
  B. ALCL.
  C. Multiple myeloma.
  D. T-PLL.
  E. HL.

40. Which of the following karyotypes is most likely to be found in a newborn female with multiple congenital abnormalities and dysmorphic features?
  A. 47,XX,+18.
  B. 46,XX,t(7;18)(q21;q21).
  C. 47,XX,+16.
  D. 47,XXX.
  E. 46,XX,inv(9)(p12q13).

41. Which woman is at greatest risk of having a child with trisomy 21 (Down syndrome)?
    A. A 30-year-old woman with a 46,XX karyotype.
    B. A woman with the karyotype 45,XX,t(21;21)(q10;q10).
    C. A woman with no family history of Down syndrome.
    D. A woman with the karyotype 45,XX,t(14;21)(q10;q10).
    E. A 35-year-old woman who had a previous child with trisomy 21.

ANSWERS

1. A. 46,XY,inv(11)(p13;q21).
Rationale: This is an apparently balanced rearrangement. If no gains or losses are detected at the breakpoints, this structural abnormality would be truly balanced and will yield a normal result with aCGH or CMA.
B. 45,XY,der(13;21)(q10;q10),+21.
Rationale: This is an unbalanced karyotype, showing trisomy 21. aCGH or CMA will show a gain of chromosome 21.
C. 47,XY,+mar.
Rationale: Marker chromosomes cannot be identified by banding methods alone. aCGH or CMA will show a gain of a chromosomal region from which this marker is derived if it contains euchromatin. Very small markers with only heterochromatin will show a normal result.
D. 46,XY,del(7)(q11.2;q11.2).
Rationale: This is a deletion on the long arm of chromosome 7. aCGH or CMA will show a loss of this region on chromosome 7.
E. 46,XY,add(11)(q23).
Rationale: This is an unbalanced rearrangement. There is an additional material of unknown origin on the distal long arm of chromosome 11. Because of this additional material, there is also a loss of chromosome material distal to band q23. aCGH or CMA will show a loss of chromosome region distal to 11q23 and a gain of the chromosomal region from which the additional material is derived.

Major points of discussion

- aCGH or CMA is a method used to detect the differences in copy number or dosage of a particular DNA segment between two different DNA samples: the patient sample and the reference DNA sample. This is a rapidly emerging technique in clinical cytogenetics.
- This method is used to detect any unbalanced chromosome abnormalities. Unbalanced abnormalities include gains and losses of (1) entire chromosomes (aneuploidy), (2) small individual segments of DNA that cannot be detected by standard chromosome analysis, (3) extra SMCs, and (4) ring chromosomes. This method is used in both constitutional and cancer cytogenetics.
- Depending on the resolution of the chip (the number of probes or oligonucleotides and the spacing between the probes or oligos across the genome), small deletions or duplications can be identified with detailed information about the genomic region involved: size, base positions, number of genes, and genomic content.
- Truly balanced chromosome rearrangements, such as inversions and balanced translocations, cannot be detected by this method.
- This method has revealed previously unappreciated normal variation in the number of copies of DNA segments known as copy number variants.[60]

2. A. Burkitt lymphoma (BL) with a poor prognosis.
Rationale: t(8;14)(q24;q32), t(8;22)(q24;q11), and t(2;8) (p11;q24) are the characteristic chromosome translocations in BL. The t(4;11) translocation is not seen in BL.
B. Myelodysplastic syndrome (MDS) with a good prognosis.
Rationale: The chromosome changes frequently seen in MDS are del(5q)/monosomy 5, del(7q)/monosomy 7, del(20q)/monosomy 20, and trisomy 8. The t(4;11) translocation is not seen in MDS.
C. Acute lymphoblastic leukemia (ALL) with a poor prognosis.
Rationale: The t(4;11)(q21;q23) translocation and the associated MLL rearrangement are seen in ALL and the prognosis is very poor.
D. ALL with a good prognosis.
Rationale: Although the t(4;11)(q21;q23) translocation and the associated MLL rearrangement are seen in acute lymphoblastic leukemia, this translocation is *not* associated with a good prognosis.
E. Acute promyelocytic leukemia (APL) with a good prognosis.
Rationale: APL is associated with chromosome translocation t(15;17)(q22;q21). The t(4;11) translocation is not seen in APL.

Major points of discussion

- Clonal karyotypic abnormalities are seen in two thirds of all newly diagnosed ALL patients. The chromosome changes involving both number and structure are seen. These include near-haploid, hypodiploid, hyperdiploid, and pseudo-diploid karyotypes.
- The chromosome changes in B-cell ALL play important roles with regard to diagnostic classification and prognosis prediction.
- A major focus concerning the pathogenetic role of chromosomal abnormalities in ALL has centered on the structural changes typical of this disease. The most commonly seen chromosome translocations in ALL are t(12;21)(p13;q22), translocations involving 11q23 with various different chromosomes, t(9;22)(q34;q11.2), and t(1;19)(q23;p13.3).
- The MLL gene at 11q23 is rearranged with multiple chromosome regions in ALL. The most frequent reciprocal translocation are t(4;11)(q21;q23), t(9;11) (p21;q23), t(6;11)(q27;q23), and t(11;19)(q23;p13). Among the MLL rearranged translocations in ALL, t(4;11) is the most common abnormality.
- The t(4;11)(q21;q23) translocation leads to a fusion between the MLL gene and AF4 (AFF1) gene at 4q21, thereby generating an MLL-AFF1 fusion transcript. This translocation is strongly associated with ALL in infants and is also seen in a small proportion of acute myelocytic leukemia cases.

- In general, leukemias with the t(4;11)(q21;q23) translocation exhibit a poor prognosis. In particular, infant ALL patients carrying t(4;11) have a high relapse rate and a poor outcome.[24,51]

3. A. Natural killer (NK)-cell leukemia and lymphoma.
Rationale: No specific chromosome translocation has been identified in NK-cell neoplasms. However, deletions of 6q and 13q are frequently seen.
B. Anaplastic large cell lymphoma (ALCL).
Rationale: The immunophenotype in this case is consistent with an ALCL. A balanced translocation between chromosome regions 2p23 and 5q35 [t(2;5)(p23;q35)], resulting in an *ALK* rearrangement, is a classic feature of ALCL.
C. Hepatosplenic T-cell lymphoma.
Rationale: An isochromosome of the long arm of chromosome 7 [i(7)(q10)] is seen in most cases of hepatosplenic T-cell lymphoma.
D. T-cell prolymphocytic leukemia (T-PLL).
Rationale: The inv(14)(q11.2q32) abnormality is seen in most cases (~65%) of T-PLL.
E. Angioimmunoblastic T-cell lymphoma.
Rationale: The classic cytogenetic feature of angioimmunoblastic T-cell lymphoma is the presence of unrelated clones. Trisomies of chromosomes 3, 5, and X are seen in most cases.

Major points of discussion

- ALCL is a T-cell lymphoma accounting for approximately 3% of adult non-HLs and approximately 5% of childhood lymphomas. ALCL frequently involves both lymph nodes and extranodal sites, including skin, bone, soft tissue, lung, and liver. ALCLs are CD30-positive, presenting with variable morphologic features. Histologically, they present with large or small lymphoid cells with horseshoe-shaped nuclei with multiple nucleoli.
- The most common chromosome translocation in ALCL, in approximately 80% of cases, is a balanced translocation between chromosome regions 2p23 and 5q35.
- The molecular consequence of the t(2;5)(p23;q35) translocation is the fusion of the nucleophosmin (*NPM*) gene at 5q35 with the *ALK* gene at 2p23, resulting in the formation of a chimeric protein with constitutive kinase activity.
- Variant translocations involving *ALK* with other partner genes on chromosomes 1, 2, 3, 17, 19, 22, and X have been reported. Examples include t(1;2)(q21-q25;p23) fusing *ATM* with *TPM3*, t(2;3)(p23;q12) leading to a *TFG-ALK* fusion, inv(2)(p23q35) leading to a *ATIC-ALK* fusion, and t(X;2)(q11;p23) leading to *MSN-ALK* fusion. All of the translocations result in up-regulation of *ALK* expression.
- The *ALK* gene encodes a receptor tyrosine kinase, which is normally silent in lymphoid-lineage cells.
- When *ALK* is rearranged in ALCL cases, it predicts a favorable prognosis, irrespective of the translocation partner, with a 5-year overall survival rate of approximately 80%.
- ALK-negative ALCL exists, which is considered as a different biologic entity from ALK-positive ALCL, and has a poor prognosis.

- The *ALK* gene is also rearranged in non–small cell lung cancer due to paracentric inversion of 2p, resulting in an *ALK/EML4* fusion gene. *ALK* is also amplified in neuroblastoma, and mutations of *ALK* predispose patients to neuroblastoma.[2,34,47]

4. A. BL, predicting a poor prognosis.
Rationale: Specific balanced chromosome translocations, such as t(8;14)(q24;q32), t(8;22)(q24;q11), and t(2;8)(p11;q24,), are the characteristic of BL. A near-haploid karyotype is not seen in BL.
B. MDS, predicting a good prognosis.
Rationale: The chromosome changes frequently seen in MDS are del(5q)/monosomy 5, del(7q)/monosomy 7, del(20q)/monosomy 20, and trisomy 8. A near-haploid karyotype is not seen in MDS.
C. ALL, predicting a poor prognosis.
D. ALL, predicting a good prognosis.
Rationale: A near-haploid karyotype is a characteristic feature of a subset of patients with ALL and is associated with a short complete remission and a poor prognosis.
E. APL, predicting a good prognosis.
Rationale: APL is associated with the following specific chromosome translocation: t(15;17)(q22;q21). A near-haploid karyotype is not seen in APL.

Major points of discussion

- Clonal karyotypic abnormalities are seen in two thirds of all newly diagnosed ALL patients. Changes involving both chromosome number and structure are seen. These include near-haploid, hypodiploid, hyperdiploid, and pseudo-diploid karyotypes.
- The chromosome changes in B-cell ALL play an important role regarding diagnostic classification and prognosis prediction.
- Ploidy groups in ALL represent well-established cytogenetic entities comprising low hyperdiploidy (46 to 49 chromosomes), high hyperdiploidy (51 to 65 chromosomes), near-triploidy (66 to 79 chromosomes), near-tetraploidy (84 to 100 chromosomes), hypodiploidy (45 chromosomes), low hypodiploidy (31 to 39 chromosomes), and near-haploid (25 to 29 chromosomes).
- Each ploidy group predicts chemotherapy responses in ALL. Overall, hyperdiploid ALL groups respond well to standard chemotherapy compared with patients with hypodiploid and near-haploid karyotytes.
- Children with ALL with hypodiploidy karyotypes have a progressively worse outcome with decreasing chromosome numbers, even after treatment with intensive protocols.
- The near-haploid karyotype is rare, and this unique ALL patient group presents more frequently in children than in adults.
- A near-haploid karyotype is defined as having 25 to 29 chromosomes, and the majority of such cases have 26 chromosomes. This chromosome loss is not random. There is a preferential retention of disomy of chromosomes 21, X, Y, 14, and 18, in this order of frequency. Structural chromosome abnormalities are rarely seen in the near-haploid group. A near-haploid clone can also be present along with a hyperdiploid karyotype, as a result of duplication of the near-haploid

karyotype. Distinguishing a hyperdiploidy clone resulting from duplication of near-haploid cells from a true hyperdiploid karyotype is extremely important, given the very different prognostic significance of these two patient groups.

■ Childhood ALL patients with a near-haploid karyotype generally have a short complete remission and a dismal prognosis.[10,24,29]

5. A. 46,XY,(8;21)(q22;q22).
Rationale: Morphologically, the majority of t(8;21)-positive AML patients display Auer rods and dysplastic features of the granulocytes. This translocation results in *RUNX1-RUNX1T1* fusion and is associated with a favorable prognosis.
B. 46,XY,inv(16)(p13q22).
Rationale: AML cases with inv(16) are morphologically classified with a variable number of eosinophils, often with nuclear blebs and Auer rods. This inversion results in a *CBFB/MYH11* fusion and is considered a favorable prognosis marker in AML.
C. 46,XY,t(4;11)(q21;q23).
Rationale: This translocation is strongly associated with ALL. However, this translocation has been described in few cases of AML. AML with t(4;11) is more common in the pediatric population, often in infant leukemias. Characteristic features of AML patients with this translocation include monocytic morphology, leukocytosis, previous chemotherapy, and poor prognosis.
D. 46,XY,t(15;17)(q24;q21).
Rationale: APL is characterized by a preponderance of abnormal promyelocytes with conspicuous granules and bundles of Auer rods. The t(15;17) translocation is considered pathognomonic for APL.
E. 46,XY,inv(3)(q21q26).
Rationale: Inversion of chromosome 3 is associated with dysplastic megakaryocytes and increased platelets. This inversion results in the activation and overexpression of the *EVI1* gene, which has been described as an independent prognostic factor within the intermediate-risk karyotypic group.

Major points of discussion
■ The incidence of acute leukemia is approximately 4/100,000 per year; 70% of these cases are AML. which is more common in adults, and its incidence rises steeply after the age of 55 to 60 years (median age is 70 years).
■ The salient pathologic features of AML include the excessive accumulation of immature myeloid blasts in the bone marrow. This maturation block, a characteristic of acute leukemias, prevents normal hematopoiesis and leads to a lack of differentiated granulocytes, monocytes, thrombocytes, and erythrocytes.
■ The World Health Organization (WHO) classification of AML includes morphologic, immunophenotypic, genetic, and clinical features. Four categories are delineated: (1) AML with recurrent translocations, which include (8;21), (15;17), and 11q23 translocations, and inversion(16)/translocation (16;16); (2) AML with multilineage dysplasia; (3) therapy-related AML (tAML) and myelodysplatic syndromes (tMDS); and (4) AML not otherwise categorized.

■ The classic t(15;17) translocation is a characteristic finding in APL and results in a *PML/RARA* gene fusion. This is an important cytogenetic diagnosis because of its responsiveness to all *trans*-retinoic acid (ATRA) therapy, which promotes differentiation of the leukemic cells.
■ About 20% to 30% of pediatric and 40% to 50% of adult AML patients do not have any cytogenetically identified chromosome abnormality. AML with normal karyotype has been shown to have various genetic abnormalities, which include submicroscopic deletions, duplications, and uniparental disomies (which can be detected by aCGH or SNP array); thus these cases are not normal at the genomic level. Mutation analysis of genes such as *FLT3*, *NPM1*, and *CEBPA* is also used in clinical practice.

6. A. BL.
Rationale: The t(8;14)(q24;q32) translocation, resulting in *MYC* rearrangement with the *IGH* locus, is the characteristic chromosomal translocation in BL. The 1q duplication, as seen in this case, is commonly seen in progressed BL.
B. Hodgkin disease.
Rationale: In contrast to non-HLs, specific chromosome translocations have not been identified in Hodgkin disease.
C. Multiple myeloma.
Rationale: The 14q32 region involving the *IGH* gene is frequently partnered with 11q13 (the *cyclin D1* gene), 4p16 (the *FGFR3* gene), 6p25 (the *cyclin D3* gene), 16q23 (the *MAF* gene), and 20q11 (the *MAFB* gene), thereby forming balanced reciprocal translocations. Other changes frequently seen in multiple myeloma are 11q23 and 6q deletions, 1q duplications, and trisomies of chromosomes 3, 5, 7, 9, 11, 15, 19, and 21.
D. Mucosa-associated lymphoid tissue (MALT) lymphoma.
Rationale: The t(11;18)(q21;q21) balanced chromosome translocation is primarily detected in MALT lymphomas.
E. MZL.
Rationale: The three distinct clinicopathologic subtypes of MZL exhibit no characteristic chromosome changes, although trisomies 3 and 18, 7q deletions, and 14q32 rearrangements with various partners are frequently seen.

Major points of discussion
■ BL is a highly aggressive neoplasm that often presents in extranodal sites or as an acute leukemia. It is composed of monomorphic medium-sized cells with characteristic vacuolization. BL occurs as endemic and sporadic forms. The endemic variant occurs in equatorial Africa, most commonly in children. The sporadic form of BL occurs in both children and young adults throughout the world.
■ The t(8;14)(q24;q32) translocation is a diagnostic feature of BL, which is seen in 75% to 85% of all such cases. This translocation results in juxtaposition of the *IGH* enhancer to the *MYC* oncogene, resulting in the latter's deregulated expression.
■ Variant translocations, such as t(8;22)(q24;q11.2) and t(2;8)(p12;q24), which involve rearrangement of the immunoglobulin light chain genes, *IGL* and *IGK*, respectively, with the *MYC* gene are seen in the remaining 15% to 25% of cases of BL.
■ None of the three types of chromosomal translocations described above are completely specific for BL. These three types of translocations can be seen rarely in almost all histologic subtypes of B-cell lymphomas.

- Secondary chromosome abnormalities are seen in approximately 60% of cases of BL and are sometimes indicators of disease progression. The most frequent structural aberration is a 1q duplication. Other common secondary changes in BL are trisomies 7 and 12.[6,7,42]

7. A. BL.
Rationale: The t(8;22)(q24;q11.2) translocation, resulting in *MYC* rearrangement with the *IGL* locus, is the characteristic chromosome translocation seen in approximately 10% of BL cases.
B. MZL.
Rationale: The three distinct clinicopathologic subtypes of MZL exhibit no particular diagnostic chromosome changes. However, the following can be seen: trisomies 3 and 18, 7q deletions, and 14q32 rearrangements with various partners.
C. Multiple myeloma.
Rationale: The 14q32 region involving the *IGH* gene is frequently partnered with 11p13 (the *cyclin D1* gene), 4p16 (the *FGFR3* gene), 6p25 (the *cyclin D3* gene), 16q23 (the *MAF* gene), and 20q11 (the *MAFB* gene), thereby forming balanced reciprocal translocations. Other changes frequently seen in multiple myeloma are 11q23 and 6q deletions, 1q duplications, and trisomies of chromosomes 3, 5, 7, 9, 11, 15, 19, and 21.
D. MALT lymphoma.
Rationale: The t(11;18)(q21;q21) balanced chromosomal translocation is primarily detected in cases of MALT lymphoma.
E. AML.
Rationale: AML is not associated with t(8;22) translocations. The most frequently identified abnormalities in AML are t(15;17)(q22;q21), t(8;21)(q22;q22), 11q23 rearrangement, and inv(16)(p13q22).

Major points of discussion
- BL is a highly aggressive neoplasm that often presents in extranodal sites or as an acute leukemia. It is composed of monomorphic medium-sized cells with characteristic vacuolization. BL occurs in endemic and sporadic forms. The endemic variant occurs in equatorial Africa, mostly commonly in children. The sporadic type of BL occurs in both children and young adults throughout the world. BL is more common in individuals infected with Epstein-Barr virus (EBV) and is also associated with human immunodeficiency virus (HIV) due to immunosuppression.
- The t(8;14)(q24;q32) translocation is a diagnostic feature of individuals with BL, which is seen in 75% to 85% of all cases.
- Variant translocations, such as t(8;22)(q24;q11.2) and t(2;8)(p12;q24), which involve rearrangement of the *MYC* gene with the immunoglobulin light chain *IGL* and *IGK* genes, respectively, are seen in 15% to 25% of cases of BL. The t(8;22) translocation results in juxtaposition of the *IGL* enhancer with the *MYC* oncogene and thereby deregulates its expression.
- The t(8;22)(q24;q11.2) translocation is not completely specific for BL. It can also be seen, albeit rarely, in almost all histologic subtypes of B-cell lymphomas and in ALL with L3 morphology.
- The t(8;22)(q24;q11.2) translocation occurs in both endemic and sporadic forms of BL.

- There is a molecular heterogeneity in terms of the breakpoints in the *MYC* gene between the t(8;14), t(8;22), and t(2;8) translocations. The *MYC* breakpoints in t(2;8) and t(8;22) are telomeric to *MYC*; in t(8;14), the breakpoint in *MYC* is centromeric.[6,42,61]

8. A. The karyotype (Figure 23-6, *A*) predicts a good prognosis.
Rationale: Standard G-band karyotype with no identifiable chromosome changes is not a useful predictor of prognosis.
B. The two copies of the *ATM* gene by interphase FISH (Figure 23-6, *B*) predict a good prognosis.
Rationale: Disomy of the *ATM* gene is a normal condition and is not indicative of any particular prognosis in CLL.
C. The G-band karyotype (Figure 23-6, *A*) and FISH (Figure 23-6, *B*) together do not predict any particular prognosis.
Rationale: Although a normal karyotype is not predictive of prognosis, deletion of one copy of *TP53* predicts a poor prognosis in CLL.
D. Heterozygous deletion of the *TP53* gene (Figure 23-6, *B*) predicts a poor prognosis.
Rationale: Deletion 17p13 (*TP53*) as a sole abnormality, or in combination with other chromosome aberrations, is associated with an unfavorable clinical outcome.
E. Heterozygous deletion of the *TP53* gene (Figure 26-3, *B*) predicts a good prognosis.
Rationale: Deletion 17p13 (*TP53*) alone, or in combination with deletion of 11q22-23 (*ATM*), is associated with an unfavorable clinical outcome in CLL.

Major points of discussion
- CLL cells harbor characteristic chromosome abnormalities and the changes can often be of diagnostic and prognostic relevance.
- Common recurrent chromosome aberrations in CLL are trisomy 12, deletion 13q14.3 (a likely target of micro RNA genes *miR-16-1* and *miR-15a*), deletion 11q22 (a likely target of the *ATM* gene), and deletion 17p13 (a likely target of the *TP53* gene).
- Specific cytogenetic abnormalities are known to be important independent predictors of prognosis. For example, deletion 13q or monosomy 13 predict a good prognosis. *TP53* (17p13) and *ATM* (11q22) deletions individually, or in combination, predict a poor response to treatment.[3,56,59]

9. A. 10% to 15%.
B. 15% to 30%.
Rationale: These incidences are far too low.
C. 30% to 45%.
Rationale: This incidence is closer to the figures quoted in earlier studies performed in the 1980s that indicated an incidence of 50%.
D. 60% to 70%.
Rationale: Although studies in the 1970s indicated the incidence of chromosome abnormalities in spontaneous abortions to be approximately 50%, more recent studies demonstrated that by selectively using chorionic villi, or by meticulously dissecting out fetal parts, the percentage of cases with abnormal karyotypes increases to 60% to 70%. This is primarily due to a reduction of maternal cell contamination (by meticulous dissection of fetal tissues) as well as improvements in culture success rates.

E. 75% to 80%.
Rationale: This incidence is far too high.

Major points of discussion

- Most chromosome abnormalities lead to fetal loss, with the majority of losses occurring very early in gestation.
- The greater the size of the chromosomal aberration (imbalance), the earlier the fetus is expected to miscarry.
- Between 10% and 15% of all recognized pregnancies end in a spontaneous abortion; of these, approximately 65% to 70% are associated with chromosome abnormalities.
- All autosomal monosomies are lethal and most trisomies lead to early fetal loss.
- Aneuploidy accounts for the largest proportion (>80%) of abnormalities observed in products of conception.
- A 46,XX result may, in some cases, reflect the maternal karyotype as a consequence of maternal cell contamination. This is largely why gender ratios from published studies are skewed to a higher proportion of female karyotypes. The use of SNP microarray analysis for cytogenomic evaluation of miscarriages offers the ability to detect maternal cell contamination as well as provide a higher-resolution analysis for genomic imbalance.[21,40,43]

10. A. Their specific bar code, the size of the centromere, and the amount of heterochromatin.
Rationale: Although the alternating light and dark bands observed on each chromosome appear like a "bar code," the correct term to use is "banding pattern," not "bar code." The centromere size is not distinguishable from one chromosome to the next, and only a few chromosomes have discrete heterochromatic blocks that vary in size in the population.
B. The size of the chromosome, the banding pattern, and the length of the telomere.
Rationale: The actual telomere is a submicroscopic, highly repetitive DNA sequence and, therefore, cannot be observed by light microscopy. The size of the chromosome and the banding pattern are used to uniquely identify each chromosome.
C. The length of the telomere, the location of the centromere, and their specific bar code.
Rationale: Although the alternating light and dark bands observed on each chromosome appear like a bar code, the correct term to use is banding pattern, not bar code. The position of the centromere is a distinguishing feature of a chromosome and is one of the factors used for identifying chromosomes.
D. The position of the centromere, the size of the chromosome, and the banding pattern.
Rationale: The position of the centromere, the size of the chromosome, and the banding pattern are the primary factors used to identify chromosomes. The centromere position of each chromosome is not variable and the size of each chromosome remains constant in relation to all the others. Each chromosome also has a unique banding pattern.
E. The location of the heterochromatin, their specific bar code pattern, and the location of the centromere.
Rationale: Only a few chromosomes have discrete heterochromatic blocks and in all cases, these heterochromatic blocks are located just below the centromere. Although the alternating light and dark bands observed on each chromosome appear like a bar code,

the correct term to use is banding pattern, not bar code. The position of the centromere is a distinguishing feature of a chromosome and is one of the factors used for identifying chromosomes.

Major points of discussion

- When the position of the centromere is located approximately midway between the chromosomal arms, the chromosome is described as a "metacentric" chromosome. The metacentric chromosomes are 1, 3, 16, 19, and 20.
- When the position of the centromere is located off-center, such that there is a distinct difference in the sizes of the chromosomal arms, the chromosome is described as a "submetacentric" chromosome. The submetacentric chromosomes are 2, 4, 5, 6, 7, 8, 9, 10, 11, 12, 17, 18, and X.
- When the position of the centromere is located at the tip of the short arm, such that the long arm comprises almost the entire chromosome, the chromosome is described as an "acrocentric" chromosome. The acrocentric chromosomes typically refer to chromosomes 13, 14, 15, 21, and 22. However, the Y chromosome can also be considered an acrocentric chromosome.
- The chromosomes that have large heterochromatic blocks are 1, 9, 16, and Y. These blocks are composed of large arrays of tandemly repeated DNA elements. Evolutionary processes acting on these DNA blocks played a role in expansion of arrays within a particular chromosomal location. As a result, the size of these blocks became polymorphic and size variations between individuals are routinely observed. The size of the heterochromatic blocks tends to be inherited in a stable manner and, therefore, is identical to the parent from which the individual has inherited the chromosome.
- GTG (**G** bands produced with **t**rypsin using **G**iemsa) banding is the most widely used staining method for producing the characteristic G bands that are used to identify each chromosome uniquely.
- C-banding stains constitutive heterochromatin around the centromeres and the large heterochromatic regions found on chromosomes 1, 9, 16, and Y. CBG (**C** bands produced with **b**arium hydroxide using **G**iemsa) banding is a common technique for producing C bands.
- Telomeres serve to stabilize chromosome ends and are composed of repeating units of the $(TTAGG)^n$ DNA sequence.[4,39,54]

11. A. L-Isoleucine.
Rationale: Isoleucine is a stable amino acid that can be added to the culture medium when it is being formulated.
B. L-Lysine.
Rationale: Lysine is a stable amino acid that can be added to the culture medium when it is being formulated.
C. L-Valine.
Rationale: Valine is a stable amino acid that can be added to the culture medium when it is being formulated.
D. L-Leucine.
Rationale: Leucine is a stable amino acid that can be added to the culture medium when it is being formulated.
E. L-Glutamine.
Rationale: L-Glutamine is unstable and breaks down on storage to D-glutamine, a form that cannot be used by cells.

ʟ-Glutamine may be kept frozen to retain its stability and should only be added to culture medium just prior to use.

Major points of discussion

- Cell culture medium contains all the necessary factors required for growth of cells targeted for cytogenetic analysis.
- Cell culture medium should be constantly monitored for sterility. Most commercial media contain a pH indicator, phenol red, which changes color when contamination is present.
- Antibiotics and antifungal agents are typically added to control growth of bacterial/fungal contaminants.
- Serum (typically fetal bovine serum) contains growth factors required for cell viability and proliferation.
- Typical cytogenetic growth media contain buffered solution with phenol red, sugars, amino acids, ions, and supplements (serum, antibiotics, antifungal agents, ʟ-glutamine).[4,35]

12. A. This result indicates a sample mix-up in the laboratory with the POC being triploid and the normal female cells coming from another specimen in the laboratory.
Rationale: Sample mix-ups can be seen in clinical laboratories; however, the mixing of samples is not common.
B. The 69,XXY cells are an artifact of tissue culture and the POC contains only normal female cells.
Rationale: Cells with a 69,XXY karyotype are not artifacts of tissue culture. Triploidy is found in approximately 2% of spontaneous abortions.
C. The POC has a 69,XXY karyotype and the cells with the 46,XX karyotype are maternal in origin.
Rationale: Overgrowth of maternal cells in culture is common from abortion/miscarriage specimens. Chromosome analysis from these specimens requires diligent cleaning away of adherent maternal tissue.
D. This is a twin pregnancy: One twin has a 69,XXY karyotype and the other twin has a 46,XX karyotype.
Rationale: This is a possibility; however, overgrowth of maternal cells in culture is the most likely scenario.
E. This represents true triploidy mosaicism; the fetus has two cell lines (69,XXY and 46,XX).
Rationale: This is a possibility; however, true triploid mosaicism is very rare and very few cases are described in the literature.

Major points of discussion

- Triploidy is found in approximately 2% of spontaneous abortions. Most triploid pregnancies are lost early in pregnancy.
- Triploidy could be diandry (two copies of the paternal genome) or digyny (two copies of the maternal genome).
- Diandry usually results from dispermy; that is, two sperm fertilizing the oocyte. In rare instances, diandry results from a complete nondisjunction in the sperm that fertilizes the oocyte. Digyny results from complete nondisjunction in the first or second meiotic division of the oocyte.
- Most diandric triploid fetuses spontaneously abort in the first trimester. The very few that survive the second trimester are partial hydatidifrom moles. Digynic triploids spontaneously abort early in the first trimester.

- There is one case report of a digynic triploid (69,XXX) coexisting with a normal twin (46,XY); however, this is very rare.
- Intrauterine survival into the third trimester is possible in cases of fetal-placental discordance; that is, the placenta is diploid and the fetus is triploid. However, this is almost invariably associated with perinatal death. Rare instances of survival for more than 1 month are known.[20,23,31]

13. A. Deletion 20q as the sole abnormality is *not* associated with myeloid neoplasms, such as MDS or AML.
Rationale: Deletion 20q as an isolated abnormality is a common recurring change in a spectrum of myeloid malignancies, such as MDS and AML.
B. Deletion 20q as the sole abnormality is associated with MDS and predicts a good prognosis.
Rationale: Deletion 20q is seen in 5% to 7% of cases of both isolated MDS and treatment-related MDS. The International Prognosis Scoring System (IPSS) classified deletion 20q as a favorable prognostic marker when it occurs as an isolated abnormality in cases of MDS.
C. Deletion 20q as the sole abnormality is diagnostic of a specific subtype of AML and predicts a poor prognosis.
Rationale: Deletion 20q is not specific to any particular FAB subtype of AML and, as an isolated abnormality, is seen in less than 1% of AML patients. In this setting, it is not a favorable cytogenetic change, as it is in MDS.
D. Deletion 20q as the sole abnormality predicts a poor prognosis in MDS.
Rationale: According to the IPSS, deletion 20q as an isolated abnormality predicts good prognosis.
E. Deletion 20q in a complex karyotype predicts a good prognosis in MDS.
Rationale: Deletion 20q in the setting of a complex karyotype is of less favorable prognostic value.

Major points of discussion

- A deletion of the long arm of chromosome 20, del(20q), is a common recurring cytogenetic abnormality in a wide variety of malignant myeloid disorders, such as MDS, AML, and myeloproliferative neoplasms.
- Deletion 20q as an isolated abnormality is seen in 5% to 7% of cases of isolated MDS and treatment-related MDS. Isolated 20q deletion is associated with a favorable outcome in MDS according to the IPSS. When deletion of 20q is the sole abnormality in MDS patients, it predicts a low risk for progression to AML and these patients have a prolonged survival.
- When MDS patients carry del(20q) as a part of a more complex karyotype, they are at risk for a poor outcome.
- Deletion 20q is also found in 1% to 2% of all cases of AML, and very few AML patients carry this as the sole chromosome change. However, deletion 20q is not specific for any particular FAB subtype of AML. In addition, the prognostic impact of del(20q) as a single chromosomal abnormality in AML is unclear.
- Deletion 20q is frequently associated with other chromosome changes in MDS and AML patients, such as del(5q), trisomy 8, and trisomy 21.[9,25,27]

14. A. Low, because the couple already has six children and none of them have Down syndrome.
Rationale: The absence of Down syndrome in multiple prior pregnancies diminishes the likelihood of inherited forms of Down syndrome due to familial balanced rearrangements. It does not diminish the risk for the most common mechanism (nondisjunction leading to simple trisomy of chromosome 21). The risk for nondisjunction increases with maternal age and the risk for this couple would actually be higher than for any of their previous pregnancies, simply because the mother is older.
B. High, as most Down syndrome cases are inherited.
Rationale: Most cases of Down syndrome (~95%) are *not* inherited and are due to nondisjunction leading to simple trisomy of chromosome 21.
C. The same as the age-related risk of the mother.
Rationale: The absence of Down syndrome in multiple prior pregnancies diminishes the likelihood of inherited forms of Down syndrome due to familial balanced rearrangements. It does not diminish the risk for the most common mechanism (nondisjunction leading to simple trisomy of chromosome 21). The risk for nondisjunction increases with maternal age and the risk for this couple would be equal to the mother's age-related risk.
D. High, because the mother of the child with Down syndrome was 22 when the child was born.
Rationale: Although the risk of having a child with Down syndrome increases with maternal age, Down syndrome children are still born to younger mothers.
E. Low, because the cousin is on the father's side of the family.
Rationale: The risk of a familial form of Down syndrome (i.e., translocation) is not influenced by which side of the family the index case occurred.

Major points of discussion
- In 1959, Down syndrome was the first medical condition shown to be caused by a chromosome abnormality.
- Down syndrome is recognized as the most common single known cause of intellectual disability.
- Down syndrome has the highest incidence at birth of any chromosome abnormality.
- The majority of Down syndrome is due to nondisjunction leading to trisomy of chromosome 21.
- The majority (~90%) of nondisjunction events reflect maternal meiotic errors.
- Approximately 75% of maternal meiotic errors occur at meiosis I and the remainder at meiosis II.[21,38,54]

15. A. 46,XY.
Rationale: This answer corresponds to the karytoype of a normal male fetus. The signal pattern with this karyotype would be:
   Probe set A: 2 red, 2 green
   Probe set B: 2 aqua, 1 green, 1 red
B. 45,XY,der(13;21)(q10;q10).
Rationale: This karytoype indicates a male fetus with a Robertsonian translocation. The signal pattern with this karyotype would be:
   Probe set A: 2 red, 2 green
   Probe set B: 2 aqua, 1 green, 1 red
C. 46,XY,der(13;21)(q10;q10),+21.
Rationale: This karyotype indicates a male fetus with a Robertsonian translocation and trisomy 21. The signal pattern with this karyotype would be:

   Probe set A: 3 red, 2 green
   Probe set B: 2 aqua, 1 green, 1 red
D. 46,XY,der(13;21)(q10;q10),+13.
Rationale: The observed signal pattern is consistent with this karyotype.
E. 46,XY,der(13;21)(q10;q10),+18.
Rationale: This karyotype indicates a male fetus with a Robertsonian translocation and trisomy 18. The signal pattern with this karyotype would be:
   Probe set A: 2 red, 2 green
   Probe set B: 3 aqua, 1 green, 1 red

Major points of discussion
- These probe sets detect the most common chromosome aneuploidies (trisomy for chromosomes 13, 21, and 18 and sex chromosome aneuploidies) that can result in a live birth.
- Interphase FISH using this probe set is routinely used for rapid detection of aneuploidies in prenatal samples. However, this probe set provides limited information.
- This probe set will not detect aneuploidies of chromosomes other than those of 13, 21, 18, X, and Y. Structural abnormalities can also not be detected because the probes are specific for either the centromeric regions or a particular locus on the chromosome.
- A full chromosome study is required to distinguish structural rearrangements; for example, the karyotypes described in choices A and B will have the same signal pattern. However, from this signal pattern, it cannot be discerned whether the fetus has a normal karyotype (46,XY) or is a carrier of a Robertsonian translocation 45, XY,der(13;21)(q10;q10).
- Karyotyping from cultured cells is required for a full chromosome study.[60]

16. A. BL.
Rationale: t(8;14)(q24;q32), t(8;22)(q24;q11), and t(2;8)(p11;q24) are the characteristic chromosome translocations in BL.
B. HL.
Rationale: In contrast to non-HLs, specific chromosome translocations have not been identified in HL.
C. Multiple myeloma.
Rationale: Both structural and numerical chromosome changes are seen in multiple myeloma. The 14q32 region involving the *IGH* gene is frequently partnered with 11q13 (the *cyclin D1* gene), 4p16 (the *FGFR3* gene), 6p25 (the *cyclin D3* gene), 16q23 (the *MAF* gene), and 20q11 (the *MAFB* gene), thereby forming balanced reciprocal translocations. Other changes frequently seen in multiple myeloma are 11q23 deletions, 6q deletions, 1q duplications, and trisomies of chromosomes 3, 5, 7, 9, 11, 15, 19, and 21.
D. MALT lymphoma.
Rationale: The t(11;18)(q21;q21) balanced chromosome translocation is primarily detected in MALT lymphoma.
E. Follicular lymphoma (FL).
Rationale: t(14;18)(q32;q21) is a characteristic feature of FL and is used as a diagnostic marker for this type of lymphoma. Other frequently seen chromosome changes in high-grade FL are deletion of 6q and trisomies of chromosomes 7, 12, and X.

Major points of discussion

- FL is a neoplasm resembling the B cells in the follicle center. Approximately 70% to 80% of FLs are characterized by the presence of a translocation between chromosomes 14 and 18 [t(14;18)(q32)]. The t(14;18) translocation results in juxtaposition of the *BCL2* gene at 18q21 with the *IHC* locus at 14q32; as a result, the *BCL2* gene is overexpressed. Rarely, 18q21 is translocated with the *ILC* gene loci at 2p12 and 22q11.
- The t(14;18)(q32;q21) translocation is a diagnostic feature of FL.
- In addition to t(14;18), other secondary chromosome alterations, such as deletions on 6q, 17p, 1p36, trisomy 7, and translocations involving 3q27 (the *BCL6* gene), are also seen in FL.
- Secondary chromosome abnormalities are sometimes indicators of disease progression, transformation to diffuse large B-cell lymphoma, or prognosis. For example, trisomy 7 and 6q and 17p deletions are associated with morphologic progression. Tumors with the 3q27 rearrangement can progress to FL. The 6q and 1p36 deletions are associated with an unfavorable outcome.[3,56,59]

17a. A. 46,XX.
Rationale: The 46,XX karyotype reflects a normal female karyotype. However, the hybridization pattern shows one green and one red signal corresponding to a male chromosome composition.
B. 47,XXY.
Rationale: The 47,XYY karyotype is for a male who has two X chromosomes and a single Y chromosome, which is consistent with a clinical diagnosis of Klinefelter syndrome. The hybridization pattern shows one green and one red signal corresponding to one copy of the X chromosome and one copy of the Y chromosome.
C. 47,XX,+18.
Rationale: The 47,XX,+18 karyotype indicates a female with an extra copy of chromosome 18; that is, trisomy 18. The hybridization pattern shows one green, one red, and two aqua signals corresponding to one copy of the X chromosome, one copy of the Y chromosome, and two copies of chromosome 18.
D. 47,XY,+18.
Rationale: The 47,XY,+18 karyotype indicates a male with an extra copy of chromosome 18; that is, trisomy 18. The hybridization pattern shows one green, one red, and two aqua signals corresponding to one copy of the X chromosome, one copy of the Y chromosome, and two copies of chromosome 18.
E. 46,XY.
Rationale: The 46,XY karyotype reflects a normal male karyotype. If all the remaining chromosomes are normal, the expected hybridization pattern for the probes indicated above should be one green, one red, and two aqua signals corresponding to one copy of the X chromosome, one copy of the Y chromosome, and two copies of chromosome 18.

17b. A. ish(DXZ1x1,DYZ3x1,D18Z1 × 2).
Rationale: "nuc ish" is always used for describing FISH results on interphase nuclei.

B. 46,XX.ish(CEP-X,CEP-Y)x1,(CEP-18) × 2.
Rationale: 46,XX.ish indicates that FISH has been performed on a metaphase spread. Probe results from the same hybridization are described in the same set of parentheses and not separately. The hybridization pattern in Figure 23-10 is also consistent with a male, not a female.
C. 46. nuc ish(CEP X,Y,18,18).
Rationale: Interphase FISH results do not indicate predicted chromosome number (unless traditional karyotyping has simultaneously been performed). Interphase FISH results should indicate the number of signals for each probe.
D. nuc ish(DXZ1x1,DYZ3x1,D18Z1 × 2).
Rationale: Interphase FISH results are designated by "nuc ish" followed by the number of signals for each probe. Probe results from the same hybridization are described in the same set of parentheses.
E. nuc ish(X,Y,18,18).
Rationale: Interphase FISH results should indicate the number of signals for each probe.

Major points of discussion

- Information of interest is designated by the symbol "nuc ish" in all FISH assays performed on interphase nuclei.
- The abbreviation "nuc ish" is followed, in parentheses, by the locus designation, multiplication sign (×), and the number of signals seen.
- If probes for two or more loci are used in the same hybridization, they follow one another in a single set of parentheses, separated by a comma (,) and a multiplication sign (×) outside the parentheses if the number of signals for each probe are the same, and inside the parentheses if the number of hybridization signals varies.
- All interphase FISH studies performed on cancer specimens should indicate the number of cells scored in square brackets [ ] following the hybridization results.
- Results from prenatal FISH studies on direct chorionic villi are typically available within 24 to 48 hours.[54]

18. A. A fetus with triploidy.
Rationale: Three signals are observed for all probes used in this assay. Given the ultrasound anomalies, the diagnosis of triploidy is the most likely explanation.
B. A fetus with tetraploidy.
Rationale: If the fetus has tetraploidy, four signals would be observed for each probe used in this assay.
C. A fetus with trisomy 13, trisomy 16, trisomy 18, trisomy 21, and trisomy 22.
Rationale: Although the fetus does indeed have trisomy of these chromosomes, multiple aneuploidy involving five chromosomes has not been reported prenatally. The three signals observed for each of these chromosomes are an indication that there is an extra set of *all* chromosomes; that is, triploidy.
D. A fetus with malignant transformation.
Rationale: Trisomy of chromosomes 13, 16, 18, 21, and 22 has not been described as a malignant event in chorionic villi obtained from a 10-week-old fetus.
E. Uncertain, because the multiple signals observed are more likely an indication of assay failure. A repeat FISH analysis is indicated.

Rationale: Multiple signals are commonly observed in FISH analyses and are not an indication of assay failure.

Major points of discussion

■ The chromosome count in triploidy is 69, which represents three copies of the human haploid chromosome number; that is, 3n = 69.

■ Diandry is the term used to describe triploidy when the extra chromosome set derives from the father.

■ The majority of diandry triploidy is caused by the fertilization of a single ovum by two sperm.

■ Digyny is the term used to describe triploidy when the extra chromosome set derives from the mother.

■ Digyny is more commonly caused by the fertilization of a diploid ovum by a single haploid sperm.

■ The great majority of triploid conceptions spontaneously abort during the first, or early second, trimester.

19. A. Inversion 16 and *CBFB* gene rearrangement are NOT diagnostic of any subtype of acute myeloblastic leukemia (AML).
Rationale: Inversion (16)(p13.1q22), t(16;16)(p13.1;q22), and deletion 16q22 are variants of each other. These changes are pathognomonic of acute myelomonocytic leukemia.
B. Inversion 16 and *CBFB* gene rearrangement are diagnostic of a specific subtype of AML and predict a good prognosis.
Rationale: Inversion 16 and the associated *CBFB* rearrangement are diagnostic of AML with monocytic and granulocytic differentiation and abnormal eosinophils. This change predicts a better prognosis and results in a longer complete remission when treated with high-dose cytarabine.
C. Inversion 16 and *CBFB* gene rearrangement are diagnostic of a specific subtype of AML and predict a poor prognosis.
Rationale: Inversion 16 is diagnostic of AML M4Eo and predictive of a high complete remission rate; therefore, this predicts a good prognosis.
D. Inversion 16 and *CBFB* gene rearrangement are diagnostic of a specific subtype of AML but have no prognostic value.
Rationale: AML with inversion 16, and its other variants, is highly responsive to treatment; therefore, this is a prognostic indicator.
E. Inversion 16 and *CBFB* gene rearrangement are diagnostic of ALL.
Rationale: Inversion 16 is not seen in ALL. B-cell ALL exhibits other characteristic chromosome changes, which are of diagnostic and prognostic value.

Major points of discussion

■ Approximately 50% to 75% of pediatric and adult AML cases harbor characteristic clonal chromosome abnormalities. The abnormalities include specific translocations, deletions, and inversions. Most common primary chromosome aberrations seen in AML are t(8;21) (q22;q22), t(15;17)(q22;q12-21), translocations involving the 11q23 (*MLL*) region, inversion between 16p/16q, trisomy 8, and deletions of chromosome arms 5q, 7q, and/or 20q.

■ The chromosome changes t(8;21)(q22;q22), t(15;17) (q22;q12-21), and inversion (16)(p13q22) are diagnostic of specific subtypes of AML and serve as prognostic indicators of treatment outcome.

■ Certain chromosome changes in AML serve as indicators of prognosis. For example, 11q123 translocations with different partner chromosomes predict a generally poor outcome.[3,32,59]

20. A. BL.
Rationale: The t(8;14)(q24;q32) translocation, resulting in *MYC* rearrangement with the *IGH* locus, is the characteristic chromosome translocation in BL.
B. HL.
Rationale: In contrast to non-HLs, specific chromosome translocations have not been identified in HL.
C. FL.
Rationale: The t(14;18)(q32;q21) translocation is a characteristic feature of FL and is used as a diagnostic marker for this type of lymphoma.
D. MALT lymphoma.
Rationale: The t(11;18)(q21;q21) balanced chromosomal translocation is diagnostic of MALT lymphoma.
E. Splenic marginal zone lymphoma (SMZL).
Rationale: Although SMZL exhibits no characteristic chromosome changes, trisomies 3 and 18, 7q deletions, and 14q32 rearrangements are frequently seen.

Major points of discussion

■ Extranodal MZL of MALT represents 50% of gastric lymphomas and is an indolent disease. Morphologically, MALT lymphomas consist of heterogeneous small B cells corresponding to marginal zone (centrocyte-like) lymphocytes and are phenotypically IgM+, CD20+, CD79a+, CD5−, and CD23−. A role for *Helicobacter pylori* in gastric MALT lymphoma has been well established, and the eradication of *H. pylori* by antibiotic treatment can cure a large proportion of patients with gastric MALT lymphomas. Bone marrow involvement is less in gastric MALT cases compared with MALT lymphomas from other sites, such as the lung and ocular adnexa.

■ Three major and mutually exclusive recurrent chromosome translocations that target activation of the *NFKB* pathway are associated with MALT lymphomas. The t(11;18)(q21;q21) translocation is seen as a sole abnormality in approximately 50% of MALT lymphomas associated with the stomach and lung. This translocation results in formation of a *BIRC3-MALT1* fusion gene.

■ The second most frequently detected translocation is t (14;18)(q32;q21), which is present in approximately 11% of MALT lymphomas. This translocation is more frequently associated with MALT lymphomas in the liver and ocular adnexa. This translocation juxtaposes the *MALT1* gene next to the *IGH* locus at 14q32. This translocation is cytogenetically identical to the t(14;18) (q32;q21) translocation seen in follicle center cell origin lymphomas; it can only be differentiated by using molecular methods (e.g., FISH and polymerase chain reaction [PCR]). The third translocation, t(1;4)(p22;q32), is detected in less than 2% of MALT lymphomas. This translocation juxtaposes the *BCL10* gene at 1q22 next to the *IGH* locus at 14q32.

■ Translocation-negative MALT lymphomas are associated with chromosomal changes leading to partial trisomy of the long arms of chromosomes 3 and 18.

■ MALT lymphomas have an indolent course and are sensitive to radiation therapy and antibiotic therapy for

H. pylori. Tumors harboring the t(11;18) translocation have a lower probability response to *H. pylori* antibiotic therapy. Occasionally, MALT lymphomas may transform into high-grade, diffuse large B-cell lymphomas.[1,19,41]

21. A. BL.
Rationale: t(8;14)(q24;q32), t(8;22)(q24;q11), and t(2;8) (p11;q24) are the characteristic chromosome translocations in BL.
B. Mantle cell lymphoma.
Rationale: Mantle cell lymphoma presents with a t(11;14) (q13;q32) translocation in virtually all cases; this translocation is used as a diagnostic marker. Although t (11;14) is seen in rare cases of multiple myeloma and chronic lymphocytic leukemia, it is not a diagnostic feature of these lymphomas.
C. MZL.
Rationale: Chromosome alterations involving the gain of the long arms of chromosomes 3 and 18 are commonly seen in MZLs.
D. MALT lymphoma.
Rationale: The chromosome change t(11;18)(q21;q21) is primarily detected in MALT lymphomas.
E. Diffuse large B-cell lymphoma.
Rationale: Approximately 30% to 40% of diffuse large B-cell lymphoma (DLCBL) cases show abnormalities at the 3q27 region involving the *BCL6* gene, with the *IHC* locus at 14q32 as the major translocation partner. Translocation t(14;18) (q32;q21) and deletion 6q are the other major chromosome changes in diffuse large B-cell lymphoma.

Major points of discussion

- Mantle cell lymphoma consists of monomorphic small to medium-sized lymphoid cells resembling centrocytes.
- Mantle cell lymphoma has a strong male predominance and is considered to be a low-grade B-cell non-HL with a progressive clinical course.
- The t(11;14)(q13;q32) translocation is the cytogenetic hallmark of mantle cell lymphoma and is considered as a primary genetic event in its genesis. At the molecular level, this translocation juxtaposes the *cyclin D1* gene at 11q23 next to the *IHC* locus at 14q32, resulting in overexpression of the *cyclin D1* gene.
- Other secondary chromosome abnormalities, such as monosomy 13/deletion 13q, trisomy 12, gain of chromosome 3q, and deletion of 9q can often be seen in the blastoid form of mantle cell lymphoma.
- Secondary chromosome abnormalities are associated with a poor prognosis in mantle cell lymphoma.[3,56,59]

22a. A. DiGeorge syndrome.
Rationale: DiGeorge syndrome is caused by a 1.5- to 3.0-Mb hemizygous deletion of the proximal long arm region of chromosome at 22q11.2. Haploinsufficiency of the *TBX1* gene is believed to be responsible for most of the physical malformations. The principal clinical features include hypocalcemia arising from parathyroid hypoplasia, thymic hypoplasia, and outflow tract defects of the heart.
B. Cat-eye syndrome.
Rationale: Cat-eye syndrome is usually associated with an SMC derived from chromosome 22. The SMC is often dicentic and bisatellited and represents an inversion

duplication of the genomic material from the proximal short arm to the proximal long arm of chromosome 22. There is great variability in the clinical features, especially the congenital malformations. The principal clinical features include coloboma of the iris, anal atresia with fistula, downslanting palpebral fissures, preauricular tags and/or pits, and the frequent occurrence of heart and renal malformations. Mental development may be near-normal or normal, with as many as 47% of cases falling within the normal range (IQ greater than 85).
C. Angelman syndrome.
Rationale: Angelman syndrome is a neurodevelopmental disorder characterized by mental retardation, movement or balance disorder, typical abnormal behaviors, and severe limitations in speech and language. Most cases are caused by the lack of a maternal contribution to the imprinted region on chromosome 15q11-q13. Approximately 70% of Angelman syndrome cases are due to a deletion of the critical genomic region on the maternally inherited chromosome at 15q11-13. Other mechanisms include mutation in the E3 ubiquitin-protein ligase gene (*UBE3A*) (5% to 10%), paternal uniparental disomy (2% to 5%), and an imprinting defect (2% to 5%). In the remainder of cases, the mechanisms are unknown.
D. Charcot-Marie-Tooth syndrome type 1A.
Rationale: Charcot-Marie-Tooth disease is a sensorineural peripheral polyneuropathy. It is the most common inherited disorder of the peripheral nervous system affecting approximately 1:2,500 individuals. Charcot-Marie-Tooth disease type 1A is caused by duplication of, or mutation in, the *PMP22* gene located on the short arm of chromosome 17 at 17p12.
E. Beckwith-Wiedemann syndrome.
Rationale: Beckwith-Wiedemann syndrome is a pediatric overgrowth disorder involving a predisposition to tumor development. The classic features include exomphalos, macroglossia, and gigantism. Clinical presentation is highly variable. Beckwith-Wiedemann syndrome is caused by mutation or deletion of imprinted genes within the chromosome 11p15.5 region. Specific genes involved include *CDKN1C*, *H19*, and *LIT1*. Cytogenetically detectable abnormalities (duplication, inversion, or translocation) involving chromosome 11p15 are found in 1% or less of affected patients. Loss or gain of methylation at the imprinting center 2 (IC2) on the maternal chromosome account for roughly 50% and 5% of cases, respectively. Paternal uniparental disomy of 11p15.5 accounts for approximately 20% of cases.

22b. A. Most markers derived from chromosome 22 are mosaic.
Rationale: The presence of mosaicism has no bearing on the ability to identify the origin of a marker chromosome.
B. Commercial chromosome 22 probes are not approved by the Food and Drug Administration (FDA).
Rationale: Most commercial probes are not FDA approved, and this has no bearing on the ability to identify the origin of a marker chromosome.
C. Chromosomes 14 and 22 share common α-satellite sequences.
Rationale: Because more than 99% of markers are centric fragments of variable size, centromere probes are the best-suited probes to identify the origin of a marker

chromosome. Every human centromere is composed of α-satellite sequences, and the commercial centromere probes are typically composed of these α-satellites sequences. The centromeres of most human chromosomes contain unique α-satellite sequences that can distinguish one chromosome from another. However, chromosomes 14 and 22 share common α-satellite sequences and, therefore, cannot be uniquely identified when using commercial centromeric probes.

D. There are no commercial probes for chromosome 22.
Rationale: There are multiple commercially available FISH probes that map to chromosome 22.

E. Most markers derived from chromosome 22 also contain chromosomal sequences from chromosome 18.
Rationale: See Major Points of Discussion.

Major points of discussion

- An SMC is an additional chromosomal fragment that lacks sufficient banding information to allow for identification of its origins by classic cytogenetic methods.
- The phenotypic consequences of having an SMC are highly variable, ranging from benign to severe. The risk of an adverse phenotypic outcome is correlated with the gene content of the SMC: The larger the gene content, the more likely is the adverse outcome.
- SMCs occur in approximately 1:3333 consecutive newborns. Their frequency in the mentally retarded population is 10 times higher, occurring in approximately 1:305 cases.
- Approximately 80% of SMCs derive from the acrocentric chromosomes (13, 14, 15, 21, and 21) and 50% of these come from chromosome 15.
- Approximately 20% of SMCs are inherited from a normal parent with no increased risk of an adverse outcome expected.
- FISH using a combination of centromere, locus-specific, or chromosome-specific probes has been used to resolve the chromosomal origin of SMCs. Currently, microarray analysis is the preferred method for identifying the chromosomal origin of SMCs because it elucidates not only the chromosomal origin but also the gene content.[13,16,39,48,55]

23a. **A. Not significantly increased over the background risk of 3% to 4%.**
Rationale: Marker chromosomes, derived from chromosome 15, that do not include the Prader-Willi/Angelman critical region (as shown by FISH in this case, which was negative for the *SNRPN* probe on the marker chromosome) are typically not associated with an adverse clinical phenotype. The finding of biparental inheritance of the normal chromosome 15 homologues effectively rules out a genomic disorder caused by uniparental disomy.

B. High, because chromosome 15 contains imprinted genes.
Rationale: Although chromosome 15 does contain imprinted genes, biparental inheritance of the normal chromosome 15 homologues effectively rules out a genomic disorder caused by uniparental disomy.

C. Negligible, because there are no imprinted genes on chromosome 15.
Rationale: Chromosome 15 does contain imprinted genes.

D. High, because the marker chromosome likely resulted from a rescue of a trisomy 15 fetus.
Rationale: Although the marker chromosome may have resulted from the rescue of a trisomy 15 fetus, the follow-up molecular studies revealed biparental inheritance of the normal chromosome 15 homologues, which effectively rules out the risk of a genomic disorder caused by uniparental disomy.

E. Unclear, because further molecular testing is required before accurate risk assessment can be made.
Rationale: In this clinical scenario, all the relevant testing has been performed to allow for an appropriate clinical interpretation.

23b. A. A balanced translocation between the short arms of chromosomes 4 and 5.
Rationale: Balanced translocations are usually not associated with any clinical phenotype unless the breakpoints occur in a critical region of a gene, thereby disrupting gene function, or there is a concomitant microdeletion or microduplication at the breakpoint sites.

B. An unbalanced translocation that always involves the proximal long arm of chromosome 22.
Rationale: Unbalanced translocations are associated with a clinical phenotype. However, chromosome 15 needs to be involved, with a net loss of the proximal long arm region, in order to result in PWS.

C. An insertion of extra chromosomal material into the distal long arm region of chromosome 17.
Rationale: Extra material inserted into another chromosome is likely to be associated with a clinical phenotype. However, chromosome 15 needs to be involved, with net loss of the proximal long arm region, in order to result in PWS.

D. A duplication of chromosomal material at the proximal region of the long arm of chromosome 7.
Rationale: A duplication of the proximal 7q region is associated with the 7q11.23 duplication syndrome, which is characterized by facial dysmorphism and prominent speech delay.

E. A deletion on the proximal region of the long arm of chromosome 15.
Rationale: A deletion, specifically of the paternally inherited chromosome 15 at 15q11.2, is associated with a clinical diagnosis of PWS.

Major points of discussion

- PWS is a genomic imprinting disorder characterized by the following:
  - Hypotonia and feeding difficulties in early infancy
  - Excessive eating in childhood, gradual morbid obesity
  - Delayed motor milestones and language development
  - Cognitive impairment
  - Temper tantrums
  - Hypogonadism, short stature, strabismus, and scoliosis
- The critical genomic region implicated in PWS is the proximal region of the long arm of chromosome 15, just below the centromere (15q11.2-q13).
- The critical genomic region implicated in PWS contains imprinted genes, which means that expression of that

gene occurs in a gender-specific manner; that is, expression only occurs from one parent's allele. The parental allele that is not expressed (i.e., is silent) is referred to as "imprinted." Thus, a maternally imprinted gene will not be expressed from the maternally inherited chromosome but will only be expressed from the paternally inherited chromosome.

■ Multiple genes in the PWS genomic region are maternally imprinted; thus, expression of those genes occurs from the paternally inherited chromosome. A deletion of this region on the *paternally inherited* chromosome results in PWS, because expression of these imprinted genes no longer occurs. The deletion is typically interstitial and is usually 5 to 6 Mb in size.

■ Maternal uniparental disomy of chromosome 15 (i.e., both copies of chromosome 15 are derived from the mother; none from the father) effectively results in the same clinical consequence (PWS) because the genes that need to be expressed are missing (i.e., no paternal contribution).

■ A minor number of PWS cases (<3%) can be caused by imprinting defects that result from epigenetic causes that demonstrate a maternal-only DNA methylation pattern despite the presence of both parental alleles (i.e., biparental inheritance). Approximately 15% of individuals with imprinting defects have a very small deletion (7.5 to 100 kb) in the PWS imprinting center region located at the 5′ end of the *SNRPN* gene and promoter.

■ Approximately 65% to 75% of PWS cases are due to a deletion of the critical genomic region on the paternally inherited chromosome at 15q11.2.

■ Approximately 20% to 30% of PWS cases are due to maternal uniparental disomy of chromosome 15.

■ Approximately 1% to 3% of PWS cases are due to imprinting defects.

■ Deletions of the same critical genomic on the *maternally* inherited chromosome at 15q11.2 or paternal uniparental disomy of chromosome 15 lead to a completely different disorder: Angelman syndrome.

■ Angelman syndrome is characterized by the following:
  ● Severe developmental delay
  ● Absent or limited speech
  ● Gait ataxia
  ● Happy demeanor with frequent inappropriate laughter, smiling, and excitability
  ● Microcephaly and seizures

■ Angelman syndrome may also be caused by defects/mutations in the imprinting center or by mutations in the *UBE3A* gene.[11,36,37]

24. A. A whole chromosome paint probe specific for chromosome 17.
Rationale: Paint probes cannot detect microdeletion syndromes. Paint probes are used to detect chromosome translocations and to determine the origin of a marker chromosome.
B. Spectral karyotyping (SKY) using multicolor chromosome paint probes for all chromosomes.
Rationale: This method is mainly used to identify structural chromosome abnormalities such as translocations and marker chromosomes. Small deletions cannot be detected by SKY.

C. A locus-specific FISH probe for the commonly deleted region on chromosome 17.
Rationale: FISH using a locus-specific probe for the SMS critical region containing the *RAI1* gene is used to detect this microdeletion on chromosome 17p11.2.
D. A centromere 17–specific FISH probe.
Rationale: Centromeric probes are used to detect the number of copies of a chromosome. Microdeletions cannot be detected by centromeric probes.
E. A subtelomeric probe for the short arm of chromosome 17.
Rationale: A subtelomeric probe cannot be used because the deletion in the SMS is in the proximal short arm. A subtelomeric probe will be useful only for distal deletion or duplication of a chromosome.

Major points of discussion
■ The diagnosis of SMS is based on clinical findings and confirmed by detection of an interstitial deletion of chromosome 17p11.2 by FISH, aCGH, or CMA.
■ All deletions associated with SMS include a deletion of the *RAI1* gene located on chromosome 17p11.2. This syndrome is characterized by distinctive facial features that progress with age, developmental delay, cognitive impairment, and behavioral abnormalities. Infants have feeding difficulties, failure to thrive, hypotonia, hyporeflexia, prolonged napping, and generalized lethargy. The majority of these individuals have a mild-to-moderate range of intellectual disability.
■ Approximately 90% of the cases with deletion of chromosome 17p11.2 can be detected using a locus-specific probe for the *RAI1* gene. Sequence analysis is used in 5% to 10% of the suspected SMS patients when FISH testing is negative for the 17p11.2 deletion.
■ Chromosome paint probes are fluorescently labeled libraries of DNA sequences derived from flow-sorted chromosomes and SKY is a FISH method that allows visualization of all the human chromosomes, each in a different fluorescent color.
■ Recently, aCGH or CMA has become the diagnostic test of choice for detecting microdeletion syndromes.[57,60]

25a. A. The karyotype shows a balanced translocation between the short arms of chromosomes 15 and 17.
B. The karyotype shows an unbalanced translocation between the short arms of chromosomes 15 and 17, which results in partial trisomy of 15p and partial monosomy of 17p.
C. The karyotype shows an unbalanced translocation between the short arms of chromosomes 15 and 17, which results in partial monosomy of 15p and partial trisomy of 17p.
D. The karyotype shows an unbalanced derivative chromosome 17 resulting from a translocated insertion of short arm material from chromosome 15p at band p13.3 into 17p11.2.
E. The karyotype shows an unbalanced derivative chromosome 17 resulting from a translocated insertion of short arm material from chromosome 15p at band p11.2 into 17p13.3.
Rationale: The karyotype does not reflect an insertion but rather an unbalanced translocation between the short arms of chromosomes 15 and 17 (the imbalance results in partial trisomy of 15p and partial monosomy of 17p.) The

abnormal chromosome is a derivative chromosome 17 that has extra material derived from the short arm of chromosome 15 (pter-15p11.2), which replaces the material deleted on chromosome 17 (17pter-p13.3).

25b. A. Sotos syndrome.
Rationale: Sotos syndrome is caused by (1) a heterozygous mutation in the *NSD1* gene or (2) a deletion in the 5q35 region including genomic sequence in addition to the *NSD1* gene. The principal clinical features include overgrowth from the prenatal stage through childhood, distinctive facial features, large head circumference, pointed chin, and mild-to-severe learning difficulties.
B. SMS.
Rationale: SMS is caused in most cases (90%) by a 3.7-Mb interstitial deletion in the 17p11.2 region. This region is closer (i.e., more proximal) to the centromere than the translocation described in the current case. The disorder can also be caused by mutations in the *RAI1* gene, which is within the Smith-Magenis 17p11.2 chromosome region. The principal clinical features include mild-to-severe learning disabilities, brachycephaly, midface hypoplasia, prognathism, hoarse voice, speech delay with or without hearing loss, psychomotor and growth retardation, and behavioral problems.
C. Cri-du-chat syndrome.
Rationale: Cri-du-chat syndrome is caused by a deletion of the short arm of chromosome 5 and is characterized by a high-pitched, monotonous cry; microcephaly; a round face; hypertelorism; epicanthic folds; micrognathia; impaired growth; severe developmental delay; and learning disability.
D. DiGeorge syndrome.
Rationale: DiGeorge syndrome is caused by a 1.5- to 3.0-Mb hemizygous deletion of the proximal long arm region of chromosome at 22q11.2. Haploinsufficiency of the *TBX1* gene is believed to be responsible for most of the physical malformations. The principal clinical features include hypocalcemia arising from parathyroid hypoplasia, thymic hypoplasia, and cardiac outflow tract defects.
E. Miller-Dieker syndrome.
Rationale: Miller-Dieker syndrome is a contiguous gene deletion syndrome involving genes on chromosome 17p13.3. Deletions or mutations in the *LIS1* gene appear to cause the lissencephaly. The principal clinical features include lissencephaly, cardiac malformations, microcephaly, wrinkled skin over the glabella and frontal suture, prominent occiput, narrow forehead, downward-slanting palpebral fissures, small nose and chin, hypoplastic male external genitalia, growth retardation, and mental deficiency with seizures and electroencephalographic abnormalities. A reduced lifespan is commonly observed.

25c. A. A sequence-based mutation because the karyotype is balanced.
Rationale: The karyotype is unbalanced with partial trisomy (extra genetic material) of the short arm of chromosome 15 and partial monosomy (missing genetic material) of the short arm of chromosome 17.
B. The missing genetic material from the short arm of chromosome 15 and the extra genetic material from the short arm of chromosome 17.

Rationale: The missing genetic material derives from the short arm of chromosome 17 and the extra genetic material from the short arm of chromosome 15.
C. The extra genetic material from the short arm of chromosome 15 and the missing genetic material from the short arm of chromosome 17.
Rationale: Although this statement reflects the genomic imbalance consistent with this karyotype, the associated phenotype is unlikely to be linked to the extra material from the short arm of chromosome 15. This is because the short arm of chromosome 15 (as well as the short arms of all the acrocentric chromosomes) contains highly variable amounts of ribosomal gene repeats; loss or gain of this genetic material is clinically insignificant because there are sufficient ribosomal genes on the remaining acrocentric short arms. The sizes of the short arms of the acrocentric chromosomes (and their resulting gene content) are highly polymorphic, with some individuals showing almost no visible short arm material and others showing extremely large short arms.
D. Only the missing genetic material from the short arm of chromosome 17.
Rationale: A deletion of the terminal region of chromosome 17 at 17p13.3 (including the *LIS1* gene) is associated with a clinical diagnosis of the Miller-Dieker syndrome, which is characterized by lissencephaly with dysmorphic features. The extra material from the short arm of chromosome 15 contains multiple ribosomal gene repeats that already exist as a polymorphic entity; thus, this is unlikely to be a contributing factor to the clinical phenotype.
E. Only the extra genetic material from the short arm of chromosome 15.
Rationale: The short arm of chromosome 15 (as well as the short arms of all the acrocentric chromosomes) contains highly variable amounts of ribosomal gene repeats; gain (or loss) of this genetic material is clinically insignificant because there are sufficient ribosomal genes on the remaining acrocentric short arms. The size of the short arms of the acrocentric chromosomes (and their resulting gene content) is highly polymorphic, with some individuals showing almost no visible short arm material and others showing extremely large short arms. In this karyotype, the gain of the short arm material is unlikely to be pathogenic and the observed phenotype is likely due to the missing material on the short arm of chromosome 17.

Major points of discussion
- Facial dysmorphism and other anomalies in Miller-Dieker patients appear to be the result of a loss of genes distal to *LIS1*.
- Approximately 80% of individuals with Miller-Dieker syndrome have a de novo deletion involving 17p13.3.
- In approximately 12% to 20% of Miller-Dieker syndrome cases, the deletion at 17p13.3 is due to a familial balanced chromosome rearrangement.
- The deletion at 17p13.3 is cytogenetically visible in approximately 70% of patients with Miller-Dieker syndrome. Some cases with isolated lissencephaly do not show visible cytogenetic deletions and are more likely to have mutations of the *LIS1* gene or tiny deletions restricted to the *LIS1* gene.
- Additional molecular cytogenetic testing should be pursued for those patients with clinical features of

Miller-Dieker syndrome that show a normal karyotype. Additional testing can be performed by FISH using a probe that maps to the *LIS1* gene region or by DNA microarray analysis.[16,17,21,33,48]

26. A. BL.
Rationale: t(8;14)(q24;q32), t(8;22)(q24;q11), and t(2;8) (p11;q24) are the characteristic chromosome translocations in BL.
B. MZL.
Rationale: Chromosome alterations involving gains of the long arms of chromosomes 3 and 18 are commonly seen in MZLs.
C. Multiple myeloma, possibly with good prognosis.
D. Multiple myeloma, possibly with poor prognosis.
Rationale: 14q32 rearrangements are seen in approximately 50% of plasma cell neoplasia cases. The t(14;20)(q32;q11.2) abnormality is characteristic of multiple myeloma, and the presence of 1q duplications is indicative of a poor prognosis.
E. MALT lymphoma.
Rationale: The chromosome change of t(11;18)(q21;q21) is primarily detected in MALT lymphomas.

Major points of discussion

- Multiple myeloma is a malignant monoclonal plasma cell proliferation of postgerminal center-cell origin. Multiple myeloma is often preceded by a premalignant condition called "monoclonal gammopathy of undetermined significance" (i.e., MGUS).
- Chromosome abnormalities are found in only approximately 30% of the cases by conventional karyotypic analysis due to the low proliferative index exhibited by multiple myeloma.
- Karyotypes are generally complex, involving both chromosome number and structure. The most common chromosomes that involve changes in chromosome number are monosomy 13 and trisomies of chromosomes 3, 5, 7, 9, 11, 15, 19, and 21. Structural chromosome abnormalities most commonly involve 14q32 (i.e., *IGH*) rearrangements, deletions at 1p, 13q, 11q22, and 17p, and duplications of the long arm of chromosome 1q. Chromosome changes are of diagnostic importance and provide critical prognostic information in multiple myeloma.
- The t(14;20)(q32;q11.2) abnormality occurs recurrently only in multiple myeloma; thus, it serves as a diagnostic cytogenetic marker.
- At least five recurrent *IGH* translocation partners have been identified in multiple myeloma. These are 11q13 (*CCND1* in 15% to 20%), 4p16 (*MMSET* and *FGFR3* in 10% to 20%), 16q23 (*MAF* in 5%), 6p21 (*CCND3* in 3%), and 20q11.2 (*MAFB* in 2%). The following *IGH* translocations are associated with short progression-free survival and decreased overall survival: t(4;14), t(14;16), and t(14;20).
- Hyperdiploidy in multiple myeloma predicts a good prognosis. Similarly, among the *IGH* translocation partners, the t(11;14)(q13;q32) translocation predicts a good prognosis.
- The structural alterations involving the 17p13 (i.e., *TP53*) deletion and the 1q21 duplication predict an adverse outcome. These cytogenetic changes frequently occur with the adverse group of *IGH* translocations.

- Thus, the specific cytogenetic aberrations can be used to define the prognostic classes in multiple myeloma.[5,8]

27. **A. High-grade B-cell non-Hodgkin lymphoma (B-NHL).**
Rationale: The t(2;8)(p11.2;q24) translocation, resulting in *MYC* rearrangement with the *IGK* locus, is seen in BL and DLBCL. A complex karyotype associated with t(2;8) is particularly seen in DLBCL and BL.
B. MZL.
Rationale: The three distinct clinicopathologic subtypes of MZL exhibit no diagnostic chromosome changes. However, trisomies 3 and 18, 7q deletion, and 14q32 rearrangements with various partners are frequently seen.
C. Multiple myeloma.
Rationale: In multiple myeloma, the 14q32 region involving the *IGH* gene is frequently partnered with 11q13 (the *cyclin D1* gene), 4p16 (the *FGFR3* gene), 6p25 (the *cyclin D3* gene), 16q23 (the *MAF* gene), and 20q11 (the *MAFB* gene), thereby forming balanced reciprocal translocations. Other changes frequently seen in multiple myeloma are deletions at 11q23 and 6q, 1q duplications, and trisomies of chromosomes 3, 5, 7, 9, 11, 15, 19, and 21.
D. MALT lymphoma.
Rationale: The t(11;18)(q21;q21) balanced translocation is primarily detected in MALT lymphoma.
E. HL.
Rationale: HL is not associated with t(2;8). Specific chromosome changes have not been reported for HL. However, chromosome deletions involving 1p, 6q, 7q, and duplications of 1q have been seen.

Major points of discussion

- The immunoglobulin (IG) loci (i.e., *IGH* at 14q32, *IGK* at 2p11.2, and *IGL* at 22q11.2) are recurrently rearranged in chromosomal translocations in different subtypes of mature B-cell lymphomas. For some specific subtypes, such as BL, the IG translocations are pathognomonic and occur in most cases (>95%). In other instances, such as DLBCL, IG translocations are detectable in approximately half of the cases, accompanied by other chromosome changes. Multiple IG translocations occur in B-cell lymphomas involving both heavy and light chain genes. The most common combinations are t(14;18)(q32;21) in FL, followed by t(8;14) or its variants, t(2;8) or t(8;22), in DLBCL.
- The t(8;14)(q24;q32) translocation and its variants, t(2;8) (p11.2;q24) and t(8;22)(q24;q11.2), are common in BL but can occur in almost any type of mature B-cell neoplasm.
- The t(2;8)(p11.2;q24) translocation, involving rearrangement of the *IGK* gene with the *MYC* gene, are seen in approximately 5% of cases of BL and rarely in DLBCL. The t(2;8) translocation results in juxtaposition of the *IGK* enhancer to the *MYC* oncogene and deregulates the latter's expression.
- The t(2;8)(p11.2;q24) translocation in DLBCL is thought to be a secondary change associated with a complex karyotype. Most recurrent chromosome aberrations in complex karyotypes are gains of chromosomes X, 1q, 3, 7, 12, and 18; losses of chromosomes 6q, 13, 15, and 17; and are associated with aggressive behavior.
- There is molecular heterogeneity regarding the breakpoints in the *MYC* gene between t(8;14) and

t(8;22)/t(2;8). The *MYC* breakpoints in t(2;8) and t(8;22) are telomeric to *MYC*; in t(8;14) the breakpoint in *MYC* is centromeric.[6,22,42]

28. A. 46,XY,del(5)(q13q33).
Rationale: This karyotype indicates deletion 5q. Deletion of chromosome 5q as a sole chromosome abnormality is also known as the 5q– syndrome and represents a distinct clinical entity. It presents with a macrocytic anemia and a normal or elevated platelet count. Abnormalities in the megakaryocytic lineage are prominent. This deletion is associated with a favorable outcome with low rates of leukemic transformation and a relatively long survival (i.e., several years).
B. 47,XY,+8.
Rationale: This karyotype indicates trisomy 8. This abnormality is seen in all MDS subgroups, both as an isolated chromosome abnormality and with other recurring chromosome abnormalities known to have prognostic significance. This abnormality is associated with a variable clinical course and is expected to be associated with intermediate prognosis.
C. 46,XY,del(20)(q11.2q13.3).
Rationale: This karyotype indicates deletion of the long arm of chromosome 20. Patients with deletion 20q have prominent dysplasia in the erythroid and megakaryocytic lineages. These patients have low disease risk (usually refractory anemia), a low rate of progression to acute leukemia, and prolonged survival (i.e., a median of 45 months versus 28 months for other MDS patients).
D. 45,X,-Y.
Rationale: This karyotype indicates loss of the Y chromosome. Loss of the Y chromosome as a sole cytogenetic abnormality in a patient with a diagnosis of MDS (clinical and bone marrow morphology findings) is associated with a favorable outcome.
E. 46,XY,del(7)(q11.2q36).
Rationale: This karyotype indicates deletion 7q. Deletion 7q or monosomy 7 is associated with poor outcome in terms of both survival and progression to acute leukemia.

Major points of discussion

■ MDS is a heterogeneous group of clonal bone marrow disorders characterized by the presence of dysplastic maturation of the hematopoietic cells and peripheral cytopenias. MDS patients have a propensity to progress to an acute leukemia.

■ The incidence of MDS increases with age; most patients are over 60 years of age. Approximately 10% to 15% of MDS cases follow treatment (therapy-related MDS [t-MDS]) with chemotherapy and radiation for both neoplastic as well as benign disorders.

■ The WHO classification of MDS is based on bone marrow, histology, blast count, and cytogenetic findings. The cytogenetic evaluation of a bone marrow sample is valuable in assessing the prognosis, the risk for progression to acute leukemia, and survival in MDS patients.

■ A normal karyotype is found in 30% to 60% of patients with MDS depending on the method used (karyotype, FISH, aCGH, or SNP array) to detect chromosome abnormalities. The international MDS risk assessment workshop found that patients with a normal karyotype fell within the favorable risk group. The median survival for these patients is 3.8 years. The time to progression to acute leukemia of 25% of this cohort was 5.6 years.

■ A complex karyotype is found in approximately 20% of patients with primary MDS and in more than 90% of patients with t-MDS. A complex karyotype is defined as the presence of three or more chromosome abnormalities. The majority of these cases show abnormal chromosomes 5 or 7. A complex karyotype is associated with poor prognosis in MDS.[25]

29. A. Astrocytomas.
Rationale: Gain of chromosome 7 and loss of chromosome 10 are common genetic changes in astrocytomas.
B. Medulloblastomas.
Rationale: An isochromosome 17q in brain tumors is pathognomonic for medulloblastoma.
C. Meningiomas.
Rationale: Loss of chromosome 22 is the most common cytogenetic aberration in meningiomas.
D. Oligodendrogliomas.
Rationale: Patients whose oligodendrogliomas have concomitant 1p and 19q deletions have a significantly longer survival than those without deletions.
E. Ependymomas.
Rationale: Deletions of chromosome 19 and 22 are recurring chromosome abnormalities in ependymomas.

Major points of discussion

■ A wide variety of cytogenetic abnormalities are found in tumors of the nervous system.

■ Astrocytomas are the best-studied adult nervous system tumors. Common gross genetic abnormalities include gain of chromosome 7 and loss of chromosome 10. Gain of epidermal growth factor receptor function is common in high-grade astrocytomas.

■ Medulloblastomas are primitive neuroectodermal tumors and are most commonly seen in children. The most common abnormality is isochromosome 17, which results in deletion of the short arm of chromosome 17p containing the *REN* and *TP53* genes and gain of the long arm of chromosome 17q.

■ In meningiomas, loss of chromosome 22 and deletion 22q are common cytogenetic abnormalities. Patients with neurofibromatosis type II (NF2) have a predisposition to meningiomas.

■ Concomitant deletions of 1p and 19q are the characteristic cytogenetic abnormalities in oligodendrogliomas. Loss of both 1p and 19q correlates with a better response to chemotherapy and radiotherapy.

■ Ependymomas are typically benign. These tumors show deletions of chromosomes 19 and 22; otherwise, they have a relatively normal karyotype.

30. A. Chromophobe-type RCC.
Rationale: Chromophobe RCCs exhibit a unique combination of chromosome losses with a modal chromosome number of 38-39. Monosomy of chromosomes 1, 2, 6, 10, 13, 17, and 21 are most frequent.

B. Renal oncocytoma.
Rationale: Loss of chromosomes 1 and 14, and the Y chromosome, along with 11q13 rearrangements are characteristic of a renal oncocytoma.
C. Papillary RCC.
Rationale: A combination of trisomy or tetrasomy of chromosome 7, trisomy 17, and loss of the Y chromosome is a frequent feature of papillary RCC. Additional trisomies of chromosomes 12, 16, and 20 are seen in aggressive tumors.
D. Conventional clear cell RCC.
Rationale: Chromosome 3p deletions involving the 3p21 region are a characteristic feature of this neoplasm.
E. Renal angiomyolipoma.
Rationale: Chromosome abnormalities are rare in renal angiomyolipomas. Trisomy 7 was reported in a few cases.

Major points of discussion

- RCC is a heterogeneous group of epithelial tumors in terms of histology and clinical behavior. RCCs are classified based on cytology, cell type of origin, and genetic changes.
- Major classes of RCC are clear cell, papillary, chromophobe, oncocytoma, collecting duct carcinomas, sarcomatoid transformation in RCC, and mucinous tubular and spindle cell carcinoma. Although most RCCs are sporadic, syndromic forms have been reported for each of the major histologic types.
- Cytogenetic alterations are highly specific to each major histologic type of RCC and are of diagnostic relevance.
- Clear cell RCC arising from mature renal tubular cells represents approximately 75% of all RCCs. Clear cell RCC is characterized by deletions on chromosome 3p. Several common regions of deletion at 3p14, 3p21, and 3p25 were identified. The 3q21 deletion is obligatory for classification as a clear cell RCC. Additional abnormalities include partial trisomy of 5q and gain of chromosomes 12 and 20.
- Papillary RCC represents about 10% of all RCCs. Trisomy or tetrasomy of chromosome 7 and trisomy 17 are characteristic features of papillary RCC. Gain of chromosomes 12, 16, and 20 is present in aggressive tumors.
- Chromophobe-type RCCs represent 5% of all RCCs. Cytogenetically, chromophobe RCC exhibits a modal chromosome number of 38-39 with frequent losses of chromosomes 1, 2, 6, 10, 13, 17, and 21.
- Renal oncotyoma is a benign neoplasm. Chromosome abnormalities are seen in approximately 50% of oncocytomas. Loss of chromosomes 1 and 14, and loss of the Y chromosome in males, are seen in one subset of tumors. In a second subset, translocations at 11q13 are seen;. 11q13 rearranges with many different chromosomes in this setting.
- Mucinous tubular and spindle cell carcinoma is a distinct form of RCC. Cytogenetic characteristics of very few cases have been reported. Loss of chromosomes 1, 14, and 15 has been described.[12,28]

31. A. Embryonal rhabdomyosarcoma.
Rationale: Embryonal rhabdomyosarcomas do not show any recurrent balanced chromosome translocations.
B. Primitive neuroectoderal tumor.
Rationale: t(11;22)(q24;q12), resulting in fusion of the *EWS* gene on 22q12 with *FLI1* at 11q24, is a classic feature of primitive neuroectoderal tumor/Ewing sarcoma and serves as a diagnostic chromosome translocation for Ewing sarcoma.
C. Giant cell tumor of bone.
Rationale: Giant cell tumor of bone shows a near-diploid range chromosomes; no diagnostic cytogenetic change has yet been identified.
D. Lipoma.
Rationale: Rearrangements of 12q13-15 regions are seen in two thirds of clonally abnormal cases, with 3q27-29 as the most common translocation partner.
E. Alveolar rhabdomyosarcoma.
Rationale: Most alveolar rhabdomyosarcoma cases exhibit characteristic chromosome translocations, such as t(2;13) (q36;q14) or t(1;13)(p36;q14). The *FOXO1* gene on 13q14 rearranges with the *PAX3* gene on 2q35 and the *PAX7* gene on 1p36 and results in formation of fusion gene products.

Major points of discussion

- Ewing sarcomas, also known as primitive neuroectodermal tumors (PNETs), are highly aggressive tumors of neural crest derivation. The cytogenetic hallmark of Ewing sarcoma is t(11;22)(q24;q12), which is seen in approximately 90% of all histologic subtypes. This translocation is diagnostic of this entity.
- The t(11;22)(q24;q12) translocation results in rearrangement of the *EWS* gene at 11q24 and the *FLI1* gene at 22q12. The translocation results in the formation of the ESW-FLI1 chimeric protein.
- Approximately 5% of Ewing sarcomas result from variant translocations involving the *EWS* gene at 11q24, resulting in t(21;22)(q12;q12)[*EWS-ERG*] and t(7;22) (p22;q12) [*EWS-ETV1*].[3,44]

32. A. Chronic myeloid leukemia (CML), predicting a poor prognosis.
Rationale: The hallmark of CML is the t(9;22)(q34;q11.2) translocation and its associated variant translocations. A high hyperdiploid karyotype is not a common feature of CML.
B. MDS, predicting a good prognosis.
Rationale: The chromosome changes frequently seen in MDS are del(5q)/monosomy 5, del(7q)/monosomy 7, del(20q)/monosomy 20, and trisomy 8. A high hyperdiploid karyotype is not a feature of MDS.
C. Pre-B-cell ALL (pre-B ALL), predicting a poor prognosis.
D. Pre-B ALL, predicting a good prognosis.
Rationale: The described immunophenotype is characteristic of pre-B ALL and a high hyperdiploid karyotype is commonly seen in a subset of pre-B ALL patients. A karyotype showing hyperdiploidy is associated with a high sensitivity to chemotherapy and a better clinical outcome, thus predicting a good prognosis.
E. AML, predicting a good prognosis.
Rationale: AML is associated with specific chromosome translocations, such as t(15;17)(q22;q21), t(16;16)(p13; q22), t(8;21)(q22;q22), and other loss or gain of chromosome regions. A high hyperdiploid karyotype is not commonly seen in AML.

Major points of discussion

- Clonal karyotypic abnormalities are seen in two thirds of all newly diagnosed ALL patients. Chromosome changes involving both number and structure are seen. Those involving chromosome number include near-haploid,

hypodiploid, hyperdiploid, and pseudo-diploid karyotypes.
- The chromosome changes in B-cell ALL play an important role with regard to diagnostic classification and prognosis prediction.
- Ploidy groups in ALL represent well-established cytogenetic entities comprising low hyperdiploidy (46 to 49 chromosomes), high hyperdiploidy (51 to 65 chromosomes), near-triploidy (66 to 79 chromosomes, near-tetraploidy (84 to 100 chromosomes), hypodiploidy (45 chromosomes), low hypodiploidy (31 to 39 chromosomes), and near-haploidy (25 to 29 chromosomes).
- Each ploidy group predicts chemotherapy responses in ALL. Overall, the hyperdiploid ALL group responds well to standard chemotherapy compared with patients in the hypodiploid and near-haploid groups.
- One third of children presenting with ALL harbor the high-hyperdiploidy karyotype (51 to 65 chromosomes). Children with high-hyperdiploid ALL respond well to standard chemotherapy regimens. Event-free survival rates are up to 80% at 5 years for this group of patients.
- High-hyperdiploid ALL is characterized by a nonrandom gain of chromosomes X, 4, 6, 10, 14, 17, 18, and 21. However, involvement of other additional chromosomes can also be seen.
- Within the high-hyperdiploid karyotype group, other variables such as gender, age, individual trisomies, and modal chromosome numbers can affect the outcome. For example, girls aged 1 to 9 years with trisomy 18, in particular, are reported to have the best event-free survival.[24,29,46]

33. A. The t(15;17)(q22;q21) translocation is commonly seen in MDS.
Rationale: Common chromosome changes associated with MDS are deletion 5q/monosomy 5, deletion 7q/monosomy 7, deletion 20q/monosomy 20, and trisomy 8.
B. The t(15;17)(q22;q21) translocation is diagnostic of CML.
Rationale: t(15;17)(q21;q22) is not associated with CML. CML is characterized by t(9;22)(q34;q11.2).
C. The t(15;17)(q22;q21) translocation is diagnostic of APL but does not predict treatment outcome.
Rationale: The t(15;17)(q22;q21) translocation is diagnostic of APL. Because these lesions exhibit high sensitivity to treatment, this predicts a good prognosis.
D. The chromosomal translocation (15;17)(q22;q21) is *not* associated with acute myelocytic leukemia.
Rationale: The t(15;17)(q22;q21) translocation is specific to the FAB M3 subtype of acute myelocytic leukemia and is pathognomonic of APL.
E. **The t(15;17)(q22;q21) translocation is diagnostic of APL and predicts a favorable treatment outcome.**
Rationale: t(15;17)(q22;q21) and the associated *PML/RARA* rearrangement is diagnostic of APL. These neoplastic cells are highly sensitive to treatment with ATRA, which acts as a differentiating agent. This translocation predicts a good prognosis in this disorder.

Major points of discussion
- The t(15;17)(q22;q21) translocation is confined to the FAB M3 morphologic subtype of APL with hypergranular promyelocytic leukemic cells.

- The t(15;17) translocation is the sole cytogenetic abnormality in approximately 75% of cases. Trisomy 8 is the most common secondary change in 10% to 15% of cases.
- Despite the remarkable specificity of t(15;17)(q22;q21) in APL, this translocation can rarely present as a secondary change during chronic myelocytic leukemia in blast crisis.
- The t(15;17)(q22;q21) translocation results in the retinoic acid receptor α (*RARA*) gene on 17q22 fusing with a nuclear regulatory factor gene (i.e., the promyelocytic leukemia or *PML* gene) on 15q22, thereby giving rise to the *PML/RARA* fusion gene, which mediates the leukemogenic process.
- APL with the t(15;17)(q22;q21) translocation exhibits a particular sensitivity to treatment with ATRA, which acts as differentiating agent. Response of APL treated with ATRA and other combinations of drugs (e.g., anthracyclines, arsenic trioxide) is highest compared with any other acute myelocytic leukemia subsets.
- Variant translocations involving 17q22 (*RARA*) and *NPM1* at 5q35, *NUMA1* at 11q13, and *ZBTB16* (previously known as *PLZF*) at 11q23 are seen in fewer than 2% of cases of APL.[15,45]

34. A. **Chromophobe-type RCC.**
Rationale: Chromophobe RCCs exhibit a unique combination of chromosome losses with a modal chromosome number of 38-39. Monosomy of chromosomes 1, 2, 6, 10, 13, 17, and 21 are most frequent.
B. Renal oncocytoma.
Rationale: Loss of chromosomes 1 and 14 and the Y chromosome, along with 11q13 rearrangements, are characteristic of a renal oncocytoma.
C. Papillary RCC.
Rationale: A combination of trisomy or tetrasomy of chromosome 7, trisomy 17, and loss of the Y chromosome is a frequent feature of papillary RCC. Additional trisomies of chromosomes 12, 16, and 20 are seen in aggressive tumors.
D. Conventional clear cell RCC.
Rationale: Chromosome 3p deletions involving the 3p21 region are a characteristic feature of this neoplasm.
E. Renal angiomyolipoma.
Rationale: Chromosome abnormalities are rare in renal angiomyolipomas. Trisomy 7 was reported in a few cases.

Major points of discussion
- RCCs are a heterogeneous group of epithelial tumors in terms of histology and clinical behavior. RCCs are classified based on cytology, cell type of origin, and genetic changes.
- Major classes of RCC are clear cell, papillary, chromophobe, oncocytoma, collecting duct carcinomas, sarcomatoid transformation in RCC, and mucinous tubular and spindle cell carcinoma. Although most RCCs are sporadic, syndromic forms have been reported for each of the major histologic types.
- Cytogenetic alterations are highly specific to each major histologic type of RCC and are of diagnostic relevance.
- Clear cell RCC arising from mature renal tubular cells represents approximately 75% of all RCCs. Clear cell RCC is characterized by deletions on chromosome 3p. Several common regions of deletion at 3p14, 3p21, and 3p25 were identified. The 3q21 deletion is obligatory for

classification as a clear cell RCC. Additional abnormalities include partial trisomy of 5q and gain of chromosomes 12 and 20.

- Papillary RCC represents approximately 10% of all RCCs. Trisomy or tetrasomy of chromosome 7 and trisomy 17 are characteristic features of papillary RCC. Gain of chromosomes 12, 16, and 20 are present in aggressive tumors.
- Chromophobe RCC represents approximately 5% of all RCCs. Cytogenetically, chromophobe RCC exhibits a modal chromosome number of 38-39 with frequent losses of chromosomes 1, 2, 6, 10, 13, 17, and 21.
- Renal oncotyoma is a benign neoplasm. Chromosome abnormalities are seen in approximately 50% of oncocytomas. Loss of chromosomes 1 and 14, and loss of the Y chromosome in males, are seen in one subset of tumors. In a second subset, translocations at 11q13 are seen; 11q13 rearranges with many different chromosomes in this setting.
- Mucinous tubular and spindle cell carcinoma is a distinct form of RCC. Cytogenetic characteristics of very few cases have been reported. Loss of chromosomes 1, 14, and 15 has been described.

35. A. Clear cell RCC.
Rationale: Deletion of chromosome 3p is a characteristic finding in clear cell RCC.
B. Papillary RCC.
Rationale: Combinations of trisomy 7 and 17 are commonly found in papillary RCC.
C. Chromophobe RCC.
Rationale: Combination monosomies (chromosomes 1, 2, 6, 10, 13, 17 and/or 21) are found in chromphobe RCC.
D. Mucinous tubular and spindle cell carcinoma.
Rationale: Loss of chromosomes 1, 14, and 15 are found in these tumors.
E. Oncocytoma.
Rationale: Renal oncotyoma is a benign neoplasm. Chromosome abnormalities are seen in approximately 50% of oncocytomas. Loss of chromosomes 1 and 14, and loss of the Y chromosome in males, are seen in one subset of tumors. In a second subset, translocations at 11q13 are seen. 11q13 rearranges with many different chromosomes in this setting.

Major points of discussion
- Although the diagnosis of the renal tumors is based on their classic histologic characteristics, a small but significant percentage of tumors have ambiguous morphologic features, and approximately 5% are reported as "unclassified" because of the overlapping morphologic characteristics. Identification of the cytogenetic abnormalities can assist in the diagnosis and prognosis of renal epithelial tumors.
- The 5-year survival and disease-free progression of RCCs varies by subtype: chromophobe RCC (100% and 94%), papillary RCC (86% and 88%), clear cell RCC (76% and 70%), and RCC unclassified (24% and 18%). Oncocytomas are benign neoplasms with very low risk of metastasis.
- SNP arrays and aCGH could resolve morphologically challenging renal tumors. These genomic methods are becoming the method of choice for comprehensive evaluation of chromosomal imbalances in RCC.

- Conventional cytogenetics is the method of choice when assessing for nonrecurrent balanced translocations, such as those present in familial non–von Hippel-Lindau clear cell RCC. FISH can be used to detect the presence of recurrent chromosomal translocations, such as those present in pediatric tumors involving the Xp11.2 locus.
- Cytogenetic analysis does not provide distinction between papillary adenomas and low-grade RCCs because of overlapping combinations of numerical chromosome abnormalities. Tumor diameter remains an important diagnostic criterion.[28,30]

36. A. 45,XX,t(13;21)(p10;p10).
Rationale: Although the correct chromosomes are shown here, the letters "der" should be used instead of "t" and the translocation breakpoint should be (q10;q10).
B. 45,XX,der(13;21)(q10;q10).
C. 46,XX,t(13;21)(p10;q10).
D. 46,XX,der(13),t(13;21)(p10;p10).
Rationale: The Robertsonian derivative always involves both chromosomes; that is, der(13;21).
E. 46,XX,der(13;21)(q10;p10).
Rationale for B, C, and E: Balanced carriers of a Robertsonian translocation have 45 chromosomes. The translocation is described as a derivative chromosome and thus the use of "der" is appropriate. The breakpoints for Robertsonian translocations are always at (q10;q10).

Major points of discussion
- A Robertsonian translocation is a special type of translocation that originates only through translocation of the acrocentric chromosomes (i.e., 13, 14, 15, 21, 22).
- The breakpoints primarily occur in the short arms, resulting in dicentric chromosomes.
- Breaks may also occur in one short arm and one long arm of the participating chromosomes. This results in a monocentric rearrangement.
- The formation of the Robertsonian translocation effectively creates a derivative chromosome, which consists primarily of the long arms of the two participating acrocentric chromosomes.
- The formation of the Robertsonian translocation also produces a derivative chromosome, which consists of the short arms of the two participating acrocentric chromosomes. This small derivative chromosome is simultaneously lost, resulting in a net chromosome number of 45. Because the short arms of the acrocentric chromosomes contain a superfluous amount of ribosomal gene repeats, loss of this small derivative fragment is clinically insignificant as there are sufficient ribosomal genes on the remaining acrocentric short arms.
- Either "rob" or "der" can be used to describe the Robertsonian translocation; that is[21,54]:
  - 45,XX,der(13;21)(q10;q10)
  - 45,XX,rob(13;21)(q10;q10)

37. A. Synovial sarcoma.
Rationale: The t(X;18) is found in almost all synovial sarcomas; this translocation results in either the *SS18-SSX1,* *SS18-SSX2,* or *SS18-SSX4* fusion genes.

B. Desmoplastic small round cell tumor.
Rationale: The characteristic translocation in this tumor is t(11;22)(p13;q12), resulting in *EWSR1-WT1* fusion transcript.
C. Embryonal rhabdomyosarcoma.
Rationale: These tumors have complex karyotypes, but no recurrent translocations have been identified.
D. Alveolar rhabdomyosarcoma.
Rationale: The cytogenetic hallmark of alveolar rhabdomyosarcomas is t(2;13)(q36;q14) and, less frequently, t(1;13)(p36;q14); these translocations result in *PAX3-FOXO1A* and *PAX7-FOXO1A* fusions, respectively.
E. Myxoid liposarcoma.
Rationale: These tumors have a t(12;16)(q13;p11), which results in a *FUS-DDIT3* chimeric gene.

Major points of discussion

- Cytogenetic and molecular studies of soft tissue sarcomas have shown specific chromosome translocations.
- The t(X;18) is a characteristic finding in synovial sarcomas. A third of these tumors show t(X;18) as a sole chromosome abnormality; the remaining show an unbalanced derivative chromosome X, resulting from t(X;18) and other complex chromosome abnormalities. Cytogenetic and molecular studies indicate that patients with simple karyotypes and the *SS18-SSX2* fusion have a better clinical outcome than patients with a complex tumor karyotype and the *SS18-SSX1* fusion.
- Chromosome analysis in desmoplastic round cell tumors usually shows a near-diploid karyotype with a few numerical and structural aberrations. Identification of t(11;22) or the *EWSR1-WT1* fusion transcript is useful in the differential diagnosis of small cell round cell tumors and may show higher sensitivity than immunohistochemical analyses.
- Although no structural chromosome abnormalities are seen in embryonal rhabdomyosarcoma, gain of several chromosomes (i.e., chromosomes 2, 8, 12, 13, 1q, 7q, 11q) and loss of chromosomes 1p, 9p, 14q, 15q, and 17p are common. Patients with embryonal rhabdomyosarcomas have a better survival than those with alveolar rhabdomyosarcoma.
- In alveolar rhabdomyosarcoma, t(2;13) and t(1;13) are often present in duplicate or triplicates; secondary numerical and structural abnormalities are common and the karyotypes are usually complex. Tumors with t(2;13), expressing *PAX3-FOXO1A*, have a higher propensity to metastasize to the bone marrow.

38. A. Embryonal rhabdomyosarcoma.
Rationale: Embryonal rhabdomyosarcomas do not show any recurrent balanced chromosome translocations.
B. Alveolar rhabdomyosarcoma.
Rationale: Alveolar rhabdomyosarcomas exhibit the following characteristic balanced chromosome translocations: t(2;13)(q36;q14) or t(1;13)(p36;q14). The *FOXO1* gene on 13q14 rearranges with the *PAX3* gene on 2q35 and the *PAX7* gene on 1p36, resulting in the formation of fusion gene products.
C. Primitive neuroectoderal tumor.
Rationale: t(11;22)(q24;q12), resulting in the fusion of the *EWS* gene on 22q12 with *FLI1* at 11q24, is a classic feature of a primitive neuroectoderal tumor/Ewing sarcoma and serves as diagnostic marker for this neoplasm.

D. Synovial sarcoma.
Rationale: The characteristic chromosome translocation in synovial sarcoma is the recombination between the Xp11.2 and 18p11.2 regions, resulting in t(X;18)(p11.2;q11.2). This translocation results in fusion genes between *SS18* (*SYT*) on 18p with one of three genes (i.e., *SSX1*, *SSX2*, or *SSX4*) in the Xp11.2 region.
E. Myxoid liposarcoma.
Rationale: The cytogenetic hallmark of a myxoid liposarcoma is a balanced translocation, t(12;16)(q13;p11.2), resulting in formation of the *FUS-DDIT3* fusion gene.

Major points of discussion

- Synovial sarcoma is a rare soft tissue tumor accounting for 5% to 8% of soft tissue sarcomas. Synovial sarcoma is prevalent in young adults, and it occurs in the para-articular regions of the extremities, the parapharyngeal region, the abdominal wall, and in lung or cardiac tissue. It presents with a biphasic epithelial and spindle cell component, as a monophasic fibrous type, or as a poorly differentiated small cell neoplasm.
- Synovial sarcoma is characterized by the presence of a reciprocal balanced translocation between chromosome regions Xp11.2 and 18q11.2 [t(12;16)(q13;p11.2)] in more than 90% of the cases.
- Rare variants have been described involving Xp11.2 alone or 18q11.2 alone, with either involved in translocations with other chromosomes.
- The molecular consequence of the t(X;18)(p11.2;q11.2) translocation is the rearrangement between synovial sarcoma translocation on chromosome 18 (i.e., *SS18*, or alternatively, *SYT*) with one of three related synovial sarcomas, X breakpoint genes (i.e., *SSX1*, *SSX2*, or *SSX4*), resulting in different fusion genes (i.e., *SS18-SSX1*, *SS18-SSX2*, or *SS18-SSX4*).
- Some synovial sarcoma cases exhibit complex karyotypes and amplification of the 12q13 region, which are associated with worse overall survival.[14,26,53]

39. A. BL.
Rationale: The t(8;14)(q24;q32) translocation, resulting in rearrangement of the *MYC* gene with the *IGH* locus, is the characteristic chromosome translocation in BL.
B. ALCL.
Rationale: A balanced translocation between chromosome regions 2p23 and 5q35 [t(2;5)(p23;q35)], resulting in *ALK* rearrangement, is a classic feature of ALCL.
C. Multiple myeloma.
Rationale: In multiple myeloma, the 14q32 region involving the *IGH* gene is frequently partnered with 11q13 (the *cyclin D1* gene), 4p16 (the *FGFR3* gene), 6p25 (the *cyclin D3* gene), 16q23 (the *MAF* gene), and 20q11 (the *MAFB* gene), thereby forming balanced reciprocal translocations.
D. T-PLL.
Rationale: The immunophenotype in the current case is consistent with a mature T-cell leukemia/lymphoma. The inv(14)(q11.2q32) cytogenetic abnormality is frequently seen (~65% of cases) in T-cell prolymphocytic leukemia.
E. HL.
Rationale: HL is not associated with inv(14). Specific chromosome changes have not been reported in HL. However, chromosome deletions involving 1p, 6q, 7q, and duplications of 1q, can be seen.

Major points of discussion

- The TCR is a heterodimer composed of either αβ or γδ chains. The genes encoding these proteins are *TCRA/D* at 14q11.2, *TCRB* at 7q34, and *TCRG* at 7p14. In mature T-cell neoplasms, TCR loci are often involved in structural rearrangements with oncogenes, resulting in deregulation of the partner genes.
- The *TCRA/D* region is frequently involved in translocations in T-PLL and in HTLV+adult T-cell lymphoma/leukemia. *TCRA/D* genes are also rarely involved in translocation rearrangements in T-cell ALL, ataxia telangiectasia, and leukemias of B lineage.
- *TCRA/D* gene translocations are seen as inv(14) (q11.2q32) or in t(14;14)(q11.2;q32) translocations, partnering with the *T-cell leukemia/lymphoma 1* (*TCL1*) gene at 14q32.
- The genetic hallmark of T-PLL is inv(14)(q11.2q32), which is present in up to 80% of cases. Its variant, t(14;14)(q11.2; q32), is detected in approximately 10% of T-PLL cases. In both types of chromosome aberrations, the *TCL1* gene at 14q32 is juxtaposed next to the *TCRA/D* locus at 14q11.2, resulting in up-regulation of TCL1 expression.
- The TCR-associated translocations are regarded as the primary oncogenic events in T-PLL.
- T-PLL is generally considered a very aggressive neoplasm among T-cell lymphomas, and they are poorly responsive to chemotherapy.[18,50,62]

40. A. 47,XX,+18.
Rationale: This karyotype shows an extra copy of chromosome 18, which is associated with a clinical diagnosis of trisomy 18. Trisomy 18 is characterized by multiple congenital abnormalities and developmental delay.
B. 46,XX,t(7;18)(q21;q21).
Rationale: This karyotype shows a balanced translocation between the long arms of chromosomes 7 and 18. Balanced translocations are not typically associated with multiple congenital abnormalities and dysmorphic features unless (1) there is an accompanying submicroscopic microdeletion/ microduplication at the breakpoint regions, or (2) the breakpoint occurs in a critical region with concomitant disruption of the gene function.
C. 47,XX,+16.
Rationale: This karyotype shows an extra copy of chromosome 16 (trisomy 16), which is always lethal in the first or second trimester.
D. 47,XXX.
Rationale: This karyotype shows an extra copy of the X chromosome, which is associated with a clinical diagnosis of the triple X syndrome. Physical development in females with XXX is generally unremarkable and there are no phenotypic abnormalities. Some may be tall, be at risk for learning disabilities, and may have fertility problems. There is a general tendency for IQ to be slightly reduced compared with siblings.
E. 46,XX,inv(9)(p12q13).
Rationale: This karyotype shows a balanced pericentric inversion of chromosome 9. Most pericentric inversions confer an increased risk for miscarriages and offspring with congenital abnormalities and/or mental retardation as a result of unbalanced segregation during gametogenesis. However, this particular inversion is a well-established benign polymorphism with no associated clinical risks.

Major points of discussion

- Trisomy 18, also known as Edward syndrome, is the second most common congenital malformation syndrome after Down syndrome.
- Trisomy 18 occurs with a frequency of 1:3333 to 1:6000 births.
- Although trisomy 18 infants can survive to term, spontaneous abortion is the more likely outcome; thus, the prevalence of this chromosome abnormality is greater at the time of chorionic villus sampling and decreases all the way to term.
- The median postnatal survival time is 14.5 days.
- Only 5% to 10% of trisomy 18 newborns survive the first year.
- Those who survive have severe mental deficiency.[21,33,43,63]

41. A. A 30-year-old woman with a 46,XX karyotype.
Rationale: Risk of trisomy 21 or Down syndrome increases with advanced maternal age. Age-associated risk for trisomy 21 at 16 weeks (amniocentesis) is 1:620 for a 30-year-old woman.
B. A woman with the karyotype 45,XX,t(21;21) (q10;q10).
Rationale: A woman with this karyotype can only have trisomy 21 or monosomy 21 conceptions.
C. A woman with no family history of Down syndrome.
Rationale: A woman with no family history may still have an age-associated risk for Down syndrome.
D. A woman with the karyotype 45,XX,t(14;21)(q10;q10).
Rationale: Female carriers of this translocation have an approximately 15% risk of trisomy 21. Nonetheless, the woman described in Case B is at a greater risk for a trisomy 21 live birth.
E. A 35-year-old woman who had a previous child with trisomy 21.
Rationale: Age-associated risk for trisomy 21 at 16 weeks (i.e., at amniocentesis) is 1:245 for a 35-year-old woman.

Major points of discussion

- Robertsonian translocations are whole-arm translocations between acrocentric chromosomes. In humans, the acrocentric chromosomes are 13, 14, 15, 21, and 22. As a result of this translocation, the derivative chromosome contains the complete long arms of the two acrocentric chromosomes fused together and this derivative chromosome lacks at least some short-arm chromatin.
- Robertsonian translocation carriers are increased risk for trisomy or monosomy because of unbalanced segregation at meiosis.
- Advanced maternal age is the most important etiologic factor in risk for aneuploidy and human reproductive failure. Association of advanced maternal age and Down syndrome was known even before the chromosomal basis of Down syndrome was discovered.
- Women with the karyotype 45,XX,t(21;21)(q10;q10) can only have only trisomy 21 or monosomy 21 conceptions. Conceptions with monosomy 21 result in spontaneous abortions. A trisomy 21 conception may survive and result in a live birth with the infant having Down syndrome.
- Female carriers of the Robertsonian translocation (14;21) are at increased risk, a 10% to 15% risk of trisomy 21. The risk for male carriers is very different; it is less than 1%.[49,52,58]

References

1. Akagi T, Motegi M, Tamura A, et al. A novel gene, MALT1 at 18q21, is involved in t(11;18) (q21;q21) found in low-grade B-cell lymphoma of mucosa-associated lymphoid tissue. Oncogene 1999;18:5785–5794.

2. Amin HM, Lai R. Pathobiology of ALK+anaplastic large-cell lymphoma. Blood 2007;110:2259–2267.

3. Atlas of Genetics and Cytogenetics in Oncology and Hematology. Available at http://AtlasGeneticsOncology.org.

4. Barch MJ, Knutsen T, et al., eds. The AGT Cytogenetics Laboratory Manual. New York: Lippincott-Raven; 1997.

5. Bergsagel PL, Kuehl WM. Molecular pathogenesis and a consequent classification of multiple myeloma. J Clin Oncol 2005;23:6333–6338.

6. Blum KA, Lozanski G, Byrd JC. Adult Burkitt leukemia and lymphoma. Blood 2004;104:3009–3020.

7. Boerma EG, Siebert R, Kluin PM, et al. Translocations involving 8q24 in Burkitt lymphoma and other malignant lymphomas: a historical review of cytogenetics in the light of today's knowledge. Leukemia 2009;23:225–234.

8. Boyd KD, Ross FM, Chiecchio L, et al. A novel prognostic model in myeloma based on co-segregating adverse FISH lesions and the ISS: analysis of patients treated in the MRC Myeloma IX trial. Leukemia 2012;26:349–355.

9. Braun T, de Botton S, Taksin AL, et al. Characteristics and outcome of myelodysplastic syndromes (MDS) with isolated 20q deletion: a report on 62 cases. Leuk Res 2011;35:863–867.

10. Brodeur GM, Williams DL, Look AT, et al. Near-haploid acute lymphoblastic leukemia: a unique subgroup with a poor prognosis? Blood 1981;58:14–19.

11. Cassidy SB, Schwartz S, Miller JL, et al. Prader-Willi syndrome. Genet Med 2012;14:10–26.

12. Cheng L, Zhang S, MacLennan GT, et al. Molecular and cytogenetic insights into the pathogenesis, classification, differential diagnosis, and prognosis of renal epithelial neoplasms. Hum Pathol 2009;40:10–29.

13. Crolla JA, Long F, Rivera H, et al. FISH and molecular study of autosomal supernumerary marker chromosomes excluding those derived from chromosomes 15 and 22: I. Results of 26 new cases. Am J Med Genet 1998;75:355–366.

14. de Leeuw B, Balemans M, Olde Weghuis D, et al. Identification of two alternative fusion genes, SYT-SSX1 and SYT-SSX2, in t(X;18) (p11.2;q11.2)-positive synovial sarcomas. Hum Mol Genet 1995;4:1097–1099.

15. de Thé H, Chen Z. Acute promyelocytic leukaemia: novel insights into the mechanisms of cure. Nat Rev Cancer 2010;10: 775–783.

16. DECIPHER (Database of Chromosomal Imbalance and Phenotype in Humans Using Ensembl Resources). Available at decipher. sanger.ac.uk.

17. Dobyns WB, Das S. LIS1-associated lissencephaly band heterotopia. 2009 Mar 3. In Pagon RA, Bird TD, Dolan CR, et al., editors. GeneReviews. Seattle, WA: University of Washington; 1993.

18. Dürig J, Bug S, Klein-Hitpass L, et al. Combined single nucleotide polymorphism-based genomic mapping and global gene expression profiling identifies novel chromosomal imbalances, mechanisms and candidate genes important in the pathogenesis of T-cell prolymphocytic leukemia with inv(14)(q11q32). Leukemia 2007;21:2153–2163.

19. Farinha P, Gascoyne RD. Molecular pathogenesis of mucosa-associated lymphoid tissue lymphoma. J Clin Oncol 2005;23: 6370–6378.

20. Gardner RJ, Sutherland GR, Shaffer LG. Down syndrome, other full aneuploidies, and polyploidies. In Chromosome Abnormalities and Genetic Counseling. 4th ed. New York: Oxford University Press; 2012, pp 277–294.

21. Gardner RJ, Sutherland GR, Shaffer LG. Down syndrome, other full aneuploidies, and polyploidies. In Chromosome Abnormalities and Genetic Counseling. 4th ed. New York: Oxford University Press; 2012.

22. Gascoyne RD. Emerging prognostic factors in diffuse large B cell lymphoma. Curr Opin Oncol 2004;16:436–441.

23. Gassner R, Metzenbauer M, Hafner E, et al. Triploidy in a twin pregnancy: small placenta volume as an early sonographic marker. Prenat Diagn 2003;23:16–20.

24. Graux C. Biology of acute lymphoblastic leukemia (ALL): clinical and therapeutic relevance. Transfus Apher Sci 2011;44:183–189.

25. Greenberg P, Cox C, Le Beau MM, et al. International scoring system for evaluating prognosis in myelodysplastic syndromes. Blood 1997;89:2079–2088.

26. Griffin CA, Emanuel BS. Translocation (X;18) in a synovial sarcoma. Cancer Genet Cytogenet 1987;26:181–183.

27. Haase D. Cytogenetic features in myelodysplastic syndromes. Ann Hematol 2008;87:515–526.

28. Hagenkord JM, Gatalica Z, Jonasch E, et al. Clinical genomics of renal epithelial tumors. Cancer Genet 2011;204:285–297.

29. Harrison CJ, Haas O, Harbott J, et al. Detection of prognostically relevant genetic abnormalities in childhood B-cell precursor acute lymphoblastic leukaemia: recommendations from the Biology and Diagnosis Committee of the International Berlin-Frankfürt-Münster study group. Br J Haematol 2010;151: 132–142.

30. Jhang JS, Narayan G, Murty VV, et al. Renal oncocytomas with 11q13 rearrangements: cytogenetic, molecular, and immunohistochemical analysis of cyclin D1. Cancer Genet Cytogenet 2004;149:114–119.

31. Jobanputra V, Esteves C, Sobrino A, et al. Using FISH to increase the yield and accuracy of karyotypes from spontaneous abortion specimens. Prenat Diagn 2011;31:755–759.

32. Johansson B, Harrison CJ. Acute myeloid leukemia. In Heim S, Mitelman F, eds. Cancer Cytogenetics. 3rd ed. Hoboken, NJ: John Wiley & Sons, 2009, pp 45–140.

33. Jones KL, Smith DW. Smith's Recognizable Patterns of Human Malformation. 6th ed. Philadelphia: Elsevier; 2006.

34. Kadin ME, Morris SW. The t(2;5) in human lymphomas. Leuk Lymphoma 1998;29:249–256.

35. Keagle MB, Gersen SL. Basic laboratory procedures. In Gersen SL, Keagle MB, eds. The Principles of Clinical Cytogenetics. Totowa, NJ: Humana Press, 2005, pp 63–80.

36. Leana-Cox J, Jenkins L, Palmer CG, et al. Molecular cytogenetic analysis of inv dup(15) chromosomes, using probes specific for the Prader-Willi/Angelman syndrome region: clinical implications. Am J Hum Genet 1994;54:748–756.

37. Ledbetter DH, Riccardi VM, Airhart SD, et al. Deletions of chromosome 15 as a cause of the Prader-Willi syndrome. N Engl J Med 1981;304:325–329.

38. Lejeune J, Gautier M. Turpin R et al. Etude des chromosomes somatiques de neuf enfants mongoliens [Study of somatic chromosomes from 9 mongoloid children]. Compt Rend 1959;248:1721–1722.

39. Levy B, Dunn TM, et al. Satellite DNA. In Creighton TE, ed. Wiley Encyclopedia of Molecular Medicine. New York: John Wiley & Sons, 2002, pp 2859–2862.

40. Levy B, Hirschhorn K, Kardon N. Chromosome abnormalities in spontaneous abortions, 2007: In Wells D, ed. Cytogenetics in Reproductive Medicine. Austin: Landes Bioscience; 2007, pp 59–66. Available at http://www.landesbioscience.com/pdf/Levy1_MC_ Report.pdf.

41. Liu H, Ruskon-Fourmestraux A, Lavergne-Slove A, et al. Resistance of t(11;18) positive gastric mucosa-associated lymphoid tissue lymphoma to *Helicobacter pylori* eradication therapy. Lancet 2001;357:39–40.

42. Lones MA, Sanger WG, Le Beau MM, et al. Chromosome abnormalities may correlate with prognosis in Burkitt/Burkitt-like lymphomas of children and adolescents: a report from

Children's Cancer Group Study CCG-E08. J Pediatr Hematol Oncol 2004;26:169–178.

43. Menasha J, Levy B, Hirschhorn K, et al. Incidence and spectrum of chromosome abnormalities in spontaneous abortions: new insights from a 12-year study. Genet Med 2005;7:251–263.

44. Mertens F, Mandahl N. Tumors of bone. In Heim S, Mitelman F, eds. Cancer Cytogenetics. 3rd ed. Hoboken, NJ: John Wiley & Sons; 2009, pp 655–674.

45. Mistry AR, Pedersen EW, Solomon E, et al. The molecular pathogenesis of acute promyelocytic leukaemia: implications for the clinical management of the disease. Blood Rev 2003;17:71–97.

46. Moorman AV, Richards SM, Martineau M, et al. Outcome heterogeneity in childhood high-hyperdiploid acute lymphoblastic leukemia. Blood 2003;102:2756–2762.

47. Morris SW, Kirstein MN, Valentine MB, et al. Fusion of a kinase gene, ALK, to a nucleolar protein gene, NPM, in non-Hodgkin's lymphoma. Science 1994;263:1281–1284.

48. OMIM (Online Mendelian Inheritance in Man). An Online Catalog of Human Genes and Genetic Disorders. Available at http://omim.org.

49. Parental age counseling and screening for fetal trisomy. In Gardner RJ, Sutherland GR, Shaffer LG, eds. Chromosome Abnormalities and Genetic Counseling. 4th ed. New York: Oxford University Press; 2012, pp 403–416.

50. Pekarsky Y, Hallas C, Croce CM. Molecular basis of mature T-cell leukemia. JAMA 2001;286:2308–2314.

51. Pui CH, Chessells JM, Camitta B, et al. Clinical heterogeneity in childhood acute lymphoblastic leukemia with 11q23 rearrangements. Leukemia 2003;17:700–706.

52. Gardner RJ, Sutherland GR, Shaffer LG. Robertsonian translocations. In Chromosome Abnormalities and Genetic Counseling. 4th ed. New York: Oxford University Press; 2012, pp 140–154.

53. Sandberg AA, Bridge JA. Updates on the cytogenetics and molecular genetics of bone and soft tissue tumors. Synovial sarcoma Cancer Genet Cytogenet 2002;133:1–23.

54. Shaffer LG, Slovak ML, Campbell LJ, eds. ISCN 2009: An International System for Human Cytogenetic Nomenclature. Basel/Unionville, CT: Karger; 2009.

55. Shuman C, Beckwith JB, Smith AC, et al. Beckwith-Wiedemann syndrome. In Pagon RA, Bird TD, Dolan CR, et al, eds. GeneReviews. Seattle: University of Washington, 1993.

56. Siebert R. Mature B- and T-cell neoplasms and Hodgkin lymphoma. In Heim S, Mitelman F, eds. Cancer Cytogenetics. 3rd ed. Hoboken, NJ: John Wiley & Sons; 2009, pp 297–374.

57. Smith ACM, Boyd K, Elsea SH, et al. Smith-Magenis syndrome. In GeneReviews at GeneTests: Medical Genetics Information Resource. Available at www.genetests.org.

58. Snijders RJM, Sebire NJ, Nicolaides KH. Maternal age and gestational age-specific risk for chromosomal defects. Fetal Diagn Ther 1995;10:356–367.

59. Swerdlow SH, Harris NL, Jaffe ES, et al. WHO Classification of Tumours of Haematopoietic and Lymphoid Tissues. 4th ed. Lyon, France: International Agency for Research on Cancer, 2008, pp 109–145, 180–232.

60. Nussbaum RL, McInnes RR, Willard HF. Tools of human molecular genetics. In Thompson & Thompson Genetics in Medicine. 7th ed. Philadelphia: Elsevier; 2007, pp 41–58.

61. Végso G, Hajdu M, Sebestyén A. Lymphoproliferative disorders after solid organ transplantation-classification, incidence, risk factors, early detection and treatment options. Pathol Oncol Res 2011;17:443–454.

62. Virgilio L, Narducci MG, Isobe M, et al. Identification of the TCL1 gene involved in T-cell malignancies. Proc Natl Acad Sci U S A 1994;91:12530–12544.

63. Wyandt HE, Tonk VS. Atlas of Human Chromosome Heteromorphisms. Dordrecht/Boston: Kluwer Academic; 2004.

INDEX

Note: Page numbers followed by *f* indicate figures and *t* indicate tables.